Tenth Edition

# SAUER'S MANUAL OF SKIN DISEASES

**Brian J. Hall, MD**

*Department of Pathology*
*University of Utah*
*Salt Lake City, Utah*

**John C. Hall, MD**

*Primary Staff*
*St. Luke's Hospital*
*Lecturer of Medicine*
*University of Missouri-Kansas City School of Medicine*
*Clinician*
*Kansas City Free Health Clinic*
*Kansas City, Missouri*

With 61 Contributing Authors

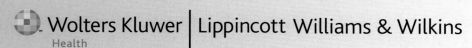

Wolters Kluwer | Lippincott Williams & Wilkins
Health

Philadelphia • Baltimore • New York • London
Buenos Aires • Hong Kong • Sydney • Tokyo

# Dedication

In memory of
Arnold and Fern Peterson,
Samantha Sue Hall,
   and Gordon Sauer, MD whose book this will always be.


Thank you, Senior Developmental Editor, Marla Sussman.

*Acquisitions Editor:* Sonya Seigafuse
*Product Manager:* Kerry Barrett
*Vendor Manager:* Bridgett Dougherty
*Senior Manufacturing Manager:* Benjamin Rivera
*Marketing Manager:* Kim Schonberger
*Creative Director:* Doug Smock
*Production Service:* MPS Limited, A Macmillan Company

© **2010 by LIPPINCOTT WILLIAMS & WILKINS, a WOLTERS KLUWER business**
**530 Walnut Street**
**Philadelphia, PA 19106 USA**
**LWW.com**

Printed in China

---

**Library of Congress Cataloging-in-Publication Data**

Hall, John C., 1947–
  Sauer's manual of skin diseases / John C. Hall; with 61
contributing authors.—10th ed.
    p. ; cm.
  Includes bibliographical references and index.
  ISBN-13: 978-1-60547-077-1 (alk. paper)
  ISBN-10: 1-60547-077-5 (alk. paper)
  1. Skin—Diseases—Handbooks, manuals, etc. I. Sauer, Gorden C.
(Gordon Chenoweth), 1921–Manual of skin diseases. II. Title. III.
Title: Manual of skin diseases.
  [DNLM: 1. Skin Diseases. WR 140 H177s 2010]
  RL74.S25 2010
  616.5—dc22

2009045124

---

Care has been taken to confirm the accuracy of the information presented and to describe generally accepted practices. However, the authors, editors, and publisher are not responsible for errors or omissions or for any consequences from application of the information in this book and make no warranty, expressed or implied, with respect to the currency, completeness, or accuracy of the contents of the publication. Application of the information in a particular situation remains the professional responsibility of the practitioner.

The authors, editors, and publisher have exerted every effort to ensure that drug selection and dosage set forth in this text are in accordance with current recommendations and practice at the time of publication. However, in view of ongoing research, changes in government regulations, and the constant flow of information relating to drug therapy and drug reactions, the reader is urged to check the package insert for each drug for any change in indications and dosage and for added warnings and precautions. This is particularly important when the recommended agent is a new or infrequently employed drug.

Some drugs and medical devices presented in the publication have Food and Drug Administration (FDA) clearance for limited use in restricted research settings. It is the responsibility of the health care provider to ascertain the FDA status of each drug or device planned for use in their clinical practice.

To purchase additional copies of this book, call our customer service department at (800) 638-3030 or fax orders to (301) 223-2320. International customers should call (301) 223-2300.

Visit Lippincott Williams & Wilkins on the Internet: at LWW.com. Lippincott Williams & Wilkins customer service representatives are available from 8:30 am to 6 pm, EST.

# TABLE OF CONTENTS

# CONTRIBUTING AUTHORS

**Sarah S. Asch, MS**
Resident
Department of Pediatrics
Children's Hospital of Pittsburgh
Pittsburgh, Pennsylvania
**Chapter 38: The Skin and Internal Disease**

**Rodney S.W. Basler, MD**
Founding Chair
Taskforce on Sport medicine
Adjunct Associate Professor
Internal Medicine
University of Nebraska Medical Center
Omaha, Nebraska
**Chapter 46: Sports Medicine Dermatology**

**Benedetta Belloni, MD**
Resident
Department of Dermatology
Klinik und Poliklinik für Dermatologie und Allergologie
am Biederstein
Technische Universität München
Munich, Germany
**Chapter 9: Immune-mediated Skin Diseases**

**Francisco G. Bravo, MD**
Associate Professor
Pathology
Universidad Peruana Cayetano Heredia
Lima, Peru
**Chapter 45: Tropical Diseases of the Skin**

**Cheryl M. Burgess, MD**
Assistant Clinical Professor
Department of Dermatology
Georgetown University Medical Center
George Washington University Hospital
Washington, DC
**Chapter 35: Skin Diseases in
Ethnic Skin**

**Antoanella Calame, MD**
Assistant Clinical Professor
Dermatology
University of Texas Southwestern
Dallas, Texas
**Chapter 24: Cutaneous Diseases Associated with Human
Immunodeficiency Virus**

**Clay Cockerell, MD**
Professor
Dermatology and Pathology
University of Texas Southwestern
Dallas, Texas
**Chapter 24: Cutaneous Diseases Associated with Human
Immunodeficiency Virus**

**Ellen de Coninck, MD**
Stanford University School of Medicine
Stanford, California
**Chapter 20: Psychodermatology**

**Daniel Aires, MD, JD**
Stiefel Professor and Division Director
Division of Dermatology
University of Kansas School of Medicine
Kansas City, Kansas
**Chapter 42: General Principles
of Skin Aging**

**Dayna Diven, MD**
Clinical Professor
Department of Dermatology
University of Texas Medical Branch Austin
Austin, Texas
**Chapter 26: Sexually Transmitted
Infections**

**Steven R. Feldman, MD, PhD**
Fellow at Dermatopathology
University of Texas Southwestern Medical Center
at Dallas
Dallas, Texas
**Chapter 47: Cutaneous Signs of Bioterrorism**

**Pascal G. Ferzli, MD, MSc, FAAD**
Dartmouth-Hitchcock Medical Center Concord
Department of Dermatology
Concord Hospital
Concord, New Hampshire
**Chapter 38: The Skin and
Internal Disease**

**Gary Goldenberg, MD**
Medical Director
Dermatology Faculty Practice
The Mount Sinai Hospital
Assistant Professor
Dermatology and Pathology
The Mount Sinai School of Medicine
New York, New York
**Chapter 37: Collagen–Vascular Diseases**

**Clifton S. Hall, MD**
Resident
Department of Dermatology
University of Texas Medical Branch Austin
Austin, Texas
**Chapter 26: Sexually Transmitted Infections**

**Nathan W. Hanson, MD**
Fellow
Mohs Micrographic and Dermatologic Surgery
Department of Dermatology
Geisinger Medical Center
Danville, Pennsylvania
**Chapter 28: Non-Melanoma Skin Cancer**

**Warren R. Heymann, MD**
Professor of Medicine and Pediatrics
Head
Division of Dermatology
Department of Medicine
UMDNJ-Robert Wood Johnson Medical School
Camden, New Jersey
**Chapter 38: The Skin and Internal Disease**

**Kimberly A. Horii, MD**
Section of Dermatology
Children's Mercy Hospitals & Clinics
Associate Professor
Department of Pediatrics
University of Missouri–Kansas City
Kansas City, Missouri
**Chapter 41: Pediatric Dermatology**

**Amy Y. Jan, MD, PhD**
Staff Dermatologist
Dermatology
Southern California Permanente Medical Group
Baldwin Park, California
**Chapter 40: Genodermatoses**

**Beverly A. Johnson, MD, FAAD**
Director
Dermatology Education
Providence Hospital
Washington, DC
Assistant Professor
Department of Dermatology
Howard University Hospital
Washington, DC
**Chapter 35: Skin Diseases in Ethnic Skin**

**Joseph L. Jorizzo, MD**
Professor, Former (Founding) Chair
Department of Dermatology
Wake Forest University School of Medicine
Winstm-Salem, North Carolina
**Chapter 37: Collagen–Vascular Diseases**

**Thelda M. Kestenbaum, MD**
Associate Professor of Medicine
University of Kansas Medical Center
Kansas City, Kansas
**Chapter 32: Diseases Affecting the Hair**

**Megan Kinney, MHAM, BS**
Baptist Medical Center
Research Assistant
Department of Dermatology
Wake Forest University
Winston-Salem, North Carolina
**Chapter 47: Cutaneous Signs of Bioterrorism**

**Christopher J. Kligora, MD**
Partner
Southeastern Pathology Associates
Rome, Georgia
**Chapter 2: Laboratory Procedures
and Tests**

**Laurie L. Kohen, MD**
Chief Resident
Dermatology
Henry Ford Hospital
Detroit, Michigan
**Chapter 39: Dermatologic Reactions to Ultraviolet
Radiation and Visible Light**

**John Koo, MD**
Director
Psoriasis Treatment Center
Vice Chairman
Department of Dermatology
University of California—San Francisco
San Francisco, California
**Chapter 20: Psychodermatology**

**Frank Custer Koranda, MD, MBA**
Associate Clinical Professor
Otolaryngology-Head and Neck Surgery
Dermatology
University of Kansas Medical Center
Kansas City, Kansas
**Chapters 5 and 6: Technologic Applications in Dermatology
and Fundamentals of Cutaneous Surgery**

**Jeffrey N. Lackey, MD**
Dermatology Resident
Dermatology Service
Walter Reed Army Medical Center
Washington, DC
**Chapter 47: Cutaneous Signs of Bioterrorism**

**W. Clark Lambert, MD, PhD**
Director
Dermatopathology
Associate Director
Dermatology Pathology and Laboratory Medicine
UMDNJ-University Hospital Newark
Newark, New Jersey
**Chapter 31: Cutaneous T-Cell Lymphoma**

**Margaret S. Lee, MD, PhD**
Attending Physician
Children's Hospital Boston
Instructor
Department of Medicine
Harvard Medical School
Boston, Massachusetts
**Chapter 30: Vascular Tumors**

**Marilyn G. Liang, MD**
Assistant
Department of Medicine
Children's Hospital Boston
Assistant Professor
Department of Dermatology
Harvard Medical School
Boston, Massachusetts
**Chapter 30: Vascular Tumors**

**Henry W. Lim, MD**
Chairman and C.S. Livingood Chair
Department of Dermatology
Henry Ford Hospital
Senior Vice President for Academic Affairs
Henry Ford Health System
Henry Ford Medical Center—New Center
Detroit, Michigan
**Chapter 39: Dermatologic Reactions to Ultraviolet
Radiation and Visible Light**

**Jasna Lipozenčić, MD, PhD**
Professor, Acting Head
University Department of Dermatology and Venerology
University Hospital Center Zagreb and School of Medicine
Zagreb, Croatia
**Chapter 10: Atopic Dermatitis**

**Deede Liu, MD, MS**
Chief Resident
Division of Dermatology
University of Kansas Medical Center
Kansas City, Kansas
**Chapter 42: General Principles of Skin Aging**

**Suzana Ljubojević, MD, PhD**
Assistant Professor
University Department of Dermatology and Venerology
Zagreb University Hospital Center, and School
of Medicine
Zagreb, Croatia
**Chapter 10: Atopic Dermatitis**

**Aaron Loyd, MD**
Resident
Department of Dermatology
Wake Forest University
Winston Salem, North Carolina
Fellow, Dermatopathology Section
New York University
New York, New York
**Chapter 37: Collagen–Vascular Diseases**

**Victor J. Marks, MD**
Section Chief and Director
Mohs Micrographic and Dermatologic Surgery
Department of Dermatology
Geisinger Medical Center
Danville, Pennsylvania
**Chapter 28: Non-Melanoma Skin Cancer**

**Brad Merritt, MD**
Mohs Surgery Fellow
Mohs Surgery Zitelli & Brodland, PC
Pittsburgh, Pennsylvania
**Chapter 33: Diseases Affecting the Nail Unit**

**Salim Mohanna, MD**
Clinical Research Associate
Instituto de Medicina Tropical "Alexander
von Humboldt"
Universidad Peruana Cayetano Heredia
Lima, Peru
**Chapter 45: Tropical Diseases of the Skin**

**Stephen J. Nervi, MD**
Dermatology and Pathology
New Jersey Medical School
Newark, New Jersey
**Chapter 31: Cutaneous T-Cell Lymphoma**

**M. Neuburg, MD**
Head, Section of Dermatologic Surgery
Froedtert Memorial Lutheran Hospital Milwaukee
Professor
Departments of Dermatology, Plastic and
Reconstructive Surgery, Otolaryngology and
Communication Sciences
Medical College of Wisconsin
Milwaukee, Wisconsin
**Chapter 44: Skin Disease in Transplant Patients**

**Scott A. Norton, MD, MPH**
Dermatology Service
Walter Reed Army Medical Center
Washington, DC
**Chapter 47: Cutaneous Signs of Bioterrorism**

**Marianne N. O'Donoghue, MD**
Associate Professor
Department of Dermatology
Rush Presbyterian—St. Luke's Medical Center
Chicago, Illinois
**Chapter 7: Cosmetics for the Physician**

**E.B. Olasz, MD, PhD**
Assistant Professor and Dermatology Section Chief
VA Hospital Milwaukee
Department of Dermatology
Medical College of Wisconsin Milwaukee
Medical College of Wisconsin
Milwaukee, Wisconsin
**Chapter 44: Skin Disease in Transplant Patients**

**Parisa Ravanfar, MD, MBA, MS**
Clinical Research Fellow
Center for Clinical Studies
Houston, Texas
**Chapter 23: Dermatologic Virology**

**Jason S. Reichenberg, MD, FAAD**
Clinical Director
Department of Dermatology
University Medical Center Brackenridge Austin
Assistant Professor
Department of Dermatology
University of Texas Medical Branch Austin
Austin, Texas
**Chapter 26: Sexually Transmitted Infections**

**Johannes Ring, MD, PhD**
Director of Clinic Director
Dean of Studies
Director der Klinik und Poliklinik Für Dermatologie und
Allergologic Biederstein
München, Germany
**Chapter 9: Immune-mediated Skin Diseases**

**Anita Satyaprakash, MD**
Resident
Division of Dermatology
Loyola University Medical Center
Maywood, Illinois
**Cahpter 23: Dermatologic Virology**

**Noah S. Scheinfeld, MD, JD**
Assistant Clinical Professor of Dermatology
Columbia University
New York, New York
**Chapter 43: Obesity and Dermatology**

**Richard K. Scher, MD, FACP**
Professor of Dermatology
University of North Carolina
Chapel Hill, North Carolina
**Chapter 33: Diseases Affecting the Nail Unit**

**Robert A. Schwartz, MD, MPH**
Professor and Chief, Dermatology
Professor of Pathology
Professor of Medicine
Professor of Pediatrics
Professor of Preventive Medicine and Community Health
New Jersey Medical School
Newark, New Jersey
**Chapter 31: Cutaneous T-Cell Lymphoma**

**Vidya Sharma, MBBS, MPH**
Professor
Department of Pediatrics
University of Missouri
Staff Physician
Section of Dermatology
Director
Performance Improvement
Department of Pediatrics
The Children's Mercy Hospital and Clinics
Kansas City, Missouri
**Chapter 41: Pediatric Dermatology**

**J. K. Shornick, MD, MHA**
Private Practice
Groton, Connecticut
**Chapter 48: Dermatoses of Pregnancy**

**Emily Stevens, BA**
Medical Student
School of Medicine
University of Kansas Medical Center
Kansas City, Kansas
**Chapter 42: General Principles of Skin Aging**

**Virginia P. Sybert, MD**
Staff Dermatologist
Dermatology Group
Health Cooperative
Clinical Professor
Division of Medical Genetics
Department of Medicine
University of Washington
Seattle, Washington
**Chapter 40: Genodermatoses**

**Crystal Thomas, MD**
Dermatopathology Fellow
Department of Dermatology
University of Texas Southwestern/Cockerell and Associates
Dallas, Texas
**Chapter 24: Cutaneous Diseases Associated with Human
Immunodeficiency Virus**

**Stephen K. Tyring, MD, PhD**
Clinical Professor
Dermatology
University of Texas Health Science Center
Houston, Texas
**Chapter 23: Dermatologic Virology**

**Kenneth R. Watson, DO**
Pathologist
Anatomic Pathology
St. Luke's Health System
Kansas City, Missouri
**Chapters 1 and 2: Structure of the Skin and Laboratory
Procedures and Tests**

**Jeffrey M. Weinberg, MD**
Director
Clinical Research
Department of Dermatology
St. Luke's-Roosevelt Hospital Center
Associate Clinical Professor
Department of Dermatology
Columbia University
New York, New York
**Chapter 14: Psoriasis**

**Robin S. Weiner, MD**
Department of Dermatology
University of Missouri Medical Center
Columbia, Missouri
**Chapter 29: Melanoma**

**Daniel West, MD**
Resident
Division of Dermatology
University of Kansas School of Medicine
Internal Medicine
University of Kansas Medical Center
Kansas City, Kansas
**Chapter 42: General Principles of Skin Aging**

**Jaeyoung Yoon, MD, PhD**
Director
Mohs Micrographic Surgery
Medicine/Dermatology
John Cochran VA Hospital
Clinical Instructor
Dermatology
St. Louis University School of Medicine
St. Louis, Missouri
**Chapter 29: Melanoma**

# Preface to the First Edition (Abridged)

Approximately 15% of all patients who walk into the general practitioner's office do so for the care of some skin disease or skin lesion. It may be for such a simple treatment as the removal of a wart, for the treatment of athlete's foot, or for something as complicated as severe cystic acne. There have been so many recent advances in the various fields of medicine that the medical school instructor can expect his or her students to learn and retain only a small percentage of the material that is taught. I believe that the courses in all phases of medicine, and particularly the courses of the various specialties, should be made as simple, basic, and concise as possible. If the student retains only a small percentage of what is presented, he or she will be able to handle an amazing number of walk-in patients. I am presenting in this book only the material that medical students and general practitioners must know for the diagnosis and the treatment of patients with common skin diseases. In condensing the material, many generalities are stated, and the reader must remember that there are exceptions to every rule. The inclusion of these exceptions would defeat the intended purpose of this book. More complicated diagnostic procedures or treatments for interesting problem cases are merely frosting on the cake. This information can be obtained by the interested student from any of several more comprehensive dermatologic texts.

This book consists of two distinct but complementary parts. The first part contains the chapters devoted to the diagnosis and the management of the important common skin diseases. In discussing the common skin diseases, a short introductory sentence is followed by a listing of the salient points of each disease in outline form. All diseases of the skin have primary lesions, secondary lesions, a rather specific distribution, a general course that includes the prognosis and the recurrence rate of the diseases, varying subjective complaints, and a known or unknown cause. Where indicated, a statement follows concerning seasonal incidence, age groups affected, family and sex incidence, contagiousness, relationship to employment, and laboratory findings. The discussion ends with a paragraph on differential diagnosis and treatment. Treatment, to be effective, has to be thought of as a chain of events. The therapy outlined on the first visit is usually different from the one given on subsequent visits or for cases that are very severe. The treatment is discussed with these variations in mind.

The second part consists of a very complete Dictionary–Index to the entire field of dermatology, defining the majority of rare diseases and the unusual dermatologic terms. The inclusion of this Dictionary–Index has a dual purpose. First, it enables me to present a concise first section on common skin diseases unencumbered by the inclusion of the rare diseases. Second, it provides rather complete coverage of all of dermatology for the more interested student. In reality, two books are contained in one.

Dermatologic nomenclature has always been a bugaboo for the new student. I heartily agree with many dermatologists that we should simplify the terminology, and that has been attempted in this text. Some of the changes are mine, but many have been suggested by others. However, after a diligent effort to simplify the names of skin diseases, one is left with the appalling fact that some of the complicated terms defy change. One of the main reasons for this is that all of our field, the skin, is visible to the naked eye. As a result, any minor alteration from normal has been scrutinized by countless physicians through the years and given countless names. The liver or heart counterpart of folliculitis ulerythematosa reticulata (ulerythema acneiform, atrophoderma reticulatum symmetricum faciei, atrophoderma vermiculatum) is yet to be discovered.

What I am presenting in this book is not specialty dermatology but general practice dermatology. Some of my medical educator friends say that only internal medicine, pediatrics, and obstetrics should be taught to medical students. They state that the specialized fields of medicine should be taught only at the internship, residency, or postgraduate level. That idea misses the very important fact that cases from all of the so-called specialty fields wander into the general practitioner's office. The general practitioner must have some basic knowledge of the varied aspects of all of medicine so that he or she can properly take care of his or her general everyday practice. This basic knowledge must be taught in the undergraduate years. The purpose of this book is to complement such teaching.

*Gordon C. Sauer, MD*

# PREFACE

This is by far the most detailed edition of *Sauer's Manual of Skin Diseases.*

I think the most important change is the addition of new chapters that greatly enhance the completeness of the text. These new chapters are on sexually transmitted diseases, non-melanoma skin cancer, vascular tumors, cutaneous T-cell lymphoma, skin diseases in ethnic skin, obesity and dermatology, skin diseases in transplant patients, and nutrition and the skin.

All of the chapters have been updated, and new authors have been recruited. These new authors are all dermatology clinicians with expertise in their chapter topics which include immunology, atopic dermatitis, malignant melanoma, and general principles of skin aging.

Updated chapters written by outstanding authors from the previous edition include structures of the skin, laboratory procedures and tests, technologic applications in dermatology, fundamentals of cutaneous surgery, cosmetics for the physician, psoriasis, psychodermatology, virology, cutaneous diseases associated with immunodeficiency virus, diseases affecting the hair, diseases affecting the nail unit, collagen–vascular diseases, the skin and internal disease, dermatologic reactions to ultraviolet light and visible light, genodermatoses, pediatric dermatology, tropical diseases of the skin, sports dermatology, cutaneous signs of bioterrorism, and dermatoses of pregnancy.

Numerous color photographs have been added to this book of dermatology, the most visual of all medical specialties.

The chapters I have retained from the previous edition remain in the basic proven structure that Dr. Sauer has been recognized for worldwide during his outstanding dermatology teaching career.

It has been a pleasure and a learning experience working with my son, who has written a chapter and done the endless work of editing and acquiring new authors.

*John C. Hall, MD*

# ACKNOWLEDGMENTS

I would like to thank Cindy Irey, a nurse par excellence, for helping with the editing. She somehow fit us into her busy schedule.

Marla Sussman was the best editor for any authors of a work of science. Her patience was endless.

The contributing chapter authors made this endeavor a true joy. They deserve kudos for the success we hope this book will achieve.

Charlotte is more than a wife. She is an inspiration, cheerleader, and friend.

Kim and Shelly, my daughters, and Tony and Tori, my grandchildren, give me my grounding and reasons for pursuit of scholarship.

My office staff kept my practice afloat while I was having fun writing. They are Christa Czysz, office manager; Kelly Howell, office administrator; Jennifer Phillips, receptionist; and Kelly Hedgens, nurse.

Thank you to Brent Johnson for his technical assistance with the photographs.

A big thank you goes to Dean Shepard, chief of photography services at St. Luke's Hospital in Kansas City, Missouri, whose photography has contributed greatly to this edition.

As brevity is the soul of wit, it is also the soul of understanding a complex subject. An overview is more priceless at the onset of learning than a mountain of detail. To stir one's interest and curiosity about a field of scientific endeavor, one needs to see that field as a whole. Therein lies the true genius of Gordon Sauer.

I frequently hear from dermatologists and nondermatologists alike that this book is their first exposure to the study of skin diseases. The tenth edition and all preceding editions are a tribute to Dr. Sauer's ability to open up the specialty of dermatology to those who wish to use its magic to help in the care of their patients.

# CHAPTER 1

# Structure of the Skin

*Kenneth R. Watson, DO*

The skin is the largest organ of the human body. It is composed of tissue that grows, differentiates, and renews itself constantly. Because the skin is a barrier between the internal organs and the external environment, it is uniquely subjected to noxious external agents and is also a sensitive reflection of internal disease. An understanding of the cause and effect of this complex interplay in the skin begins with knowledge of the basic structure of this organ.

## Layers of the Skin

The skin is divided into three distinct layers. From the external surface inward, they are the epidermis, dermis, and subcutaneous tissue (Fig. 1-1). There are regional variations of these layers that probably represent adaptations to different functions, such as:

1. a thickened keratin layer of the epidermis on the palms and soles,
2. numerous nerve fibers within the fingertips for improved tactile function,
3. increased numbers of sebaceous glands on the face, and
4. thickened dermis on the back

### Epidermis

The epidermis is the most superficial of the three layers of the skin and averages in thickness about the width of the mark of a sharp pencil (<1 mm). It contains several types of cells including keratinocytes, dendritic cells (melanocytes and Langerhans cells), and Merkel cells.

The keratinocytes, or keratin-forming cells, are by far the most common and develop into four identifiable layers of the epidermis (Fig. 1-2). From inside out, they are as follows:

Basal layer  
Spinous layer  } Living epidermis  
Granular layer  
Keratin layer  Dead end-product

The basal layer lies next to the dermis. This layer can be thought of as the stem cell layer of the epidermis, which is capable of progressive maturation into cell forms higher in the epidermis. It normally requires 3 or 4 weeks for the epidermis to replicate itself by the processes of division and differentiation. This cell turnover is greatly accelerated in diseases

such as psoriasis in which the turnover rate may be as short as 2 to 3 days.

The spinous layer, or stratum malpighii, is made up of several layers of epidermal cells, which have a polyhedral shape. The cells of this layer are connected by intercellular bridges, which may be seen in routine sections.

The granular layer is composed of flatter cells containing protein granules called *keratohyalin granules*. In lichen planus, the granular cell layer is focally increased.

The outermost layer of the epidermis is the *keratin (cornified) layer*. It is made up of stratified layers of dead keratinized cells that are constantly shedding (Fig. 1-3). The protein in these cells is called *keratin* and is capable of absorbing vast amounts of water. This is readily seen during bathing, when the skin of the palms and the soles becomes white, swollen, and wrinkled. The keratin layer provides a major barrier of protection for the body. Mucous membranes, such as the oral and vaginal mucosa, do not have granular or keratin layers.

Immediately beneath the basal layer is the interface between the epidermis and the dermis known as the basement membrane zone or dermal–epidermal junction. It is difficult to visualize in routine hematoxylin and eosin stained sections but can clearly be seen as a thin band with periodic acid schiff (PAS) stains, due to the presence of mucopolysaccharides. Ultrastructurally, the basal cells are attached to the basement membrane by hemidesmosomes. Beneath the basal cells is an electron-clear layer known as the lamina lucida. Below this is a more electron-dense layer known as the lamina densa, which consists predominantly of type IV collagen. Anchoring filaments extend through the basement membrane zone to connect the surface membranes of the basal cells to the lamina densa. There are anchoring fibrils that attach the lamina densa to the papillary dermis.

Several blistering diseases occur due to defects in the basement membrane zone. Bullous pemphigoid antigens are present within the hemidesmosomes of the basement membrane zone. Circulating IgG antibodies bind to these antigens, resulting in the subepidermal blistering disease bullous pemphigoid. Epidermolysis bullosa represents a heterogeneous group of noninflammatory blistering disorders that can be divided into three subtypes based on the location of the blister. In epidermolysis bullosa simplex, the blister usually occurs through the basal cell layer. In the junctional

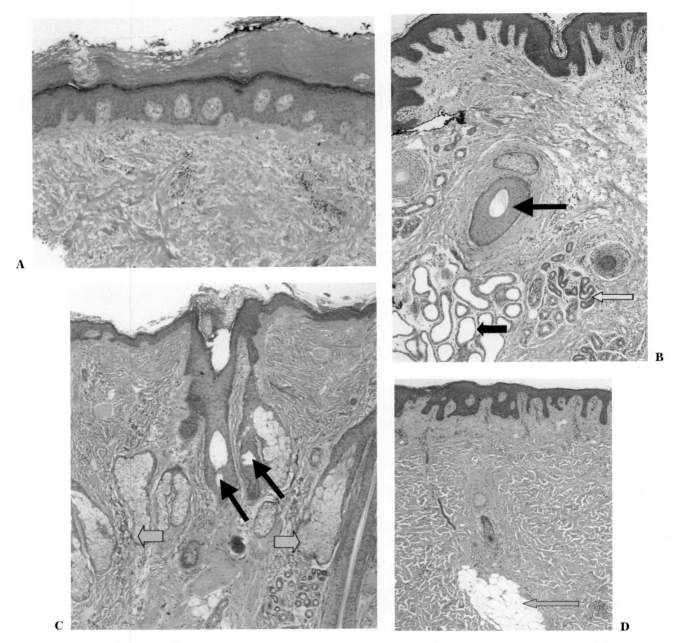

**FIGURE 1-1** ■ Histology of the skin. Photomicrographs from four different areas of the body: palm **(A)**, axilla **(B)**, face **(C)**, and back **(D)**. Note the variations in the histologic features: thickened keratin layer from the palm (Fig. A), multiple (Fig. B) glandular elements from the axilla (hair follicle, *thin black arrow*; apocrine gland, *thick black arrow*; eccrine gland, *yellow arrow*), (Fig. C) numerous pilosebaceous units from the face (hair follicles, *thin arrows*; sebaceous glands, *thick arrows*), and (Fig. D) thick dermis from the trunk (subcutaneous fat, *arrow*). *(Courtesy of Dr. K. Watson.)*

form, it occurs between the basal cells and the lamina lucida, probably due to a defect in the hemidesmosomes. In the dermolytic form, the blister occurs beneath the lamina densa in the area of the anchoring fibrils.

The *melanin-forming cells*, or *melanocytes*, are sandwiched between the more numerous keratin-forming cells in the basal layer. In routine hematoxylin and eosin stained sections, melanocytes have small, dark nuclei and clear cytoplasm, which is the result of shrinkage artifact. Approximately 10%

of the cells in the basal layer are melanocytes. However, this varies depending on the body site and ethnic background of the individual. These melanocytes are dopa-positive because they stain darkly after contact with a solution of levorotatory 3,4-dihydroxyphenylalanine, or *dopa*. This laboratory reaction closely simulates physiologic melanin formation, in which the amino acid tyrosine is oxidized by the enzyme tyrosinase to form dopa. Dopa is then further changed, through a series of complex metabolic processes, to melanin. In

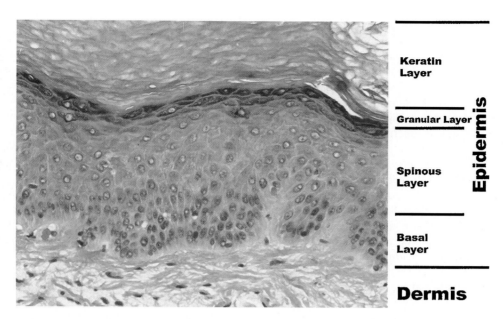

FIGURE 1-2 ■ Histology of the epidermis. A photomicrograph from the palm. *(Courtesy of Dr. K. Watson.)*

dermatopathology practices, melanocytes are most commonly recognized by showing positive immunoreactivity for S-100 protein, HMB-45, and Melan-A (MART-1), which may be useful in the diagnosis of melanocytic tumors such as malignant melanoma. Melanocytes may also be recognized using silver stains due to the fact that melanin is both argyrophilic and argentaffin. For example, the Fontana–Masson histochemical stain results in black cytoplasmic granules within melanocytes because of the ability of melanin to reduce ammoniated silver nitrate. Melanin may also be bleached, which is useful in identifying the neoplastic melanocytes that are obscured in heavily pigmented tumors.

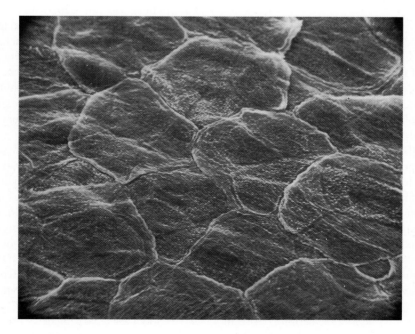

FIGURE 1-3 ■ Keratin-layer cells. Underside of the top layer of epidermal keratin-layer cells on Scotch tape stripping is seen with Cambridge Mark II Stereoscan at 1000X. *(Courtesy of Drs. J. Arnold, W. Barnes, and G. Sauer.)*

Melanin pigmentation of the skin, whether increased or decreased, is influenced by many local and systemic factors (see Chapter 30). Melanocyte-stimulating hormone from the pituitary is the most potent melanizing agent. Melanin is transferred from melanocytes to basal keratinocytes. Skin color is largely related to the amount of melanin present in basal cells. Exposure to ultraviolet light results in increased melanocyte concentration and function.

*Langerhans cells* are found scattered evenly throughout the epidermis. They are bone marrow–derived mononuclear cells. They are involved in cell-mediated hypersensitivity, antigen processing and recognition, stimulation of immune-competent cells, and graft rejection. Sunlight suppresses their immune function. Their number is decreased in certain skin diseases, such as psoriasis. Staining with membrane adenosine triphosphatase and monoclonal antibodies such as S-100 protein and CD-1 a can be done for identification. Electron microscopy reveals that these cells contain characteristic racquet-shaped Birbeck granules. These cells proliferate in the disease Langerhans cell histiocytosis (formerly known as histiocytosis X), which may be isolated to the skin or may be part of a larger systemic process.

*Merkel cells* are located within the basal layer but may also be found within hair follicles and sweat ducts. They are assumed to function as touch receptors and are associated with fine unmyelinated nerve fibers. They are inconspicuous in routine sections. They may be recognized using immunostains for the neuroendocrine markers neuron-specific enolase, chromogranin, and synaptophysin. Ultrastructurally, they contain dense core neurosecretory granules. They give rise to primary neuroendocrine carcinoma of the skin (Merkel cell carcinoma).

## Dermis

The dermis consists of connective tissue, cellular elements, and ground substance. It has a rich vascular and nerve supply and contains pilosebaceous, apocrine, and eccrine structures. Anatomically, it is divided into two compartments. The first contains thin collagen fibers, delicate elastic fibers, numerous capillaries, and abundant ground substance, which form a thin layer beneath the epidermis (papillary dermis) and surrounding adnexal structures (periadnexal dermis). Together, these are regarded as a single unit called the *adventitial dermis.* This is an important unit because it is altered together with the adjacent epithelium in many inflammatory diseases. The second compartment, known as the *reticular* or *deep dermis,* is composed of thick collagen bundles with intertwined elastic fibers. The reticular dermis is thick and comprises the bulk of the dermis. It contains less ground substance, vascular spaces, and cellular elements than the thin adventitial dermis.

The *connective tissue* component of the dermis consists of collagen fibers, including reticulin fibers, and elastic fibers. These fibers contribute to the support and elasticity of the skin.

Two different types of collagen are present within the dermis. Type I collagen is predominantly found within the thick fibers of the reticular dermis. Type III collagen, also known as *reticulin,* is largely found within the thin fibers of the papillary and periadnexal dermis. These reticulin fibers are not visible in routine hematoxylin and eosin stained sections but can be identified with silver stains. They are abundant in certain pathologic conditions such as granulomas, syphilis, sarcoidosis, and some mesenchymal tumors. The proteins present in collagen fibers are responsible for nearly one-fourth of a person's overall protein mass. If tannic acid or the salts of heavy metals, such as dichromates, are combined with collagen, the result is leather.

Elastic fibers are thinner than most collagen fibers and are entwined among them. They are composed of the protein elastin. Elastic fibers do not readily take up acidic or basic stains, such as hematoxylin and eosin, but they can be identified with the Verhoeff–van Gieson stain.

Cellular elements of the dermis include fibroblasts, endothelial cells, mast cells, and a variety of miscellaneous cells, including smooth muscle, nerve, and hematopoietic cells. The hematopoietic cells include lymphocytes, histiocytes (macrophages), eosinophils, neutrophils, and plasma cells. These hematopoietic cells are increased in numerous inflammatory diseases of the skin.

Fibroblasts form collagen and produce ground substance. They are involved in immunologic and reparative processes. Fibroblasts are increased in numerous different skin disorders.

Mast cells are derived from bone marrow stem cells. They are present in normal skin in small numbers and are usually concentrated around blood vessels, particularly post-capillary venules. They have intracytoplasmic basophilic metachromatic granules containing heparin and histamine. The granules do not stain with routine hematoxylin and eosin but may be seen with colloidal iron, toluidine blue, and Alcian blue stains. Mast cells are increased in many different inflammatory dermatoses but play a particularly important role in urticarial eruptions. Urticaria occurs when mast cells and basophils are degranulated, resulting in vascular permeability and tissue edema. Mast cell degranulation also plays a role in activating other inflammatory cells to the area of tissue injury.

Neoplastic proliferations of mast cells may form papules, plaques, and nodules within the skin, known as cutaneous mastocytosis (*urticaria pigmentosa*). They may also have a telangiectatic appearance, as in telangiectasia macularis eruptiva perstans (TMEP). In addition to metachromatic staining mentioned in the previous paragraph, these proliferations of mast cells show positive immunoreactivity for human mast cell tryptase and CD117, which may be useful in differentiating mast cell proliferations from other cutaneous neoplasms, such as Langerhans cell histiocytosis and leukemia cutis.

Histiocytes (macrophages) are present in only small numbers in the normal skin. However, in pathologic conditions, they migrate to the dermis as tissue monocytes. They play a predominant role in the phagocytosis of particulate matter and bacteria. Under special pathologic conditions, they may form giant cells. They are also involved in the immune system by phagocytizing antigens.

Lymphocytes and plasma cells are found in only small numbers in normal skin, but are significantly increased in pathologic conditions, such as increased plasma cells in syphilis.

The *ground substance* of the dermis is a gel-like amorphous matrix not easily seen in routine sections, but it may be identified with colloidal iron and Alcian blue stains. It is found in greatest concentration within the adventitial dermis, particularly around adnexal structures. There are variable amounts of ground substance in different areas of the body, with increased concentrations within the fingers and toes. The ground substance contains proteins, mucopolysaccharides, soluble collagens, enzymes, immune bodies, and metabolites. It has the capacity to bind water, allowing the movement of nutrients through the dermis, and it provides bulk, contributing to the malleability of the skin.

## Subcutaneous Tissue

The subcutaneous tissue constitutes the largest volume of adipose tissue in the body. The adipose tissue is organized into lobules by fibrous septa, which contain most of the blood vessels, nerves, and lymphatics. The thickness of the subcutaneous fat varies from one area of the body to another. It is especially thick in the abdominal region and thin in the eyelids and scrotum. The subcutaneous tissue serves as a receptacle for the formation and storage of fat as well as a site of highly dynamic lipid metabolism for nutrition. It also provides protection from physical trauma and insulation to temperature changes.

Most of the fat in the body consists of white adipose tissue (**Fig. 1-4**). The white fat cells are derived from mesenchymal cells, as are fibroblasts. They store triglycerides, which can be broken down into fatty acids and used for energy by

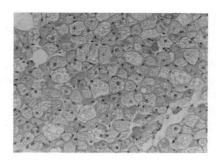

**FIGURE 1-5** ■ Brown adipose tissue. *(Courtesy of Dr. K. Watson.)*

other tissues such as muscle. White adipose tissue is increased in obesity.

There is a second distinct type of adipose tissue, known as brown fat, which is found predominantly in human newborns and also hibernating animals (**Fig. 1-5**). Brown fat cells have a different appearance than white fat cells. They are smaller, contain multiple small lipid droplets, and have increased numbers of mitochondria. Recent studies using fluorodeoxyglucose positron emission tomography (PET) suggest that a significant percentage of adult humans have active brown adipose tissue. Brown fat has a different function than white fat. It is involved in energy expenditure that is responsible for generating heat, protecting body temperature in human newborns without shivering. It may also be useful in protecting against obesity. Brown fat may develop from a common precursor to skeletal myocytes.

Lipomas are benign tumors composed of mature fat cells identical to white adipose tissue in the subcutaneous fat. Hibernoma is a benign tumor composed of fat cells resembling brown fat.

## Vasculature

The skin contains a rich vascular network that provides blood volume far exceeding its nutritional needs. In fact, the vascularization is so extensive that it has been postulated that its main function is to regulate heat and blood pressure of the body, with providing nutrition to the skin a secondary function. The vascular plexus arises from thick arteries within the subcutaneous fat. There are two major plexuses, which run parallel to the epidermis, one within the deep dermis near the dermal–subcutaneous junction and one within the superficial (papillary) dermis. There are vertically oriented perforating branches that connect the two plexuses and provide blood to surrounding dermal appendages. Perivascular inflammation surrounding the superficial and deep plexuses occurs in many types of "dermatitis," and this pattern of inflammation may be used as a method of classification of inflammatory disorders of the skin. Inflammatory reactions involving the superficial vascular plexus may result in erythema.

The vascular plexuses consist of a mixture of arterioles, venules, and capillaries. Most of the exchange of water, oxygen,

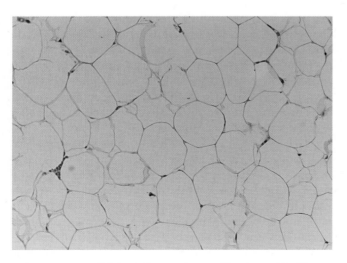

**FIGURE 1-4** ■ White adipose tissue. *(Courtesy of Dr. K. Watson.)*

and nutrients with the skin occurs through thin capillaries and venules. The skin also contains an extensive lymphatic network that is independent of the vascular plexus. No blood vessels or lymphatics are present within the epidermis.

A special vascular body, the glomus, deserves mention. The glomus body is most commonly seen on the tips of the fingers and toes and under the nails. Each glomus body consists of a venous and arterial segment, called the *Sucquet–Hoyer canal*. This canal represents a short-circuit device that connects an arteriole with a venule directly, without intervening capillaries. The result is a marked increase in the blood flow through the skin. If this body grows abnormally, it forms an often painful, red, benign glomus tumor, commonly beneath the nail.

## Nerve Supply

The skin is a major sensory organ with millions of nerve endings receiving stimulation from the surrounding environment. Sensory and autonomic nerves within the peripheral nervous system permeate the dermis with tiny nerve fibers, which may be myelinated or unmyelinated. These tiny nerve fibers are not visible in routine hematoxylin and eosin stained sections. Only larger myelinated nerve fibers and specialized nerve-end organs are discernable. Special stains are required to visualize the small nerve-fibers, such as silver impregnation techniques (Bielschowsky or Bodian stains) or immunoperoxidase stains such as neurofilament protein, which stains axons, and S-100 protein, which stains Schwann cells. The nerve fibers are variably distributed, resulting in regional variations in sensation. They are very prominent on the palms, soles, and fingers, and within mucocutaneous areas.

Numerous tiny unmyelinated sensory nerves with free nerve endings are present within the papillary dermis and surrounding hair follicles. They mediate the sensations of temperature, touch, pain, and itching. Some of the free nerve endings extend into the basal epidermis and contact Merkel cells.

---

### SAUER'S NOTES

*Itching* is the most important presenting symptom of an unhappy patient. It may be defined simply as the desire to scratch. Itching apparently is a mildly painful sensation that differs from pain in having a lower frequency of impulse stimuli. The release of proteinases (such as follows itch-powder application) may be responsible for the itch sensation. The pruritus may be of a pricking or burning type and can vary greatly from one person to another. Sulzberger called abnormally sensitive people *itchish*, analogous to *ticklish*. Itching can occur without any clinical signs of skin disease or from circulating allergens or local superficial contactants. The skin of atopic or eczema patients tends to be more itchy. Scratching makes the itching worse. This results in a perpetual itch–scratch cycle.

---

Sensory nerves in hairless skin, such as the palms and soles, and at the mucocutaneous junction terminate in specialized end organs, known as Meissner corpuscles, Vater–Pacini corpuscles, and mucocutaneous end organs. Meissner corpuscles are most numerous on the fingertips, palms, and soles, where they sense touch and vibration. They are composed of S-100–positive laminated, flattened Schwann cells. Vater–Pacini corpuscles are most numerous within the deep dermis and subcutaneous fat of the feet and hands, and they sense pressure and tension. They are large, measuring up to 1 mm in diameter, and are composed of outer spherical layers of perineurial cells and an inner nerve fiber with accompanying Schwann cell.

Sympathetic autonomic nerve fibers supply blood vessels, arrector pili muscles, apocrine glands, and eccrine glands. Adrenergic fibers carry impulses to the arrector pili muscles, which produce gooseflesh if they are stimulated. This is caused by traction of the muscle on the hair follicles to which it is attached. Cholinergic fibers, if stimulated, increase sweating and may cause a specific type of hives called *cholinergic urticaria* (see Chapter 11). Sebaceous glands do not contain autonomic fibers but are controlled by endocrine stimulation.

## Appendages

The appendages of the skin include both the cornified appendages (hairs and nails) and the glandular appendages.

### Hair Follicles

Hairs are produced by the hair follicles, which develop from germinative cells of the fetal epidermis. Because no new hair follicles are formed after birth, the different types of body hairs are manifestations of the effect of location as well as external and internal stimuli. Hormones are the most important internal stimuli influencing the various types of hair growth. There are three main types of hairs: (1) *Lanugo hairs:* fine, lightly pigmented hairs covering the body of the fetus, (2) *Vellus hairs* ("peach fuzz"): short, fine hairs that replace lanugo hairs and cover most of the body but are barely noticeable, and (3) *Terminal hairs:* long, coarse hairs present in the adult, which are prominent on the scalp, beard, pubic, and axillary regions. Terminal hairs convert into vellus hairs in male pattern baldness. Vellus hairs develop into terminal hairs in hirsutism. The palms, soles, lips, and some genital areas do not contain hair follicles.

Hair growth is cyclic, with a growing (anagen) phase (Fig. 1-6) and a resting (telogen) phase. The *catagen cycle* is the transition phase between the growing and resting stages and lasts only a few weeks. The duration of hair growth varies in different areas of the body. Approximately 90% of normal scalp hairs are in the growing (anagen) stage, which can last between 3 to 6 years or more, depending on the location. Ten percent of hairs are in the resting (telogen) stage, which lasts approximately 60 to 90 days. However, systemic stresses, such as childbirth, or systemic anesthesia may cause

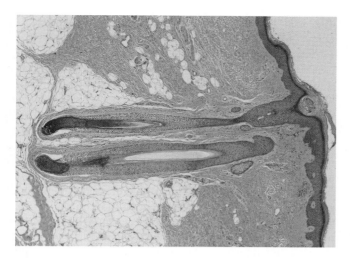

**FIGURE 1-6** ▪ Anagen hairs with hair bulb and matrix cells. *(Courtesy of Dr. K. Watson.)*

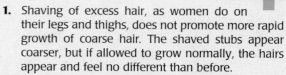
hairs to enter a resting stage prematurely. This *postpartum* or *postanesthetic effect* is noticed most commonly in the scalp when these resting hairs are depilated during combing or washing, and the thought of approaching baldness causes sudden alarm.

Hair follicles may be thought of as an invagination of the epidermis, with its different layers of cells. The hair follicle can be divided into three areas: (1) *infundibulum,* which extends from the follicular orifice to the entrance of the underlying sebaceous gland, (2) *isthmus,* which extends from the orifice of the sebaceous gland to the insertion of the erector pili muscle, and (3) *inferior segment,* which consists of the follicle below the insertion of the erector pili muscle.

The inferior portion of the follicle includes the hair bulb, which contains matrix cells. These cells perform a similar function to the basal cells of the epidermis. They are responsible for the development of the hair shaft. Melanocytes are present in the matrix and determine the color of hair.

There are approximately 100,000 anagen follicles on the normal scalp with tremendous protein-synthesizing capacity. At the rate of scalp hair growth of 0.35 mm/d, more than 100 linear feet of scalp hair is produced daily. The density of hairs in the scalp varies from 175 to 300 hairs per square centimeter. Up to 100 hairs may be normally lost daily.

### Nail Unit

The nail unit consists of a nail plate and the surrounding soft tissues, which include the nail matrix, proximal and lateral nail folds, nail bed, cuticle, and hyponychium (Fig. 29-1). The nail plate covers the dorsal distal aspect of the fingers and toes and ranges between 0.3 and 0.75 mm in thickness. It inserts into grooves in the skin that are present proximally and laterally. The plate is produced by the nail matrix, which is located at the proximal end of the plate insertion, ventral to the proximal nail fold. The matrix extends distally to the lunula, which is a crescent-shaped white area under the proximal nail plate, particularly prominent on the thumb and less prominent on the remaining fingers. The nail plate lies on the nail bed. The epithelium of the nail bed produces a small amount of keratin, which tightly adheres to the overlying nail plate. The dermis of the nail bed is richly vascular, resulting in a pink appearance and blanching when compressed. Glomus bodies are also present, which aid in temperature control of the digits. The cuticle represents the cornified layer of the proximal nail fold and serves to seal off and protect the nail matrix. The hyponychium consists of cornified epidermis located at the distal end of the nail bed beneath the distal free edge of the nail plate.

The nail unit is an invagination of the epidermis, similar to the hair follicle. Both have a matrix that produces the protein keratin. The nail plate consists almost entirely of keratin, similar to the hair shaft and cornified layer of the epidermis. Unlike hair growth, which is periodic, nail growth is continuous. Nail growth proceeds at about one-third of the rate of hair growth, or about 0.1 mm/d. It takes about 3 months to restore a removed fingernail and about three times that long for the regrowth of a new toenail. Nail growth can be inhibited during serious illnesses or in old age, increased through nail biting or occupational trauma, and altered due to a variety of diseases and medications.

### Glandular Appendages

The three types of glandular appendages of the skin are the sebaceous glands, apocrine glands, and eccrine glands (Fig. 1-7).

The *sebaceous glands* are present everywhere on the skin, except the palms and the soles. In most areas they are associated with hair follicles. There are sebaceous glands that are

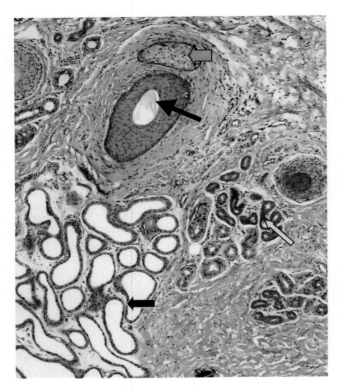

**FIGURE 1-7** ■ Histology of the glands of the skin. A photomicrograph from the axilla (hair follicle, *long black arrow*; apocrine glands, *short black arrow*; sebaceous gland, *short blue arrow*; eccrine glands, *yellow arrow*). *(Courtesy of Dr. K. Watson.)*

not associated with hair follicles, such as the buccal mucosa and vermillion border of the lip, nipple and areola of the breast, labia minora, and eyelids (meibomian glands). The sebaceous glands are holocrine glands, forming their secretions through the disintegration of the entire glandular cell. The secretion from these glands is evacuated through the sebaceous duct to a follicle that may contain either a large terminal hair or a vellus hair. This secretion, known as *sebum*, is not under any neurologic control but is a continuous outflow of the material of cell breakdown. The sebum covers the skin with a thin lipoidal film that is mildly bacteriostatic and fungistatic and retards water evaporation. The scalp and the face may contain as many as 1,000 sebaceous glands per square centimeter. The activity of the gland increases markedly at the age of puberty, and, in certain people, it becomes plugged with sebum, debris, and bacteria to form the blackheads and pimples of acne.

*Apocrine glands* are found in the axillae, genital region, breast, external ear canal (ceruminous glands), and eyelid (Moll's glands). They do not develop until the time of puberty. They consist of a coiled secretory gland located in the deep dermis or subcutaneous fat and a straight duct that usually empties into a hair follicle. The function of the secretions is unknown; however, they may act as pheromones. They are responsible for the production of body odor (the infamous "BO"). Any emotional stresses that cause adrenergic sympathetic discharge produce apocrine secretion. This secretion is sterile when excreted but undergoes decomposition when contaminated by bacteria from the skin surface, resulting in a strong and characteristic odor. The purpose of the many cosmetic underarm preparations is to remove these bacteria or block the gland's excretion. The apocrine glands are involved in *hidradenitis suppurativa*, an inflammatory process that results from follicular obstruction and retention of follicular products, which usually occurs in patients with the acne–seborrhea complex.

*Eccrine sweat glands* are distributed everywhere on the skin surface, with the greatest concentration on the palms, soles, and forehead. They develop as a downgrowth from the primitive epidermis. They are composed of coiled secretory glands, a coiled duct, a straight duct, an intraepidermal coil, and an eccrine pore. The eccrine sweat glands and the vasculature of the skin serve in the maintenance of stable internal body temperature, despite marked environmental temperature changes. They flood the skin surface with water for cooling, and the blood vessels dilate or constrict to dissipate or conserve body heat. Their prime stimulus is heat, and their activity is under the control of the nervous system, usually through the hypothalamus. Both adrenergic and cholinergic fibers innervate the glands. Blockage of the eccrine ducts results in the disease known as *miliaria* (*prickly heat*). If eccrine glands are congenitally absent, as in *anhidrotic ectodermal dysplasia*, a life-threatening hyperpyrexia may develop.

## Acknowledgment

We acknowledge the valuable assistance of Dean Shepard from St. Luke's Hospital photographic services.

## Suggested Readings

Ackerman BA. *Histologic Diagnosis of Inflammatory Skin Diseases.* Philadelphia: Lea & Febiger; 1978.

Barnhill RL. *Textbook of Dermatopathology.* New York: McGraw-Hill; 1998.

Briggaman RA. Epidermal-dermal junction: structure, composition, function and disease relationships. *Prog Dermatol.* 1990;24(2):1.

Farmer RE, Hood AF. *Pathology of the Skin.* Norwalk, CT: Appleton & Lange; 1990.

Fleischer AB. *The Clinical Management of Itching: Therapeutic Protocols for Pruritis.* London: Parthenon Publishing Group; 1998.

Goldsmith L. *Physiology, Biochemistry, and Molecular Biology of the Skin.* New York: Oxford University Press; 1991.

Hurwitz RM, Hood AF. *Pathology of the Skin: Atlas of Clinical-Pathological Correlation.* Stamford, CT: Appleton & Lange; 1997.

Lever WE, Schaumburg-Lever G. *Histopathology of the Skin.* 7th ed. Philadelphia: JB Lippincott; 1990.

Murphy GF, Elder EE. *Atlas of Tumor Pathology: Non-melanocytic Tumors of the Skin.* Washington, DC: Armed Forces Institute of Pathology; 1991.

Nedergaard J, Bengtsson T, Cannon B. Unexpected evidence for active brown adipose tissue in adult humans. *Am J Physiol Endocrinol Metab.* 2007;293:E444–E452.

Nickolof BJ. *Dermal Immune System.* Boca Raton, FL: CRC Press; 1993.

Rosen T, Martin S. *Atlas of Black Dermatology.* Boston: Little, Brown and Company; 1981.

Seale P, Bjork B, Yang W, et al. PRDM16 controls a brown fat/skeletal muscle switch. *Nature.* 2008;454:947–948.

# CHAPTER 2

# Laboratory Procedures and Tests

*Christopher J. Kligora, MD and Kenneth R. Watson, DO*

In addition to the usual laboratory procedures used in the workup of medical patients, certain special tests are of importance in the field of dermatology. These include skin tests, fungus examinations, biopsies, and immunologic diagnosis. For special problems, additional testing methods are suggested in the sections on the various diseases.

## Skin Tests

There are three types of skin tests:

- Intracutaneous
- Scratch
- Patch

The intracutaneous tests and the scratch tests can have two types of reactions: either an immediate wheal reaction or a delayed reaction. The immediate wheal reaction develops to a maximum in 5 to 20 minutes and is elicited in testing for the cause of urticaria, atopic dermatitis, and inhalant allergies. This is a type I or anaphylactoid type of immunity. The immediate wheal reaction test is seldom used for determining the cause of skin diseases.

The delayed reaction to intracutaneous skin testing is exemplified best by the tuberculin skin test. Tuberculin is available in two forms—as the purified protein derivative test and as a tuberculin tine test. The purified protein derivative test is performed by using tablets that come in two strengths and by injecting a solution of either one intracutaneously. If there is no reaction after the test with the first strength, then the second strength may be employed.

The tuberculin tine test (Mantoux) is a simple and rapid procedure using OTK. Nine prongs, or tines, covered with OTK are pressed into the skin. If at the end of 48 or 72 hours there is more than 2 mm of induration at the site of any prong insertion, the test is positive.

Patch tests are used commonly in dermatology and offer a simple and accurate method of determining whether a patient is allergic to any of the testing agents. There are two different reactions to this type of test: a primary irritant reaction and an allergic reaction. The primary irritant reaction occurs in most of the population if they are exposed to agents (in appropriate concentrations) that have skin-destroying properties. Examples of these agents include soaps, cleaning fluids, bleaches, "corn" removers, and counterirritants. The allergic reaction indicates that the patient is more sensitive than normal to the agent being tested. This test reaction is idiosyncratic and not necessarily related to concentration or dose. It also shows that the patient has had a previous exposure to that agent or a cross-sensitizing agent. This is a type IV or delayed type of immunity. It is often very helpful in cases of contact dermatitis.

The technique of the patch test is simple, but the interpretation of the test is not. For example, consider a patient presenting with dermatitis on top of the feet. It is possible that shoe leather or some chemical used in the manufacture of the leather is causing the reaction. The procedure for a patch test is to cut out a half-inch square piece of the material from the inside of the shoe, moisten the material with distilled water, place it on the skin surface, and cover it with an adhesive band or some patch-test dressing. The patch test is left on for 48 hours. When the patch test is removed, the patient is considered to have a positive patch test if there is any redness, papules, or vesiculation under the site of the testing agent. Delayed reactions to allergens can occur, and, ideally, a final reading should be made after 96 hours (4 days), that is, 2 days after the patch is removed.

The patch test can be used to make or confirm a diagnosis of poison ivy dermatitis, ragweed dermatitis, or contact dermatitis caused by medications, cosmetics, or industrial chemicals. Fisher (1995) and Adams (1990) compiled lists of chemicals, concentrations, and vehicles to be used for eliciting the allergic type of patch test reaction. Most tests can be performed very simply, however, as in the case of the shoe leather dermatitis. One precaution is that the patch must not be allowed to become wet in the 48-hour period. A patch test kit, T.R.U.E. Test (Glaxo), includes ready-to-apply self-adhesive allergen tapes. There are other more extensive patch test trays available.

A method of testing for food allergy is to use the Rowe elimination diet. The procedure is to limit the diet to the following basic foods, which are known to be hypoallergenic: lamb, lemon, grapefruit, pears, lettuce, spinach, carrots, sweet potatoes, tapioca, rice and rice bread, corn sugar, maple syrup, sesame oil, gelatin, and salt. The patient is to remain on this basic diet for 5 to 7 days. At the end of that time, one new food can be added every 2 days. The following foods can be added early: beef, white potatoes, green beans, milk (along with butter and American cheese), and white bread with puffed wheat. If there is a flare-up of the dermatitis, which should occur within 2 to 8 hours after ingestion of an offending food,

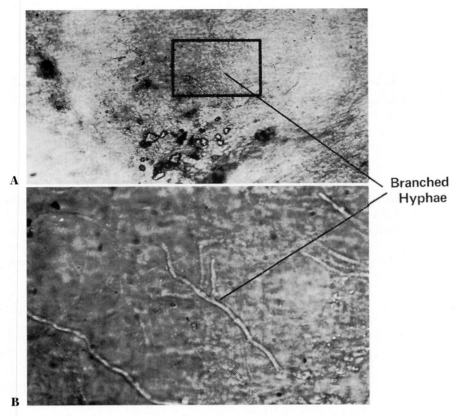

**Branched Hyphae**

**FIGURE 2-1** ■ Fungi from a skin scraping as seen with microscope in a KOH preparation. **(A)** Low-power lens (100X) view. **(B)** High-power lens (450X) view of area outlined above. *(Courtesy of Dr. D. Gibson.)*

the new food should be discontinued for the present. More new foods are added until the normal diet, minus the allergenic foods, is regained.

Keeping a "diet diary" of all foods, medicines, oral hygiene items, or anything injected or inhaled can sometimes be a retrospective way of identifying an allergen. The skin reaction usually occurs less than 8 hours after ingestion.

## Fungus Examinations

The KOH preparation is a simple office laboratory procedure for the detection of fungal organisms present in skin and nails. It is performed by scraping the diseased skin and examining the material with the microscope. The skin scrapings are obtained by abrading a scaly diseased area with a scalpel. If a blister is present, the underside of the blister is examined. The material is deposited on a glass slide and then covered with 20% aqueous potassium hydroxide solution and a coverslip. The preparation can be gently heated or allowed to stand at room temperature for 15 to 60 minutes. The addition of dimethyl sulfoxide to the KOH preparation eliminates the need to heat the specimen. A diagnostically helpful pale violet stain can be imparted to the fungi if the 20% KOH solution is mixed with an equal amount of Parker Super Quik permanent blue-black ink. Other staining

solutions are available. The slide is then examined microscopically for fungal organisms (**Fig. 2-1**).

For culture preparation, a portion of the material from the scraping can be implanted on several different types of agar, including mycobiotic agar, inhibitory mold agar (IMA), BHI (brain hear infusion) with blood, chloramphenicol, gentamicin agar, and Sabouraud's glucose agar. A white or variously colored growth is noted in approximately 1 to 3 weeks (**Fig. 2-2**).

The species of fungus can be identified by morphology on the culture plate, biochemical characteristics, and microscopic morphology with a lactophenol cotton blue stain of a smear from the fungal colony. A culture media is available that changes color when a pathogen is cultured.

## Biopsies

The biopsy and microscopic examination of a questionable skin lesion may be invaluable. A definitive diagnosis is nearly always rendered with most pigmented lesions and other cutaneous tumors. In the case of inflammatory lesions, histologic findings may or may not be diagnostic, depending on the disease process, the age of the lesion, clinical description of the lesion(s) including extent of involvement, other symptoms and/or medical conditions, and a differential diagnosis.

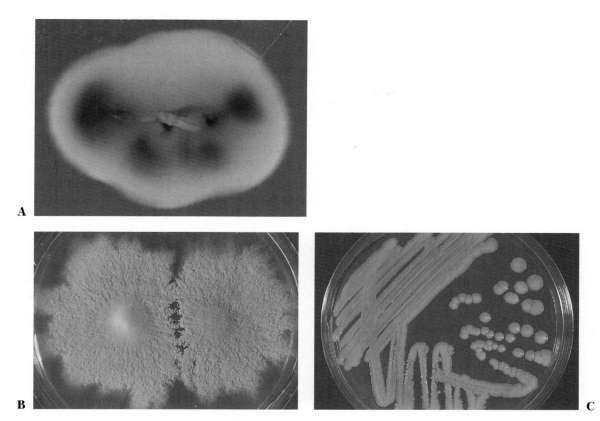

**FIGURE 2-2** ■ Fungus cultures: subcultures grown on potato dextrose agar. **(A)** *Trichophyton rubrum.* **(B)** *Microsporum gypseum.* **(C)** *Candida albicans. (Courtesy of Dr. K. Watson.)*

In cases where histologic findings are not diagnostic, at the very least, many pertinent diagnoses on the clinical differential can be excluded. In addition to diagnosis, other useful parameters can be obtained with cutaneous lesions, such as depth of invasion, lymphovascular space invasion, perineural involvement, and adequacy of surgical margins. The quintessential example is malignant melanoma, where most of these factors plus several others may only be assessed histologically and are essential for staging and prognosis.

There are four principle techniques for performing skin biopsies:

1. Surgical excision with suturing
2. Punch biopsy
3. Excision with scissors
4. Shave biopsy

---

**SAUER'S NOTES**

1. The skin biopsy specimen must include adequate tissue for proper interpretation by the pathologist.
2. Communication between a pathologist knowledgeable in this disease and the clinician is mandatory for accurate tissue diagnosis.

---

The decision in favor of one method depends on factors such as location of the biopsy, desired cosmetic result, depth of the diseased tissue, type of lesion to be removed (flat or elevated), and simplicity of technique. For example, vesicles should be completely excised in an attempt to keep the roof intact. Scalp biopsy specimens should extend into the subcutis to include the bulbs of terminal follicles. The instruments and materials needed to perform a skin biopsy are discussed in Chapter 6.

### Surgical Excision

The technique of performing surgical excision biopsies with suturing of the skin is well-known. In general, this type of biopsy is performed if a good cosmetic result is desired and if the entire lesion is to be removed. The disadvantage is that this procedure is the most time consuming of the three techniques, and it is necessary for the patient to return for removal of the sutures. Absorbable sutures can eliminate the need for a return visit. It is important that a sharp scalpel be used to reduce compression artifact and that care is taken not to crush the specimen with the forceps.

### Punch Biopsy

Punch biopsies can be done rather rapidly, with or without suturing of the wound. A punch biopsy instrument of appropriate size is needed. Disposable biopsy punches are available. A local anesthetic is usually injected at the site. The operator rotates the instrument until it penetrates to the subcutaneous level. The circle of tissue is then removed. Bleeding can be stopped with pressure or by the use of one or two sutures. An elliptical, like as compared better than versus a circular wound results in a neater scar after suturing. The elliptical punch can be produced by stretching the skin perpendicular to the desired suture line before the punch is rotated. Punch biopsies may be inadequate for evaluation of vesiculobullous diseases and must be deep enough to include subcutaneous fat if used for diagnosis of panniculitis or tumors in a subcutaneous location. In most instances, pigmented lesions should not be punched unless they can be completely excised.

### Scissors Biopsy

The third way to remove skin tissue for a biopsy specimen is to excise the piece with sharp pointed scissors and stop the bleeding with light electrosurgery, Monsel solution, or aluminum chloride solution. This procedure is useful for certain types of elevated lesions and in areas in which the cosmetic result is not too important. The greatest advantage of this procedure is the speed and the simplicity with which it can be done.

### Shave Biopsy

A scalpel or razor blade can be used to slice off a lesion. This can be performed superficially or deeply. Hemostasis can be accomplished by pressure, light electrosurgery, Monsel solution, or aluminum chloride solution. This method is generally not recommended for excision of melanocytic lesions or other potentially malignant tumors where margin assessment is required. However, it can be used for initial evaluation of pigmented tumors if done deep and wide enough.

### Biopsy Handling

The biopsy specimen must be placed in an appropriate fixture, usually 10% formalin. If the specimen tends to curl, it can be stretched out on a piece of paper or cardboard before fixing. Mailing specimens in formalin during winter may result in freezing artifact. This can be avoided by the addition of 95% ethyl alcohol, 10% by volume. For some procedures, fresh tissue should be taken directly for pathologic processing (fresh tissue, Mohs surgery, direct immunofluorescence), put in sterile saline (for culture of fungi and bacteria, including acid-fast bacteria), viral transport media (for viral culture), Michel's solution (direct immunofluorescence), and occasionally sent frozen on dry ice for special procedures.

## Cytodiagnosis

The Tzanck test is useful in identifying bullous diseases such as pemphigus and vesicular virus eruptions (herpes simplex and herpes zoster). The technique and choice of lesions are important. For best results, select an early lesion. In the case of a blister, remove the top with a scalpel or sharp scissors.

Blot the excess fluid with a gauze pad, and then gently scrape the floor of the blister with a scalpel blade. Try not to cause bleeding. Make a thin smear of the cells on a clean glass slide. If you are dealing with a solid lesion, squeeze the material between two slides. The slide may be air dried, but it can also be fixed by placing it in 95% ethanol for 15 seconds. Stain the slide with Wright–Giemsa stain (stain for 30 seconds, rinse with water, let dry, and then observe under high-power oil immersion) or hematoxylin and eosin. Pap smear technique can also yield good results.

In addition to skin testing, fungus examination, biopsies, and cytodiagnosis, there are certain tests for specific skin conditions that are discussed in connection with their respective diseases.

## Additional Studies

The deposition of immunoglobulin and complement may be detected by direct immunofluorescence. This is an extremely valuable technique for the diagnosis of lupus erythematosus and autoimmune bullous diseases. It is performed on a frozen section; therefore, the biopsy specimen must be received fresh or in Michel's solution.

Immunohistology is particularly helpful in the accurate diagnosis and classification of neoplasms. It is possible to identify specific antigens in a routinely processed tissue section by attaching a labeled antibody. For example, malignant melanoma may be identified using antibodies directed against S-100 protein as well as other more sensitive melanoma-specific antigens, such as MART-1 and tyrosinase (**Fig. 2-3**). Different cytokeratin subtypes may be used to

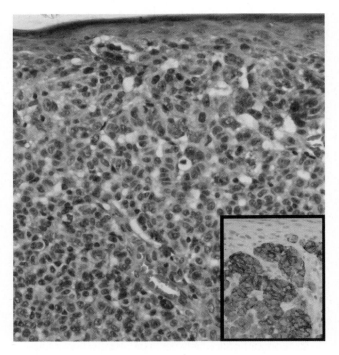

**FIGURE 2-3** ■ Photomicrograph of malignant melanoma with positive immunoreactivity for Mart-1 (*inset*). *(Courtesy of Dr. K. Watson.)*

help differentiate certain epithelial tumors that are histologically similar. For example, cytokeratin 7 helps to differentiate metastatic small cell carcinoma of the lung from primary Merkel cell carcinoma of the skin, as well as both mammary and extramammary Paget's disease from squamous cell carcinoma in situ (Bowen's disease). Mesenchymal tumors, such as dermatofibroma, are generally immunoreactive for the intermediate filament vimentin, as well as a host of other markers, depending on the tumor type and cell origin. Leukocyte common antigen labels most lymphomas and leukemias. Multiple other antibodies can be used to distinguish the cell line, diagnosis, and prognosis. CD3, CD4, CD8, CD5, and CD7 are all T-cell markers that can be used to distinguish patch-stage mycosis fungoides from benign mimics, such as small plaque parapsoriasis and other forms of eczema.

DNA technology may be very useful. In situ hybridization allows recognition of specific DNA or RNA sequences using a gene probe in frozen or paraffin tissue sections. For example, a variety of different viruses, including herpes simplex, cytomegalovirus, and a human papillomavirus, can be identified using this technique.

Flow cytometry is another method of identifying specific cell antigens and is generally only useful with lymphomas and leukemias. This test is most commonly performed on lymph nodes, peripheral blood, and bone marrow, but may also be performed on solid organs, such as skin, provided the abnormal cell population is of sufficient quantity. A fresh specimen is needed. Following manipulation of the tissue to tease out the abnormal cells into a liquid media, the individual cells are labeled with antibodies (up to four at once) and passed through a light-scattering source that is able to measure cell size as well as antigen expression. The main advantage that flow cytometry has over tissue immunohistochemistry is the ability to characterize small populations of abnormal cells and to establish monoclonality via the analysis of immunoglobulin light chain expression. Polymerase chain reaction (PCR) may now also be used to establish monoclonality in both fresh and paraffin-embedded tissue. Disadvantages include lengthy time to diagnosis, high cost, and extreme sensitivity to DNA carryover/contamination problems from other specimens. PCR is able to pick up very small populations of clonal cells that may not be truly neoplastic or malignant.

## Acknowledgments

We acknowledge the assistance of Dr. Cindy Essmeyer and members of her staff, Marcella Godinez, M.T., Katrin Boese, M.T., and Tammy Thorne, M.T., in preparation of the section on fungus examination. We also acknowledge the valuable assistance of Dean Shepard, from St. Luke's Hospital photographic services.

## Suggested Readings

Ackerman AB. *Histopathologic Diagnosis of Inflammatory Skin Diseases.* Philadelphia: Lea & Febiger; 1978:149.

Adams RM. *Occupational Skin Disease.* Orlando: Grune & Stratton; 1990.

Beare JM, Bingham EA. The influence of the results of laboratory and ancillary investigations in the management of skin disease. *Int J Dermatol.* 1981;20:653–655.

Epstein E, Epstein E Jr. *Skin Surgery.* 6th ed. Philadelphia: WB Saunders; 1987.

Fisher AA. *Contact Dermatitis.* 4th ed. Philadelphia: Lea & Febiger; 1995.

Hurwitz RM, Hood AF. *Pathology of the Skin: Atlas of Clinical–Pathological Correlation.* Stamford, CT: Appleton & Lange; 1998.

Isenberg HD, ed. *Essential Procedures for Clinical Microbiology.* Washington, DC: ASM Press; 1998.

Koneman EW, Roberts GD. *Practical Laboratory Mycology.* 3rd ed. Baltimore: Williams & Wilkins; 1985.

Lever WF, Schaumburg-Lever G. *Histopathology of the Skin.* 7th ed. Philadelphia: JB Lippincott; 1990.

Vassileva S. Immunofluorescence in dermatology. *Int J Dermatol.* 1990;332:153.

CHAPTER 3

# Dermatologic Diagnosis

*John C. Hall, MD*

This chapter will discuss how to describe primary and secondary skin lesions, common dermatologic conditions associated with different anatomic locations, seasonal skin diseases, military dermatoses, and dermatoses found in patients of color.

## Primary and Secondary Lesions

Most skin diseases have some characteristic primary lesions. It is important to examine the patient closely to find the primary lesion. Commonly, however, secondary lesions that are a direct result of overtreatment, excessive scratching, or infection have obliterated the primary lesions. Even in these cases, it is usually possible, through careful examination, to find some primary lesions at the edge of the eruption or on other, less irritated areas of the body (Fig. 3-1). Combinations of primary and secondary lesions also frequently occur.

### Primary Lesions

- *Macules:* Up to 1 cm and are circumscribed, flat discolorations of the skin (Fig. 3-2A). Examples include freckles, flat nevi, and some drug eruptions.
- *Patches:* Larger than 1 cm and are circumscribed, flat discolorations of the skin. Examples include vitiligo, some drug eruptions, senile freckles, melasma, and measles exanthem.
- *Papules:* Up to 1 cm and are circumscribed, elevated, superficial, solid lesions (Fig. 3-2B). Examples include elevated nevi, some drug eruptions, warts, and lichen planus. A *wheal* (hive) is a type of papule that is edematous and transitory (present <24 hours). Causes of wheals include drug eruptions, food allergies, numerous underlying illnesses, and insect bites.
- *Plaques:* Larger than 1 cm and are circumscribed, elevated, superficial, solid lesions. Examples include mycosis fungoides and lichen simplex chronicus.
- *Nodules:* Range in size (up to 1 cm) and are solid lesions with depth. They may be above, level with, or beneath the skin surface (Fig. 3-2C, D). Examples are nodular secondary or tertiary syphilis, basal cell cancers, dermatofibromas, and xanthomas.
- *Tumors:* Larger than 1 cm and are solid lesions with depth. They may be above, level with, or beneath the skin surface (Fig. 3-2E). Examples include tumor

stage of mycosis fungoides and larger basal cell cancers.
- *Vesicles:* Up to 1 cm in size and are circumscribed elevations of the skin containing serous fluid (Fig. 3-2F). Examples include poison ivy, early chickenpox, herpes zoster, herpes simplex, dyshidrosis, and contact dermatitis.
- *Bullae:* Larger than 1 cm and are circumscribed elevations containing serous fluid. Examples include pemphigus, bullous pemphigoid, poison ivy, and second-degree burns.

### SAUER'S NOTES

1. One of the dermatologist's tools of the trade is a magnifying lens. *Use it.*
2. A complete examination of the entire body is a necessity when confronting a patient with a diffuse skin eruption or an unusual localized eruption.
3. Touch the skin and skin lesions. You learn a lot by palpating, and patients appreciate that you are not afraid of "catching" the problem. (For the uncommon contagious problem, use precaution.)
4. When in doubt of the diagnosis, verify your clinical impression with a biopsy. The most frequent reason for a successful malpractice suit in dermatology is failure to diagnose.
5. Do not underestimate the importance of adequate lighting.
6. Dermoscopy is a new tool that is mainly used to evaluate pigmented lesions. It combines diascopy and magnification and is useful in diagnosing melanoma as well as deciding which tumors need a biopsy. Diascopy is a test to observe change in color after compression of a skin condition with a clear plastic or glass slide. If an observer has significant experience in dermoscopy, it is useful when deciding whether a lesion is truly benign or not.
7. There are computerized systems that will soon be available to evaluate multiple variables of pigmented tumors in vivo to decide whether a biopsy is necessary.
8. Serial photography systems have been shown by some authors to be useful when determining which pigmented tumors have changed significantly enough over time to warrant a biopsy.

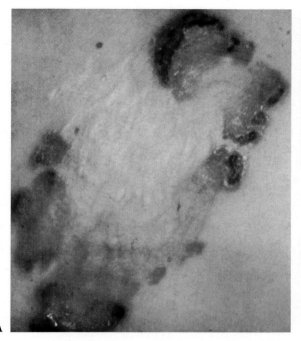
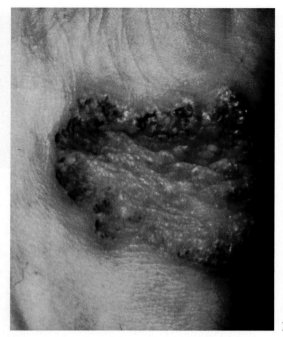

A                                                                        B

**FIGURE 3-1** ■ Nodular lesions. **(A)** Grouped nodular lesions with central scarring (tertiary syphilis). **(B)** Grouped warty, nodular lesions with central scarring (tuberculosis verrucosa cutis). *(Courtesy of Marion B. Sulzberger, Folia Dermatologica, No. 1, Geigy Pharmaceuticals.)*

■ *Pustules:* Vary in size and are circumscribed elevations of the skin containing purulent fluid (**Fig. 3-2G**). Examples include acne, pustular psoriasis, and impetigo.

■ *Petechiae:* Range in size (up to 1 cm) and are circumscribed deposits of blood or blood pigments. Examples are thrombocytopenia, vasculitis, and drug eruptions.

■ *Purpura:* A circumscribed deposit of blood or blood pigment that is larger than 1 cm in the skin. Examples include senile purpura, drug eruptions, bleeding diatheses, chronic topical and systemic corticosteroid use, and vasculitis.

## Secondary Lesions

■ *Scales:* Shedding, dead epidermal cells that may be dry or greasy. Examples are seborrhea (greasy) and psoriasis (dry).

■ *Crusts:* Variously colored masses of skin exudates of blood, serum, pus, or any combination of these (**Fig. 3-3A**). Examples include impetigo, infected dermatitis, nummular eczema, or any area of excoriation.

■ *Excoriations:* Abrasions of the skin, usually superficial and traumatic. Examples are scratched insect bites, scabies, eczema, and dermatitis herpetiformis.

■ *Fissures:* Linear breaks in the skin, sharply defined with abrupt walls. Examples include congenital syphilis, interdigital tinea pedis, and hand eczema.

■ *Induration:* Woodiness or hardness as seen in infiltrating tumors such as dermatofibrosarcoma

protuberans, cutaneous metastasis, lymphoma, scleroderma, or hypertrophic scars.

■ *Ulcers:* Variously sized and shaped excavations in the skin extending into the dermis or often deeper that usually heal with a scar. Examples include stasis ulcers of legs, ischemic leg ulcers, pyoderma gangrenosum, and tertiary syphilis.

■ *Scars:* Formations of connective tissue replacing tissue lost through injury or disease. Examples are discoid lupus, lichen planus in the scalp, and third-degree burns.

■ *Keloids:* Hypertrophic scars beyond the borders of the original injury (**Fig. 3-3B**). They are elevated, can be progressive, and usually are the result of some sort of trauma in the skin. Keloids are more common in darker-skinned people. They are common on the upper torso, neck, and with body piercing (especially with piercings of the earlobe). Rarely, keloids can occur spontaneously. Any type of full-thickness skin trauma can heal with a keloidal scar. They are unsightly and can be numb, pruritic, or painful.

■ *Lichenification:* A diffuse area of thickening and scaling with a resultant increase in skin lines and markings (**Fig. 3-3C**). It is often seen in atopic dermatitis or any area chronically rubbed or scratched.

Several combinations of primary and secondary lesions commonly exist on the same patient. Examples are *papulosquamous lesions* of psoriasis, *vesiculopustular lesions* in contact dermatitis, and *crusted excoriations* in scabies.

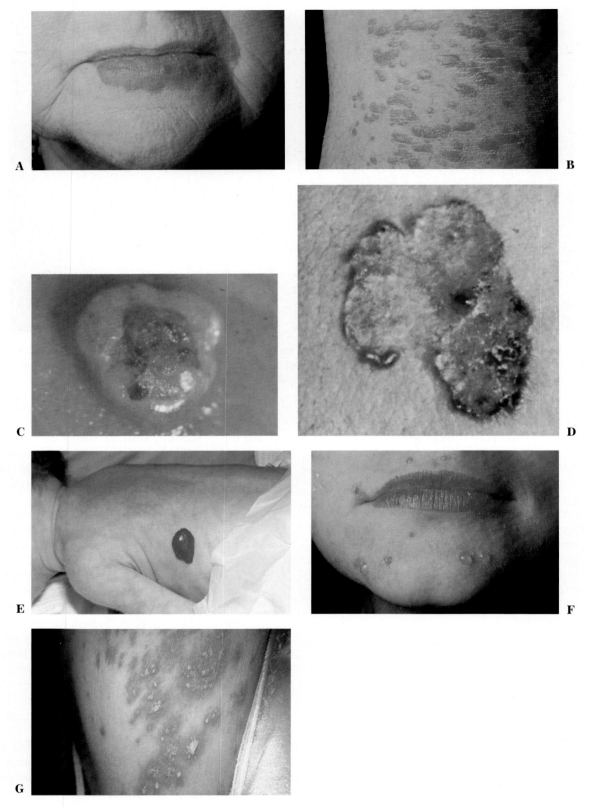

**FIGURE 3-2** ■ Primary skin lesions. **(A)** Patch on lip (port wine hemangioma). **(B)** Papules on knee (lichen planus). **(C)** Nodule on lower eyelid (basal cell carcinoma). **(D)** Polycyclic nodular lesion (superficial basal cell carcinoma). **(E)** Tumor on the left side of an infant (hemangioma). **(F)** Vesicles on chin (pemphigus vulgaris). **(G)** Pustules, pretibial (pustular psoriasis). *(Courtesy of Geigy Pharmaceuticals.)*

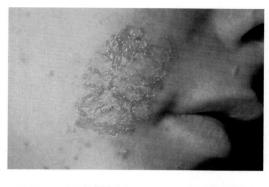
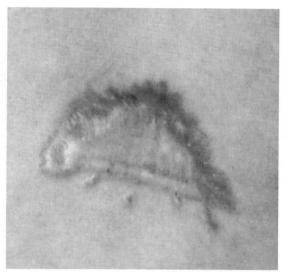
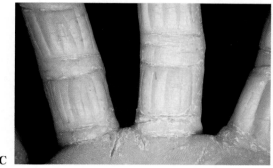

**FIGURE 3-3** ■ Secondary lesions. **(A)** Crust on cheek (impetigo). **(B)** Keloid. **(C)** Lichenification of flexor fingers in a patient with chronic eczema.

## Special Lesions

Some primary lesions, limited to a few skin diseases, can be called *specialized lesions.*

- *Burrows:* Very thin and short (in scabies) or tortuous and long (in creeping eruption) tunnels in the epidermis.
- *Comedones* or *blackheads:* Plugs of whitish (whiteheads or closed comedones) or blackish (blackheads or open comedones) sebaceous and keratinous material lodged in the pilosebaceous follicle, usually seen on the face, chest, or back and, rarely, on the upper part of the arms. Examples include acne and Favre–Racouchot on sun-damaged skin in the temporal areas. These are a hallmark of chloracne. Chloracne is caused by exposure to hydrocarbons such as those found in cutting oils and Agent Orange.
- *Cutaneous horn:* A localized spike-shaped area of marked overgrowth of keratin that can stick above the skin half an inch or more. It is quite localized (usually 0.5 to 1 cm in width or less). It most commonly overlies actinic keratoses, but can overlie seborrheic keratoses, squamous cell carcinomas, warts, porokeratoses, or, less likely, hyperkeratotic basal cell cancers.
- *Flagellate:* Linear whiplike red lesions most often associated with bleomycin therapy but also reported with peplomycin therapy, dermatomyositis, adult-onset Still's disease, and Shiitake mushroom dermatitis associated with eating this particular mushroom.

- *Follicular plugs:* Keratin plugs in the hair follicle that are 1 to 3 mm in size and most characteristically seen in lupus erythematosus ("carpet tack sign" seen on the underside of the scale) and lichen planus (more flask-shaped plugs).
- *Mal perforans ulcer:* Seen in diabetics and leprosy patients. There is an associated neuropathy, so the ulcers are painless despite being deep and destructive. They are circular and sharply marginated or "punched out." These ulcers are usually associated with vasculitis; however, ischemic (very painful) and factitial ulcers can also have the same appearance.
- *Milia:* Whitish papules, 1 to 2 mm in diameter, that have no visible opening onto the skin surface. Examples are found in healed burns or superficial trauma sites, healed bullous disease sites, or newborns. They are not uncommon on the face of adults and can become more widespread in newborns.
- *Chancre:* Rounded, usually single, erosions or ulcers often with an exudative surface. These include the following: anthrax, atypical mycobacterium, blastomycosis (primary cutaneous type), chancroid, coccidioidomycosis (primary cutaneous type), cowpox, cutaneous diphtheria, erysipeloid, furuncle, milker's nodule, orf, rat-bite fever (sodoku), sporotrichosis, syphilis (genital but also extragenital), tuberculosis (primary inoculation type), tularemia, and vaccinia.
- *Striae cutis distensae:* Red, resolving to white, linear areas of atrophy that may be indented. They are seen mainly on the thighs, buttocks, and breasts. They can be seen during rapid weight loss, prolonged use

of topical or systemic corticosteroids, bodybuilding (especially with androgen ingestion), Cushing's disease, and pregnancy, where it is most pronounced over the abdomen.

■ *Telangiectasias:* Dilated superficial blood vessels. Examples include spider hemangiomas, chronic radiodermatitis, basal cell cancer, sebaceous hyperplasia, prolonged chronic sun exposure, necrobiosis lipoidica diabeticorum, and rosacea.

In addition, distinct and often diagnostic changes can occur in the nail plates and the hairs. These are discussed in the chapters relating to these appendages.

## Diagnosis by Location

A physician is often confronted with a patient with skin trouble localized to one part of the body (**Figs. 3-4 to 3-7**). The following list of diseases with special locations is meant

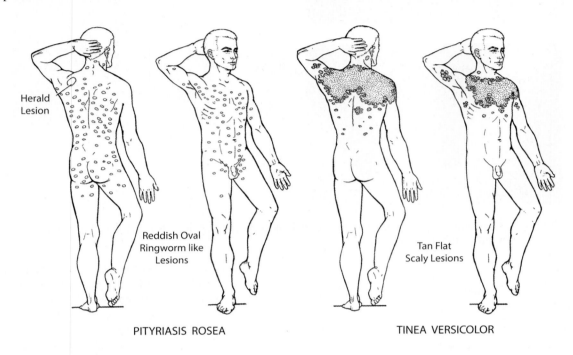

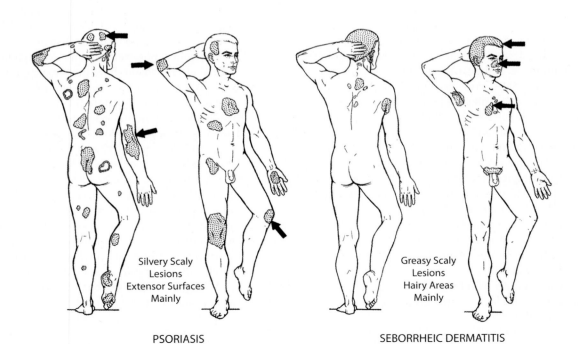

**FIGURE 3-4** ■ Dermatologic silhouettes. Diagnosis by location.

to aid in the diagnosis of such conditions, but this list should not be considered exclusive. Generalizations are the rule, and many rare diseases are omitted. For further information concerning each particular disease, consult the Dictionary-Index located at the end of the book.

- *Scalp:* Seborrheic dermatitis, contact dermatitis, seborrheic keratoses, pilar cysts, psoriasis, folliculitis, pediculosis, and hair loss due to the following: male or female pattern alopecia areata, lichen

planopilaris, tinea, chronic discoid lupus erythematosus, telogen effluvium (postpartum alopecia), or trichotillomania.
- *Ears:* Seborrheic dermatitis, psoriasis, atopic eczema, lichen simplex chronicus, actinic keratoses, melanoma, varix, seborrheic keratoses, and squamous cell carcinomas.
- *Face:* Acne, rosacea, impetigo, contact dermatitis, seborrheic dermatitis, folliculitis, herpes simplex, lupus erythematosus, dermatomyositis, nevi,

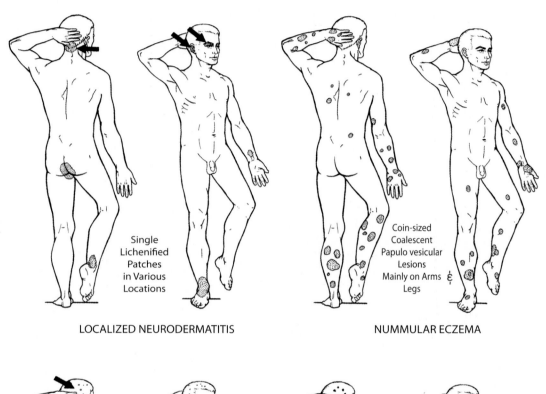

Single Lichenified Patches in Various Locations

LOCALIZED NEURODERMATITIS

Coin-sized Coalescent Papulo vesicular Lesions Mainly on Arms & Legs

NUMMULAR ECZEMA

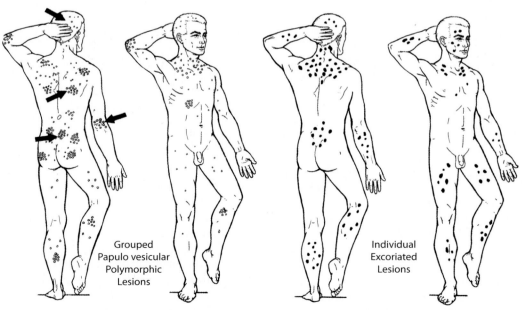

Grouped Papulo vesicular Polymorphic Lesions

DERMATITIS HERPETIFORMIS

Individual Excoriated Lesions

NEUROTIC EXCORIATIONS

**FIGURE 3-5** ■ Dermatologic silhouettes. Diagnosis by location.

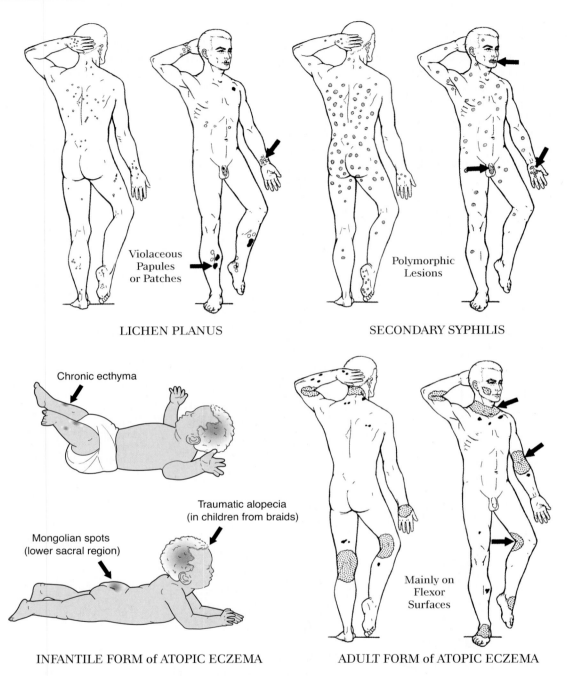

Violaceous
Papules
or Patches

LICHEN PLANUS

Polymorphic
Lesions

SECONDARY SYPHILIS

Chronic ecthyma

Traumatic alopecia
(in children from braids)

Mongolian spots
(lower sacral region)

INFANTILE FORM of ATOPIC ECZEMA

Mainly on
Flexor
Surfaces

ADULT FORM of ATOPIC ECZEMA

FIGURE 3-6 ■ Dermatologic silhouettes. Diagnosis by location.

**SAUER'S NOTES**

In diagnosing a rather generalized skin eruption, the following three mimicking conditions must be considered first and ruled in or out by an appropriate history or examination:

1. Drug eruption
2. Contact dermatitis
3. Infectious diseases, such as acquired immunodeficiency syndrome, other viral exanthems, and secondary syphilis

melasma, melanoma (especially lentigo maligna melanoma), basal cell cancer, actinic keratosis, seborrheic keratosis, squamous cell carcinoma, seborrheic keratosis, milia, and sebaceous hyperplasia.

■ *Eyelids:* Contact dermatitis due to cosmetics, especially fingernail polish or hair sprays, dermatomyositis, seborrheic dermatitis, atopic eczema, skin tags, syringomas, and basal cell cancer.

■ *Posterior neck:* Neurodermatitis (lichen simplex chronicus), seborrheic dermatitis, psoriasis, folliculitis, contact dermatitis, cutis rhomboidalis

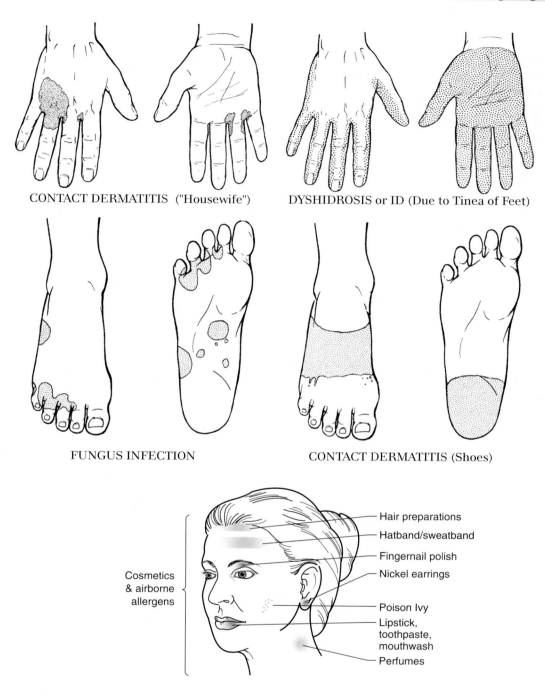

CONTACT DERMATITIS ("Housewife")    DYSHIDROSIS or ID (Due to Tinea of Feet)

FUNGUS INFECTION    CONTACT DERMATITIS (Shoes)

Hair preparations
Hatband/sweatband
Fingernail polish
Nickel earrings
Cosmetics & airborne allergens
Poison Ivy
Lipstick, toothpaste, mouthwash
Perfumes

CONTACT DERMATITIS

**FIGURE 3-7** ■ Dermatologic silhouettes. Diagnosis by location.

nuchae, and acne keloidalis nuchae especially in darker-skinned patients.

■ *Mouth:* Aphthae, herpes simplex, geographic tongue, syphilis, lichen planus, traumatic fibromas, erythema multiforme, oral hairy leukoplakia, squamous cell cancer, candidiasis, and pemphigus.

■ *Axillae:* Contact dermatitis, seborrheic dermatitis, hidradenitis suppurativa, erythrasma, acanthosis nigricans, and Fox–Fordyce disease.

■ *Chest and back:* Tinea versicolor, pityriasis rosea, acne, seborrheic dermatitis, psoriasis, secondary syphilis, epidermoid cysts of the back, seborrheic keratoses, senile or cherry angiomas, nevi, and melanomas, especially on the backs of men.

■ *Groin and crural areas:* Tinea infection, candida infection, bacterial intertrigo, scabies, pediculosis, granuloma inguinale, warts, skin tags, hidradenitis suppurativa, folliculitis, seborrhea, and inverse psoriasis.

- *Penis:* Contact dermatitis, fixed drug eruption, condyloma acuminata, candida balanitis, chancroid, herpes simplex, primary, actinic keratoses, secondary syphilis, scabies, balanitis xerotica obliterans, warts, psoriasis, seborrhea, and pearly penile papules.
- *Hands:* Contact dermatitis, id reaction to fungal infection of the feet, atopic eczema, psoriasis, verrucae, pustular psoriasis, nummular eczema, erythema multiforme, secondary syphilis (palms), fungal infection, dyshidrotic eczema, warts, and squamous cell carcinoma of the dorsal hands.
- *Cubital fossae and popliteal fossae:* Atopic eczema, contact dermatitis, and folliculitis.
- *Elbows and knees:* Psoriasis, xanthomas, dermatomyositis, granuloma annulare, and atopic eczema.
- *Feet:* Fungal infection, primary or secondary bacterial infection, contact dermatitis from footwear or foot care, atopic eczema, verrucae, psoriasis, erythema multiforme, dyshidrotic eczema, and secondary syphilis (soles of feet).

## Seasonal Skin Diseases

Certain dermatoses have an increased incidence in various seasons of the year. In a busy dermatologist's office, a clinician can see "epidemics" of atopic eczema, pityriasis rosea, psoriasis, and winter itch, among others. Knowledge of this seasonal incidence associated with some skin conditions is helpful from a diagnostic standpoint. It is sufficient simply to list these seasonal diseases here, because more specific information concerning them can be found elsewhere in this text. Remember that there are always exceptions to every rule.

### Winter

- Atopic eczema
- Irritant contact dermatitis of the hands
- Psoriasis
- Seborrheic dermatitis
- Nummular eczema
- Winter itch and dry skin (xerosis)
- Ichthyosis

### Spring

- Pityriasis rosea
- Erythema multiforme
- Acne (flares)
- Viral exanthems

### Summer

- Contact dermatitis due to poison ivy
- Tinea of the feet and the groin
- Candida intertrigo
- Miliaria or prickly heat
- Impetigo and other pyodermas
- Polymorphous light eruption

- Insect bites
- Tinea versicolor (noticed after suntan)
- Darier's disease (uncommon)
- Epidermolysis bullosa (uncommon)

### Fall

- Winter itch
- Senile pruritus
- Atopic eczema
- Acne (less sun, more stress with school starting)
- Pityriasis rosea
- Contact dermatitis due to ragweed
- Seborrheic dermatitis
- Tinea of the scalp (schoolchildren)
- Viral exanthems

## Military Dermatoses

Certain parts of the world continue to be at war, and under its ravages, the lack of good personal hygiene, the lack of adequate food, and the presence of overcrowding, injuries, and pestilence can result in the aggravation of any existing skin disease. In this setting, there is an increased incidence of the following skin diseases:

- Scabies
- Pediculosis
- Syphilis and other sexually transmitted diseases
- Bacterial dermatoses
- Tinea of the feet and the groin
- Pyoderma
- Miliaria
- Leishmaniasis (Middle East)

## Dermatoses of Dark-skinned Patients

The following skin diseases are seen with greater frequency in people of color than in light-skinned patients (Figs. 3-8 and 3-9):

- Keloids
- Dermatosis papulosa nigra (variant of seborrheic keratoses that are dark, small, multiple, facial, and more common in women)
- Pigmentary disturbances from many causes, both hypopigmented and hyperpigmented
- Traumatic marginal alopecia (traction alopecia) (from braids and from heated irons used in hair straightening)
- Seborrheic dermatitis of the scalp, aggravated by grease on the hair
- Ingrown hairs of the beard (pseudofolliculitis barbae)
- Acne keloidalis nuchae
- Annular form of secondary syphilis
- Granuloma inguinale
- Mongolian spots
- Acral lentiginous melanomas
- Tinea capitis (in children who braid their hair)

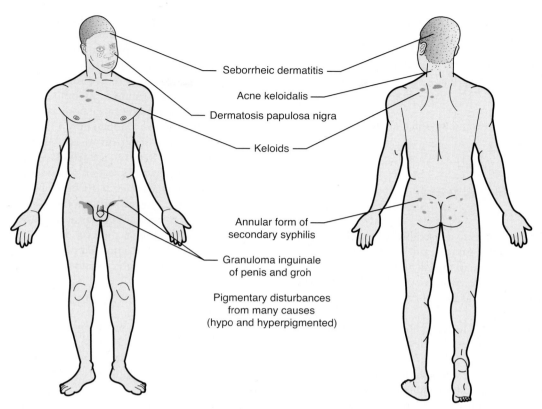

FIGURE 3-8 ■ Dermatologic silhouettes. Conditions more common among dark-skinned patients.

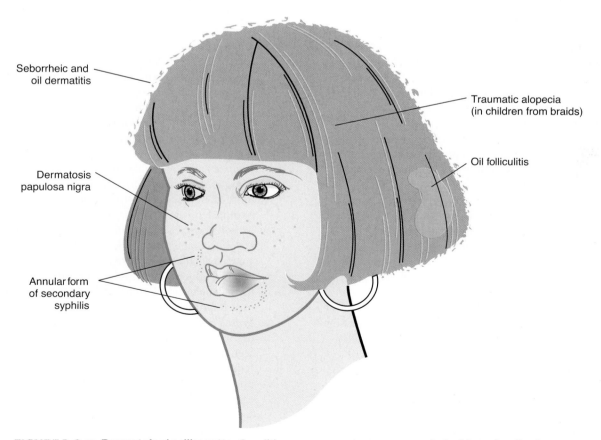

FIGURE 3-9 ■ Dermatologic silhouette. Conditions more common among dark-skinned patients.

On the other hand, certain skin conditions are rarely seen in dark-skinned people:

- Squamous cell or basal cell carcinomas
- Actinic keratoses
- Porokeratosis
- Psoriasis
- Superficial spreading, nodular, and lentigo maligna melanoma
- Scabies

## Descriptive Terms Often Used in Dermatology

- *Acneiform:* Refers to a resemblance of acne as seen in acne, folliculitis, rosacea, and some drug eruptions such as those due to topical and systemic corticosteroids. It can also be seen with ingestion of iodides or bromides and as part of chloracne due to hydrocarbon exposure.
- *Agnimated:* refers to aggregated in a group such as a clustered group of blue nevi or agnimated blue nevi.
- *Annulare* or *arciform lesions:* Refer to a peripheral circular curving of the lesions seen in diseases such as erythema annulare centrifugum, erythema chronica migrans of Lyme disease, erythema marginatum of Scarlet fever, erythema gyratum perstans (which can be associated with underlying malignancy), tinea, impetigo, and psoriasis.
- *Atrophic:* Refers to a thinning of the skin as seen in mycosis fungoides with fine superficial "cigarette paper" wrinkling atrophy or deep with a resultant scarring formation as in discoid lupus erythematosus or third-degree burns.
- *Color alterations*
  *Hyperpigmented:* Increased pigment as seen in postinflammatory hyperpigmentation and residual lesions of lichen planus or dermatitis herpetiformis.
  *Hypopigmented:* Decreased pigment as seen in pityriasis alba, tinea versicolor after a tan, and postinflammatory hypopigmentation.
  *Depigmented:* Loss of pigment as in vitiligo or scar.
  *Violaceous:* Reddish-purple discoloration as seen in vasculitis and the tumors of mycosis fungoides.
  *Apple-jelly colored:* Reddish-brown color seen most often in sarcoidosis, particularly upon pressing the skin with a clear glass slide. This is called diascopy.
  *Porcelain-white:* Stark white color that can be seen in morphea, generalized cutaneous scleroderma, Degos disease, and atrophie blanche or livedoid vasculopathy.
  *Heliotrope:* Refers to violaceous color as seen on upper eyelids in dermatomyositis.

*Cayenne pepper:* Tiny reddish-brown spots due to hemosiderin staining of the skin, seen most often in the pigmented purpuric dermatoses.
- *Cushingoid:* An appearance seen in patients on high-dose, long-term systemic corticosteroids in which the face has a round or moonlike appearance and there is increased central body fat particularly over the back with a "buffalo hump." Acne, striae, rosacea, and hirsutism are also often seen.
- *En cuirasse:* Refers to a shieldlike induration usually at the chest wall as seen in scleroderma and infiltrated malignancies, particularly breast cancer.
- *Exophytic:* Protruding from the skin such as in some squamous cell carcinomas, warts, advanced cutaneous lymphoma, and keloids.
- *Filiform:* Refers to tiny filamentous projections that come from a tumor, usually indicative of a filiform wart.
- *Forme fruste:* Refers to an atypical or partial example of a skin disease.
- *Herpetiform:* Means "in a group" and is seen in the blisters of herpes simplex, herpes zoster, varicella, and the autoimmune blistering diseases of dermatitis herpetiformis and impetigo herpetiformis (herpes gestationis).
- *Incognito:* Refers to a hidden skin disease such as in scabies patients who frequently bathe, in dermatitis herpetiformis that is so excoriated that no primary skin lesions can be seen, or in some cases of cutaneous T-cell lymphoma.
- *Keratotic:* Thickening of the horny layer causing dry, heaped up, hard skin such as in keratotic actinic keratosis, squamous cell cancer, keratoderma palmaris et plantaris, chronic palm and sole psoriasis, or eczema (especially lichen simplex chronicus).
- *Linear:* In a line as in poison ivy dermatitis, coup de sabre type of morphea, lichen striatus, and excoriations.
- *Leonine facies:* A lionlike look to the face with thickening of the normal furrows over the entire face, most often described with cutaneous T-cell lymphoma, leprosy, or tertiary syphilis.
- *Morbilliform:* Usually used to refer to a measles-like eruption that is symmetric, macular, and consists of 1 cm or smaller, usually red, macules that can become confluent. This is seen most often in morbilliform drug eruptions and viral exanthems, including measles, rubella, and HIV exanthem, among others.
- *Peau d' orange:* A bulging of the skin with an orange-peel look that has a mottled texture and is seen in cutaneous mucinosis such as myxedema, lymphoma of the skin such as T-helper cell lymphoma, other cutaneous malignancies such as breast cancer, and elephantiasis nostra verrucosa such as seen in chronic lymphedema of the lower extremities.
- *Pedunculated:* Ab narrow stalklike attachment to the skin as in skin tags.

- *Perifollicular:* Eruptions that seem to be around the hair follicle. This term is often used to describe folliculitis, keratosis pilaris, and follicular eczema.
- *Poikiloderma:* Has three components—fine "cigarette paper" wrinkling atrophy, alternating or lacey hyper- and hypopigmentation, and telangiectasias. This is seen as a result of radiation dermatitis, chronic corticosteroid use topically or systemically, and chronic sun exposure most often seen as poikiloderma of Civatte on the sides of the neck. It is also found in collagen–vascular disease (most commonly lupus erythematosus) as well as in dermatomyositis. It can be a generalized eruption, in which case it is called *poikiloderma atrophicans vasculare* and is considered by most authorities to be a cutaneous T-cell lymphoma.
- *Psoriasiform:* Resembling psoriasis, as in psoriasis or a psoriasiform plaque of cutaneous T-cell lymphoma.
- *Punched out:* Circular with sharply demarcated edges and full-thickness skin loss and is most often used in relation to an arterial ischemic ulcer, vasculitic ulcer, or mal perforans ulcer.
- *Purpuric:* Purple areas due to bleeding under the skin or purpura. This can be seen in vasculitis, pyoderma gangrenosum, drug eruptions, and brown recluse spider bites.
- *Reticulate:* A lacy distribution of skin lesions as seen in oral lichen planus, the pigmentation of poikiloderma, and the pigmentation seen in erythema ab igne. This can also be referred to as weblike.
- *Scalloped edges:* Circinate or rounded edges as in impetigo and ruptured blisters in bullous diseases.
- *Sclerodermoid:* Indurated skin, often with loss of pigment, and characteristic of scleroderma, scleredema, bleomycin injection sites, pentazocine (Talwin) injection sites, and chronic cutaneous graft-versus-host disease.
- *Telangiectatic:* Covered with telangiectasias as in rosacea, lupus erythematosus.
- *Umbilicated:* A tumor or plaque that has a central indentation or dell. This is often used to describe molluscum contagiosum and can also be seen in sebaceous hyperplasia, basal cell carcinoma, and sometimes in viral blisters such as in herpes simplex or herpes zoster.
- *Varicelliform:* To resemble chickenpox such as in smallpox, chickenpox, herpes zoster, Kaposi's varicelliform eruption, or pityriasis lichenoides et varioliformis of Muccha and Habermann.
- *Varioliformis:* to resemble smallpox as in pityriasis lichenoides et varioliformis acuta or smallpox.
- *Verrucous:* wartlike in appearance such as in a verrucous keratoacanthoma, squamous cell carcinoma, or wart.
- *Zosteriform:* refers to the distribution of cutaneous disease in a nerve root distribution. This is seen in herpes zoster, some epidermal and other hamartomatous nevi, and occasionally vitiligo, lichen planus, and others.

## Suggested Readings

Archer CB, Robertson SJ. *Black and White Skin Diseases: An Atlas and Text.* Oxford, UK: Blackwell Science; 1995.

Bouchier IAD, Ellis H, Fleming PR. *French's Index of Differential Diagnosis.* 13th ed. London, UK: Butterworth-Heinemann; 1996.

Callen JP. *Color Atlas of Dermatology.* 2nd ed. Philadelphia: W.B. Saunders; 1999.

Du Vivier A. *Atlas of Clinical Dermatology.* 3rd ed. Philadelphia, PA: W.B. Saunders; 2002.

Eliot H, Ghatan Y. *Dermatological Differential Diagnosis and Pearls.* London: Parthenon; 1998.

Fleischer AB Jr., Feldman S, McConnell C, et al. *Emergency Dermatology.* Columbus, OH: McGraw-Hill; 2002.

Goodheart HP. *Goodheart's Photoguide to Common Skin Disorders.* 2nd ed. Philadelphia, PA: Lippincott Williams & Wilkins; 2003.

Habif TP. *Clinical Dermatology.* 4th ed. St. Louis: Mosby; 2004.

Habif TP, Campbell JL Jr., Chapman MS, et al. *Skin Disease: Diagnosis and Treatment.* St. Louis: Mosby; 2001.

Helm KF, Marks JG. *Atlas of Differential Diagnosis in Dermatology.* Philadelphia, PA: W.B. Saunders; 1998.

Ramos-e-Silva M. Ethnic hair and skin: what is the state of science? *Clin Dermatol.* 2002;20:321–324.

Hunter J, Savin J, Dahl M. *Clinical Dermatology.* 3rd ed. Oxford, UK: Blackwell Publishing; 2003.

Jackson R. *Morphological Diagnosis of Skin Disease.* Lewiston, NY: Manticore; 1999.

Johnson BL, Moy RL, White GM. *Ethnic Skin: Medical and Surgical.* St. Louis: C.V. Mosby; 1998.

Kerdel FA, Jimenez-Acosta, F. *Dermatology: Just the Facts.* New York: McGraw-Hill; 2003.

Lawrence CM, Cox NH. *Physical Signs in Dermatology.* 2nd ed. St. Louis: Mosby; 2001.

Provost TT, Flynn JA. *Cutaneous Medicine: Cutaneous Manifestations of Systemic Disease.* Hamilton, Ontario: BC Decker; 2001.

Poyner TF. *Common Skin Diseases.* Oxford, UK: Blackwell Science; 1999.

Rotstein H. *Principles and Practice of Dermatology.* 3rd ed. Newton, MA: Boston Publishing Co; 1993.

Rycroft RJG, Robertson SJ. *A Color Handbook of Dermatology.* London: Manson; 1999.

Steigleder GK. *Pocket Atlas of Dermatology.* 2nd ed. New York: Theime; 1993.

Sybert VP. Skin manifestations in individuals of African or Asian descent. *Pediatr Dermatol.* 1996;13:163–164.

White GM, Cox NH. *Diseases of the Skin: A Color Atlas and Text.* St. Louis: Mosby; 2000.

# CHAPTER 4

# Dermatologic Therapy

*John C. Hall, MD*

Many hundreds of medications are available for use in treating skin diseases. Most physicians, however, have a few favorite prescriptions that they prescribe day in and day out. These few prescriptions may then be altered slightly to suit an individual patient or disease. Prescription pads printed with commonly used preparations can help save the clinician time and are always legible for the patient. Prescription pads that cannot be photocopied are mandatory.

Treatment of most of the common skin conditions is simpler to understand when the physician is aware of three basic principles:

1. The first principle is to treat the skin lesion by its *type of skin lesion,* more than the cause, influences the kind of local medication used. The old adage "If it's wet, dry it with a wet dressing, and if it's dry, wet it with an ointment" is true in most cases. For example, to treat a patient with an acute oozing, crusting dermatitis of the dorsum of the hand, whether due to poison ivy or soap, the physician should prescribe wet soaks. For a chronic-looking, dry, scaly patch of psoriasis on the elbow, an ointment is indicated because it holds moisture in the skin; an aqueous lotion or a wet dressing is more drying. Bear in mind, however, that the type of skin lesion can change rapidly under treatment. The patient must be followed closely after beginning therapy. An acute oozing dermatitis treated with water soaks can change, in 2 or 3 days, to a dry, scaly lesion that requires an ointment. Conversely, a chronic dry patch may become irritated with greasy ointment and begin to ooze.

2. The second basic principle in treatment is *first do no harm* and never overtreat. It is important for the physician to know which of the chemicals prescribed for local use on the skin are the greatest irritants and sensitizers. It is no exaggeration to say that a commonly seen dermatitis is actually due to patient overtreatment before coming to the office *(overtreatment contact dermatitis).* The patient, many times has gone to the neighborhood drugstore, or to a friend, and used any, and many, of the medications available for the treatment of skin diseases. It is certainly not unusual to hear the patient tell of using an athlete's foot salve for the treatment of the lesions of pityriasis rosea.

3. The third principle is to *instruct the patient adequately regarding the application of the medicine prescribed.* The patient does not have to be told how to swallow a pill,

but does have to be told how to put on a wet dressing. Most patients with skin disorders are ambulatory, so there is no nurse to help them; they are their own nurses. The success or the failure of therapy rests on adequate instruction of the patient or person responsible for the care. Even in hospitals, particularly when wet dressings or aqueous lotions are prescribed, it is wise for the physician to instruct the nurse regarding the procedure.

With these principles of management in mind, let us now turn to the medicine used. It is important to stress that we are endeavoring to present here only the most basic material necessary to treat most skin diseases. For instance, there are many solutions for wet dressings, but Domeboro solution is our preference. Other physicians have preferences different

---

**SAUER'S NOTES**

### SKIN DISEASES ASSOCIATED WITH SMOKING (THERAPY IS QUITTING)

1. Smoker's wrinkles—deep facial wrinkles
2. Poor wound healing—especially for flaps and grafts
3. Psoriasis—especially associated with pustular psoriasis
4. Severity of skin cancer—increased risk of basal cancers becoming morpheaform
5. Atopic dermatitis in children whose mothers smoke
6. Arteriosclerotic vascular disease—Buerger's disease, ischemic leg ulcers
7. Leukoplakia and squamous cell cancer of the lip and oral mucosa
8. Condyloma and cervical cancer
9. Increased severity of Raynaud's phenomena and ischemic ulcers
10. Increased neuropathy (especially in diabetics) with mal perforans ulcers
11. Embolic phenomena—blue toes, livedo reticularis, necrosis with ulcers
12. Decreased effectiveness of antimalarials for cutaneous lupus erythematosus
13. Crohn's disease (15% with associated skin disease) incidence and activity
14. Increased nonlymphocytic leukemia systemically including skin
15. Possibly less incidence of aphthous ulcers and acne

from the drugs listed and their choices are respected, but to list all of them does not serve the purpose of this book.

Two factors have guided us in the selection of medications presented in this formulary. First, the medication must be readily available in most drugstores; second, it must be a very effective medication for one or several skin conditions. The medications listed in this formulary also are listed in a complete way in the treatment section for the particular disease. Instructions for more complete use of the medications, however, are as described in this formulary.

## Formulary

A particular topical medication is prescribed to produce a specific beneficial effect.

---

### SAUER'S NOTES

### LOCAL THERAPY

1. The type of skin lesion (oozing, infected, or dry), more than the cause, should determine the local medication that is prescribed.
2. Do no harm. Begin local therapy for a particular case with mild drugs. The strength of the treatment can be increased if the condition worsens.
3. Do not begin local corticosteroid therapy with the "biggest gun" available, particularly for chronic dermatoses.
4. Carefully instruct the patient or nurse regarding the local application of salves, lotions, wet dressings, and baths. Thin coats of topical medications save money and are as effective as thick coats. Numbers of applications are more important than how thickly the medication is put on. Also, applying medications after hydration such as baths, showers, and hand washing increases penetration and makes topical therapy more effective. Effectiveness can also be increased by occlusion with Saran wrap or occlusions with cotton socks or cotton dermal gloves.
5. Prescribe the correct amount of medication for the area and the dermatosis to be treated. This knowledge comes with experience.
6. Change the therapy as the response indicates. If a new prescription is indicated and the patient has some of the first prescription left, instruct the patient to alternate using the old and new prescriptions.
7. If a prescription is going to be relatively expensive, explain this fact to the patient.
8. For many diseases, "therapy plus" is indicated. Advise the patient to continue to treat the skin problem for a specified period after the dermatosis has apparently cleared. This may prevent or slow down recurrences.
9. Instruct the patient to telephone you, your nurse, nurse practitioner, medical assistant, or physician assistant if there are any questions or if the medicine appears to irritate the dermatosis.

---

## Effects of Locally Applied Drugs

*Anesthetic agents* are used in the skin to decrease pain when injections, laser, cryotherapy, electrolysis, excisions, or other procedures are performed. These include lidocaine hydrochloride 3% cream (LidaMantle), 30% to 40% lidocaine compounded in Velvachol or Acid Mantle cream, EMLA cream or disc (2.5% lidocaine and 2.5% prilocaine), and ethyl chloride spray. Anesthetic agents for mucous membranes are used to temporarily ameliorate discomfort from mucous membrane diseases. They include viscous solution of lidocaine (2%) and Hurricaine liquid or gel spray (20% benzocaine); for ophthalmic use, Alcaine solution (0.5% proparacaine) and Pontocaine (0.5% tetracaine) are used.

*Antipruritic agents* relieve itching in various ways. Commonly used chemicals include menthol (0.25%), phenol (0.5%), camphor (2%), pramoxine hydrochloride (1%), sulfur (2% to 5%), and coal tar solution (liquor carbonis detergens [LCD]) (2% to 10%). These chemicals are added to various bases for the desired effect. Numerous safe and unsafe proprietary preparations for relief of itching are also available. The unsafe preparations are those that contain sensitizing antihistamines, benzocaine, and related—*caine* derivatives. Itch-X gel and spray is over the counter (OTC) and contains 1% pramoxine hydrochloride and 10% benzyl peroxide (Itch-X lotion is OTC, 1% hydrocortisone).

*Keratoplastic agents* tend to increase the thickness of the horny layer. Salicylic acid (1% to 2%) is an example of a keratoplastic agent that will thicken the horny layer.

*Keratolytics* remove or soften the horny layer. Commonly used agents of this type include salicylic acid (4% [Salex lotion and cream] to 10%), resorcinol (2% to 4%), urea (20% to 50%), and sulfur (4% to 10%). A strong destructive agent is trichloroacetic acid. Urea in 5% to 10% concentration (Eucerin Plus lotion and Carmol) is moisturizing, whereas in 20% to 50% (Vanamide, Keralac, Carmol) concentration, it is keratolytic. Urea is also available in a nail stick applicator, Kerastick (50%), for onychoschizia and in a Redi-Cloth (Kerol [42%]). α-Hydroxy acids (lactic acid [Lac-Hydrin 5% or 12% cream and lotion or AmLactin and AmLactin XL 12% cream or lotion]), which are sold over the counter, and glycolic acid (Aqua Glycol is sold OTC in various concentrations and is available as facial cleanser, toner, face cream, shampoo, body cleanser, hand lotion, and body lotion) in 5% to 12% concentrations are moisturizers, whereas in higher concentrations up to 80%, are keratolytic and can be used in the office for facial peeling, with caution. Some moisturizers combine ureas and α-hydroxy acids such as U-Kera E (40% urea, 2% glycolic acid) and Eucerin Plus. Kerol Topical Suspension (50% urea with lactic acid and salicylic acid) is keratolytic and can be massaged into callosities for 60 seconds after bath or shower.

*Antieczematous agents* remove oozing and vesicular excretions by various actions. Soaks for 10 minutes twice a day or clean towels soaked in a solution for 10 minutes twice a day are very effective. The commonest agents include water soaks or compresses (lukewarm to cool), Domeboro solution packets or dissolvable tablets that are nonprescription, coal tar solution (2% to 5%), hydrocortisone 0.5% to 2% (0.5% and 1% are available without a prescription), and more potent corticosteroid derivatives incorporated in solutions, foams, and creams.

*Antiparasitic agents* destroy or inhibit living infestations. Examples include permethrin (Elimite or Acticin) cream for scabies, γ-benzene hexachloride (Kwell) cream and lotion for scabies and pediculosis, crotamiton (Eurax) for scabies, and permethrin (Nix) for pediculosis. For scabies and lice, 10% sulfur can be mixed in petrolatum and is effective and very safe, even in infants and pregnant women, but is malodorous and stains.

*Antiseptics* destroy or inhibit bacteria, fungi, and viruses. Alcohol hand sanitizers are effective on hands and clorox-containing cleansers are very effective on inanimate fomites such as counters, floors, exam tables, and so on.

*Antibacterial topical medications* include gentamicin (Garamycin), retapamulin ointment (Altabax), mupirocin (Bactroban), bacitracin (recently found to cause a significant number of cases of contact dermatitis), Polysporin, and neomycin (Neosporin), which causes an appreciable (at least 1%) incidence of allergic contact sensitivity. Soaps, such as Lever 2000 and Cetaphil antibacterial soap, can have extra antibacterial additives.

*Antifungal and anticandidal topical agents* include miconazole (Micatin, Monistat-Derm), clotrimazole (Lotrimin, Mycelex), ciclopirox (Loprox), econazole (Spectazole), oxiconazole (Oxistat), naftifine (Naftin), ketoconazole (Nizoral), butenafine hydrochloride (Mentax, Lotrimin Ultra), and terbinafine (Lamisil). Sulfur (3% to 10%) is an older but effective antifungal and anticandida agent. Nystatin is anticandida but not antifungal.

*Antiviral topical agents* are acyclovir (Zovirax) ointment or cream and penciclovir (Denavir).

*Emollients* soften and moisturize the skin surface. Nivea oil, mineral oil, and white petrolatum are good examples. Newer emollients are more cosmetically elegant and effective.

*Ointments* moisturize the skin. Examples include Vaseline Petroleum Jelly, Lanolin, Aquaphor, Cetaphil, and Eucerin.

*Creams* dry the skin but are more cosmetically acceptable than ointments because they do not feel greasy and do not leave oil marks on paper products. Examples are Dermovan and Acid Mantle cream. Newer moisturizers attempt to restore the normal skin barrier for protection and to increase penetration of other topicals applied on top of these agents. Three examples are Mimyx, Atopiclair, and CeraVe.

## Types of Topical Dermatologic Medications

*Baths*

1. Tar bath

   Coal tar solution (USP, LCD) 120.0 ml
   *Or* Cutar bath oil
   *Sig:* Add 2 tbsp to a tub of lukewarm water, 6- to 8-in deep.

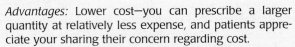

*Actions:* Antipruritic and antieczematous

2. Starch bath

   Limit or Argo starch, small box
   *Sig:* Add half box of starch to a tub of cool water, 6- to 8-in deep.
   *Actions:* Soothing; antieczematous and antipruritic
   *Indications:* Generalized itching and urticaria

3. Aveeno (regular and oilated) colloidal oatmeal bath

   *Sig:* Add 1 cup to the tub of water.
   *Actions:* Soothing and cleansing
   *Indications:* Oilated for generalized itching and dryness of skin, winter, and senile itch. Regular for oozing, draining, wet dermatitis.

4. Oil baths (see section on oils and emulsions) for dry skin.

5. Bleach baths and compresses. For baths, add 1 cup of bleach to full tub of water to soak for several minutes, and add 1 tablespoonful to 1 quart of water to use as compresses for several minutes b.i.d. to treat recurrent recalcitrant *Staphylococcus aureus* folliculitis and secondary infection in atopic dermatitis.

*Soaps and Shampoos*

1. Dove soaps, Neutrogena soaps, Cetaphil, Basis

   *Action:* Mild cleansing agents
   *Indications:* Dry skin or winter itch

2. Dial soap, Lever 2000, Cetaphil antibacterial soap

   *Actions:* Cleansing and antibacterial
   *Indications:* Acne, pyodermas

3. Capex shampoo 120.0
   *Sig:* Shampoo as needed.
   *Actions:* Anti-inflammatory, antipruritic, and cleansing
   *Indications:* Dandruff, psoriasis of scalp
   *Comment:* Contains fluocinolone acetonide, 0.01%

4. Selsun Suspension or Head and Shoulders Intensive Treatment shampoo 120.0

*Sig:* Shampoo hair with two separate applications and rinses. You can leave the first application on the scalp for 5 minutes before rinsing off. Do not use another shampoo as a final cleanser. Contains selenium sulfide.

*Actions:* Cleansing and antiseborrheic

*Indications:* Dandruff, itching scalp (not toxic if used as directed but poisonous if swallowed, so keep out of reach of small children).

**5.** Tar shampoos: Tarsum (can be applied overnight or for several hours as a scalp oil and then shampooed out), Polytar, T/Gel (regular and maximum strength), Pentrax, Ionil T, and so on

*Sig:* Shampoo as necessary, even daily.

*Actions:* Cleansing and antiseborrheic

*Indications:* Dandruff, psoriasis, atopic eczema of the scalp

**6.** Nizoral shampoo 120.0 or Loprox shampoo

*Sig:* Shampoo two or three times a week.

*Actions:* Anticandidal and antiseborrheic

*Indication:* Dandruff, tinea versicolor, and tinea capitis infection

*Comment:* Nizoral is available as 1% OTC or as 2% with a prescription.

Loprox shampoo is similar, with ciclopirox as the active ingredient

**7.** T-Sal, Salex, and other salicylic acid shampoos

*Indications:* Psoriasis and seborrheic dermatitis

### Wet Dressings or Soaks

**1.** Burow's solution, 1:20

*Sig:* Add 1 Domeboro tablet or packet to 1 pint of tap water. Cover affected area with sheeting wet with solution and tie on with gauze bandage or string. Do not allow any wet dressing to dry out. It can also be used as a solution for soaks.

*Actions:* Acidifying, antieczematous, and antiseptic

*Indications:* Oozing, vesicular skin conditions

**2.** Vinegar solution

*Sig:* Add ½ cup of white vinegar to 1 quart of water for wet dressings or soaks, as described for Burrow's solution.

*Indications:* Antieczematous, antiyeast, antifungal, antibacterial including antipseudomonas

**3.** Salt solution

*Sig:* Add 1 tbsp of salt to 1 quart of water for wet dressings or soaks, as above.

*Indications:* Antieczematous, cleansing

### Powders

**1.** Purified talc (USP), ZeaSORB powder, or ZeaSORB-AF powder 60 (contains miconazole)

*Sig:* Dust on locally b.i.d. (supply in a powder can)

*Actions:* Absorbent, protective, and cooling

*Indications:* Intertrigo, diaper dermatitis

**2.** Tinactin powder, Micatin powder, ZeaSORB-AF powder, or Desenex powder

*Sig:* Dust on feet in the morning

*Actions:* Absorbent, antifungal, and antiyeast

*Indications:* Prevention and treatment of tinea pedis and tinea cruris as well as candida intertrigo

*Comment:* These powders are available OTC.

**3.** Mycostatin powder 15.0

*Sig:* Dust on locally b.i.d.

*Action:* Anticandida

*Indication:* Candida intertrigo

### Shake Lotions

**1.** Calamine lotion (USP) 120

*Sig:* Apply locally to affected area t.i.d. with fingers or brush.

*Actions:* Antipruritic and antieczematous

*Indications:* Widespread, mildly oozing, inflamed dermatoses

**2.** Nonalcoholic white shake lotion

   a. Zinc oxide 24.0
   b. Talc 24.0
   c. Glycerin 12.0
   d. Distilled water q.s. ad 120.0

**3.** White shake lotion

   a. Zinc oxide 24.0
   b. Talc 24.0
   c. Glycerin 12.0
   d. Distilled water q.s. ad 120.0

**4.** Proprietary lotions

   a. Sarna lotion (with menthol and camphor), Sarna for Sensitive Skin contains pramoxine
   b. Cetaphil lotion
   c. Aveeno anti-itch lotion (contains pramoxine)

### Oils and Emulsions

**1.** Zinc oxide, 40%

Olive oil q.s. 120.0

*Sig:* Apply locally to affected area by hand or brush t.i.d.

*Actions:* Soothing, antipruritic, and astringent

*Indications:* Acute and subacute eczematous eruptions

---

### SAUER'S NOTES

**1.** Shake lotions 1, 2, and 3 are listed for physicians who desire specially compounded lotions. One or two pharmacists near your office will be glad to compound them and keep them on hand.

**2.** To these lotions you can add sulfur, resorcinol, menthol, phenol, and so on, as indicated.

**2.** Bath oils

Nivea skin oil, Alpha-Keri, Cutar bath oil (contains tar)

*Sig:* Add 1 to 2 tbsp to a tub of water. *Caution:* Avoid slipping in tub.

*Actions:* Emollient and lubricant

*Indications:* Winter itch, dry skin, atopic eczema

**3.** Hand and body emulsions: A multitude of products are available OTC. Some have petrolatum or phospholipids (Moisturel), some have urea or α-hydroxy acids (Lac-Hydrin lotion 5% OTC, Lac-Hydrin cream and lotion 12% prescription, and AmLactin 12% cream and lotion OTC), Vaseline, (Curel) ceramides (CeraVe and EpiCeram Skin Body Emulsion), phospholipids (Moisturel), shea butter (Cetaphil hand cream), lanolin (Eucerin, Nivea, and Aquaphor), and some are lanolin free.

*Sig:* Apply locally as necessary.

*Actions:* Emollient and lubricant

*Indications:* Dry skin, winter itch, atopic eczema

**4.** Scalp oil

Derma-Smoothe/FS oil (fluocinolone acetonide 0.01%) 120.0

*Sig:* Moisten scalp hair and apply lotion overnight; wear a plastic cap

*Indications:* Scalp psoriasis, lichen simplex chronicus, severe seborrheic dermatitis

**5.** Baker's P and S Liquid (phenol and sodium chloride)

*Sig:* Apply overnight under shower cap as needed for scaling

*Indications:* Thick scaling psoriasis

### Tinctures and Aqueous Solutions

**1.** Povidone–iodine (Betadine) solution (also in skin cleanser, shampoo, and ointment) 15

*Sig:* Apply with swab t.i.d.

*Actions:* Antibacterial, antifungal, and antiviral

*Indication:* General antisepsis

**2.** Gentian violet solution

Gentian violet, 1%

Distilled water q.s. 30.0

*Sig:* Apply with swab b.i.d.

*Actions:* Antifungal and antibacterial

*Indications:* Candidiasis, leg ulcers

**3.** Antifungal solutions

a. Lotrimin, Mycelex, Loprox, Tinactin, Micatin, Monistat-Derm, and Lamisil spray, among others 30.0

*Sig:* Apply locally b.i.d.

b. Fungi-Nail 30.0

*Sig:* Apply locally b.i.d.

*Comment:* Contains resorcinol, salicylic acid, parachlorometaxylenol, and benzocaine in a base with acetic acid and alcohol

c. Penlac nail lacquer (contains ciclopirox)

*Sig:* Apply thin coat two times a week; contains ciclopirox

d. Castellani's paint (can get as uncolored): Used for intertrigo

### Pastes

**1.** Zinc oxide paste (USP)

*Sig:* Apply locally b.i.d.

*Actions:* Protective, absorbent, and astringent

*Indications:* Localized crusted or scaly dermatoses

### Creams and Ointments

A physician can write prescriptions for creams and ointments in two ways: (1) by prescribing proprietary creams and ointments already compounded by pharmaceutical companies or (2) by formulating one's own prescriptions by adding medications to certain bases, as indicated for the particular patient being treated. For the physician who uses the second method, two different types of bases are used:

**1.** *Water-washable cream bases:* These bases are pleasant for the patient to use, nongreasy, and almost always indicated when treating intertriginous and hairy areas. Their disadvantage is that they can be too drying. A number of medications, as specifically indicated, can be added to these bases (i.e., menthol, sulfur, tars, hydrocortisone, and triamcinolone).

   a. Unibase
   b. Vanicream
   c. Acid Mantle cream
   d. Dermovan
   e. Unscented cold cream (not water washable)

**2.** *Ointment bases:* These petroleum jelly–type bases are, and should be, the most useful in dermatology. Although not as pleasant for the patient to use as the cream bases, their greasy quality alleviates dryness, removes scales, and enables the medicaments to better penetrate skin lesions. Disadvantages are that they can flare or cause folliculitis, acne, or rosacea, and they are less cosmetically acceptable because of the greasy feel. Any local medicine can be incorporated into these bases.

   a. White petrolatum (USP)
   b. Zinc oxide ointment (USP), very protective
   c. Aquaphor (contains lanolin)
   d. Eucerin (contains lanolin)
   e. Moisturel (may sting when first applied)

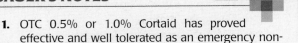

### SAUER'S NOTES

**1.** OTC 0.5% or 1.0% Cortaid has proved effective and well tolerated as an emergency nonprescription treatment.

**2.** Do not use group I topical agents for longer than 2 weeks or more than a 45 g tube per week. A rest period must follow for 2 weeks.

**3.** Do not overuse the more potent topical steroids because of possible side effects.

## SAUER'S NOTES

## COMPOUND PREPARATIONS

Compound proprietary preparations are frequently prescribed, particularly by family practice physicians and nondermatologic specialists. Physicians should know the ingredients in these compound preparations and should know the side effects. Here are some popular compounds:

*Mycolog II cream:* Contains Nystatin and triamcinolone. *Beware:* It is not beneficial for fungus (tinea) infections; the triamcinolone after long-term use can cause atrophy, striae, and telangiectasia of the skin, especially in intertriginous areas and on the face.

*Lotrisone cream:* Contains clotrimazole and betamethasone dipropionate. *Beware:* The betamethasone with long-term use can cause atrophy, striae, and dilated vessels, especially in intertriginous areas and on the face. It also can have significant enough absorption to cause systemic corticosteroid side effects.

*Iodoquinol–hydrocortisone cream (Vytone):* Contains iodoquin plus 1% hydrocortisone. *Beware:* The iodoquin causes a moderate yellow stain on skin and clothing.

*Cortisporin ointment:* Contains 1% hydrocortisone with neomycin, Polysporin, and bacitracin. *Beware:* Neomycin allergies can occur infrequently and bacitracin has now also become a significant allergen.

For the physician who wishes to prescribe ready-made, proprietary preparations, these are listed in groups:

3. *Antifungal ointments and creams:* Lotrimin cream, Lotrimin Ultra cream, Mycelex cream, Spectazole cream, Loprox cream, Tinactin cream, Lamisil cream, Oxistat cream, Naftin cream, Nizoral cream, Mentax cream, and others

   *Action:* Antifungal

4. *Antibiotic ointments and creams:* Bactroban ointment or Centany ointment (can get generic mupirocin) and cream, Altabax (retapamulin) ointment, gentamicin ointment and cream, Neosporin ointment, Mycitracin ointment, and Polysporin ointment (antibiotic solutions are discussed in Chapter 13 under Acne Treatment)

5. *Antiviral ointments for herpes simplex virus infections:* acyclovir ointment and penciclovir cream

6. *Corticosteroid ointments and creams*

   a. Hydrocortisone preparations (0.5% and 1% hydrocortisone creams and ointments are available OTC and generically)
      - Hytone 1% and 2.5% cream and ointment
   b. Desonide preparations (can be written generically)
      - Tridesilon cream and ointment
      - DesOwen cream and ointment
   c. Triamcinolone preparations (0.5%, 0.1%, 0.025%, 0.01%)
      - Kenalog ointment and cream
      - Aristocort ointment and creams
      - Also available generically

   d. Other fluorinated corticosteroid preparations (see Table 4-1 for a listing of these preparations, which are ranked according to potency)

7. *Corticosteroid antibiotic ointments and creams:* Cortisporin ointment

8. *Corticosteroid antifungal–antiyeast preparations:*

   a. Lotrisone (anticandidal and antifungal), contains betamethasone and clotrimazole
   b. Mycolog II cream and ointment (anticandida), contains triamcinolone and nystatin; generic available

9. *Antipruritic creams and lotions:*

   a. Eurax cream
   b. Sarna lotion
   c. Prax lotion
   d. PrameGel
   e. Doxepin (Zonalon) cream (may cause drowsiness)
   f. Aveeno anti-itch lotion
   g. Eucerin calming cream
   h. Eucerin anti-itch spray

10. *Retinoic acid products:*

    a. Retin-A cream (0.025%, 0.05%, 0.1%) and Retin-A gel (0.01% and 0.025%), Retin-A Micro (0.04% and 0.1%), Retin A Micro Pump (0.04% and 0.01%), and Renova (0.02%)

    *Actions:* Antiacne comedones and small pustules (especially the gel) and antiphotoaging
    *Indications:* Acne of comedonal and small pustular type; aging wrinkles on face; removal of mild actinic keratoses and prevention of actinic keratoses, and treatment of freckles, molluscum contagiosum, and flat warts

    b. Differin (adapalene gel and cream 0.1% and 0.03%)
    *Action:* Retinoic acid receptor binder
    *Indications:* Acne of comedonal and small pustular type
    c. Avita (tretinoin 0.025%) cream may be less drying
    *Action:* Antiacne
    *Indications:* Acne of comedonal and small pustular type
    d. Tazorac (tazarotene) 30 g 0.1% cream, 100 g 0.05% gel, and 100 g 0.1% gel
    *Action:* Used for treatment of acne, psoriasis, prevention and treatment of actinic keratoses, and prevention of skin cancer
    *Comment:* Expensive and may be irritating
    e. Avage (0.1% tazarotene) cream 30 g
    *Action:* Approved for acne and may be milder than the same concentration of Tazorac

11. *Miscellaneous creams, ointments, and gels:*
    a. MetroGel (metronidazole 0.75%) 15.0
    Noritate cream (metronidazole 1%) 30.0
    *Indications:* Rosacea, perioral dermatitis
    b. Dovonex ointment (also comes as cream and scalp solution) 30.0 or 100.0
    *Action:* Antipsoriatic
    *Comment:* Moderately expensive

**TABLE 4-1** ▪ **Potency Ranking of Some Commonly Used Topical Corticosteroids\***

**Group I**

Cordran tape
Diprolene AF cream 0.05%
Diprolene ointment 0.05%
Diprolene gel 0.05%
OLUX-E foam
Temovate cream 0.05%
Temovate ointment 0.05%
Temovate gel 0.05%
Temovate emollient 0.05%
Temovate solution 0.05%
Ultravate cream 0.05%
Ultravate ointment 0.05%
Vanos (fluocinonide) 0.1% cream

**Group II**

Cyclocort ointment 0.1%
Diprolene AF cream 0.05%
Diprosone ointment 0.05%
Halog cream 0.1%
Halog ointment 0.1%
Halog solution 0.1%
Halog-E cream 0.1%
Lidex cream 0.05%
Lidex gel 0.05%
Lidex ointment 0.05%
Lidex solution 0.05%
Maxiflor ointment 0.05%
Psorcon cream 0.05%
Psorcon ointment 0.05%
Topicort cream 0.25%
Topicort gel 0.05%
Topicort ointment 0.25%

**Group III**

Aristocort cream 0.5%
Aristocort ointment 0.5%
Aristocort A cream 0.5%
Aristocort A ointment 0.5%
Betamethasone ointment 0.1%
Cutivate ointment 0.005%
Cyclocort lotion 0.1%
Diprosone cream 0.05%
Elocon ointment 0.1%
Kenalog cream 0.5%
Kenalog ointment 0.5%
Maxiflor cream 0.05%
Topicort LP cream 0.5%

**Group IV**

Aristocort ointment 0.1%
Cordran ointment 0.05%
Cyclocort cream 0.1%
Desonide ointment 0.2%
Elocon cream 0.1%
Elocon lotion 0.1%
Fluocinolone ointment 0.025%
Fluocinolone cream 0.2%
Halog cream 0.025%
Halog ointment 0.025%
Kenalog cream 0.1%
Kenalog ointment 0.1%
Topicort LP cream

**Group V**

Aristocort cream 0.1%
Betamethasone valerate cream 0.1%
Betamethasone valerate lotion 0.1%
Cloderm cream 0.1%
Cordran cream 0.05%
Cordran lotion 0.5%
Cordran ointment 0.025%
Cutivate cream 0.1%
Dermatop cream 0.1%
DesOwen ointment 0.05%
Fluocinolone cream 0.025%
Kenalog cream 0.1%
Kenalog lotion 0.1%
Kenalog ointment 0.025%
Locoid cream 0.1%
Locoid ointment 0.1%
Tridesilon ointment 0.05%

**Group VI**

Aclovate cream 0.05%
Aclovate ointment 0.05%
Aristocort cream 0.1%
Betamethasone valerate 0.1%
DesOwen cream 0.05%
DesOwen ointment 0.05%
DesOwen lotion 0.05%
Fluocinolone cream 0.01%
Fluocinolone solution 0.01%
Kenalog cream 0.025%
Kenalog lotion 0.025%
Locoid solution 0.1%
Tridesilon cream 0.05%

**Group VII**

Epifoam 1.0%
Fluocinolone cream 1.0%, 2.5%
Hydrocortisone cream 1.0%, 2.5%
Hydrocortisone lotion 1.0%, 2.5%

\*Group I is the superpotency category. Potency descends with each group, to group VII, which is the least potent (groups II and III are potent corticosteroids; IV and V are midstrength corticosteroids; VI and VII are mild corticosteroids). There is no significant difference between agents within groups II through VII. The compounds are arranged alphabetically within the groups. In group I, Temovate cream or ointment is most potent. *(Courtesy of the late Dr. Richard B. Stoughton and Dr. Roger C. Cornell.)*

c. Aczone (5% avlosulfone [dapsone])

*Action:* Antiacne and antirosacea

*Comment:* Some authors think a G6PD deficiency test should be done before therapy is initiated

12. *Scabicidal and pediculicidal preparations:*

a. Eurax cream and lotion (crotamiton)

*Action:* Scabicidal

*Comment:* It is antipruritic

b. Kwell (lindane) lotion and cream

*Actions:* Scabicidal and pediculicidal

c. Elimite or Acticin cream

*Action:* Scabicidal

d. Nix Crème rinse

*Indications:* Head lice, nits

e. Ovide (malathion) topical

*Action:* Pediculicidal

*Indications:* Head lice, nits

f. Ivermectin oral

*Action:* Scabicidal

*Indications:* Scabies

13. *Sunscreen creams and lotions:* Para-aminobenzoic acid (PABA) and its esters, such as octyl dimethyl PABA (padimate O), octocrylene, octyl salicylate, methyl anthranilate, avobenzone (Parsol 1789), cinnamates (octyl-methoxycinnamate), oxybenzone (benzophenone-3) are effective ultraviolet light absorbers. Zinc oxide and titanium oxide are light blockers. There are many products on the market. Any sunscreen with a sun protective factor (SPF) of 30 or above offers effective sun-damage protection against short-wavelength ultraviolet light or UVB (290 to 310 nm), if used correctly. There is no equivalent SPF number in the United States for long-wavelength ultraviolet light or UVA, which is also important in photoaging, development of skin precancers and skin cancers, lupus erythematosus, and porphyrias and is usually the most important wavelength for photoallergic reactions. Therefore, titanium dioxide, zinc oxide, or avobenzone (Parsol 1789) and probably the two best sunscreens, Antiehelios (Mexoryl SX[expensive] and Helioplex sufficiently screen out UVA and UVB in a possibly more cosmetically acceptable base.

*Sig:* Apply to exposed areas before going outside. This should be done at least a half hour in advance for the best effect. Reapplication is important if exposure to water or significant sweating occurs. After 1 hour, reapplication is advisable. Too thin of an application is a common mistake.

*Action:* Screening out ultraviolet rays

*Indications:* Polymorphous light eruption, photoaging, systemic and chronic lupus erythematosus, some cases of dermatomyositis, photoallergy from systemic or topical medications, some types of porphyria, and prevention of skin precancers and skin cancers, especially in light-complexioned people

14. *Antiyeast:* All products listed under *Antifungal* as well as products containing nystatin, which can be used orally,

as a cream, as an ointment, with 0.1% triamcinolone (Mycolog II cream and ointment, which can be obtained generically), with various powders (ZeaSORB-AF, which also comes as a drying gel), and with any product which causes skin drying such as Domeboro compresses or ZeaSORB powder.

### Aerosols and Foams

Various local medications have been incorporated in aerosol and foam-producing containers. These include corticosteroids (OLUX foam, LUXIQ foam), antibiotics (Evoclin foam), antiacne agents (Ovace foam), antirosacea agents (Ovace foam), antifungal agents (Lamisil spray), Retin A pump, antipruritic medicines (Eucerin spray), and so on. Clobex spray is a class 1 topical corticosteroid.

Kenalog spray (63-g can) and Diprosone aerosol are effective corticosteroid preparations for scalp psoriasis and seborrhea.

Triamcinolone (LUXIQ) and clobetasol (OLUX) are corticosteroid foams and Ovace foam is sodium sulfacetamide foam used for seborrhea, acne, and rosacea. Evoclin is erythromycin foam used to treat acne. Rogaine comes as a foam for hair loss and Verdeso (desonide 0.05%) is a class VI steroid now available as a foam.

### Corticosteroid Medicated Tape

1. Cordran tape (also comes as a patch)

   *Indications:* Small areas of psoriasis, neurodermatitis, lichen planus

### Medicated Skin Patches

Several are available for transdermal delivery of such agents as nitroglycerin, EMLA patch, and lidocaine patch for topical anesthesia, nicotine antismoking patches, and hormones. More will be developed.

### Imiquimod

Imiquimod (Aldara) is used topically for superficial basal cell cancers, actinic keratoses, cutaneous Kaposi's sarcoma, molluscum contagiosum, genital warts, and other warts under occlusion. It is being used experimentally for other skin diseases such as Bowen's disease, elastosis perforans serpiginosa, cutaneous leishmaniasis, alopecia areata, and lentigo maligna melanoma. Other indications may well become approved with more experience with this topical medication. See section on actinic keratosis therapy in Chapter 28 and wart therapy in Chapter 23.

### Local Agents for Office Use

1. Podophyllum in compound tincture benzoin

   Podophyllum resin (USP) 25%

   Compound tincture benzoin q.s. ad 30.0

   *Sig:* Apply small amount to warts with cotton-tipped applicator every 4 or 5 days until warts are gone.

Excess amount may be washed off in 3 to 6 hours of application to prevent irritation.

*Action:* Removal of venereal warts

*Comment:* Other podophyllum proprietary preparations such as podofilox (Condylox) are marketed.

**2.** Trichloroacetic acid solution (saturated) or bichloracetic acid

*Sig:* Apply with caution with cotton-tipped applicator (have water handy to neutralize within a few seconds).

*Indications:* Warts on children, seborrheic keratoses, xanthelasma, sebaceous hyperplasia

**3.** Modified Unna's boot

   a. Dome-Paste bandage

   b. Gelocast

   c. Compression gelatin bandage with zinc oxide and glycerin then wrap with Coflex flexible wrap

*Indications:* Stasis ulcers, localized neurodermatitis (lichen simplex chronicus)

**4.** Ace bandage, 3- or 4-in wide

*Indications:* Stasis dermatitis, leg edema

## Local Therapy Rules of Thumb

Students and general practitioners state that they are especially confused by dermatologists' reasons for using one chemical for one skin lesion and not another or one chemical for unrelated skin diseases. The answer to this dilemma is not easily given. More often than not, the major reason for our preference is that experience has taught us and those before us that the particular drug works. Some drugs do have definite chemical actions, such as anti-inflammatory, antipruritic, antifungal, or keratolytic actions, and these have been listed in the formulary. But there is no definite scientific explanation for the beneficial effect of some of the other drugs, such as tar or sulfur in cases of psoriasis.

In an attempt to solve this apparent confusion, here are some generalizations summarizing our experience.

---

**SAUER'S NOTES**

1. You can compound preparations with LCD, sulfur, resorcinol, and salicylic acid.
2. These chemicals can be used to complement the corticosteroids in a mixture.
3. When prescribing one of these chemicals, always begin with the lower percentage or potency of the drug. Increase the percentage or potency only when a stronger action is desired and no irritation has occurred with the concentration already tried.
4. I am quite aware of the arguments against the use of pharmacy-compounded prescriptions. They have worked exceptionally well for me and for my patients.

---

*Tars (coal tar solution [LCD], 3% to 10%; crude coal tar, 1% to 5%; anthralin, 0.1% to 1%).*

These products have the 3 Ss: sting, stain, and stink.
Consider for use in cases of:

Atopic eczema
Psoriasis
Seborrheic dermatitis
Lichen simplex chronicus
Avoid in intertriginous areas (can cause a folliculitis and irritation)

*Sulfur (sulfur, precipitated, 3% to 10%)*

Consider for use in cases of:

Tinea of any area of the body
Acne vulgaris and rosacea
Seborrheic dermatitis
Pyodermas (combine with antibiotic salves)
Psoriasis
Insect bites in children

*Resorcinol (resorcinol monoacetate, 1% to 5%)*

Consider for use in cases of:
Acne vulgaris and rosacea (usually with sulfur)
Seborrheic dermatitis
Psoriasis

*Salicylic acid (1% to 5%, higher with caution)*

Consider for use in cases of:

Psoriasis
Lichen simplex chronicus, localized thick form
Tinea of feet or palms (when peeling is desired)
Seborrheic dermatitis
Avoid use in intertriginous areas.

*Menthol (0.25%); phenol (0.5% to 2%); camphor (1% to 2%)*

Consider for use in any pruritic dermatoses. Avoid use over large areas of the body.

*Hydrocortisone and related corticosteroids (hydrocortisone powder) (0.5% to 2%) and triamcinolone (0.1%, 0.025%, and 0.01%)*

Consider for use in cases of:

Contact dermatitis of any area
Seborrheic dermatitis
Intertrigo of axillary, crural, or inframammary regions
Atopic eczema
Lichen simplex chronicus
Avoid use over large areas of the body and for prolonged periods.

*Fluorinated corticosteroids, locally*

These chemicals are not readily available as powders for personal compounding, but triamcinolone, fluocinolone, and others are available as generic creams and ointments. Consider for use with or without occlusive dressings, in cases of:

Psoriasis, localized to small area (see Chapter 14)
Lichen simplex chronicus (see Chapter 11)
Lichen planus, especially hypertrophic type

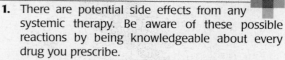

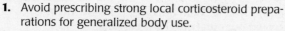

Also anywhere that hydrocortisone is indicated, but limit duration of therapy.

Avoid use over large areas of the body. Class I topical corticosteroids should be used for no more than 14 consecutive days.

## Quantity of Cream or Ointment to Prescribe

Several factors influence any general statements about dosage: the severity of the dermatosis, whether it is acute or chronic dermatosis, the base of the product (a petrolatum-based ointment spreads over the skin farther than a cream and is more moisturizing), whether it is dispensed in a tube or jar (patients use less from tubes), and the intelligence of the patient.

- 15 g of a cream used b.i.d. treats a mild hand dermatosis for 10 to 14 days.
- 30 g of a cream used b.i.d. treats an arm for 14 days.
- 60 g of a cream used b.i.d. treats a leg for 14 days.
- 480 to 960 g or 1 to 2 lb of a cream used b.i.d. treats the entire body for 14 days. This is seldom a practical prescription, but unmedicated white petrolatum or a cream base is economical to use over a large surface area. Other therapeutic agents should be used to make the dermatoses less extensive (i.e., internal corticosteroids).

## Specific Internal Drugs for Specific Diseases

As in all fields of medicine, certain diseases can be treated best by certain specific systemic drugs. These drugs may not be curative, but they should be considered when beginning to outline a course of management for a particular patient.

Many factors influence the decision to use or not use such a specific drug. Here follows a list of skin diseases and some systemic medicines considered specific (or as specific as possible) for the disease. For proper dosage and contraindications, check the appropriate sections in this book or in current books on therapy.

- *Acne vulgaris or rosacea in the scarring or severe stage:* antibiotics, Nicomide, generic nicotinic acid, and in women, spironolactone and birth control pills. For severe cases of cystic acne in men or women without indication of or risk of pregnancy, isotretinoin (Accutane) is indicated.
- *Acquired immunodeficiency syndrome (AIDS):* Many systemic drugs are used, directed as specifically as possible against opportunistic organisms, tumors, and the human immunodeficiency virus (HIV). Highly active antiretroviral therapy (HAART) is the most effective therapeutic regimen for AIDS. Because of its expense, only 10% of HIV-infected patients worldwide are treated with HAART. This is a critical problem on the African continent.
- *Alopecia areata:* corticosteroids in any of four forms—rarely IM or PO corticosteroids.
- *Atrophie blanche vasculopathy:* pentoxifylline (Trental), anticoagulants such as aspirin, clopidogrel (Plavix), dipyridamole (Persantine), and less commonly warfarin (Coumadin).
- *Bullous pemphigoid:* systemic and group I topical corticosteroids, tetracycline in combination with niacinamide, dapsone, methotrexate, azathioprine, intravenous immunoglobulin, other immunosuppressives.
- *Creeping eruption:* thiabendazole, topical or oral.
- *Darier's disease:* vitamin A, for controlled periods of time, and possibly isotretinoin and acitretin.
- *Dermatitis herpetiformis:* dapsone and sulfapyridine.
- *Dermatomyositis:* systemic and topical corticosteroids; immunosuppressive agents. Methotrexate, hydroxychloroquine (Plaquenil), and, when other therapies have failed, intravenous IgG.
- *Granuloma annulare:* intralesional corticosteroids.
- *Herpes simplex:* acyclovir (Zovirax) topical, oral, or intravenous; famciclovir oral (Famvir); valacyclovir

oral (Valtrex); foscarnet sodium intravenous (Foscavir). Suppressive therapy for 1 year is advocated by some to reduce diseases severity and transmission. Foscarnet can be used intravenously for resistant cases.

- *Herpes zoster:* acyclovir oral or intravenous, famciclovir oral, and valacyclovir oral.
- *Kawasaki's syndrome:* intravenous γ-globulin and aspirin.
- *Lichen simplex chronicus:* intralesional corticosteroids, topical corticosteroids with or without occlusion.
- *Lupus erythematosus:* for systemic lupus erythematosus, use corticosteroids or immunosuppressive agents with care; for discoid form, use topical and intralesional corticosteroids and hydroxychloroquine or related antimalarials (beware of eye damage). Intravenous IgG can be tried when other treatments have failed.
- *Mycosis fungoides* (T helper cell lymphoma or cutaneous T-cell lymphoma [CTCL]): psoralens and ultraviolet light (PUVA), narrow band UVB, corticosteroids, antimetabolites, retinoids (bexarotene [Targretin]), denileukin diftitox (for CD25-positive tumors), topical nitrogen mustard, topical bischloroethylnitrosourea (BCNU), electron beam radiation, extracorporeal photophoresis, bone marrow transplant (for end-stage disease when all other therapy has failed), and $\alpha_{2b}$-interferon.
- *Necrobiosis lipoidica diabeticorum:* topical and intralesional corticosteroids.
- *Pemphigus:* corticosteroids systemically, cyclosporine, intravenous immunoglobulin, and antimetabolites. Monoclonal antibodies such as Rituximab have had some reported success.
- *Pruritus from many causes:* antihistamines (topical and oral) and tranquilizer-like drugs. Doxepin (Zonalon) cream may be beneficial but can cause drowsiness when used over large areas. Selected cases can be treated with oral corticosteroids.
- *Psoriasis, localized:* intralesional and topical corticosteroids, tar, Dovonex (calcipotriene), especially in combination with topical corticosteroids. Occasionally oral antibiotics such as sulfasalazine or tetracycline or oral antiyeast medications such as ketoconazole are used.
- *Psoriasis, severe:* corticosteroids topically, PUVA, narrow band UVB, methotrexate, cyclosporine (Neoral), and, in men or postmenopausal or sterile women, acitretin (Soriatane). A whole new class of drugs called *biologicals which block lymphokines produced by T-8 lymphoctyes* are now available. These include infliximab (Remicade) intravenously, etanercept (Enbrel) subcutaneously, and alefacept (Amevive) intramuscularly. Etanercept, adalimumab, and infliximab are especially helpful in patients with accompanying psoriatic arthritis.

> **SAUER'S NOTES**
>
> Real-time teledermatology as well as store-and-forward teledermatology are proven advances in providing care to areas of the United States and the world where dermatologic care by dermatologists would not otherwise be accessible.

These biologicals are all related to TNF-α (tumor necrosis factor alpha) blockade, except efalizumab, which blocks the CD11a receptor site. Two IL (interleukin) 12, 23 blockers will soon be available.

- *Pyodermas of skin:* systemic antibiotics are valuable, when indicated.
- *Sarcoidosis:* topical, intralesional, and systemic corticosteroids; antimalarials; and, when severe and recalcitrant, methotrexate. Early reports with infliximab and related TNF-α blockers have been promising. Pentoxyphylline (Trental) can be tried.
- *Sporotrichosis:* saturated aqueous solution of potassium iodide orally and ketoconazole orally.
- *Syphilis:* penicillin or other antibiotics.
- *Tinea of scalp, body, crural area, nails:* topical imidazoles, ciclopirox or allylamines (oral and topical); or orally griseofulvin and, for selected cases, orally ketoconazole (Nizoral) and itraconazole (Sporanox).
- *Toxic epidermal necrolysis (TEN) or Stevens–Johnson syndrome:* Stop offending drug and life support measures. Systemic corticosteroids early in high doses may be beneficial but this is controversial and later in the disease may be contraindicated. Cyclosporine or intravenous IgG have been advocated by some authors.
- *Tuberculosis of the skin:* dihydrostreptomycin, isoniazid, p-aminosalicylic acid, and rifampin.
- *Urticaria:* oral antihistamines (H1 and H2), oral corticosteroids and, when severe, intramuscular and intravenous corticosteroids, sulfasalazine, dapsone, and combinations of these medications. When associated with other signs of anaphylaxis, such as shortness of breath, subcutaneous epinephrine (this can be used by patients in an emergency as EpiPen).

## Suggested Readings

Arndt KA, Bowers KE. *Manual of Dermatologic Therapeutics.*6th ed. Philadelphia: Lippincott Williams & Wilkins; 2002.

Bronaugh RL, Maibach HI. *Topical Absorption of Dermatological Products.* New York: Marcel Dekker; 2002.

Buchanan P. *Prescribing in Dermatology.* Cambridge: Cambridge University Press; 2006

Drake LA, Dinehart SM, Farmer ER, et al. Guidelines of care for the use of topical glucocorticosteroids. *J Am Acad Dermatol.* 1996;35:615–619.

el-Azhary RA. Azathioprine: Current status and future considerations. *Int J Dermatol.* 2003;42:335–341.

Katz HI. *Dermatologist's Guide to Adverse Therapeutic Interactions.* Philadelphia: Lippincott–Raven; 1997.

Lebwohl MG, Heymann WR, Berth-Jones J, et al. *Treatment of Skin Disease: Comprehensive Therapeutic Strategies.* St. Louis: Mosby; 2008.

Levine N. *Dermatology: Diseases and Therapy.* Cambridge: Cambridge University Press; 2007.

Levine N, Levin CC. *Dermatology Therapy: A to Z Essentials.* New York: Springer; 2004.

Loden M, Maibach HI. *Dry Skin and Moisturizers.* London: Taylor and Francis, 2006.

Olsen EA. A double-blind controlled comparison of generic and trade-name topical steroids using the vasoconstriction assay. *Arch Dermatol.* 1991;127:197–201.

*Physicians' Desk Reference.* Oradell, NJ: Medical Economics; 2005.

Scheman AJ, Severson DL. *Pocket Guide to Medications Used in Dermatology.* 8th ed. Philadelphia: Lippincott Williams & Wilkins; 2003.

Shelley WB, Shelley ED. *Advanced Dermatologic Therapy II.* Philadelphia: WB Saunders; 2001.

Wakelin SH. *Handbook of Systemic Drug Treatment in Dermatology.* London: Manson Publishing; 2002.

Wolverton SE. *Comprehensive Dermatologic Drug Therapy.* Philadelphia: WB Saunders; 2007.

# CHAPTER 5

# Technologic Applications in Dermatology

*Frank Custer Koranda, MD, MBA*

The therapeutic options of dermatologists have widely expanded with advances in technology. Most of these technologies can be employed in an office setting. Some of the more common technologic applications include lasers, intense pulsed light (IPL), photodynamic therapy, radiofrequency devices, liposuction, lipotransfer, fat autograft mesenchymal injection (FAMI), Botox injections, tissue fillers, and augmentation.

## Lasers

Laser is an acronym for light (L) amplification (A) by the stimulated (S) emissions (E) of radiation (R). The characteristics of laser light are that the light is monochromatic (a single wavelength), collimated (the rays are parallel or nondivergent), and coherent (the rays are in phase so that they can pass over distances without loss of energy).

### Carbon Dioxide Laser

When laser light contacts the skin, the light energy is absorbed. The energy causes thermal coagulation or, with greater energy, tissue vaporization. The carbon dioxide ($CO_2$) laser has a wavelength of 1600 nm in the mid-infrared spectrum, which is invisible. The $CO_2$ laser is absorbed by water in the tissue. It is an ablative laser, causing damage to all tissue because the water content is the laser target. When the $CO_2$ laser is used in a focused mode, it can be used as a cutting instrument with a width of 0.2 mm as compared with the 0.25 mm width of a #15 scalpel blade. As the $CO_2$ laser cuts, it vaporizes the tissue. In a defocused mode, the $CO_2$ laser's effect is that of tissue coagulation, and in this mode it can seal blood vessels 0.5 mm or smaller in diameter. The $CO_2$ laser produces thermal damage that can spread beyond the target tissue.

The depth of penetration of the $CO_2$ laser is controlled by the power output measured in watts and by the time on target. Fluence is the measurement of the energy density to the target and is expressed as joules per square centimeter.

Because the $CO_2$ laser is invisible, it is coupled and coaxially aligned with a low-power laser in the visible spectrum that serves as an aiming device. The helium-neon-aiming laser produces a red light.

The initial $CO_2$ lasers were of a continuous wave output unless deactivated by the foot control. In the early 1990s, pulsed focused $CO_2$ lasers were introduced. The goal of pulsing the laser was to decrease the thermal damage to surrounding nontargeted skin. The initial pulsed $CO_2$ lasers were of 0.1 to 1.0 seconds in duration. To further reduce thermal transfer, ultrapulsed $CO_2$ lasers were developed to deliver high-energy output over a very short duration. The Coherent UltraPulse $CO_2$ laser can deliver 250 to 500 W of power in less than a 1-millisecond pulse.

The ultrapulsed laser reduces tissue damage by timing the pulse duration to approximate the tissues' thermal relaxation time, that is, the time for a tissue to significantly cool by heat conduction. The principles of selective photothermolysis apply to most lasers: first, there is selective absorption of the laser energy or light by the target tissue; second, with the use of a brief pulse at high enough power, effective energy may be transmitted to the target with limited heat dispersal beyond the target. The $CO_2$ laser is used for a wide variety of treatments and conditions:

- Resurfacing of the face for rejuvenation of the skin and reduction of wrinkles
- Vaporization of actinic cheilitis
- Planning for rhinophyma (Fig. 5-1), angiofibromata of tuberous sclerosis, sebaceous hyperplasia
- Removal of common warts and condylomata accuminatum
- Removal of keloids and hypertrohic scars (Fig. 5-2)
- Incisional surgery requiring more precision and when hemostasis by methods other than electrocoagulation is needed

These examples are a limited list of the applications of the $CO_2$ laser.

The $CO_2$ laser was one of the first lasers to have been widely employed for a variety of cutaneous conditions. Today there are hosts of other lasers with different wavelength outputs and other characteristics such as pulsed modes, pulsed durations, and pulsed repetitions. Each laser has different uses depending on the absorption spectrum of the target tissues. The wavelength of the laser is matched to the absorption peaks of the target tissues.

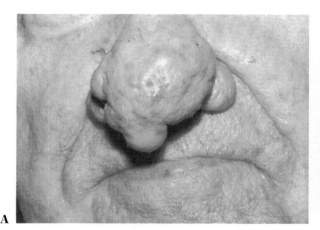
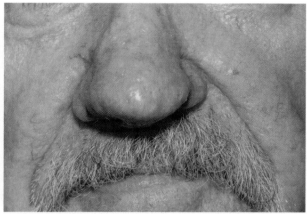

**FIGURE 5-1** ■ Rhinophyma before **(A)** and after **(B)** nasal planing with the Coherent $CO_2$ Ultrapulse laser.

These other lasers have wavelengths in the visible (400 to 700 nm) to near-infrared (700 to 1200 nm) spectra. In general, as the wavelength of the light increases, the depth of penetration into the skin increases and so does the depth at which the energy is absorbed. In addition to identifying the absorption spectrum of the targeted structure, the depth of the structure in the skin also influences the selection of a laser with the appropriate wavelength output. The wavelength must also be different from the absorption peaks of any intervening tissue that could absorb the laser light before it reaches its target tissue.

### Pulsed Dye, Nd:YG, Q-switched, and Diode Lasers

The pulsed dye laser, usually with a 585-nm wavelength and a 450-microsecond or 0.45-millisecond pulse, has been used extensively for congenital hemangiomas, particularly port wine stains (**Fig. 5-3**). Multiple treatments, sometimes more than 20, are required. The necessity for retreatment 5 to 8 years after apparently successful treatment is not unusual. Recurrence may be due to blood vessels at a depth beyond the reach of the 585-nm wavelength laser.

For deeper penetration, a neodymium:yttrium aluminum garnet (Nd:YAG) laser at 1064 nm can be directed toward deeper vasculature while sparing the overlying melanin. This

type of laser has also been used for deeper and larger leg vein treatments (**Fig. 5-4**).

Q-switched (QS) lasers have a pulse duration of 10 to 20 nanoseconds. QS lasers are most frequently used for tattoo removal by heating and fracturing the ink pigment particles. The fragmented particles are extruded through the epidermis and cleared by the lymphatic system. Usually six or more treatments are required and often all the remnants of the tattoo cannot be removed. Some residual scarring or pigmentary changes in the skin are common. The selection of the proper laser depends on the color of the tattoo. Green pigment is best removed by a red light laser; red pigment, by a green light laser; and yellow pigment is poorly removed by all lasers. The QS Ruby (694 nm) and QS Alexandrite (77 nm) lasers are used for blue and green inks, the QS Nd:YAG (1064 nm) for black ink, and the QS Nd:YAG/2 (532 nm) for red inks. Most professional tattoos require the use of different lasers for effective treatment because of the multicolors. Homemade tattoos with India ink are easier to remove than professional tattoos (**Fig. 5-5**).

Hair removal lasers are usually in the 694- to 1064-nm wavelengths so that there is sufficient depth of penetration for absorption by the melanin in the hair follicle. The 800-nm diode laser is also effective for hair removal. This laser contains a cooling system to afford additional protection against

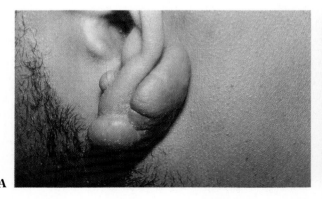
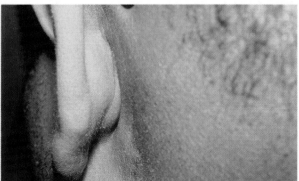

**FIGURE 5-2** ■ Keloid of the ear before **(A)** and after **(B)** removal with the Coherent $CO_2$ Ultrapulse laser.

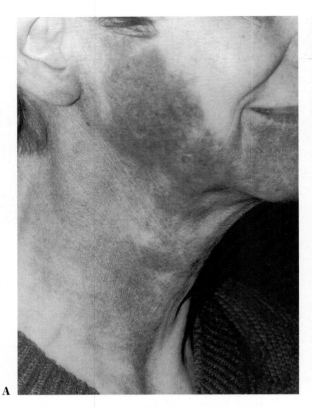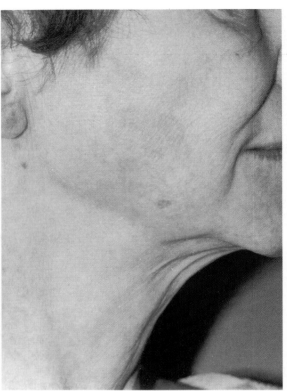

**FIGURE 5-3** ■ Congenital port wine stain hemangioma before **(A)** and after **(B)** treatment with candela-pulsed tuneable 585-nm dye laser.

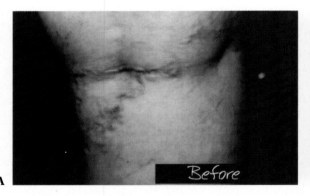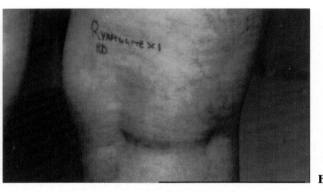

**FIGURE 5-4** ■ Varicose veins of the leg before **(A)** and after **(B)** treatment with Lumenis Vasculite laser.

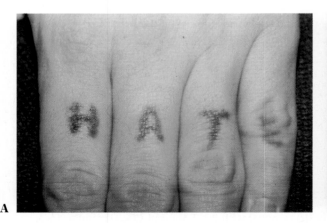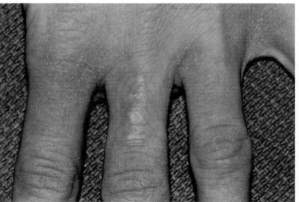

**FIGURE 5-5** ■ Homemade tattoo before **(A)** and after **(B)** laser removal.

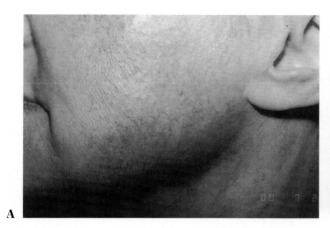 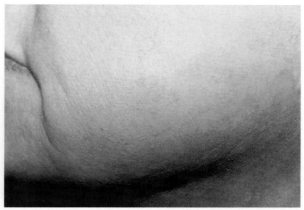

A                                                                                          B

FIGURE 5-6 ■ Facial telangiectasias before (**A**) and after (**B**) treatment with Lumenis Photoderm IPL.

injury to the overlying skin. Although the lasers have been touted for permanent removal of hair, more truly this is a process for the progressive reduction of hair. This process requires several treatments and often follow-up treatments in ensuing years. Usually laser treatment is only effective for pigmented hair, since melanin is the target. The most common side effects are hyper- or hypopigmentation. The darker the skin and the higher the fluences applied to the tissue, the more aptly these effects may develop.

### Fractional Laser Therapy

Fractional laser therapy is based on the principle of selective photothermolysis. A specific wavelength of light is selected, which is matched to a target in the skin such as hemoglobin, water, and melanin. It is then delivered rapidly enough to limit thermal damage to the target before it diffuses out to the surrounding tissue. With the fractional laser a microarray of laser energy is delivered, creating zones or microscopic tunnels of thermal damage in the epidermis and dermis separated by intervening areas of undamaged tissue. In other words, only a fraction of the area is treated. This allows for more rapid healing and for less risk of adverse outcomes. Fractional laser therapy is used for photodamaged skin, melasma, atrophic acne scars, and surgical scars. Two of the

popular fractional lasers are the Fraxel SR laser, which is an erbium-doped 1550-nm device with fluences from 35 to 40 mJ per microthermal zone, and the Palomar Lux 1540 Fractional laser, which is an erbium-doped 1540-nm device with fluences of 70 mJ per microthermal zone. Since only a fraction of the area is treated at one time, treatments are carried out every 3 to 4 weeks for four to eight times.

### Intense Pulsed Light

IPL is a noncoherent, broad band of wavelengths from 515 to 1,200 nm generated by a high-energy flash lamp. For treatment, wavelengths of light are selected by the use of optical cut-off filters that eliminate wavelengths less than the filter's wavelength of light transmission. The first IPL device was the Photoderm system by Lumenis. There are other good systems available, such as the Palomar. Initially in the mid-1990s, the IPL was promoted for the treatment of leg veins, but the indications for IPL have greatly expanded and leg veins are the least indication. IPL is very effective for:

- Facial telangiectasias (Fig. 5-6)
- The vascular component of rosacea
- Poikiloderma of Civatte
- Mottled facial pigmentation from actinic damage (Fig. 5-7)

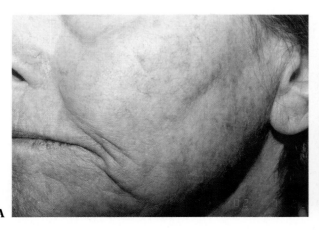 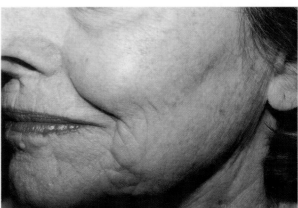

A                                                                                          B

FIGURE 5-7 ■ Actinically damaged facial skin before (**A**) and after (**B**) treatment with Lumenis Photoderm IPL.

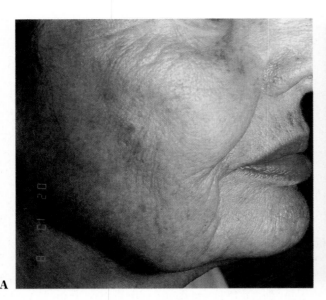
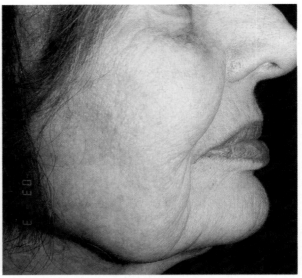

**A**                                                                                                          **B**

FIGURE 5-8 ■ Photoaged skin of the face before **(A)** and after **(B)** one treatment with Lumenis Photoderm IPL.

In treating these conditions, it was observed that there was also an improvement in skin tone and a decrease in fine wrinkling (**Fig. 5-8**). Now a major indication is for facial rejuvenation. The photorejuvenation process is done as a series of four to six IPL treatments at 3- to 4-week intervals.

## Photodynamic Therapy

The basis of photodynamic therapy (PDT) is that a photosensitizing drug is taken up by tissue that is then exposed to light sources whose wavelength matches the absorption spectrum of the photosensitizing drug. The photosensitized tissue is excited by the light and destroyed. This phenomenon was first observed in 1900 when *Paramecium caudatum* in acridine orange solution was exposed to light and then died quickly. Starting over 30 years ago, extensive experimentation was carried out with the intravenous administration of hematoporphyrin derivative (HpD) to patients with various types of cancers. The cancer cells tend to take up the HpD more selectively than the normal cells. The cancers were exposed to appropriate wavelength light sources. The photoreaction which would occur was in theory to destroy the cancer cells. Results were variable.

In 1999, the US Food and Drug Administration (FDA) approved the use of a topical photosensitizer, δ-aminolevulinic acid (ALA) for the treatment of actinic keratoses. ALA is a precursor to protoporphyrin IX (PpIX), which is formed when ALA is absorbed into the skin. Because cancerous and precancerous cells have a higher turnover rate than normal cells, there is enhanced absorption of ALA over normal cells. The epidermis of dysplastic tissue is also a less effective barrier to penetration.

Peak absorption of PpIX is at 409 nm (the Soret band). PpIX also has markedly less absorption peaks at 509, 544, 584, and 635 nm. When the PpIX-laden cells are exposed to

the appropriate light source, singlet oxygen phototoxic reactions occur, leading to cell death. The Blu-U light, with a peak output at 417 nm, but with a range of 410 to 417 nm, is often used for treatment of actinic keratoses.

It has been observed that moderately severe acne responds well to PDT with Blu-U light. IPL with output above 560 nm and lasers with 585- or 595-nm output provide deeper penetration of the light and might provide an even more enhanced effect on the sebaceous gland, which is the focus of acne development.

Following PDT, the skin is red, peels, and may crust in some areas depending on the intensity of the reaction. Because ALA is a photosensitizing drug and there is some residual amount in the skin after treatment, it is imperative that the patient avoid direct exposure to outside light. The patient is instructed to stay indoors for the first 36 hours, continue to stay out of direct sunlight for the next 2 weeks, and remain indoors as much as possible. When outdoors, a wide-brimmed hat should be worn for the next week. Daily application with an effective UVA block is required. A micronized zinc oxide sunscreen provides the best protection.

IPL has been used for photorejuvenation of the face, resulting in a decrease in fine wrinkling, smoothing of texture, decrease in telangiectasias, and evenness of coloration. IPL photorejuvenation may be enhanced by combining it with the application of ALA. Enhanced IPL photorejuvenation is usually done as a series of three treatments every 3 to 4 weeks. After treatment, the same precautions against sun exposure as with other PDTs are mandatory.

## Radiofrequency Devices

The radiofrequency (RF) device is an attempt to nonablatively (cause no damage to the skin surface) rejuvenate the facial skin. The Thermage ThermaCool TC or Thermalift

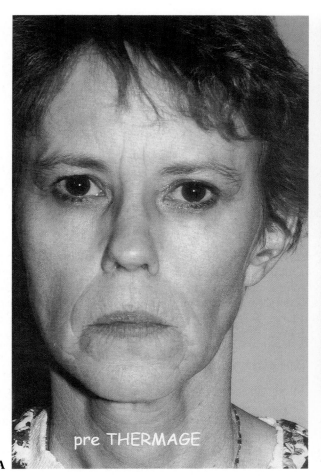

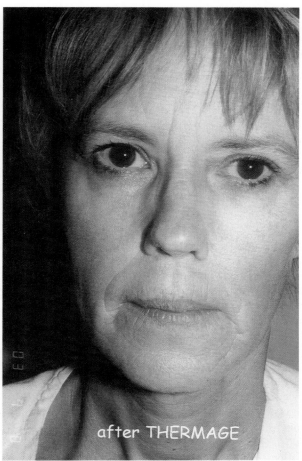

pre THERMAGE

after THERMAGE

**A**                                                                                    **B**

FIGURE 5-9 ■ Facial wrinkling before (**A**) and after (**B**) treatment with Thermage ThermaCool TC.

system was granted FDA clearance in 2002. With this method, the epidermis is protected by cryogen cooling as the RF energy is delivered into the dermis. As the RF energy is absorbed, the collagen fibers contract. Later and ongoing for 4 to 6 months, collagen synthesis occurs in response to this thermal energy.

The initial protocol of the Thermage system was to apply a single pass of high-energy levels of RF to the facial skin with several hundred impulses delivered. This was quite uncomfortable despite the use of topical anesthetic creams. The most severe side effect, which was not common, was waffling or an unevenness of the skin surface after treatment, probably owing to fat atrophy.

Some patients have achieved significant improvement after RF treatment (Fig. 5-9). However, in the majority of patients, the improvement was so subtle or nonexistent that it did not justify the cost.

In order to eliminate the severe discomfort and potential complications and to improve the results, Thermage changed the treatment protocol. Now, multiple passes are made over the skin with the delivery of lower levels of RF energy. The discomfort is now minimal and tolerable, and in our series of patients, the waffling of the skin has been eliminated. However, the degree of improvement is widely variable, from no improvement, to little improvement, to noticeable improvement. The improvement is usually never what is seen in the advertisement photographs.

My partner, Dr. Colleen Reisz, and I have tried to identify characteristics in the subset of patients who do show a response to RF. These patients usually have some manifestation of a forme fruste of Ehlers–Danlos syndrome. Usually the manifestation is some type of hypermobility of joints. Because Ehlers–Danlos has a variability of expression, it may often be undiagnosed and the incidence may be as high as 1 in 5,000 people. However, there is still variability in these patients in their response to RF treatment.

Multiple companies now have RF devices: Palomar Star-Lux IR, Cutera Titan, Sciton BBL Skin Tyte, Syneron Polaris and ReFirme, Lumenis Aluma, Alma Accent.

Although there are advertisements by some physicians and spas that RF is a face-lift without surgery, RF is not a replacement or substitute for face-lifts, chemical peels, or laser resurfacing.

Conceptually, RF devices have potential, but that potential has not been reliably achieved at present. Until RF devices give consistent, predictable results, "caveat emptor" should be observed by both physician and patient.

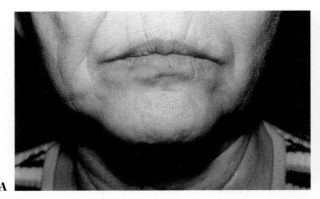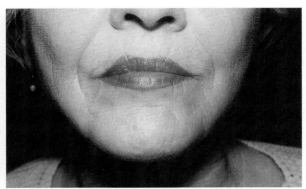

**A**    **B**

FIGURE 5-10 ■ Jowling of the face and neck fullness before **(A)** and after **(B)** liposuction.

## Liposuction

Liposuction is a technique for recontouring or sculpturing various body areas by fat extraction through various-sized cannulas to which suction is applied. The technique was developed in the late 1970s by Dr. Yves-Gerard Illouz of Paris, France. The earlier methods of performing liposuction were the "dry methods" carried out under general anesthesia. With large volumes of fat removal (greater than 1500 mL), these procedures were associated with fluid balance problems, necessitating fluid replacement and the need for homologous blood transfusions, and then modified by using autologous blood transfusions. Dr. Eugene Courtiss in *Plastic and Reconstruction Surgery,* in 1992, noted that 44% of 108 patients undergoing large-volume liposuction required hospitalization after the procedure.

In 1986, a dermatologist, Dr. Jeffrey Klein, revolutionized the technique and the safety of liposuction with his work on tumescent liposuction by the infiltration of a large volume of diluted lidocaine with epinephrine saline solution into the areas of liposuction. With this tumescent technique, blood loss is minimal and it is possible to perform liposuction without general anesthesia. Another dermatologist, Dr. Patrick Lillis, advanced the tumescent technique by demonstrating the safety of using greater amounts of lidocaine.

Although liposuction is most commonly done on the abdomen, thighs, and arms, it is a significant adjunct in the rejuvenation of the jowls (Fig. 5-10) and the neck (Fig. 5-11). Tumescent liposuction is performed on an outpatient basis. Intravenous sedation or general anesthesia may also be employed if the patient desires, but it is usually not necessary.

## Botulinum Toxin Type A

Botulinum toxin (BT) type A is a neurotoxin from the organism *Clostridium botulinum*, which is the causative agent of botulism. Botulism is associated with food poisoning from improperly sterilized canned goods. BT acts at the presynaptic terminal of motor nerves to block the release of acetylcholine. Death from botulism is caused by paralysis of the diaphragmatic muscles.

In 1980, minute doses of BT injected into eye muscle were reported to correct strabismus. Soon BT was used for neurologic conditions. A husband and wife, Dr. Alastair Caruthers, a dermatologist, and Dr. Jean Carruthers, an ophthalmologist, first used BT for cosmetic purposes in 1988. Dr. Jean Carruthers observed a loss of wrinkles in patients she was treating with BT for blepharospasm.

In cosmetic use, BT is better known by its registered name, Botox. BT injections are one of the cosmetic

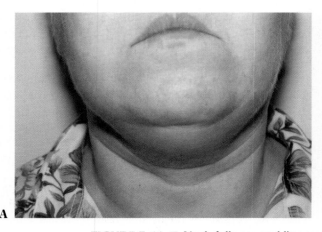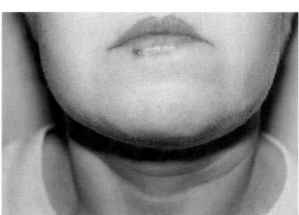

**A**    **B**

FIGURE 5-11 ■ Neck fullness and lipomatosus before **(A)** and after **(B)** liposuction.

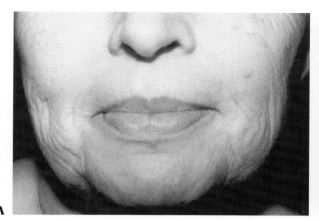
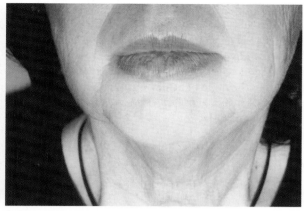

**FIGURE 5-12** ■ Periorbital area before **(A)** and after **(B)** BT injection.

procedures most commonly performed. The cosmetic use of BT is best indicated for the upper third of the face to erase horizontal forehead folds, smooth out the vertical and horizontal furrows of the glabella, ablate the "crow's feet" of the lateral orbit, and lift the eyebrows by blocking the depressor muscles (Fig. 5-12). The effect of BT usually lasts about 4 months and then needs to be repeated if the individual wishes to maintain the effect. BT has also been used to efface the vertical rhytides of the upper lip, weaken platysmal neck bands, and blunt the marionette line effect of the depressor labii muscle. Some patients being treated cosmetically with BT have also noticed improvement and lessening of migraine headaches.

## Lipotransfer and Fat Autograft Mesenchymal Injection

With aging and photodamage, there is a thinning of the epidermis and fracturing and atrophy of dermal collagen. The subcutaneous fat also atrophies. This leads to deepening furrows, particularly in the nasolabial folds and in the marionette lines. But the atrophy is not just skin deep. Muscles atrophy and shorten, and bone is reabsorbed. The face becomes more narrowed and hollowed compared to the youthful appearance of a full, rounded face. Correcting this atrophy with a face-lift pulls the skin up and tightens it but does not address the problem of volume loss. Volume loss must be replaced.

The transfer of autologous fat or fat grafting was first reported in 1893 to fill out scars. Since then, fat grafting or lipotransfer has gone in and out of popularity because of problems with viability and survival of fat grafts. Fat should be the ideal volume filler since it is readily and widely available on most individuals, it is living tissue, and it is nonallergenic.

Donor sites for fat grafting include the abdomen, the flanks, the thigh, and the knee. Gentle harvesting of the fat is important and is accomplished by low-pressure aspiration of the fat into a blunt cannula attached to a 10-mL syringe. Once the cannula is introduced into the area of fat harvest, the plunger on the syringe is slowly pulled back creating a low-pressure vacuum. Centrifugation of the fat separates out three layers: a supranatant layer of oily fluid, a middle layer of fat, and an infranatant layer of blood and fluid. The fat is then transferred to 1-mL tubes for injection. Only blunt cannulas are used both for harvesting fat and for the lipotransfer process. The blunt tips reduce the risk of intravascular injection.

Dr. Roger Amar, a French plastic surgeon, has further refined the process of lipotransfer with his emphasis on injecting the fat into the facial muscles. Muscle tissue is an ideal recipient bed since it is well vascularized. Dr. Amar has developed a set of cannulas with different configurations to best accommodate the facial muscles being injected. He has also established a precise protocol for this method for which he coined the term fat autograft muscle injection (FAMI) (Fig. 5-13).

Various authors have observed what appears to be a regeneration of muscles and bone in areas of fat grafting. Adipose tissue has been determined to have a higher

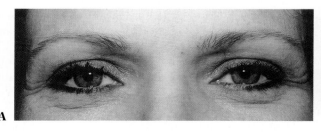
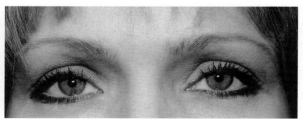

**FIGURE 5-13** ■ Aging face before **(A)** and after **(B)** FAMI.

concentration of stem cells or mesenchymal cells than any other body tissue. The transfer of stem cells along with the fat cells may explain this rejuvenation. Since these stem cells are from the individual, the ethical problem associated with embryonic stem cells does not arise. Dr. Amar has adjusted his method in the hope of achieving a higher concentration of stem or mesenchymal cells. FAMI now stands for fat autograft mesenchymal injection.

## Engineered Materials for Soft Tissue Fillers and Augmentation

### Injectable Bovine Collagen

This product was introduced in 1979 as Zyderm and ushered in the present era of tissue fillers. This injectable bovine collagen has been used for:

- Filling out of wrinkles and rhytides
- Filling of depressed scars
- Ablation of the nasolabial folds
- Augmentation of the lips

Injectable bovine collagen has an allergic potential; skin testing is required prior to use. A negative test does not rule out the possibility of an immunologic response, which can include swelling or edema, erythema, and firmness in the area of injection. The incidence is about 2%. A rarer response is that of an abscess-type reaction, which may lead to scarring.

The collagen is injected through a 30-gauge needle. Collagen is not permanent. The average duration is 4 to 6 months. This short duration may be an asset in a patient who is not sure whether he or she wants the effect of fuller lips.

The original Zyderm I bovine collagen has been modified to Zyderm II, which contains double the weight of bovine collagen, and to Zyplast, which contains cross-linked collagen. Zyplast is intended for deeper placement into the mid and deep dermis to fill out deeper contours such as the mesolabial folds and to augment the lip.

Zyplast is contraindicated in the glabellar folds because of an associated case of blindness that may have been caused by the material entering a blood vessel because of the deeper placement. However, blindness has even been reported with steroid injections about the eyes and with topical lidocaine with epinephrine on nasal packs after intranasal surgery.

Because the collagen is from cattle, patients may have a concern about prion-type diseases. There is reassurance in that the collagen comes from protected herds.

### Injectable Porcine Collagen

Evolence is a ribose cross-linked porcine collagen that may last up to a year. Skin testing is not required.

### Injectable Collagen from Human Source

Cosmo Derm I and II and CosmoPlast are harvested from cell cultures from the foreskin of newborns. There is no need for allergy testing. Duration is short-lived and at times may not last to 3 months.

Cymetra is human collagen derived from cadavers. Cymetra is a micronized form of Alloderm. It may last up to a year.

### Injectable Hyaluronic Acid

The hyaluronic acid products are the most commonly used injectable fillers at present. They are approved for the filling out of facial wrinkles and folds such as the nasolabial fold. They are frequently used for augmenting the lips. No allergy testing is required.

The Restylane group of products of injectable hyaluronic acid are produced from streptococcal bacteria. Hyaluronic acid is not a protein. It is a polysaccharide and is part of the ground substance of connective tissue. Hyaluronic acid is hydrophilic, and there may be some increased edema about the injection site in the immediate posttreatment days. Restylane comes in three forms:

- Restylane Fine Lines for superficial wrinkles,
- Restylane for all-purpose use, and
- Perlane for filling of deeper contours, nasolabial folds, marionette lines, and for augmentation of the lips.

The difference in the three types is the molecular size. Restylane Fine Lines has the smallest molecules and Perlane, the largest. Hyaluronic acid is injected through a 27-guage needle. Injection into the lips and perioral area is painful. It is best to regionally anesthetize these areas with infraorbital and mental nerve blocks. Use only a small amount of lidocaine so the tissue to be filled is not distorted. Although swelling, bruising, erythema, and discomfort may occur at the sites of injection, they last only a few days. Longer-term difficulties, persistent erythema, edema, acneiform eruption, and induration are rare. The longer maintenance of effect and its nonallergic nature have made hyaluronic acid one of the most popular options for a soft tissue filler. Restylane usually lasts for 6 to 9 months, and Perlane may last well over a year. Other hyaluronic acids are Hylaform derived from rooster combs and Juvederm derived from bacterial strains.

### Injectable Calcium Hydroxylapatite Microparticles

Radiesse is an injectable filler containing calcium hydroxylapatite (CaHA) microspheres varying from 25 to 45 $\mu$m suspended in an aqueous gel with lidocaine. It is FDA approved for filling moderate and severe wrinkles and folds and for HIV (human immunodeficiency virus)-associated lipoatrophy. Collagen forms about the microspheres, and the suspension gel is gradually absorbed. In time, the microspheres undergo degradation. Duration of effect is for at least a year or longer. The safety profile is good. The microspheres of CaHA are radiopaque and visible on x-ray. CaHA is not indicated for lip augmentation because of a tendency for nodule formation.

### Injectable Polymethylmethacrylate Microparticles

Artefill is an injectable filler containing polymethylmethacrylate (PMMA) microspheres, which are round, smooth, uniform, and not less than 20 $\mu$m, suspended in bovine collagen with lidocaine. Artefill is the third generation of this product. Artecoll was the second generation. Artefill has greater uniformity of microparticle size and the amount of particles less than 20 $\mu$m has been reduced to less than 1%. Microparticles less than 20 $\mu$m stimulate phagocytosis, which was associated with adverse effects observed with the earlier generations of this product. Artefill is classed as a permanent filler. A foreign body response to the PMMA leads to collagen deposition. The bovine collagen suspension is gradually absorbed so that over 3 months a significant amount of the correction is lost. Complete stabilized correction will require two to four treatments separated by 3 to 4 months.

The safety profile now is relatively good. There is one report from Germany of a patient undergoing interferon therapy who had a sarcoidal granulomatous response in the area of PMMA. She had had Artecoll, a second-generation PMMA, injected into her face 10 years earlier. However, interferon can be, on rare occasion, associated with cutaneous sarcoidosis.

### Injectable Poly-L-Lactic Acid Microparticles

Sculptra (poly-L-lactic acid [PLLA]) is used for HIV-related lipoatrophy and as a volume filler rather than a line filler for facial rejuvenation. Allergy testing is not required. PLLA is deposited at the dermal–subcutaneous border and in the superficial subcutaneous fat. In areas where the skin is thinner, periorbital rim, temporal hollow, and zygomatic arch, it is deposited just above the periosteum. PLLA stimulates fibroblast and collagen generation. Concave areas are filled out to give a fuller, rounded face of youth. For facial rejuvenation two or more injection sessions are required. Treatment sessions are separated by 4 to 6 weeks in order to evaluate the response. Sculptra is diluted to 6 mL for the lower two thirds of the face. For injection into areas of thinner skin, a more diluted solution is preferable. A topical anesthetic applied for 45 minutes prior to injection minimizes discomfort significantly. There is also lidocaine in the Sculptra solution. Injection is usually performed as the needle is withdrawn, taking care to deposit an even line of PLLA. Small papules may develop if injected too superficially. Deep nodules may develop if bolus depositions occur. These are palpable in the subcutaneous tissue but not visible. Massaging the injected areas three or four times a day for the next week will help to more evenly distribute the PLLA. Sculptra has a long-lasting effect of 18 to 24 months.

### Expanded Polytetrafluoroethylene Facial Implants

Expanded polytetrafluoroethylene (e-PTFE), better known as Gore-Tex, is a nonabsorbable, permanent substance that has been used in abdominal and vascular surgery for 30 years. For at least 15 years, it has been used to augment soft tissue.

e-PTFE is nonallergenic, biocompatible, and usually noninflammatory. e-PTFE has micropores that allow for the ingrowth of some tissue, which serves to anchor it. This ingrowth may make an e-PTFE more difficult to remove. Capsule formation about the implant has usually not been a problem. e-PTFE is supplied in sheets of various sizes, in oval and circular hollow tubes, in multistrands, and in implants shaped for the chin, nose, and malar areas.

Softform and UltraSoft tubular e-PTFE implants are innovative methods of coupling the e-PTFE hollow tube to an insertion trocar. This system is used for augmentation of the nasolabial folds and the upper and the lower lips.

The procedure is done under local anesthesia or with nerve blocks. A small stab incision is made at both ends of the site where the tube will be placed. The trocar is usually inserted into the inferior incision for the nasolabial fold augmentation and the lateral incision for upper lip augmentation. The trocar is tunneled under the dermis and passed out through the incision at the other end. The attached e-PTFE tube is pulled through the tunnel. Using scissors, the e-PTFE is cut with a downward bevel. The total length of the e-PTFE tube is left slightly longer than the distance between the incisions. A small pocket is formed with the scissors below the inferior incision and above the superior incision so that the ends of the tube can be buried away from the incision. The incision sites are closed with one or two stitches of 6-0 nylon (Fig. 5-14).

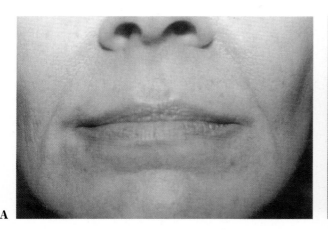
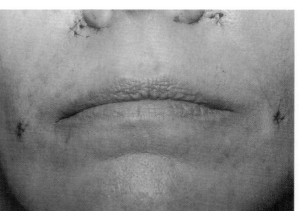

**A**                                                                 **B**

FIGURE 5-14 ▪ Nasolabial folds before **(A)** and after **(B)** insertion of UltraSoft tubular e-PTFE implant.

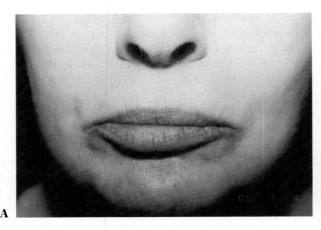
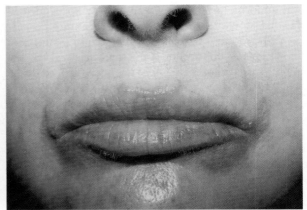

**FIGURE 5-15** ■ Upper lip before **(A)** and after **(B)** insertion of UltraSoft tubular e-PTFE implant.

When the tubular system is used to augment the lip, a single tube is run along the entire length of the lower lip. However, two tubes are used for the upper lip in order not to efface the "cupid's bow" of the philtrum and to accentuate it.

In the upper lip, the e-PTFE tube is placed from the corner of the mouth to the high point of the cupid's bow on each side (Fig. 5-15). Although the e-PTFE tubes can nicely fill out the nasolabial folds and augment the lips, the tubes are palpable. Infection has not been a problem. Because of their superficial subdermal placement, the e-PTFE tubes may excite some reactivity at the incision site with drainage and inflammation. At times, this may necessitate the removal of the tube. In some patients the tube may also contract by a third or more.

## Tempered Optimism

We physicians have the opportunity and the ability to improve the human condition. Technologic advances continue to enhance this capability. But medical treatments have potential risks as well as benefits. With any treatment or procedure or material used, there will always be some patients who have unanticipated and untoward sequelae and

### SAUER'S NOTES

New technologies in all fields of medicine are driven not only for the betterment of man but for financial gain. The medical–industrial complex is a multibillion business. In promoting these technologies, photos of the best results and data highlighting the positive results are featured. There is an admonition in the military that is wise to remember: "Never believe what you hear, and only half of what you see."

difficulties despite the best of evaluation, precautions, equipment, and technique. Biologic systems have an inherent unpredictability.

## Suggested Readings

Gold, MH. Photodynamic therapy. *Dermatol Clin.* 2007;25 (1):1–125.
Gordon, ML. A conservative approach to the nonsurgical rejuvenation of the face. *Dermatol Clin.* 2005;23:365–371.
Sherman, RN. Sculptra: the new three-dimensional filler. *Clin Plast Surg.* 2006;33:539–550.

# CHAPTER 6

# Fundamentals of Cutaneous Surgery

*Frank Custer Koranda, MD, MBA*

Skin, "the gift wrap of life" is the barrier between us and a hostile environment. Skin is the largest organ of the body. Sooner or later, most physicians will have to deal with a tear, cut, or incision into this barrier that will need to be repaired.

## Instrument Selection

Quality instruments are expensive but are usually worth the price. For most cutaneous surgery, smaller needle holders are best, such as the Webster, Halsey, or smooth-jawed needle holders used in neurosurgery (Fig. 6-1A). Smooth jaws are less traumatic than precise needles and less apt to cut 5-0 or 6-0 sutures than serrated jaws. For very delicate surgery and for very fine sutures such as 7-0, the Castroviejo needle holder may be preferred (Fig. 6-1B). The amount of motion necessary to lock and unlock the Castroviejo is less than that required for the standard type of needle holder.

Skin should be handled as atraumatically as possible. Very gentle handling requires the use of skin hooks such as the single-hook Frazier or the fine double-hook Tyrell. If using pickups to handle tissue, use Adson forceps with fine teeth or Micro-Adson forceps. A finer type of forceps is the Bishop-Harmon with teeth (Fig. 6-1C).

For scissors dissection, a Littler is well designed for most situations (Fig. 6-1E). For finer work, a Stevens scissors is a good choice (Fig. 6-1E).

If larger scissors are desired, the Metzenbaum, Malis, or Ragnell scissors may be used (Fig. 6-1D). For precise cutting of sutures and for suture removal, the Gradle scissors may be used (Fig. 6-1F).

The no. 3 scalpel handle is used with the nos. 10, 11, and 15 blades. For precise incisions, the 15C blade is best. This blade was originally designed for periodontal surgery.

A basic cutaneous surgical pack may include the following:

- Webster or neurosurgery smooth-jawed needle holder
- Adson delicate forceps with teeth or Micro-Adson forceps with teeth
- No. 3 scalpel handle
- Littler scissors
- Fine suture scissors
- Utility sutures for cutting dressings
- Mosquito hemostats (two)
- Towel clips, 3½ in
- Gauze sponges, 4 × 4 in (ten)
- Several round toothpicks for skin marking (toothpicks dipped in methylene blue) make a finer line than the standard marking pens and are less expensive
- Cotton-tipped applicators as an option for point control of bleeding

## Suture Selection

The two general groups of suture are absorbable and nonabsorbable. The common absorbable sutures are:

- Plain gut
- Chromic gut
- Polyglactin 910 (Vicryl)
- Polyglycolic acid (Dexon)
- Polydioxanone (PDS)
- Polyglyconate (Maxon)
- Poliglecaprone (Monocryl)

Gut suture is made from the submucosal layer of the small intestine of sheep and the serosal layer of cattle and undergoes degradation by phagocytosis, creating a foreign body response in the patient. Plain gut gradually looses its tensile strength over 2 weeks. Chromic gut suture is coated with chromic salts to delay degradation. It has a slightly prolonged tensile strength over plain gut.

Fast-absorbing plain gut is a modification of plain gut that is designed to break down in 4 to 7 days and is used as a skin stitch. It comes in 6-0 and 5-0 sizes. The 6-0 fast-absorbing plain gut usually does break down in 6 to 7 days, but the 5-0 often persists for 10 to 15 days. The 6-0 fast-absorbing suture can usually be wiped out of the incision with a moistened Q-tip or with antibiotic ointment on the Q-tip. The disadvantage is that there may be more of an inflammatory reaction to this material than to nylon.

Synthetic absorbable sutures undergo degradation by hydrolysis. Synthetic sutures usually produce less of an

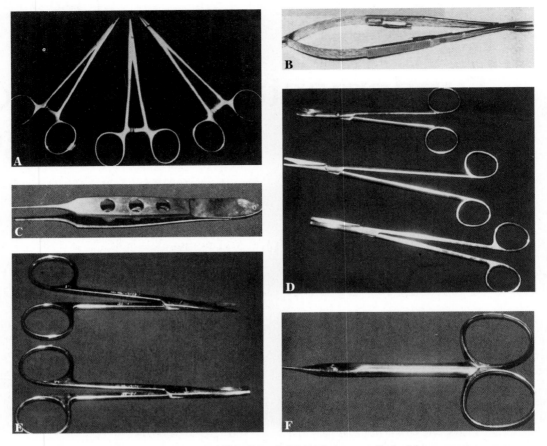

**FIGURE 6-1** ▪ Surgical instruments. **(A)** Left to right: Webster needle holder, neurosurgery needle holder, and Halsey needle holder. **(B)** Castroviejo needle holder. **(C)** Bishop-Harmon ophthalmic forceps. **(D)** Top to bottom: Metzenbaum, Malis, and Ragnell scissors. **(E)** Top to bottom: Stevens scissors and Littler scissors. **(F)** Gradle scissors.

inflammatory response in the subcutaneous tissue than do the gut sutures. Vicryl and Dexon are similar, but Vicryl has a better tensile strength profile, maintaining 75% at 2 weeks and 50% at 3 weeks. The hydrolysis and absorption of Vicryl is also significantly faster than that of Dexon. PDS and Maxon maintain their tensile strength longer—70% at 3 weeks, 50% at 4 weeks, and 25% at 6 weeks. Hydrolysis occurs between 180 and 210 days.

Monocryl maintains 50% to 60% of its tensile strength at 1 week and 20% to 30% at 2 weeks. It is a good choice for a facial subcutaneous suture since it produces less of an inflammatory response than Vicryl or Dexon. Monocryl usually requires five to six throws on the knot or there may be slippage.

The major nonabsorbable sutures are silk, nylon, and polypropylene. Silk suture is frequently used on the eyelids and lips since it is soft and not irritatingly sharp.

Monofilament nylon suture such as Ethilon is a general-purpose skin suture. Polypropylene or Prolene is a monofilament suture with an increased memory and high tensile strength. It requires six throws to a knot.

For subcutaneous sutures on the face, usually a 4-0 or 5-0 size suture is used. For skin sutures on the face, usually a 5-0 or 6-0 size suture is used. For more delicate work, 7-0 size may be indicated.

For skin and fascia, use a reverse cutting needle. With the reverse cutting needle, the cutting edge is on the outside of the curve. For facial surgery or for other fine cutaneous surgery, precision point needles are best. There is reduced tissue drag and trauma with these supersmooth, highly honed needles. In the Ethicon product line, these needles have the code prefix P, PS, or PC (for plastic or plastic surgery or plastic cosmetic) and in the Davis & Geck line, PR or PRE (for plastic reconstructive). The number after the prefix indicates the size of the curvature. The P3 needle has good utility for the face. For general cutaneous surgery, an FS (for skin) reverse cutting needle may be used, but there is considerable drag and tissue resistance compared with the precision needle.

## Types of Stitches

### Buried Subcutaneous Stitch

The buried subcutaneous stitch is used to close the dead space to prevent hematoma and a nidus for infection (**Fig. 6-2**). It also reduces the tension on the skin. Burying the knot deep in the tissue decreases the amount of tissue reaction in the

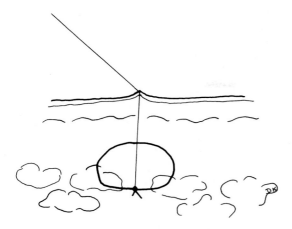

FIGURE 6-2 ■ Buried subcutaneous stitch.

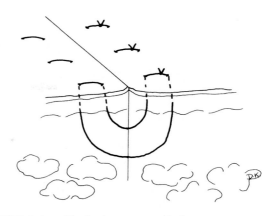

FIGURE 6-4 ■ Vertical mattress stitch.

more superficial part of the wound so that the major inflammatory response is away from the surface of the incision and less apt to disrupt it.

To bury the knot, the needle first enters through the deep portion of the wound and exits more superficially on the same side. It then enters superficially on the other side of the wound and exits through the deeper tissue on that side of the wound. This is usually an absorbable suture.

Many texts recommend that interrupted subcutaneous sutures be used in case a suture breaks. However, multiple buried sutures, each with a knot, will place a greater mass of foreign body in the tissue and produce a greater inflammatory response. Running a subcutaneous suture poses no difficulty even if the suture should break since the friction on the suture and the edema of the tissue secure it.

## Simple Skin Stitch

With the simple skin stitch, the suture is passed through the epidermis and dermis from one side to the other (**Fig. 6-3**). The exit and entry points are usually 2 to 3 mm from the incision edge. A greater "bite" of tissue should be taken more deeply than superficially to help evert the wound edges.

The simple skin stitch functions to approximate and evert the wound edges and to adjust the height of the wound edges so that they are even. If one side of a wound is lower than the other side, a slightly deeper bite should be taken on the lower side for the initial wound height adjustment. The knot is then placed on the lower side of the wound to further finely adjust the height of the wound edges.

## Vertical Mattress Stitch

The vertical mattress stitch tents up the skin edges (**Fig. 6-4**). This eversion of the edges compensates for contracture that later occurs in the wound which may produce a linear depression. If with simple interrupted stitches or with a simple running stitch the wound is not everted sufficiently, vertical mattress stitches may be placed in the areas not everted.

## Horizontal Mattress Stitch

The horizontal mattress stitch is used for the closure of a wound under tension. It can cause strangulation of the skin (**Fig. 6-5**). Therefore, it may be used with a bolster such as a small piece of a red Robinson catheter through which the

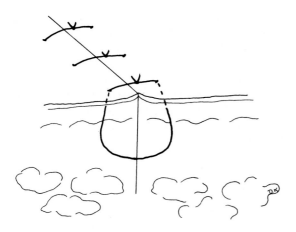

FIGURE 6-3 ■ Simple stitch.

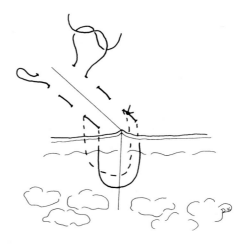

FIGURE 6-5 ■ Horizontal mattress stitch.

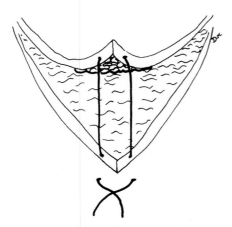

**FIGURE 6-6** ▪ Corner stitch (tip stitch, half-buried mattress stitch).

exposed suture passes to reduce the pressure on the skin. In general it is not a preferred stitch for facial surgery.

## Corner Stitch (Tip Stitch)

The corner stitch is used for v-shaped corners, to prevent necrosis of the skin tip. It is inserted vertically down through the main segment of skin and out through the dermis. It then enters horizontally through the dermis in the tip of the flap and out and then back up through the main segment of skin (Fig. 6-6). The suture should enter and leave the flap tip in the same dermal plane that it exits and reenters the dermis of the main body of skin for an even wound.

## Running Simple Stitch

The running simple stitch is a continuously repeated over-and-over stitch that is a rapid method of closure (Fig. 6-7). This stitch can evenly distribute tension along the wound. By adjusting the depth of bite of tissue with each placement of the suture, the height of the wound edges may be adjusted. This stitch is easier and less traumatic to remove than multiple interrupted stitches.

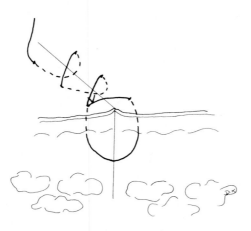

**FIGURE 6-7** ▪ Running simple stitch.

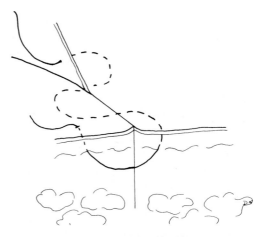

**FIGURE 6-8** ▪ Running intradermal stitch.

## Running Intradermal Stitch

The running intradermal stitch is placed in the dermis and may be left in place for an extended period without causing cross-hatching of the skin (Fig. 6-8). The suture used may be a permanent type such as Prolene because of its memory and strength or an absorbable type such as PDS or Monocryl depending on the stress on the wound. The suture enters the skin at a point 4 to 5 mm beyond the edge of the incision. From this point it is brought into the wound and then into the dermis on one side and crosses to the other side. The stitch is continued in a running S pattern staying in the same plane of the dermis from one side to the other. In a long running intradermal stitch that is to be removed, it is wise to have it periodically come through the surface of the skin and then back in through the skin. This allows for removal of the suture in short segments facilitating later removal since the friction on the suture and the healing process tend to secure the suture. With PDS or Monocryl, the need for removal can be avoided.

Although the running intradermal stitch nicely coapts the wound edges, further approximation may be accomplished with a tissue adhesive to the surface of the skin edges.

## Suture Tying

Sutures should be tied so that they lie down as square knots. The sutures should be tied to coapt the wound edges but not to strangulate. Most err by tying too tightly. One way of avoiding too tightly tied knots is to not snug down the second throw of the suture. Leaving this throw slightly loose also compensates for the tissue edema that develops in wounds. Tying too tightly is a major cause of suture track marks on the skin. Leaving sutures in too long is another factor. Granulomas or microcysts may form along the suture tract if the suture is left in too long.

## Hemostasis

Hemostasis is essential to good wound healing. A rule of thumb on controlling bleeders is that named vessels should be clamped and ligated, and unnamed vessels may be electrocoagulated. In tying off vessels, use the smallest suture that is practical, usually a 4-0 or 5-0 on the face. The suture should be cut on the knot to leave the least amount of material in the wound that might cause a foreign body reaction.

A biterminal device is usually used for electrocoagulation. The current enters the patient through an active or coagulating electrode. When tissue contact is made, heat is generated and coagulation occurs. The current passes through the patient and out via the dispersing electrode, the grounding pad. The patient usually becomes part of the current circuit.

The grounding pad should be placed as close as possible to the surgical site. If possible, the heart should not be between the active electrode and the grounding pad because it then becomes part of the current pathway. The area of coagulation should be kept dry with sponging or with suction; bleeding into the area disperses the current and diminishes the coagulation effect.

Biterminal coagulation is not bipolar coagulation. Bipolar coagulation is the system in which a single electrode contains both terminals. With bipolar coagulation forceps, the current passes between the tines of the forceps, coagulating the tissue between the tines. Bipolar coagulation is more precise, produces less tissue damage, and does not involve current transmission through the patient.

True electrocautery is essentially a red-hot branding iron that seals blood vessels by the direct application of heat. An electrocautery system uses either low-frequency alternating current or direct current. The current remains in the electrode tip and does not pass into the patient. There are a variety of disposable battery-powered cautery pens.

In the preoperative evaluation, it is important to ask whether the patient has any implanted electrical devices such as a pacemaker, vagus nerve stimulator, or other neurostimulator. The majority of newer pacemakers are defibrillating. With the defibrillating pacemakers, electrocoagulation should not be used until proper protective measures have been undertaken. The manufacturers have toll-free numbers to call for instructions. In the event that there is a question, the cautery pens should be safe because they seal the blood vessels by direct heat and not by electricity.

## Patient Information on Potential Complications or Side Effects of Skin Surgery

1. *Scar formation:* Scars form whenever there is injury to the skin. Some scars are more noticeable than others. Some individuals are more prone to thickened or keloid scars. Scars in areas of high sebaceous gland concentration and activity such as the nose and forehead are more likely to be widened and become depressed. Postoperative treatment of the scar may be necessary.
2. *Pain:* Postoperative pain will depend on the extent of surgery and also on the particular individual. Pain medications are prescribed and may be taken after surgery if needed. With pain medications, do not drive, operate machinery, or make important decisions. Alcohol can amplify the effects of pain medications. It is best to eat something solid before pain medications since they may irritate the stomach and cause nausea.
3. *Bleeding:* Bleeding after surgery can usually be controlled with pressure applied to the wound for 15 to 20 minutes and with ice compresses. Some oozing is to be expected. In the case of severe or persistent bleeding, please call the doctor.
4. *Swelling:* Various degrees of swelling will occur. Cold compresses on for 20 minutes and off for 10 minutes for the first 24 to 48 hours will lessen swelling. Elevation of the head at 15 to 20 degrees when lying down or sleeping will help to reduce edema. A reclining chair usually provides a good angle of head elevation.
5. *Bruising:* Bruising around the surgery site will resolve. With surgery of the anterior scalp, forehead, or around the eyes, a black eye may develop within 12 to 72 hours after surgery. Sometimes the eye will swell shut.
6. *Hematoma:* This is a lump that forms under the skin from bleeding after the surgery. It represents a collection of blood.
7. *Infection:* With any injury to the skin or surgery, infection is possible. Therefore, an antibiotic ointment, and sometimes antibiotic tablets, may be prescribed at the time of surgery. Wound infections usually occur 4 days after surgery. If you suspect an infection, please call the doctor.
8. *Numbness:* It is common to have numbness in the area of surgery because there are always sensory nerves running through the skin. Usually this numbness will go away in 6 to 12 months. But in some instances, it may be permanent.
9. *Paralysis of nerve:* If a cancer extends into the area of a nerve that controls the movement of muscles, temporary or permanent paralysis may occur. The greatest areas of risk on the face are the temple area where the nerve to the eyebrow and eyelid runs and  the lower cheek where the nerve to the lower lip runs.
10. *Wound dehiscence:* In straightforward terms, this means the wound separates or pulls apart. This can happen anywhere, but it is most prone to occur when the wound overlies an area of muscle mass such as on the back or the extremities. If a body movement seems to tug on the wound, stop the movement and relax.
11. *Wound healing:* Not all skin wounds heal ideally. At times a skin repair, graft, or flap may fail to heal well or the wound may seem to lift up or protrude. This may affect part of the wound or the whole wound. Most often, the wound will still heal adequately with treatment. Sometimes additional surgery is required.

## Patient Instructions for Surgery

1. If you are taking prescribed medications, continue to take them unless instructed otherwise.
2. If you are taking Plavix (clopidogrel) or Coumadin (warfarin) because of a heart attack, atrial fibrillation,

blood clot, heart stent, stroke, or transient ischemic attack (TIA), you will usually be able to continue on the medication, although you will probably bleed more and may have a greater chance of postoperative bleeding. If you are taking Coumadin, you may require a blood test international normalized ratio (INR) within a week of surgery.

3. If you are routinely taking aspirin or ibuprofen products such as Motrin, Aleve, or Advil for headaches, pain, or preventive measures, please stop 10 days before surgery. These products may cause more bleeding during and after surgery. Aspirin and ibuprofen may be in various products. For instance aspirin is in Pepto-Bismol and Alka-Seltzer. Aspirin may be listed as salicylate or salicylic acid. If you have arthritis, celecoxib (Celebrex), an anti-inflammatory drug that does not have an effect on bleeding, may be prescribed. It is used with caution in patients who have cardiovascular disease or risk factors for cardiovascular disease.

4. If you have a pacemaker, it is important that you inform the doctor and specify its type and whether it is a defibrillating pacemaker so that proper precautions may be taken. Please also mention if you have a neurostimulator implant such as a vagus nerve stimulator.

5. If you have any joint replacement implants you may need antibiotics prior to surgery. If you have had carditis, mitral valve prolapse, or heart valve replacement, you will be prescribed preoperative antibiotics.

6. Two weeks before surgery, stop taking vitamin E and supplements such as garlic, ginger, ginkgo biloba, ginseng, and ephedra. In general, it is best to stop all supplements 2 weeks prior to surgery.

7. Stop smoking for 2 weeks before and for 2 weeks after surgery. It is well documented that smoking causes poor wound healing.

8. Wash your hair the night before or morning of surgery.

9. Shower and wash your face the morning of surgery.

10. Someone should come with you or be available to drive you home.

11. Please arrive at the designated time.

12. If you decide to cancel surgery, please let your surgeon know in enough time so that another patient can be scheduled. However, doctors do understand that illness may occur unexpectedly.

13. If you are apprehensive and require an antianxiety medication, it may be prescribed. However, you must sign your operative consent ahead of time or before taking the medication.

## Patient Safety

Whether doing surgery in a hospital, in an ambulatory surgery center, or in the office, a protocol for preventing wrong site, wrong procedure, and wrong person surgery should be instituted. This protocol is referred to as "time out." Time out includes all persons involved in the surgery, which can vary depending on the location (i.e., the hospital vs. the office). In the hospital, it would involve the surgeon, the anesthesiologist, the circulating nurse, and the surgical ("scrub nurse") technician or nurse. In office surgery, it will usually only involve the surgeon and the nurse or medical assistant. Time out is a verification procedure.

The site of surgery should be marked. If multiple surgeons are doing procedures in the same facility, the surgeon's initials will also be placed with a skin marker. The person performing the surgery should mark the site. Marking should occur with the patient involved, awake, and aware, if possible, for cross verification.

Patient's identity should be verified with two identifiers such as name and birth date. In the operating area, the nurse will again verify the patient's identity, procedure to be done, surgical site, patient's position (if appropriate), and any other pertinent information such as the presence of a pacemaker or other implants. This is done in the presence of the entire surgical team who are to acknowledge that the information is correct. This is similar to a pilot's preflight checklist.

## Skin Preparation for Surgery

It is best to shave as little hair as possible; do not shave the eyebrows because they grow very slowly. Prep the skin with Betadine or Hibiclens; do not use Hibiclens around the eye. Use Betadine or Shur-Clens (poloxaner 188) around the eye. Prepare a large enough surgical field so that one may see not only the immediate surgical site but also the relationship to the surrounding anatomic landmarks to be sure that the closure of the wound is not distorting some other structure such as the nose, lip, or eyelid.

Incision lines are marked out before any distortion by infiltrative anesthesia. Round toothpicks dipped in methylene blue or Bonney's blue make a more exact line than most skin marking pens.

## Anesthesia

Most cutaneous surgery requires only infiltrative or regional block anesthesia. The standard agent, 1% lidocaine, is a safe, rapidly acting, short-duration anesthetic to which allergic reactions are exceedingly rare. By the addition of epinephrine, systemic absorption of lidocaine is lessened, duration of action is significantly prolonged, and a local hemostatic effect is achieved. Optimal vasoconstriction usually occurs in 15 minutes. The available commercial preparations may combine lidocaine with 1:100,000 epinephrine. Patients may react to epinephrine with apprehension, body tremors, diaphoresis, palpitations, tachycardia, and increased blood pressure. These side effects can be decreased or eliminated by diluting the epinephrine to 1:200,000 or even 1:400,000 without significantly changing its efficacy.

The maximum recommended dosage of lidocaine is 500 mg, the equivalent of 50 mL of a 1% lidocaine solution. The earliest sign of toxicity is on the central nervous system (CNS) with mild sedation, which may proceed to seizure activity. Cardiac toxicity usually occurs at twice the level.

Warming the anesthetic agent to room temperature and buffering the lidocaine decreases the discomfort of the injection. Lidocaine is buffered by diluting it 10% with 8.4% sodium bicarbonate.

At the end of the procedure, a longer acting anesthetic 0.25% bupivacaine diluted to 1:400,000 may be injected for a more prolonged anesthesia of 5 to 8 hours. Even after sensation returns, there may be an analgesia that will persist for some time. Toxic limit for bupivacaine is 3 mg/kg. Bupivacaine can cause cardiac toxicity at the same levels needed to cause CNS toxicity. Bupivacaine can bind tightly to myocardial tissue and may trigger dysrhythmias. This is more of a problem in a highly vascular area such as the tonsillar bed. However, intravascular injection should be avoided.

Ropivacaine is another long-acting anesthetic with less potential for cardiac toxicity than bupivacaine. Ropivacaine has a toxic limit of 3 mg/kg. Epinephrine does not decrease its systemic absorption as with lidocaine and bupivacaine.

## Placement of Incisions

Incisions should be planned so that they are as parallel to or within wrinkle, smile, and expression lines as can be. When there is a lack of definite wrinkles, place the incisions in the direction of relaxed skin tension lines. These lines run at right angles to the contractions of the underlying muscle.

Incision scars may also be camouflaged by placing them at the boundaries of aesthetic and anatomic areas, such as the vermilion junction, the paranasal fold (the junction of the nose and the cheek), the submandibular area, the submental area, the preauricular sulcus, and along the eyebrow or within the hairline.

## Skin Incisions

Incisions should be made vertical to the skin surface. Obliquely angled incisions do not coapt as well. An exception to this rule is in the area adjacent to the eyebrows or in the hair. Incisions placed here should be at an angle that parallels the angle of the hair shaft as it emerges from the skin to avoid transection of the hair follicle.

Even small wounds benefit from undermining equal to the width of the wound to reduce tension. Undermining may be done with a scissor or a scalpel. On the face, the level of undermining is usually just under the dermal plexus. On the scalp, the most effective mobilization of the skin is by undermining between the aponeurosis of Galen and the periosteum, which is a relatively blood-free plane. However, this is below the sensory nerves.

## Excisions

The standard excision is fusiform in shape. If the length-to-width ratio is less than 4:1 or if one side is longer than the other, redundant tissue will develop at the corners or ends of the closure. These so-called dog-ears or standing cones of tissue, if small, level out and flatten as the wound undergoes contracture. If large, they should be removed by tenting up

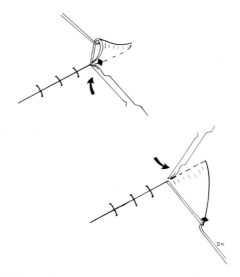

**FIGURE 6-9** ■ Tenting up corner of wound with skin hook to define extent of dog-ear.

the corner of the wound with a skin hook to define the extent of the dog-ear. The dog-ear is incised along its base on one side or the other. The final wound curves toward the side on which the incision is placed. After making the incision along one side of the base of the dog-ear, the flap of tissue that is created is pulled across the incision. Where the base of the redundant tissue crosses the incision, it is transected. The dog-ear is eliminated and closure of the wound is completed (Fig. 6-9).

## Wound Dressings

In the first hours after the incision, a coagulum forms over the wound. Between 12 and 72 hours, there are two spurts of mitotic activity, and epidermal cells begin migrating across the wound. However, if a dried crust forms, it is a barrier to the epidermal migration. Rather than being able to migrate straight and level across the gap between the wound edges, the epidermal cells must find a plane of migration beneath the dried crusts. This leads to a shallow, linear depression in the healed incision.

To prevent wound crusting and the resultant linear trough in the healed wound, an occlusive dressing such as Bio-Occlusive or Tegaderm may be used. Another option is Dermicel tape, which is hypoallergenic. It is applied directly to the wound with no ointment applied. Its adhesive has some bacteriostatic properties. If an antibiotic ointment such as mupirocin is applied to the wound, it is covered with Xeroform or Vaseline gauze. Mastisol is applied to the surrounding skin and the dressing is secured with flexible cloth adhesive Band-Aids.

A moist environment develops under these dressings, which inhibits the formation of a crust and accelerates epidermal regeneration. Because of the abundant blood supply of the face, infection is not a problem.

The dressing is removed at 2 to 3 days postsurgery. Because of the increased incidence of methicillin-resistant

*Staphylococcus aureus* (MRSA) in the community, mupirocin ointment three times a day to the wound or retapamulin ointment (Altabax) twice a day to the wound is usually prescribed.

## Suture Removal

There are no hard-and-fast rules for suture removal. If there is doubt about whether the sutures should be removed, cut every other or third stitch and observe for another day or so. Some guidelines for the timing of suture removal are:

- Face: 5 to 7 days
- Neck: 7 to 12 days
- Back: 10 to 14 days
- Abdomen: 7 to 10 days
- Extremities: 10 to 18 days

Wound infections are most apt to develop 4 to 5 days after surgery.

To avoid disrupting the wound, the sutures should be cut with a fine scissor such as a Gradle or with a no. 11 scalpel blade. Pull the suture toward the incision to remove. Pulling the suture away from the incision places traction on the incision line.

Warn the patient to treat the area gently and continue to apply the antibiotic ointment for another week or so. Fibroplasia is just beginning at this point, and the epidermal bridging is the only thing holding the wound. The incision line may be reinforced with Steri-strips or with tissue adhesive. If this is done, antibiotic ointment is discontinued.

## Wound Dynamics

### Wound Healing

Wound healing is divided into four phases:

- Inflammatory
- Fibroblastic
- Proliferative
- Remodeling

These phases overlap and blend into each other. During the early inflammatory phase, there is vasoconstriction with platelet aggregation. After 5 to 10 minutes of vasoconstriction, there is active venule dilatation and increased vascular permeability, lasting about 72 hours. Within a few hours of these vascular responses, a cellular response occurs. Polymorphonuclear leukocytes migrate into the area. There is a diapedesis of monocytes that transform into tissue macrophages. The macrophage is the dominant cell for the first 3 to 4 days. It initiates the fibroblastic phase.

While the inflammatory phase is still proceeding, the proliferative phase commences. Epidermal cells undergo changes and begin migrating into the wound. By the third day, migration of epidermal cells across an apposed incision is complete. Fibroblasts within the dermis begin to proliferate at 25 to 36 hours after the initial injury. By the fourth day, the fibroblastic phase is heralded by the synthesis of collagen and proteoglycans by the proliferating fibroblasts. Collagen fibers are laid down in a random pattern without orientation.

Overlapping with and toward the latter part of the fibroblastic phase, the remodeling phase begins. This is a phase of differentiation, resorption, and maturation. Fibroblasts disappear from the wound, and collagen fibers are modeled into organized bundles and patterns. This phase may go on for a year or longer.

### Wound Contraction

In an open wound healing by second intention, there is an active drawing of the full thickness of the surrounding skin toward the center of the wound. Wound contraction begins during the proliferative phase of wound healing. There is a differentiation of fibroblasts to myofibroblasts, which are responsible for this activity. Wound contraction usually proceeds until the wound is closed or until surrounding forces on the skin are greater than the contractile forces of the myofibroblasts.

### Wound Contracture

All wound scars undergo contracture with a resultant shortening along their axes. This process of contracture is due to collagen cross-linking, which occurs during the remodeling phase. Contracture is distinct and different from wound contraction. Intralesional steroids counter the collagen cross-linking.

### Wound Strength

By 2 weeks, the wound has gained 7% of its final strength; by 3 weeks, 20%; by 4 weeks, 50%. At full maturation, the healed wound regains about 80% of the strength of the original intact skin.

## Documentation and Assessment

Although success or failure in cutaneous surgery may be readily apparent, it is important to document results with objective photography. After surgery, patients tend to scrutinize their faces and will see asymmetries and blemishes that were always there but did not receive any notice. But the patients may now attribute these imperfections to the surgery.

With consistent, standardized photographs, one may judge progress and analyze techniques and methods. Preoperative and postoperative photographs are essential, as are intraoperative photographs. Photographs are a method of self-assessment and serve as a stimulus and direction for improvement.

## Mohs Micrographic Surgery for Targeted Removal of Skin Cancers

Skin cancer is the most common type of malignancy in the United States. The major causes of skin cancers are ultraviolet light exposure, ionizing radiation, and chemicals such as

## SAUER'S NOTES

1. One of the more common complaints after skin surgery is a numbness or altered sensation in the area. This is not a complication but an anticipated result of cutting through the skin. It is best to warn patients of this possibility before surgery and that this alteration in sensation may last for 6 to 12 months and sometimes may be permanent.

2. In areas of high sebaceous gland activity such as the T area of the face and in patients with acne and rosacea, incisions tend to spread and widen no matter how meticulous and precise the surgery. This is a phenomenon of wound healing. "What the patient is told before surgery is informed consent; what is told after surgery may be taken as an excuse."

3. Beware of the temporal branch of the facial nerve. As it exits the parotid gland at the superior border, it runs a superficial course over the zygomatic arch and into the temporal area. Transection of this branch causes paralysis of the frontalis muscle on that side and drooping of the eyebrow. With any excision in the temporal area, this is a possibility. Forewarn the patient. A drooping eyebrow may be corrected with a browpexy.

4. Beware of the spinal accessory nerve in the posterior triangle of the neck. The spinal accessory nerve pierces through the posterior border of the sternocleidomastoid muscle a little above its midpoint and enters the posterior triangle. The spinal accessory nerve then travels superficially, just below the subcutaneous fat in the investing fascia covering the posterior triangle. There is also a chain of lymph nodes intimately associated with the spinal accessory nerve along its course in the posterior triangle. Paralysis of this nerve causes an inability to raise the arm above the horizontal position. This nerve has been transected by those aware of its superficial location as well as by those unaware. "Good judgment is based on experience, which is based on bad judgment."

5. No matter how careful and diligent the surgeon, the response of biologic systems is not always predictable; and the outcome not always anticipated or desired. "If one wants to be a surgeon, be prepared to cry and to pray."

arsenic. The yearly incidence of skin cancer is over 1.5 million in Americans. Basal cell carcinoma is the most common type and accounts for 75% to 80% of skin cancers. Squamous cell carcinoma is the next most common form and accounts for 15% to 20%. However, squamous cell carcinoma is more common in immunosuppressed patients, black patients, patients with cancer on the lips and hands, and in patients treated with PUVA (psoralens and UVA light).

## Mohs Surgery

Mohs surgery is a precise surgical method combined with histologic mapping for a targeted removal of skin cancer. This procedure was developed by Dr. Frederic Mohs of the University of Wisconsin, Madison.

Mohs surgery provides the greatest assurance of cancer removal along with the most conservative margins of resection. It has the highest cure rates for skin cancer: 97% to 99% for primary skin cancers and 95% to 96% for recurrent skin cancers.

While a medical student at Wisconsin in the 1930s, Frederic Mohs was a Brittingham research assistant in the zoology department. He was studying the inflammatory response of normal tissue and cancerous tissue in rats that were injected with different irritants. He observed that the injection of 20% zinc chloride produced necrosis in the tissue, but that on microscopic examination, histologic detail was preserved. He stated his "eureka" observation: "The chemical had produced fixation in situ."

Over the years, this observation led to his development of a method of skin cancer removal guided by microscopic control. He published his first article on this method in 1941, entitled "Chemosurgery: a microscopically controlled method of cancer excision." However, chemosurgery with the application of a zinc chloride paste to the skin cancer and subsequent cancer removal and microscopic checking would usually be a several-day ongoing procedure.

In the early 1950s, Dr. Mohs did begin to remove eyelid cancers without the zinc chloride fixation and was still able to microscopically control the excision. In 1974, Dr. Theodore Tromovitch and Dr. Samuel Stegman reported on a significant number of skin cancer patients having microscopically controlled excision routinely using a fresh tissue technique without the zinc chloride fixation. Their study ushered in the present era of Mohs surgery not requiring an in vivo tissue fixation and making it possible to remove most skin cancers during 1 day of surgery.

Mohs surgery is most commonly used for basal and squamous cell carcinomas, but it has found application in the removal of other types of skin cancers and some oropharyngeal cancers.

Prior to the surgery, a definitive diagnosis is established by biopsy. Most procedures may be accomplished under local anesthesia. Photo documentation is commonly done.

## Mohs Surgery Method

The mass of clinically evident cancer is removed either by scalpel or curette or both (**Figs. 6-10** and **6-11**). An advantage of curettage is that cancerous tissue is usually less resistant to the action of the curette than normal tissue. The mechanical resistance of normal tissue helps to define the extent of the cancer. After the apparent cancer mass has been removed, the first stage of Mohs surgery is performed.

With the scalpel, a thin underlying layer of tissue is excised from the bed of the cancer along with a 2 to 3 mm

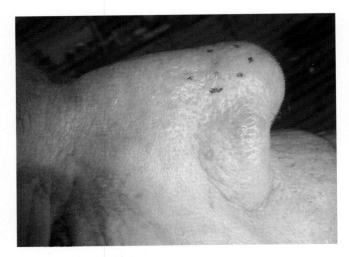

FIGURE 6-10 ■ Basal cell carcinoma, outlined on right tip of the nose.

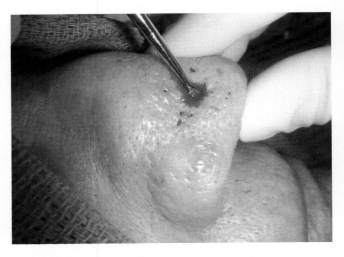

FIGURE 6-11 ■ Curettage of basal cell carcinoma on right tip of the nose.

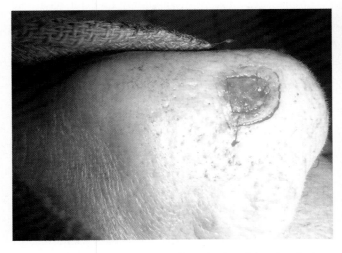

FIGURE 6-12 ■ Area of cancer: right tip of the nose, incised for removal of tissue layer for processing with Mohs technique.

perimeter margin (Fig. 6-12). The edges of the excision are beveled at 45 degrees in order to facilitate the histologic processing. Prior to the excision, small hash or reference marks are placed at various points along the perimeter of the excision and into the excision specimen for more precise histologic orientation. A saucerized type of excision is then performed (Fig. 6-13).

The excised specimen is subdivided into smaller pieces as necessary for tissue processing. An excised Mohs surgery layer may consist of one piece or multiple pieces, depending on the size of the cancer. The specimen is laid on grid paper with the patient's name and the specimen's orientation marked (Fig. 6-14). A map of the specimen's shape, subdivisions, reference marks, color coding, and position on the face or other area is drawn (Fig. 6-15).

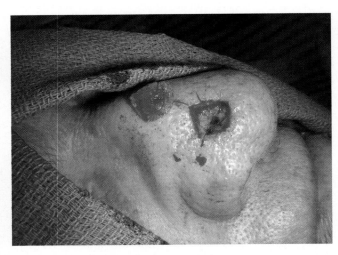

FIGURE 6-13 ■ Tissue layer removed and lying directly above excision site on right tip of the nose.

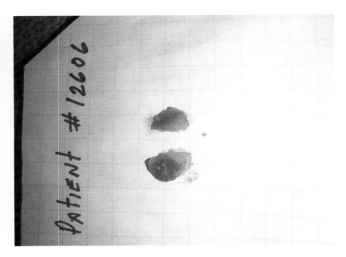

FIGURE 6-14 ■ The specimen of tissue layer that has been subdivided is laid on grid paper with the patient's number for identification and for orientation of specimen as to superior and inferior, left and right.

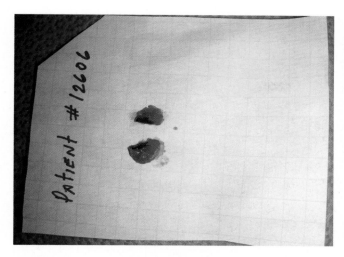

FIGURE 6-15 ■ The specimen on grid paper with color coding applied to the subdivided edges.

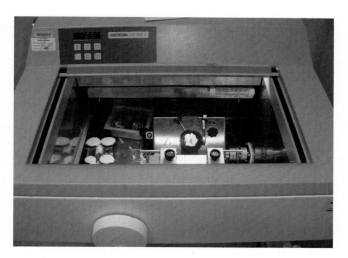

FIGURE 6-17 ■ Cryostat with specimen on chuck.

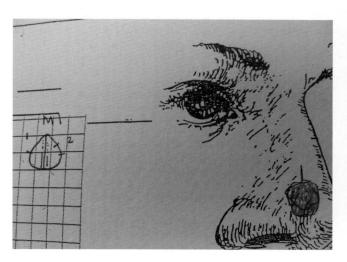

FIGURE 6-16 ■ Map of specimen to the left and diagram of the nose with the area of cancer marked to the right.

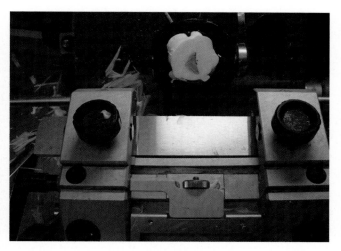

FIGURE 6-18 ■ Close-up of specimen on chuck in cryostat. The microtome blade is below the chuck.

A temporary dressing is applied to the patient, and the patient is escorted to the waiting area while the specimen is processed in the laboratory. The specimen is transferred to the laboratory where color coding is applied to the edges for further orientation and correlation with the map (Fig. 6-16). Each specimen piece is then inverted and compressed so that the edges are in the same plane as the deep margin. The specimen piece is placed on a cryostat chuck for cutting horizontal microscopic sections and the chuck is fixed in the cryostat (Figs. 6-17 and 6-18). The microscopic sections are usually cut at 4 to 14 μm in thickness depending on the characteristics of the tissue.

The horizontally cut microscopic slides of the excised layers from the perimeter and base of the cancer are the sine qua non of this procedure. To accomplish this requires well-trained technicians.

The processing of the specimens for Mohs surgery requires finely practiced skill to ensure that the specimen's deep and perimeter margins are in the same plane. This skill is time and energy demanding.

Various devices have been designed to facilitate this processing. The innovative CryoHist invented by the late Dr. David Rada is a sophisticated apparatus that uses vacuum compression with freezing of the specimen to achieve consistent horizontal cuts (Fig. 6-19).

The microscopic sections are mounted on glass slides and stained, usually with hematoxylin and eosin. After placing cover slips on the labeled slides, they are ready to be examined under the microscope (Fig. 6-20).

The Mohs surgeon serves two roles—first as the surgeon excising the cancer and second as the dermatopathologist microscopically examining the slides of the excised cancer. Because of the need for extensive training in dermatopathology, most Mohs surgeons are dermatologists.

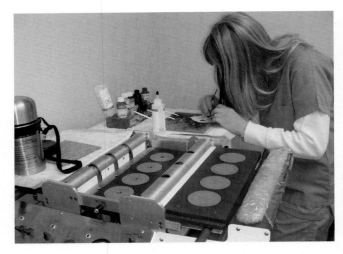

FIGURE 6-19 ■ Rada CryoHist in foreground with a technician preparing the specimen in the background.

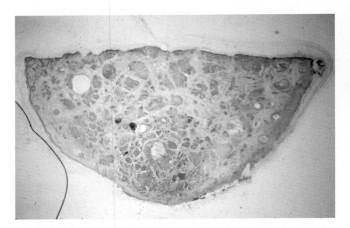

FIGURE 6-20 ■ Microscopic slide of compressed, horizontal section. Along the curved edge of the border is the epidermis. The straight-edged portion of the specimen is where it has been subdivided. There is blue color coding along part of the straight edge, indicating the superior half of the specimen, and red color coding along the other part, indicating the inferior half of the specimen. The area between the curved edge and straight edge is the deep margin of the excision.

There is basal cell carcinoma in the central area with close proximity to the middle part of the skin edge. Thus, another layer of excision is required from this area.

The Mohs surgeon examines the specimen under the microscope and correlates the findings with the map of the excised specimen. If no cancer remains, the patient is ready for either immediate or delayed reconstruction. If residual cancer is identified, the location of the cancer seen on the slide is correlated with the map and the position of the cancer is plotted. A further layer of Mohs surgery is performed in the targeted area of remaining cancer. The process of microscopic processing of horizontal compressed specimens and microscopic examination is repeated. The layered

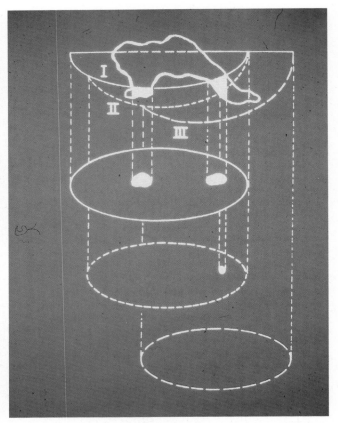

FIGURE 6-21 ■ Diagram of the concept of Mohs surgery with a layer excision of the residual cancer guided by microscopic control.

resection of tissue is repeated as is needed in each patient until the perimeter and deep margins are totally clear of cancer cells (Fig. 6-21).

## Indications for Mohs Surgery

Various methods are used to treat skin cancers: (1) cryosurgery, (2) curettage and electrodessication (scraping and burning), (3) topical creams, (4) radiation therapy, (5) excision, (6) Mohs surgery.

Mohs surgery may be used for most skin cancers, but there are situations when it should be the major consideration for the method of removal.

1. Recurrent skin cancers (Figs. 6-22 to 6-28)
2. Skin cancers greater than 2 cm in clinical measurement (Figs. 6-29 to 6-32)
3. Morphea and sclerosing basal cell carcinomas (Figs. 6-33 to 6-35)
4. Cancers with ill-defined borders (Figs. 6-36 and 6-37)
5. Skin cancers in areas with high recurrence rates: ears, nose, eyelids, and scalp (Figs. 6-38 and 6-39)
6. Cancers induced by radiation therapy
7. Cancers induced by immunosuppression
8. Histologically aggressive cancers: poorly differentiated squamous cell carcinoma, cancer with perineural invasion,

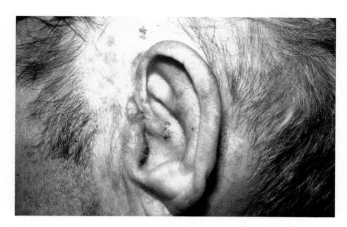

FIGURE 6-22 ■ Recurrent basal cell carcinoma of the left ear. This cancer had been removed on three previous occasions by other doctors.

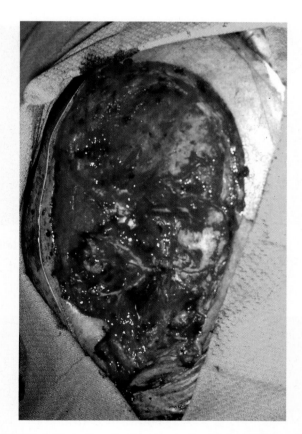

FIGURE 6-23 ■ Resultant wound after Mohs surgery with parotidectomy with facial nerve dissection and mastoidectomy. The facial nerve with its upper and lower divisions is seen in the center area of the wound.

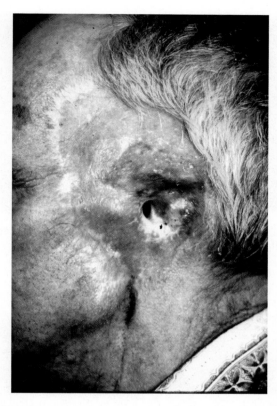

FIGURE 6-24 ■ Area of left ear after full thickness skin graft.

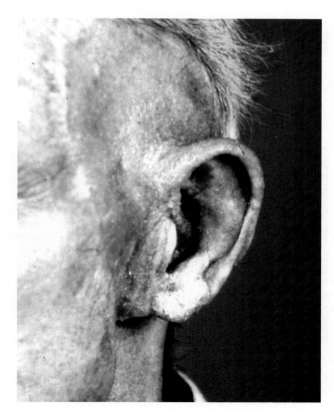

FIGURE 6-25 ■ Prosthetic ear in place.

metatypical basal cell carcinoma, infiltrating basal cell carcinoma

9. Cancers in critical areas: perioral, genital, hands, feet (Figures 6-40 to 6-43)

10. Cancers where maximum tissue preservation is required

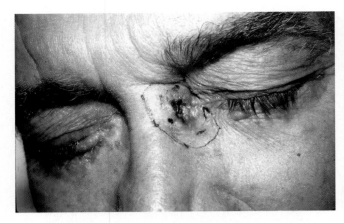

FIGURE 6-26 ▪ Recurrent basal cell carcinoma in medial canthus of the left eye.

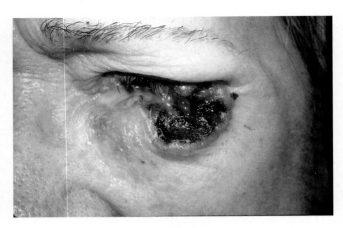

FIGURE 6-29 ▪ Primary basal cell carcinoma, greater than 2 cm in size, of the left eyelid and extending onto the bulbar conjunctiva.

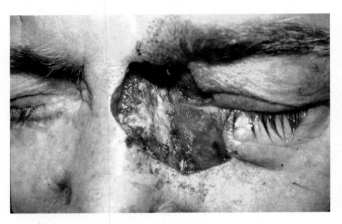

FIGURE 6-27 ▪ Wound of medial canthus of the left eye after Mohs surgery.

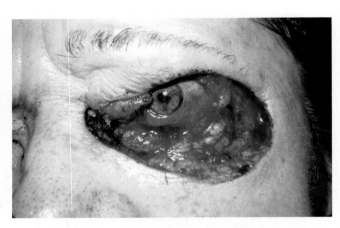

FIGURE 6-30 ▪ Extent of basal cell carcinoma of the left eyelid and bulbar conjunctiva after Mohs surgery.

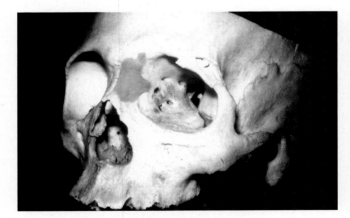

FIGURE 6-28 ▪ Skull with red putty, representing the extent of the cancer in Figure 6-26. Cancer of the medial canthus tends to extend along the medial wall of the orbit toward the lamina papyracea. At the lamina papyracea, the cancer may penetrate into the ethmoid sinus.

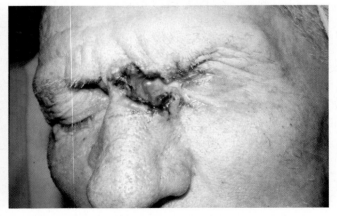

FIGURE 6-31 ▪ Primary basal cell carcinoma, greater than 2 cm in size, of the medial canthus infiltrating into the eye and the orbit.

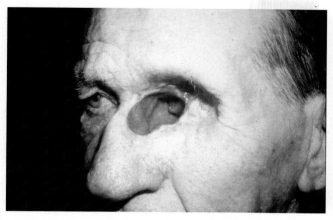

FIGURE 6-32 ▪ Extent of cancer in Figure 6-31 after Mohs surgery with orbital exenteration of the eye and ethmoidectomy.

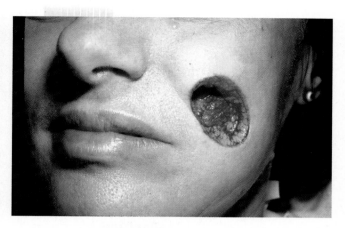

FIGURE 6-35 ▪ Extent of morphea basal cell carcinoma in Figure 6-33 after Mohs surgery.

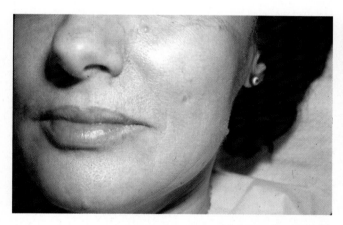

FIGURE 6-33 ▪ Morphea basal cell carcinoma of the cheek.

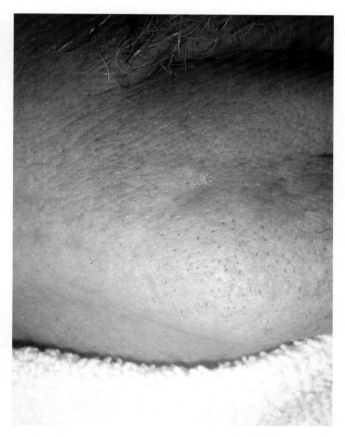

FIGURE 6-36 ▪ Basal cell carcinoma of the right chin with ill-defined clinical borders.

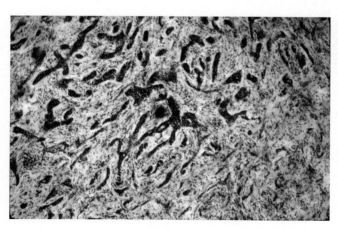

FIGURE 6-34 ▪ Histology slide of morphea type of basal cell carcinoma displaying an infiltrating, sclerotic pattern with Indian filing of the cancer cells.

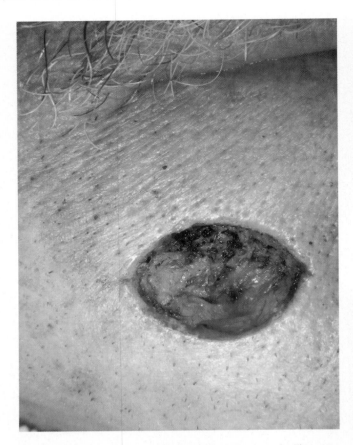

FIGURE 6-37 ■ Extent of basal cell carcinoma in Figure 6-36 after Mohs surgery.

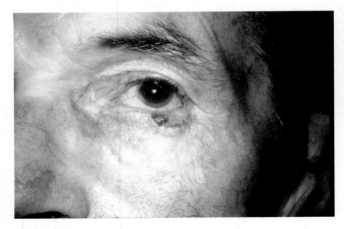

FIGURE 6-38 ■ Primary basal cell carcinoma of the left lateral lower eyelid.

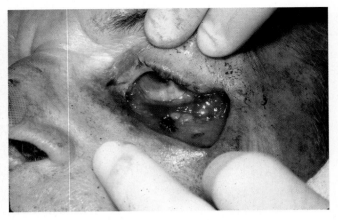

FIGURE 6-39 ■ Extent of cancer in Figure 6-38 after Mohs surgery.

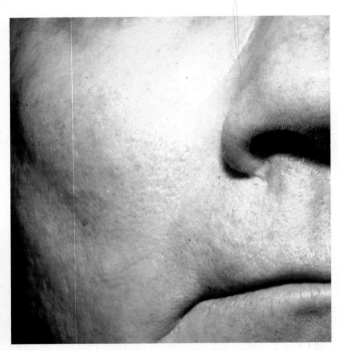

FIGURE 6-40 ■ Basal cell carcinoma of the upper lip at the junction of the ala nasi and nasal sill.

## Advantages of Mohs Surgery

1. The horizontal compressed frozen sections allow for microscopic examination of the entire perimeter and of all the deep margins.
2. The mapping with microscopic control allows for accurate targeting of residual cancer.
3. There is maximum assurance of cancer removal with minimal sacrifice of normal tissue.

### A Personal Note on Frederic E. Mohs, M.D.

Dr. Mohs spent his entire career at the University of Wisconsin in Madison from undergraduate school until his death on July 1, 2002 (Fig. 6-44). He treated his first patient with chemosurgery on June 23, 1936 at the University of Wisconsin Hospital. Today Dr. Mohs' name and his procedure are synonymous. Mohs surgery is practiced throughout the world.

Dr. Mohs was a very quiet man, but he was focused on his life's mission, which was to continue to improve and

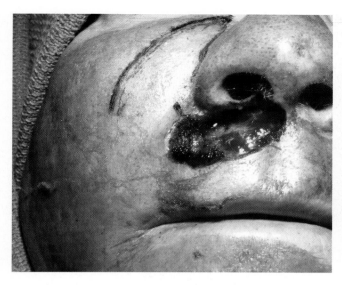

**FIGURE 6-41** ■ Extent of cancer in Figure 6-40 after Mohs surgery.

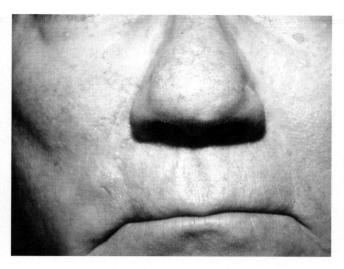

**FIGURE 6-43** ■ Healed reconstructed lip from Figure 6-42.

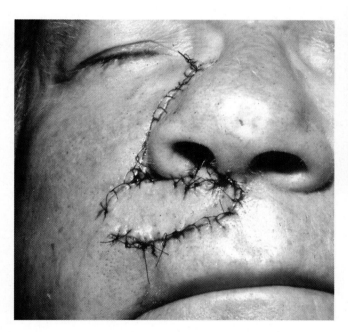

**FIGURE 6-42** ■ Reconstruction of the wound in Figure 6-41 a with nasolabial transposition flap.

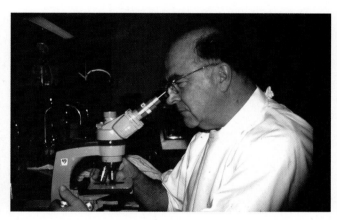

**FIGURE 6-44** ■ Frederic E. Mohs, M.D. in his laboratory at the University of Wisconsin.

perfect his technique, to apply it wherever appropriate, and to teach it to all who were interested (Fig. 6-44). He never wavered from his goal. I first met Dr. Mohs when I referred a patient with a recurrent skin cancer to him. I went to Madison with the patient to see exactly what Mohs surgery was. For the next year, I would travel back to Madison for a week every 3 to 4 months to learn more. Dr. Mohs invited me to be his Brittingham fellow, which I accepted. Dr. Mohs pointed out that the Brittingham grant was the same one he had had and that was how micrographic surgery had begun.

He loved the University of Wisconsin and being from Wisconsin. During one January blizzard, I had mushed on into the hospital and was operating with Dr. Mohs. He commented on how great it was to live in Wisconsin and have to deal with such elements. I thought he was joking, but he was serious. The most severe rebuke I ever heard Dr. Mohs give when someone whined or complained was "You're not from Wisconsin, are you?"

## Suggested Readings

Gross KG, Steinman HK, Rapini RP. *Mohs Surgery: Fundamentals and Techniques.* St. Louis: Mosby; 1999.

McGregor IA, McGregor AD. *Fundamental Techniques of Plastic Surgery.* Edinburgh: Churchill Livingstone; 1999.

Mohs, FE. Chemosurgery: a microscopically controlled method of cancer excision. *Arch Surg.* 1941; 42:279–295.

Mohs FE. *Chemosurgery: Microscopically Controlled Surgery for Skin Cancer.* Springfield: CC Thomas; 1978.

Tromovitch TA, Stegman SJ. Microscopically controlled excision of skin tumors: chemosurgery (Mohs): fresh tissue technique. *Arch Dermatol.* 1974;110:231–232.

Weerda H. *Reconstructive Facial Plastic Surgery.* Stuttgart: Thieme; 2001.

# CHAPTER 7

# Cosmetics for the Physician

*Marianne N. O'Donoghue, MD*

As physicians, especially dermatologists, our patients with cosmetic concerns often confront us. We need to explain the preferred methods of cleansing and moisturizing, safe hair care products, nail products, and skin-enhancing practices. It is important to know how cosmetics function, which products cause adverse reactions, and how we can recommend them for the better care of our patients.

The U.S. Food and Drug Administration (FDA) defines cosmetics as "(1) articles intended to be rubbed, poured, sprinkled, or sprayed on, introduced into, or otherwise applied to the human body or any part thereof for cleansing, beautifying, promoting attractiveness, or altering the appearance, and (2) articles intended for use as a component of any such article: except that such term shall not include soap." The cosmetic manufacturers do not regulate cosmetics as strictly as drugs, but there is a voluntary registration. Cosmetic Ingredient Review is an independent panel of expert scientists and physicians established to examine all published and voluntarily submitted industry data and summarize them in a safety monograph for each individual cosmetic ingredient or class of cosmetic ingredient.

In the United States, the regulation for labeling cosmetics is that the manufacturer should label all ingredients in descending order of concentration for all ingredients greater than 1% of the product. Ingredients that compose less than 1% of the product may be listed in any order. The labels need only be on the outside wrapping.

Products intended for retail sale need a statement of identity, net quantity of content, name and place of business and the manufacturer or distributor, declaration of ingredient statement, any necessary warning statements, and directions for use. If not intended for retail sale (e.g., cosmetics in a beauty salon) these specifications need not be met.

---

### SAUER'S NOTES

1. Simple, honest cosmetic advice is expected by your patients.
2. If cosmetic questions are not answered by the physician, then they will be answered by someone whose interest lies beyond giving the cheapest, safest, and most practical answers.

---

This means that the physician can trace the origin of any product to which a patient has an adverse reaction. The research and development departments of most cosmetic companies are helpful and knowledgeable, especially if the inquiring physician is not argumentative. The cosmetic industry has worked very hard to be helpful to the dermatologist.

## Classification of Cosmetics

Cosmetics can be classified into toiletries, skin care products, fragrance products, and makeup or color products.

### Toiletries

These include soaps (cleansers), shampoos, hair rinses and conditioners, hair dressings, sprays and setting lotions, hair color preparations, waving preparations, straightening (relaxing) agents, deodorants, antiperspirants, and sun protective agents.

### Cleansers

The purpose of cleansing is to remove sebum that attracts dirt, desquamate the skin, remove airborne pollutants, remove pathogenic organisms, and remove any existing makeup.

The classic cleanser, and the one that has been present for decades, is soap. Soap consists of a substance made up of fatty acid in oil or fat and an alkaline substance. Clear or transparent soap permits better control of the alkaline residue and rinses off more easily. Hard-milled soaps have been considered elegant for many years. Synthetic detergents (syndets) are shaped like soap in bars but consist of anionic surfactants, such as sodium lauryl sulfate that can have a more acidic pH. This makes the syndet easier to rinse off in hard water, and the product can be adjusted to be less irritating to the skin. Special soaps can include medicaments, granules, emollients, or fragrance. Soaps and synthetic detergents have been tested for irritancy, transepidermal water loss, pH, and many other qualities. All of these products have their advantages and disadvantages.

Liquid cleansers have become more popular than ever. To produce a liquid cleanser, water is added and then preservatives (often formaldehyde releasers) later to prevent pseudomonas infections. These products can become more irritating than bar soap.

Shower gels have become as popular in the United States as they are in Europe. They may have potassium lauryl sulfate as their anionic surfactant or many other ingredients. Many contain the ingredient cocamidopropyl betaine that has become a very common sensitizer. These shower gels appear to rinse off well but may be a little more irritating in some individuals. Perfumed liquid gels using peppermint and pineapple scents have caused many cases of contact and irritant dermatitis in the past seven or so years.

Cleansing cloths impregnated with a body wash–type cleanser are the newest cleansing technology. The fibered facial cloths have a textured side, which induces exfoliation, and a smooth rinse side, which leaves behind petrolatum. This allows cleansing, exfoliation, and moisturization to occur in one product.

## Shampoos

Shampoos have three major components—water, detergent, and a fatty material. Like body cleansers, the soap shampoos contain alkali plus oil and fat. Because these may leave a precipitate on the hair shaft with hard water, soap shampoos are rarely used anymore.

Most shampoos are soapless and are made of sulfonated oil. They consist of (1) principal surfactants for detergent and foaming power, (2) secondary surfactants to condition the hair, and (3) additives to complete the formulation and special effects. Because most of the damage to the hair shaft is from chemicals that have a high pH, such as color and permanent or straightening agents, many shampoos are formulated today with an acidic or neutral pH. Because shampoo contains a large amount of water, preservatives (which will be considered later) must be added. Formaldehyde is the most common preservative in shampoo. Because shampoo is only left on the hair for a short period of time, contact dermatitis does not usually occur. Hairdressers, however, are often confronted with that problem. Some of the other additives besides preservatives, such as color, fragrance, and newer essential oils, occasionally can cause allergic reactions.

The major therapeutic agents added to shampoos are tar, salicylic acid, zinc pyrithione, sulfur, and by prescription ketoconazole, cycloallamine, clobetasol, and fluocinonide. It is important for physicians to know that these ingredients do not necessarily harm the hair or strip the color. The formulation of these therapeutic shampoos can contain as many conditioners and beautifying ingredients as nontherapeutic shampoos. They can even be recommended for color-treated, permed, or African-American hair. The formulation must simply be selected for the type of hair (e.g., dry, oily, fine, or coarse).

## Conditioners

Because of the trauma to the hair shaft from sun, wind, chemical treatments, and water, conditioners are a necessary

hair grooming product for both men and women. The original rinses to remove the soap shampoo film were lemon and vinegar. These substances are still helpful when a person is "roughing it" in the wild or simply not supplied with real conditioners. The other rinses coat the hair shaft so it does not become tangled with the hair shaft next to it. These products contain wax and paraffin, and they allow the hair to shine without static cling. Balsam is a product in that category.

The major conditioners for traumatized hair are cationic surfactant conditioners. Quaternary ammonium compounds, especially stearalkonium ammonium chloride, have been used for many years to make the hair manageable. It is possible to attach a polymer (such as polyvinylpyrrolidone) or other film formers to the quaternary ammonium compounds. These not only condition the hair, they add extra volume or body. There are even conditioners that contain sunscreens to protect the hair color. Occasionally, too-frequent use of any of these conditioners can cause a buildup on the hair shaft so that the hair becomes too soft. This can be counteracted with an anionic shampoo to strip off the buildup so that the hair is fresh and more easily managed.

Protein-based conditioners consist of amino acids and small polypeptide fragments of hydrolyzed protein. These can be incorporated into the cortex of the hair shaft when the hair has just been processed with color or permanent waving or has been under a heat cap. This is advisable for hair that has been damaged through processing, wind, swimming, or sun. There have been reports of contact urticaria to the protein components of hair conditioners such as quaternary derivatives of hydrolyzed bovine collagen protein.

Styling aids consist of lotions, gels, mousses, or hair spray. Most of these products contain water, copolymers, polyvinylpyrrolidone, quaternary salts, and fragrance. They waterproof the hair so that perspiration or mild rain does not upset the style.

## Permanent Waves and Relaxers

The three natural wave patterns of hair are straight, wavy, and kinky. To allow the hair to be curled differently, straightened, or become slightly wavy, a chemical reaction involving the breaking of disulfide bonds of the hair with heat, high pH, or thioglycolates must take place. For straightening, it is broken with sodium hydroxide, guanidine hydroxide, lithium hydroxide, heat, or thioglycolates. The hair is placed over rods or curlers, treated with the appropriate chemical until the shape of the hair shaft is changed, then neutralized with hydrogen peroxide with sodium perborate or potassium bromate. Some of the disulfide bonds are never repaired, so this process can be very hard on the hair shaft.

The mildest form of hair curling is the acid permanent—glycerol monothioglycolate. This is appropriate for fine or for color-treated hair. There are more cases of allergic contact dermatitis due to this chemical than to the other curling or straightening agents. This permanent wave must be administered in a professional salon.

The midstrength permanent wave is ammonium thioglycolate. This can be used on healthy hair for curling or on kinky hair for straightening. This may be performed at home because of its safety.

The strongest chemicals for these procedures are for resistant kinky hair and include lye (with the higher pH) or sodium, lithium, or calcium hydroxide. Professionals must apply these products. If the chemicals are left on too long, the hair shaft may break. They can also burn the skin.

The most common hair loss in African Americans today is central centrifugal cicatricial alopecia (CCCA). Often this is caused by straightening procedures or the frequent use of extensions. It is important for the dermatologist to ask specific questions regarding these procedures. A good physician must recognize that these procedures must take place. He or she must just advise the patient about the strength of chemicals, frequency of use, or the exact form of extensions the patient is using. CCCA can be treated with topical potent steroids if caught early enough. If not, intralesional steroids may be given. Another cause of breakage of hair in these patients is straightening the hair too frequently. If the hair at the nape of the neck is broken at about 1 cm length, the patient may be straightening his or her hair every 6 weeks instead of 8 weeks as recommended.

*Hair Coloring*

The five major types of hair coloring are temporary, gradual, natural, semipermanent, and permanent.

The *temporary colors* are textile dyes. These dyes lie on the top of the cuticle and come off easily with perspiration or rain. Their advantage is they let the individual try a color and not cause any permanent change. These are safe and do not cause allergic reactions. The disadvantage is that the color can come off easily onto one's face or clothes.

The *gradual colors* consist of metallic salts. The hair can go from gray to brown or black by the action of lead acetate and sulfur. These salts precipitate on the outside of the hair shaft and allow a gradual change in color. Unfortunately, the hair looks very lusterless and can have a characteristic sulfur odor. The metal precipitate also precludes any other hair processing, such as permanent or other coloring procedures. The hair must grow out or have a stripping process before other cosmetic procedures may take place.

*Natural coloring* with henna from *Lawsonia inermis* is rarely used anymore. This is a vegetable dye that has no concern regarding carcinogenicity. It imparts red highlights to hair. This substance can precipitate asthma and allergies. Henna also stains gray hair an unpleasant orange color.

*Semipermanent dyes* are a nice first step for a person going from gray to a darker color. The active ingredients are low molecular weight dyes specifically synthesized for hair coloring. Because the molecules are small, they can penetrate the cuticle and go into the cortex. These dyes leave the hair shiny and attractive. Because these same molecules can slip

out of the cuticle just as easily, the color only lasts for four to six shampoos. These dyes have low allergenicity, are easy to apply, and cause only minimal hair shaft damage. Because there is no peroxide used, the colors can only go darker, not lighter.

By far the most common products for hair color in men and women today are the *permanent hair color dyes*. In permanent or oxidative hair coloring, the formation of colorless molecules from their precursors occurs inside the cortex as a result of oxidation by hydrogen peroxide. The reaction is $p$-phenylenediamine + $H_2O_2$ : amines: amines + couplers : indo dyes. The indo dye molecules are so large that they cannot slip out of the cortex of the hair shaft. This color lasts for 4 to 6 weeks, until the new growth of scalp hair at the base becomes visible. The correct procedure then is simply to color the 1 or l.5 cm of new growth.

*Frosting or highlighting* of the hair consists of taking strands of the hair and selectively bleaching them with the same procedure using 30 or 40 volumes percent for hydrogen peroxide (instead of 20 volumes percent, as in normal color).

For a real brunette to become a platinum blond, two processes must be used: first, a removal of all the color with peroxide, and second, a dying of the hair as outlined previously. This is the most traumatic procedure that can be performed on the hair. With all of these chemical processes, the hair can be broken off at any point on the shaft. Table 7-1 provides a summary of these color techniques.

## Skin Care Products

According to the North American Contact Dermatitis Group, skin care products cause the greatest number of adverse reactions in cosmetics. These can be irritant dermatitis, allergic dermatitis, acne cosmetica, or folliculitis. To understand these products more thoroughly, it is important to study the types of ingredients compounded for these products. These consist of emollients, humectants, surfactants, preservatives, and fragrance.

*Emollients*

Emollients are film-forming materials that add substance to cosmetic preparations and function on the skin to retard water loss. Six categories of emollients are hydrocarbons, waxes, natural lipid polyesters, lightweight esters and ethers, silicone, and ceramides.

The *hydrocarbons* that are most familiar are mineral oil and petrolatum. Because these products contain no water, there is no need to add preservatives to them. It has been shown by tagging $C^+$ atoms that petrolatum actually penetrates into the intercellular substance of the epithelium. These hydrocarbons are heavy and may not be as aesthetically pleasing as other moisturizers. In the temperate zones in the winter, however, they are ideal for hands, feet, and other very dry areas on the body. They probably are too occlusive for facial skin. Cosmetic grade petrolatum has been a more frequently used ingredient of facial cosmetics in the last few years. This grade is noncomedogenic.

**TABLE 7-1 ■ Coloring Products and Their Key Characteristics***

| Type of Coloring Product | Recognition | Skill Involved | Type of Dye | Color Change Range | Site of Action | Lasting Quality | Overall Performance | Degree of Abuse of Hair Structure | Potential for Dermatologic Complaints |
|---|---|---|---|---|---|---|---|---|---|
| Temporary color rinses | Multiple-use package | Minimal; apply and dry | High molecular weight acid dyes as used in textiles, and certified food colors in a hydro-alcoholic suspension | Covers gray | Surface of shaft | Poor; removed by shampooing | Poor | Negligible | Negligible |
| Semi-permanent | Single- or multiple-use package; more viscous than no. 1 to prevent dripping off hair | Moderate; apply to freshly shampooed hair and leave in place for 15–40 min; skin patch test required | Low molecular weight dyes: nitrophenylene-diamines, nitroamino-phenols, aminoanthro-quinones in shampoo vehicle or a solvent system | Covers gray; one to three shades on dark side of normal hair color | Penetrates to cortex | Gradually lost through three to five shampoos | Fair | Negligible | Negligible |
| Permanent oxidation type | | | | | | | | | |
| Single process | Two-unit system for mixing just before use | Moderate; skin patch test required | Several classes of dyes including PPD† intermediates in an alkaline peroxide "shampoo" | Covers gray; two or three shades on each side of normal | Cortex | Permanent; new growth touch-up every 4–8 weeks | Excellent | Moderate | Modest |
| Double process | Same as above | Professional attention necessary | As above, but hair must be previously decolorized (stripped) | Unlimited | Cortex | As above | Excellent | Significant | Moderate; hair breakage; local and systemic peroxide reactions |
| Progressive | Multiple-use package | None | Metallic salts particularly lead, in solution, cream, or pomade form | Discolors hair only | Surface and some beneath cuticle | As long as product is used regularly | Poor | Minimal | Negligible; a public health problem; incompatible with other chemical hair services |
| Vegetable | For all practical purposes, this does not exist and is not available. | | | | | | | | |
| Henna | Although true henna is a vegetable dye, its color properties and lasting abilities make it unacceptable. Products are being marketed currently with this name but are actually henna coloring in the second and third categories above. | | | | | | | | |

*The late Dr. Earl Brauer compiled this chart for previous editions of this book.

†p-Phenylenediamine.

*Waxes* consist of beeswax, synthetic beeswax, cholesterol, and lanolin. These substances usually cause no adverse reaction themselves, but esters of lanolin can occasionally be comedogenic (cause comedonal acne).

The *natural lipid polyesters* retard water loss by integrating with the proteins of the stratum corneum. Short-chain acids such as coconut oil, capric or caprylic triglycerides, esters of lanolin, and synthesized unsaturated fatty acid esters such as sorbitol oleate or lanolin linoleate can be comedogenic because of their interaction with the stratum corneum. Long-chain polyesters are less likely to be comedogenic because of their molecular size.

*Lightweight esters and ethers,* such as isopropyl myristate, also can be comedogenic. They are acceptable if they comprise less than 2% of the formulation. Some of these products act as preservatives at lower concentrations.

By far the most helpful emollient today is *silicone.* This inert product has been pulverized into tiny particles and then added to many products for "slip." It has replaced many of the acnegenic ingredients in facial cosmetics and has performed excellently. Silicone is lubricating, protective, and water repellant. It can be soothing in patients with hypersensitive skin, such as acne rosacea patients. There is no absorption of silicone topically, so concerns of safety with this product are absent. It has no adverse reaction regarding allergenicity or comedogenicity.

*Ceramides* have been a new addition to our moisturizing armamentarium. The stacking of corneocytes in the stratum corneum has been held together by a lipid moiety. We describe atopic patients or people with severe xerosis as not having enough mortar in a "bricks and mortar" epithelium. The extracellular matrix contains ceramides, free sterols (cholesterol), and free fatty acids. Ceramides make up the majority of the matrix (40% to 50%) and consist of a fatty acid and sphingoid base. Dr. Peter Elias has done major research to prove the worth of ceramides in dermatology. These ingredients have provided a nongreasy emollient for many of our patients.

## Humectants

Humectants are used to preserve moisture content of materials and attract and absorb water from their environment. Most of these products are cosmetically more pleasing to use. They are especially valuable in climates in which there is more humidity. Examples of humectants are glycerin, sodium pyroglutamic acid, sorbitol, urea, lactic acid, and propylene glycol.

Urea and lactic acid are very helpful ingredients for conditions of hyperkeratosis, such as ichthyosis, keratosis pilaris, Darier's disease, and severe dry skin. They can occasionally cause irritation or stinging but are not sensitizing.

Propylene glycol is one of the favorite solvents for topical steroids. It is present in at least two thirds of the topical steroid cream products and in many of the ointments. It can be an irritant and occasionally cause contact dermatitis.

## Surfactants

Surfactants are surface-active ingredients that make it easier to mix the oil phase and water phase in an emulsion and effect a smoother contact between two surfaces. These substances can cause the skin to be more penetrable by lowering the barrier properties of the skin and allowing themselves or other ingredients to penetrate the surface and cause irritation or sensitization.

The four major types of surfactants are anionic, nonionic, cationic, and amphoteric.

The *anionic surfactants* are the principal ingredients in shampoos and synthetic detergent liquid soap. Sodium lauryl sulfate is an excellent cleanser, and it is the major workhorse for liquid facial cleansers as well as shampoos. Other anionics are alpha olefin sulfonates, Na/K stearate, triethanolamine (TEA)-lauryl sulfate, and sulfosuccinates.

The *nonionic surfactants* are gentler than the anionics. They allow for the removal of minerals from hard water and increase the viscosity and solubility of shampoos. They behave as emulsifiers. These include sorbitan fatty acids, polysorbates, polyethylene glycol (PEG) lipids, and lauramine oxide.

The *cationic surfactants* function largely as conditioners for hair, thickeners for shampoo, and hair grooming aids. These include stearalkonium chloride, quaternary ammonium salts, quaternary fatty acids, and amino acids.

The *amphoteric surfactants* contain a balance of positive and negative charges. These are not as aggressive products as the anionic surfactants and are the chief ingredients in baby shampoo. Examples of these surfactants are *N*-alkyl-amino acids, betaines, and alkyl imidazoline compounds. These surfactants became more popular in the late 1990s. Cocamidopropyl betaine has been used in shampoos and shower gels more frequently. The use of cocamidopropyl betaine is widespread in the United States. Allergic contact dermatitis to these products has been reported many times in the past few years.

## Preservatives

Preservatives are second only to fragrance in causing contact dermatitis. They are absolutely necessary, however, to keep the products fresh and safe. The more water there is in a product, the more important is the content of preservatives.

Preservatives are classified into three categories: antimicrobials, ultraviolet light absorbers, and antioxidants. The allergenicity of preservatives is variable. The variables include

Inherent sensitizing potential
Concentration in the final product
The type-wash-off or leave on
The duration of the skin contact
The state of the epidermal surface when applied
The body region

Of all these variables, the first two are the most important. Preservatives are mixed and matched depending on whether there is a concern of gram-positive or gram-negative organisms, *Candida* sp, *Pityrosporum ovale,* or fungus.

The following is a review of four of the most commonly used groups of preservatives, their efficacies, and their disadvantages.

***Formaldehyde and Formaldehyde Releasers.*** Free formaldehyde is present, especially in shampoos, because of its efficacy against *Pseudomonas aeruginosa.* Because it is left on for such a short time, patients usually have no reaction to it. However, hairdressers who shampoo their clients all day are likely to experience a contact or an irritant dermatitis from it. Formaldehyde treatment of cornstarch in surgeons' gloves has been implicated as a potential source of sensitization. Formaldehyde-allergic people must avoid permanent press or wrinkle-resistant garments. They should wash all new clothing items before wearing and wear protective undergarments when able.

Of the formaldehyde releasers, *quaternium 15* is number one and *imidazolidinyl urea* is number two in causing contact dermatitis. Other formaldehyde releasers include *BNPD (Bronopol), diazolidinyl urea (Germall II),* and *DMDM hydantoin (Glydant).* All of these products are very effective against Pseudomonas.

***Parabens.*** Parabens are the least allergenic and most popular of all the preservatives. They are very effective against fungi and gram-positive bacteria. They are relatively water insoluble, so are not effective against *Pseudomonas* sp. Combining two parabens in the same formulation enhances efficacy. Cross-reaction between individual parabens is the rule. As with the formaldehyde releasers, parabens are more likely to react with dermatitic skin, but sensitization is not common with these preservatives.

***Antioxidants.*** Antioxidants are less frequently used. These include butylated hydroxyanisole (BHA), butylated hydroxytoluene (BHT), triclosan, and sorbic acid. BHA and BHT are important for the prevention of spoilage. These are present in lipstick and sunscreens. Their widest use is in foods. Triclosan is a disinfectant and preservative in deodorants, shampoo, and soap. Sorbic acid is used often in creams and lotions. It is fungistatic but has poor bacterial inhibition.

***Kathon CG (Methylchloroisothiazoline and Methylisothiazolinone).*** This organic preservative was considered the most complete and safest preservative until the 1990s. It is an odorless and colorless biocide that exhibits microbicidal activity against a wide spectrum of fungi and gram-positive and gram-negative bacteria.

More than 80 publications in the 1990s have reported allergic contact dermatitis to cleansing cream, hair tonics, hair balsam, wash softeners, cosmetics, and moist toilet paper. When these reports came in, a more serious study of Kathon CG took place. According to the North American Contact Dermatitis Group, the incidence of allergy is 1.9%. As long as the concentration is below 15 ppm in rinse-off products and less than 7.5 ppm in leave-on products, this substance is acceptable.

## Fragrance and Fragrance Products

Fragrance as an ingredient in skin care products is the highest allergen. In one study, it accounted for 149 of 536 reactions. Together, fragrance and preservatives accounted for half of all the reactions to cosmetics.

Fragrance products include perfume, cologne, toilet water, bathwater additives, bath powder, and aftershave lotions.

The most common reaction to fragrance is allergic contact dermatitis, followed by photodermatitis, contact urticaria, irritation, and depigmentation.

The common fragrance allergens are

Cinnamic alcohol
Cinnamic aldehyde
Hydroxycitronellal
Isoeugenol
Oak moss absolute

The most common photoallergen is musk ambrette. This substance is currently not used as often. Balsam of Peru as a patch test is a good screening agent for fragrance. In the past, oil of bergamot found in Shalimar perfume was the most common photoallergen. Now, those perfumes that contain oil of bergamot contain the bergapten-free variety, so there are fewer photodermatitis reactions.

## Makeup (Color) Products

Color cosmetics include foundation, eye makeup (shadow, liner, mascara), lipstick, rouge, blush, and nail enamel.

The use of color cosmetics is likened to an artist painting a picture on a canvas. *Foundation* is used to give a simple flawless complexion on which other color cosmetics can be applied.

Spot coverage can be achieved with several products before foundation is applied. For patients with defects after surgery, telangiectasias, or lentigines, an erase stick or a heavier concealer product is applied before foundation. For patients with rosacea, some products with a green-tinted lotion or cream, with or without sulfur, may be used. Acne patients can use tinted spot sticks containing sulfur, salicylic acid, or benzoyl peroxide. For patients with scar tissue, laser resurfacing or face peeling may be helpful. A green or lavender tint prefoundation may be used before the regular foundation is applied.

The types of foundation vary with coverage and cream or moisture content. The concealing or covering quality varies with the amount of titanium dioxide and not the density of the product. Foundation can be transparent, imparting only color, translucent, offering more cover, or opaque, offering total coverage. This increasing amount of coverage does not affect the comedogenicity of the product.

Foundation can be divided into oil-based foundation, water-based foundation, oil-free foundation, and water-free or anhydrous foundation.

Water-based foundations are oil-in-water emulsions. The pigment is emulsified in a small amount of oil. The primary emulsifier is a soap, for example, TEA or a nonionic surfactant. These are best for normal skin.

Oil-free foundations contain no animal, vegetable, or mineral oils. They contain dimethicone or cyclomethicone as an emollient. These are for people with oily skin and are noncomedogenic, nonacnegenic, and hypoallergenic.

Water-free or anhydrous foundations are all waterproof. They contain vegetable oil, mineral oil, lanolin alcohol, and synthetics to form the oil phase. Waxes may be added to make it a cream. High concentrations of pigments may be added to these preparations. Titanium dioxide, iron oxides, and ultramarine blue are added to them.

These products are the best camouflage cosmetics. They may be combined with high quantities of powder. Under these foundations, green or mauve tints can be added to improve red or yellow discoloration. This is important for acne rosacea, laser therapy, and post cosmetic surgery. With the clever use of highlighting with concealer, asymmetry, scleroderma, heavy cheeks, or an unclear jaw line can be concealed. It is not necessarily a physician's place to demonstrate this to the patient, but the physician should know where to send a patient who needs help to normalize his or her appearance. Even tattooing of burned or scarred skin can aid in normalizing a patient's appearance.

## Powders

These can set the foundation and make it last longer. According to Zoe Draelos, M.D., the covering ability of face powder ingredients in the order of increasing opacity is: titanium dioxide, kaolin, magnesium carbonate, magnesium stearate, zinc stearate, prepared chalk, zinc oxide, rice starch, precipitated chalk, and talc.

Dermatologists are interested in the amount of cream or moisturizer in foundation. For teenagers, a shake lotion–type foundation is less likely to contribute to acne. For 20- to 50-year-old women, heavier makeup that is labeled noncomedogenic or oil-free may be appropriate. For most women 50 years or older, any kind of moisturizing foundation is acceptable as long as they are not prone to adult acne.

The ingredients that are more likely to be comedogenic are

- Isopropyl myristate
- Isopropyl ester
- Oleic acid
- Stearic acid
- Petrolatum (not cosmetic grade)
- Lanolin (especially acetylated lanolin alcohols and lanolin fatty acids)

The products that have been substituted for the above ingredients, and that are less likely to be comedogenic, are low-dose mineral oil, octyl palmitate, isostearyl neopentanoate, cottonseed oil, corn oil, safflower oil, propylene glycol, spermaceti, beeswax, and sodium lauryl sulfate.

The final product, however, must be tested to decide if the compound is truly comedogenic or not. This is best tested on the face or back of patients who are acne prone.

*Blush* adds color and the look of good health to the patient's appearance. Cream blush can be comedogenic and hard to apply. Older patients who have dry skin may be the best patients to use it. Powder blush seems to be the best choice. It should be applied in the same areas that children flush when exercising. Usually, these products do not cause adverse reactions.

*Lipsticks* are made of waxes that are usually nonallergenic and noncomedogenic. When eosin dyes were used for long-lasting lipsticks, there were cases of photodermatitis. They are used less frequently now. Sunscreens or castor oil may be the only ingredients that cause allergic reactions.

For women who have vertical lines above and below the vermilion border, the use of a lead lipstick pencil or liner can be helpful. This stops the waxy lipstick from "bleeding" into the vertical furrows when the patient eats or drinks. Lip liner is also recommended for women with asymmetry of their lips owing to removal of a tumor, other lip surgery, or lips that are too thin. The desired outline of the lips can be drawn with the pencil or line and then the color can be filled in.

*Eye makeup*—shadow, liner, mascara—can be used to enlarge, brighten, or accentuate the eyes. Because of the need to prevent infection, most eye makeup contains preservatives. These preservatives are listed on the outside of the package and patients can check to see if they have had an adverse reaction to them. Generally, the preservatives are Ethlenediamine tera acetate (EDTA), British antilewisite (BAL), thimerosal, parabens, quaternium 15, or phenylmercuric acetate/nitrate. Usually, each cosmetic company formulates its products with its specific preservatives. Therefore, a patient who cannot use one company's eye product may be able to use another company's product. Most American eye cosmetics are formulated without fragrance and with the simplest hypoallergenic formula.

*Eye shadow* can function to conceal flaws or enlarge the eye. Usually, if the patient has an allergic reaction to cream eye shadow, a powder eye shadow is a good substitute.

*Eyeliner* may help to change the shape of the eye as well as accentuate it. These products usually are waxes and therefore have no adverse reaction. Pencil eyeliner is preferred to liquid eyeliner for a more natural appearance.

*Mascara* can be water based or waterproof. The water-based products are healthier for the eyelashes because they can be removed easily with soap and water. Products with lengtheners, however, may add lacquer and may require special solvents to remove the old mascara. Waterproof mascara may have a lower concentration of preservatives and may therefore be less allergenic for some patients. It is necessary to use an eye makeup remover to take mascara off. The use of the special remover may be more traumatic to the eyelashes. Because of this, patients with fragile lashes (e.g., patients with alopecia areata) should wear water-washable mascara.

*Eyelash curlers* can be used to give the illusion of longer lashes and conceal blepharochalasis. The patient who is allergic to nickel or rubber should not use this instrument. If the eyelash curler is to be used, it must be used before the mascara is applied.

*Nail enamels,* including base coats and top coats, have similar composition:

*Film former:* nitrocellulose
*Resin:* toluene sulfonamide/formaldehyde resin, alkyl resins, acrylates, vinyls, polyesters
*Plasticizers:* camphor, dibutyl phthalate, dioctyl phthalate, tricresyl phosphate
*Solvents:* alcohol, toluene, ethyl acetate, butyl acetate
*Colorants:* (optional)
*Pearlizers:* guanine, bismuth oxychloride (optional)

The major ingredient that causes allergic contact dermatitis is toluene sulfonamide. Butyl and ethyl methacrylate, which are in the glue used for sculptured nails, press-on nails, and nail mending, can also cause contact dermatitis. Cuticle remover (sodium or potassium hydroxide) is left on the cuticle to dissolve dead skin. If left on too long, this product becomes an irritant. The entire nail can be separated from the nail bed by too vigorous use of cuticle remover.

## Cosmeceuticals

This term is an unofficial way to describe cosmetic-type products that are promoted with aggressive claims to have a favorable impact on the condition of the skin. These products include retinoids, antioxidants (vitamins), $\alpha$-hydroxy acids, $\beta$-hydroxy acids, antiperspirants, sunscreens, and self-tanners.

### Retinoids

In 1984, L.H. Kligman demonstrated that connective tissue could be repaired in the rhino mouse with tretinoin. Subsequently, this was established in humans with a multicenter, double-blind study over a 48-week period. This ushered in a new method of skin care for photoaging, cancer, and cosmetic reasons. The gold standard for the reversal of photoaging is tretinoin, but because of its irritant potential, many other products have been studied.

#### Older Retinoids: First Generation

Since 1984, many preparations of tretinoin have been made. The first products with concentrations of 0.1% were irritating to the skins of many patients. Since that time, formulations of 0.025% and 0.01% have been incorporated into creams and gels. These products have been demonstrated in biopsies, photographs, and clinical observations to truly rejuvenate the skin. Cosmetic chemists have taken the formulations even further by incorporating tretinoin into microsponges and special polymers, and adding moisturizers. The tretinoin products are truly the best for rejuvenation. There is even a 4-week treatment with tretinoin in a solution of 50% ethanol and 50% propylene glycol 400 that was studied by D.E. Kligman and Z.D. Draelos for rapid retinization of photoaged facial skin. Almost all subjects improved on all measures of clinical grading (fine lines, mottled pigmentation, and surface texture/roughness) by 4 weeks. The newer tools for accessing skin changes—digital cameras, consistent lighting, and computers—have allowed for greater accuracy in observations.

#### Retinoids: Second Generation

Adapalene 0.1 cream and gel is less irritating than tretinoin. This product has been used for photoaging but is used more for acne therapy. Tazarotene cream 0.1% has been compared with tretinoin emollient cream 0.05% for efficacy. The results were similar, but the tazarotene cream demonstrated quicker efficacy at weeks 12 and 20. The main side effect of this retinoid is irritation.

### First-generation Cosmeceuticals

For patients who cannot tolerate retinoids, new products are discovered daily. The first sets of these products consist of vitamins, other naturally occurring antioxidants, plant antioxidants, $\alpha$-hydroxy and $\beta$-hydroxy acids.

#### Antioxidants

Antioxidants are products that quench or offset free radicals. These free radicals occur because of exposure to sunlight, pollution, and heavy metals; stress; drugs; and normal metabolism. Free radicals have a role in skin carcinogenesis, inflammation, and aging. The mechanism by which they disturb homeostasis is the combination of oxygen with other molecules, leaving an odd number of electrons. Oxygen with an unpaired electron is reactive because it takes electrons from vital components, leaving them damaged. DNA, cytoskeletal elements, and cellular membranes may all be adversely affected. Antioxidants couple with unpaired electrons to disarm or offset the free radicals.

Naturally occurring antioxidants include vitamins A, $B_3$ (niacinamide), $B_5$ (panthenol), C, and E. Other naturally occurring antioxidants include $\alpha$-lipoic acid, $\beta$-carotene, catalase, glutathione, superoxide dismutase, ubiquinone (coenzyme $Q_{10}$), and plant antioxidants such as green tea polyphenols, silymarin, soy isoflavones, and furfuryladenine. These ingredients have been incorporated into many products over the past 10 to 14 years. Their success at a cellular level has been assessed with biopsies, photographs, and sun testing. The model for testing most of the antioxidants is the use of these products before, during, and after sun exposure. The results were a lack of erythema, sunburn cell production, or other signs of ultraviolet damage. The scientists also tested the ability of the skin to keep its immunity. Sun can cause immunosuppression, which can stop cancer surveillance. These antioxidants can prevent the immunosuppression from occurring.

All of these antioxidants have been put into formulations to treat fine and coarse wrinkling, dyspigmentation, and erythema. The gold standard of improving skin quality is still tretinoin in whatever formulation it occurs. Some patients cannot tolerate the irritation from tretinoin. For those individuals the antioxidant cosmetics are appropriate.

It is important for the physician to understand some of the nuances of the current products.

*Niacinamide* in aging human skin cells in vitro increases synthesis of collagen, involucrin, filaggrin, and keratin. It increases the biosynthesis of ceramides and other stratum corneum lipids, therefore leading to an improved epidermal barrier and a decrease of transepidermal water loss.

*Dexapanthenol* is a stable alcohol form of pantothenic acid converted in the skin. It acts as a humectant. It is also used in healing ointments.

*Vitamin C* promotes collagen synthesis, has antioxidant properties, and has photoprotection from both UVA and UVB. It is anti-inflammatory, lightens hyperpigmentation, and reduces postlaser resurfacing erythema.

*Vitamin E* is the major antioxidant in scavenging lipid peroxyl radicals. It plays a major role in photoprotection and acts as a humectant. The combination of vitamins C and E is synergized to have a more efficient role in photoprotection and rejuvenation.

*Idebenone* is a synthetic form of ubiquinone and has been demonstrated to be very effective as an antioxidant.

*The plant antioxidants* have been demonstrated to act as photoprotectors and network antioxidants and to help with dyspigmentation. The major ones are green tea polyphenol, silymarin, soy isoflavones, and furfuryladenine (Kinerase).

*Rosemary* is a substance that is better known as a spice but is a potent antioxidant due to its phenolic deterpines. It has been shown to suppress tumorigenesis in the two-stage cancer model in mice. It also exhibits photoprotection in mice.

*Oatmeal* is a substance that has always been soothing and anti-inflammatory. It can repair skin and hair damage from ultraviolet radiation, smoke, bacteria, and free radicals.

*Olive oil* contains polyphenolic compounds that protect against inflammation. It is found in soaps, lip balms, shampoos, and moisturizers. Extra-virgin olive has protected mice after ultraviolet exposure.

Grape seed extract is an antioxidant because of its oligomeric proanthocyanides. These compounds are in the flavonoid family, which is most famous for green and black tea. This extract helps vascular endothelial growth factor expressed in keratinocytes, which fosters wound healing. It also scavenges free radicals for vitamins C and E.

*Tea tree oil* is a compound that has been widely used in hair and skin products because of its activity against *Propionibacterium acnes* and trichophytic dermatophytosis. It is very popular in beauty salon products. It has the highest rate of contact dermatitis of the cosmeceuticals. Many reports have come from Great Britain. Its efficacy in antidandruff shampoos needs to be proved.

*Coffeeberry extract* has been included with green tea since they both contain polyphenols. Green tea is anti-inflammatory and a photoprotector. Coffeeberry is supposed to have more antioxidants than the tea.

### α-Hydroxy Acids

Dermatologists have used lactic acid for many years. The research by Van Scott has ushered the rest of the α-hydroxy acids into widespread use. These natural fruit acids exert their influence by diminishing corneocyte cohesion. The most commonly used ingredients are

- *Glycolic acid*: sugarcane
- *Lactic acid*: sour milk
- *Malic acid*: apples
- *Citric acid*: citrus fruits
- *Tartaric acid*: grapes

Leyden (1994) outlines the functions of these α-hydroxy acids clearly.

1. They bind water in the skin; therefore, the stratum corneum becomes more flexible.
2. They normalize desquamation of corneocytes from the stratum corneum. This may occur by interaction with stratum corneum lipids.
3. They release cytokines locally.
4. They cause a thickening of the epidermis.
5. They increase production of hyaluronic acid within the dermis. This may be due to the increased production of transforming growth factor-β.
6. In both ichthyosis and the thickened stratum corneum of dry skin, the α-hydroxy acids make the skin thin down toward normal.

The α-hydroxy acids have been incorporated into cosmetic formulations for shampoos, soaps, face creams, and body creams. The difficulty in formulating these products is the need to be buffered. A 5% concentration in one product may not be as effective as a 5% concentration in another. Glycolic acid peels have also been unpredictable because of this lack of standardization. These products are being improved daily.

### β-Hydroxy Acids

In the search for a less irritating and stinging compound for creams and peels, β-hydroxy acids have become very popular. There is only one ingredient in this category, salicylic acid. Dermatologists have known about this keratolytic agent for years chiefly as an exfoliant for acne at concentrations of 2% to 3% and a therapy for warts at concentrations of 10% to 15% in creams and 40% in pastes. Salicylic acid appears to have an anti-inflammatory component and may have less sting and irritancy than glycolic acid.

β-Hydroxy acid face peels have also become popular for patients who cannot tolerate glycolic or trichloroacetic acid peels.

### Second-generation Cosmeceuticals

These products have been developed from wound healing and skin repair studies. They are usually dermally active compounds. These increase fibroblast activity, increase protein and collagen syntheses, produce antioxidant enzymes, and are less irritating than retinoids. There are three categories of these cosmeceuticals—copper peptides, human growth factors, and pentapeptides.

### Copper Peptides

These products have been shown to enhance wound healing especially in Mohs and laser procedures and in the therapy of diabetic ulcers. They promote vascular formation, promote collagen and elastin, and are a catalyst for antioxidants.

In a poster exhibit at the AAD (February 2002), Leyden et al. presented a case study involving 67 patients. Most patients improved in fine lines and wrinkles, surface roughness, and increased skin density. At this point, copper peptide products are only available in private doctors' offices.

### Human Growth Factors

These products are safe; there is no inflammatory reaction. They cause increased protein production. They are usually obtained from placental extracts or are growth factors bioengineered from human foreskin. The before and after photographs of patients using these products are very impressive. The downsides of human growth factors are that they are very expensive, and they have a very unpleasant odor.

### Pentapeptides

It was discovered in vitro in 1993 that a subfragment of type I collagen could stimulate type I, type III, and fibronectin. Ex vivo studies in full thickness human skin biopsies demonstrated stimulation of collagen I. Pentapeptides consisted of five amino acids that when combined with palmitic acid could penetrate the skin (palmitoyl pentapeptide-3 Pal-KTTKS). When this product was compared with retinol, it decreased wrinkles in depth and volume. In vitro studies demonstrate stimulation of collagen IV and glucosaminoglycans including hyaluronic acid. The advantages of pentapeptides are that they stimulate matrix formation and are not irritating. These products are available over the counter and appear to be successful for both wound healing and rejuvenation.

## Antiperspirants

Antiperspirants are considered drugs (cosmeceutical) because of their physical interaction in the sweat duct. These products, which contain aluminum salts, act by causing a precipitation in the duct itself to block the secretion of sweat. They must have a specific amount of aluminum salts and in laboratory tests must reduce sweat by at least 20% in half the people tested.

Deodorants contain bacteria-killing agents such as triclosan, bacteria-retarding ingredients, and fragrance. They are a cosmetic because they do not change the function of the skin but just mask body odor.

For efficacy, roll-on products are best, then the sticks, and then the spray products.

## Sunscreens

Sunscreens are the most important of the cosmetics that men and women can use. Because these prevent skin cancer, they are considered a drug or cosmeceutical. These products are usually calibrated according to the sun protective factor (SPF). The SPF value for UVB is the ratio of the UVB dose required to produce the minimal erythema reaction through the applied sunscreen product (2 mg/cm$^2$) compared with the UVB dose required to produce the same degree of minimal erythema reaction without sunscreen.

Sunscreens consist of physical sunblocks, chemical UVB sunblocks, and chemical UVA sunblocks.

*Zinc oxide* has been used by lifeguards and children for many years on noses, ear tips, upper cheeks, and shoulders. The advantage of this substance is that it is inert and therefore not allergenic. The disadvantage is that it is messy. With the newer ability to pulverize this chemical, very elegant and superior products have been synthesized. The spectrum of microfine zinc oxide extends from 290 to 400 nm. This is the most complete sunscreen available.

*Titanium dioxide* has also been added to products for hypoallergenic coverage as well as a complete block. Without using the microfine type, patients may look like they have a purple cast to their skin. With the advent of microfine titanium dioxide, the coverage extends from 290 to 350 nm.

Both of these physical sunblocks have good coverage and no allergic or photoallergic reactions; they are waterproof, chemical free, superior coverage for UVA and good coverage for UVB. The disadvantages are that they can give a masklike or opaque appearance and may give the skin a violet color.

### Chemical Absorbers UVB

*p-Aminobenzoic acid (PABA) and PABA esters* (Padimate O, Padimate A, glycerol PABA) were the major sunblocks in the United States until the mid-1980s. Their advantages are that they protect against the 290 to 320 nm wavelength, they are easy to work with cosmetically, the esters are non-staining, and they bind to the horny layer. If a patient applied these 3 days in a row, he or she might still have protection on the fourth day. The disadvantages are the lack of protection for UVA, cross-sensitivity with benzoin and *p*-phenylenediamine, and that PABA itself may stain. Today, only Padimate O is readily available. This is used primarily in hair products.

*Cinnamates (octyl methoxycinnamate and cinoxate)* have largely replaced PABA in many products. These are incorporated in face makeup in which an SPF of 6 to 12 may be desired. These are easy to work with and rarely sensitizing. These are the most common ingredients in cosmetic products for sun protection.

*Salicylates (homomenthyl, octyl, triethanolamine)* only have an SPF of 3.5 but are excellent additions to formulations to increase SPF protection. Rarely, they may cause photodermatitis.

*Octocrylene and phenylbenzimidazole sulfonic acid* are two other excellent UVB chemical sunscreens. They can even stabilize avobenzone (Parsol 1789), so are helpful in combination sunscreens.

### Chemical Absorbers: UVA

**Benzophenones.** Benzophenones were the chief UVA blockers until recently. Oxybenzone and dioxybenzone have a broad absorption spectrum of 300 to 350 nm. These ingredients are incorporated into compounds easily and are less allergenic than the PABA derivatives. There are many reports of photocontact dermatitis from oxybenzone and occasional reports of contact dermatitis and contact urticaria from dioxybenzone. The most common occurrence of the photocontact dermatitis from these products occurs with intense and very warm sun exposure such as is found near the equator. Many patients can use these products in temperate zones but react while on vacation. Physical sunblocks should then be substituted.

**Parsol 1789 (Avobenzone).** Parsol 1789 has been available since about 1989 in the United States. It has a spectrum of 310 to 400 nm, with a peak at 358 nm. Because of this spectrum, it is the sunblock of choice for all patients with special UVA needs. Of course, it must be combined with a UVB block for total protection. Cinnamates did not combine well with this ingredient. Now, octocrylene is the ingredient that stabilizes Parsol and allows the attainment of a complete chemical sunblock, but by itself it doesn't last as long. Newer UVA protectors have now come to the forefront. L'Oreal developed Mexoryl containing ecamsule. Neutrogena developed Helioplex, and L'Oreal developed Ecamsule. All of these products protect the avobenzone, allowing the sunblock to last 3 to 4 hours. They have been tested in patients with polymorphous light eruption and lupus erythematosus. The physical sunblocks, microfine zinc oxide and titanium dioxide, are used very commonly in patients with UVA sensitivity. They also may be added in combination with these new special sunblocks.

Vitamins C and E can synergize with the chemical sunblocks. They may be in many sunblocks in the future.

### Tanning Product Categories

Self-tanning lotions consist primarily of dihydroxyacetone (DHA). These have a protein-staining effect from the DHA in the stratum corneum of the skin. These products used to be orange and streaky but have been perfected to an even-colored tone by the addition of silicone to the vehicle. They have been formulated into sprays available at salons to cover the entire body. Although these are nontoxic, they may accentuate freckles and seborrheic keratosis and therefore be unattractive. When using these products, patients should sand themselves with a loofah or cleansing granules before the application to make the color even.

Bronzing gels consist of henna, walnut, juglone, and lawsone. These are water-soluble dyes to stain the skin. They can be messy on clothes and have the stickiness of a gel but usually look good on the face. They are also noncomedogenic.

Tanning promoters, such as 5-methoxypsoralen, have been well documented to be highly phototoxic and carcinogenic. 5-Methoxypsoralen is not available over the counter in the United States.

Tanning pills consist of canthaxanthin and are toxic to both the skin and eyes. These are not available over the counter in the United States.

## How to Test for Cosmetic Allergy

The standard test and the T.R.U.E. test (the cosmetics section includes imidazolidinyl urea, wool (lanolin) alcohols, *p*-phenylenediamine, thimerosal, formaldehyde, colophony, quaternium l5, balsam of Peru, and cinnamic aldehyde).

The cosmetics that can be tested without dilution are antiperspirants, blushes, eyeliners, eye shadow, foundations, lipstick, moisturizers, perfumes, and sunscreens.

The cosmetics that are volatile and need to be allowed to dry on the patch or chamber before 48-hour occlusion are liquid eyeliner, mascara, and nail enamel.

The cosmetics that need to be diluted for testing are soaps, shampoos, shaving preparations, hair dyes, and permanent solution. These may need open patch testing or usage testing.

## Suggested Readings

Adams RM, Maibach HI. A five-year study of cosmetic reactions. *J Am Acad Dermatol*.1985;13:1062–1069.

Darr D, Combs S, Dunston S, et al. Topical vitamin C protects porcine skin from ultraviolet radiation-induced damage. *Br J Dermatol*. 1992;127: 247–253.

DeLeo V, Clark S, Fowler J, et al. A new ecamsule-containing SPF 40 sunscreen cream for the prevention of polymorphous light eruption (PMLE): a double-blind randomized, controlled study in maximized, outdoor conditions. *Cutis*. 2009;83:95–103.

Draelos ZD. Alpha-hydroxy acids and other topical agents. *Dermatol Ther*. 2000;13:154–158.

Draelos ZD. Cosmetics and cosmeceuticals. In: Bolognia JL, Jorizzo JL, Rapini RP, eds. *Dermatology*. 2nd ed. St. Louis: Mosby; 2008:2304.

Elmets CA, Singh D, Tubesing K, et al. Cutaneous photoprotection from ultraviolet injury by green tea polyphenols. *J Am Acad Dermatol*. 2003; 44:425–432.

Emerit I, Packer L, Auclair C. *Antioxidants in Therapy and Preventative Medicine*. New York: Plenum Press;1990:594.

Guin JD. Reaction to cocamidopropyl hydroxysultaine, an amphoteric surfactant and conditioner. *Contact Dermatitis*. 2000;42:284.

Jackson EM. Tanning without sun: accelerators, promoters, pills, bronzing gels, and self-tanning lotions. *Am J Contact Dermat*. 1994;5:38.

Kligman AM, Dogadkina D, Lavker RM. Effects of topical tretinoin on non-sun-exposed protected skin of the elderly. *J Am Acad Dermatol*. 1993; 29:25–33.

Kligman DE, Draelos ZD. High-strength tretinoin for rapid retinization of photoaged facial skin. *Dermatol Surg*. 2004;30:864–866.

Larsen WG. Perfume dermatitis. *J Am Acad Dermatol*. 1985;12:1–9.

Leyden J. Alpha-hydroxy acids. *Dialog Dermatol*. 1994;34:3.

Maibach HI, Engasser PG. Dermatitis due to cosmetics. In: Fischer AA, ed. *Contact Dermatitis*. 3rd ed. Philadelphia: Lea & Febiger; 1986; 2986:368–393.

O'Donoghue MN. Hair care products. In: Olsen EA. *Disorders of Hair Growth, Diagnosis and Treatment*. 3rd ed. New York/Chicago: McGraw-Hill; 2003: 481–496.

O'Donoghue MN, guest editor, Cosmeceuticals: bleaching agents and the controversy of hydroquinone. *Dermatol Ther*. 2007;20:307–376.

Olsen EA, Katz HI, Levin N, et al. Tretinoin emollient cream for photodamaged skin: results of 48-week, multicenter, double-blind studies. *J Am Acad Dermatol*. 1997;37:217–226.

Pathak MA. Sunscreens and their use in the preventative treatment of sunlight-induced skin damage. *J Dermatol Surg Oncol*. 1987;13:739–750.

Pinnell SR. Cutaneous photodamage, oxidative stress, and topical antioxidant protection. *J Am Acad Dermatol*. 2003;48:1–19.

# CHAPTER 8

# Dermatologic Allergy

*John C. Hall, MD*

This chapter will discuss contact dermatitis, industrial dermatoses, atopic eczema, and drug eruptions because of their obvious allergenic factors. However, it is important to keep in mind that some cases of contact dermatitis and industrial dermatitis are caused by irritants. Nummular eczema will also be discussed in this chapter because it resembles some forms of atopic eczema and may even be a variant of atopic eczema.

## Contact Dermatitis

Contact dermatitis (Figs. 8-1 to 8-4), or dermatitis venenata, is a very common inflammation of the skin caused by the exposure of skin to either primary irritant substances, such as soaps, or allergenic substances, such as poison ivy resin. Industrial dermatoses are also included at the end of this section.

### Presentation

#### Primary Lesions

Any of the stages, from mild redness, edema, or vesicles to large bullae with a marked amount of oozing, can be seen in primary lesions. This is usually limited to sites where the contactant touches the skin. However, when the reaction is severe, it can flare beyond these sites of contact. With poison ivy, oak, and sumac, a black stain on skin or clothing can sometimes be seen.

#### Secondary Lesions

Crusting from a secondary bacterial infection, excoriation, or lichenification occurs in secondary lesions. When the local site is severely affected, a generalized eruption can occur in a symmetrical and widespread distribution. This is called an id or autoeczematous eruption. It commonly causes vesicles on the palms, soles, and sides of the fingers and toes. It can be generalized and is symmetric. It is also very pruritic.

#### Distribution and Causes

Any agent can affect any area of the body. However, certain agents commonly affect certain skin areas.

- *Face and neck* (Fig. 8-5): cosmetics, soaps, insect sprays, ragweed, perfumes or hair sprays (sides of neck), fingernail polish (eyelids), hat bands (forehead), mouthwashes, toothpaste, lipstick (perioral), nickel metal (under earrings), necklaces and collars (neck), industrial oil (facial chloracne).
- *Hands and forearms:* soaps, hand lotions, wristbands, industrial chemicals, poison ivy, and a multitude of other agents. Irritation from soap often begins under rings as do allergic reactions from nickel (common) (dimethylglyoxime testing can be used to see if nickel is present in a metal object such as jewelry) or gold (rare). Latex from gloves can cause a contact dermatitis and contact urticaria. It can be associated with life-threatening anaphylaxis and is becoming an increasing danger because of the increased use of latex gloves and latex contraceptives.
- *Axillae:* deodorants, dress shields, detergents, bleaching agents, fabric softeners, antistatic agents, and dry cleaning solutions.
- *Trunk:* clothing that is new and not previously cleaned (because it contains a formaldehyde resin), clothing with rubber or metal attached to it (commonly seen on the central abdomen from the metal clasp found in jeans), and transdermal drug patches from the adhesive or the drug.
- *Anogenital region:* douches, dusting powder, diapers in infants or adults, contraceptives, colored toilet paper, topical hemorrhoid preparations, poison ivy, or topicals for treatment of pruritus ani, candida, and fungal infections.
- *Feet:* shoes, foot powders, topical agents for athlete's foot infections.
- *Generalized eruption:* volatile airborne chemicals (paint, spray, ragweed), medicaments locally applied to large areas, bath powders, or clothing (especially if not previously washed).

### Course

Duration can be very short (sometimes only days) or quite long (weeks, months, or even years). As a general rule, successive recurrences become more chronic and more severe (e.g., seasonal ragweed dermatitis can evolve into a year-round dermatitis). Once established in patients, hypersensitivity reactions are seldom lost. However, years of exposure without a reaction may occur before sensitization takes

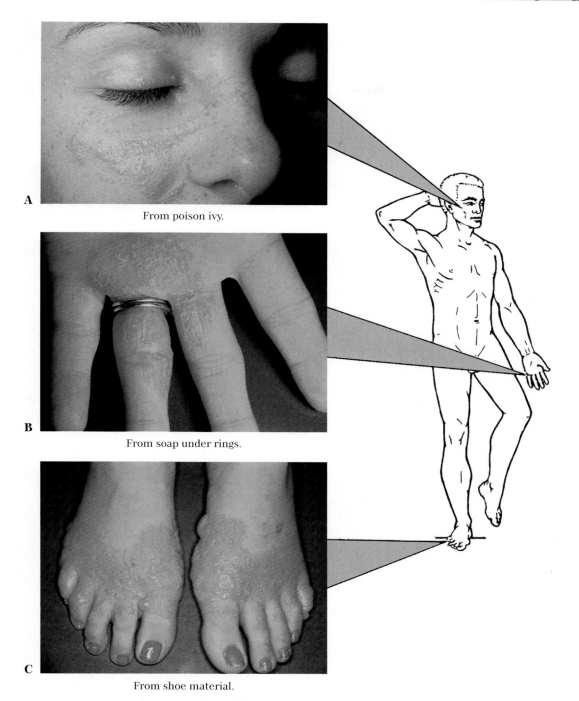

A

From poison ivy.

B

From soap under rings.

C

From shoe material.

**FIGURE 8-1** ■ Contact dermatitis. **(A)** From poison ivy. **(B)** From soap under rings. **(C)** From shoe material. *(Courtesy of Burroughs Wellcome Co.)*

place. Also, certain people are more susceptible to allergic and irritant contact dermatoses than others. This is particularly true in patients who already have inflamed skin. An example of this is how irritants commonly cause contact dermatitis in patients with eczema. A very careful seasonal history regarding the onset, especially in chronic cases, may lead to the discovery of an unsuspected causative agent such as ragweed.

An eczematous reaction (e.g., the blister fluid of poison ivy) contains no allergen that can cause the dermatitis in another person or in other areas on the same person. However, if the poison ivy oil or other allergen remains on the clothes of the affected person, contact with those clothes of a susceptible person could cause a contact dermatitis. Smaller amounts of oil can cause a dermatitis even weeks after exposure and may make the patient think the allergen is systemic

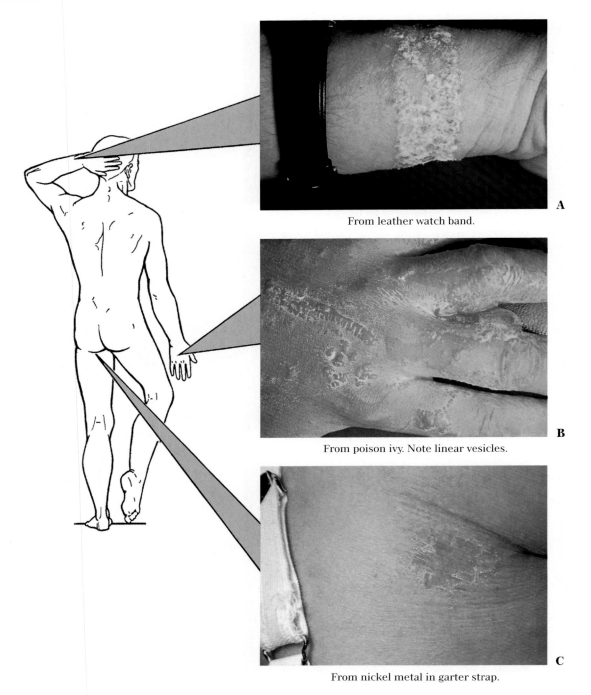

From leather watch band.

**A**

From poison ivy. Note linear vesicles.

**B**

From nickel metal in garter strap.

**C**

**FIGURE 8-2** ■ Contact dermatitis. **(A)** From a leather watchband. **(B)** From poison ivy. Note linear vesicles. **(C)** From nickel metal in a garter strap. *(Courtesy of Burroughs Wellcome Co.)*

or bloodborne. The hair or fur of animals, as well as utensils used in hunting or gardening, can also transfer the allergenic oleoresin of poison ivy.

*Laboratory Findings*

Patch tests (see Chapter 2) are valuable in eliciting the cause of a contact dermatitis. However, careful interpretation is required by the clinician.

Differential Diagnosis

A contact reaction must be considered and ruled in or out in any case of eczematous or oozing dermatitis on any body area.

Treatment

Two of the most common contact dermatoses seen in the physician's office are poison ivy (or poison oak or sumac)

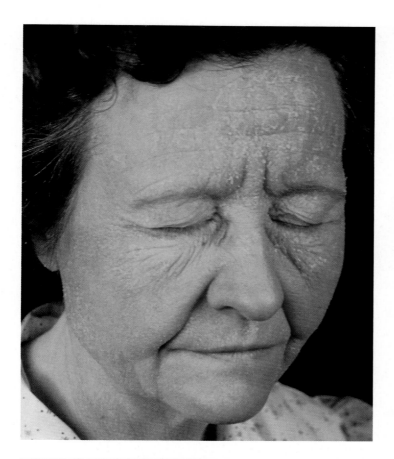

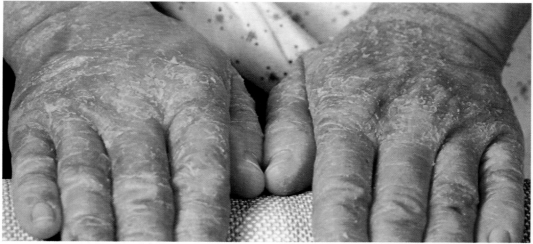

**FIGURE 8-3** ■ Contact dermatitis in a nurse due to chlorpromazine. The hands and face were involved most severely. This eruption was aggravated following exposure to sunlight. *(Courtesy of K.U.M.C.; Burroughs Wellcome Co.)*

and hand dermatitis. The treatments for these two conditions will be discussed separately.

### Treatment of Contact Dermatitis Owing to Poison Ivy

*Case Example:* A patient comes to the office with a linear, vesicular dermatitis of the feet, hands, and face. He states that he spent the weekend fishing and that the rash broke

out the following day. The itching is rather severe but not enough to keep him awake at night. He had "poison ivy" 5 years ago.

***First Visit.***

1. There are several mistaken notions about poison ivy dermatitis. Assure the patient that he cannot pass on the

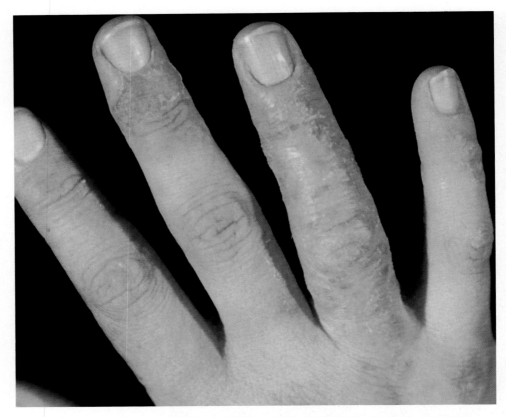

FIGURE 8-4 ■ Contact dermatitis of the hand. This common dermatitis is usually due to continued exposure to soap and water. *(Courtesy of K.U.M.C.; Burroughs Wellcome Co.)*

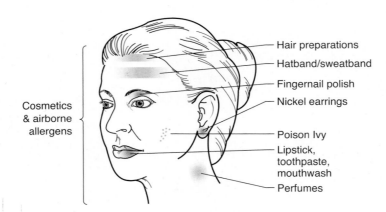

FIGURE 8-5 ■ Contact dermatitis of the face.

dermatitis to his family or spread it on himself from the blister fluid. The flexor fingers or palms have a very thick keratin layer that the allergen cannot penetrate. However, the allergen can be spread over the rest of the body, from the fingers to other areas of the body.

2. Suggest that the clothes worn while fishing need to be washed in warm soapy water to remove the allergenic resin.

3. Prescribe Burow's solution wet packs.

    *Sig:* Add one packet of powder (Domeboro) to 1 quart of cool water. Apply sheeting or toweling, wet with the solution, and apply to the blistered areas for 20 minutes twice a day. The wet packs need not be removed during the 20-minute period. (For a more widespread case of poison ivy dermatitis, take cool baths with a half box of Aveeno [colloidal oatmeal] or soluble starch in a tub. This will give considerable relief from the itching.)

4. 1% Hydrocortisone lotion q.s. 60.0 (1% Hytone [available OTC] lotion, 1% hydrocortisone (HC) Pramosone lotion (contains the antipruritic antihistamine pramoxine) among others. Cheaper OTC pramoxine-containing topicals can also be used.

*Sig:* Apply t.i.d. and PRN for itching on affected areas.

5. Chlorpheniramine maleate tablets, 4 mg 60 (many other antihistamines are available as sedating or nonsedating [probably not as effective] varieties; some are OTC).

*Sig:* Take 1 tablet t.i.d. (for relief of itching).

*Comment:* Warn patient about the side effect of drowsiness. This drug is available OTC and is less expensive than if written as a prescription.

6. Use cortisone-type injection IM. Short but rapid-acting corticosteroids are moderately beneficial, such as betamethasone (Celestone Soluspan) (8 mg/mL in a dose of 1 to 2 mL subcutaneously), or dexamethasone (Decadron-LA) (8 mg/mL in a dose of 1 to 1.5 mL IM). Triamcinolone (Kenalog) 20 to 40 mg IM can also be given. Caution the patient about a possible change in insulin requirements in diabetics as well as possible mood alterations with insomnia and jitteriness.

### Subsequent Visits.

1. Continue the wet packs only as long as there are blisters and oozing. Extended use is too drying for the skin.
2. After 3 or 4 days of use, the lotion may be too drying. Substitute fluorinated corticosteroid emollient cream q.s. 60.0.

*Sig:* Apply a small amount locally t.i.d., or more often if itching is present.

### Severe Cases of Poison Ivy Dermatitis.

An oral corticosteroid is indicated in severe cases of poison ivy dermatitis: prednisone, 10 mg #30.

*Sig:* Take 5 tablets each morning for 2 days, 4 tablets each morning for 2 days, 3 tablets each morning for 2 days, 2 tablets each morning for 2 days, and 1 tablet each morning for 2 days. Take with food in the morning. Repeat if not improving sufficiently.

The use of a poison ivy vaccine orally or IM is contraindicated during an acute episode. Desensitization may occur after a long course of oral ingestion of graduated doses of the allergen, but pruritus ani, generalized pruritus, and urticaria probably make the treatment worse than the disease. Desensitization does not occur after a short course of IM injections of the vaccine, and this form of prophylactic therapy is worthless. Barrier creams may decrease dermatitis if applied before exposure; examples include Hydropel and Ivy Block.

A window of up to 2 hours may exist where washing the skin with a surfactant (e.g., Dial soap) and oil-removing compound (e.g., soap or Goop) or a chemical inactivator (e.g., Tecnu) may ameliorate or prevent the contact dermatitis.

### Treatment of Contact Dermatitis of the Hand Owing to Soap

*Case Example:* A young housewife states that she has had a breakout on her hands for 5 weeks. The dermatitis developed about 4 weeks after the birth of her last child. She states that she had a similar eruption after her previous two pregnancies. She has used a lot of local medication of her own, and the rash is getting worse instead of better. The patient and her immediate family never had any asthma, hay fever, or eczema.

Examination of the patient's hands reveals small vesicles on the sides of all of her fingers, with a 5-cm area of oozing and crusting around her left ring finger.

### First Visit.

1. Assure the patient that the hand eczema is not contagious to her family.
2. Inform the patient that soap irritates the dermatitis and that it must be avoided as much as possible. A homemaker will find this avoidance very difficult. One of the best remedies is to wear protective gloves when extended soap-and-water contact is unavoidable. Rubber gloves

alone produce a considerable amount of irritating perspiration, but this is absorbed when thin white cotton gloves are worn under the rubber gloves. Lined rubber gloves are not as satisfactory because the lining eventually becomes dirty and soggy and cannot be cleaned easily. Bluettes is an excellent protective glove with a cotton lining.

3. For body and hand cleanliness, a mild soap, such as Dove, can be used, or any of the following: Cetaphil soapless cleanser, Basis soap, and Neutrogena soaps.

4. Tell the patient that these prophylactic measures must be adhered to for several weeks after the eruption has apparently cleared, or there will be a recurrence. Injured skin is sensitive and needs to be pampered for an extended time.

5. Burow's solution soaks.

   *Sig:* Add 1 packet of powder (Domeboro) to 1 quart of cool water. Soak hands for 15 minutes twice a day.

6. Fluorinated corticosteroid ointment (see Formulary in Chapter 4) 15.0 gms

   *Sig:* Apply sparingly, locally, q.i.d. especially after shower and hand washing

### Resistant, Chronic Cases.

1. To the corticosteroid ointment add, as indicated, sulfur (3% to 5%), coal tar solution (3% to 10%), or an antipruritic agent such as menthol (0.25%) or camphor (2%).

2. Oral corticosteroid therapy. A short course of such therapy rapidly improves or cures a chronic dermatitis. Attempt to avoid repeating more than is absolutely necessary.

3. Prevention of flares of contact dermatitis can be accomplished by frequent use of emollient preparations. Curel, Cetaphil hand cream, Eucerin Plus lotion, CeraVe, and Neutrogena Norwegian hand cream are examples. Bag Balm or Udder Cream are odiferous and less cosmetically acceptable choices.

## Occupational Dermatoses

Sixty-five percent of all the industrial diseases are dermatoses. The most common cause of these skin problems is contact irritants, of which cutting oils are the worst offenders. Lack of adequate cleansing is a big contributing factor to cutting oil dermatitis. On the other hand, harsh or abrasive cleansers can aggravate the dermatitis.

It is not possible to list the thousands of different chemicals used in the hundreds of varied industrial operations that have the potential of causing a primary irritant reaction or an allergic reaction on the skin surface. Excellent books on the subject of occupational dermatitis are listed in the bibliography section at the end of this chapter.

### Management of Industrial Dermatitis

*Case Example:* A cutting-tool laborer presents with a pruritic, red, vesicular dermatitis of 2 months' duration on his hands, forearms, and face.

1. Obtain a careful, detailed history of his type of work and any recent change, such as use of new chemicals or new cleansing agents or exposure at home with hobbies, painting, and so on. Question him concerning remission of the dermatitis on weekends or while on vacation.

2. Question the patient concerning the first aid care given at the plant. Too often, this care aggravates the dermatitis. Bland protective remedies should be substituted for potential sensitizers such as sulfonamide and neomycin salves, antihistamine creams, benzocaine ointments, nitrofuran preparations, and strong or sensitizing antipruritic lotions and salves.

3. Treatment of the dermatitis with wet compresses, bland lotions, or salves is the same as for any contact dermatitis (see previous discussion). Unfortunately, many of the occupational dermatoses respond slowly to therapy. This is due in part to the fact that most patients continue to work and are exposed, repeatedly, to small amounts of the irritating chemicals, even though precautions are taken. Also, certain industrial chemicals, such as chromates, beryllium salts, and cutting oils, injure the skin in such a way as to prevent healing for months and years and result in a chronic eczema or chronic psoriasis (Koebner phenomena) in prone individuals.

4. Transferring a patient to a new job in the same work setting where exposure is less intensive may be helpful. Protective clothing such as gloves (being sure not to make the patient too awkward around dangerous machines) or protective creams (Tetrix, EpiCeram skin barrier emulsion) or sprays (Pro Q topical, OTC aerosol foam) can be beneficial. Barrier creams include Hollister Moisture Barrier, Mentor Shield Skin, Hydrogel, Uniderm, and Dermofilm.

5. The legal complications with compensation boards, insurance companies, the industry, and the injured patient can be discouraging, frustrating, and time consuming. However, most patients are not malingerers, and they do expect and deserve proper care and compensation for their injuries.

A comprehensive paper by Gordon C. Sauer on the percentages of skin impairment is entitled "A Guide to the Evaluation of Permanent Impairment of the Skin" (*Arch Dermatol.* 1968;97:566). A similar guide published by the American Medical Association in 1990 is listed in the bibliography section at the conclusion of this chapter.

## Atopic Eczema

Atopic eczema (**Figs. 8-6 to 8-10; Table 8-1**), or atopic dermatitis, is a rather common, markedly pruritic, chronic skin condition that occurs in two clinical forms: infantile and adult.

### Clinical Lesions

- *Infantile form:* blisters, oozing, and crusting, with excoriation.

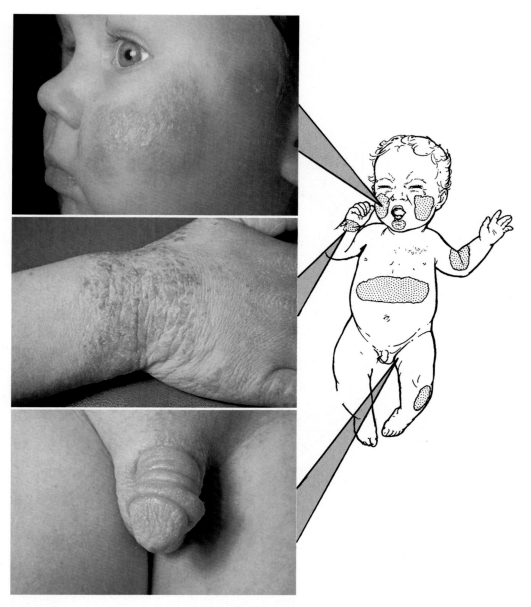

**FIGURE 8-6** ■ Atopic eczema (infant). *(Courtesy of Dome Chemicals.)*

- *Adolescent and adult forms:* marked dryness, thickening (lichenification), excoriation, and even scarring.

## Distribution

- *Infantile form:* on the face, scalp, arms, legs, or generalized. The diaper area is usually clear, probably because of occlusion of the area and urea exposure from urine.
- *Adolescent and adult forms:* on the cubital and popliteal fossae and, less commonly, on the dorsa of the hands and feet, ears, or generalized. Atopic eczema of the soles of the feet is quite common in adolescents. In adults, there is a more chronic, localized disease, especially involving the genitalia, posterior scalp, and ankles (often referred to as *lichen simplex chronicus* [LSC]). Pruritus is severe and paroxysmal.

## Course

The course varies from a mild single episode to severe chronic, recurrent episodes resulting in the "psychoitchical" person. Eczema is referred to as "the itch that rashes." The infantile form usually becomes milder or even disappears after the age of 3 or 4 years, and approximately 70% of cases clear by puberty. During puberty and the late teenage years, flare-ups or new outbreaks can occur. Adult-onset eczema, once thought to be rare, is actually quite common. Young housewives or househusbands may have their first recurrence of atopic eczema since childhood because of their new jobs of

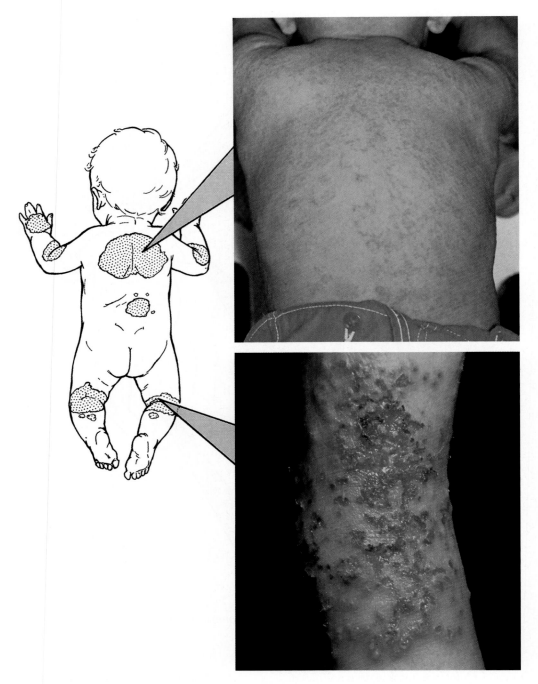

**FIGURE 8-7** ■ Atopic eczema (infant). *(Courtesy of Roche Laboratories.)*

dishwashing and child care. Thirty percent of patients with atopic dermatitis eventually develop allergic asthma or hay fever, penicillin allergy, hives, or marked reaction to insect bites.

## Causes

The following factors are important:

■ *Heredity* is the most important single factor. The family history is usually positive for one or more

of the triad of allergic diseases: asthma, hay fever, or atopic eczema. Penicillin allergy, hives, and a marked reaction to insect bites are also a part of the atopic diathesis, which is called type 1 or anaphylactoid immunity. Determination of this history in cases of hand dermatitis is important because it often enables the physician, on the patient's first visit, to prognosticate a more drawn-out recovery than if the patient had a simple contact dermatitis.

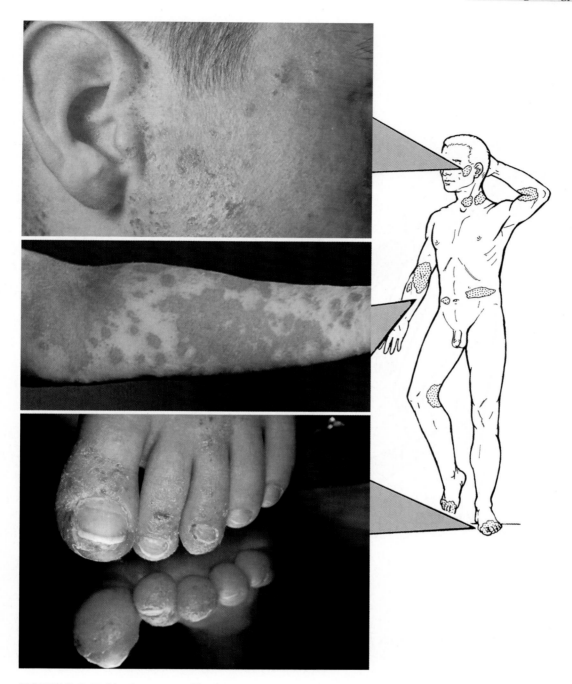

**FIGURE 8-8** ■ Atopic eczema. The bottom photograph, by the use of a mirror, demonstrates the undersurface of the toes. *(Courtesy of Sandoz Pharmaceuticals.)*

■ *Dryness* of the skin is important. Most often, atopic eczema is worse in the winter owing to the decrease in home or office and outdoor humidity. For this reason, the use of soap and water should be reduced and hot water avoided. Emollients (lanolin free) can be applied after bathing.

■ *Wool* and *lanolin* (wool fat) commonly irritate the skin of these patients. Wearing wool or silk clothes

may be another reason for an increased incidence of atopic eczema in the winter. Cotton clothes and bed clothing are preferred.

■ *Allergy to foods* is a factor that is often overstressed, particularly with the infantile form. The mother's history of certain foods causing trouble should be a guide for eliminating foods. This can be tested by adding the incriminated foods to the diet, one new

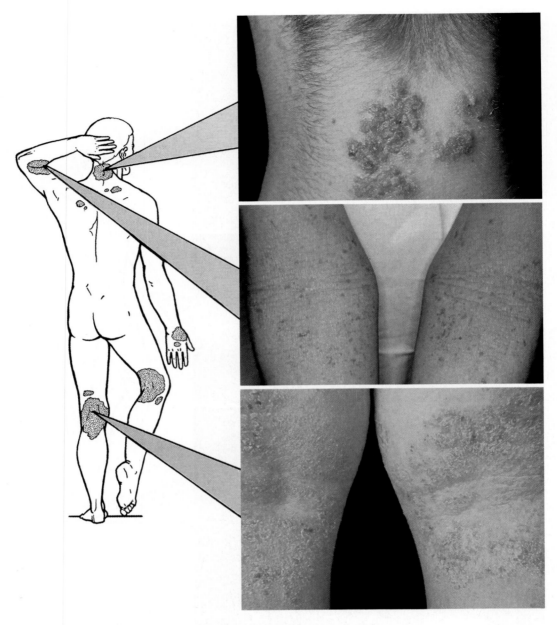

**FIGURE 8-9** ■ Atopic eczema. *(Courtesy of Geigy Pharmaceuticals.)*

food every 48 hours, when the dermatitis is stable. Scratch tests and intracutaneous tests uncover very few dermatologic allergens.

■ *Emotional stress* and *nervousness* aggravate any existing conditions such as itching, duodenal ulcers, or migraine headaches. Therefore, this "nervous" factor is important but not causative enough to label this disease *disseminated neurodermatitis.*

■ *Concomitant bacterial infection* of the skin, particularly with *Staphylococcus aureus,* is common. Cultures may be helpful to guide antibiotic choices. Community-acquired methicillin resistant *Staphylococcus aureus* (CA-MRSA) has become ubiquitous.

### Differential Diagnosis

■ *Dermatitis venenata* (contact dermatitis to plants): positive history, usually of contactants; no family allergic history; distribution rather characteristic where the allergen has touched the skin and often with characteristic streaking.

■ *Psoriasis:* patches localized to extensor surfaces, mainly knees and elbows, with characteristic thick silvery-white scales (see Chapter 14). Nail involvement is not uncommon.

■ *Seborrheic dermatitis in infants:* absence of family allergy history; lesions scaly and greasy and often seen in the diaper or intertriginous areas (see Chapter 13).

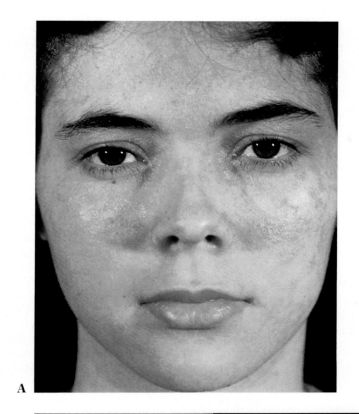

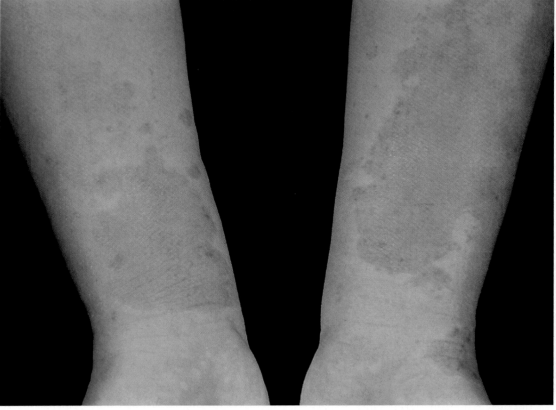

**FIGURE 8-10** ■ Atopic eczema. This case of facial atopic eczema **(A)** resembled acute lupus erythematosus. The arm eruption **(B)** is on another patient and exemplifies the chronic lichenified form of atopic eczema. *(Courtesy of K.U.M.C.; Dome Chemicals.)*

**TABLE 8-1 ■ Hanifin and Rajka Criteria for Diagnosis of Atopic Dermatitis**

| Major Criteria | Minor Criteria |
|---|---|
| Pruritus | Xerosis |
| *Adults:* flexural lichenification or linearity | Ichthyosis, palmar hyperlinearity |
| | Keratosis pilaris |
| *Children:* facial or extensor involvement | Type I skin test reactivity Elevated serum IgE |
| Chronic or chronically relapsing dermatitis | Early age of onset Tendency toward skin infections |
| | Nipple eczema |
| Atopic history, personal or familial | Cheilitis |
| | Recurrent conjunctivitis |
| | Dennie–Morgan fold (accentuated skin line on the lower eyelids) |
| | Keratoconus |
| | Anterior subcapsular cataracts |
| | Orbital darkening |
| | Facial pallor/facial erythema |
| | Pityriasis alba |
| | Anterior neck folds |
| | Pruritus with perspiration |
| | Intolerance to wool and lipid solvents |
| | Perifollicular accentuation (especially in people of color) |
| | Food intolerance |
| | Course influenced by environmental/emotional factors |
| | White dermatographism/ delayed blanch |

*Note:* Three major plus four or more minor criteria should be present.

## General Management for Atopic Eczema

Inform the patient or family that this is usually a chronic problem, that this is an inherited condition, that skin tests usually are not helpful, and that relief can occur from the dermatitis and the itch, but there is no "cure" except time.

### Treatment of Infantile Form

*Case Example:* A child, aged 6 months, presents with mild oozing, red, excoriated dermatitis on face, arms, and legs.

***First Visit.***

1. Follow a regular diet except for the avoidance of any foods that the parent believes aggravated the eruption.
2. Avoid exposure of the infant to excessive bathing with soaps and to contact with wool and products containing lanolin. Use mild soap sparingly. Cool to lukewarm bath water.
3. Coal tar solution (liquor carbonis detergens [LCD]) or Cutar (topical, OTC) bath oil 120.0

    *Sig:* Add ½ tbsp to the lukewarm bath water. Be sure to lubricate skin after each bath.
4. Hydrocortisone ointment, 1%, 30.0

    *Sig:* Apply sparingly b.i.d. to affected areas.
    *Comment:* 1% Hytone ointment is in a petrolatum base without lanolin. Other proprietary corticosteroid preparations are listed in the Formulary in Chapter 4.
5. Diphenhydramine (Benadryl) elixir 90.0

    *Sig:* Take 1 tsp b.i.d.
    *Comment:* Warn the parent that this drug may paradoxically stimulate the child.
6. If infection is present, treat with the appropriate systemic antibiotic, such as erythromycin, cephalexin, or cloxacillin. For MRSA, treat with liquid clindamycin or Bactrim DS (generic).
7. Pimecrolimus (Elidel) cream and tacrolimus (Protopic) ointment in 0.03% and 0.1% are the most significant recent advances in topical therapy for eczema. They can be used as monotherapy or as a corticosteroid-sparing drug (this is the author's preference) in conjunction with topical corticosteroids. They do not cause cutaneous atrophy and striae, which are not insignificant problems with topical corticosteroids. Also, systemic absorption of corticosteroids is particularly of concern in infants.

***Subsequent Visits.*** Add coal tar solution such as LCD (3% to 10%) to the above ointment.

***Severe or Resistant Cases.***

1. Restrict diet to milk only; after 3 days, add one different food every 24 hours. An offending food causes a flare-up of the eczema in several hours.
2. Hydrocortisone liquid: Cortef (oral) 90.0

    *Sig:* Take 1 tsp (10 mg) q.i.d. for 3 days, then 1 tsp t.i.d. for 1 week.
    *Comment:* Decrease the dose or discontinue as improvement warrants. Base the dosage on the weight of the child.
3. Hospitalization with a change of environment may be necessary for a severe case. This may be necessary in a case of parental negligence.

***Treatment of Adult Form*** *Case Example:* A young adult presents with dry, scaly, lichenified patches in the cubital and popliteal fossae.

***First Visit.***

1. Counsel the patient to avoid stress, excess soap for bathing, lanolin preparations locally, and contact with wool.

2. Coal tar solution (LCD) 5%

   Fluorinated corticosteroid ointment or emollient cream (see Chapter 4) q.s. 30.0

3. Hydroxyzine, 25 mg #90

   *Sig:* Take 1 tablet t.i.d.

   *Comment:* Available generically. Warn the patient about the side effect of drowsiness.

4. Elidel and Protopic are topical corticosteroid-sparing drugs.

***Subsequent Visits.***

1. Gradually increase the concentration of the coal tar solution in the previously mentioned salve up to 10%.

2. Increase the potency of the corticosteroid ointment or emollient cream.

3. For patients with infected crusted lesions (many patients have an element of infection), an antibiotic such as erythromycin, 250 mg, may be prescribed b.i.d. or t.i.d. for several weeks.

4. Systemic corticosteroid therapy may be indicated for severe and resistant cases.

5. Topical doxepin hydrochloride (Zonalon) cream

   *Sig:* Spread a thin coat q.i.d. on pruritic areas.

   *Comment:* Can cause drowsiness with overuse on large surface areas and may sting or burn when therapy is first initiated.

6. Leukotriene inhibitors have been shown to be of benefit recently by some authors. An example is zafirlukast (Accolate).

   *Sig:* Take 20 mg/tablet; 1 tablet by mouth b.i.d.

7. Recombinant human interferon-$\gamma$ has shown some benefit in some studies; 50 $\mu g/m^2$ is given subcutaneously daily. This is primarily experimental.

8. Rarely, immunosuppressive therapy such as methotrexate may have to be employed in recalcitrant, life-altering disease.

9. Various forms of ultraviolet (UV) light therapy can be helpful, including psoralens and UVA (PUVA), narrow band UVB (TL-01), UVB, UVA, and UVA II. Increased risk of skin cancer and photoaging are to be considered.

10. Omalizumab (Xolair) given subcutaneously has been reported to be beneficial in cases of severe eczema.

## Nummular Eczema

Nummular eczema (Fig. 8-11) is a moderately common, very pruritic, distinctive, eczematous eruption characterized by coin-shaped (nummular) papulovesicular patches, mainly on the arms and the legs of young adults and elderly patients.

### Presentation

*Primary Lesions*

Coin-shaped patches of vesicles and papules are usually seen on the extremities and occasionally on the trunk.

*Secondary Lesions*

Lichenification and bacterial infection do occur.

*Course*

This is very chronic, particularly in older people. Recurrences are common, especially in fall and winter.

*Subjective Complaints*

Itching is usually quite severe.

*Causes*

Nothing is definite, but these factors are important:

- History is usually positive for asthma, hay fever, or atopic eczema, particularly in the young adult.
- Bacterial infection of the lesions may occur.
- The low indoor humidity of winter causes dry skin, which intensifies the itching, particularly in elderly patients.

### Differential Diagnosis

- *Atopic eczema:* mainly in the antecubital and popliteal fossae, not coin-sized lesions (see preceding section).
- *Psoriasis:* not vesicular; see scalp and fingernail lesions (see Chapter 14).
- *Contact dermatitis:* will not see coin-shaped lesions (see beginning of this chapter).

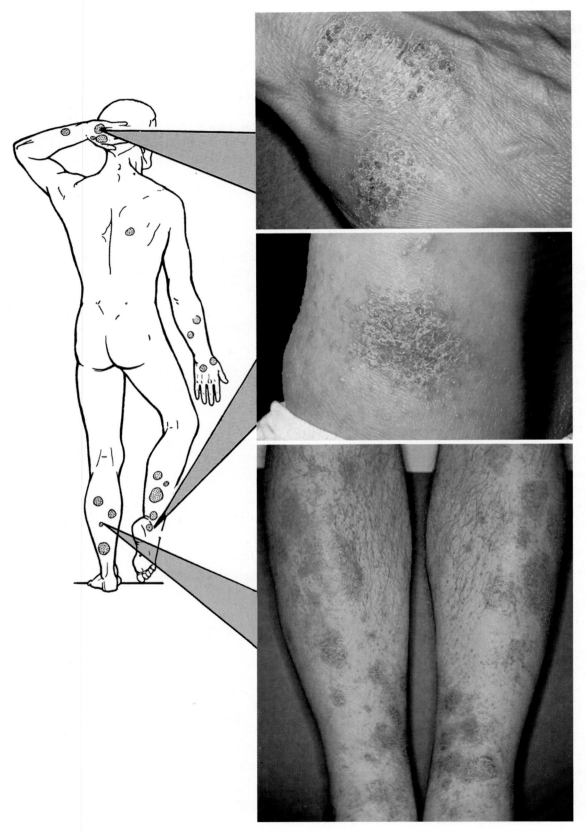

**FIGURE 8-11** ▪ Nummular eczema. *(Courtesy of Schering Corp.)*

■ *Id reaction* from stasis dermatitis of the legs or a localized contact dermatitis: impossible to differentiate this clinically, at times, from nummular eczema, but patient will have a history of previous primary localized dermatitis that suddenly became aggravated and widespread.

*Treatment*

*Case Example:* An elderly man presents in the winter with five to eight distinct, coin-shaped, excoriated, vesicular, crusted lesions on the arms and the legs.

### First Visit.
1. Instruct the patient to avoid excessive use of soaps.
2. Use superfatted soaps such as Dove or Cetaphil, and lubricate the skin immediately after every bath or shower. Use water as cool as is tolerable to bathe.
3. Corticosteroid ointment 60.0

   *Sig:* Apply t.i.d. locally.
   *Comment:* The use of an ointment base is particularly important in the therapy for nummular eczema. I find adding a mild tar such as MG 217 in a 19% concentration is helpful.
4. Diphenhydramine, 50 mg #15 (another inexpensive OTC generic is clemastine 1.34 or 2.68 mg q.d.)

   *Sig:* Take 1 capsule h.s. for antipruritic and sedative effect.
   *Comment:* Available generically and OTC.
5. Consider Elidel and Protopic as topical nonsteroid alternatives.

### Resistant Cases.
1. Add coal tar solution (LCD), 3% to 10%, to the previously mentioned salve.
2. Oral antibiotic therapy may be beneficial. Prescribe erythromycin, 250 mg, t.i.d. for several weeks.
3. A short course of oral corticosteroid therapy is effective, but relapses are common.

   Rarely, methotrexate can be employed. Watch for liver and hematologic toxicity.

## Drug Eruptions

It can be stated almost without exception that any drug administered systemically is capable of causing a skin eruption (Figs. 8-12 to 8-14).

To jog the memory of patients, I often ask, "Do you take any medicine for any condition? What about medicated toothpaste, laxatives, vitamins, aspirin, and tonics? Have you received any shots in the past month? Have you been treating a cold, headache, sinus condition, painful joints, or cramps from your menses?"

Any of the larger dermatologic texts has extensive lists of common and uncommon drugs, with their common and uncommon skin reactions. These books must be consulted

for the rare reactions, but the following paragraphs cover 95% of these idiosyncrasies.

Photosensitivity reactions from drugs are covered in Chapter 39. Hepatic drug metabolism pathway involving cytochrome P-450 enzymes defines the most significant and largest group of drug-drug interactions. Adverse drug interactions must always be considered.

### Drugs and Associated Dermatoses

Drug eruptions are usually not characteristic for any certain drug or group of drugs, but experience has shown that certain clinical pictures commonly follow the use of certain drugs. Common drugs causing skin eruptions are given in Table 8-2, and common skin eruptions caused by drugs are given in Table 8-3.

### Course

The course of drug eruptions depends on many factors, including the type of drug, severity of the cutaneous reaction, systemic involvement, general health of the patient, and efficacy of corrective therapy. Most cases with bullae, purpura, or exfoliative dermatitis have a serious prognosis and a protracted course. Urticarial reactions may herald the onset of anaphylaxis, and questioning about shortness of breath or trouble swallowing may be important in these patients.

### Treatment

1. Eliminate the drug. This is the single most important therapeutic intervention. This simple procedure is often delayed, with resulting serious consequences, because a careful history is not taken. If the eruption is mild and the drug necessary, discontinuation of the drug may not be mandatory. But if it is a serious drug eruption, all drugs should be stopped as a potentially lifesaving intervention.
2. Further therapy depends on the seriousness of the eruption. Morbilliform drug eruptions (measles-like) are the most common type and may resolve with no therapy. An itching drug eruption should be treated to relieve the itch. Cases of exfoliative dermatitis or severe erythema

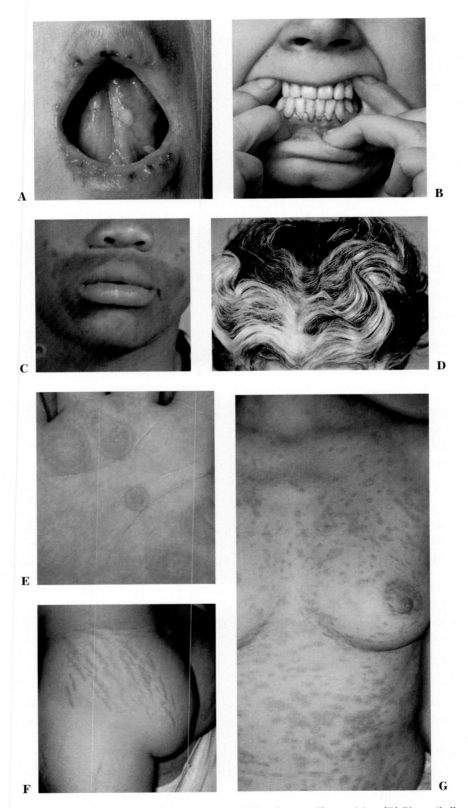

**FIGURE 8-12** ■ Drug eruptions. **(A)** Erosions of the tongue and lips from sulfonamides. **(B)** Bismuth line of the gums. **(C)** Phenolphthalein fixed eruption of the lips of an African-American boy. **(D)** Whitening of scalp hair from chloroquine therapy for lupus erythematosus. **(E)** Erythema multiforme-like eruption of the palm from oral antibiotic therapy. **(F)** Striae of the buttocks of a 30-year-old man following 9 months of corticosteroid therapy. **(G)** Papulosquamous eruption of the chest from phenolphthalein. *(Courtesy of E.R. Squibb.)*

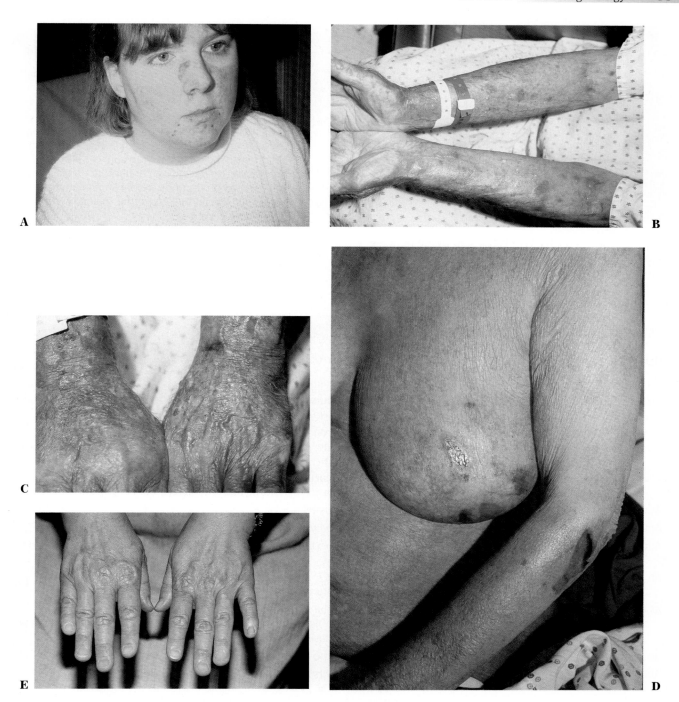

**FIGURE 8-13** ■ Side effects of topical corticosteroid abuse. **(A)** Steroid rosacea. **(B)** Atrophy, telangiectasias, milia. **(C)** Purpura, atrophy. **(D)** Fragility with tearing and cigarette paper wrinkling atrophy. **(E)** Hydroxyurea dermopathy mimicking dermatomyositis.

multiforme-like lesions require corticosteroid and other supportive therapy.

3. Toxic epidermal necrolysis and Stevens–Johnson syndrome can be treated with high-dose intravenous immunoglobulin G and intensive supportive hospital care. High-dose systemic corticosteroids are controversial and, if used, should be given as early as possible. Discontinuation of the offending drug in a timely manner is the most important prognostic factor and can be lifesaving and vision-saving.

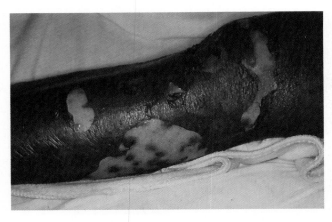

**FIGURE 8-14** ■ Positive Nikolsky's sign of the right leg: sheets of skin peeling off with very light pressure. This was due to secondary therapy with a sulfur-related drug.

### SAUER'S NOTES

1. When confronted with any diffuse or puzzling eruption, routinely question the patient regarding *any* medication taken by *any* route.
2. Ask: "Are you taking any vitamins, laxatives, nerve pills, and so forth?" This jogs the patient's memory.
3. Remember, any ingested chemical agent can cause an eruption, such as toothpaste, mouthwash, breath freshener, and chewing gum.
4. Antiseizure medications, antibiotics, sulfa and sulfa-related drugs, nonsteroidal anti-inflammatory drugs, and allopurinol cause the majority of cutaneous drug eruptions.

**TABLE 8-2** ■ **Drugs and the Dermatoses they Cause**

| Drug | Dermatosis/Comments |
| --- | --- |
| Accutane | See *isotretinoin* |
| Acetaminophen (Tylenol) | Infrequent cause of drug eruption; urticaria and erythematous eruptions are noted. Also fixed drug eruption. |
| Adrenocorticotropic hormones (ACTH, prednisone, IM triamcinolone) | Cushing's syndrome, hyperpigmentation, acneiform eruptions, rosacea, striae, perioral dermatitis, seborrheic dermatitis–like eruptions, and hirsutism |
| Allopurinol (Zyloprim) | Erythema, maculopapular rash, and severe bullae (including Stevens–Johnson syndrome and toxic epidermal necrolysis) |
| Amantadine | Livedo reticularis |
| Amiodarone | Photosensitivity reaction and blue-gray discoloration of the skin |
| Amphetamine (Benzedrine) | Coldness of extremities; redness of the neck and shoulders; increased itching in LSC |
| Ampicillin | See *antibiotics;* flare of morbilliform eruption in over half of patients with infectious mononucleosis |
| ACE inhibitors | Maculopapular eruption with eosinophilia, pemphigus, a bullous pemphigoid–like eruption, angioedema, rosacea, urticaria, and possibly flare of psoriasis |
| Antabuse | Redness of the face and acne |
| Antibiotics | Various agents have different reactions, but in general: *candida overgrowth* in oral, genital, and anal orifices results in pruritus ani, pruritus vulvae, and generalized pruritus; candida skin lesions may spread out from these foci. Urticaria, morbilliform, and erythema multiforme-like eruptions, particularly from penicillin |
| | *Ampicillin:* generalized maculopapular rash, very common in patients with infectious mononucleosis |
| | *Sulfa derivatives:* particularly a problem in HIV+ patients. See *streptomycin* and the later section on photosensitivity reactions |
| Anticoagulants | *Coumadin* and *heparin:* severe hemorrhagic skin infarction and necrosis |
| Antineoplastic agents | Skin and mucocutaneous reactions, including alopecia, stomatitis, radiation recall reaction, and erythema |
| Apresoline (see *hydralazine*) | *Immediate reaction:* pruritus, urticaria, and sweating |
| Atabrine hydrochloride | *Delayed serum sickness reaction:* urticaria, redness, purpura |

**TABLE 8-2** ■ (*Continued*)

| Drug | Dermatosis/Comments |
|---|---|
| Aspirin and salicylates (a multitude of cold, flu, and antipain remedies; e.g., Pepto-Bismol) | Urticaria, purpura, bullous lesions |
| Atabrine | Universal yellow pigmentation; blue macules on the face and mucosa; lichen planus–like eruption |
| Atropine | Scarlet fever–like rash |
| Barbiturates | Urticarial, erythematous, bullous, or purpuric eruptions; fixed drug eruptions |
| Beta-blockers | Alopecia; psoriasis flare |
| Cetuximab (monoclonal antibody that binds the epidermal growth factor receptor) | Acneiform eruption 3 weeks posttherapy in 90% of patients; can consider prophylactic therapy with tetracycline. Used to treat solid tumors. Follicular eruption (80%), painful fissures of fingers and toes (60%), paronychia (30%), telangiectasias, alterations of hair growth and hypopigmentation |
| Bleomycin | *Antitumor antibiotic:* gangrene, erythema, sclerosis, nail changes, characteristic striate lesions |
| Captopril | Pemphigus-like eruption; see *ACE inhibitors* |
| Chloroquine (Aralen) | Follicular eruption (⅓ of patients); acneiform eruptions, seborrheic eruptions, nail bed changes |
| Chemotherapy agents | See *antineoplastic agents;* also see specific drug |
| Chloral hydrate | Urticarial, papular, erythematous, and purpuric eruptions |
| Chloroquine (Aralen) | Erythematous or lichenoid eruptions with pruritus and urticaria; ocular retinal damage from long-term use of chloroquine and other antimalarials can be irreversible |
| Cimetidine | Petechial and purpuric eruptions, especially of the legs; see section on photosensitivity reactions |
| Chlorpromazine (Thorazine) | Maculopapular rash, increased sun sensitivity, purpura with agranulocytosis, and icterus from hepatitis |
| | *Long-term therapy:* slate-gray to violet discoloration of the skin |
| Cimetidine | Dry, scaly skin |
| Codeine and morphine | Erythematous, urticarial, or vesicular eruption |
| Collagen (bovine) injections | Skin edema, erythema, induration, and urticaria at implantation sites |
| Contraceptive drugs | Chloasma-like eruption, erythema nodosum, hives; some cases of acne are aggravated |
| Cortisone and derivatives | Allergy (rare); see *ACTH* |
| Coumadin | See *anticoagulants* |
| Cyclosporin | Hypertrichosis, sebaceous hyperplasia, acne, folliculitis, epidermal cysts, Kaposi's sarcoma, skin precancers and cancers, gingival hyperplasia, follicular keratosis, palmoplantar paresthesias, and dysesthesias associated with temperature change |
| Dapsone (avlosulfone) | Red, maculopapular, vesicular eruption with agranulocytosis occurs, occasionally resembling erythema nodosum |
| Diltiazem | Rare. Photodistributed hyperpigmentation, subacute cutaneous LE, toxic epidermal necrolysis, Stevens–Johnson syndrome, photosensitivity, vasculitis, pruritus, urticaria, and maculopapular dermatitis |
| Dextran (used in peritoneal dialysis) | Urticarial reactions |
| Diethylpropion hydrochloride (Tenuate, Tepanil) | Measles-like eruption |
| Dilantin | See *phenytoin* |
| Epidermal growth factors | See *cetuximab, erlotinib* |

(*continued*)

**TABLE 8-2** ■ *(Continued)*

| Drug | Dermatosis/Comments |
|------|---------------------|
| Erlotinib | Follicular eruption (60%), painful fissures in the fingers and toes (40%), paronychia (40%), alterations of hair growth (30%), telangiectasias, and hyperpigmentation |
| Docetaxel | *Cutaneous reactions:* up to 70% incidence, beginning usually 2–4 days after treatment with 80% pain or itching; purple-red macules or plaques, often acral, that may peel in 3–4 weeks; if worse with repeated doses, this drug may have to be stopped; local hypothermia may be ameliorative; extravasation necrosis, nail loss, supravenous discoloration, subungual abscess, skin sclerosis |
| | *Acral erythrodyesthesia with desquamation:* in a few weeks; may worsen each episode and may limit dosage |
| | *Diffuse:* (10%) mild scaly erythema with follicular accentuation; does not necessarily recur |
| | *Intertrigo eruption:* due to friction from clothing; loose-fitting clothes may help |
| | *Melanotic macules:* on trunk or extremities; stomatitis; radiation and sunburn recall |
| | *To ameliorate reactions:* 99% DMSO four times a day, oral antioxidants (vitamins E, C, A, and selenium), and oral misoprostol (prostaglandin E, analog) |
| Estrogenic medications | Edema of the legs with cutaneous redness progressing to exfoliative dermatitis |
| Feldene | See *piroxicam* |
| Flagyl | See *metronidazole* |
| Furosemide | Bullous hemorrhagic eruption |
| Gold | Eczematous dermatitis of the hands, arms, and legs, or a pityriasis rosea–like eruption; also, seborrheic-like eruption, urticaria, and purpura |
| Heparin | See *anticoagulants* |
| Hydralazine (Apresoline) | SLE-like reaction |
| Hydroxyurea | Dermopathy mimicking cutaneous findings of dermatomyositis; atrophic, erythematous dermatitis over the back of the hands that may be photo-induced; leg ulcers; hyperpigmentation, especially nails (longitudinal bands) and palms |
| Ibuprofen (Nuprin, Motrin, Advil) | Bullous eruptions, including erythema multiforme, Stevens–Johnson syndrome, toxic epidermal necrolysis, urticaria, photosensitivity, fixed drug reactions, morbilliform reactions |
| IVIG (intravenous IgG infusion) | Pompholyx (dyshidrosis)-like eruption 5–7 days after treatment can evolve into a generalized eczematous eruption |
| Icodextrin (used in peritoneal dialysis) | Psoriasiform dermatosis, acute generalized exanthematous pustulosis |
| Imipramine | Slate-gray discoloration of the skin |
| Insulin | Urticaria with serum sickness symptoms; fat atrophy at the injection site |
| Iodides | See *bromides;* papular, pustular, ulcerative, or granulomatous lesions mainly on acne areas or the legs; administration of chloride hastens recovery |
| Isoniazid | Erythematous and maculopapular, generalized, purpuric, bullous, and nummular eczema–like; acne aggravation |
| Isotretinoin | Dry red skin and lips (common); alopecia (rare) |
| Lasix | See *furosemide* |
| Lamotrigine | At least 10% with cutaneous drug reactions; may be similar to phenytoin cutaneous drug reactions |

**TABLE 8-2** ■ *(Continued)*

| Drug | Dermatosis/Comments |
|---|---|
| Lithium | Acne-like lesions on the body; psoriasis exacerbation |
| Meclizine hydrochloride (Antivert) | Urticaria |
| Meprobamate | Small purpuric lesions, erythema multiforme-like eruption |
| Metronidazole (Flagyl) | Urticaria, pruritus |
| Minocycline | Skin (muddy skin syndrome), teeth, and scar discoloration |
| | *Rare:* hypersensitivity, sickness-like reaction, drug-induced lupus erythematosus, SLE-like syndrome, autoimmune hepatitis, *p*-ANCA–positive cutaneous polyarteritis nodosa, elastosis perforans serpiginosum, localized cutis laxa, pseudoxanthoma elasticum, anetoderma (primary anetoderma has been associated with antiphospholipid syndrome), bullous pemphigoid |
| Pentazocine venous | When used as an abused substance it causes deep ulcers along venous access sites with surrounding hyperpigmented woody induration, fibrous myopathy, and puffy hand syndrome |
| Phenolphthalein (found in 4-way Cold Tablets, ex-lax, bile salts, and pink icing on cakes) | *Rare syndrome:* hepatitis, exfoliative dermatitis, fever, lymphadenopathy, eosinophilia, lymphocytosis |
| Morphine | See *codeine;* lichen planus–like eruption; fixed drug eruption, photosensitivity |
| Nevirapine | Unusually high incidence of potentially life-threatening Stevens–Johnson syndrome; urticaria, erythema multiforme-like eruption, toxic epidermal necrolysis |
| Penicillin | See *antibiotics* |
| Procainamide | Lupus-like rash, lichen planus–like rash, pemphigus foliaceus |
| Psoralens | *Fixed drug eruption:* hyperpigmented or purplish, flat or slightly elevated, discrete, single or multiple patches |
| | See section on photosensitivity reactions |
| Phenytoin (Dilantin) | Hypertrophy of gums, erythema multiforme-like eruption; pseudolymphoma syndrome, morbilliform reaction |
| | *Fetal hydantoin syndrome:* organ defects plus nail hypoplasia |
| | *Note:* one of the most common causes of toxic epidermal necrolysis or Stevens–Johnson syndrome along with other antiseizure medications |
| Propranolol (Inderal) | *Rare:* drug eruption; See *beta-blockers* |
| Sirolimus | Acneiform eruption that may be recalcitrant to therapy |
| Psoralens | See section on photosensitivity reactions |
| Quinidine | Edema, purpura, scarlatiniform eruption; may progress to exfoliative dermatitis |
| Quinine | Diffuse eruption (any kind) |
| Rauwolfia alkaloids (reserpine) | Urticaria, photosensitivity reactions, petechial eruptions |
| Rifampin | Pruritus, urticaria, acne, bullous pemphigoid, mucositis, exfoliative erythroderma, red urine, reddened soft contact lenses |
| Salicylates | See *aspirin* |
| Streptomycin | Urticaria; erythematous, morbilliform, and purpuric eruptions |
| Sulfonamides | Urticaria, scarlatiniform eruption, erythema nodosum, eczematous flare of exudative dermatitis, erythema multiforme-like bullous eruption, fixed eruption; see later section on photosensitivity reactions, morbilliform reaction |
| | *AIDS patients:* develop allergic drug eruptions quite often; one of the most common causes of toxic epidermal necrolysis and Stevens–Johnson syndrome |

*(continued)*

**TABLE 8-2** ■ (*Continued*)

| Drug | Dermatosis/Comments |
|---|---|
| Sulfonylureas | See *sulfonamides* and section on photosensitivity reactions |
| Suramin | Cutaneous reaction (80%), especially morbilliform, UV light recall (skin eruptions at sites of previous UV exposure), urticaria, "suramin keratoses" |
| Taxanes (paclitaxel, docetaxel) | Scleroderma-like skin changes, fixed drug, onycholysis, acral erythema, erythema multiforme, pustular eruptions |
| Tyrosine kinase inhibitors (cetuximab [Erbitux], gefitinib [Iressa], erlotinib [Tarceva], imatinib [Gleevec] | Persistent folliculitis with attributes of both acne and pemphigus in 75% of patients. |
| Testosterone and related drugs | Acne-like lesions, alopecia in scalp, hirsutism |
| Tetracycline | Fixed drug eruption, photosensitivity, serum sickness–like reaction patient < 8 years old: teeth staining; see *antibiotics* |
| Thalidomide | Erythroderma, pustulosis, toxic epidermal necrolysis |
| Thiazides | See section on photosensitivity reactions |
| Trimethoprim | Rarely incriminated in drug eruptions |
| Vitamin A | *Long-term, high-dose therapy:* scaly, rough, itchy skin with coarse, dry, scant hair growth, and systemic changes including liver toxicity |
| Vitamin D | Skin lesions rare, but headache, nausea, diarrhea, increased urination, and sore gums and joints can be present |
| Vitamin B group | Urticaria, pruritic redness, and even anaphylactic reactions can occur after IM or IV administration |
|  | *Nicotinic acid:* red flush (common—warn patient to eliminate unnecessary alarm), pruritus (common), hives (rare, within 15–30 min of oral ingestion of 50–100 mg) |
| Warfarin sodium | See *anticoagulants* |

*Abbreviations:* ACTH, adrenocorticotropic hormone; LSC, lichen simplex chronicus; ACE, angiotensin-converting enzyme; SLE, systemic lupus erythematosus; UV, ultraviolet.

**TABLE 8-3** ■ **Dermatoses and the Drugs that Cause Them**

| Dermatosis | Drug(s) | Comments |
|---|---|---|
| Acne-like or pustular lesions | Bromides, iodides, lithium, testosterone, corticosteroids | |
| Acral erythema | Redness, pain, and swelling of the hands and feet associated with various chemotherapeutic agents including cyclophosphamide, cytosine arabinoside, docetaxel, doxorubicin, fluorouracil, hydroxyurea, mercaptopurine, methotrexate, and mitotane | Most commonly cytarabine, doxorubicin, and fluorouracil<br><br>Chemotherapy can be continued or briefly interrupted with use of topical corticosteroids |
| Actinic keratosis inflammation occurring in patients on systemic chemotherapy | First described with fluorouracil; also doxorubicin, cisplatin, fludarabine, dactinomycin, dacarbazine, and vincristine sulfate | |
| Alopecia | Amethopterin (methotrexate) and other antineoplastic agents; colchicine, clofibrate, testosterone and other androgens; tricyclic antidepressants; beta-blockers; heparin; progesterone derivatives; coumarin derivatives; isotretinoin | |

**TABLE 8-3** ■ (Continued)

| Dermatosis | Drug(s) | Comments |
|---|---|---|
| Angioedema | Aspirin, NSAIDs, ACE inhibitors | |
| Baboon syndrome | Mercury (most often); also ampicillin, amoxicillin, nickel, erythromycin, heparin, and food additives | Systemic contact dermatitis owing to ingestion, inhalation, or percutaneous absorption; symmetric diffuse acute light red exanthema on the buttocks, anogenital area, major flexural areas of the extremities; peaks at day 2–5 of exposure to the involved drug; resolves within 1 week |
| DIDMOHS (drug-induced delayed [3–6 weeks] multiorgan hypersensitivity syndrome of Sontheimer and Houpt; also called DRESS [drug rash with eosinophilia and systemic symptoms of Bocquet and Roujeau]) | Dapsone, carbamazepine, phenobarbital, minocycline, trimethoprim, sulfamethoxazole, procarbazine, allopurinol, terbinafine | Exanthematous or papulopustular febrile eruption with hepatitis (also possible lung, renal, thyroid involvement), lymphadenopathy, and eosinophilia |
| Eczematous eruption | Quinine, antihistamines, gold, mercury, sulfonamides, penicillin, organic arsenic | |
| Erythema annulare centrifugum | Salicylates, antimalarials, amitriptyline, gold, etizolam | Proximal extremities and trunk with red advancing circinate plaques that may have a dry fine adherent scale in the inner spreading edge. Can be associated with underlying infections, hormonal abnormalities, and underlying malignancies |
| Erythema multiforme–like eruption | Penicillin and other antibiotics, sulfonamides, phenolphthalein, barbiturates, phenytoin, meprobamate | |
| Erythema nodosum–like eruption | Sulfonamides, iodides, salicylates, oral contraceptives, dapsone | |
| Exfoliative dermatitis | Particularly owing to arsenic, penicillin, sulfonamides, allopurinol, barbiturates | In the course of any severe generalized drug eruption |
| Fixed drug eruption | Phenolphthalein, acetaminophen, barbiturates, organic arsenic, gold, salicylates, sulfonamides, tetracycline, many others | *Fixed drug eruption:* hyperpigmented or purplish; flat or slightly elevated; discrete, single, or multiple patches. Occurs at the same sites on drug challenge |
| Hyperpigmentation | Contraceptives, atabrine, chloroquine, minocycline, chlorpromazine, amiodarone, bismuth, and gold, silver salts, ACTH, estrogen, adriamycin, AZT, methotrexate | |
| Hypertrichosis | Oral minoxidil, phenytoin, cyclosporine<br>*Less severe:* oral contraceptives, systemic corticosteroids, psoralens, streptomycin sulfate | |
| Ichthyosis | Cimetidine, clofazimine, hydroxyurea, cholesterol-lowering agents, nicotinic acid, coenzyme A reductase inhibitors, triparanol | |
| Keratoses and epitheliomas | Arsenic, mercury, PUVA therapy, immunosuppressive agents | |
| Lichen planus–like eruption | Atabrine, arsenic, naproxen, gold, others | |
| Lupus erythematosus | Minocycline, hydralazine, procainamide, isoniazid, chlorpromazine, diltiazem, quinidine | |

(continued)

**TABLE 8-3** ■ *(Continued)*

| Dermatosis | Drug(s) | Comments |
|---|---|---|
| Linear IgA bullous dermatosis | Vancomycin (most common), furosemide, captopril, lithium, amiodarone, diclofenac, cefamandole, somatostatin, rifampin, topical iodine, phenytoin, trimethoprim, sulfamethoxazole, penicillin G, IL-2, interferon-γ | |
| Lipoatrophies from injections | Corticosteroids (e.g., triamcinolone), insulin, vasopressin, human growth hormone, iron dextran, diphtheria–pertussis–tetanus (DPT) immunization serum, antihistamines, Talwin injection usually due to abuse | |
| Lipodystrophy | *Partial:* proteinase inhibitors used to treat AIDS–indinavir or ritonavir plus saquinavir cause decreased subcutaneous fat on the face (cadaveric or cachectic facies) and extremities (pseudomuscular appearance) with increased prominence of the superficial veins, central adiposity with increased abdominal girth (pseudo-obesity), enlargement of breasts, increased dorsal-cervical fat pads (buffalo hump or pseudo-Cushing's syndrome) | Increased triglyceride and LDL cholesterol and low HDL cholesterol also occurs. |
| Measles-like eruption | Barbiturates, arsenic, sulfonamides, quinine, many others | |
| Mucous membrane lesions | *Pigmentation:* bismuth<br><br>*Hypertrophy:* phenytoin<br><br>*Erosive lesions:* sulfonamides, antineoplastic agents, many other drugs | |
| Nail changes | *Onycholysis* (distal detachment): tetracycline, apparently owing to a phototoxic reaction | |
| Neutrophilic eccrine hidradenitis | Bleomycin, chlorambucil, cyclophosphamide, cytarabine, doxorubicin, lomustine, mitoxantrone | |
| Nicolau syndrome (embolia cutis medicamentosa) | Diclofenac, ibuprofen, iodine, benzathine penicillin, vitamin K, DPT immunizations, antihistamines, interferon-α, corticosteroids | At IM injection site; see Dictionary–Index |
| Nummular eczema–like eruption | Combination of isoniazid and *p*-aminosalicylic acid | |
| Necrosis of the skin | *Localized:* coumarin and heparin derivatives (subcutaneous or intravenous); recombinant interferon-γ<br><br>*Distant:* coumarin and heparin derivatives | |
| Ochronosis, exogenous | Topical phenol, quinine injections, topical resorcinol<br><br>*With prolonged use:* topical hydroquinone, mainly in dark-skinned patients at the site of application only | |

**TABLE 8-3** ■ (Continued)

| Dermatosis | Drug(s) | Comments |
|---|---|---|
| Palmoplantar erythrodysesthesia | Chemotherapeutic agents, especially doxorubicin, docetaxel, fluorouracil and cytarabine. Also, epidermal growth factor inhibitors such as sunitinib | Clinically there is tender erythema and swelling of the fingers, toes, palms, and soles. Sometimes there are blisters. Histologically there may be eccrine syringosquamous metaplasia, neutrophilic eccrine hidradenitis or changes similar to graft-vs-host disease |
| Pemphigoid-like lesions | Furosemide, penicillin, sulfasalazine, ibuprofen | |
| Pemphigus-like lesions | Rifampin, penicillamine, captopril, pyrazolone derivatives | |
| Photosensitivity reaction | *Sulfonamides:* sulfonylurea | Several of the newer drugs and some of the older ones cause a dermatitis upon exposure to sunlight. These skin reactions can be urticarial, erythematous, vesicular, or plaque-like. The mechanism can be either phototoxic or photoallergic, but this distinction can be difficult to ascertain. This list of *photosensitizing drugs* is rather complete, but also see Chapter 39 |
| | *Hypoglycemics:* tolbutamide (Orinase), chlorpropamide (Diabinese) | |
| | *Antibiotics:* demethylchlortetracycline (Declomycin), doxycycline (Doryx, Monodox, Vibramycin), griseofulvin (Fulvicin, Grifulvin, Gris-PEG), maxaquin (Lomefloxacin), nalidixic acid (NegGram), tetracycline | |
| | *Benzofurans:* amiodarone | |
| | *Chlorothiazide diuretics:* chlorothiazide (Diuril); hydrochlorothiazide; methyclothiazide | |
| | *Phenothiazines:* chlorpromazine (Thorazine); prochlorperazine (Compazine); promethazine (Phenergan) | |
| | *Psoralens:* methoxsalen (Oxsoralen); trioxsalen (Trisoralen) | |
| | *Oxicams:* piroxicam (Feldene) | |
| Pityriasis rosea-like eruption | Bismuth, gold, barbiturates, antihistamines also see Chapter 39 | |
| Porphyria cutanea tarda exacerbation | Estrogen, iron, ethanol ingestion, hexachlorobenzene, chlorinated phenols, polychlorinated biphenyls; possibly pravastatin | |
| Pseudolymphoma | Antidepressants, diphenylhydantoin, α-agonists, ACE inhibitors, anticonvulsants, antihistamines, benzodiazepine, beta-blockers, calcium channel blockers, lipid-lowering agents, lithium, NSAIDs, phenothiazines, procainamide, estrogen, progesterone | |

*(continued)*

**TABLE 8-3** ▪ (*Continued*)

| Dermatosis | Drug(s) | Comments |
|---|---|---|
| Pseudoporphyria cutanea tarda (PCT) | NSAIDs (naproxen, nabumetone, oxaprozin, ketoprofen, mefenamic acid, diflunisal), nalidixic acid, tetracycline, chlorothalidone, furosemide, hydrochlorothiazide/triamterene, isotretinoin, etretinate, cyclosporine, 5-fluorouracil, pyridoxine, amiodarone, flutamide, dapsone, aspirin | Skin findings but no biochemical abnormalities. May persist for months after offending drug is stopped, mimics skin findings and skin biopsy of PCT |
| Psoriasis exacerbation | Lithium, beta-blockers, ACE inhibitors, antimalarials, NSAIDs, terbinafine | |
| Purpuric eruptions | Barbiturates, salicylates, meprobamate, organic arsenic, sulfonamides, chlorothiazide diuretics, corticosteroids (long-term use) | |
| Pustulosis, AGEP | Antibiotics (mainly β-lactam); many others | |
| Radiation recall | Chemotherapeutic agents, antituberculous medications, Simvastatin, interferon alpha 2b | |
| Rheumatoid nodulosis, accelerated | Methotrexate | Painful nodules mainly on the hands in longstanding rheumatoid arthritis patients. Dissipates after the drug is stopped. |
| Scarlet fever–like eruption or "toxic erythema" | Arsenic, barbiturates, codeine, morphine, mercury, quinidine, salicylates, sulfonamides, others | |
| Seborrheic dermatitis–like eruption | Gold, ACTH | |
| Stevens–Johnson syndrome | Lamotrigine, valproic acid, penicillin, barbiturates, diphenylhydantoin, sulfonamides, rifampin, NSAIDs, salicylates | |
| Subacute cutaneous lupus erythematosus | Hydrochlorothiazide, ACE inhibitors, calcium channel blockers, interferons, statins | |
| Urticaria | Penicillin, salicylates, serums, sulfonamides, barbiturates, opium group, contraceptive drugs, Rauwolfia alkaloids, ACE inhibitors | |
| Vesicular or bullous eruptions | Sulfonamides, penicillin, mephenytoin | |
| Whitening of the hair | Chloroquine, hydroxychloroquine | In blonde- or red-haired people |

*Abbreviations:* NSAID, nonsteroidal anti-inflammatory drugs; ACE, angiotensin-converting enzyme; AGEP, acute generalized exanthematous pustulosis; ACTH, adrenocorticotropic hormone; PUVA, psoralens and ultraviolet light; HDL, high-density lipoprotein; LDL, low-density lipoprotein; .

## Suggested Readings

Abramovitz W. Atopic dermatitis. J *Am Acad Dermatol.* 2005;53(1 Suppl 1):S86–S93.

American Medical Association. *Guides to the Evaluation of Permanent Impairment.* 3rd ed. Chicago: AMA; 1990.

DiCarlo JB, McCall CO. Pharmacologic alternatives for severe atopic dermatitis. *Int J Dermatol.* 2001;40:82–88.

Eichenfield LF, Hanifin JM, Luger TA, et al. Consensus conference on pediatric atopic dermatitis. *J Am Acad Dermatol.* 2003;49:1088–1095.

Kanerva L, Elsner P, Wahlberg J, et al. *Condensed Handbook of Occupational Dermatology.* New York: Springer; 2003.

Litt JZ. *Litt's Drug Eruption Reference Manual Including Drug Interactions.* 5th ed. Philadelphia: Taylor & Francis; 2009.

*Physicians' Desk Reference to Pharmaceutical Specialties and Biologicals.* Oradell, NJ: Medical Economics; 2008.

Rietschel R, Fowler JF. *Fisher's Contact Dermatitis.* 5th ed. Philadelphia: Lippincott, Williams & Wilkins; 2000.

Roujeau JC, Stern RS. Severe adverse cutaneous reactions to drugs. *N Engl J Med.* 1994;331:1272–1285.

Warshaw EM. Latex allergy. *J Am Acad Dermatol.* 1998;39:1–24.

Williams HC. *Atopic Dermatitis: The Epidemiology, Causes, and Prevention of Atopic Eczema.* Cambridge, UK: Cambridge University Press; 2000.

# CHAPTER 9

# Immune-mediated Skin Diseases

*Johannes Ring, MD, PhD and Benedetta Belloni, MD*

## Introduction: The Skin as an Immune Organ

Not only the skin is the largest organ of the body, the barrier against noxious influences from the environment, a sensory organ, and a metabolic organ, but it is also an immune organ: all the necessary constituents to produce an immune response are present in the skin. Epidermal dendritic cells (Langerhans cells) lie immediately under the stratum corneum and represent the outermost "sentinel" of our immune system. Furthermore, the skin contains different types of lymphocytes and dendritic cells in the dermis. In addition, the dermis homes mast cells and bystander cells, acting as effector cells. Keratinocytes have been shown to produce all kinds of cytokines and chemokines that play an important role in the immune response. Furthermore, there is ample capacity of innate immune responses like antimicrobial peptides (e.g., defensins) or dendritic cells with various pathogen reaction pattern receptors (e.g., toll-like receptors [TLRs]) to attract inflammatory cells such as neutrophilic leukocytes among others.

Under normal, healthy circumstances, this immune system is not sleeping; it is constantly regulated to stay in balance. Dendritic cells of the epidermis as well as regulatory T cells play an important role in this regulation and balance.

There are several ways in which this homeostatic balance can be disturbed—either by disruption of natural tolerance against self-antigens (autoimmunity) or by pathogenic immune reactions against foreign substances, be it small chemicals (haptens) or proteins leading to allergic skin diseases.

## Allergic Skin Diseases

Allergy is defined as an immunologically mediated hypersensitivity reaction leading to disease and can be classified into several pathogenic types of immune reactions (modified according to Coombs and Gell):

Type I   Immediate hypersensitivity, Immunoglobulin E (IgE)-mediated (urticaria, angioedema, anaphylaxis, allergic rhinoconjunctivitis, extrinsic bronchial asthma, atopic eczema (AE))

Type II   Cytotoxic immune reactions (thrombocytopenic purpura, other hematologic allergies)

Type III   Immune complex reactions (serum sickness, leukocytoclastic vasculitis, immune complex anaphylaxis, urticaria)

Type IV   Cellular hypersensitivity

Type IVa   T-helper-cells type1 (Th1)-mediated allergic contact dermatitis, delayed-type hypersensitivity

Type IVb   T-helper-cells type2 (Th2)-mediated, atopic eczema (see also type I)

Type IVc   CD8-mediated exanthematous and bullous drug eruptions

Type IVd   Th17-mediated pustular drug eruptions (acute generalized exanthematous pustulosis [AGEP])

Type V   Granulomatous skin reactions (e.g., to bovine collagen, tattoo reactions)

Type VI   Stimulating–neutralizing reaction (autoantibodies against IgE or Fcε receptor in chronic urticaria)

No other organ shows a similar wide spectrum of different pathophysiologic mechanisms as well as clinical manifestations of allergic reactions like the skin (Table 9-1).

**TABLE 9-1 ■ Various Types of Pathogenic Immune Reactions Manifesting on the Skin**

| Clinical Manifestations | Possible Pathomechanism |
| --- | --- |
| Urticaria | IgE, serum sickness (type I) |
| Purpura (thrombocytopenic) | Cytotoxic (type II) |
| Purpura (vasculitis) | Immune complex (type III) |
| Atopic eczema | IgE + Th2 (type I + type IVb) |
| Allergic contact dermatitis | Th1 (type IVa) |
| Maculopapular exanthema | Type IV |
| Exfoliative dermatitis | Type IVa (CD4) |
| Lymphohistiocytic infiltration | Possibly type IV |
| Vesiculobullous and fixed drug eruption | Type IVc (CD8) |
| Toxic epidermal necrolysis (Lyell's syndrome) | Possibly type IVc (CD8) |
| Granulomatous reaction (e.g., bovine collagen) | Type V |
| Autoimmune urticaria | Type VI? |

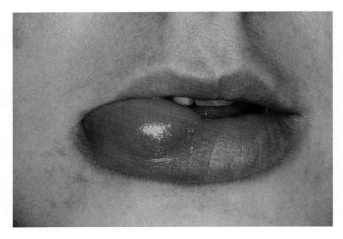

**FIGURE 9-2** ■ Swelling of a large portion of the lower lip illustrative of angioedema.

In the following text, the most important allergic skin diseases will be briefly described. It has to be mentioned that all of the allergic diseases—whether they are in the skin or in the respiratory tract—can also be induced by nonimmune reactions (pseudoallergic reactions or "intrinsic" types), whereby these terms are negatively defined by the absence of detectable specific immune reactions.

## Urticaria, Angioedema, Anaphylaxis

Urticaria (Fig. 9-1) is defined as the occurrence of wheals, which generally stay for one to several hours, in rare cases up to 2 or 3 days (urticaria vasculitis). The classical example of urticaria is the histamine-induced wheal, which develops after 10 to 15 minutes of injection of histamine into the skin via prick or intradermal test and leads to a wheal and flare reaction associated with itch. The basis is an increased capillary permeability (edema), vasodilatation (redness), and an axon

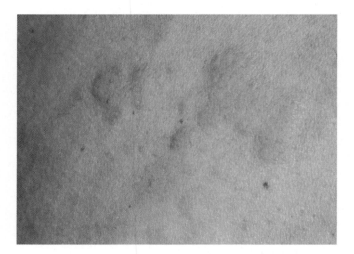

**FIGURE 9-1** ■ Typical wheals or urticaria with elevated well-demarcated erythematous plaques that were evanescent.

reflex leading to further vasodilatation (flare) (Lewis' triad or triple response of Lewis).

Angioedema (Fig. 9-2) is often regarded as the subcutaneous form of urticaria with large and deep swellings, particularly in soft tissues (eyelids, lips, genital area). Urticaria and angioedema can occur in any part of the body (also on palms and soles, where patients feel pain instead of itch). Urticarial skin lesions, although itchy, are never scratched so that blood appears, but rather rubbed superficially. There are obviously different qualities of the itch sensation, which can be felt but not clearly described in our language.

Urticaria can be classified into acute (wheals occurring over a period of less than 6 weeks) and chronic (wheals appearing over a period longer than 6 weeks), which can be either intermittent or chronically relapsing with wheals appearing almost every day.

Acute urticaria is most often associated with acute infection and/or an allergic stimulus (e.g., food, drug). Chronic urticaria is also often called idiopathic when trigger factors cannot be detected. These trigger factors can be either allergens or infectious diseases of internal organs. Additives in foods can give rise to pseudoallergic type I reactions in a subgroup of chronic urticaria patients.

Autoantibodies against IgE or the high-affinity IgE receptor have been found that lead to mast cell degranulation; this phenomenon can be shown in the autologous serum test when a wheal develops after injection of a 1/10 dilution of autologous serum (Greaves' test) (see also type VI). Another subgroup of chronic urticaria when the wheals persist over several days shows leukocytoclastic vasculitis in the dermatohistopathology and is called urticarial vasculitis. This disease is sometimes associated with autoimmune diseases (lupus erythematosus).

## Management

Antihistamines are the drugs of choice; sedating antihistamines can be given overnight, sometimes also having a beneficial effect on underlying stress reactions with psychosomatic involvement. During the day, the modern nonsedating histamine H1 antagonists are helpful. When urticaria recurs, an allergy workup or workup for an underlying infection may be beneficial. Psychosomatic counseling often is helpful in chronic urticaria. A subgroup of physical urticaria, where wheals are induced by mechanical stimuli (urticaria factitia, dermographism, pressure), temperature (cold or warm), or radiation (solar urticaria), is difficult to treat. Dapsone (avlosulfone) has been proven helpful in some cases.

Urticaria and angioedema may always be the first signs of anaphylaxis. Therefore, they have to be taken seriously. Patients with acute, severe urticaria should be observed at least 1 hour after the onset of therapy (best intravenous or intramuscular) of antihistamines and/or steroids to make sure that no further symptoms of anaphylaxis develop.

## Thrombocytopenic Purpura

This is a classical type II reaction in the skin, where antibodies against substances (mostly drugs) on the surface of platelets lead to thrombocytopenia and noninflammatory purpura. This rather rare condition can be elicited by analgesics or hypnotics. The idiopathic form can be treated with intravenous immunoglobulin (IVIG).

## Allergic Leukocytoclastic Vasculitis

This is the prototype of a type III allergic reaction in the skin, where immune complexes lead to attraction of neutrophils with activation of proteases and mast cells, leading to destruction of vessels and vessel walls. Most often, infectious (hepatitis) or neoplastic diseases are elicitors; however, food allergens and drugs can also induce allergic leukocytoclastic vasculitis (Fig. 9-3). In the course of serum sickness (the allergic condition inspiring Clemens von Pirquet to create the term "allergy" over 100 years ago), urticaria goes along with fever and lymph node swelling in an acute type III reaction.

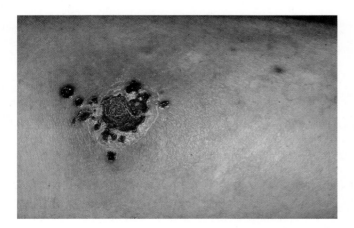

**FIGURE 9-3** ■ Hemorrhagic confluent papules with ill-defined erythema fading from the center, indicative of leukocytoclastic vasculitis.

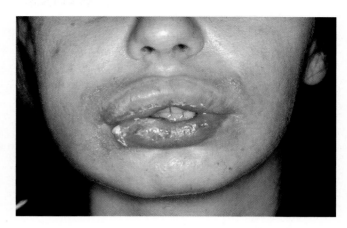

**FIGURE 9-4** ■ Severe swelling of the lips with surrounding erythema with vesicles, typical of a contact dermatitis to toothpaste, mouthwash, chewing gum, or food.

## Allergic Contact Dermatitis

Allergic contact dermatitis (ACD) (Fig. 9-4) is the most common occupational disease in many countries of the Western world. The dermatopathology of ACD shows acanthosis, parakeratosis, spongiosis (intercellular edema in the epidermis with intact desmosomes looking like a sponge), and lymphocytic infiltrations in the upper dermis. The terms "dermatitis" and "eczema" are used interchangeably in the dermatologic literature and are defined as:

"Non-contagious epidermo-dermitis with characteristic clinical (synchronous or metachronous polymorphology) and dermato-pathological characteristics (acanthosis, parakeratosis, spongiosis) occurring mostly on the basis of hypersensitivity."

There are several types of eczema/dermatitis diseases (Table 9-2).

Seborrheic dermatitis may represent a hyperergic reaction to skin microflora (*Malassezia* species) and show a little spongiosis.

ACD develops against small chemicals (haptens) taken up by epidermal dendritic cells (Langerhans cells) and then presented to lymphocytes that polarize into Th1 cells, leading to the inflammation in the skin. Dendritic cells attract these cells when

**TABLE 9-2** ■ **Classification of Eczema/Dermatitis**

Contact dermatitis
- Allergic
- Irritant

Atopic eczema (atopic dermatitis, eczema)
- Intrinsic atopic eczema
- Extrinsic atopic eczema

Nummular eczema

Seborrheic dermatitis

Others

carrying the cutaneous lymphocyte antigen (CLA). Major cytokines produced by these lymphocytes are interleukin-2, tumor necrosis factor alpha (TNF-$\alpha$), and interferon gamma (IFN-$\gamma$), giving rise to keratinocyte apoptosis and spongiosis.

The most common contact allergens are tested in standard series, constantly updated by international or regional contact dermatitis research groups (ICDRG, American CDRG, European CDRG, etc.). A current standard is shown in Table 9-3.

ACD is very common in the population (15%, not only in hospital series but also in population-based studies). Nickel and fragrances seem to be the most common contact

**TABLE 9-3** ■ **Standard Patch Test Series of the German Contact Dermatitis Research Group (2006)**

| Test Substance | Vehicle | Concentration (%)* |
|---|---|---|
| Potassium dichromate | P | 0.5 |
| Thiuram mix[†] | PP | 1.0 |
| Cobalt (II) chloride 6H$_2$O | P | 1.0 |
| Balsam of Peru | P | 25.0 |
| Colophony (rosin) | P | 20.0 |
| N-isopropyl-N-phenyl-p-phenylenediamine | P | 0.1 |
| Wool wax alcohol | P | 30.0 |
| Mercapto mix[‡] | P | 1.0 |
| Epoxy resin | P | 1.0 |
| Nickel (II) sulfate 6H$_2$O | P | 5.0 |
| p-tert-Butylphenol formaldehyde resin | P | 1.0 |
| Formaldehyde | W | 1.0 |
| Fragrance mix I[§] | P | 8.0 |
| Turpentine | P | 10.0 |
| (Chlor-)methylisothiazolinone | W | 100 ppm |
| Paraben mix|| | P | 16.0 |
| Cetyl stearyl alcohol | P | 20.0 |
| Zinc diethyldithiocarbamate | P | 1.0 |
| Dibromodicyanobutane | P | 0.3 |
| Propolis | P | 10.0 |
| Bufexamac | P | 5.0 |
| Compositae mix[¶] | P | 5.0 |
| Mercaptobenzothiazole | P | 2.0 |
| Lyral (fragrance) | P | 5.0 |
| Fragrance mix II[#] | P | 14.0 |
| Bronopol (2-bromo-2-nitro-1,3-propandiol | P | 0.5 |

*Note: para*-Phenylenediamine has been removed from the German standard series due to the risk of active sensitization. It is tested only if it is suspected of being a relevant allergen in an individual patient.

*If not otherwise specified.

[†]Thiuram mix, 1%: tetramethylthiurammonosulfide, 0.25%; tetramethylthiuramdisulfide, 0.25%; tetraethylthiuramdisulfide, 0.25%; and dipentamethylenethiuramdisulfide, 0.25%.

[‡]Mercapto mix, 1%: N-cyclohexylbenzothiazylsulfenamide, 0.33%; dibenzothiazyldisulfide, 0.33%; morpholinylmercaptobenzothiazole, 0.33%.

[§]Fragrance mix I, 18.0%: cinnamic alcohol, 1.0%; cinnamic aldehyde, 1.0%; eugenol, 1.0%; amyl cinnamic aldehyde, 1.0%; hydroxycitronellal, 1.0%,; geraniol, 1.0%; isoeugenol, 1.0%; oak moss, 1.0%.

||Paraben mix, 16.0%: butyl-, ethyl-, methyl-, propyl-p-oxybenzoic acid, each 4.0%.

[¶]Compositae mix, 5%: *Tanacetum vulgare,* 1.0%; *Arnica montana,* 0.5%; parthenolide, 0.1%; *Chamomilla romana,* 2.4%, *Achillea millefolium,* 1.0%.

[#]Fragrance mix II, 14%: $\alpha$-hexal cinnamic aldehyde, 5%; citral, 1%,; citronellol, 0.5%; coumarin, 2.5%; farnesol, 2.5%; hydroxymethylpentylcyclohexencarboxaldehyde, 2.5%.

*Abbreviations:* P, white petrolatum; W, water; ppm, parts per million.

allergens. For special occupations, specific test series have been developed (hairdressers, bricklayers, bakers, etc.). Careful diagnosis and avoidance of eliciting allergens is the mainstay of therapy. This often leads to changes in profession since currently there is no way to induce tolerance for ACD as there is in IgE-mediated disease (allergen-specific immunotherapy [ASIT]). Symptomatic treatment is performed with topical (rarely systemic) glucocorticosteroids, together with ultraviolet (UV) therapy (e.g., topical psoralens and ultraviolet light [PUVA] in allergic hand dermatitis). Recently, in chronic hand eczema, alitretinoin (Panretin) has been introduced as a therapeutic novelty.

## Atopic Eczema/Atopic Dermatitis

AE (also called atopic dermatitis or eczema) is the most common inflammatory skin disease in childhood (Fig. 9-5) (10% to 20% of children affected in some Western countries), but it can also occur in adults with increasing frequency.

There are several diagnostic criteria that comprise major and minor features (Hanifin and Rajka, UK working party). Simple diagnostic criteria are shown in Table 9-4.

In over 80% of cases, AE typically starts in the first years of life, sometimes as early as 6 to 12 weeks after birth. It shows a typical predilection of affected body sites according to age, with the extensor surfaces in the face in the infantile phase and the big flexors in children and young adults, ending in chronic lichenified lesions on hands and feet and, later, prurigo nodules (prurigo-type) all over the body.

The condition is extremely itchy. The skin is scratched until bleeding, often bed clothes are bloody, and the quality of life is highly disturbed, not only for patients but also for the families. The famous slogan "If I don't sleep, nobody

| TABLE 9-4 ■ **Simplified Criteria for Atopic Eczema** |
|---|
| Typical morphologic changes for age |
| Typical age-dependent localization |
| Pruritus |
| Stigmata of atopy |
| Personal or family history of atopy |
| IgE-mediated sensitization |

*Note:* When four out of six criteria are positive, the diagnosis of atopic eczema may be made.

*Source:* From Ring J, Przybilla B, Ruzicka T, eds. *Handbook of Atopic Eczema.* 2nd ed. Berlin: Springer; 2006. With kind permission of Springer Science+Business Media.

sleeps" contains a lot of truth. A hallmark in the pathophysiology of AE is the barrier disturbance, which most likely is due to a mutation in the filaggrin gene. Filaggrin is a relevant protein forming the cornified envelope leading to the correct attachment of keratin filaments in lipids in the stratum corneum. When filaggrin is defective (15% of the European population), the skin is "dry" and shows epidermal barrier dysfunction, associated with a higher risk of AE (Odds ratio [OR] 3-4).

Pathophysiologically, AE corresponds to a type IVb reaction, which is a mixture of IgE and Th2 at the onset of disease, but in the chronic phase Th1 activity predominates. There are a few diseases with similarly elevated IgE levels in the serum. Not all sensitizations against food or aeroallergens are clinically relevant.

For a long time, these IgE-mediated sensitizations were only regarded as epiphenomenon since the patients also suffered from hay fever and asthma. However, recently, it has become clear that IgE-inducing allergens can induce eczema on the uninvolved skin, as shown in the atopy patch test (APT). The most frequent allergens eliciting positive APT reactions are house-dust mites, pollen, and animal epithelium (cat). These reactions most often manifest in air-exposed body areas (face, arms, and hands).

In many patients, foods can also trigger AE, more often in children than in adults. The gold standard to prove the relevance of a given food allergen is the double-blind placebo-controlled food challenge (DBPCFC), which is a tedious but important test to help avoid unnecessary dietary restrictions. We have seen many harmed children suffering from malnutrition because parents were following a very restrictive, irrational, and not at all indicated diet.

## Management

Management of AE includes a careful allergy history to identify individual provocation factors that can be avoided. Acute treatment is done with antipruriginous and anti-inflammatory agents. Topical glucocorticosteroids (mild to moderate) are the mainstay. Many patients or parents are reluctant to use corticosteroids (corticophobia). It takes time to explain the whole process of management and reduce baseless fears.

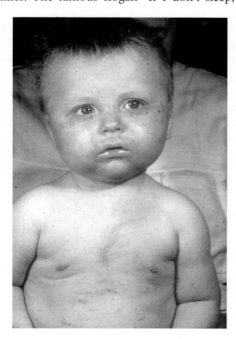

**FIGURE 9-5** ■ Marked atopic dermatitis in an infant with oozing crusted dermatitis under the eyes and over the trunk.

**TABLE 9-5 ■ Morphologic Variants of Cutaneous Drug Eruptions**

| Morphology | Elicitor (Examples) |
|---|---|
| Urticarial eruptions | See "Foods, Drugs" |
| Erythematovesicular eruptions | See "Contact Dermatitis" |
| Purpura/hemorrhagic eruptions | See "Cytotoxic Reactions" and "Immune Complex Reactions" |
| Erythema multiforme | Barbiturates |
|  | Sulfonamides |
|  | Hydantoin |
|  | Hydralazine |
|  | Carbamazepine |
|  | Diuretics |
|  | NSAIDs |
| Erythema nodosum | Anticonceptives |
|  | Halogens |
|  | Sulfonamides |
| Macular and maculopapular | Penicillin |
|  | Ampicillin |
|  | Allopurinol |
|  | Sulfonamides |
|  | NSAIDs |
| Exfoliative dermatitis | Antiepileptics |
|  | Phenylbutazone |
|  | Heavy metals (e.g., arsenic) |
| Fixed drug eruption | Barbiturates |
|  | Analgesics |
|  | NSAIDs |
|  | Tetracycline |
|  | Sulfonamides |
|  | Anticonceptives |
|  | Hydantoin |
|  | Laxants |
|  | Metronidazole |
| Lichenoid drug eruptions | Thiazides |
|  | Phenothiazine |
|  | Captopril |
|  | Gold |
|  | Sulfonamides |
| Acneiform drug eruptions | Steroid hormones |
|  | Halogens |
|  | Lithium isoniazid |
|  | Vitamins (B) |
|  | Hydantoin |
| Lymphocytic infiltration | Analgesics (plus alcohol?) |

**TABLE 9-5 ■ (continued)**

| Morphology | Elicitor (Examples) |
|---|---|
| Psoriasiform eruptions | Beta-blockers |
|  | Gold salts |
|  | Lithium |

For some years, topical calcineurin inhibitors (TCI) such as tacrolimus and pimecrolimus have been in use. They have anti-inflammatory effects without the classical steroid side effects (like skin atrophy). They also have special antipruritic effects. In the United States, there is currently a black box warning indicating a risk of cutaneous lymphoma with these medications. Most experts however think this is unwarranted, and there are efforts to have this warning removed.

Until recently, acute exacerbation was treated and, after symptoms subsided, emollients only were used until the next relapse occurred. Now, many authors have changed to a so-called proactive strategy, whereby low-potency steroids or TCIs are given once or twice weekly over longer periods in order to prevent the next exacerbation.

Not all AE cases are associated with IgE reactions; there are cases of so-called "intrinsic" AE, which clinically is very similar but no IgE antibodies are found. This intrinsic type is more common in childhood and in females.

Basic skin care (better treatment of the disturbed barrier function) with emollients and oil baths is the mainstay in topical dermatotherapy. There is no miracle pill or ointment, but individual approaches can be found for each patient.

UV therapy has proven helpful, especially the long-wave UVA-1 modalities. For very severe cases, climate therapy (high altitude) above 1,500 m (e.g., Davos, Switzerland) has proven helpful.

Contrary to psoriasis, where the new biologics have tremendously enriched the therapeutic armamentarium, in AE there is only limited experimental hope from occasional studies with anti-IgE, anti-IL-5, anti-CD20, or others.

Psychosomatic involvement in AE is considerable. Many patients suffer from exacerbations due to psychic stress. Coping strategies and stress management techniques can be helpful (autogenous training, progressive muscle relaxation, etc.). Therefore, educational programs have been developed—"eczema schools," which work well and are reimbursed by insurance in some countries.

### Exanthematous Drug Eruptions

Exanthematous drug eruptions can be classified according to either pathophysiology (Table 9-1) or morphology (Table 9-5). They can occur after many different drugs; the rule is: at the beginning, every bystander is a suspect. Even rare elicitors can be responsible in a single individual. Of course, there are hit lists of drugs eliciting cutaneous drug eruptions in a typical morphology more often than others. However, in single cases, the history has to be taken very carefully. Drugs that have been introduced recently are more suspect than others; however, severe cutaneous drug eruptions have been attributed to drugs that have been taken over years.

Maculopapular eruptions can also be induced by viral infections. Sometimes they require the combination of a virus and a drug, like the ampicillin rash where Epstein–Barr virus infection together with ampicillin induces the rash in almost 100% of patients. Maculopapular exanthema is most often benign; however, it can progress to bullous-type eruptions.

A severe complication is the drug-related eosinophilia with systemic symptoms (DRESS) or drug-induced delayed multiorgan system hypersensitivity syndrome (DIDMOHS), where maculopapular exanthema together with fever and eosinophilia goes along with serious internal organ involvement (elicitors include antiepileptics, Human immunodeficiency virus [HIV] medication, etc.).

The most serious cutaneous adverse reaction is toxic epidermal necrolysis (TEN), also called drug-induced Lyell's syndrome, where the whole skin can "swim off" like in a severe burn (syndrome of burning skin). In staphylococcal scalded skin syndrome (SSSS), the blister is subcorneal, whereas in TEN, the blister forms in the lower parts of the epidermis with total necrosis of keratinocytes and conspicuously little inflammation.

Hit lists of elicitors of TEN are

- Allopurinol
- Carbamazepine
- Cotrimoxazole
- Lamotrigine
- Nevirapine
- Nonsteroidal anti-inflammatory drugs (NSAIDs)
- Phenobarbital
- Phenytoin
- Sulfonamides

There are registers of severe cutaneous reactions in some countries, which continuously update and identify the most common triggers of this severe condition.

Even under the best treatment conditions (intensive care, burn wards, isolated room), the lethality of this condition is still between 20% and 30%. Most often affected are elderly individuals with polypragmatic pharmacotherapy (10 to 15 different drugs), which makes the identification of the elicitors often very difficult.

There is controversy regarding treatment with glucocorticosteroids. Most authors recommend a short (4 days), high-dose steroid treatment, while others prefer IVIG. Cyclosporine has been advocated by some authors. Due to the dramatic nature of the disease, controlled clinical trials are very difficult to perform. The involvement of the mucosa including the conjunctiva of the eye makes careful ophthalmologic care mandatory.

Erythema exsudativum multiforme can be either virus- (herpes simplex) or drug-induced. If it affects more than 10% of the body surface and goes along with a mucosal involvement, it is called Stevens–Johnson syndrome, which can eventually progress to TEN.

Although some drugs more often induce a specific reaction pattern such an exanthematous drug eruption (e.g., gold salts inducing lichenoid eruptions), the morphology of the skin eruption does not identify the elicitor. A common drug, like penicillin, can elicit all kinds of pathogenic immune reactions (from urticaria and anaphylaxis to contact dermatitis and exanthematous eruptions) via different mechanisms.

## Autoimmune Skin Diseases

Autoimmunity develops through a loss of tolerance to self-proteins, which normally evolves during embryonic life, leading to reactions against self-proteins or nucleic acids. There are two major groups of autoimmune skin diseases:

- Connective tissue diseases (also called collagenoses)
- Autoimmune blistering diseases

### Connective Tissue Diseases

Connective tissue diseases are systemic diseases with involvement of the skin and other organs with many symptoms and overlap stages. Characteristically, patients develop autoantibodies against self-substances and deposits of immune complexes in tissue. The most common connective tissue diseases are

- Lupus erythematosus (LE)
- Scleroderma
- Dermatomyositis

LE represents a spectrum of diseases that range from acute life-threatening systemic disease (acute SLE) to mild variants like subacute cutaneous LE (SCLE) and discoid LE (DLE), which is usually only in the skin. There are many overlaps of these extremes.

SLE is characterized by autoantibodies and immune complexes (Table 9-6) against substances from cell nuclei (nucleic acids, nucleoproteins, etc.). The prevalence of SLE is 15 to 50 per 100 000, with a female preponderance. Seven percent of patients with SLE have skin symptoms, which typically include a butterfly rash (Fig. 9-6) (symmetrical erythema in the face, often photo-aggravated). On the trunk, there are maculopapular skin eruptions, on the dorsum of the fingers, red partly keratotic patches, and hyperkeratosis of the eponychium and finger tips. Systemic symptoms include fever, weight loss, and arthralgia. Serous surfaces can be inflamed as pleuritis or pericarditis. Glomerulonephritis is a severe complication in 70% of patients. Psychiatric and neurologic symptoms can occur. For the diagnosis, the criteria of the American Rheumatism Association (ARA) are helpful (Table 9-7).

Dermatopathologic findings are hyperkeratosis of the epidermis, hydropic degeneration of basal keratinocytes with thickening of the basal membrane, increased dermal mucin, as well as lymphocytic inflammatory infiltrate along the vessels and adnexa in the dermis (so-called "interface dermatitis"). In immunofluorescence, deposits of IgG and IgM as well as C3 are found at the dermo-epidermal junction (Fig. 9-7).

**TABLE 9-6 ■ Antinuclear Antibodies and Clinical Manifestation of Lupus Erythematosus**

| Autoantigen | Molecule | Clinical Relevance |
|---|---|---|
| dsDNA | Native DNA | Severe SLE |
| Sm | Ribonucleoprotein | Severe SLE with renal involvement |
| U1-RNP | Ribonucleoprotein | Mild SLE, overlap syndromes |
| rRNP | Ribosomal protein | Overlap syndromes, SLE with cerebral involvement |
| Ro (SSA) | Ribonucleoprotein | SCLE, Sjögren syndrome, neonatal LE |
| La (SSB) | Ribonucleoprotein | SCLE, Sjögren syndrome, neonatal LE |
| Ku | Repair protein | SLE with polymyositis |
| Histone | Histone | Drug-induced LE |

### Subacute Cutaneous Lupus Erythematosus

SCLE shows a strong photosensitivity and is characterized by the presence of antibodies against cytoplasmic proteins Ro/SS-A (Table 9-6). There is less systemic involvement.

### Discoid Lupus Erythematosus

DLE is a chronic relapsing skin disease, predominantly in the light-exposed areas (face), with discoid red squamous plaques with atrophy and hyperkeratosis. In DLE, autoantibodies are often absent. In dermatopathology, an atrophic epidermis with hyperkeratosis and keratotic plaques as well as vacuolization of basal cells, edema, and thickening of the basal membrane are characteristic, together with a perivascular and perifollicular lymphocytic infiltrate. Rare forms include lupus erythematosus profundus, also called lupus panniculitis, with deep subcutaneous painful nodules as well as drug-induced LE, where autoantibodies against histones are characteristic.

### Management

Since UV is often an aggravating factor, photoprotection is mandatory, which involves anti-inflammatory treatment with systemic or topical glucocorticosteroids, sometimes as high as 100 to 200 mg prednisolone per day. Sometimes immunosuppressives, like azathioprine or cyclophosphamide, are added. Milder forms can be treated by hydroxychloroquine (ophthalmologic control). In more cutaneous forms, topical therapy with glucocorticosteroids is essential.

### Scleroderma

Scleroderma can be subdivided into circumscript scleroderma (also called morphea) and systemic scleroderma or progressive systemic scleroderma (PSS). Scleroderma is a disease of the connective tissue with fibrosis, vascular changes, and inflammation.

***Progressive Systemic Scleroderma.*** PSS is a rare disease with a preponderance of women between 40 and 50 years. There are different clinical subtypes:

- Limited systemic scleroderma, also called acrosclerotic type, with mild involvement of internal organs

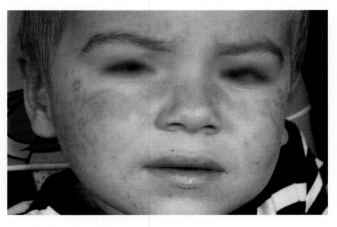

**FIGURE 9-6 ■** Classic butterfly erythema of acute cutaneous lupus erythematosus over the central face of a child.

**TABLE 9-7 ■ Criteria of the American College of Rheumatology (ACR) for diagnosis of SLE**

Malar rash (butterfly rash)

Discoid rash

Photosensitivity

Oral ulcers

Arthritis

Serositis (pleura, pericardium)

Renal disorders

Neurologic disorders

Hematologic disorder (leukopenia, anemia, thrombocytopenia)

Immunologic disorder

Antinuclear antibodies

*Note:* If 4 of the criteria are positive, the diagnosis of SLE is made.

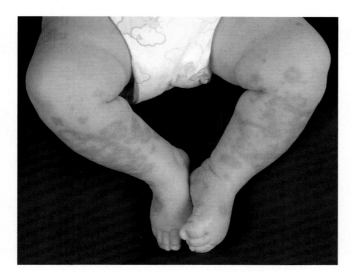

**FIGURE 9-7** ■ Neonatal lupus erythematosus with atrophic white centers and surrounding circinate erythema.

- CREST syndrome (calcinosis cutis, Raynaud's syndrome, esophageal stenosis, sclerodactyly, telangiectasias)
- Diffuse systemic sclerosis with rapid progression and massive involvement of internal organs

Clinically, characteristic signs are sclerosis of the skin, small face and loss of mimic movement, microstomia, and microcheilia. Frenulum sclerosis of the tongue is common. Acrosclerosis (Fig. 9-8) goes along with necrosis of the fingertips. Internal organ involvement shows esophageal stenosis with dyskinesia, interstitial fibrosis of the lung with restrictive ventilatory insufficiency, nephritis with proteinuria and hypertension, interstitial fibrosis of the heart with myocardial insufficiency, and secondary pulmonary hypertension. Antinuclear antibodies comprise antibodies against RNA polymerase and DNA topoisomerase (Scl 70); in CREST syndrome, anticentromere antibodies are typical.

The treatment is difficult; in acute inflammatory phases, systemic glucocorticosteroids and immunosuppressives are

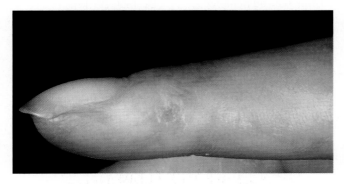

**FIGURE 9-8** ■ Stellate calcific scar of the distal side of a sclerotic finger in a patient with scleroderma.

given (azathioprine, cyclophosphamide). Fibrosis has been treated with D-penicillamine or intravenous penicillin, sometimes together with UVA. Vasodilatory strategies include pentoxifylline, ACE inhibitors, and calcium antagonists. New treatment options with endothelin receptor antagonists have proven to be effective in reducing pulmonary hypertension and fingertip necrosis. Regular and careful physiotherapy is important.

***Localized Scleroderma (Morphea).*** Morphea is a connective tissue disease with patchy fibrosing plaques slowly spreading with a slight erythematous surface and a lilac-colored border (lilac ring). The sclerotic areas later become atrophic and lose hair and sweat capabilities; some show hyper- or hypopigmentation.

Dermatopathologically, dense lymphocytic infiltrates are found in the superficial and deep dermis together with edema and, in progressive stages, fibrosis. Fibrotic entrapment of the eccrine sweat glands is characteristic.

There are different clinical subtypes of morphea:

- Plaque-like morphea
- Disseminated morphea
- Linear morphea, most spectacular as "en coup de sabre" from forehead to cheeks (this sometimes shows connections to progressive hemifacial atrophy (Parry–Romberg), which goes along with disfiguration and involvement of the subcutaneous fat and the bone)
- Disabling pansclerotic morphea of children (in this very serious disease, joint contractions and mutilating changes are prominent)

Treatment is started with topical glucocorticosteroids, UV therapy may also help, as well as topical vitamin D3 analogs (calcipotriene) or intravenous penicillin. Regular physical therapy is very important.

### Dermatomyositis

Dermatomyositis is an autoimmune disease affecting the skin and the skeletal muscles as well as the internal organs. In some patients it represents a paraneoplasia. Most commonly affected are females between 30 and 50 years.

Dermatomyositis manifests typically in the face with lilac-colored erythema and swellings, leading to characteristic depressive facies (Fig. 9-9). On the dorsum of the digits, red papules, lichenoid and atrophic (Gottron signs), are typical, as well as periungual telangiectasia (Fig. 9-10) and pain. Sometimes poikiloderma can occur with calcinosis in the subcutaneous tissue.

The first symptom is often weakness of the proximal muscles (trying to elevate the arms or climb the stairs). Myositis goes along with elevated creatine kinase values in the serum, abnormal electromyography, and inflammation in the muscular tissue. Autoantibodies comprise Anti nuclear antibodies (ANA) as well as antibodies against Jo1 (histidyl tRNA-synthetase) and Mi2 (nucleoprotein).

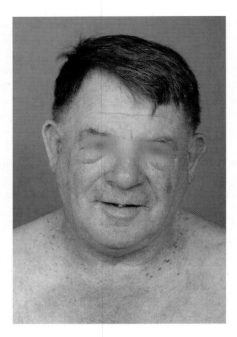

**FIGURE 9-9** ■ Swelling and redness over the eyelids and a photodistributed erythematous eruption over the chest in a patient with dermatomyositis.

Differential diagnosis comprises SLE as well as overlap syndromes and other muscular diseases such as fibromyalgia or myasthenia gravis, and trichinosis.

In adults, screening for tumors is essential before starting therapy, which consists of high doses of glucocorticosteroids given systemically in the initial phase and slowly tapered down to safer doses. Often, immunosuppressive treatment with azathioprine, methotrexate, or cyclosporin is indicated. IVIG is sometimes beneficial. If underlying neoplasias are found, disease-directed treatment will often diminish symptoms. Childhood dermatomyositis generally has a better prognosis.

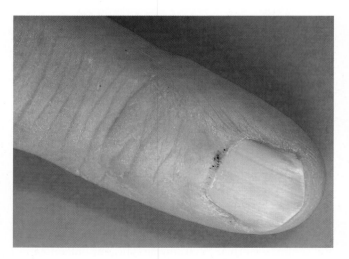

**FIGURE 9-10** ■ Sausage-shaped capillary telangiectasias and hemmorrhages of the proximal nail fold seen most often in dermatomyositis.

## Autoimmune Blistering Disease

The immunologically mediated blistering diseases can be classified into three groups:

- Pemphigus group
- Pemphigoid group
- Dermatitis herpetiformis (DH) and IgA linear dermatoses

The three groups differ both in clinical manifestations as well as in pathophysiology and dermatopathology (Table 9-8).

### Pemphigus Group

The blistering in pemphigus occurs via acantholysis, that is, loss or dysfunction of desmosomes through antibodies against desmogleins 1 and 3. Desmogleins are transmembrane proteins (cadherin family) that are crucial for keratinocyte adhesion.

***Pemphigus Vulgaris.*** Pemphigus vulgaris often starts in the mucosa (Fig. 9-11) (oral or genital), at the umbilicus or the scalp. Characteristic are soft blisters that are rapidly destroyed and leave erosions and crusting. In an acute phase, it is possible to induce a blister by tangential pressure on the skin (Nikolski's phenomenon 1).

In a smear, rounded keratinocytes are found (Tzanck test) as a demonstration of acantholysis. In dermatopathology, the blister is intraepidermal with leukocyte infiltrates and deposits of IgG and complement in the intercellular areas of epidermis. Autoantibodies are directed against desmoglein 3.

**TABLE 9-8** ■ **Autoantibodies in Blistering Autoimmune Diseases**

| Disease | Autoantigen |
|---|---|
| Pemphigus vulgaris | Desmoglein 3 |
| Pemphigus vegetans | Desmoglein 3 |
| Pemphigus foliaceus | Desmoglein 1 |
| Pemphigus seborrhoicus | Desmoglein 1 |
| Pemphigus erythematosus | Desmoglein 1, nuclear antigens |
| Drug-induced pemphigus | Desmoglein 1, desmoglein 3 |
| Paraneoplastic pemphigus | Desmoglein 3 (also desmoplakin 1 and 2, BP 230) |
| Bullous pemphigoid | BP180 (collagen type XVII), BP 230 |
| Pemphigoid gestationis | BP 180, BP 230 |
| Linear IgA dermatosis | BP 180, LAD 1 |
| Mucous membrane pemphigoid | BP 180, laminin 332 and 331, $\alpha6\ \beta4$-integrin |
| Epidermolysis bullosa acquisita | Type VII collagen |

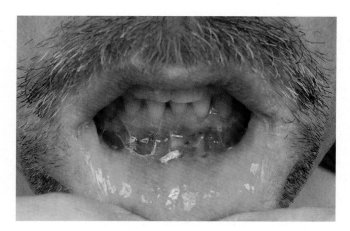

**FIGURE 9-11** ■ An oral erosion of the mucous membranes in a patient with pemphigus.

*Therapy:* systemic glucocorticosteroids in rather high doses (1 to 2 mg prednisolone/kg/d) slowly tapered down. Sometimes, additional immunosuppression with azathioprine, cyclophosphamide, methotrexate, cyclosporin A, and plasmapheresis are considered. A hopeful new treatment is the biologic anti-CD20 (rituximab).

***Pemphigus Vegetans.*** Pemphigus vegetans is a special form of pemphigus vulgaris, where the blisters and erosions are followed by papillomatous proliferations of tissue, especially in the intertriginous areas.

***Pemphigus Foliaceus.*** Pemphigus foliaceus is mediated through antibodies against desmoglein 1, which is more prominent in the upper epidermis; therefore, the blisters are more superficial and often immediately scaly and crusty (like foils) (Fig. 9-12).

A subtype of endemic pemphigus foliaceus in Brazil is called "fogo selvagem" (wild fire) and has been associated with some insect bites. Pemphigus erythematosus (pemphigus seborrhoicus, Senear–Usher syndrome) is a variant of pemphigus foliaceus that occurs together with LE and shows pemphigus antibodies plus ANAs in the laboratory; this is a very rare disease.

***Paraneoplastic Pemphigus.*** Paraneoplastic pemphigus is seen in association with certain malignant neoplasias (lymphoma, thymoma, and other cancers). It is a subtype of pemphigus and occurs with autoantibodies against desmoplakin I and II as well as bullous pemphigoid antigen in the hemidesmosomes in basal keratinocytes. Clinically, there is a polymorphous skin eruption with erythematous areas, blisters, and target-like lesions as well as erosions with mucosal involvement. Pemphigus paraneoplasticus often does not respond well to classical therapy.

*Pemphigoid Group*

***Bullous Pemphigoid.*** Bullous pemphigoid (BP) is a disease of the elderly and the most common autoimmune bullous

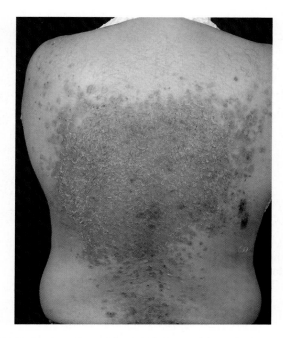

**FIGURE 9-12** ■ Pemphigus foliaceus with typical "foil-like" scaling.

disease in the Western world (4/100,000). Clinically, large, tense, serum-containing and pressure-resistant blisters mushroom out of normal skin or on a red base. The blisters can be moved within the skin by tangential pressure (Nikolski's sign 2 or Asboe-Hansen sign). The disease is extremely itchy and starts often with urticarial plaques for some months before blisters appear. On dermatohistopathology, the blister is subepidermal with infiltrates of eosinophils. Immunofluorescent linear subepidermal deposits of C3 or IgG are typical. The autoantibodies are directed against proteins in the hemidesmosomes (BP 180 and BP 230). BP 180 has been recently identified as collagen XVII.

There are some subtypes or variants of BP such as *localized BP* on the shins or on the scalp, *dyshidrosiform BP* on the palmoplantar surface, and *pemphigoid vegetans* with eroded plaques and vegetations in the intertriginous areas.

The treatment consists of systemic corticosteroids (lower doses than for pemphigus vulgaris, 0.5 mg/ kg daily) in elderly patients; sometimes topical therapy with high-potency steroids (clobetasol) alone is also effective. Dapsone as well as erythromycin has been tried, when there is a contraindication for systemic steroids.

***Pemphigoid Gestationis (Herpes Gestationis).*** Herpes gestationis (Fig. 9-13) is a self-limited variant of BP during pregnancy. Typically, pemphigoid gestationis is extensively pruritic in herpetiform eruptions with or without little blistering occurring mostly in the third trimester. After birth, the eruption usually clears within months. The disease will commonly recur during the following pregnancy and may have a more severe course.

There is no increased risk of fetal malformations; however, there may be a tendency toward an increased incidence

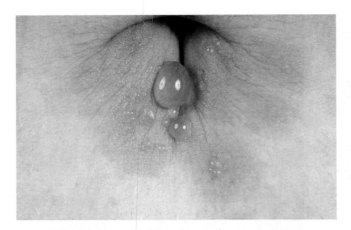

**FIGURE 9-13** ■ Cluster of periumbilical blisters on an erythematous base in a patient with pemphigoid gestationis.

of early births. Therapy includes topical steroids in mild cases or short-term systemic steroids. Occasionally, skin eruptions can occur in the newborn, evolving from transplacental transfer of maternal autoantibodies.

***Cicatricial Mucosal Membrane Pemphigoid.*** Cicatricial or mucosal membrane pemphigoid is a chronic dermatosis with a predilection for mucosal membranes, including ocular and conjunctival, and is regarded as a cicatricial variant of BP. Autoantibodies IgG are directed against collagen XVII, laminin 332 (formerly laminin 5), epiligrin, kalinin, nicein, or collagen VII.

The disease is very resistant to therapy; corticosteroids are often not effective, and sometimes, they are used intralesionally. Sulfones, retinoids, and immunosuppressives have been tried. Major problems include ocular synechiae.

***Epidermolysis Bullosa Acquisita.*** Epidermolysis bullosa acquisita (EBA) is a rare disease with noninflammatory blistering on mechanically irritated skin areas and increased skin fragility and scarring. Autoantibodies are directed against type VII collagen and sometimes antibodies are of the IgA class.

Systemic corticosteroids, cyclosporine, and dapsone can be tried. The disease is rather resistant to therapy. In the differential diagnosis, bullous SLE and DH of Duhring also have to be considered.

### Dermatitis Herpetiformis (Duhring's Disease)

Dermatitis herpetiformis is regarded as a skin manifestation of celiac disease. The clinical manifestations include herpetiform skin eruptions with small blisters and burning sensations. Sites of predilection are the knees, elbows, scalp, and buttocks. Almost all DH patients also have celiac disease, but not vice versa. Few DH patients have symptoms of celiac disease and are surprised when a gluten-free diet is recommended.

In dermatopathology, subepidermal blisters with papillary microabscesses are characteristic. Direct immunofluorescence IgA deposits in the papillary dermis in perilesional skin are typical. The disease does not respond to corticosteroids. Dapsone is the treatment of choice. Anemia is common, and a G6PDH deficiency test should be conducted in these patients before therapy to avoid extreme hemolysis. Concomitant use of cimetidine may make anemia less severe. Sulfapyridine, although sometimes difficult to obtain, is as effective as dapsone and can have less severe side effects.

### Linear IgA Dermatosis

In this rare disease, pruritic erythematous papules and plaques are followed by dense vesicles and blisters, sometimes in a linear or herpetiform pattern. Dermatopathologically, subepidermal blisters with rich neutrophilic infiltrates are seen. In immunofluorescence, linear deposits of IgA at the dermal–epidermal junctions are characteristic. In children, the prognosis is usually good. In adults, the disease is more chronic. Therapy of choice is dapsone; systemic steroids are not very effective.

## Suggested Readings

Bieber T. Atopic dermatitis. *N Engl J Med.* 2008;358:1483–1494.
Frosch P, Menné T, Lepoittevin JP, eds. *Contact Dermatitis.* 4th ed. Berlin: Springer; 2006.
Greaves M. Chronic urticaria. *J Allergy Clin Immunol.* 2000;105:664–672.
Joly P, Mouquet H, Roujeau JC, et al. A single cycle of rituximab for treatment of severe pemphigus. *N Engl J Med.* 2007;357:545–552.
Karpati S. Dermatitis herpetiformis: close to unravelling a disease? *J Dermatol Sci.* 2004;34:83–90.
Mockenhaupt M, Viboud C, Dunant A, et al. Stevens-Johnson syndrome and toxic epidermal necrolysis: assessment of medication risks with emphasis on recently marketed drugs. The EuroSCAR-Study. *J Invest Dermatol.* 2008;128:35–44.
Ring J. *Allergy in Practice.* Berlin: Springer; 2005.
Ring J, Przybilla B, Ruzicka T, eds. *Handbook of Atopic Eczema.* 2nd ed. Berlin: Springer; 2006.
Staab D, Diepgen TL, Fartasch M, et al. Age-related structured educational programmes for the management of atopic dermatitis in children and adolescents: multicentre, randomised controlled trial. *BMJ.* 2006;332:933–938.
Stanley JR, Amagai M. Pemphigus, bullous impetigo, and the staphylococcal scalded-skin syndrome. *N Engl J Med.* 2006;355:1800–1810.
Weidinger S, Illig T, Baurecht H et al. Loss-of-function variations within the filaggrin gene predispose for atopic dermatitis with allergic sensitizations. *J Allergy Clin Immunol.* 2006;118:214–219.

# CHAPTER 10

# Atopic Dermatitis

*Jasna Lipozenčić, MD, PhD and Suzana Ljubojević, MD, PhD*

## Introduction

Atopic dermatitis (AD) is a chronic inflammatory skin disease, characterized by severe pruritus and typical age-specific clinical picture (scaly, and oozing plaques on the forehead and face, neck, hands, and flexural area) and is frequently associated with other genetic predisposed atopic diseases such as asthma and/or allergic rhinitis. The prevalence of AD is rather high, mostly involving children, and affects 2% to 5% of the general population with 10% to 20% or more occurrences in infants and children and 1% to 3% in adults. There is wide variation in the prevalence of AD in different populations of the world, and it appears to be increasing.

The course of the disease is characterized by exacerbations and remissions that cannot always be etiologically explained. Complete remission has been estimated to occur in one third of patients after 2 years of age and in another one third after 5 years of age. However, many patients with infantile AD or juvenile AD experience discomforts up to their adult age.

Self-healing, the susceptibility to allergy, and the characteristic immune profile of lesional skin and peripheral blood are hallmarks of AD. They, together with the two different types of AD (intrinsic and extrinsic), require new definitions and reassessments. According to the recent findings of a search for susceptibility genes, it appears that nonatopic dermatitis should be considered a distinct entity of childhood eczema. The affected youngsters show dry ichthyosiform and eczematous skin changes at an early age with absence of sensitization to common allergens, and 33% of them should be clear of skin lesions by the age of 5 years of age without skin lesions.

The terminology of AD is controversial, with many different names used in different countries, among them neurodermitis, flexural eczema, Besnier's prurigo, constitutionalis atopica, and atopic eczema. Johansson and colleagues and the European Academy of Allergology and Clinical Immunology (EAACI) proposed a new term, "atopic eczema/dermatitis syndrome" (AEDS), which was divided into nonallergic and allergic types, the latter applying to immunoglobulin (Ig) E–associated allergic AEDS. They revised the nomenclature of AD and atopy and called only the IgE-associated forms of the diseases true AD. It is hoped that the term "eczema" will replace the current term AD.

## Genetic Aspects

Several genetic analyses have identified different chromosome regions with a linkage to AD features: Th2 cell cytokine genes on *5q31–33, on 1q21, 3q21, 17q25,* and *20p* which are closely related to some major psoriasis loci. Further genetic regions associated with AD features include gene polymorphisms, activator of transcription *(STAT)-6;* the proximal promoter of regulated on activation, T-cell expressed and secreted (RANTES); interleukin (IL)-4, IL-4 R$\alpha$; and transforming growth factor (TGF)-$\beta$. An association of one region intron 2 polymorphisms *(rs 324011)* with total serum IgE and a STAT-6 risk haplotype for elevated IgE in white adults was also proven. Candidate genes found in regions *(3q21, 5q31–33, and 11q13)* code for various immunomodulators, including costimulatory proteins (CD80 and CD86) involved in T-cell activation *(3q21);* IL-3, 4, 5, and 11; granulocyte–macrophage colony-stimulating factor (GM-CSF) *(5q31–33);* and the beta subunit of the high-affinity IgE receptors *(11q13).* Finally, a genetic linkage was shown to contribute to immunologic abnormalities of AD pathogenesis. Atopic constitution is more frequently transmitted by maternal inheritance.

## Immunologic Background

AD is frequently associated with immunodeficiency (selective IgA and IgM). Numerous factors are implicated in the onset of the disease. Hyperimmunoglobulinemia E is characteristic of atopic diseases; however, AD is also a consequence of immune response type IV. The cells infiltrating the skin are predominated by Th2 cell types that produce IL-4/IL-10/IL-13 and enable differentiation of B lymphocytes and production of IgE and eosinophilia. It has been demonstrated that Langerhans cells (LCs), dendritic cells (DC) of the dermis, and peripheral blood monocytes of atopic patients can bind monomeric IgE via high-affinity IgE receptors (Fc$\varepsilon$RI), representing allergen-binding molecules on antigen-presenting cells. In the same way, they translate and present the allergen to T lymphocytes. Mastocytes also play a major role in the genesis of AD, via allergen stimulation of the secretion of mediators (histamine, prostaglandins, and cytokines including IL-3, IL-4, IL-5, IL-6, and tumor necrosis factor alpha [TNF-$\alpha$]). Thus, the function of suppressor

(CD8) lymphocytes is impaired due to the underlying gene defect. There are activated Th1 cells with increased production of interferon (IFN)-γ in acute AD skin lesions binding to keratinocytes and, consequently, inflammatory skin changes in the disease. A relative imbalance between Th1 and Th2 subsets of CD4+ T cells producing cytokines are indicative of prominent immune disorders in AD. Autoreactivity to human proteins in patients with AD has been postulated as a decisive pathogenetic factor for AD. Several investigations have looked into the question of whether the stress-inducible enzyme, manganese superoxide dismutase (MnSOD) of human and fungal origin, might act as an autoallergen in AD. The findings on T cells with regulatory features as well as on IgE-mediated autoreactivity will give insight into the defective tolerance of AD patients. Imbalance of Th1 and Th2 in AD depends on polymorphism in the IL-18 gene on peripheral mononuclear cells, which reacts after stimulation with superantigens through upregulation of IL-18 and downregulation of IL-12. Substance P, nerve growth factor (NGF), and vasoactive intestinal polypeptides (VIP) are increased in the blood of AD patients. Cytokines and chemokines are also key factors in the pathogenesis of AD.

There is a Th2 cytokine profile of IL-4, IL-5, and IL-13 in the skin in the acute phase of AD, while Th1/0 with IFN-γ, IL-12, and GM-CSF prevail in the chronic phase. There is significant coordination between AD disease activity and skin eosinophilic cationic protein (ECP) deposition. Moreover, ECP and IL-16 are elevated in the acute AD phase, and IL-10 plays an important immunoregulatory role in atopic as well as nonatopic eczema. In lesional AD skin, there are two types of the high-affinity receptors for IgE-bearing myeloid dendritic cells (DC) (i.e., LCs and inflammatory dendritic epidermal cells [IDECs]), each of which displays a different function in the pathophysiology of AD. Specifically, LCs play a predominant role in the initiation of the allergic immune response and conversion of prime naïve T cells into T cells of the Th2 type with high amounts of IL-4. Furthermore, stimulation of high-affinity receptors for IgE on the surface of LCs by allergens induces the release of chemotactic signals and recruitment of IDECs and T cells in vitro. Stimulation of high-affinity IgE receptors (FcεRI) on IDECs leads to the release of high amounts of proinflammatory signals, which contribute to the allergic immune response. Keratinocytes play a role in innate immunity by expressing toll-like receptors and by producing antimicrobial peptides in response to invading microbes. AD keratinocytes secrete a unique profile of chemokines and cytokines. Apoptosis of keratinocytes is a crucial event in the formation of eczema (spongiosis in AD). The expression of different immunologic parameters has been studied in AD patients since immune dysregulation is a possible key defect in AD. Regulatory T cells (Tregs) or Th3 cells (CD25+/CD4+) can suppress Th1 as well as Th2 cells. Superantigens of *Staphylococcus aureus* cause defects in Tregs function and promote the skin inflammation. Autoallergens (e.g., Homs 1–5 and DSF 70) are atopy-related autoantigens (ARA) in the setting of AD and other atopic diseases. IgE autoreactivity appears very early (during the first year of life) and is associated with flares in AD. Adhesion molecules may play an important role in the homing of T-cell subsets into allergen-exposed skin of atopic individuals. High expressions of adhesion molecules, especially intracellular adhesion molecules (ICAM)-1 and ICAM-3, E-selectin, and L-selectin, in skin lesions of AD patients revealed that they may play an important role in the pathogenesis of AD and may be of clinical relevance for the management of AD. AD is a product of an interaction between various susceptibility genes, host and environmental factors, infectious agents, defects in skin barrier function, and immunologic responses.

## Skin Barrier Dysfunction

AD is characterized by dry skin and increased transepidermal water loss even in nonlesional skin, and fewer ceramides in the cornified envelope of lesional and nonlesional skin are found in AD patients. Changes in the stratum corneum pH in AD skin may impair lipid metabolism in the skin. Such alterations allow the penetration of and increase susceptibility to irritants and allergens, triggering the inflammatory response, cutaneous hyperreactivity, inflammation, and skin damage characteristic of AD. Filaggrin deficiency leads to mild or severe ichthyosis vulgaris. Impaired keratinocyte differentiation and barrier formation allow increased transepidermal water loss and the entry of allergens, antigens, and chemicals from the environment in AD.

## Environmental Factors

The importance of environmental factors in the development of AD has been increasing. The majority (40% to 65%) of AD patients experience deterioration in the winter, probably due to decreased humidity of the air outdoors (due to cold) as well as indoors due to heating. The aggravation by sun exposure is probably due to a nonspecific intolerance of heat caused by impaired function of sweating in affected skin and induction of itch sweating. Outdoor pollution seems to be one of the major causes of the dramatic increase of atopy in recent years. Chemical compounds and exhaust particles as well as pollen are released into the air and may have indirect effects on the allergic sensitization. AD is major contributing factor to occupational irritant or allergic contact dermatitis. Irritants, such as soaps, detergents, and disinfectants, and prolonged exposure to water have an excitatory effect on the impaired barrier layer of atopic skin. Daily washing with soap and water or noxious agent may elicit an irritant contact reaction in atopic individuals. Saliva frequently induces perioral eczema. Contact with wool is a common trigger of irritant contact dermatitis in AD. Other textiles, especially synthetics or dyed fabrics, are sometimes incriminated. Tobacco smoke is also a potent irritator of atopic skin. Nutritive allergens are primarily important in AD in children. The most common allergens in children are egg whites, cow's milk, peanuts, soya, shellfish, and flour. The prevalence of food allergy in AD varies widely from 25% to 60% according to different studies. There are also nonspecific irritant reactions predominantly to acid fruit (citrus fruit, tomatoes) and salty or spicy foods. Aggravation of eczema may also be provoked by food additives.

Among airborne allergens, the most important are grass, weeds, and tree pollen allergens, animal epidermis, dander allergens, and house-dust mites. Airborne allergy in AD varies widely according to different studies. Great attention has been paid to skin colonization and infection with *S. aureus*. This bacterium can be isolated in nostrils and intertriginous regions in 5% to 15% of normal individuals but is found in 64% to 100% of skin lesions in AD patients. It influences the course of the disease via different mechanisms: exotoxins, enzymes, superantigen, and protein A. Bacterial toxins act as superantigens aligned along MHC II and can directly stimulate massive T-cell proliferation. This discovery has entailed introduction in AD treatment of antistaphylococcal antibiotics. *Malassezia furfur (Pityrosporum ovale)* yeast may produce positive skin prick reactions in a higher rate (49%) in patients with AD of the head, scalp, and neck region. It can also be detected in the serum (specific IgE to *P. ovale*) and can provoke positive patch-test reaction. *M. furfur* can induce an eczematous reaction in sensitized AD patients and may be a trigger factor for AD. Patients with AD do not have a major deficiency in defending against viruses. However, some viral skin infections can have a dramatic course. Kaposi's herpetiform (**Figs. 10-1 and 10-2**) and varicelliform eruptions caused by the spread of herpes and varicella viruses, Epstein–Barr virus, parainfluenza virus, respiratory syncytial virus, and cytomegalovirus infections have been reported to trigger exacerbation of AD. Atopic patients often respond to stress, frustration, embarrassment, or other upsetting events with increased pruritus and scratching. When the higher cortical centers are activated by stress, there is an increased secretion of substance P from the adrenal glands. They serve as brain peptides that are easily released by psychosocial stress,

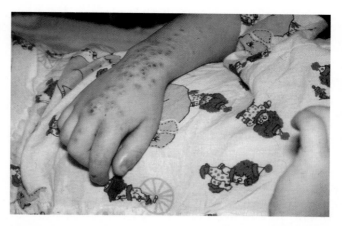

**FIGURE 10-2** ■ The same patient as in Figure 10-1 with vesicular eruption over the arm.

triggering or exacerbating itching, especially in patients with AD. Histamine is not believed to be the essential mediator of itch in AD. Proteases, kinins, prostaglandins, neuropeptides, acetylcholine, cytokines, and opioids can cause itch or potentiate histamine release into atopic skin.

## Clinical Features

AD is a multifaceted disease. The clinical picture, morphology, and distribution of the skin lesion vary greatly depending on the age of the patient, the ethnic group he or she belongs to, the course and duration of the disease, aggravating factors, and possible complications such as superinfection (Fig. 10-3). Its manifestations range from very mild to severe disease.

There are three classical stages of disease—infantile, childhood, and adulthood—each of which may show acute, subacute, and/or chronic skin reactions. Acute lesions are characterized by intensely pruritic, erythematous papules and vesicles over erythematous skin, erosions, and serous exudates. Subacute lesions form erythematous, excoriated scaly papules, whereas chronic lesions show skin thickening with pronounced skin markings (lichenification) (Fig. 10-4) and nodular papules. All three stages of skin lesions may frequently be present in the same patient.

In infancy, the characteristic lesions consist of symmetrical, dry, erythematous, scaly plaques with follicular papules on the face, mostly involving the cheeks, forehead, and scalp but not the perioral region. When a child starts to crawl, the lesions extend to the upper trunk, extensor aspect of the upper and lower extremities, and the dorsal aspects of the hands and feet. The diaper region is usually spared due to the moisture retention of diapers. The childhood phase, during the second and third years of life, shows a modified clinical picture with characteristic papules and plaques localized primarily in large joint flexures, especially on the neck, elbows, wrists, knees, and ankles. Later in childhood and in adolescence, lesions involving flexural areas persist, including the eyelids, hands, and feet, where pustules are frequently observed. Many children develop a "nummular" pattern of AD. In

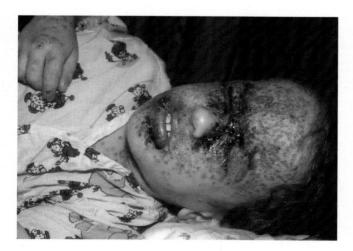

**FIGURE 10-1** ■ Eczema herpetiformis (Kaposi's varicelliform eruption) in a six-year-old boy with a long history of eczema and exposure to herpes simplex on the lip. Excellent response was seen with intravenous acyclovir.

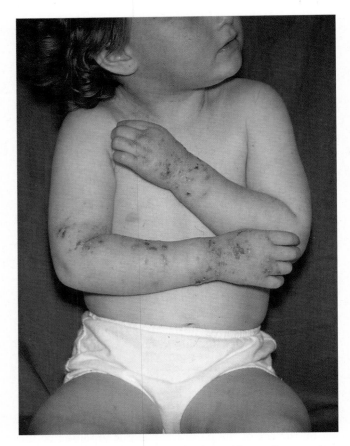

FIGURE 10-3 ▪ Secondary infection with crusting, oozing oval lesions over the forearms of a child with childhood eczema.

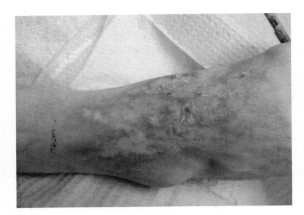

FIGURE 10-5 ▪ Well demarcated lichenified plaque of lichen simplex chronicus over anterior ankle.

adults, the disease is characterized by lichenification, chronic course, thickened areas in flexures, on the neck and eyelids, and chronic facial edema. Localized patches of AD can occur on the nipples, especially in adolescent and young women. The disease has a chronic or chronic-relapsing course, with alternating periods of regression and exacerbation of skin changes with pruritus. In some patients, a seasonal variant of

the disease is present, with exacerbations occurring mostly in spring and autumn. Severe pruritus is the main characteristic of AD. It worsens in the evening, during sweating, and by wearing wool clothing.

## Differential Diagnosis

Keratosis pilaris (Fig. 10-5) is seen most commonly during childhood and presents as small, rough, raised lesions (papules). Xerosis is considered to be the most common dermatosis of atopic individuals. It can persist for life, independent of the activity of atopic symptoms. Pityriasis alba is a benign chronic skin disorder that affects some children, usually between the ages of 6 and 12 but may occur up to age 20 to 30. Sometimes pityriasis alba can be confused with vitiligo. When an ichthyosis vulgaris patient has severe pruritus of flexural involvement, he or she usually has atopic dermatitis. Dennie–Morgan lines are symmetrical, prominent folds, extending from the medial aspect of the lower lid. The sign is present in about 70% of atopic children. Palmoplantar hyperlinearity is found in people with AD who frequently have a thickening of the skin on the palms and soles with an increase in the number of lines in the skin (hyperlinearity). Cheilitis is noted as a persistent scaliness, usually restricted to the vermilion, but often extending onto the perioral skin. The biggest group of patients with cheilitis have severe AD or at least an atopic diathesis with persistent nodules.

Nipple dermatitis is noted in 12% to 23% of patients with AD. It is most common in postpubertal girls. The very sensitive areolar skin koebnerizes with the slightest rubbing or friction of clothing.

## Histologic Features

Acute eczematous lesions are characterized by marked epidermal intercellular edema (spongiosis). Chronic lichenified lesions are characterized by an acantholytic epidermis with elongation of the rete ridges, parakeratosis, and only minimum spongiosis. Those chronic lesions have an increased

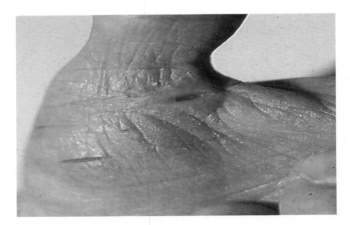

FIGURE 10-4 ▪ Dramatic lichenification (increased markings of normal skin) over the dorsal surface of the hand in an eczema patient.

number of IgE-bearing LCs and IDECs in the epidermis, and macrophages dominate the dermal mononuclear cell infiltrate. These lesions also contain eosinophils.

## Diagnosis

Well-defined diagnostic criteria are important in the diagnosis of AD, and diagnostic criteria developed by Hanifin and Rajka (see Table 8-1) are widely accepted. Skin biopsies are not essential for the diagnosis, but they can exclude other diagnoses in adults. In the differential diagnosis, combination forms with components of atopic, contact, and irritative eczema are important. Atopic eczema of the hands and the feet must be differentiated from psoriasis, from keratodermas in the palms and soles, and from tinea. The differential diagnosis of acute AD with intense erythema of the skin, together with exudation or blistering, for example, differs from differential diagnoses of the chronic lichenified form. Elements contributing to the establishment of the diagnosis of AD are compiled from patient history, clinical findings, skin tests, and laboratory investigations. Hanifin and Rajka were the first to attempt a systematic approach toward the standardization of the diagnosis of AD by proposing 4 major and 23 minor criteria for AD in 1980. The Lillehammer criteria of 1994 are based on the idea that the distribution of the AD may differ in the infantile, childhood, and adult phases. Diagnostic Lillehammer criteria are visible eczema in at least one of the regions, at least one positive anamnestic laboratory criteria, and at least three of the clinical, anamnestic, or laboratory criteria. In addition, as a fourth criterion, the skin disease should always have a duration of at least 6 weeks in the infantile phase or 3 months in the childhood and adult phases.

## Laboratory Findings

Laboratory tests are chosen according to history data and physical examination. The investigation of exacerbating factors in AD involves a patient history, specific skin and blood tests, and challenge tests, depending on the degree of disease severity and on the suspected factors involved. The atopy patch test (APT) was introduced to assess sensitization to inhalant allergens in AEDS patients. Fuiano and Incorvaia recently confirmed the high value of APT in patients with mite-induced AEDS and suggested that its routine use might also improve the diagnosis of respiratory allergy to housedust mites. Cytokine responses to allergens can be detected in cord blood mononuclear cells (CBMC), suggesting allergen priming in utero.

The APT is primarily a tool for investigating the mechanisms of eczema in the skin. It can, however, also reveal sensitization in patients with AD and might identify a subgroup of AD patients. Sensitization to inhalant allergens (e.g., dust, mites, animal dander, and pollen) can be detected by skin prick tests (SPTs) (if the skin is free from eczema) or by measuring specific IgE antibodies.

Contact sensitization to topical medications frequently occurs in AD patients, especially in adults. The possibility of contact allergy needs to be ruled out by patch testing.

## Treatment

Successful management of AD requires a different approach involving skin care, identification and elimination of flare factors, and anti-inflammatory treatment. General measures of prevention and treatment of AD include avoiding those factors that have been identified as potential causes of disease exacerbations. This implies avoidance of skin contact with wool, synthetic materials, and foods that can induce irritation (e.g., citrus fruit or tomatoes). Patients are advised to avoid staying in smoky areas and to reduce exposure to house dust, feather, and animal hair. Staying in mountains 1,500 m above sea level is useful. Staying at the seaside, sea bathing, and sun exposure usually prove beneficial in AD patients. However, skin sun protection is necessary, such as avoiding most intensive sun exposure (between 11:00 AM and 5:00 PM), along with application of sun protecting preparations and daily skin care. Skin care includes appropriate skin hygiene, which is of paramount importance. Patients with hypersensitivity to a nutritive allergen are recommended to comply with an appropriate dietary regimen. When prescribing diets for children, it should be borne in mind that inappropriate diet may lead to malnutrition while even a minimal dietary deficit may cause changes in immune response.

It should be emphasized that hypersensitivity to food allergens is mostly diagnosed in children, whereas hypersensitivity to inhalant allergens and development of contact allergic dermatitis predominate in older patients.

### Topical Therapy

Skin care preparation should be applied over the skin within 3 minutes (3-minute rule) of bathing; otherwise, bathing will lead to skin drying instead of desirable skin hydration. Bathing is also important because the penetration of corticosteroids into the hydrated skin is best after bathing. Soaps with minimum defatting activity and a neutral pH are preferred. The use of oily baths followed by neutral preparations for skin ointment and hydration (creams, ointments, and emulsions) several times a day and continuously, is necessary in most AD patients. The higher the degree of skin dryness, the greater the frequency of preparation usage. Preparations with the addition of urea, omega fatty acids, lipids, zinc, and copper are used for this purpose. Local therapy for AD is tailored to the stage of disease: in acute stage, indifferent creams and bases (hydrophilic creams, oil/water emulsions); in subacute stage, mild antiphlogistic creams and soft pastes; and in chronic stage, water/oil ointments and tar preparations are used. Keratolytics and rehydrating ointments (salicylic acid, urea) applied by occlusive technique for 4 to 12 hours are used for hyperkeratoses/rhagades. Water–alcohol compresses, soft zinc pastes, or zinc oil are applied in cases of moist, macerated lesions, whereas oil baths and occasional use of corticosteroid preparations are recommended for all stages. Local corticosteroid preparations remain the most important agents in the management of AD patients for their anti-inflammatory and antipruritic action. The potent corticosteroids should be avoided on the face, the genitalia, and the intertriginous area. With mild disease activity, a small amount of topical corticosteroids two to three times weekly (monthly amounts in the mean range of 15 g in infants, 30 g in children, and up to 60 to 90 g in adolescents and adults) achieves good maintenance. Emollients containing polidocanol are effective in reducing pruritic symptoms. Topical calcineurin inhibitors are steroid-free preparations and include tacrolimus (Protopic cream 0.1% and 0.03%) and pimecrolimus (Elidel 1% ointment), which have an immunomodulatory effect. They are both indicated for the short-term or intermittent long-term treatment of AD in patients older than 2 years of age who are unresponsive to conventional therapy. Their main advantage over corticosteroids is that these agents do not cause skin atrophy and telangiectasia because they do not affect collagen synthesis. They are especially useful for facial and intertriginous lesions. Tar preparation may have antipruritic and anti-inflammatory effects on the skin. Protopic, Elidel, and tar preparations are all useful in reducing the potency of topical corticosteroids required in chronic maintenance of AD. Tar preparations should not be used on acutely inflamed skin, since this often results in skin irritation. Capsaicin 0.025% cream acts on substance P release and has an antipruritic effect. In case of localized pyodermal lesions, local antibiotics, mostly mupirocin, are applied. The yeast *P. ovale* is efficiently eliminated by use of a ketoconazole shampoo or with miconazole alone or in combination with hydrocortisone.

## Systemic Management

### Infectious Agents

Skin infections with *S. aureus* are rather common in AD patients (Fig. 10-3). Therefore, therapy with oral antibiotics, mostly erythromycin, azithromycin, and cephalosporin preparations, is quite frequently justified. Infection with herpes simplex virus is a severe and life-threatening complication of AD and requires acyclovir (e.g., valacyclovir).

### Antihistaminics

Systemic antihistamines are widely used in acute flares against itch. They may be helpful to decrease pruritus and permit sleep during flares. Antihistamine H1 receptor antagonists, especially those with sedative effect (diphenhydramine) are frequently prescribed for AD patients; however, their efficacy is variable. These agents (hydroxyzine, terfenadine, loratadine [desloratadine], astemizol, cetirizine, fexofenadine) are efficacious in the control of pruritus generated by mastocyte degranulation but not of T-lymphocyte–mediated inflammatory processes. Nonsedating antihistamines seem to have only very modest value in AD. Tricyclic antidepressants, high-potency antagonists (doxepine, amitriptyline), are also useful. Leukotriene inhibitors have received considerable word-of-mouth testimonial support.

### Systemic Corticosteroids

The use of systemic corticosteroids is only advised in a short course for acute flare-ups. In children they are used seldom and only during the acute phase.

### Phototherapy

Natural sunlight is frequently beneficial to patients with AD. However, if the sunlight occurs in the setting of high heat and humidity, thereby triggering sweating and pruritus, it may be deleterious to patients. Heliomarinotherapy (sun and sea therapy) is also useful. UVB or combined UVA and UVB exposure is efficacious in AD patients. High daily doses of UVA1 (340 to 400 nm) are even more efficacious. Photochemotherapy with oral photosensitizer methoxypsoralen (MOP) (Meladinin tablets) followed by UVA exposure (PUVA therapy) may be indicated in patients with severe, widespread AD with failure of topical steroid therapy or significant corticosteroid side effects. Topical application of 0.3% 8-MOP ointment (PUVA cream therapy) could be used to treat palmoplantar AD lesions.

### Cyclosporine

Cyclosporine is a potent immunosuppressive drug that acts primarily on T-cell receptors by suppressing cytokine transcription. Severe AD patients, refractory to topical corticosteroid therapy, can benefit from treatment with oral cyclosporine (3 to 5 mg/kg/day for 8 weeks or 3 months). Discontinuation of treatment frequently results in rapid relapse of skin disease.

### Interferon Therapy

INF-$\gamma$ is known to suppress IgE responses and downregulate Th2 proliferation and function. The treatment with recombinant INF-$\gamma$ results in clinical improvement and decreases total circulating eosinophil counts (10 to 100 $\mu$g/m$^2$).

### Extracorporeal Photopheresis

This treatment consists of the passage of psoralen-treated leukocytes through an extracorporeal UVA light system. It could be used in severe AD patients who are resistant to therapy.

### Allergen Immunotherapy

Available evidence of the effectiveness of immunotherapy with aeroallergens in the treatment of AD is mixed. The efficacy of immunotherapy with aeroallergens must be proven in the treatment of AD.

### Other

Systemic immunosuppressants such as azathioprine (1 to 3 mg/kg/3 months) and mycophenolate mofetil (MMF) are indicated in the management of resistant forms of AD and are behind cyclosporin in AD management. MMF has a better safety profile than cyclosporine or azathioprine, but controlled studies are needed to prove efficacy. Thalidomide (25 to 200 mg/d) is efficacious in resistant cases of AD, even in children. Phosphodiesterase inhibitors are agents intended for generalized forms of the disease.

### Leukotriene Antagonists

Leukotriene antagonists (montelukast and zafirlukast) are useful for the treatment of asthma and allergic rhinitis. In AD therapy they are not fully elucidated. Zafirlukast is approved in AD and asthma for adolescents and adults. In chronic AD, montelukast achieved little success. Montelukast administrated 5 mg daily for 4 weeks in a clinical double-blind study of moderate to severe AD in young patients (6 to 16 years) showed a significant decrease in severity, but in another study with severe AD and different doses (5, 10, and 20 mg), there was only partial improvement (relief of pruritus and erythema) in very few patients. AD patients failed to show any benefit from leukotriene receptor antagonist therapy.

### Bioengineered Immunomodulators

Most of the new approaches aim at inhibiting components of the allergic inflammatory response, including cytokine modulation (e.g., TNF inhibitors), blockade of inflammatory cell recruitment (chemokine receptor antagonists, cutaneous lymphocyte antigen [CLA] inhibitors), and inhibition of T-cell activation (alefacept and efalizumab). Bioengineered immunomodulators are in the clinical trial phase for AD treatment. They change the immune profile from Th1 to Th2 or block cytokines. These agents are currently in clinical trials for psoriasis and psoriatic arthritis.

### IgE-blocking Antibody

IgE-blocking antibody omalizumab (Xolair) is a recombinant human monoclonal antibody. Omalizumab works by binding free serum IgE and avoids binding to Fc$\varepsilon$RI receptors as well as Fc$\varepsilon$RII (CD23) receptors on mast cells, basophils, and antigen-presenting cell surfaces, which stops the release of proinflammatory mediators.

Omalizumab is for use in adults and children older than 12 years with asthma and AD for months; subcutaneous injections of 0.016 mg/kg/IgE (UI/ml) and 0.03 mg/kg/ IgE (UI/ml) per 4 weeks fortnightly or monthly. The role of omalizumab in dermatology and for AD is probably best directed toward patients who have high levels of IgE and in whom the IgE is an etiologic factor for their disease.

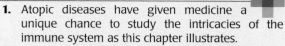

**SAUER'S NOTES**

1. Atopic diseases have given medicine a unique chance to study the intricacies of the immune system as this chapter illustrates.
2. An increase in atopic illness, most notably asthma and eczema, continues to be a major health problem of the new century.
3. Do not underestimate the importance of a well-maintained doctor–patient relationship in dealing with patients and their families in this very chronic and often frustrating group of diseases.

## Conclusion

AD develops as a consequence of complex etiology and pathogenesis. The severity and extent of skin lesions and deviation in laboratory parameters, especially immunologic ones, may greatly differ from patient to patient. A consensus will have to be established in the near future on the new criteria defining AD, based on the model set 25 years ago by Hanifin and Rajka. The increasing prevalence of this disease worldwide underlines the role of prevention, recognition, and optimal treatment of the many patients with AD.

## Suggested Readings

Akdis CA, Akdis M, Bieber T, et al. Diagnosis and treatment of atopic dermatitis in children and adults: European Academy of Allergology and Clinical Immunology/American Academy of Allergy, Asthma and Immunology/PRACTALL Consensus Report. *Allergy.* 2006;61:969–87.

Cookson WO, Moffatt MF. The genetics of atopic dermatitis. *Curr Opin Allergy Clin Immunol.* 2002;2:383–387.

Hanifin J, Rajka G. Diagnostic features of atopic dermatitis. *Acta Derm Venereol (Stockh).* 1980;92(suppl):44–47.

Lipozenčić J, Ljubojević S. Atopic dermatitis. *Rad. Medical Sciences.* 2008; 449 (32):77–103.

Lipozenčić J, Wolf R. Atopic dermatitis: an update and review of the literature. *Dermatol Clin.* 2007;25:605–612.

Möhrenschlager M, Darsow U, Schnopp C, et al. Atopic eczema: what's new? *J Eur Acad Dermatol Venereol.* 2006;20:503–13.

Novak N, Bieber T, Leung DY. Immune mechanisms leading to atopic dermatitis. *J Allergy Clin Immunol.* 2003;112:S128–S139.

Pastar Z, Lipozencić J, Ljubojevic S. Etiopathogenesis of atopic dermatitis—an overview. *Acta Dermatovenerol Croat.* 2005;13:54–62.

Ring J, Huss-Marp J. Atopic eczema. *Karger Gazette.* 2004;67:7–9.

Scheinfeld NS, Tutrone WD, Weinberg JM, et al. Phototherapy of atopic dermatitis. *Clin Dermatol.* 2003;21:241–248.

Schultz Larsen F, Hanifin JM. Epidemiology of atopic dermatitis. *Immunol Allergy Clin North Am.* 2002;22:1–24.

# CHAPTER 11

# Pruritic Dermatoses

*John C. Hall, MD*

Pruritus, or itching, brings more patients to the physician's office than any other skin disease symptom. Itchy skin is not easily cured or even alleviated. Decreased quality of life due to pruritus can be as significant as with pain. Many hundreds of proprietary over-the-counter and prescription drugs are touted as effective anti-itch remedies, but none is 100% effective. Many are partially effective, but it is unfortunate that the most effective locally applied chemicals frequently irritate or sensitize the skin.

Pruritus is a symptom of many of the common skin diseases, such as contact dermatitis, atopic eczema, seborrheic dermatitis, hives, scabies, insect bites, some drug eruptions, and many other dermatoses. Relief of itching is of prime importance in treating these diseases.

In addition to the pruritus that occurs as a symptom of many skin diseases, there are other clinical forms of pruritus that deserve special consideration. These special types include *generalized pruritus* of the winter, senile, and essential varieties and *localized pruritus* of the lichen simplex type, which affects the ears, anal area, lower legs in men, back of the neck in women, and genitalia. Localized pruritus of unknown etiology should alert one to the possibility of underlying peripheral nerve or central nervous system pathology.

## Generalized Pruritus

Diffuse itching of the body without perceptible skin disease usually is due to winter dry skin or senile skin.

### Winter Pruritus

Winter pruritus, or pruritus hiemalis, is a common form of generalized pruritus, although most patients complain of itching confined mainly to their legs. Every autumn, a certain number of elderly patients, and occasionally young ones, walk into the physician's office complaining bitterly of the rather sudden onset of itching of their legs. Men often also itch around the waist. These patients have dry skin caused by the low humidity in their furnace-heated homes, or occasionally from the low humidity resulting from cooling air conditioning. Clinically, the skin shows excoriations and dry, curled, scaling plaques resembling a sun-baked, muddy beach at low tide. The dry skin associated with winter itch is to be differentiated from *ichthyosis*, a congenital, inherited dermatosis of varying severity, which is also worse in the winter.

> **SAUER'S NOTE**
>
> When the presenting complaint is generalized itching of the skin, always stroke the skin on the forearm with your nail or a tongue depressor. After 5 minutes or so, if there is a wheal reaction at the stroking site, you have a diagnosis of dermographism. This is a common problem that is easily overlooked.

Treatment of winter pruritus consists of the following:

1. Bathing should involve as cool water as possible and as little soap as possible. Soap can be limited to the face, axillae, groin, genitalia, hands, and feet.
2. A bland soap, such as Dove, Oilatum, Cetaphil, or Basis, is used sparingly.
3. An oil is added to the bath water, such as Lubath, RoBathol, Nivea, or Alpha Keri. (The patient should be warned to avoid slipping in the tub.) The oil can be rubbed on after a shower.
4. Emollient lotions are beneficial, such as Complex 15 (phospholipid), CeraVe (ceramides), Curel (petrolatum), Eucerin, Aquaphor (esterified lanolin, quite greasy), Pen Kera, or Moisturel (not as greasy and noncomedogenic). $\alpha$-Hydroxy acid preparations include AmLactin 12% cream and lotion (over the counter), Lac-Hydrin 5% (over the counter), Lac-Hydrin 12% (prescription only), and Eucerin Plus. Urea products (in these higher concentrations may be irritating except on palms or soles) that are beneficial include Kera Lotion (35%), Keracream (40%), Vanamide (40%), Carmol 40 cream and lotion (40%), and Eucerin Plus lotion (also has lactic acid as an $\alpha$-hydroxy acid). Lubricants should be applied immediately after bathing for the most benefit.
5. A low-potency corticosteroid ointment applied twice daily is effective. Triamcinolone ointment 0.1% is midpotency and very inexpensive. A 1% hydrocortisone can be mixed with any of the mentioned moisturizers or used as a nonspecific ointment.
6. Oral antihistamines are sometimes effective, such as chlorpheniramine (Chlor-Trimeton), 4 mg h.s. or q.i.d, or diphenhydramine (Benadryl), 50 mg h.s. There are newer nonsedating antihistamines such as Claritin 10 mg q.d.

(over the counter), Clarinex 10 mg q.d., Zyrtec (may be slightly sedating and also more effective) 10 mg q.d., and Allegra 60 or 180 mg q.d. Some dermatologists do not think the nonsedating antihistamines are as effective as the sedating antihistamines. A commonly used sedating antihistamine is hydroxyzine, 10 mg every 8 hours while awake. The dose can be titrated to 25 mg, 50 mg, or rarely 100 mg. The soporific effect, or drowsiness, often becomes less severe with prolonged use.

7. Doxepin (Sinequan) starting at 10 mg/d and working up to 50 mg/d has been used with some success but can be sedating.

8. Neurontin (gabapentin) 300 mg/d and over weeks to months working up to doses as high as 1,800 mg/d in divided doses has been shown to be successful by some authors.

9. Ultraviolet light in the form of psoralens and ultraviolet light (PUVA) (increases risk of skin malignancy) and narrow band UVB may be beneficial.

## Senile Pruritus

Senile pruritus is a resistant form of generalized pruritus in the elderly patient. It can occur at any time of the year and may or may not be associated with dry skin. There is some evidence that these patients have a disorder of keratinization. This form of itch occurs most commonly on the scalp, shoulders, sacral areas, and legs. Clinically, some patients have no cutaneous signs of the itch, but others may have linear excoriations. *Scabies* should be ruled out, as well as the diseases mentioned under the next form of pruritus to be considered, essential pruritus.

Treatment is usually not very satisfactory. In addition to the agents mentioned previously in connection with winter pruritus, the injection of 40 mg of triamcinolone acetonide suspension (Kenalog-40) intramuscularly every 4 to 6 weeks for two or three injections is quite beneficial. I do not like to repeat this more often than three to four times a year to avoid systemic corticosteroid side effects. Topical antipruritic agents can be used, such as pramoxine hydrochloride (Pramosone with either 1% or 2.5% hydrocortisone is a prescription or Aveeno Anti-itch lotion, which is available over the counter). Menthol (0.5%), phenol (0.5%), or sulfur (2% to 5%) can be added to any appropriate base (see Chapter 4).

## Essential Pruritus

Essential pruritus is the rarest form of the generalized itching diseases. No person of any age is exempt, but it occurs most frequently in the elderly patient. The itching is usually quite diffuse, with occasional "bites" in certain localized areas. All itching is worse at night, and no exception is made for this form of pruritus. Before a diagnosis of essential pruritus is made, the following diseases must be ruled out by appropriate studies:

- Drug reaction
- Diabetes mellitus
- Uremia

- Lymphoma (mycosis fungoides, leukemia, or lymphoma [especially Hodgkin's disease]), as a paraneoplastic syndrome from any metastatic underlying malignancy
- Primary sclerosing cholangitis, which has very severe pruritus
- Liver disease (especially hepatitis B or C even without jaundice)
- Bullous pemphigoid before the blisters are present
- AIDS and other immunosuppressed states
- Stress or more severe psychiatric illness such as psychosis or parasitophobia
- Hyperthyroidism
- Post–brain tissue damage such as a stroke, brain cancer, or trauma
- Intestinal parasites
- Intrahepatic cholestasis of pregnancy—early diagnosis in the second half of pregnancy with elevation of total serum bile acids should prompt early treatment with ursodeoxycholic acid
- Telangiectasia macularis eruptiva perstans (may need skin biopsy to find)
- Cutaneous T-cell lymphoma "incognito" (may need skin biopsy to find)
- Drugs, especially opiates such as morphine

Treatment is the same as for senile and winter pruritus. Narrow band UVB is a safe and sometimes effective nonspecific treatment for pruritus. For more recalcitrant severe cases, here is a list of other therapies that can be tried: psychotherapy (including hypnosis), acupuncture, in dialysis patients more intense dialysis and magnesium-free dialysis, systemic metronidazole (primary sclerosing cholangitis), ursodeoxycholic acid (primary biliary cirrhosis), sertraline (75 to 100 mg daily), naltrexone (12.5 mg to start and up to 50 mg daily), rifampicin (150 mg t.i.d.), ondansetron (8 mg t.i.d.), gabapentin, nalfurafine, ketotifen, cholestyramine (liver and gallbladder disease), oral activated charcoal, thalidomide, intravenous lidocaine, bupropion, doxepin (10 to 30 mg h.s.), and pimozide.

# Localized Pruritic Dermatoses

## Lichen Simplex Chronicus

Other common terms for lichen simplex chronicus (LSC) include *localized neurodermatitis* and *lichenified dermatitis*. There are pros and cons for all the terms.

LSC (**Fig. 11-1**) is a common skin condition characterized by the occurrence of single or, less frequently, multiple patches of chronic itching and thickened, scaly, dry skin in one or more of several classic locations. It is unrelated to atopic eczema according to some experts, but others feel it is an adult form of eczema.

### *Primary Lesions*

This disease begins as a small, localized, well-demarcated, pruritic papule or patch of dermatitis that might have been

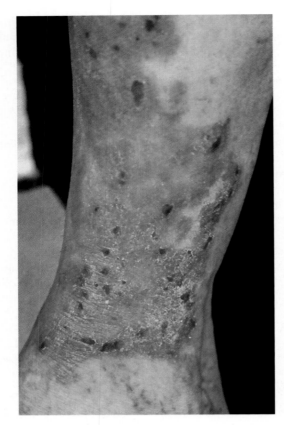

**FIGURE 11-1** ■ Localized LSC of the leg. This is a common location. Note the lichenification and excoriations owing to the marked pruritus. *(Courtesy of K.U.M.C.; Duke Labs, Inc.)*

an insect bite, chigger bite, contact dermatitis, or other minor irritation that may or may not be remembered by the patient. Because of various etiologic factors, a cycle of itching, scratching, more itching, and more scratching supervenes, and achronic dermatosis develops. Emotional stress is thought to lower the itch threshold and cause exacerbation of the disease. The itching is intense and paroxysmal in nature.

### Secondary Lesions

These include excoriations, lichenification, and, in severe cases, marked verrucous thickening of the skin, with pigmentary changes. In severe cases, healing is bound to be followed by some scarring.

### Presentation and Characteristics

**Distribution.** This condition is seen most commonly at the hairline of the nape of the neck and on the wrists, the ankles, the ears (see external otitis), anal area (see pruritus ani), and so on (**Fig. 11-2**).

**Course.** This disease is chronic and recurrent. Most cases respond quickly to potent topical corticosteroid treatment, but some can last for years and defy all forms of therapy.

**Subjective Complaints.** The primary symptom is intense itching, often paroxysmal, that is usually worse at night, occurs even during sleep, and may awaken the patient.

**Causes.** The initial cause (a bite, stasis dermatitis, contact dermatitis, seborrheic dermatitis, tinea cruris, psoriasis) may be very evanescent, but it is generally agreed that the chronicity of the lesion is due to the nervous habit of scratching. It is a rare patient who does not volunteer the information or admit, if questioned, that the itching is worse when he or she is upset, nervous, or tired. Why some people with a minor skin injury respond with the development of a lichenified patch of skin and others do not is possibly due to the personality of the patient or in an atopic patient due to an increased release of antihistamines with an exaggerated triple response of Lewis beginning the chronic itch–scratch cycle.

**Age Group.** It is very common to see localized neurodermatitis of the posterior neck in menopausal women. Men often prefer the lower leg or ankle. Other clinical types of neurodermatitis are seen at any age.

**Family Incidence.** This disorder may be unrelated to allergies in the patient or family, thus differing from atopic eczema. Atopic people are more "itchy," however, and, as mentioned, some authors feel the two diseases are a continuum.

**Related to Employment.** Recurrent exposure and contact to irritating agents at work can lead to LSC.

### Differential Diagnosis

■ *Psoriasis:* Several patches on the body in classic areas of distribution; family history of disease; classic silvery whitish scales; sharply circumscribed patch; itching may be intense, especially in the scalp and perianal areas, but it is often minimal (see Chapters 14 and 15).
■ *Atopic eczema:* Allergic history in patient or family; multiple lesions; classically seen in cubital and popliteal areas and face (see Chapter 8).
■ *Contact dermatitis:* Acute onset; contact history positive; usually red, vesicular, and oozing; distribution matches site of exposure to contactant; may be acute contact dermatitis overlying LSC owing to overzealous therapy (see Chapter 8).
■ *Lichen planus, hypertrophic form on anterior tibial area:* Lichen planus in mouth and on other body areas; biopsy specimen usually characteristic (see Chapter 15).
■ *Seborrheic dermatitis of scalp:* Does not itch as much; is better in summer; a diffuse, scaly, greasy eruption (see Chapter 15).

### Treatment

*Case Example:* A 45-year-old woman presents with a severely itching, scaly, red, lichenified patch on the back of the neck at the hairline.

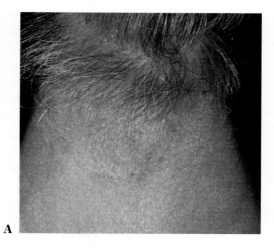

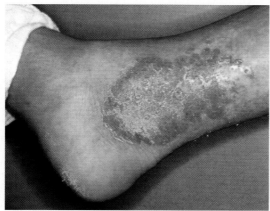

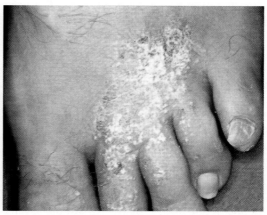

**FIGURE 11-2** ■ Localized LSC in occipital area of the scalp (**A**), of the medial aspect of ankle following lichen planus of the area (**B**), and on the dorsum of the foot (**C**). *(Courtesy of Duke Labs, Inc.)*

***First Visit.***

1. Explain the condition to the patient, and tell her that the medicine is directed toward stopping the itch. If this can be done, and if she cooperates by keeping her hands off the area, the disease will disappear. Emphasize the effect of scratching by stating that if both arms were broken, the eruption would be gone when the casts were removed. However, this is not a recommended form of therapy. Do not blame the patient for this disease in your zeal to explain the importance of keeping hands off.

2. For severe bouts of intractable itching, prescribe ice-cold Burow's solution packs.

   *Sig:* Add 1 packet of Domeboro powder to 1 quart of ice-cold water. Apply cloth wet with this solution for 15 minutes PRN.

3. A moderate-potency corticosteroid ointment or emollient cream 15.0.

   *Sig:* Apply q.i.d., or more often, as itching requires.

   The moderate-potency fluorinated corticosteroid creams (Synalar, Cordran, Lidex, Diprosone, Cutivate) can be used under an occlusive dressing of plastic wrap on extremity lesions. The dressing can be left on overnight.

*Warning:* Long-term occlusive dressing therapy with corticosteroids can cause atrophy of the skin.

***Subsequent Visits.***

1. Add menthol (0.25%) or coal tar solution (3% to 10%) to above ointment or cream for greater antipruritic effect.

2. Intralesional corticosteroid therapy is a very effective and safe treatment. The technique is as follows: use a 1-in-long No. 26 needle or $30\frac{1}{2}$ needle and a Luer-Lok–type tuberculin syringe. Inject 3 or 5 mg/cc of triamcinolone parenteral solution (Kenalog-10 or Aristocort intralesional suspension diluted with normal saline or xylocaine with or without epinephrine) intradermally or subcutaneously, directly under the skin lesion. Do not inject all the solution in one area, but spread it around as you advance the needle. Usually 1 cc or less is injected each time. The injection can be repeated every 3 or 4 weeks as necessary to eliminate the patch of dermatitis.

*Warning:* A complication of an atrophic depression at the injection site can occur. This usually can be avoided if the concentration of triamcinolone in one area is kept low, and when it occurs, it usually disappears after months.

***Resistant Cases.***

1. An antihistamine or antianxiety agent orally.
2. Prednisone 10 mg.
   *Sig:* 1 tablet q.i.d. for 3 days, then 2 tablets every morning for 7 days.
3. Dome-Paste boot or Coban wrap. Apply in office for cases of neurodermatitis localized to the arms and legs. This is a physical deterrent to scratching. Leave on for 1 week at a time.
4. Psychotherapy is of questionable value and patients may be offended by the suggestion.

## External Otitis

*External otitis* is a descriptive term for a common and persistent dermatitis of the ears owing to several causes. The agent most frequently blamed for this condition is "fungus," but pathogenic fungi are rarely found in the external ear. The true causes of external otitis, in order of frequency, are as follows: seborrheic dermatitis (which is now felt to be related to *Pityrosporum ovale* yeast infection), LSC, contact dermatitis, atopic eczema, psoriasis, *Pseudomonas* bacterial infection (which is usually secondary to other causes) and, lastly, fungal infection, which also can be primary or secondary to other factors. For further information on the specific processes, refer to each of the diseases mentioned.

### Treatment

Treatment should be directed primarily toward the specific cause, such as care of the scalp for seborrheic cases or avoidance of jewelry for contact cases. When the primary cause has been addressed, however, certain special techniques and medicines must be used in addition to clear up this troublesome area.

*Case Example:* An elderly woman presents with an oozing, red, crusted, swollen left external ear, with a wet canal but an intact drum. A considerable amount of seborrheic dermatitis of the scalp is confluent with the acutely inflamed ear area. The patient has had itching ear trouble off and on for 10 years, but in the past month, it has become most severe.

***First Visit.***

1. Always inspect the canal and the drum with an otoscope. If excessive wax and debris are present in the canal, or if the drum is involved in the process, the patient should be treated for these problems or referred to an ear specialist. An effective liquid to dry up the oozing canal is as follows:

   Hydrocortisone powder 1%
   Burow's solution, 1:10 strength q.s. 15.0
   *Sig:* Place 2 drops in ear t.i.d.
2. Burow's solution wet packs
   *Sig:* Add 1 packet of Domeboro powder to 1 quart of cool water. Apply wet cloths to external ear for 15 minutes t.i.d.
3. Corticosteroid ointment 15.0
   *Sig:* Apply locally to external ear t.i.d., not in canal.

***Subsequent Visits.*** Several days later, after decreased swelling, cessation of oozing, and lessening of itching, institute the following changes in therapy:

1. Decrease the soaks to once a day.
2. Sulfur, ppt. (parts per thousand) 5%
   Corticosteroid ointment q.s. 15.0
   *Sig:* Apply locally t.i.d. to ear with the little finger, not down in the canal, with a cotton-tipped applicator.

For persistent cases, a short course of oral corticosteroid or antibiotic therapy often removes the "fire" so that local remedies are effective.

## Pruritus Ani

Itching of the anal area is a common malady that can vary in severity from mild to marked. The patient with this very annoying symptom is apt to resort to self-treatment and therefore delay the visit to the physician. Usually, the patient has overtreated the sensitive area, and the immediate problem of the physician is to quiet the acute contact dermatitis. The original cause of the pruritus ani is often difficult to ascertain.

Pruritic diseases common in this area are seborrheic dermatitis, psoriasis, lichen sclerosis et atrophicus, candidiasis, tinea, pin worms (especially in children), and hemorrhoids in adults.

### Presentation and Characteristics

***Primary Lesions.*** These can range from slight redness confined to a very small area to an extensive contact dermatitis with redness, vesicles, and oozing of the entire buttock.

***Secondary Lesions.*** Excoriations from the intense itching are very common, and after a prolonged time, they progress toward lichenification. A generalized papulovesicular id eruption can develop from an acute flare-up of this entity.

***Course.*** Most cases of pruritus ani respond rapidly and completely to proper management, especially if the cause can be ascertained and eliminated. Every physician, however, will have a patient who will continue to scratch and defy all therapy.

***Causes.*** The proper management of this socially unacceptable form of pruritus consists in searching for and eliminating

---

**SAUER'S NOTES**

1. Many cases of acute ear dermatitis are aggravated by an allergy to the therapeutic cream, such as Neosporin, or the ingredients in the base.
2. A corticosteroid in a petrolatum base eliminates this problem.
3. Use 1% Hytone ointment, DesOwen ointment, or Tridesilon ointment. Author likes Cloderm cream.

## SAUER'S NOTES

1. Do not prescribe a fluorinated corticosteroid salve for the anogenital area. It can cause telangiectasia and atrophy of the skin after long-term use.

2. One of my favorite medications for pruritus ani or genital pruritus is 1% Hytone ointment applied sparingly locally two or three times a day. The petrolatum base is well tolerated.

3. If the anogenital pruritus is resistant to therapy and especially if the involvement is unilateral, a biopsy should be performed to rule out Bowen's disease or extramammary Paget's disease. Although psychologically disconcerting to the patient, this is a simple area to biopsy with curved iris scissor after local anesthesia has plumped up the skin. It heals rapidly and can be extremely important to be sure a serious malignancy has not been missed.

4. A short burst of systemic corticosteroids may be necessary to break the itch–scratch cycle. An example of this would be 10 days of prednisone beginning with 50 mg each morning and decreasing by 10 mg every 2 days until gone. Thirty 10 mg tablets is the full 10-day course and no refills should be given.

the several factors that contribute to the persistence of this symptom complex. These factors can be divided into general and specific etiologic factors.

### General Factors

- *Diet:* The following irritating foods should be removed from the diet: chocolate, nuts, cheese, and spicy foods. Coffee, because of its stimulating effect on any form of itching, should be limited to 1 cup a day. Rarely, certain other foods are noted by the patient to aggravate the pruritus.

- *Bathing:* Many patients have the misconception that the itching is caused by uncleanliness. Therefore, they resort to excessive bathing and scrubbing of the anal area. This is harmful and irritating and must be stopped.

- *Toilet care:* Harsh toilet paper contributes greatly to the continuance of this condition. Cotton or a proprietary cleansing cloth (e.g., Tucks) must be used for wiping. Mineral oil or Balneol lotion can be added to the cotton if necessary. Rarely, an allergy to the pastel tint in colored toilet tissues is a factor causing pruritus.

- *Scratching:* As with all the diseases of this group, chronic scratching leads to a vicious cycle. The chief aim of the physician is to give relief from this itching, but a gentle admonishment to the patient to keep hands off is indicated. With the physician's help, the itch–scratch cycle can be broken. The emotional and mental personality of the patient regulates the effectiveness of this suggestion.

### Specific Etiologic Factors

- *Oral antibiotics:* Pruritus ani from oral antibiotic therapy is seen frequently. It may or may not be due to an overgrowth of Candida organisms. The physician who automatically questions patients about recent drug ingestion will not miss this diagnosis.

- *LSC:* It is always a problem to know which comes first, the itching or the "nervousness." In most instances, the itching comes first, but there is no denying that once pruritus ani has developed, it is aggravated by emotional tension and "nerves." However, only the rare patient has a "deep-seated" psychologic problem.

- *Psoriasis:* In this area, psoriasis is common. Usually, other skin surfaces are also involved.

- *Atopic eczema:* Atopic eczema of this site is rather unusual. A history of atopy in the patient or family is helpful in establishing this cause.

- *Fungal infection:* Contrary to old beliefs, this cause is quite rare. Clinically, a raised, sharp, papulovesicular border is seen that commonly is confluent with tinea of the crural area or buttocks. If a scraping or a culture reveals fungi, then local or systemic antifungal therapy is indicated for cure.

- *Worm infestation:* In children, pinworms can often be implicated. A diagnosis is made by finding eggs on morning anal smears, by applying scotch tape to the anal orifice and viewing the worms under the microscope, or by seeing the small white worms when the child is sleeping. Worms are a rare cause of adult pruritus ani.

- *Hemorrhoids:* In the layperson's mind, this is undoubtedly the most common cause. Actually, it is an unimportant primary factor but may be a contributing factor. Hemorrhoidectomy alone is rarely successful as a cure for pruritus ani.

- *Cancer:* This is a very rare cause of anal itching, but a rectal or proctoscopic examination may be indicated, especially in men who have sex with men.

### Treatment.

*Case Example:* A patient states that he has had anal itching for 4 months. It began after a 5-day course of an antibiotic for the "flu." Many local remedies have been used; the latest, a supposed remedy for athlete's foot, aggravated the condition. Examination reveals an oozing, macerated, red area around the anus.

### First Visit.

1. Initial therapy should include removal of the general factors listed under *Causes* and giving instructions as to diet, bathing, toilet care, and scratching.

2. Burow's solution wet packs

   *Sig:* Add 1 packet of Domeboro to 1 quart of cool water. Apply wet cloths to the area b.i.d. while lying in bed for 20 minutes, or more often if necessary for severe itching. Ice cubes may be added to the solution for more anti-itching effect.

3. Low-potency corticosteroid cream or ointment q.s. 15.0

   *Sig:* Apply to area b.i.d.

4. Diphenhydramine, 50 mg

   *Sig:* 1 capsule h.s. (for itching and sedation).
   *Comment:* Available over the counter.

**Subsequent Visits.**

1. As tolerated, add increasing strengths of sulfur, coal tar solution, or menthol (0.25%) or phenol (0.5%) to the above cream, or to Vytone cream with hydrocortisone 1% and iodoquinol (can be given in a cheaper generic formulation).

2. Intralesional corticosteroid injection therapy is very effective. Usually, the minor discomfort of the injection is quite well tolerated because of the patient's desire to be cured. The technique is described in the section on LSC. Use only 3 mg/cc triamcinilone or lower concentration.

## Genital Pruritus

Itching of the female vulva or the male scrotum can be treated in much the same way as pruritus ani if the special considerations discussed in this section are borne in mind.

### Vulvar Pruritus

Etiologically, vulvar pruritus is caused by *Candida* or *Trichomonas* infection; contact dermatitis from underwear, douche chemicals, contraceptive jellies and diaphragms; chronic cervicitis; neurodermatitis; menopausal or senile atrophic changes; lichen sclerosus et atrophicus; bacillary vaginosis; or leukoplakia. Pruritus vulvae is frequently seen in patients with diabetes mellitus and during pregnancy.

Treatment can be adapted from that for pruritus ani (see preceding section) with the addition of a daily douche, such as 2 tbsp of vinegar to 1 quart of warm water.

*Vulvodynia* is a difficult problem to manage. The sensation of burning and pain in the vulvar area is not uncommon and requires careful etiologic evaluation. Most cases can be managed as a contact dermatitis, but there is a strong psychologic element. A minimal dose of haloperidol (Haldol), 1 mg b.i.d., amitriptyline (Elavil), 10 mg h.s., or (doxepin) (Sinequan), 10 mg h.s. is occasionally indicated and effective. Larger doses may be necessary. Scrotodynia is a similar variant in men and pudendal nerve disease should

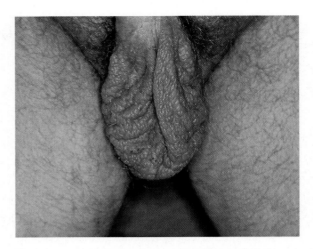

**FIGURE 11-3** ■ Localized LSC of the scrotum, with marked lichenification and thickening of the skin. *(Courtesy of Duke Labs, Inc.)*

be considered in the differential diagnosis especially in bicycle enthusiasts.

### Scrotal Pruritus

Etiologically, scrotal pruritus is due to tinea infection; contact dermatitis from soaps, powders, or clothing; or LSC (**Fig. 11-3**). Treatment is similar to that given for pruritus ani in the preceding section.

## Notalgia Paresthetica

Notalgia paresthetica is a moderately common localized pruritic dermatosis that is usually confined to the middle upper back or scapular area off to one side of the spine. A pigmented patch may be formed by the chronic rubbing. Spinal nerve impingement has been suggested as the etiology by some authors. Zonalon cream four times a day may be helpful, but when applied over large areas, it may cause drowsiness. Some evidence exists for a hereditary factor. EMLA anesthetic cream and capsaicin (Zostrix) cream may be beneficial.

## Suggested Readings

Fleischer A. *The Clinical Management of Itching.* New York: Parthenon Publishing Group; 2000.
Kam PC, Tan KH. Pruritus—itching for a cause and relief? *Anaesthesia.* 1996;51(12):1133–1138.
Yosipovitch G, David M. The diagnostic and therapeutic approach to idiopathic generalized pruritus. *Int J Dermatol.* 1999;38:881–887.
Yosipovitch G, Greaves MW, Fleischer A, et al. *Itch: Basic Mechanisms and Therapy.* New York: Marcel Dekker; 2004.

# CHAPTER 12

# Vascular Dermatoses

*John C. Hall, MD*

Urticaria, erythema multiforme and its variants, and erythema nodosum are included under the heading of vascular dermatoses because of their vascular reaction patterns. Stasis dermatitis is included because it is a dermatosis owing to venous insufficiency in the legs. Vasculitis is due to inflammation on the arterial side of the vascular tree in small or large vessels. Pigmented purpura is due to microvascular capillary leakage of red blood cells and hence hemosiderin staining in a prone patient. It is called a benign hemosiderosis in contrast to the "malignant" type of hemosiderosis seen in hemochromatosis, where internal organs (especially the liver) may be involved. Pyoderma gangrenosum is an ulcerative inflammatory disease, mainly of the lower extremities. Cutaneous necrosis is end-stage vascular compromise with gangrenous disease.

## Urticaria

The commonly (10% to 25% of population at some time in life) seen entity of urticaria (Fig. 12-1), or hives, can be acute or chronic and due to known or unknown causes. Numerous factors, both immunologic and nonimmunologic, can be involved in its pathogenesis. The urticarial wheal results from liberation of histamine from tissue mast cells and from circulating basophils.

*Nonimmunologic* factors that can release histamine from these cells include

- chemicals,
- various drugs (including morphine and codeine),
- ingestion of fish (especially shellfish), nuts (especially peanuts), and other foods,
- bacterial toxins, and
- physical agents.

An example of the type of wheal caused by physical agents is the linear wheal produced by light stroking of the skin, known as *dermographism.* (Consult the Dictionary–Index at the end of the book for the triple response of Lewis reaction.)

*Immunologic* mechanisms are probably involved more often in acute than in chronic urticaria. The most commonly considered of these mechanisms is the type I hypersensitivity state, which is triggered by polyvalent antigen bridging that involves two specific immunoglobulin (Ig) E molecules that are bound to the mast cell or basophil surface (see Chapter 9).

### Lesions

Pea-sized red papules to large circinate patterns with red borders and white centers that can cover an entire side of the trunk or the thigh may be noted. Vesicles and bullae are seen in severe cases, along with hemorrhagic effusions. A severe

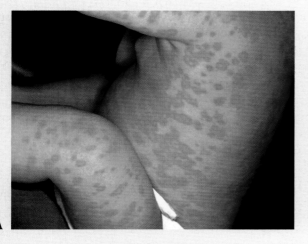
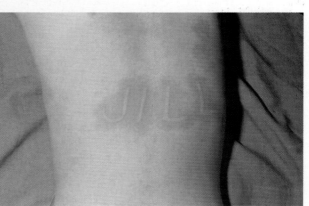

A          B

**FIGURE 12-1** ■ **(A)** Acute urticaria from penicillin in a 6-month-old child. **(B)** Dermographism on flexor wrist. *(Courtesy of Dermik Laboratories, Inc.)*

form of urticaria is labeled *angioedema*. It can involve an entire body part, such as the lip or the hand. Edema of the glottis and bronchospasm are serious complications and are true medical emergencies.

## Presentation and Characteristics

### Course

Acute cases may be mild or explosive but usually disappear with or without treatment in a few hours or days. The chronic form has remissions and exacerbations for months or years. One definition of chronic urticaria is one episode at least twice weekly for 6 weeks.

### Causes

After careful questioning and investigation, many cases of hives, particularly of the chronic type, are concluded to result from no apparent causative agent. Other cases, mainly the acute ones, have been found to result from the following factors or agents:

- *Drugs or chemicals:* Penicillin and derivatives are probably the most common causes of acute hives, but any other drug, whether ingested, injected, inhaled, or, rarely, applied on the skin, can cause the reaction (see Chapter 8).
- *Foods:* Foods are a common cause of acute hives. The main offenders are seafood, nuts, chocolate, strawberries, cheeses, pork, eggs, wheat, and milk. Chronic hives can be caused by traces of penicillin in milk products (Fig. 12-1A).
- *Insect bites and stings:* Insect bites, stings from mosquitoes, fleas, or spiders, and contact with certain moths, leeches, and jellyfish may cause hives.
- *Physical agents:* Hives can result from heat, cold, radiant energy vibration, water, and physical injury. *Dermographism* is a term applied to a localized urticarial wheal produced by scratching the skin in certain people (Fig. 12-1B).
- *Inhalants:* Nasal sprays, insect sprays, dust, feathers, pollens, and animal dander are some common offenders.
- *Infections:* A focus of infection is always considered, sooner or later, in chronic cases of hives, and in unusual instances it is causative. The sinuses, teeth, tonsils, gallbladder, and genitourinary tract should be checked.
- *Internal disease:* Urticaria has been seen with liver disease, intestinal parasites, cancer, rheumatic fever, lupus erythematosus, vitiligo, pernicious anemia, rheumatoid arthritis, and others.
- *"Nerves":* After all other causes of chronic urticaria have been ruled out, there remain a substantial number of cases that appear to be related to nervous stress, worry, or fatigue. These cases benefit most from the establishment of good rapport between the patient and the physician.

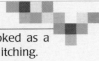

**SAUER'S NOTE**

Dermographism is commonly overlooked as a cause of the patient's "welts" or vague itching.

- *Contact urticaria syndrome:* This uncommon response can be incited by local contact on the skin of drugs and chemicals, foods, insects, animal hair or dander, and plants.
- *Cholinergic urticaria:* Clinically, small papular welts are seen that are caused by heat (hot bath), stress, or strenuous exercise.

## Differential Diagnosis

- *Erythema multiforme:* Systemic fever, malaise, and mouth lesions are noted in children and young adults (see the next section of this chapter).
- *Dermographism:* A common finding in young adults, especially those who present complaining of welts on their skin or vague itching of the skin with no residual lesions. To make the diagnosis, stroke the skin firmly to see if an urticarial response develops. The course can be chronic, but hydroxyzine, 10 mg b.i.d. or t.i.d., is quite helpful. (Warn the patient about the possibility of drowsiness.) Nonsedating antihistamines can also be tried.
- *Urticarial vasculitis:* Lesions may last more than 24 hours, may be painful, leave a bruise or hyperpigmentation, and be associated with hypocomplementemia and systemic lupus erythematosus. Skin biopsy is confirmatory.

## Treatment

*Case Example:* A patient presents for a case of acute hives due to penicillin injection 1 week previously for a "cold."

1. Colloidal bath
   *Sig:* Add 1 cup of starch or oatmeal (Aveeno) to 6 to 8 in of lukewarm water in the tub. Bathe for 15 minutes once or twice a day.
2. Sarna lotion, Aveeno Anti-itch lotion, or PrameGel or any pramoxine-containing topical over the counter (OTC).
   *Sig:* Apply PRN locally for itching.
3. Hydroxyzine (Atarax), 10 mg #30
   *Sig:* Take 1 tablet t.i.d., a.c. (warn of drowsiness).
4. Diphenhydramine (Benadryl), 50 mg
   *Comment:* Available OTC
5. Nonsedating antihistamines can also be used.
6. Betamethasone sodium phosphate (6 mgms/cc Celstone Soluspan), 3 mg/cc
   *Sig:* Inject 1 to 1.5 cc intramuscularly.

For a more severe case of acute hives:

1. Diphenhydramine injection
   *Sig:* Inject 2 mL (20 mg) subcutaneously, *or*

2. Epinephrine hydrochloride

   *Sig:* Inject 0.3 to 0.5 mL of 1:1,000 solution subcutaneously, *or*

3. Prednisone tablets, 10 mg #30

   *Sig:* Take 5 tablets every 2 days and decrease by 1 tablet every 2 days for a 10-day course.

For treatment of a patient with chronic hives of 6 months' duration when cause is undetermined after careful history and examination:

1. Hydroxyzine (Atarax), 10 to 25 mg #60

   *Sig:* Take 1 tablet t.i.d. depending on drowsiness and effectiveness. Continue for weeks or months.
   Clemastine (Tavist) 1.34 or 2.68 mg #30
   *Sig:* Take 1 tablet b.i.d., available OTC.
   Cyproheptadine (Periactin) 4 mg #60
   *Sig:* One tablet by mouth t.i.d.

2. Loratadine (Claritin) now OTC 10 mg #30

   *Sig:* Take 1 tablet once a day.
   Cetirizine (Zyrtec) 5 mg or 10 mg #30
   *Sig:* Take 1 tablet once a day.
   Fexofenadine (Allegra), 60 mg or 180 mg #30
   *Sig:* Take 1 tablet once a day.

3. Cimetidine (Tagamet), 300 mg #60

   *Sig:* Take 1 tablet t.i.d. (200 mg, 400 mg, or 800 mg).
   *Comment:* This H2 blocker is of benefit in some cases and can be added to H1 blockers.

4. Suggest avoidance of seafood, nuts, chocolate, cheese and other milk products, strawberries, pork, excessively spicy foods, and excess of coffee or tea.

5. Keep a diet diary of everything ingested (including all foods, all medicines, even OTC, candy, menthol cigarettes, chewing gum, chewing tobacco, mouthwash, breath fresheners) and then see what items were used 12 to 24 hours before the episode of hives occurred.

6. A mild sedative or tranquilizer such as meprobamate, 400 mg t.i.d., or chlordiazepoxide (Librium), 5 mg t.i.d., may help.

7. Doxepin (Sinequan) 10 mg #60

   *Sig:* 1 tablet t.i.d.
   *Comment:* This is a tricyclic antidepressant with potent antihistaminic properties. It can cause drowsiness, dry mouth, and other side effects of this classification of drugs.

8. Immunosuppressive drugs such as prednisone are unfortunately necessary in severe cases.

9. Zaditor (ketotifen fumarate) is a mast-cell stabilizer with benefits in severe cases, but I have not used this drug.

10. Sulfasalazine (500 mg increased up to 4,000 mg by increasing by 500 mg each week) has been reported in chronic idiopathic urticaria to be a steroid-sparing or steroid-replacing drug in one report.

## Erythema Multiforme

The term *erythema multiforme* introduces a flurry of confusion in the mind of any student of medicine. It is our purpose in this section to attempt to dispel that confusion. Erythema multiforme, as originally described by Hebra, is an uncommon, distinct disease of unknown cause characterized by red iris-shaped or bull's eye–like macules, papules, or bullae confined mainly to the extremities, the face, and the lips (Fig. 12-2). It can be accompanied by mild fever, malaise, and arthralgia. It occurs usually in children and young adults in the spring and the fall, has a duration of 2 to 4 weeks, and frequently is recurrent for several years.

The only relation between Hebra's erythema multiforme and the following diseases or syndromes is the clinical appearance of the eruption.

- *Stevens–Johnson syndrome* is a severe and rarely fatal variant of erythema multiforme. It is characterized by high fever, extensive purpura, bullae, ulcers of the mucous membranes, and, after 2 to 3 days, ulcers of the skin. Eye involvement can result in blindness. It can be related to drugs and its severest form is considered by some to be the same as toxic epidermal necrolysis (see Chapter 18).
- *Erythema multiforme bullosum* is a severe, chronic, bullous disease of adults (see Chapter 18). There is an opinion that this syndrome is completely separate from erythema multiforme. More macular truncal lesions and more epidermal necrosis and less infiltrate may be seen in Stevens–Johnson syndrome (toxic epidermal necrolysis). Sulfonamides, anticonvulsant agents, allopurinol, chlormezanone, and nonsteroidal anti-inflammatory drugs commonly cause erythema multiforme bullosum.
- *Erythema multiforme–like drug eruption* is frequently due to phenacetin, quinine, penicillin, mercury, arsenic, phenylbutazone, barbiturates, trimethadione, phenytoin, sulfonamides, and antitoxins (see Chapter 8).
- *Erythema multiforme–like eruption* is caused rather commonly as part of a herpes simplex outbreak and in conjunction with rheumatic fever, pneumonia,

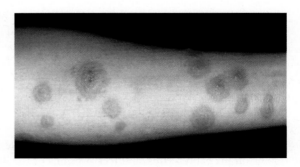

**FIGURE 12-2** ■ Erythema multiforme–like eruption on the arm during pregnancy. *(Courtesy of Dermik Laboratories, Inc.)*

meningitis, measles, Coxsackievirus infection, pregnancy, and cancer. It also occurs after deep x-ray therapy and as an allergic reaction to foods.

## Differential Diagnosis

■ The *erythema perstans* group, or figurate erythemas, includes over a dozen clinical entities with impossible-to-remember names. (See Dictionary–Index under *erythema perstans*.) All have various-sized erythematous patches, papules, or plaques with a definite red border and a less active center, forming circles, half circles, groups of circles, and linear bands. Multiple causes have been ascribed, including tick bites; allergic reactions; fungal, bacterial, viral, and spirochetal infections; and internal cancer. The duration of and the response to therapy vary with each individual case.

■ *Erythema chronicum migrans* is the distinctive cutaneous eruption of the multisystem tick-borne spirochetosis Lyme disease. The deer tick, *Ixodes dammini,* is the vector for this spirochete. Early therapy with doxycycline or ampicillin may prevent late manifestations of the disease (see Chapter 22).

■ *Reiter's syndrome* is the triad of conjunctivitis, urethritis, and, most important, arthritis, that occurs predominantly in men and lasts about 6 months. The skin manifestations consist of psoriasiform dermatitis, which is called *balanitis circinata* on the penis and *keratoderma blennorrhagica* on the palms and soles.

■ *Behçet's syndrome* consists of the triad of genital, oral, and ophthalmic ulcerations seen most commonly in men; it can last for years, with recurrences. Other manifestations include cutaneous pustular vasculitis, synovitis, and meningoencephalitis. It is more prevalent in eastern Mediterranean countries and Japan. Skin hypersensitivity to trauma or pathergy is observed with sterile pustular formation 24 to 48 hours after an intradermal needle prick.

■ *Urticaria:* Clinically, urticaria may resemble erythema multiforme, but hives are associated with only mild systemic symptoms. It can occur in any age group; iris lesions are unusual. Usually, it can be attributed to penicillin or other drug therapy, and it responds rapidly but often not completely to antihistamine therapy (see first part of this chapter). It is evanescent and dissipates or moves to a new area in less than 24 hours.

## Treatment

*Case Example:* A 12-year-old boy presents with bull's eye–like lesions on his hands, arms, and feet, erosions of the lips and mucous membranes of the mouth, malaise, and a temperature of 101°F (38.3°C) orally. He had a similar eruption last spring.

1. Order bed rest and increased oral fluid intake.
2. Acetaminophen (Tylenol), 325 mg OTC
   *Sig:* Take 1 to 2 tablets q.i.d., *or*
   Prednisone, 10 mg #16
   *Sig:* Take 2 tablets stat and then 2 tablets every morning for 7 days.
3. For severe cases, such as the Stevens–Johnson form, hospitalization is indicated, where intravenous corticosteroid therapy (debatable), intravenous fluid replacement infusions, immunoglobulin, and other supportive measures can be administered.

## Erythema Nodosum

Erythema nodosum is an uncommon reaction pattern seen mainly on the anterior tibial areas of the legs (Fig. 12-3). It appears as erythematous nodules in successive crops and is preceded by fever, malaise, and arthralgia.

### Presentation and Characteristics

*Primary Lesions*

Bilateral, red, tender, rather well-circumscribed nodules are seen mainly on the pretibial surface of the legs and, rarely, on the arms and the body. Later, the flat, indurated lesions may become raised, confluent, and purpuric. Only a few lesions develop at one time.

*Secondary Lesions*

The lesions never suppurate or form ulcers but can heal with a bruise.

*Course*

The lesions last several weeks, but the duration can be affected by therapy directed to the cause, if it is known. Relapses are related to the cause. The lesions can be idiopathic and have a chronic course.

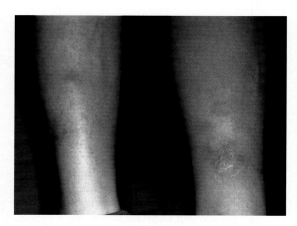

**FIGURE 12-3** ■ Erythema nodosum on the legs. *(Courtesy of Dermik Laboratories, Inc.)*

*Causes*

Careful clinical and laboratory examinations are necessary to determine the cause of this toxic reaction pattern. The following tests should be performed:

- Complete blood cell count
- Erythrocyte sedimentation rate
- Urinalysis
- Strep screen, serum pregnancy test, angiotensin-converting enzyme, tuberculin skin test
- Serologic test for syphilis
- Chest x-ray
- Specific skin tests, as indicated

The causes of erythema nodosum are

- Streptococcal infection (rheumatic fever, pharyngitis, scarlet fever, arthritis)
- Fungal infection (coccidioidomycosis, trichophyton infection)
- Pregnancy or oral contraceptives
- Sarcoidosis
- Lymphogranuloma venereum
- Syphilis
- Chancroid
- Drugs (contraceptive pills, sulfonamides, iodides, bromides, echinacea herbal therapy)
- Hepatitis C
- HIV infection
- Celiac disease
- Carcinoid syndrome
- Tuberculosis

It is rare in children, but when it occurs, group A β-hemolytic streptococcal infection (which may be occult) is the most common cause. Oral contraceptives are a common cause in adult women. It is not uncommon to be unable to find a cause.

*Age and Gender Incidence*

The disorder occurs predominantly in adolescent girls and young women.

*Laboratory Findings*

Histopathologic examination reveals a nonspecific but characteristically localized inflammatory infiltrate in the subcutaneous tissue and in and around the veins.

## Differential Diagnosis

- *Erythema induratum:* Chronic vasculitis of young women that occurs on the posterior calf area and often suppurates; biopsy shows a tuberculoid-type infiltrate, usually with caseation. A tuberculous causation has been suggested.
- *Necrobiosis lipoidica diabeticorum:* A cutaneous manifestation of diabetes mellitus, characterized by well-defined patches of reddish-yellow atrophic skin, often with overlying telangiectasias primarily on anterior areas of the legs. The lesions can ulcerate; biopsy results are characteristic, but biopsy may not be indicated because of the possibility of poor healing and the characteristic clinical presentation (see Chapter 38).
- *Periarteritis nodosa:* A rare, sometimes fatal, arteritis that most often occurs in men. Twenty-five percent of patients show painful subcutaneous nodules and purpura, mainly of the lower extremities, which often show livedo reticularis. It is a multiorgan system disease; renal failure is often a component. There is a cutaneous variety. (+) p-ANCA blood test is needed for diagnosis.
- *Superficial thrombophlebitis migrans (Buerger's disease):* An early venous change of Buerger's disease commonly seen in male patients, with painful nodules of the anterior tibial area. Biopsy is of value. Smoking has been suggested as an important contributing factor.
- *Nodular panniculitis or Weber–Christian disease:* Occurs mainly in obese middle-aged women. Tender, indurated, subcutaneous nodules and plaques are seen, usually on the thighs and the buttocks. Each crop is preceded by fever and malaise. Residual atrophy and hyperpigmentation occur.
- *Leukocytoclastic vasculitis:* Includes a constellation of diseases, such as allergic angiitis, allergic vasculitis, necrotizing vasculitis, and cutaneous systemic vasculitis. Clinically, palpable purpuric lesions are seen, most commonly on the lower part of the legs. In later stages, the lesions may become nodular, bullous, infarctive, and ulcerative. Various etiologic agents have been implicated, such as infection, drugs, and foreign proteins. Treatment includes bed rest, pentoxifylline (Trental), corticosteroids, and other immunosuppressive drugs (see Chapter 9).

For completeness, the following five rare syndromes with *inflammatory nodules of the legs* are defined in the Dictionary–Index:

1. Subcutaneous fat necrosis with pancreatic disease
2. Migratory panniculitis
3. Allergic granulomatosis
4. Necrobiotic granulomatosis
5. Embolic nodules from several sources

## Treatment

1. Treat the cause, if possible.
2. Rest, local heat, and aspirin are valuable. The eruption is self-limited if the cause can be eliminated.
3. Chronic cases can be disabling enough to warrant a short course of corticosteroid therapy. Some cases have benefited from naproxen (Naprosyn), 250 mg b.i.d. (or other nonsteroidal anti-inflammatory drugs), for 2 to 4 weeks.

## Stasis (Venous) Dermatitis and Ulcers

Stasis dermatitis is a common condition owing to impaired venous circulation in the legs of older patients (Fig. 12-4). Almost all cases are associated with varicose veins, and because the tendency to develop varicosities is a familial characteristic, stasis dermatitis is also familial. The medial malleolar area of the ankle is the most common location. Stasis ulcers can develop in the impaired skin. They are commonly accompanied by brownish discoloration, pruritus, excoriations, and dry, fine adherent scales. Late in the disease edema may be accompanied by lymphedematous blebs (elephantiasis verrucosa) and leakage of a serous thick yellow lymph fluid. Numerous conditions are associated with stasis dermatitis (Table 12-3).

### Presentation and Characteristics

#### Primary Lesions

Early cases of stasis dermatitis begin as a red, scaly, pruritic patch that rapidly becomes vesicular and crusted owing to scratching and subsequent secondary infection. Bacterial infection may be responsible for the spread of the patch and the chronicity of the eruption. Edema of the affected ankle area results in a further decrease in circulation and, consequently, more infection. The lesions may be unilateral or bilateral.

#### Secondary Lesions

Three secondary conditions can arise from untreated stasis dermatitis:

- *Hyperpigmentation:* This is inevitable following the healing of either simple or severe stasis dermatitis of the legs. This reddish-brown increase in pigmentation is slow to disappear, and in many elderly patients it never does so.
- *Stasis ulcers:* These can occur as the result of edema, trauma, deeper bacterial infection, or improper care of the primary dermatitis.

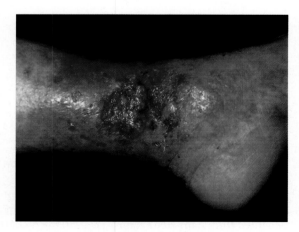

**FIGURE 12-4** ■ Stasis dermatitis. *(Courtesy of Dermik Laboratories, Inc.)*

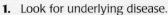

**SAUER'S NOTE**

Leg ulcer mantras

1. Look for underlying disease.
2. Look for an underlying malignant tumor, that is, basal cell cancer, squamous cell cancer, melanoma.
3. Look for clotting disorders.
4. Look for causes of ischemia, that is, arteriosclerotic vascular disease.
5. Look for an infection (primary or secondary).
6. Look for contact dermatitis.
7. Always consider a skin biopsy as part of the evaluation.

- *Infectious eczematoid dermatitis:* This can develop on the legs, the arms, and even the entire body, either slowly or as an explosive, rapidly spreading distant, symmetric, autoeczematous, or "id" eruption (see Chapter 21).

#### Course

The rapidity of healing of stasis dermatitis depends on the age of the patient and other factors listed under *Causes.* In elderly patients who have untreated varicose veins, stasis dermatitis can persist for years with remissions and exacerbations. If stasis dermatitis develops in a patient in the 40- to 50-year age group, the prognosis is particularly bad for future recurrences and possible ulcers. Once stasis ulcers develop, they can rapidly expand in size and depth. Healing of the ulcer, if possible for a given patient, depends on many factors. Ulcers less than 1 year old, less than 5 cm², and ulcers that show significant healing after 3 weeks are more likely to heal by compression and bioocclusive dressings alone. Grafting procedures may be necessary for other venous leg ulcers. Negative pressure devices have shown promise.

#### Causes

Poor venous circulation owing to the sluggish blood flow in tortuous, dilated varicose veins with incompetence of the venous valves in the distribution of the greater saphenous vein (medial ankle) is the primary cause. If the factors of obesity, congestive heart failure, renal failure, lack of proper rest or care of the legs, pruritus, secondary infection, low-protein diet, and old age are added to the circulation problem, the result can be a chronic, disabling disease. Table 12-1 lists tests for nonhealing ulcers.

#### Differential Diagnosis

- *Contact dermatitis:* Taking a careful history is important especially regarding nylon hose, new socks, contact with ragweed, high-top shoes, and so on, appears where contactant has touched the skin; no venous insufficiency is noted.

**TABLE 12-1 ■ Tests for Hypercoagulability in Nonhealing Leg Ulcers**

Activated partial thromboplastin time (aPTT)

Anticardiolipin antibody

Antithrombin III

CBC

Cryoglobulins

Factor II (prothrombin)

Factor V (Leiden)

Homocysteine (methylenetetrahydrofolate reductase)

Immunoglobulin electrophoresis

Lupus anticoagulant

Prothrombin time (PTT)

Protein C and protein S

Sickle cell

Thrombin time

- *Lichen simplex chronicus:* Thickened, dry, very pruritic plaque; no venous insufficiency is found (see Chapter 11).
- *Atrophie blanche:* Characterized by small ulcers that heal with irregular white scars; seen mainly over the ankles and legs. Telangiectasis and hyperpigmentation surround the scars. This arterial vasculopathy can respond to pentoxifylline (Trental). Another name for it is segmental hyalinizing vasculopathy. Anticoagulants such as aspirin, Plavix (clopidogrel), Trental (pentoxifylline), Persantine (dipyramidol), and Coumadin may be beneficial. Underlying clotting disorders need to be searched for with a hypercoagulability panel.
- *Arterial or ischemic ulcers:* These are usually more punched out and painful. Intermittent claudication and nighttime pain are relieved by exercise. Arterial duplex ultrasound or arteriography may be necessary to diagnose these ulcers. Revascularization procedures may be indicated, and compression therapies can be counterproductive.
- *Drug eruptions:* These are often worst and first on lower legs and usually sudden in appearance. Recent use of a new drug is a helpful indication, but the eruption can be from a drug that has been taken for a longer period of time. The clinical manifestations are protean.

Differential diagnosis for stasis ulcers includes

- Pyodermic ulcers
- Arterial ulcers (such as mal perforans of diabetes)
- Periarteritis nodosa
- Necrobiosis lipoidica ulcers
- Pyoderma gangrenosum
- Malignancies (especially squamous cell carcinoma)

- Ulcers from autoimmune diseases especially lupus erythematosus
- Vasculitis

Blood tests, cultures, and biopsies help to establish the type of ulcer. Never underestimate the value of a good history and physical. Imaging studies such as a venous and/or arterial Doppler study or angiography are often necessary.

## Treatment of Stasis Dermatitis

*Case Example:* A 55-year-old laborer presents with scaly, reddish, slightly edematous, excoriated dermatitis on the medial aspect of the left ankle and leg of 6 weeks' duration.

1. Prescribe rest and elevation of the leg as much as possible by lying in bed. The foot of the bed should be elevated 4 in by placing two bricks under the legs. Attempt to elevate the leg when sitting. Avoid prolonged standing or sitting with the legs bent. Taking time to walk on a long train, car, or plane trip is a good idea. Work restrictions may be necessary.
2. Burow's solution wet packs
   *Sig:* Add 1 packet of powder to 1 quart of warm water. Apply cloths wet with this solution for 30 minutes b.i.d.
3. An antibiotic and corticosteroid ointment mixture q.s. 30.0
   *Sig:* Apply to leg t.i.d.

For more severe cases of stasis dermatitis with oozing, cellulitis, and 3-pitting edema, the following treatment should be ordered, in addition:

1. Hospitalization or enforced bed rest at home for the purpose of (1) applying the wet packs for longer periods of time and (2) strict rest and elevation of the leg.
2. A course of an oral antibiotic.
3. Prednisone, 10 mg #36
   *Sig:* Take 2 tablets b.i.d. for 4 days, then 2 tablets in the morning for 10 days.
4. Ace elastic bandage, 4-in wide, no. 8

After the patient is discharged from the hospital and ambulatory, give instructions for the correct application of an ace bandadge or a properly measured pressure garment to the leg before arising in the morning. This helps to reduce the edema that could cause a recrudescence of the dermatitis. Pressure dressing should either be knee-high or thigh-high.

## Treatment of Stasis Ulcer

As for any chronic difficult medical problem, there are many methods touted for successful management.

*Case Example:* Consider a 75-year-old obese woman on a low income who has a 4-cm ulcer on her medial right ankle area with surrounding dermatitis, edema, and pigmentation.

1. *Manage the primary problem or problems:* Attempt to remedy the obesity, make sure there is adequate nutrition, and treat systemic or other causes of the ulcer.

2. *Correct the physiologic alterations:* Control the edema with adhesive flexible bandages of adequate width (4-in-wide usually) and with correct application from foot up to knee. A Jobst-type support stocking or pump may be indicated in resistant cases.

3. *Treat contributing factors:* Control the dermatitis, itching, and infection.

4. *Promote healing:* Occlusion of the ulcer has been proven to accelerate healing. Unna's boots, adhesive flexible bandage dressings, and polyurethane-type films have been used with success. Enzymatic granules have their proponents as do collagen granules and Granulex. Accuzyme, which contains papain and urea, that is an example of a topical debriding agent.

5. *Skin grafting may be indicated in deep, stubborn ulcers:* Artificial skin substitutes such as Apligraf may be used.

6. *Hyperbaric oxygenation:* This may be helpful for many different types of ulcers where available but is usually used for ischemic ulcers. Claustrophobia and tympanic membrane rupture are two significant side effects.

7. *Topical negative pressure devices:* This is also called vacuum-assisted closure and consists of a fenestrated evacuation tube embedded in a foam dressing and covered with an airtight dressing. Then a vacuum source attached to the tube applies continuous or intermittent subatmospheric pressure at 100 to 125 mm Hg. The wound needs debridement before beginning this therapy, and the gauze should be changed at least every other day.

8. *Alginate dressings (Kaltostat, Sorbsan, Tegagen, AlgiSite, Aquacel Hydrofiber):* These are derived from brown seaweed and are very absorbent. They are available as ropes or pads. Care must be taken not to overdry the ulcer.

9. *Foams:* Foams (3M Adhesive foam, Lyofoam C, Allevyn hydrocellular dressing, Allevyn cavity dressing) and hydrocolloids (Tegasorb, DuoDERM CGF, Comfeel Plus) can be used when moderate absorption is desired.

10. *Collagen products:* Collagen products such as Promogran, Oasis wound matrix, and Cymetra are sometimes used for recalcitrant leg ulcers.

11. *Silver ion dressings:* Silver ion dressings (silver sulfadiazine, Aquacel Ag Hydrofiber, Acticoat 7, Actisorb Silver 220, Silverlon wound contact dressing, SilvaSorb, Silvercel), although causing discoloration and some irritation, are helpful in ulcers where infection is suspected.

12. *Regranex:* This is a topical recombinant human platelet growth factor touted by some authors.

13. *"Short-contact" tretinoin solution (0.05%):* This can cause irritation but has been used to attempt to increase granulation tissue.

14. *Hydrogels:* Hydrogels (Restore hydrogel, Carrasyn hydrogel, SAF-gel, Curagel, XCell cellulose dressing) are mainly helpful in hydrating wounds.

15. *Topical options:* The array of topical options for ulcers is confusing, and they are often very expensive. The author frequently uses Johnson & Johnson advanced healing adhesive pads, which are cheap and easy to use (the pad is left on until it falls off in a few days). Be sure the wound is not infected and has been debrided either mechanically or with debriding pad topicals.

Here is the technique we would use for this case example. The diagnosis is stasis or venous ulcer.

1. Advise a multiple vitamin and mineral supplement tablet once a day, including zinc and magnesium.

2. Elevate the leg as much as possible when lying down prone.

3. Erythromycin, 250 mg #100

   *Sig:* Take 2 to 3 tablets a day until ulcer is healed.
   *Comment:* Infection is common.

4. Prednisone, 10 mg #60

   *Sig:* Take 1 tablet every morning.
   *Actions:* Antipruritic, anti-inflammatory

5. Apply an *occlusive dressing* in the office. If there is a lot of drainage and debris, the frequency of dressing changes should be every 3 to 4 days at first, then weekly. Use a footrest stand for the leg. Keep a record of the size of the ulcer.

   a. Apply Bactroban ointment to a Telfa dressing.
   b. Place gauze squares in four layers over the Telfa dressing.
   c. Apply adhesive flexible bandage wrap over the gauze, down to the foot arch and up to below the knee, more firmly wrapped distally. Do not apply too tightly at first.
   d. Wrap an adhesive flexible bandage, 4-in-wide, over the Coban.
   e. Leave the dressing on for 3 to 7 days, and then reapply.

6. Pentoxifylline (Trental) at a dosage of 1,200 to 2,400 mg and divided into three doses per day with food has been shown to be beneficial. Gastrointestinal upset is common.

7. Another variant of occlusive dressing is as follows:

   a. ZeaSORB powder on the ulcer.
   b. Midstrength cortisone cream around the ulcer.
   c. Zinc oxide wrap around the entire leg with a tighter wrap distally.
   d. Flexible adhesive bandage as a second wrap. Change every week, and keep dry.

No management of a venous stasis ulcer is 100% effective, but this routine with modifications is the one we use. If an ulcer is stable or decreasing in size after 4 weeks the current treatment should be continued. If it is enlarging, then alternate therapy, including surgery, should be considered.

After the ulcer has healed, which takes many weeks, advise the patient to wear an elastic bandage or support hose constantly during the day, primarily as protection against injury of the damaged and scarred skin and to decrease recurrent edema.

## Purpuric Dermatoses

Purpuric lesions are caused by an extravasation of red blood cells into the skin or mucous membranes. The lesions can be distinguished from erythema and telangiectasia by the fact

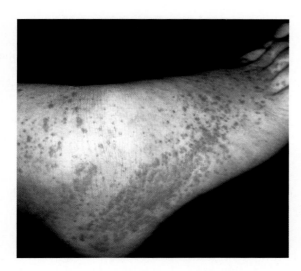

**FIGURE 12-5** ■ Acute purpura, of unknown origin, in a 12-year-old boy. *(Courtesy of Dermik Laboratories, Inc.)*

that purpuric lesions do not blanch under pressure applied by the finger or by a clear glass slide (diascopy) (Fig. 12-5)

- *Petechiae* are small, superficial purpuric lesions. These are most often a sign of platelet deficiency or malfunction.
- *Ecchymoses*, or bruises, are more extensive, round or irregularly shaped purpuric lesions often seen in the elderly (senile purpura), patients on chronic topical or systemic corticosteroids, and patients on anticoagulants.
- *Hematomas* are large, deep, fluctuant, tumorlike hemorrhages in the skin.

The purpuras can be divided into the *thrombocytopenic* forms and the *nonthrombocytopenic* forms.

- *Thrombocytopenic purpura* may be idiopathic or secondary to various chronic diseases or to a drug sensitivity. The platelet count is below normal, the bleeding time is prolonged, and the clotting time is normal, but the clot does not retract normally. This form of purpura is rare.
- *Nonthrombocytopenic purpura* is more commonly seen. *Henoch–Schönlein purpura* is a form of non-thrombocytopenic purpura most commonly seen in children that is characterized by recurrent attacks of purpura accompanied by arthritis, hematuria, IgA glomerulonephritis, and gastrointestinal disorders. Approximately 75% of the time it involves the skin only. If the skin biopsy is done at precisely the correct time, leukocytoclastic vasculitis and IgA can be seen deposited in the vessel wall if the biopsy is done at precisely the correct time.

The ecchymoses, or *senile purpura,* seen in elderly patients after minor injury are very common. Ecchymoses are also seen in patients who have been on long-term systemic corticosteroid therapy and also occur after prolonged use of the high-potency corticosteroids locally and from corticosteroid nasal

inhalers. Anticoagulants make these more common. Another common purpuric eruption is that known as *stasis purpura.* These lesions are associated with vascular insufficiency of the legs and occur as the early sign of this change, or they are seen around areas of stasis dermatitis or stasis ulcers. Frequently seen is a petechial drug eruption owing to chlorothiazide diuretics.

## Pigmented Purpuric Eruptions

A less common group of cases are those seen in middle-aged adults, classified under the name *pigmented purpuric eruptions.* They are usually asymptomatic, but some cases of pigmented purpuric eruptions are pruritic. The cause is unknown. Most cases have a positive tourniquet test, but other bleeding tests are usually normal. Clinically, these patients have grouped nonblanchable petechial lesions that begin on the legs and extend up to the thighs, and occasionally up to the waist and onto the arms. They turn into a brown cayenne pepper—like nonpalpable discoloration that fades over weeks to months.

Some clinicians are able to separate these pigmented purpuric eruptions into

- Purpura annularis telangiectodes (Majocchi's disease)
- Progressive pigmentary dermatosis (Schamberg's disease)
- Pigmented purpuric lichenoid dermatosis (Gougerot and Blum disease)

Majocchi's disease commonly begins on the legs but slowly spreads to become generalized. Telangiectatic capillaries become confluent and produce annular or serpiginous lesions. The capillaries break down, causing purpuric lesions. Schamberg's disease is a slowly progressive pigmentary condition of the lower part of the legs that fades after a period of months but may recur. The Gougerot and Blum form is accompanied by severe itching and eczematous changes. Otherwise, it resembles Schamberg's disease.

### Treatment

For these pigmented purpuric eruptions, therapy may not be necessary. Occlusive dressing therapy with a corticosteroid cream can be beneficial, or support garments can be used for prevention. For resistant cases, prednisone, 10 mg, 1 to 2 tablets in the morning for 3 to 6 weeks is indicated.

## Pyoderma Gangrenosum

Pyoderma gangrenosum is a painful ulcerative disease, usually of the lower extremities.

### Lesions

It begins as a pustule but, over days to weeks, turns into a boggy, bluish-black ulcer with rolled edges. There are sometimes satellite pustules that then also ulcerate. The edges are erythematous and undermined, and the extent of the ulcer is often more extensive than what is first suspected. It exhibits pathergy, which means it can occur at any site of trauma.

## Presentation and Characteristics

It is usually relentless and chronic unless treated aggressively and may occur at sites other than the lower extremities and around ostomy sites. Treatment of the underlying condition can, but does not always, result in resolution of the disease.

### Causes

Inflammatory bowel disease (50% of the time it is associated with Crohn's and 50% of the time it is associated with ulcerative colitis) is an underlying association in one third of cases. Approximately 1.5% to 5% of inflammatory bowel disease patients have pyoderma gangrenosum. In 7% to 10% of pyoderma gangrenosum cases there is an associated underlying malignancy. Leukemia is the commonest and is a bad prognostic sign, with 25% of cases being fatal within 12 months after the diagnosis of pyoderma gangrenosum. In polycythemia vera, if pyoderma gangrenosum develops there is an increased chance of leukemia developing. Waldenström's macroglobulinemia, multiple myeloma, myelofibrosis, lymphoma, and metastatic solid tumors can also be underlying diseases.

Sporadic associations with other underlying illnesses include chronic active hepatitis, thyroid disease, hidradenitis suppurativa, cystic acne, sarcoidosis, diabetes mellitus, systemic lupus erythematous, rheumatoid arthritis, AIDS, and Takayasu's arteritis.

Certain clinical subtypes are more apt to be related to certain underlying conditions.

1. *Ulcerative:* Most common, usually associated with underlying disease, especially inflammatory bowel disease. Very painful, spreads rapidly, and needs aggressive therapy. May be associated with arthritis (especially large joint and monoarticular) and increased IgA (up to 10%).
2. *Pustular:* Grouped pustules on a red base. Toxic patients with acute inflammatory bowel disease. May clear if inflammatory bowel disease is controlled.
3. *Bullous:* Superficial bullae and superficial ulcer with surrounding erythema associated with myeloproliferative disease especially leukemia. Systemic treatment is required.
4. *Vegetative:* It is relatively painless, vegetative, relatively superficial single, relatively slow progression without undermining border and without underlying illness. Treatment is less aggressive and sometimes can be achieved with local modalities only.

## Differential Diagnosis

- *Brown recluse spider bite:* Rapid (within hours) necrosis without ulceration. No underlying illness. Single lesion. More common in the midwestern part of the United States, that is, Missouri spider.
- *Purpura fulminans:* Toxic patient with widespread areas of necrosis without ulceration. Underlying

disseminated intravascular coagulopathy (DIC). Rapid decline and often fatal.

- *Stasis ulcer:* Stasis dermatitis of the lower extremities over the medial malleolus (distribution of greater saphenous vein) with varicosities, edema, and dyspigmentation. Slow in onset and chronic course with little or no pain even though size can be large and depth can be to the tendon of the ankle.
- *Necrotizing fasciitis:* Patient may be very toxic, especially as disease progresses. There are deep gangrenous plaques that may be very painful or anesthetic with rapid spread. It is not infrequently fatal.
- *Vasculitis:* Clinically with palpable purpura and histologically with vasculitis (fibrinoid necrosis of vessel walls and perivascular neutrophils with leukocytoclasis). May not ulcerate or ulcerate much later (weeks to months).

## Treatment

### Local

1. Avoid aggressive debridement and skin grafting since pathergy may occur.
2. Intralesional corticosteroid (4 to 6 mg/cc triamcinolone) around and under ulcers can help stop spread and start healing.
3. Class I (clobetasol ointment under occlusion) may be beneficial, and topical tacrolimus has been tried.

### Systemic

1. High-dose systemic corticosteroids (40 to 60 mgms of prednisone daily; taper off over weeks depending on response to therapy).
2. Begin a corticosteroid-sparing agent such as minocycline (100 mg b.i.d.), avlosulfone (100 mg/d), sulfapyridine (500 mg b.i.d.), sulfasalazine (500 mg b.i.d.), azathioprine (50 mg b.i.d.), mycophenolate mofetil, methotrexate, cyclosporine, and tacrolimus.

Biologic agents that have been used with success (most notably etanercept and adalimumab).

## Telangiectasias

Telangiectasias are abnormal, dilated small blood vessels. Telangiectasias are divided into *primary forms*, in which the causes are unknown, and *secondary forms*, which are related to some known disturbance. The primary telangiectasias include the simple and compound hemangiomas of infants, essential telangiectasias, and spider hemangiomas (see Chapter 37). Diseases with numerous telangiectasias include

- Cirrhosis of the liver
- Osler–Weber–Rendu disease, which also has mucous membrane involvement
- Lupus erythematosus
- Scleroderma
- Dermatomyositis
- Cutaneous polyarteritis

- Metastatic carcinoid syndrome
- Ataxia telangiectasia
- Angiokeratoma corporis diffusum
- Telangiectasia macularis eruptiva perstans
- Rosacea
- Overlying basal cell cancers and sebaceous hyperplasia
- Overlying necrobiosis lipoidica diabeticorum

Unilateral nevoid telangiectasia syndrome can be congenital or acquired. The acquired form appears when increased estrogen levels occur in women during puberty or pregnancy or in cirrhosis. C3, C4, and trigeminal dermatomes are most commonly involved.

Hereditary benign telangiectasia is an uncommon autosomal dominant disorder with generalized telangiectasias at an early age, especially on sun-exposed areas. There is no mucosal involvement.

Secondary telangiectasia is very commonly seen on the fair-skinned person as a result of aging, chronic topical and systemic corticosteroid use, and chronic sun exposure. X-ray therapy and burns can also cause telangiectasias.

Treatment for secondary telangiectasias can be accomplished quite adequately with very light electrosurgery to the vessels, which is usually tolerated without anesthesia, or for many extensive lesions, use of laser therapy or intense pulsed light therapy is helpful. Injectable sclerosing agents are available for therapy on the lower legs as are endovascular laser and vessel ligation.

## Vasculitis

Inflammation of the blood vessels (vasculitis) (Fig. 12-6) commonly affects the skin and has numerous underlying causes. It can be cutaneous only (Gougerot's and Ruiter's type), but often involves other organs, most commonly the joints, kidney, and gastrointestinal tract and rarely the nervous system, eye (temporal arteritis), heart, and respiratory tract. Diagnosis is confirmed by biopsy and then appropriate tests need to be done to look for underlying causes (Table 12-2). Vasculitis classification (Table 12-3) is complex, but it can be helpful in trying to find an underlying cause (Table 12-4). Laboratory evaluation is important (Table 12-5).

### Presentation and Characteristics

*Primary Lesions*

Palpable purpura is the classic clinical appearance. Varying shades of bluish-red discoloration may be firmly indurated or difficult to feel. Lesions can be large (many centimeters) or quite small (several millimeters) with a petechial look. The dependent areas are the location where they are most commonly seen—legs on ambulatory patients and the buttocks and back in bedridden patients.

*Secondary Lesions*

As the vascular damage progresses, blisters, nodules, ulcers, necrosis, and gangrene may occur. Livedo reticularis (see

Dictionary–Index) is a bluish-red, netlike appearing condition that can be associated with vasculitis.

*Course*

The disease may be very chronic and long lasting, such as in lupus erythematosus, or acute and self-limited, such as in Henoch–Schönlein purpura (see Chapter 38). Early diagnosis and therapy can prevent renal failure or bowel necrosis.

*Causes*

See Table 12-2.

### Differential Diagnosis

- *Urticaria:* Evanescent, very pruritic.
- *Thrombophlebitis:* There are varicosities and stasis changes and positive Doppler studies in this localized distribution of a vein almost always in the lower extremity below the knee.
- *Erythema nodosum:* May be impossible to tell without a deep skin biopsy, especially in female patients. A deep nodule is present, usually only in a pretibial location.
- *Petechia:* Small, uniform, single-color, nonpalpable lesions associated with decreased platelets.
- *Schamberg's disease* (benign pigmented purpura, benign hemosiderosis): Cayenne pepper–colored tiny lesions. No underlying illness. Skin biopsy differentiates. Usually below the knees, but it can rarely be generalized. For several variations, see hemosiderosis in the Dictionary–Index and discussion under petechiae in this chapter.
- *Panniculitis:* Lesions very deep and nodular. May have elevated amylase and lipase when associated with pancreatitis.
- *Cellulitis:* Lesions warm and tender. Elevated white blood cell count with fever. May have proximal, tender, red, linear lymphatic involvement. Lymph nodes may be enlarged.
- *Insect bites:* Very pruritic. History of exposure to insects; acute in onset. Can be excoriated and can be chronic.

### Treatment

Systemic corticosteroids are the mainstay of early therapy. Corticosteroid-sparing drugs including colchicine, dapsone, azathioprine, methotrexate, Cytoxan (drug of choice for Wegener's granulomatosis), intravenous γ-globulin, antimalarials, and plasmapheresis have all been used.

## Livedo Vasculopathy (Atrophie Blanche, Segmental Hyalinizing Vasculopathy)

This disease was at one time thought to be a vasculitis of immune origin and occasionally mimics a true vasculitis. The pathogenesis begins with the deposition of fibrin within the vessel walls without inflammation or immune complex

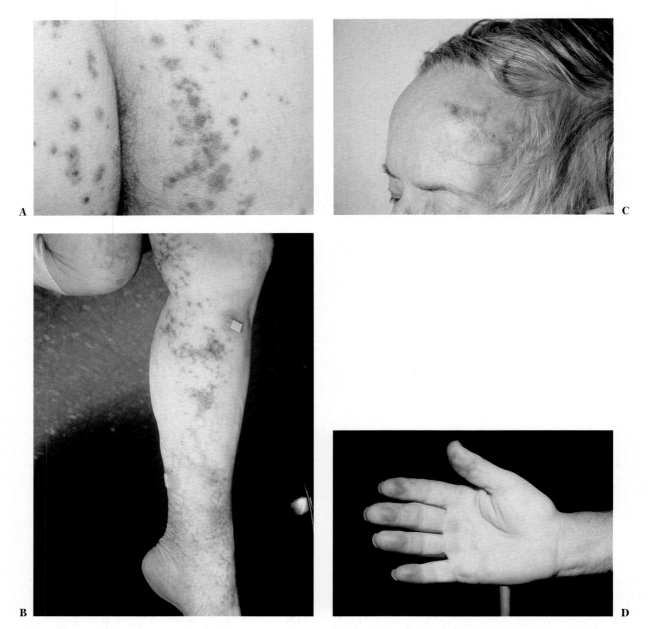

**FIGURE 12-6** ▪ Forms of vasculitis. **(A)** Vasculitis on the buttock of a patient with renal and gastrointestinal vasculitis. Bedridden patient often erupts first on the buttock. **(B)** Vasculitis of the lower extremity owing to mixed cryoglobulinemia. Patient was worse in cold weather. **(C)** Temporal arteritis. Systemic corticosteroids were used to prevent blindness. **(D)** Fingers showing vasculitis in a patient with Wegener's granulomatosis.

deposition. Later biopsy specimens show a secondary vasculitis. Therefore, biopsy of early disease is essential for correct diagnosis and, subsequently, the correct therapy. Livedo vasculopathy may be seen in association with stasis dermatitis or collagen–vascular disease.

### Presentation and Characteristics

#### Primary Lesions

There are recurrent, chronic, painful, stellate-shaped ulcers over lower extremities (especially over the lower medial ankles and malleoli). They heal slowly with characteristic porcelain-colored, stellate-shaped atrophic scars with surrounding ectatic blood vessels and reddish-brown hyperpigmentation.

#### Secondary Lesions

Cellulitis with pain, swelling, redness, and warmth of surrounding skin can occur.

#### Course

The disease is very chronic and without proper therapy can slowly progress to involve larger areas of the lower extremities

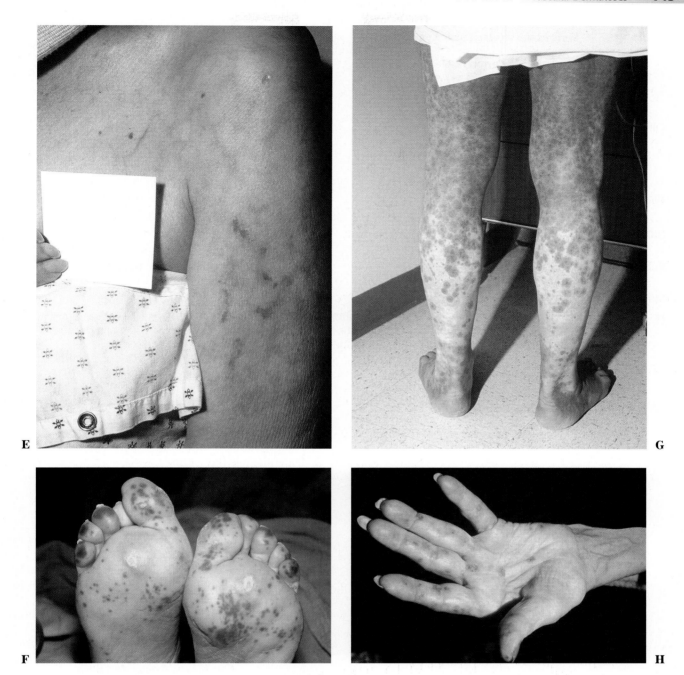

E

G

F

H

**FIGURE 12-6** ■ (*continued*) (**E**) Livedo reticularis pattern of vasculitis. This patient has systemic lupus erythematosus. (**F**) Vasculitis of the feet. Lower extremities are the location where it is most common in ambulatory patients. (**G**) Widespread, drug-induced vasculitis owing to ampicillin. (**H**) Vasculitis of the hand in a patient with rheumatoid arthritis.

but is rare above the knee. Although treatment can halt the disease ulcers and pain, the scars and dilated vessels as well as the hyperpigmentation remain.

### Cause

A disorder of coagulation with elevated fibrinopeptide, decreased plasminogen activator, and abnormal platelet functions are all considered possibilities.

### Differential Diagnosis

- *Stasis dermatitis:* Stellate scar less common; does have dramatic hyperpigmentation following eczematous dermatitis, often with edema and varicosities. Vasculitis more widespread and can be multisystem. Different biopsy with true vasculitic inflammatory changes seen early in course. Atrophie blanche scars less common.

**TABLE 12-2 ■ Venous versus Ischemic Leg Ulcers**

|  | **Venous Ulcers** | **Ischemic Ulcers** |
| --- | --- | --- |
| Symptoms | Itching | Pain (often severe with tenderness) |
|  | Asymptomatic |  |
| Clinical | Stasis dermatitis | Induration, redness |
|  | Scaling | Pulses diminished or absent |
|  | Hyperpigmentation | Intermittent claudication |
|  | Edema, varicosities | Decrease pain upon exercise |
| Ulcer Appearance | Ragged edge | Sharp edge, "punched out" |
|  | Exudative base | Dry crusted or clean base |
| Ulcer Location | Medial malleolus (distribution of greater saphenous vein) | Pretibial |
| Radiographic | Abnormal venous Doppler | Abnormal arterial Doppler and arterial angiogram |
| Mainstay of Therapy | Pressure dressing | Arterial surgical repair |
| History | Thrombophlebitis, obesity, diabetes, vein or lymphatic obstruction or disruption from blood clots, infection or surgery | Arteriosclerotic vascular disease including heart, cerebrovascular, and peripheral arterial vascular disease |

**TABLE 12-3 ■ Types of Vasculitis**

I. Leukocytoclastic vasculitis (hypersensitivity angiitis or allergic vasculitis)

   A. Idiopathic

   B. Drug induced

   C. Hypocomplementemic vasculitis (often urticarial)

   D. Essential mixed cryoglobulinemia

   E. Hyperglobulinemic purpuras (Waldenström's macroglobulinemia)

II. Rheumatic Vasculitis

   A. Systemic lupus erythematosus

   B. Rheumatoid Vasculitis

   C. Dermatomyositis

III. Granulomatous Vasculitis

   A. Allergic granulomatous vasculitis (Churg–Strauss)

   B. Wegener's Granulomatosis

   C. Lymphomatoid Granulomatosis

IV. Polyarteritis nodosa

   A. Classic type

   B. Cutaneous type

V. Giant cell arteritis

   A. Temporal arteritis

   B. Takayasu's disease

## Treatment

First visit

1. Aspirin, 81 mg/d with food
2. Dipyridamole (Persantin)
3. Pentoxifylline (Trental), 400 mg b.i.d. with food
4. Any combination of the first three

Second visit

1. Warfarin is probably the best choice of more aggressive anticoagulation therapy
2. Can combine warfarin with 1, 2, or 3 from the previous list
3. Heparin can be given subcutaneously, but it is expensive and has greater risk of bleeding
4. More experimental therapies include tissue plasminogen activator and fluindione

**TABLE 12-4 ■ Conditions Associated with Stasis Ulcers**

Previous surgery (including joint replacements, vessel harvesting, fracture)

Diabetes mellitus

Venous insufficiency and thrombophlebitis

Anemia

Prolonged standing or sitting with legs bent

Obesity

Poor nutrition (lack of sufficient vitamins A, C, E, selenium, zinc, copper, thiamine, pantothenic acid, manganese)

Neuropathy

Immunosuppression

**TABLE 12-5 ▪ Basic Laboratory Evaluation of Vasculitis**

Urine analysis (most crucial test because early asymptomatic renal disease can be detected and progression to renal failure prevented)

Stool screen for occult blood (stool Guaiac)

Complete blood count with platelets and coagulation screen

Hypercoagulability studies may be indicated such as anticardiolipin and antiphospholipid antibodies, complement levels, homocysteine, factor V Leiden, that is, hypercoagulability screen and hematology consult

Antinuclear antibody, rheumatoid factor, liver enzymes, hepatitis screen, cryoglobulins, cryofibrinogen, and immunoglobulins

Antineutrophil cytoplasmic antibody (ANCA) that is positive in Wegener's granulomatosis (c-ANCA)

Polyarteritis nodosa (p-ANCA)

## Acute Cutaneous Necrosis

This group of diseases (Figs. 12-7 to 12-17) can be defined by sudden onset, painful areas of full-thickness skin loss and gangrene. They have a variety of causes but a similar looking end-stage of black, necrotic, gangrenous tissue.

### Presentation and Characteristics

*Primary Lesions*

These are most commonly seen in the lower extremities. The center is dusky gray or black with induration and often severe pain. An advancing edge of erythema indicates areas of eventual spread of the tissue destruction. Debridement of tissue is often very extensive, and sometimes amputation is required.

*Secondary Lesions*

Ulcerations with or without secondary infections may occur, and significant scar formation is the rule.

*Course*

Systemic disease is not uncommon and a lethal outcome may result. Early, aggressive therapy can ameliorate mortality and morbidity in some cases.

*Causes*

The causes include Coumadin necrosis, calciphylaxis, spider bite (most commonly the brown recluse in the United States), hypercoagulability states, necrotizing fasciitis, pyoderma gangrenosum, vasculitis, *Mycobacterium ulcerans* (tropical areas), purpura fulminans, embolic phenomena, arteriosclerotic occlusive disease (Buerger's disease is an example), ecthyma gangrenosum (usually due to pseudomonas sepsis), and *Vibrio vulnificus* infection.

**TABLE 12-6 ▪ Underlying Conditions Associated with Cutaneous Necrosis**

| Diseases | Underlying Condition |
| --- | --- |
| Coumadin necrosis | Obesity, female, decreased amount or function of protein C or S in all cases |
| Heparin necrosis | Heparin-induced thrombocytopenia, heparin-induced antiplatelet antibodies |
| Calciphylaxis | End-stage renal disease (almost all cases) |
| Spider bites | Outpatient setting, patient not ill |
| Hypercoagulability states | See Table 12-2, clotting disorders, polycythemia, cryoglobulinemia, Waldenström's macroglobulinemia, hyperimmunoglobulinemia |
| Necrotizing fasciitis | Cellulitis (most often group A streptococci) in all cases, postop, rarely pregnancy, diabetes (40%–50%), underlying cancer +/− chemotherapy, varicella (especially in children), renal dialysis, use of NSAIDs, AIDS, traumatic wound |
| Pyoderma gangrenosum | See earlier in this chapter |
| Vasculitis | See earlier in this chapter |
| *Mycobacterium ulcerans* | Endemic tropical African infection |
| Purpura fulminans | DIC in almost all cases usually caused by sepsis, may have abnormalities of protein C or S |
| Embolic phenomena | Associated with orthopaedic, arterial, or cardiac procedures |
| Arteriosclerotic occlusive disease | Arteriosclerotic disease elsewhere (heart, kidney, brain, peripheral arteries), smoking, obesity, diabetes, hyperlipidemia, family history, sedentary lifestyle, hypertension |
| Echthyma gangrenosum | *Pseudomonas aeruginosa* sepsis in almost all cases, HIV, chemotherapy, neutropenia, predisposing antibiotic, underlying cancer, IV drug abuse, agammaglobulinemia |
| *Vibrio vulnificas* infection | Always swimming in contaminated water (via aspiration, swallowing, or a wound) or eating contaminated raw shellfish (especially oysters), often on systemic corticosteroid treatment and alcoholic liver disease |

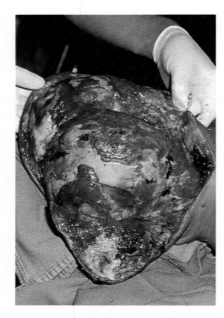

**FIGURE 12-7** ■ Necrotizing fasciitis of the scalp showing extensive necrosis that eventually went even beyond the margins shown here. Group A beta streptococci was cultured. The patient walked out of the hospital with full recovery.

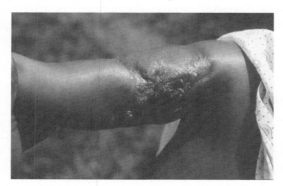

**FIGURE 12-8** ■ *Mycobacterium ulcerans* in an African child at the time of debridement. *(Courtesy of Dennis Palmer, M.D.)*

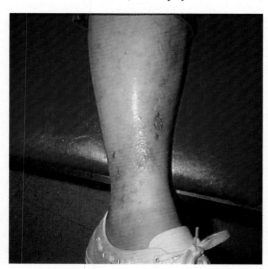

**FIGURE 12-9** ■ Necrotic ulcer on the leg in a patient with antiphospholipid syndrome.

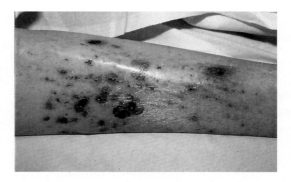

**FIGURE 12-10** ■ Emboli with necrosis on the leg of an elderly male after arteriogram of the iliac artery.

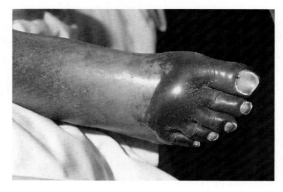

**FIGURE 12-11** ■ Coumadin necrosis on day 3 of Coumadin therapy resulting in partial amputation of the foot.

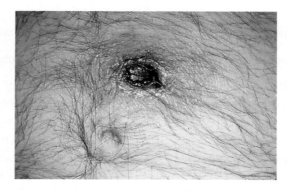

**FIGURE 12-12** ■ Echthyma gangrenosum on the umbilicus of a patient with pseudomonas sepsis.

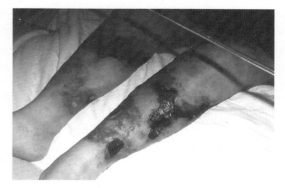

**FIGURE 12-13** ■ Calciphylaxis in an elderly woman who refused further hemodialysis due to the severity of her pain and died of renal failure.

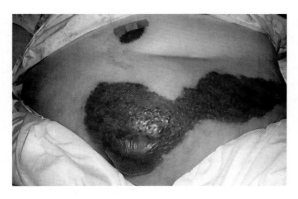

FIGURE 12-14 ■ Heparin necrosis at a subcutaneous heparin injection site on the abdomen of a pregnant woman. Heparin is given as prophylaxis to prevent thrombophlebitis.

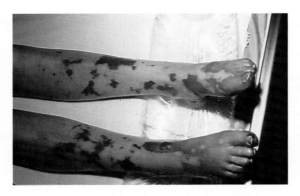

FIGURE 12-15 ■ Purpura fulminans (symmetrical peripheral gangrene) in a woman with DIC due to sepsis. Partial amputation of both feet was required.

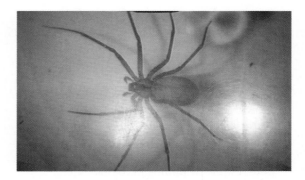

FIGURE 12-16 ■ *Loxosceles reclusus* (brown recluse) spider with characteristic violin on the dorsal surface.

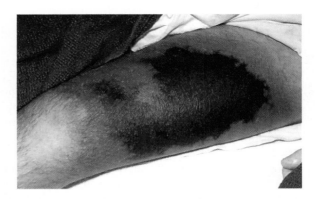

FIGURE 12-17 ■ Necrotic type of vasculitis on the anterior thigh in an HIV patient.

## Differential Diagnosis

- *Coumadin necrosis (Fig. 12-11):* Over 90% of cases occur between days 3 and 5 after Coumadin therapy has been started. It can occur with any Coumadin derivative. It occurs most often on areas with large amounts of subcutaneous fat. Only one or two areas are usually involved. Biopsy with fibrin thrombi and minimal inflammation is useful.
- *Heparin necrosis (Fig. 12-14):* Usually occurs within weeks of beginning heparin. Occurs most often at subcutaneous injection sites but can be widespread at sites distant to both IV and subcutaneous heparin. Seen with any type of heparin as part of HIT (heparin-induced thrombocytopenia) syndrome with antiplatelet antibodies present.
- *Calciphylaxis (Fig. 12-13):* Seen in end-stage renal patients, usually on the lower extremities. Exquisite pain with large areas are involved and there is at least 50% mortality.
- *Spider bites:* Occurs in ambulatory patients without underlying disease. Mainly affects lower extremities, and spider (especially brown recluse in the United States [Fig. 12-16]) is usually not seen. Patient is ambulatory and usually not toxic.
- *Hypercoagulability states:* Often asymmetric with small, multiple distal sites and livedo reticularis.
- *Necrotizing fasciitis (Fig. 12-7):* Patient is very toxic with a marked increase in CPK. May have a history of trauma. The disease may be very painful early and anesthetic late. Affects a single, very large area with rapid spread over hours. Common in groin or genital area (Fournier's gangrene).
- *Pyoderma gangrenosum:* Primarily an ulcerative disease. It is a marker of underlying disease. See earlier in the chapter.
- *Vasculitis:* Often not gangrenous. Palpable purpura also present. See earlier in the chapter.
- *M. ulcerans (Fig. 12-8):* Endemic in tropical Africa. Not painful, and patient is not toxic. It is not usually life threatening.
- *Purpura fulminans (Fig. 12-15):* Patient is toxic and usually septic. There is symmetrical peripheral gangrene with rapid downhill course and DIC.
- *Emboli:* There are multiple, small distal lesions with livedo reticularis and a history of cardiac or orthopedic procedure. Watch for related renal embolic phenomena with renal failure (blood in urine and increased creatinine).

- *Arteriosclerotic vascular occlusion:* Necrosis follows distribution of artery. Angiographic studies may be diagnostic. History of arteriosclerosis.
- *Ecthyma gangrenosum (Fig. 12-12):* Septic patient with blood culture positive for *Pseudomonas aeruginosa* in most cases. May have single or multiple sites of involvement. Likes anogenital site.
- *Vibrio vulnificus infection:* Very toxic patient with a history of raw ingestion by eating raw shellfish, by swallowing infected water, or through an open wound while swimming in coastal waters.

## Treatment

Following these patients with surgical as well as medical consultation is warranted.

1. *Coumadin necrosis:* Can continue Coumadin but would not restart. May need to debride later.
2. *Heparin necrosis:* Stop heparin immediately and permanently. May need to debride later.
3. *Calciphylaxis:* Take IV sodium thiosulfate (12.5 to 50 gm three times a week). If hyperparathyroid consider parathyroidectomy. Hyperbaric oxygen, increased low calcium dialysis, bisphosphonates, and cinacalcet have all been tried.
4. *Spider bites:* Prednisone (50 mg each arm for 2 days and decrease by 10 mg every 2 days for a 10-day course) or dapsone (100 mg each day for 3 to 5 days) can be tried. Debride late, if at all. Ace wrap, ice compresses, and elevation are the old standby.
5. *Hypercoagulable state:* See if your hematologist is in the office and perform a hypercoagulability screen.
6. *Necrotizing fasciitis:* Emergency, aggressive debridement and emergency IV antibiotics of vancomycin and/or clindamycin (while awaiting cultures) are undertaken. Hyperbaric oxygenation, if available, has been used.
7. *Pyoderma gangrenosum:* See earlier in the chapter. Take systemic corticosteroids early and begin steroid-sparing drug for long-term use.
8. *Vasculitis:* See earlier in the chapter. Take systemic corticosteroids early to save skin and renal function.
9. *M. ulcerans:* Debridement and possible anti-mycobacterium therapy (may be unavailable in jungle) can be undertaken.
10. *Purpura fulminans:* Treat DIC and sepsis or other underlying condition. Debride as needed.
11. *Embolic phenomena:* Anticoagulation may be helpful. Renal compromise may be unavoidable.
12. *Arteriosclerotic occlusive disease:* Consider arterial repair and then consider anticoagulation.
13. *Ecthyma gangrenosum:* Treat sepsis early and debride later if necessary.
14. *Vibrio vulnificus:* Emergency debridement and emergency IV antibiotics, especially tetracyclines and penicillins (cephalosporins and chloramphenicol have also been used).

## Suggested Readings

Cherry G. *The Oxford European Wound Healing Course Handbook.* Oxford: Oxford University Press; 2002.

Ghersetich I, Panconesi E. The purpuras. *Int J Dermatol.* 1994;33:1.

Greaves MW, Kaplan AP. *Urticaria and Angiodema.* New York: Marcel Dekker; 2004.

Hairston BR, Davis MD, Pittelkow MR, et al. Livedoid vasculopathy: further evidence for procoagulant pathogenesis. *Arch Dermatol.* 2006;142:1413–1418.

Henz BM, Zuberbier T, Grabbe J, et al. *Urticaria: Clinical, Diagnostic, and Therapeutic Aspects.* New York: Springer-Verlag; 1998.

Kaplan AP, Greaves MW. Angioedema. *J Am Acad Dermatol.* 2005;53(3):373–388.

Nussinovitch M, Prais D, Finkelstein Y, et al. Cutaneous manifestations of Henoch–Schönlein purpura in young children. *Pediatr Dermatol.* 1998;15:426–428.

Ollert MW, Thomas P, Korting HC, et al. Erythema induratum of Bazin. Evidence of T-lymphocyte hyperresponsiveness to purified protein derivative of tuberculin: report of two cases and treatment. *Arch Dermatol.* 1993;129:469–473.

Reichrath J, Bens G, Bonowitz A, et al. Treatment recommendations for pyoderma gangrenosum: an evidence-based review of the literature based on more than 350 patients. *J Am Acad Dermatol.* 2005;53(2):273–283.

Stein SL, Miller LC, Konnikov N. Wegener's granulomatosis: case report and literature review. *Pediatr Dermatol.* 1998;15:352–356.

Valencia IC, Falabella A, Kirsner RS, et al. Chronic venous insufficiency and venous leg ulceration. *J Am Acad Dermatol.* 2001;44:401–421.

Zimmet SE. Venous leg ulcers: modern evaluation and management. *Dermatol Surg.* 1999;25(3):236–241.

# CHAPTER 13

# Seborrheic Dermatitis, Acne, and Rosacea

*John C. Hall, MD*

Seborrhea dermatitis, acne, and rosacea all tend to occur in patients with oily skin. They occur in areas where the oil glands are the largest and most plentiful such as the scalp, face, central chest, and upper back. Response to therapy is better with substances that remove oil and are worsened by substances that are oily. Many therapies are beneficial for all three diseases.

## Seborrheic Dermatitis

*Seborrheic dermatitis,* in our opinion, is a synonym for *dandruff.* The former is the more severe manifestation of this dermatosis. Seborrheic dermatitis is exceedingly common on the scalp, but less common on the other areas of predilection: ears, face, sternal area, axillae, intergluteal area, and pubic area (**Figs. 13-1 and 13-2**). It occurs as part of the acne seborrhea complex. Dandruff is spoken of as oily or dry, but it is all basically oily. If dandruff scales are pressed between two pieces of tissue paper, an oily residue is expressed, leaving a mark on the tissue.

Certain misconceptions that have arisen concerning this common dermatosis needs to be corrected. Seborrheic dermatitis cannot be cured, but remissions for varying amounts of time do occur naturally or as the result of treatment. Seborrheic dermatitis does not cause permanent hair loss or baldness unless it becomes grossly infected. Seborrheic dermatitis is not contagious. The cause is unknown, but an important etiologic factor is the yeast *Pityrosporum ovale.*

Seborrheic dermatitis in AIDS patients can be widespread and recalcitrant to therapy. It can be severe and is common in patients with Parkinson's disease.

### Presentation and Characteristics

#### Primary Lesions

Redness and scaling appear in varying degrees. The scale is of the greasy type (see Fig. 13-1).

#### Secondary Lesions

Rarely seen are excoriations from severe itching and secondary bacterial infection. Lichen simplex chronicus can follow a chronic itching and scratching habit.

#### Course

Exacerbations and remissions are common, depending on the season, treatment, and age and general health of the patient. A true cure is impossible.

#### Seasonal Incidence

This condition is worse in colder weather, presumably due to lack of summer sunlight.

#### Age Incidence

Seborrhea occurs in infants (called *cradle cap*), but usually disappears by the age of 6 months (**Fig. 13-3**). It may recur again at puberty.

### Differential Diagnosis

#### Scalp Lesions

- *Psoriasis:* Sharply defined, silvery-white, dry, scaly patches; typical psoriasis lesions on the elbows, knees, nails, or elsewhere (see Chapter 14).
- *Lichen simplex chronicus:* Usually a single patch on the posterior scalp area or around the ears; intense itching; excoriation; thickening of the skin (see Chapter 8).
- *Tinea capitis:* Usually occurs in a child; broken-off hairs, with or without pustular reaction; some types fluoresce under Wood's light; positive culture and potassium hydroxide mount (see Chapter 25).
- *Atopic eczema:* Usually occurs in infants (where it spares the diaper area) or children; diffuse dry scaliness; eczema also on face, arms, and legs; atopic personal and family history (see Chapter 8).

#### Face Lesions

- *Systemic lupus erythematosus:* Faint, reddish, slightly scaly, "butterfly" eruption, aggravated by sunlight, with fever, malaise, arthritis, Raynaud's and positive antinuclear antibody test (see Chapter 37).

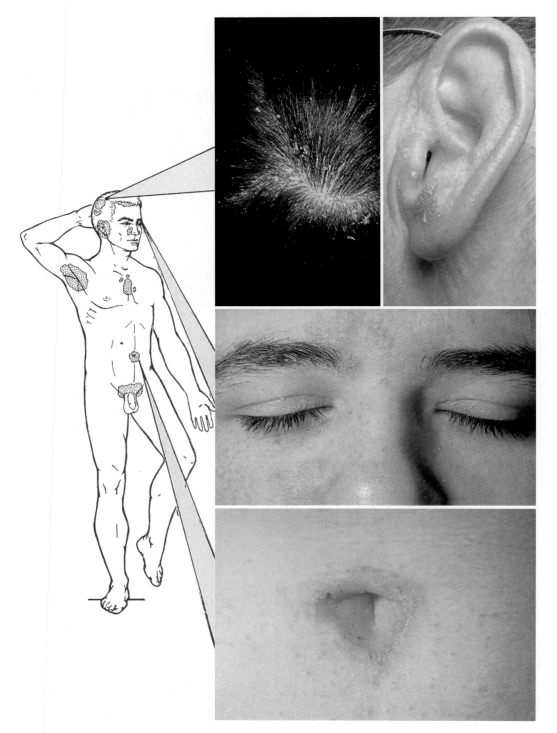

**FIGURE 13-1** ■ Seborrheic dermatitis. *(Courtesy of Owen Laboratories, Inc.)*

■ *Chronic discoid lupus erythematosus:* Sharply defined, red, scaly, atrophic areas with large follicular openings with keratotic plugs, resistant to local therapy, often leaves scars (see Chapter 37).

### Body Lesions

■ *Tinea corporis* (see Chapter 25)
■ *Psoriasis* (see Chapter 14)

■ *Pityriasis rosea* (see Chapter 15)
■ *Tinea versicolor* (see Chapter 15)

### Treatment

*Case Example:* A young man presents with recurrent red, scaly lesions at the border of the scalp and forehead and diffuse, mild, whitish scaling throughout the scalp.

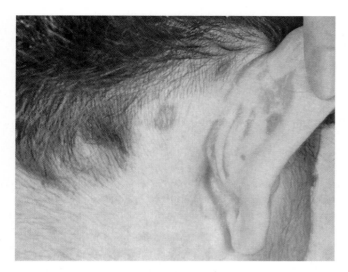

**FIGURE 13-2** ■ Seborrheic dermatitis behind the ear and at the border of the scalp. *(Courtesy of Smith Kline & French Laboratories.)*

1. Management of cases of dandruff must include explaining the disease and stating that it is not contagious, that there is no true cure, that it does not cause baldness, and that there are seasonal variations. Therapy can be very effective, but only for keeping the dandruff under control.
2. With this information in mind, tell the patient that shampooing offers the best management. There are several shampoos available, and the patient may have to experiment to find the most suitable one. The following types can be suggested:

    Selenium sulfide 2½% suspension (Selsun; Head and Shoulders Intensive Treatment, which is available over the counter; Selseb prescription shampoo, which also contains urea and zinc pyrithione) 120.0.
    *Sig:* Shampoo as frequently as necessary to alleviate itching and scaling. Use no other soap. Refill prescription p.r.n.

    Additional shampoos:
    - Tar shampoos, such as Ionil T, Tarsum, Reme-T, Pentrax, X Seb T, T-Gel, and T-Sal (a salicylic acid shampoo).
    - Zinc pyrithione shampoos, such as Zincon, Head & Shoulders, and DHS Zinc.
    - Ketoconazole (Nizoral) shampoo (over the counter) and as a higher percentage it is available as a prescription, Loprox shampoo, Capex shampoo (contains fluocinolone, by prescription) or Clobex shampoo (contains clobetasol and should be used Monday, Wednesday, and Friday by prescription).
    *Sig:* Shampoo as frequently as necessary to keep scaling and itching to a minimum.
3. Triamcinolone (Kenalog) spray, 63 mL.
    *Sig:* Apply sparingly to scalp at night. Squirt the spray through a plastic tube that is supplied.
    *Comment:* A spray is less messy on the scalp than a corticosteroid solution, but solutions are available.
4. A low-potency corticosteroid cream 15.0.
    *Sig:* Apply b.i.d. locally to body lesions. A good combination is 1% HC and 2% sulfur in Acid Mantle cream. Generic Vytone cream is another safe therapy.
5. Ketoconazole 2% cream 15.0 (available over the counter).
    *Sig:* Apply b.i.d. on scalp or body lesions.
    *Comment:* This is a corticosteroid-sparing agent. Ciclopirox (Loprox shampoo) and sodium sulfacetamide (Ovace) wash, used as a shampoo, may also be used.
6. 5% LCD (liquor carbonis detergens), 3% salicylic acid in betamethasone solution is another example to apply twice a day to the scalp.
7. Fluocinolone 0.01% solution is popular because it is mixed in propylene glycol, which kills yeast.
8. Pimecrolimus (Elidel) cream and tacrolimus ointment 0.1% and 0.3% (Protopic) can be used in a thin coat b.i.d. without topical corticosteroid side effects.
9. Foam preparations such as sodium sulfacetamide foam (Ovace), betamethasone valerate (Luxiq) foam, or clobetasol (Olux) foam may be beneficial b.i.d. and after shampooing. Avoid overuse of triamcinolone and especially clobetasol.

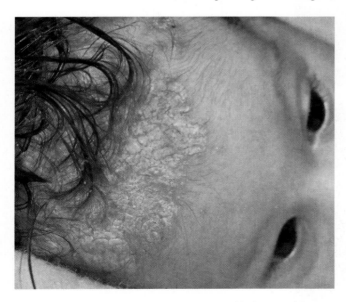

**FIGURE 13-3** ■ Seborrheic dermatitis of infancy. This is one of the causes of "cradle cap." *(Courtesy of Smith Kline & French Laboratories.)*

---

**SAUER'S NOTES**

1. Do not prescribe a fluorinated corticosteroid cream for long-term use on the face or in intertriginous areas.
2. Reiterate that there is no cure for seborrheic dermatitis; long-term management is necessary.
3. Reassure the patient that seborrheic dermatitis does not cause permanent hair loss.

## Acne

Acne vulgaris is a common skin condition of adolescents and young adults. It is characterized by any combination of comedones (blackheads and whiteheads), pustules, cysts, and scarring of varying severity (**Figs. 13-4 to 13-6**).

Severe cystic acne is called *acne conglobata*. When accompanied by systemic symptoms such as arthralgia, leukocytosis, and fever, the term *acne fulminans* is used. *Hidradenitis suppurativa*, also termed *acne inversa*, is a debilitating disease of deep undermining cysts and fistulas in the axillary, inguinal, and perirectal areas. Treatment is difficult and includes surgery, antibiotics, and isotretinoin (Accutane).

Dissecting cellulitis of the scalp (perifolliculitis capitis abscedens et suffodiens) is an inflammatory disease of the scalp with undermining cysts and fistulas of the scalp resulting in scarring alopecia. Treatment is difficult but antibiotics, surgery, laser, x-ray, isotretinoin, azathioprine, dapsone, colchicine, methotrexate, and systemic and intralesional corticosteroids may be helpful.

Acne conglobata, hidradenitis suppurativa, and dissecting cellulitis of the scalp have been referred to as the *follicular occlusion triad*. Pilonidal sinus is added by some authors to make this a tetrad.

### Presentation and Characteristics

#### Primary Lesions

Comedones, papules, pustules, and, in severe cases, cysts occur.

#### Secondary Lesions

Pits and scars are evident in severe cases. Excoriations of the papules are seen in some adolescents, but most often they appear as part of the acne of women in their 20s and 30s. When severe, it is called *acne excoriae des jeunes filles*. This disease may have few or no primary acne lesions. It is difficult to treat, but some authors recommend selective serotonin reuptake inhibitors as antiobsessive-compulsive therapy.

#### Distribution

Acne occurs on the face and neck and, less commonly, on the back, chest, and arms. More rare locations are the scalp, buttocks, and upper legs.

#### Course

The condition begins at ages 8 to 12 years, or later, and lasts, with new outbreaks, for months or years. It subsides in most cases by the early 20s, but occasional flare-ups may occur for

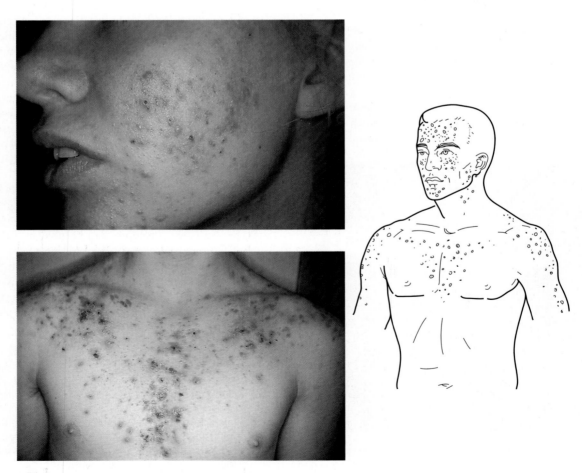

**FIGURE 13-4** ■ Acne of the face and chest.

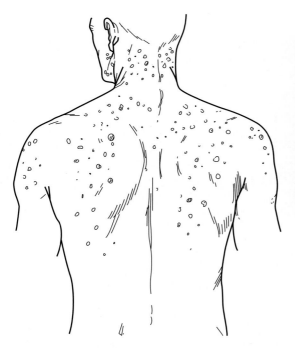

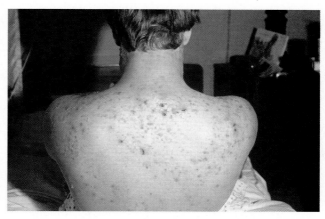

**FIGURE 13-5** ■ Acne of the neck and back.

years. Cases tend to start earlier and be more prolonged in women. This variation between sexes is most likely hormonally related. The residual scarring varies with severity of the case, individual susceptibility, and response to treatment.

*Subjective Complaint*

Tenderness of the large pustules and itching may be reported (rarely). Emotional upset is common as a result of the unattractive appearance.

*Causes*

The following factors are important:

■ Heredity
■ Hormonal balance

■ Increased heat and sweat such as with increased exercise
■ A hot, humid environment due to climate, workplace, or place of exercise
■ Diet (high glycemic diets may play a role)
■ Use of oily cosmetics
■ Sometimes exposure to oils at the workplace

In a case of severe adult acne, one should rule out an endocrine disorder. Hirsutism or abnormal menstrual periods in women are clues. Androgen abuse in male athletes can be causative.

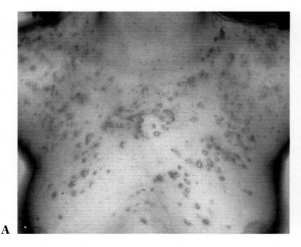

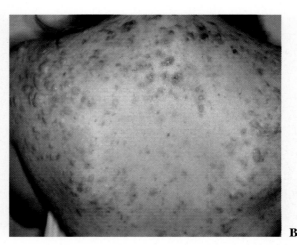

**FIGURE 13-6** ■ Severe acne vulgaris of the chest (**A**) and back (**B**) of a 15-year-old girl. *(Courtesy of Hoechst-Roussel Pharmaceuticals, Inc.)*

## Season

Most cases are better during the summer due to ultraviolet light exposure.

## Contagiousness

Acne is not contagious.

## Differential Diagnosis

- *Drug eruption:* Note history of ingestion of lithium, corticosteroids, iodides, bromides, trimethadione, antiestrogens used to treat estrogen receptor–positive breast cancer, testosterone (including anabolic steroids used by athletes and body builders), lithium and corticosteroids administered topically, orally, and intramuscularly (see Chapter 8).
- *Contact dermatitis from industrial oils* (see Chapter 8).
- *Perioral dermatitis* (**Fig. 13-7**): Red papules, small pustules, and some scaling on chin, upper lip, and nasolabial fold found almost exclusively in women. There is a perioral halo of clear skin. The cause is unknown. Corticosteroid creams locally, initially improve but eventually aggravate the eruption and usually should not be prescribed. Tetracycline, orally, as for acne, is the therapy of choice. Metronidazole gel (MetroGel) is an alternative local therapy for children under 12 years of age. Also, topical erythromycin and topical clindamycin formulations may be helpful. Some authors think this should be called *periorificial dermatitis* because it can occur around the eyes, the nares, and in the diaper area often associated with topical corticosteroid abuse. With time the eruption can become granulomatous.
- *Adenoma sebaceum:* Rare; associated with epilepsy and mental deficiency. There are 2- to 4-mm papules over central face without comedones, pustules, or cysts.

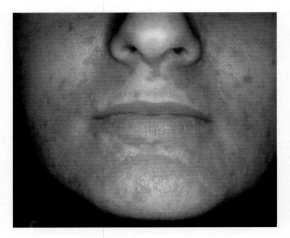

**FIGURE 13-7** ■ Perioral dermatitis. *(Courtesy of Hoechst-Roussel Pharmaceuticals, Inc.)*

## Treatment

*Case Example:* An 11-year-old patient presents with a moderate amount of facial blackheads and pustules.

### First Visit.

1. Give instructions regarding skin care (see Patient Education Sheet, "What You Should Know About Acne"). Stress to the patient and the parent that not one factor but several (heredity, hormones, diet, stress, season of the year, and greasy cosmetics) influence acne breakouts. Some of these factors cannot be altered.

2. *Bar soap:* The affected areas should be washed twice a day with a washcloth and a noncreamy soap, such as Dial, Neutrogena for acne-prone skin, or Purpose.

3. Sulfur, ppt., 6%
   Resorcinol, 4%
   Colored alcoholic shake lotion (see Formulary in Chapter 4) q.s. 60.0.
   *Sig:* Apply locally at bedtime with fingers.
   *Comment:* Proprietary products similar to the above lotion include Sulfacet-R, Novacet lotion, Klaron lotion, Ovace cream, gel and cleanser, Plexion cream and cleanser, and Seba-Nil liquid and cleanser.

4. Benzoyl peroxide preparations
   Benzoyl peroxide gel (5% or 10%) as in Benzagel, Desquam-X, Benzac-W, Panoxyl, Persa-Gel, Brevoxyl, Zoderm (also contains urea to decrease dryness), Benziq (with glycerin to decrease drying, comes as a wash and gel [5.25%] or LS Gel [2.75%]), and others. Some of these are also available as emollient gels.
   *Sig:* Apply locally once a day.
   *Comment:* Some dryness of skin is to be expected. Fabric can be bleached by the benzoyl peroxide.

5. Tretinoin (Retin A) gel (0.01% or 0.025%) or cream (0.025%, 0.05%, or 0.1%) is available generically, tretinoin (Retin A Micro 0.04% and 0.1%), tretinoin (Avita). Retin A micro is also available in a pump formula of 0.1% and 0.04%.
   *Sig:* Apply locally once a day at night. Patient toleration varies considerably.
   *Comment:* Especially valuable for comedonal acne.

6. Local antibiotic solutions, pledgets, and gels.
   Clindamycin 1% (also as a gel called Clindagel) or erythromycin 2% lotion q.s. 30.0.
   *Sig:* Apply locally once or twice a day.

7. Adapalene (Differin) 0.1% q.s. 15 g (Differin Gel [0.3%] can be used if irritation is a problem).
   *Sig:* Thin coat each night.
   *Comment:* May be less irritating and more effective than Retin A.

8. Remove the blackheads with a comedone extractor (**Fig. 13-8**) in the office.

9. Sulfur preparations with low incidence of odor or drying such as Klaron, Novacet, Ovace (cream, gel, foam, or

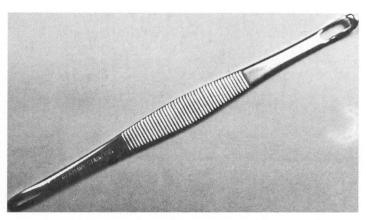

**FIGURE 13-8** ▪ Comedone extractor. The most frequently used instrument in my office. Firm but gentle pressure with the smaller end over a comedone forces the comedone out of the sebaceous gland opening. Gentle opening of the pimple with an 11 Bard Parker blade before using the comedone extractor may be helpful.

cleanser), Plexion TS (also comes as a cleanser), thin coat b.i.d.

10. Benzoyl peroxide plus antibiotic; lasts longer if kept refrigerated. Can bleach fabric. Benzamycin (benzoyl peroxide plus erythromycin), Benzaclin (benzoyl peroxide plus clindamycin), thin coat b.i.d.; and Duac (benzoyl peroxide plus clindamycin), thin coat b.i.d. It does not need to be refrigerated.

11. Akne-mycin ointment and Cleocin T lotion may be good options in patients with dry sensitive skin.

12. Ziana (clindamycin phosphate 1.2% and tretinoin 0.25%) Gel 30 and 60 g tubes. Thin coat q.h.s. This is a combination of antibiotic and retinoid, which may be more convenient than two different applications.

13. (Epiduo) Adapalene-BPO is a single daily application of 0.1% adapalene and 2.5% benzoyl peroxide in a gel base. Irritation potential is similar to adapalene alone.

14. Vanoxide HC has 5% benzoyl peroxide and is in a moisturizing lotion with 0.5% hydrocortisone to decrease irritation.

## WHAT YOU SHOULD KNOW ABOUT ACNE*

Acne is a disorder in which the oil glands of the skin are overactive and the duct of the oil gland is unable to drain the extra oil. It usually involves the face and frequently the chest and the back, because these areas are the richest in oil glands. When an oil gland opening becomes plugged, a blackhead is formed and irritates the skin in exactly the same way as any other foreign body, such as a sliver of wood. This irritation takes the form of red pimples or deep, painful cysts. This inflammation may destroy tissues and, when healed, may result in permanent scars.

The tendency to develop acne runs in families, especially those in which one or both parents have oily skin. Acne is aggravated by certain foods (especially highly glycemic foods, which contain large amounts of refined sugar), improper care of the skin, lack of adequate sleep, and nervous tension. In girls, acne is usually worse before a menstrual period. Even in boys, acne flares on a cyclic basis. Any or all of these factors can exaggerate the tendency of the oily skin to develop acne. Therefore, the prevention of acne depends on correcting not one but several of these factors.

Because acne is so common, is not contagious, and does not cause loss of time from school or work, many people tend to ignore it or regard it as a necessary part of growing up. We disagree with this.

### REASONS FOR TREATING ACNE

There are at least two very important reasons for seeking medical care for acne. The first is to prevent the scarring mentioned. Once scarring has occurred, it is permanent. Then a patient must go through the rest of life being embarrassed and annoyed by the scars, even though active pimples are no longer present. This scarring may vary from tiny little pits, which are frequently mistaken for enlarged pores, to deep, large, disfiguring pockmarks.

The second reason for starting active treatment for acne, even without scarring, is that the condition may become the source of much psychological disturbance to a patient. Even though the acne may appear to others to be mild and inconspicuous, it may seem very noticeable to the patient and lead to embarrassment, worry, and nervousness.

### TREATMENT MEASURES TO BE CARRIED OUT BY THE PATIENT

### Cleaning Measures

Your face is to be washed twice a day with soap. Do not scrub too roughly. The physician may suggest a particular soap for use. Do not use any face cream, cold cream, cleansing cream, nourishing cream, or any other kind of grease on the face. This includes the avoidance of so-called "pancake-type" makeup, which may contain oil, grease, or wax. Acne is related to excessive oiliness. You may think your face is dry because of the flakes on it, but these are actually flakes of dried oil or the greasy scaling of seborrhea. Later, when the treatment begins to take effect, your skin will actually become dry, even to the point where it is chapped and tender, especially around the mouth and the sides of the chin. When this point is reached, you will be advised as to suitable corrective measures for this temporary dryness.

*(continued)*

If the skin becomes red and uncomfortable between office visits, the applied remedy may be discontinued for one or two nights.

Girls may use face powder, dry rouge or blush (not cream rouge), and lipstick, but no face creams. Boys with acne should shave as regularly as necessary and should not use oils, greases, pomades, or hair tonics, except those that may be recommended by the physician. Hair should be dressed only with water.

Many cases of acne are associated with oily hair and dandruff and, for these cases, suitable local scalp applications and shampoos will be prescribed by the physician.

Plenty of rest is important. You should have at least 8 hours of sleep each night. Exercise is usually accompanied by increased activity of the oil glands and an acne flare. Wiping the skin off with a cool damp cloth and showering as soon as possible may be helpful. Moderate sun tanning is beneficial for acne, but a sunburn does more harm than good and all sun exposure adds to the cumulative risk of skin cancer. When you get out in the sun, do not use oily or greasy suntan preparations.

## Diet

Recent studies have indicated that high glycemic-load carbohydrates may worsen acne. This is controversial, but I think for completeness and for the patient who wants to try diet therapy, it is important to list the diet. It is advisable to avoid or limit the following foods.

### Nuts

Especially avoid peanuts, peanut butter, Brazil nuts, and coconuts. Almonds, walnuts, and pecans can be eaten in moderation.

### Milk Products

Avoid whole milk (homogenized) and 2% butterfat milk. You can drink up to two glasses of skim milk a day. Avoid sour cream, whipped cream, butter, margarine (allowed in moderation), rich creamy cheeses, ice cream, and sharp cheeses. Cottage and cheddar cheese are permitted. Sherbet can be eaten.

### Fatty Meats

Avoid meats such as lamb, pork, hamburgers, and tender steaks. Fish, chicken, and turkey can be eaten unless fried in coconut oil or animal fat. Mazola oil or other corn oils should be used in cooking. French fried potatoes should be avoided.

### Spicy Foods

Reduce as much as possible the use of spicy sauces, Worcestershire sauce, chili, catsup, spicy smoked meats, delicatessen products, and pizzas.

### Soft Drinks

Avoid soft drinks particularly ones with high sugar content.

Following this diet does not mean that you should starve yourself. Eat plenty of lean meats, fresh and cooked vegetables, fruits (and their juices), and all breads. Drink plenty of water (4 to 6 glasses) daily. One of the most important things to do is to avoid foods that are highly glycemic.

## Medical Treatment of Acne

In addition to the prescribed treatment you apply yourself; there are several aspects of the treatment of acne that must be carried out by the physician or the nurse.

One important method of treatment is the proper removal of blackheads. This is often part of the physician's job. Pimples that have pus in them and are ready to open should be opened by the physician or the nurse. This is done with surgical instruments that are designed for the purpose and do not damage tissue or cause scars. Picking of pimples by the patient can cause scarring and should be avoided. When the blackheads are removed and the pustules opened in the physician's office, the skin heals faster and scarring is minimized.

Tetracycline or other antibiotics are frequently prescribed for the acne patient who is developing scars or pits. This antibiotic therapy may be continued by the physician for many months or even years. Occasionally, one develops an upset stomach, diarrhea, or a genital itch from an overgrowth of yeast organisms. Oral fluconazole (Diflucan) has made control of vaginal yeast infection much easier. If these problems develop, stop the medication and call the physician.

Here are other important comments about oral tetracycline therapy:

1. Tetracycline may make the skin more sensitive to sunlight. Therefore, if you go skiing or to a sunny climate it may be necessary to lower the dosage or stop the tetracycline 4 days before the trip. This sun sensitivity is more common with doxycycline and less common with minocycline.

2. If a woman is on birth control pills and also on tetracycline, there is the remote possibility that the birth control pills may be less effective. Additional birth control measures are indicated at possible times of conception.
3. Do not take tetracycline or a similar antibiotic if you become pregnant because after the fifth month of pregnancy, it can permanently discolor the teeth of the child.
4. The effectiveness of the tetracycline medication is decreased if iron or milk products are ingested at the same time as the tetracycline capsules. The best rule is for you to take tetracycline 30 minutes before meals or 2 hours after a meal.
5. Serious side effects from long-term therapy are almost nonexistent, but if there is any question concerning an illness and the taking of the antibiotic, call your physician. Do not continue taking an antibiotic unless you are under the continued care of your physician. Stop the antibiotic for acne while taking an antibiotic for another condition.

Other internal medications may be prescribed by the physician for acne, such as vitamin A. For very severe cases of cystic scarring acne, isotretinoin can be prescribed, with suitable precautions. Women of childbearing age should be aware of the fact that isotretinoin can cause birth defects if the woman is or becomes pregnant during therapy.

Ultraviolet light treatments are also beneficial for some cases, but the danger of photodamage must be considered. Newer, long-wave ultraviolet light called intense pulsed light (IPL), blue light and red light therapy appears to be safe and beneficial.

Do not take any other medicines internally while under acne therapy without informing your physician.

## CONCLUSION

Do not become discouraged! Treatment is effective in at least 95% of all cases. It may be 4 to 6 weeks before noticeable improvement appears. There may be occasional mild flare-ups, but eventually your skin will improve and you and your friends will notice the difference.

It is very important for you and your parents to realize that your physician cannot shorten the length of time it takes for your oil glands to work normally. This maturing process of your skin can take several years, even into the 20s, 30s, or, for a few persons (especially women) longer.

*This information is from an instruction sheet that I give to my acne patients. I am well aware of differences of opinion regarding the role of diet in acne, but I am presenting my belief.

---

15. Atralin Gel (0.05% tretinoin) is a very low concentration of tretinoin used to decrease irritation.
16. Aczone (5% dapsone) Gel 30 g tube
*Sig:* Thin coat twice a day.
17. Acanya Gel (clindamycin phosphate 1.2% and benzoyl peroxide 2.5%).
*Sig:* Thin coat once a day.

### Treatment for a Case of Scarring Acne

1. Tetracycline, or similar antibiotic, 250 or 500 mg #100
*Sig:* Take 1 capsule q.i.d. for 3 days, then 1 capsule b.i.d. This dose can be continued for weeks, months, or years, or the dose can be lowered to 1 capsule a day for maintenance, depending, of course, on the extent of the involvement. Severe cases respond to 3 to 6 capsules a day.
Tetracycline should be taken 30 minutes before meals or 2 hours after a meal, and not concurrently with iron or calcium for optimal absorption.
*Comment:* Minocycline (Solodyn) is also available as time released at once daily dosing (1 mg/kg) at 45-, 90-, and 135-mg tablets. Other effective antibiotics include erythromycin, 250 mg b.i.d. or t.i.d.; minocycline, 100 mg/d; doxycycline (Monodox is doxycycline monohydrate with a decreased chance of esophageal inflammation; Doryx is a preparation that only needs to be given once a day with a decreased gastrointestinal upset and less photosensitivity),

100 mg b.i.d.; and minocycline (Minocin may be better absorbed), 100 mg b.i.d. Other antibiotics include clindamycin 150 or 300 mg b.i.d. and trimethoprim 100 mg b.i.d. Azithromycin (Zithromax) pulse in a 5-day dose pack 500 mg the first day, 250 mg for 4 days (Z-pack) can be used monthly or bimonthly (low dose doxycycline hyclate [20 mg] is subantimicrobial and may eliminate many side effects of larger doses).

### SAUER'S NOTES

1. For local acne medications, one product can be applied in the morning and a different product at night.
2. To ensure compliance, start with milder agents, increasing the strength as indicated and tolerated.
3. Acne flare-ups occur in cycles—hormonal (females) and seasonal (fall and spring). Keep reminding your patient of these natural flare-ups.
4. "Prom pills." The high school prom (or a wedding or a job interview) is in 1 week. The following will clear much of that inflammatory acne:
Prednisone, 10-mg tablets #14
*Sig:* Take 2 tablets each morning for 7 days.
5. Unfortunately, an appreciable number of men and women continue to have acne into the 20s, 30s, and even later years. Explain this fact to your patients.

2. Other treatments
   a. Vitamin A (water-soluble synthetic A), 50,000 #100
      *Sig:* Take 1 capsule b.i.d. for 5 months, then not for
      2 months to prevent liver toxicity. Avoid if preg-
      nancy is a possibility.
   b. Abrasive cleansers are recommended by some physi-
      cians, but the author does not personally recommend
      them and thinks they can actually make acne worse.
   c. Large papules or early cysts. Intralesional corticos-
      teroid can be injected with care. Dilute triamcinolone
      suspension (4 mg/mL) with equal part of saline or
      lidocaine (Xylocaine) with epinephrine, and inject
      about 0.1 mL into the lesion. Atrophy can result if too
      large a quantity or too high a concentration is injected.
   d. Incision of fluctuant acne cysts: *never* incise these
      widely, but if you believe the pus must be drained, do
      it through a very small incision and possibly an acne
      stylet. A zero or ear curette can be useful.
   e. Short-term prednisone systemic therapy is effective
      for severe cystic acne, especially for acne fulminans,
      an acute, disabling form of acne.
   f. Isotretinoin: For severe, scarring, cystic acne this ther-
      apy has proved very beneficial. The usual dosage is
      1 mg/kg/d given for 4 to 5 months. There are many
      minor and major side effects with this therapy (no-
      tably teratogenic effects in pregnant women), so
      isotretinoin should only be prescribed by those knowl-
      edgeable in its use. Depression may also be a side
      effect. Some authors have concluded that a lower dose
      of 20 mg/d can be efficacious with fewer side effects
      than higher doses for moderate acne. LASIK eye
      surgery should probably not be done until 6 months
      after isotretinoin therapy stopped or 6 months before
      isotretinoin therapy is started. The IPLEDGE program
      for following patients is mandatory.
3. The residual scarring of severe acne (**Fig. 13-9**) can
   be lessened by diamond fraise, or laser resurfacing.

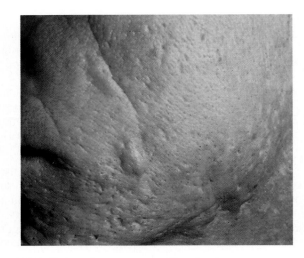

FIGURE 13-9 ■ Acne scars on the cheek.

There are many other surgical treatments available (see
Chapter 5). These procedures are being done by many
dermatologists and plastic surgeons.

4. Nicomide, 1 b.i.d. is a vitamin therapy that may be helpful.
5. Spirinolactone 25 or 50 mg b.i.d. may be beneficial in
   women especially if they flare during the last week of
   their menstrual cycle.
6. Long-wave ultraviolet light in the form of blue or red
   light or a combination of the two or IPL therapy. It appears to be safe and can be helpful.
7. Photodynamic therapy with a topical levulenic acid
   preparation and red light activation.

## Rosacea

A common pustular eruption with flushing and telangiectasias on the butterfly area of the face may occur in adults
especially in the 40- to 60-year-old age group (**Fig. 13-10**).

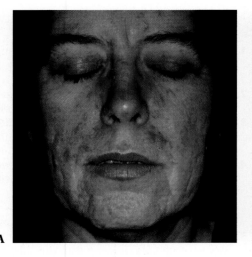

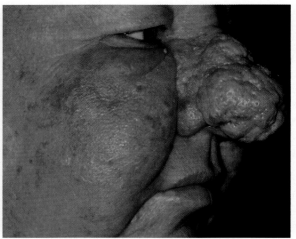

A                                                              B

FIGURE 13-10 ■ **(A)** Rosacea of a 47-year-old woman. **(B)** Rosacea, chronic, with rhinophyma. *(Courtesy of Hoechst-Roussel Pharmaceuticals, Inc.)*

## Presentation and Characteristics

### Primary Lesions

Diffuse redness, papules, pustules, and, later, dilated venules, mainly of the nose, cheeks, and forehead, are seen.

## Secondary Lesions

Severe, longstanding cases eventuate into the bulbous, greasy, hypertrophic nose characteristic of rhinophyma.

### Course

The pustules are recurrent and difficult to heal. Rosacea keratitis of the eye may occur. Rosacea is rare in children, but there is a risk of significant eye disease in this population.

### Causes

Several factors influence the disease:

1. Heredity (oily skin)
2. Excess ingestion of alcoholic beverages, hot drinks, and spicy foods
3. *Demodex* mites (may be causative)
4. Increased exercise
5. Increased exposure to hot or cold environment
6. Topical or systemic corticosteroids

Excess sun exposure and emotional stress can aggravate some cases of rosacea.

## Differential Diagnosis

- *Systemic lupus erythematosus:* No papules or pustules; positive antinuclear antibody (ANA) blood test (see Chapter 37).
- *Boils:* Usually only one large lesion; can be recurrent but may occur sporadically; an early case of rosacea may look like small boils. Bacterial culture shows *Staphylococcus aureus* or group A β-hemolytic streptococci. Responds to anti-*Staphylococcus* antibiotics (see Chapter 20).
- *Iodide or bromide drug eruption:* Clinically similar, but drug eruption usually is more widespread; history positive for drug (see Chapter 8).
- *Seborrheic dermatitis:* Pustules uncommon; red and scaly; also in scalp.
- *Rosacea-like tuberculid of Lewandowsky:* Mimics small papular rosacea clinically and tuberculids histologically, rare; biopsy helpful.
- *Flushing:* Carcinoid pheochromocytoma, mastocytosis, medullary thyroid carcinoma, climacterium in menopausal women and some medications (especially nicotinic acid).

## Treatment

*Case Example:* A 44-year-old man presents with redness and pustules on the butterfly area of the face.

1. Prescribe avoidance of these foods: chocolate, nuts, cheese, cola drinks, iodized salt, seafood, alcohol, spices, and very hot drinks.
2. Metronidazole gel (MetroGel, Metrocream, Metrolotion, or Noritate cream).
   *Sig:* Apply thin coat b.i.d. Response to therapy is slow, taking 4 to 6 weeks to benefit.
3. Sulfur, ppt. 6%
   Resorcinol 4%
   Colored alcoholic shake lotion q.s. 60.0
   *Sig:* Apply to face h.s.
   Similar proprietary lotions are Sulfacet-R lotion Rosac cream (contains a sunscreen), Rosula (contains urea to decrease irritation), sodium sulfacetamide topical preparations, Plexion topical preparations, Novacet lotion, and Avar Green (contains green tint to hide redness).
4. Tetracycline, 250-mg capsules.
   *Sig:* Take 1 capsule q.i.d. for 3 days, then 1 capsule b.i.d. for weeks, as necessary for benefit. Other antibiotics that can be used, as for acne, include doxycycline, minocycline, and erythromycin.
5. Therapy for *Helicobacter pylori* in the same treatment regimens as for peptic ulcer disease has been tried with some benefit in severe cases.
6. Azeleic acid (Azelex and Finacea) in thin coat b.i.d.
7. Crotamiton (Eurax) lotion in thin coat b.i.d.
8. Subantimicrobial doses of antibiotics (i.e., Oracea [40-mg doxycycline] one each day with food) may be safer (less vaginal yeast infections, less superinfections, less upset stomach, and less photosensitivity) and still be effective.
9. Oral zinc sulfate 100 mg three times a day is safe and has shown benefit according to some authors.
10. Other remedies used include topical tretinoin (may worsen redness), topical tacrolimus, oral sulfate (100 mg b.i.d.), and oral Nicomide (combination of vitamins and minerals).
11. Sun protection may be helpful.

## Suggested Readings

Cordain L, Lindeberg S, Hurtado M, et al. Acne vulgaris: A disease of Western Civilization. *Arch Dermatol.* 2002;138:1584–1590.
Gollnick H, Gunliffe W, Berson D, et al. Management of acne: A report from a Global Alliance to Improve Outcomes in Acne. *J Am Acad Dermatol.* 2003;49(1 Suppl):S1–S37.

# CHAPTER 14

# Psoriasis

*Jeffrey M. Weinberg, MD*

## Psoriasis

Psoriasis is a hereditary, papulosquamous skin disorder that affects 1.5% to 2% of the population in Western societies. In the United States, there are 3 to 5 million people with psoriasis, which affects men and women equally. Psoriasis can have multiple clinical presentations and varies widely among different individuals. It is typically a chronic and recurring disease that is best characterized by well-demarcated erythematous plaques with scaling. The plaques can be localized, which is the most common presentation, and confined to only certain delineated areas of the body. Most commonly plaques are seen on the elbows, knees, and the scalp. There are other variants of psoriasis. In palmoplantar psoriasis, lesions are limited to the soles of the feet and palms of the hands. In contrast, generalized pustular psoriasis and generalized erythrodermic psoriasis can involve the entire body and be a life-threatening condition, even necessitating hospitalization when seen in association with acute respiratory distress syndrome.

### Primary Lesions

*Plaque psoriasis:* The lesions are well-demarcated, salmon-colored papules and plaques with thick silvery scaling that typically bleeds when removed (Auspitz's sign). Lesions can vary greatly in size and shape in addition to distribution, which may be localized or generalized.

*Pustular psoriasis:* The lesions are typically yellow pustules that can coalesce and evolve into dark-red crusty lesions.

### Secondary Lesions

Secondary lesions are less common but can include excoriations, lichenification, (thickening) oozing, and secondary infection.

### Distribution

Psoriatic patches most commonly occur on the elbows, knees, and scalp, although involvement can occur on any area of the body, including palms, soles, and even nails.

### Course

Psoriasis is typically a chronically recurring disease, although cases of complete resolution do occur. The onset of the disease can occur at any age, but the peaks of onset are in the 20s and 50s.

### Causes

While the exact etiology of psoriasis is unknown, there is clearly a hereditary component. When one parent has psoriasis, a child has an 8% chance of having the disease. If both parents have psoriasis, the child's chance of developing psoriasis increases to as high as 41%. Specific human leukocyte antigen (HLA) types have been noted to have a higher frequency of association with psoriasis, specifically HLA-B13, HLA-B17, HLA-Bw57, and most notably HLA-Cw6.

An acute form of guttate psoriasis, which characteristically develops in children and younger adults, often follows a streptococcal infection and has characteristic smaller sized, drop-shaped lesions.

Triggering factors include physical trauma, which can elicit the lesions, or any type of excessive rubbing or scratching, which can stimulate the proliferative process. Aggravating factors include psychologic stress and certain medications such as systemic glucocorticoids, oral lithium, antimalarial drugs, systemic interferon, beta-blockers, and potentially angiotensin-converting enzyme inhibitors. Alcohol and smoking may also aggravate psoriasis.

### Subjective Complaints

Thirty percent of patients present with a complaint of pruritus, especially when psoriasis involves the scalp and anogenital area. Also common are complaints of joint pain, termed psoriatic arthritis, found in 5% to 8% of patients with psoriasis. Interestingly, 10% of patients with psoriatic arthritis have no skin manifestations of the disease. Finally, in a rare acute onset of generalized pustular psoriasis called von Zumbusch syndrome, there is associated weakness, chills, and fever.

### Season

Exacerbation is typically seen in the winter, most likely due to the lack of sunlight and low humidity. Natural ultraviolet light typically causes psoriatic symptoms to improve.

### Age Group

The disease can occur at any age. However, the average onset is typically bimodal, with one peak at approximately 23 years (although in children, mean onset is 8 years) and another at age 55.

## Contagiousness

Psoriasis is not contagious.

## Relation to Employment

Psoriatic lesions occur more typically in areas of skin injury or repeated skin stress or pressure. This is known as the Koebner phenomenon.

## Laboratory Findings

The diagnosis of psoriasis is usually made on clinical grounds, and biopsy is not necessary. If biopsy is performed, histologic findings include the following:

1. Acanthosis: thickening of the skin
2. Increased mitosis of keratinocytes, fibroblasts, and endothelial cells
3. Inflammatory cells in the dermis and epidermis

## Differential Diagnosis

1. *Seborrheic dermatitis:* Lesions more yellowish and greasy than those of psoriasis. In the scalp, the scale is usually less thick than in psoriasis. Seborrheic dermatitis and psoriasis can often coexist in some patients.
2. *Lichen simplex chronicus:* Usually fewer patches than psoriasis, with less of a thick scale.
3. *Tinea corporis:* Usually a single lesion, with outer scale and central clearing. Potassium hydroxide preparation and fungal culture are positive for fungi.
4. *Psoriasiform drug eruptions:* Check medication history.
5. *Pityriasis rosea:* "Christmas tree" configuration of oval, papulosquamous lesions. Herald patch usually precedes the wider eruption.
6. *Atopic eczema:* Ask about family history of asthma, allergic rhinitis, and eczema. Involvement typically occurs on flexural surfaces, face, and neck.
7. *Secondary or tertiary syphilis:* These can appear psoriasiform. Inquire regarding history of sexually transmitted diseases and recent symptoms. Check syphilis serology if indicated.
8. *Mycosis fungoides:* Biopsy in chronic cases, especially with involvement of the bathing trunk area.
9. *Nail dystrophy:* Psoriasis is in the differential diagnosis of nail dystrophy. Other entities to consider include onychomycosis, trauma, and lichen planus.

## Treatment

While there is no definitive cure for psoriasis there are many methods of management that can greatly improve and sometimes almost completely eradicate its skin manifestations, leading to a much improved quality of life. There are many new therapies available or in development for the treatment of the disease.

*First Visit of a Patient Presenting with Mild to Moderate Localized Lesions on the Body, Face, or Scalp*

### For Body Lesions.

1. Medium- to high-potency fluorinated corticosteroid cream or ointment
   *Sig:* Apply b.i.d. to body lesions.
2. Calcipotriene (Dovonex) ointment
   *Sig:* Apply b.i.d. to body lesions.
3. Calcipotriene and betamethasone dipropionate (Taclonex) ointment q.d.
4. Tazarotene (Tazorac) gel or cream, 0.05% or 0.1%
   *Sig:* Apply q.h.s. to body lesions.
5. Intralesional triamcinolone 10 mg/cc
   *Sig:* Apply subcutaneously to body lesions. This treatment can be very valuable for discrete, recalcitrant lesions.

### For Facial (Less Common) and Intertriginous Lesions.

1. Low-potency corticosteroid cream or ointment
   *Sig:* Apply b.i.d. to facial lesions.
2. Pimecrolimus (Elidel) cream 0.1% or tacrolimus (Protopic) ointment 0.03% or 0.01%
   *Sig:* Apply b.i.d. to facial lesions.

### For Scalp Lesions.

1. Tar shampoo
   *Sig:* Shampoo frequently.
2. Topical corticosteroid lotion (Clobex, Diprolene), solution (Cormax, Lidex), or foam (Olux, Luxiq)
   *Sig:* Apply b.i.d. to scalp.
3. Derma-Smoothe/FS scalp oil
   *Sig:* Apply overnight to scalp as directed.
4. Calcipotriene (Dovonex scalp solution) 0.0005%
   *Sig:* Apply b.i.d. to scalp.
5. Tazarotene (Tazorac) gel 0.05 or 0.1%
   *Sig:* Apply q.h.s. to scalp.
6. Excimer (Xtrac) laser twice weekly for 4 to 10 treatments

*Subsequent Visits of a Patient with Mild to Moderate Localized Psoriasis*

1. For body lesions, the potency of the corticosteroid utilized can be increased.
2. Occlusive dressings with corticosteroid can be applied at night and left overnight.
   a. Intralesional corticosteroid therapy can be given whereby individual small lesions are injected with intralesional triamcinolone as discussed previously.
3. Tazarotene (Tazorac) gel or cream, 0.05 or 0.1% as mentioned previously.
   a. Ultraviolet therapy: Options include broadband or narrowband ultraviolet B, each three times per week,

and oral PUVA (psoralen and ultraviolet A), two to three times per week. PUVA has been associated with an increased risk of squamous cell carcinoma and, with long-term use, melanoma.

4. Excimer (Xtrac) laser twice weekly for 4 to 10 treatments.

*First Visit of a Patient with Moderate to Severe Generalized Psoriasis*

1. Topical therapies listed for mild to moderate disease are utilized, possibly in combination with other therapies listed below.
2. Broadband or narrowband ultraviolet B, three times per week.
3. PUVA, two to three times per week.
4. Biologic therapies.
   a. Alefacept (Amevive) 15 mg IM for 12 weeks. A second, subsequent course can be initiated after 12 weeks off the drug. T-cell counts must be monitored biweekly.
   b. Efalizumab (Raptiva) 1 mg/cc SQ q. week. This drug can be given as continuous therapy after a conditioning dose of 0.7 mg/cc. Platelet counts should be intermittently checked. Efalizumab has shown success in the treatment of palmoplantar psoriasis. Worsening of psoriasis has been noted on abrupt discontinuation of the drug.
   c. Etanercept (Enbrel) 50 mg b.i.w. SQ for 3 months, followed by 25 mg b.i.w. This drug can be given as continuous therapy in the long term and is beneficial for psoriatic arthritis. Injection site reactions have been observed. A purified protein derivative (PPD) skin test should be checked prior to therapy. Exercise caution in patients with multiple sclerosis, congestive heart failure, tuberculosis exposure, and lupus erythematosus.
   d. Infliximab (Remicade) 5 mg/kg at weeks 0, 2, and 6, and then every 8 weeks. Infliximab is approved for psoriasis and psoriatic arthritis. As for etanercept, a PPD should be checked prior to therapy. Exercise caution in patients with multiple sclerosis, congestive heart failure, tuberculosis exposure, and lupus erythematosus.
   e. Adalimumab (Humira) 80 mg SQ as a loading dose, followed 1 week later by 40 mg SQ, and then 40 mg SQ every other week. As for other TNF (tumor necrosis factor)-inhibitors, a PPD should be checked prior to therapy. Exercise caution in patients with multiple sclerosis, congestive heart failure, tuberculosis exposure, and lupus erythematosus.
   f. Ustekinumab, an antibody to IL (interleukin)-12/23, is an intermittent biologic therapy currently under review by the FDA (as of March 2008).
5. Methotrexate: This oral drug can be used weekly. This drug has potential side effects, including liver and pulmonary toxicity. Patients should be monitored closely.
6. Acitretin (Soriatane) therapy 10 to 25 mg q.d. This drug is especially useful in cases of palmoplantar, erythrodermic, and pustular psoriasis. This drug is teratogenic, and a woman cannot become pregnant until 3 years after the

drug is discontinued. There are several other potential side effects, including alopecia, bone loss, and hyperlipidemia. Patients should be monitored closely. This drug can be combined with PUVA (Re-PUVA: combination retinoid and PUVA therapy).

*Subsequent Visits of a Patient with Moderate to Severe Generalized Psoriasis*

1. Continue or rotate therapies as per first visit.
2. Occasionally some of these therapies can be combined. Check the package inserts and published data before combining different systemic therapies.
3. Cyclosporine (Neoral): This oral immunosuppressive therapy is highly effective for short-term, rapid treatment of severe psoriasis. It has many potential toxicities, including hypertension and renal toxicity. Patients should be monitored closely.
4. Other biologic therapies: If a patient is nonresponsive to one or more biologic agents, transition to a different agent.
5. Mycophenolate mofetil (CellCept). This oral immunosuppressive drug has been reported to be effective in some patients with psoriasis. There is less organ toxicity with this than with methotrexate or cyclosporine. There

---

### SAUER'S NOTES

### MANAGEMENT OF PSORIASIS

1. Education and support are keys to the treatment of psoriasis. Give written information to the patient regarding the disease and potential treatment options. Carefully counsel patients as to the risks and benefits of their therapies. Encourage the patient to join the National Psoriasis Foundation, which provides comprehensive patient support.
2. Encourage the patient not to pick or scratch their skin or scalp. This can aggravate their psoriasis (Koebner phenomenon).
3. With the use of topical corticosteroids, observe closely for the development of striae and skin atrophy. Avoid high-potency steroids on the face and intertriginous areas.
4. When considering biologic or systemic therapy, patient selection is critical. Take a thorough medical history and review of systems.
5. Remain cognizant of the quality of life and emotional toll of psoriasis. Provide referrals for counseling when appropriate.
6. Psoriasis has been associated with comorbidities that include metabolic syndrome and increased cardiovascular risk. These entities share etiologic features and health outcomes that directly correlate with the severity of psoriatic disease. Therefore these considerations should be part of the evaluation and management of psoriasis patients. Appropriate counseling and/or referral should be made to address potential comorbidities.

is a small increased risk of lymphoma with chronic use of the drug.

## Suggested Readings

Christophers E. Comorbidities in psoriasis. *Clin Dermatol.* 2007;25:529–534.

Kimball AB, Gordon KB, Langley RG, et al. Safety and efficacy of ABT-874, a fully human interleukin 12/23 monoclonal antibody, in the treatment of moderate to severe chronic plaque psoriasis: results of a randomized, placebo-controlled, phase 2 trial. *Arch Dermatol.* 2008;144:200–207.

Krueger GG, Langley RG, Leonardi C, et al. A human interleukin-12/23 monoclonal antibody for the treatment of psoriasis. *N Engl J Med.* 2007;356:580–592.

Lebwohl M, Bagel J, Gelfand JM, et al. From the Medical Board of the National Psoriasis Foundation: monitoring and vaccinations in patients treated with biologics for psoriasis. *J Am Acad Dermatol.* 2008;58:94–105.

Menter A, Griffiths CE. Current and future management of psoriasis. *Lancet.* 2007;370:272–284.

Naldi L, Griffiths CE. Traditional therapies in the management of moderate to severe chronic plaque psoriasis: an assessment of the benefits and risks. *Br J Dermatol.* 2005;152:597–615.

Weinberg, JM, ed. *Treatment of Psoriasis.* Basel: Birkhauser Verlag; 2008.

Weinberg JM, Bottino CJ, Lindholm J, et al. Biologic therapy for psoriasis: an update on the tumor necrosis factor inhibitors infliximab, etanercept, and adalimumab, and the T-cell-targeted therapies efalizumab and alefacept. *J Drugs Dermatol.* 2005;4:544–555.

# CHAPTER 15

# Other Papulosquamous Dermatoses

*John C. Hall, MD*

Papulosquamous eruptions, as indicated by the name, infer elevation and desquamation of the skin. Seborrhea (Chapter 13), the only one of these conditions with a greasy scale, and psoriasis (Chapter 14) are the most common. Most of these conditions are inflammatory, but tinea versicolor is included here due to the similarity of its clinical appearance to the other papulosquamous conditions. Lichen nitidus (see Dictionary–Index) and lichen striatus (see Dictionary–Index) are also considered in the category of papulosquamous skin diseases.

## Pityriasis Rosea

Pityriasis rosea is a moderately common papulosquamous eruption, mainly occurring on the trunks of young adults (**Figs. 15-1 to 15-3**). It is mildly pruritic and occurs most often in the spring and fall.

### Presentation and Characteristics

#### Primary Lesions

Papulosquamous, oval erythematous discrete lesions are seen. A larger "herald patch" resembling a patch of "ringworm" may precede the general rash by 2 to 10 days. A collarette of fine scaling is seen around the edge of the lesions. It begins just inside the pink plaque.

#### Secondary Lesions

Excoriations are rare. Secondary lesions are the effect of overtreatment or contact dermatitis from topical treatment.

#### Distribution

The lesions appear mainly on the chest and trunk along Langer's lines of cleavage in the skin. Many cases have the oval lesions in a "Christmas tree branches" pattern over the back. In atypical cases, the lesions are seen in the axillae and the groin only. This is sometimes referred to as *inverse pityriasis rosea*. Facial lesions are rare in light-skinned adults but are rather commonly seen in children and people of color.

#### Course

After the development of the herald patch, new generalized lesions continue to appear for 2 to 3 weeks. The entire rash most commonly disappears within 6 to 8 weeks. Recurrences are rare. There are recurrent and long-lasting variants.

#### Subjective Complaints

Itching varies from none to severe but is usually mild. Hot showers or baths may exacerbate the itching.

#### Cause

The cause is unknown. Some authors have incriminated human herpesvirus 6 (HHV-6) and human herpesvirus 7 (HHV-7).

#### Season

Spring and fall "epidemics" are common.

#### Age Group

Young adults and older children are most often affected.

#### Contagiousness

The disease is not contagious.

### Differential Diagnosis

- *Tinea versicolor:* Lesions are tannish and irregularly shaped; fungi are seen on scraping and fine, dry, adherent scale becomes apparent when the physician scratches the area with the fingernail.
- *Drug eruption:* No herald patch; positive drug history for gold, bismuth, or sulfa (see Chapter 8).
- *Secondary syphilis:* No itching (99% true); history or presence of genital lesions; positive blood serology; palmar lesions present (see Chapter 26).
- *Psoriasis:* Usually on elbows, knees, and scalp; lesions have a thick, adherent, silvery-white scale.
- *Seborrheic dermatitis:* Greasy, irregular, scaly lesions on the sternum, central face, external auditory

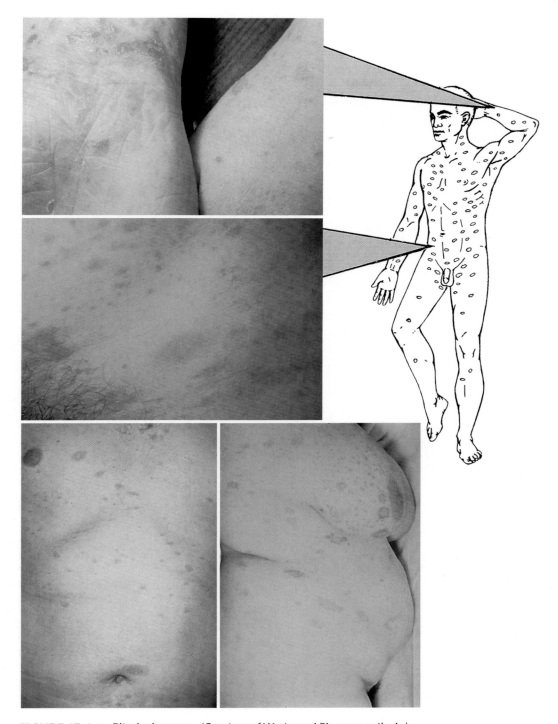

**FIGURE 15-1** ■ Pityriasis rosea. *(Courtesy of Westwood Pharmaceuticals.)*

canals, scalp, between the buttocks, and on the genitalia (see Chapter 13).

■ *Lichen planus:* Lesions are more papular and violaceous; found on the mucous membranes of the mouth and lip; very pruritic and common on flexor wrists.

■ *Parapsoriasis:* Rare; chronic form may have fine "cigarette paper" atrophy; can develop into mycosis fungoides (cutaneous T-cell lymphoma [CTCL]).

## Treatment

### First Visit

1. Reassure the patient that he or she does not have a "blood disease," that the eruption is not contagious, and that it would be rare to get it again.

2. Colloidal bath

   *Sig:* Add 1 packet of Aveeno oatmeal preparation to the tub containing 6 to 8 in lukewarm water.

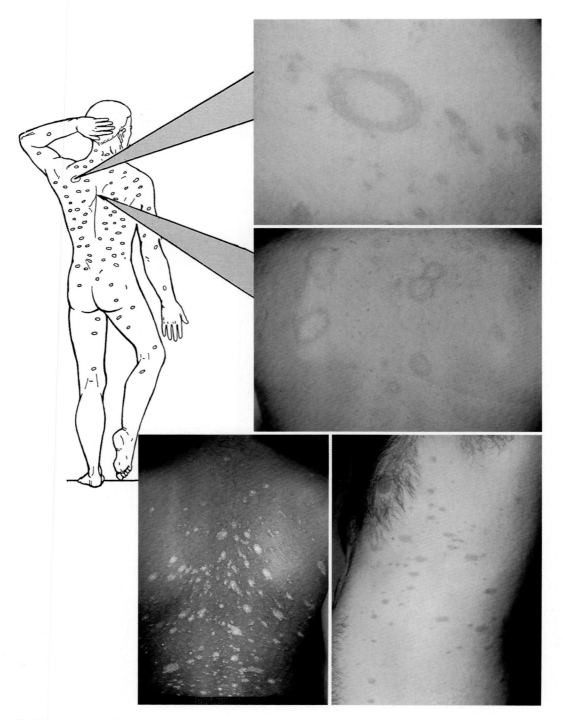

**FIGURE 15-2** ■ Pityriasis rosea. Bottom left photograph is of an African-American patient. *(Courtesy of Westwood Pharmaceuticals.)*

Bathe for 10 to 15 minutes every day or every other day.

*Comment:* Avoid soap and hot water as much as possible to reduce any itching.

**3.** Use nonalcoholic white shake lotion or Calamine lotion q.s. or any topical with pramoxine (Pramosone lotion, cream, or ointment and, over the counter, Sarna for sensitive skin, among many others)

*Sig:* Apply b.i.d. locally to affected areas.

**4.** If there is itching, prescribe an antihistamine. Cyproheptadine (Periactin), 4 mg #60

*Sig:* Take 1 tablet a.c. and h.s.

**5.** UVB therapy in increasing suberythema doses once or twice a week may be given. The severity is decreased, but itching and disease duration are probably not altered.

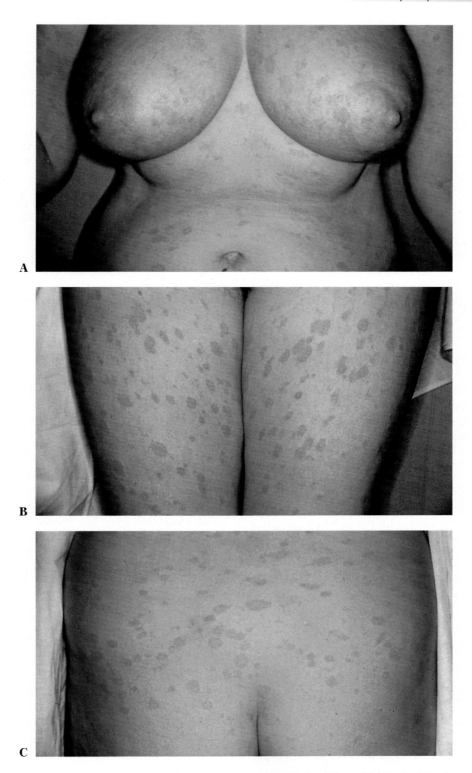

**FIGURE 15-3** ▪ Pityriasis rosea of the chest (**A**), thighs (**B**), and buttocks (**C**) of one patient. *(Courtesy of Syntex Laboratories, Inc.)*

*Subsequent Visits*

1. If the skin becomes too dry from the colloidal bath and the lotion, stop the lotion or alternate it with

   Hydrocortisone cream or ointment, 1% q.s. 60.0
   *Sig:* Apply b.i.d. locally to dry areas.

2. Continue the ultraviolet treatments.

*Severely Pruritic Cases*

1. In addition to the above, add

   Prednisone, 5 mg #40
   *Sig:* Take 1 tablet q.i.d. for 3 days, then 1 tablet t.i.d. for 4 days, then 2 tablets every morning for 1 to 2 weeks, as symptoms of itching demand.

2. Some authors found that acyclovir, 800 mg five times a day for 1 week, early in the course of the disease helps to hasten resolution.

## Tinea Versicolor

Tinea versicolor is a moderately common skin eruption with tannish-colored, well-demarcated, circular, scaly patches that cause no discomfort and are usually located on the upper chest and back (**Fig. 15-4**). It is caused by a lipophilic yeast. Dry scaling can be revealed by stroking the skin with a fingernail (coup d'ongle).

### Presentation and Characteristics

#### Primary Lesions

Papulosquamous or maculosquamous, tan, circular, well-demarcated lesions occur.

#### Secondary Lesions

Relative depigmentation results because the involved skin does not tan when exposed to sunlight. Skin not exposed to ultraviolet light is slightly hyperpigmented. The hypopigmentation cosmetic defect, obvious in the summer since the yeast is a monoamine oxidase inhibitor and does not allow tanning, often brings the patient to the office. Hence the name versicolor (varied color).

#### Distribution

The upper part of the chest and the back, neck, and arms are affected. Rarely are the lesions on the face or generalized.

#### Course

The eruption can persist for years unnoticed. Correct treatment is readily effective, but the disease usually recurs.

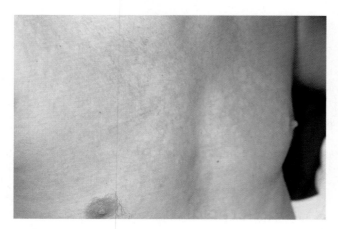

**FIGURE 15-4** ■ Tinea versicolor on the chest. The dark areas of the skin are the areas infected with the fungus. *(Courtesy of K.U.M.C.; Sandoz Pharmaceuticals)*

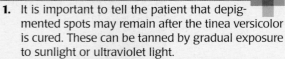

### SAUER'S NOTES

1. It is important to tell the patient that depigmented spots may remain after the tinea versicolor is cured. These can be tanned by gradual exposure to sunlight or ultraviolet light.
2. A topical imidazole cream (clotrimazole, econazole, ketoconazole, miconazole) twice a day topically for 2 weeks, with or without a sulfur soap, can be used. Terbinafine spray (Lamisil) twice a day for 1 week can also be used.
3. Ketoconazole (Nizoral) orally in various short-term regimens and itraconazole (Sporanox) 200 mg orally for 1 week have been used.

#### Cause

The causative agent is a lipophilic yeast, *Pityrosporum orbiculare*, which has a hyphal form called *Pityrosporum* or *Malassezia furfur*.

#### Contagiousness

The disease is not contagious and is not related to poor hygiene.

#### Laboratory Findings

A scraping of the scale placed on a microscopic slide, covered with a 20% solution of potassium hydroxide and a coverslip, shows the hyphae. Under the low-power lens of the microscope, very thin, short, mycelial filaments are seen. Diagnostic grapelike clusters of spores are seen best with the high-power lens. The appearance of spores and hyphae is referred to as "spaghetti and meatballs." The dimorphic organism does not grow on routine culture media.

### Differential Diagnosis

- *Pityriasis rosea:* Acute onset; lesions oval with a collarette of fine, adherent, dry scale (see earlier in this chapter).
- *Seborrheic dermatitis:* Greasy scales mainly in hairy areas (see Chapter 13).
- *Mild psoriasis:* Thicker scaly lesions on the trunk and elsewhere (see Chapter 14).
- *Vitiligo:* Because tinea versicolor commonly manifests with hypopigmentation of the skin, many cases are misdiagnosed as vitiligo. This is indeed unfortunate because tinea versicolor is quite easy to treat and has a much better prognosis than vitiligo (see Chapter 36). There is no pigment (depigmentation) in vitiligo and decreased pigment (hypopigmentation) in tinea versicolor. There are no scales in vitiligo.
- *Secondary syphilis:* Lesions are more widely distributed and present on the palms and soles (see Chapter 22).

## Treatment

1. Selenium (Selsun or Head & Shoulders intensive treatment) suspension 120.0

    *Sig:* Bathe and dry completely. Then apply medicine as a lotion to all the involved areas, usually from the neck down to the pubic area. Let it dry. Bathe again in 24 hours and wash off the medicine. Repeat the procedure again at weekly intervals for four treatments. This can be irritating.

2. Topical imidazole creams such as miconazole (available over the counter), ketoconazole (available over the counter), clotrimazole (available over the counter), econazole (Spectazole), and oxiconazole (Oxistat) twice a day for 2 weeks. Compounding 2% to 5% sulfur may add to the efficacy.

3. If lesions are extensive, 200 mg of ketoconazole orally twice a day for 5 days to cause a remission and on the first day of each month for 6 months beginning April 1 can be used to prevent summer recurrences, which are common in warm, humid climates.

*Comment:* Recurrences are rather common and can be easily retreated.

## Lichen Planus

Lichen planus is an uncommon, chronic, pruritic disease characterized by violaceous flat-topped papules that are usually seen on the wrists and the legs (**Figs. 15-5** to **15-8**; see also Fig. 3-1B). The 5 "Ps" are pruritic, polygonal, planar, purple, papules. If you would like to make it 6, you could add persistent. Mucous membrane lesions on the cheeks or lips are milky white and netlike. Erosions and ulcers on oral mucous membranes are seen in more severe disease, which can make eating and dental hygiene difficult.

### Presentation and Characteristics

*Primary Lesions*

Flat-topped, violaceous papules and papulosquamous lesions appear. On close examination of a papule, preferably after the lesion has been wet with an alcohol swipe, intersecting small white lines or papules (Wickham's striae) can be seen. These confirm the diagnosis. Uncommonly, the lesions may assume a ring-shaped configuration (especially on the penis) or may be hypertrophic (especially pretibial), atrophic, or bullous. On the mucous membranes, the lesions appear as a whitish, lacy network. When mucous membrane involvement is severe, ulcerations may occur and there is an increased occurrence of squamous cell cancer. There is a severe ulcerative form that can occur in the vulvovaginal and

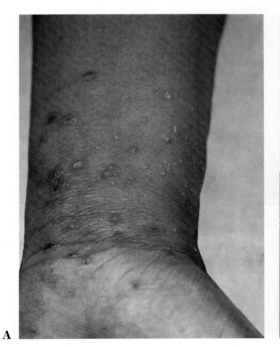
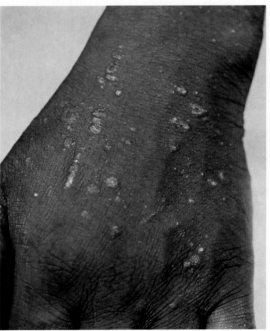

A          B

**FIGURE 15-5** ■ Lichen planus on the wrist (**A**) and the dorsum of the hand (**B**) in an African-American patient. Note the violaceous color of the papules and the linear Koebner phenomenon on the dorsum of the hand. *(Courtesy of E.R. Squibb.)*

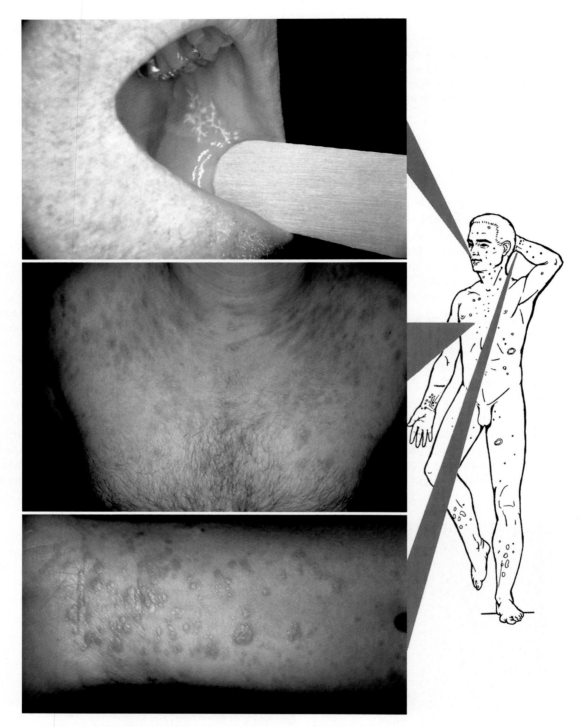

**FIGURE 15-6** ■ Lichen planus. *(Courtesy of Johnson & Johnson.)*

rectal area in women and on the soles of the feet in both sexes.

### Secondary Lesions

Excoriations and, on the legs, thick, scaly, lichenified patches have been noted. Lesions are often rubbed rather than scratched because scratching is painful.

### Distribution

Most commonly, the lesions appear on the flexural aspects of the wrists and the ankles, the penis, and the oral mucous membranes, but they can be anywhere on the body or become generalized.

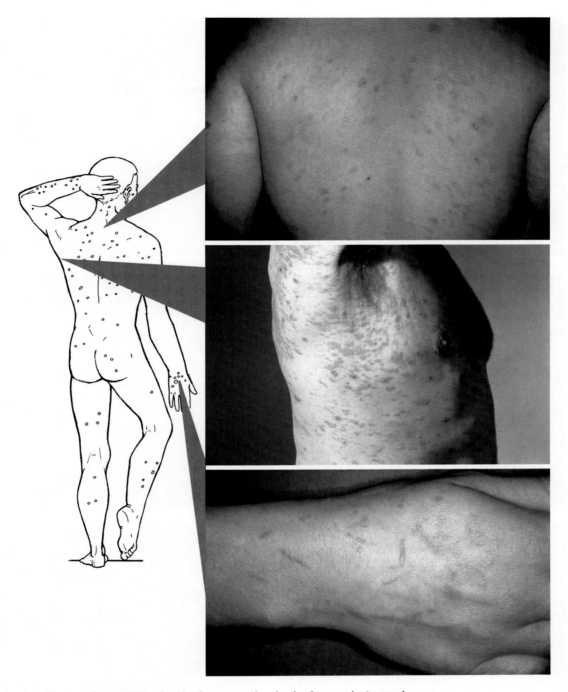

**FIGURE 15-7** ■ Lichen planus. Note the Koebner reaction in the lower photograph.

### Course

Outbreak is rather sudden, with the chronic course averaging 9 months in duration. Some cases last several years. There is no effect on the general health except for itching. Recurrences are moderately common (approximately 20%).

### Cause

The cause is unknown. The disorder is rather frequently associated with nervous or emotional upsets. It may represent an autoimmune process, and some cases have a distinct pattern on direct immunofluorescence. Hepatitis C or hepatitis B is present in some cases (possibly up to 20%). This is more common when associated with HIV. There is a rare form flared by the sun (lichen planus actinicus).

### Subjective Complaints

Itching varies from mild to severe (severe is more common).

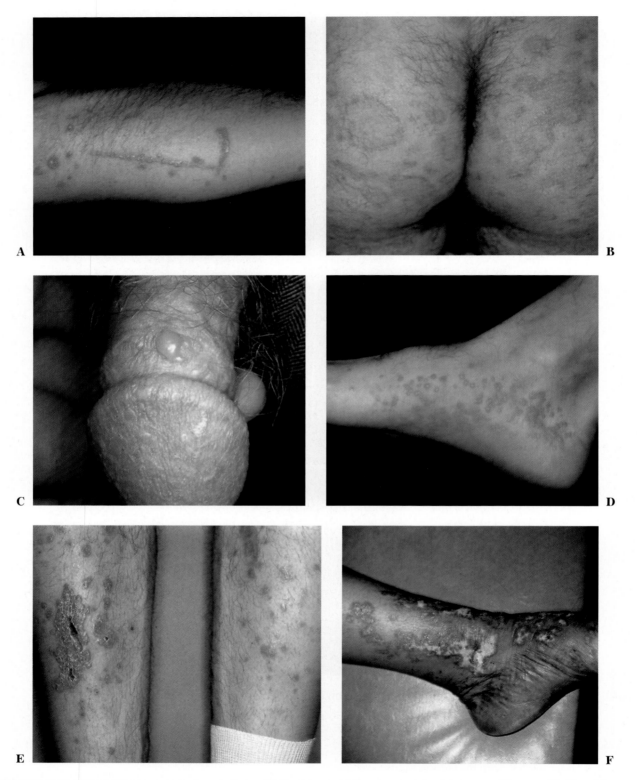

**FIGURE 15-8** ■ Lichen planus, unusual variations. (**A**) Koebner reaction in scratched areas on the arm. (**B**) Atrophic scarring lesions on the buttocks. (**C**) Bullous and vesicular lesions on the penis. (**D**) Lichen planus on the sole of the foot. (**E**) Hypertrophic lesions on the anterior tibial area of the legs. (**F**) Hypertrophic lesions on the leg of an African-American woman. *(Courtesy of Neutrogena Corp.)*

## Contagiousness

Lichen planus is not contagious.

## Relation to Employment

As in psoriasis, the lichen planus lesions can develop in scratches or skin injuries (Koebner phenomenon).

## Laboratory Findings

Microscopic section is quite characteristic.

## Differential Diagnosis

- *Secondary syphilis:* No itching; blood serology positive (see Chapter 22).
- *Drug eruption:* History of taking atabrine, arsenic, or gold (see Chapter 8).
- *Psoriasis:* Lesions more scaly, whitish on the knees and elbows (see Chapter 14).
- *Pityriasis rosea:* Herald patch mainly on the trunk (see earlier in this chapter).

Lichen planus on the leg may resemble neurodermatitis (usually one patch only; intensely pruritic; no mucous membrane lesions; excoriations; see Chapter 8) or keloids (secondary to injury with no Wickham's striae).

## Treatment

*Case Example:* A patient presents with generalized papular eruption and moderate itching.

### First Visit.

1. Assure the patient that the disease is not contagious, is not a blood disease, and is chronic but not serious. Explain that a hepatitis screen is necessary since up to 20% of patients may have hepatitis B or hepatitis C.
2. Tell the patient to avoid excess bathing with soap.
3. Suggest a low-potency corticosteroid cream 60.0

   *Sig:* Apply locally b.i.d.
4. Recommend an over-the-counter antihistamine such as chlorpheniramine, 4 mg #60

   *Sig:* Take 1 tablet b.i.d. for itching.

   *Comment:* Warn the patient of drowsiness at the onset of therapy.

### Subsequent Visits

1. Occlusive dressing with corticosteroid therapy. This is quite effective for localized cases. I have also found that if occlusive dressings are applied only to the lichen planus on the legs, the rest of the body lesions improve.
2. Meprobamate, 400 mg #100

   *Sig:* Take 1 tablet t.i.d., *or*
   Chlordiazepoxide (Librium), 5 mg
   *Sig:* Take 1 tablet t.i.d.
3. It is important in some resistant cases to rule out a focus of infection in teeth, tonsils, gallbladder, genitourinary system, and so on.
4. Corticosteroids orally or by injection are of definite value for temporarily relieving the acute cases that have severe itching or a generalized eruption.
5. Intralesional corticosteroids, especially for localized hypertrophic disease. I use this for oral mucous membrane, vulvovaginal, and rectal disease also.
6. Griseofulvin on rare occasions can decrease disease severity.
7. Treating hepatitis when present can benefit the disease (specifically hepatitis C).
8. Hydroxychloroquine sulfate (Plaquenil) orally can sometimes be helpful. See an ophthalmologist every 6 months to check for retinal toxicity.
9. Topical 0.1% pimecrolimus (Tacrolimus) t.i.d. has shown moderate benefit in one study.
10. Sulfasalazine (500 mg b.i.d.) has been used with success by some authors.

## Suggested Readings

Boyd AS, Neldner KH. Lichen planus. *J Am Acad Dermatol.* 1991;25:593–619.

Cribier B, Frances C, Chosidow O. Treatment of lichen planus. *Arch Dermatol.* 1998;134:1521–1530.

Eisen D. The clinical features, malignant potential, and systemic association of oral lichen planus: a study of 723 patients. *J Am Acad Dermatol.* 2002;46:207–214.

Gonzalez LM, Allen R, Janniger CK, et al. Pityriasis rosea: an important papulsquamous disorder. *Int J Dermatol.* 2005;44:757–764.

Fox BJ, Odom RB. Papulosquamous diseases: a review. *J Am Acad Dermatol.* 1985;12:597–624.

Sunenshine PJ, Schwartz RA, Janniger CK. Tinea versicolor. *Int J Dermatol.* 1998;37:648–655.

# CHAPTER 16

# Granulomatous Dermatoses

*John C. Hall, MD*

When considered singularly, granulomatous diseases are uncommon, but when all of them are considered together, they form a group that is interesting, varied, and ubiquitous.

A *granuloma* is a focal chronic inflammatory response to tissue injury manifested by a histologic picture of an accumulation and proliferation of leukocytes, principally of the mononuclear type and its family of derivatives, the mononuclear phagocyte system. The immunologic components in granulomatous inflammation originate from cell-mediated or -delayed hypersensitivity mechanisms controlled by thymus-dependent lymphocytes (T lymphocytes). Five groups of granulomatous inflammations have been promulgated:

- Group 1 is the *epithelioid granulomas*, which include sarcoidosis, tuberculosis in certain forms, tuberculoid leprosy, tertiary syphilis, zirconium granuloma, beryllium granuloma, mercurial granuloma, and lichen nitidus.
- Group 2, *histiocytic granulomas*, includes lepromatous leprosy, histoplasmosis, and leishmaniasis.
- Group 3 is the group of *foreign body granulomas*, including endogenous products (e.g., hair, fat, keratin), minerals (e.g., tattoos, silica, talc), plant and animal products (e.g., cactus, suture, oil, insect parts), and synthetic agents such as synthetic hair and filler substances.
- Group 4 is the *necrobiotic/palisading granulomas*, such as granuloma annulare, necrobiosis lipoidica, rheumatoid nodule, rheumatic fever nodule, catscratch disease, and lymphogranuloma venereum.
- Group 5 is the *mixed inflammatory granulomas*, including many deep fungal infections such as blastomycosis and sporotrichosis, mycobacterial infections, granuloma inguinale, and chronic granulomatous disease.

Most of these diseases are discussed with their appropriate etiologic classifications in the Dictionary–Index. Two of these granulomatous inflammations are discussed in this chapter: *sarcoidosis*, which is in group 1, and *granuloma annulare*, which is in group 4. A classification of granulomas based on etiology is listed in Table 16-1.

## Sarcoidosis

Sarcoidosis is an uncommon systemic granulomatous disease of unknown cause that affects the skin, lungs, lymph nodes, liver, spleen, parotid glands, and eyes. Less commonly involved organs that indicate more severe disease include the central nervous system, heart, bones, and upper respiratory tract. Any or all of these organs may be involved with sarcoidal granulomas. Lymphadenopathy is the single most common finding. People of color are affected more often than white patients (14:1). Only the skin manifestations of sarcoidosis are discussed here (**Fig. 16-1**; see also Fig. 38-15).

### Presentation and Characteristics

#### Primary Lesions

Cutaneous sarcoidosis is a great mimicker of other skin diseases. Superficial lesions consist of reddish papules, nodules, and plaques that may be multiple or solitary and of varying size and configuration. Annular forms of skin sarcoidosis are common. These superficial lesions usually involve the face, shoulders, and arms. Infiltration of sarcoidal lesions frequently occurs at scar sites. Subcutaneous nodular forms and telangiectatic, ulcerative, erythrodermic, and ichthyosiform types are rare. Sarcoidosis is often associated with a chronic systemic disease.

#### Secondary Lesions

Central healing can result in atrophy and scarring.

#### Course

Most cases of sarcoidosis run a chronic but benign course with remissions and exacerbations. Spontaneous "cure" is not unusual. Erythema nodosum is characteristic of acute benign sarcoidosis (see Chapter 12). Lupus pernio (indurated violaceous lesions on the ears, nose, lips, cheeks, and forehead) and plaques are characteristic of chronic, severe, systemic disease. It is seen most often in women and girls of color.

#### Causes

The cause of sarcoidosis is unknown.

**TABLE 16-1 ▪ Granulomatous Diseases of the Skin by Etiology**

**Infectious**

| | |
|---|---|
| Deep fungal | Coccidioidomycosis, paracoccidioidomycosis (South American blastomycosis), blastomycosis (North American blastomycosis), histoplasmosis, sporotrichosis, Majocchi's granuloma (deep dermatophyte infection) |
| Bacterial | Tuberculosis, leprosy, atypical mycobacteria, tertiary syphilis, granuloma inguinale, lymphogranuloma venereum, catscratch disease |
| Parasitic | Leishmaniasis |

**Noninfectious**

| *Diagnosis* | *Etiology* |
|---|---|
| Necrobiosis lipoidica diabeticorum | Five out of six patients will have or will acquire diabetes |
| Granuloma annulare | Generalized form may be associated with diabetes |
| Wegener's granulomatosis | Granulomatous vasculitis with renal, lung, and other internal organ involvement |
| Rheumatoid nodule | Rheumatoid arthritis |
| Lymphomatoid granulomatosis | Angiocentric lymphoma especially with lung involvement but also renal, skin, and CNS involvement |
| Chronic granulomatous disease | Defect of phagocyte NADPH oxidase, which leads to inability to destroy organisms after phagocytosis. Infections with bacteria and fungi occur in skin, lungs, bones, and joints, and sepsis is common |
| Foreign body granuloma | Many causative agents (see earlier in the chapter) |
| Granulomatous rosacea | Deep form of rosacea |
| Granulomatous perioral dermatitis | Deep form of perioral dermatitis |
| Crohn's disease | Inflammatory bowel disease that can rarely involve the skin |
| Churg–Strauss disease (allergic granulomatous angiitis) | Asthma, eosinophilia, and vasculitis in the skin as well as respiratory tract, kidney, GI tract, heart, and nerves |

*Laboratory Findings*

The histopathologic appearance of sarcoidosis is quite characteristic and consists of epithelioid cells surrounded by Langerhans' giant cells, CD4 lymphocytes, some CD8 lymphocytes, and mature macrophages. No acid-fast bacilli are found, and caseation necrosis is absent. The Kveim test, using sarcoidal lymph node tissue, is positive after several weeks. This is no longer used. Tuberculin-type, candida, and other skin tests are negative (anergic). The total blood serum protein is high and ranges from 7.5 to 10.0 g/dL, mainly because of an increase in the globulin fraction.

Angiotensin-converting enzyme deficiency may be noted.

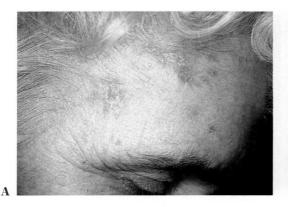
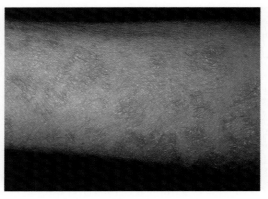

A                                                                                    B

FIGURE 16-1 ▪ **(A)** Sarcoid of the forehead. **(B)** Sarcoid on the forearm. (*Courtesy of Hoechst-Roussel Pharmaceuticals Inc.*)

Differential Diagnosis

- *Other granulomatous diseases:* These can be ruled out by biopsy, culture, and other appropriate studies.
- *Silica granulomas:* Histologically similar; a history of such injury can usually be obtained.

Treatment

For localized skin disease, intralesional corticosteroids (4 to 8 mg/cc triamcinolone) are the treatment of choice at 1- to 2-month intervals. Time appears to cure or cause remission of most cases of sarcoidosis, but corticosteroids and immunosuppressant drugs may be indicated for extensive cases, especially ones involving the lung, joints, or eye. Hydroxychloroquine and methotrexate may be beneficial. Anecdotal use of allopurinol has been reported. Doxycycline (100 mg b.i.d.) or minocycline (100 mg b.i.d.) has shown benefit in some studies. Other therapies showing some promise are pentoxifylline, isotretinoin, leflunomide, and laser.

## Granuloma Annulare

Granuloma annulare is a moderately common skin problem. The usually encountered ring-shaped, red-bordered lesion is often mistaken for ringworm by inexperienced examiners (Fig. 16-2), but there is no scaling. Several clinical variations exist. The two most common are the *localized form* and *generalized form*. There is also an annular form often seen on the glans of the penis and tongue, a rare linear form, a subcutaneous deep form, a papular variety, and a perforating form mimicking a perforating folliculitis. Some authors have described a subtle patch type of disease, which is very rare.

Women and girls with granuloma annulare predominate over men and boys in a ratio of 2.5 to 1. No ages are exempt, but the localized form is usually seen in patients in the first three decades of life and the generalized form in patients in the fourth through seventh decades. A granuloma annulare–like eruption has been reported in HIV-positive and chronic Epstein–Barr virus positive patients.

Presentation and Characteristics

*Primary Lesions*

In both the localized and generalized forms, the lesion is a red, asymptomatic papule with no scaling. The papule may be solitary. Most frequently, the lesion assumes a ring-shaped or arcuate configuration of papules that tends to enlarge centrifugally. Rarely are the rings over 5 cm in diameter. In the localized form of granuloma annulare, the lesions appear mainly over the joints on the hands, arms, feet, and legs. In the much less common generalized form, there may be hundreds of the red or tan papular circinate lesions on the extremities and on the trunk. This is the most common form in HIV-positive patients. Diabetes may be increased in this form.

*Secondary Lesions*

On healing, the red color turns to brown before the lesions disappear.

*Course*

Both forms of granuloma annulare can resolve spontaneously after one to several years, but the generalized form is more long lasting. It does not lead to scar formation.

*Causes*

The cause is unknown. An immune-complex vasculitis, cell-mediated immunity, and trauma have all been proposed as factors in the disease.

*Laboratory Findings*

The histopathologic appearance of granuloma annulare is quite characteristic. The middle and upper dermis have focal areas of altered collagenous connective tissue surrounded by an infiltrate of histiocytic cells and lymphocytes. In some cases, these cells infiltrate between the collagen bundles, giving a palisading effect. *Necrobiosis* has been used to describe these changes.

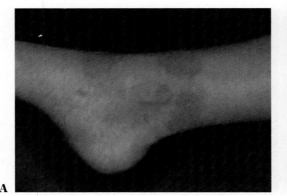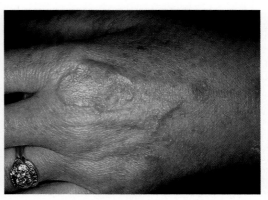

**A**    **B**

**FIGURE 16-2** ■ **(A)** Granuloma annulare on ankle area. **(B)** Granuloma annulare on the dorsum of the hand. (*Courtesy of Hoechst-Roussel Pharmaceuticals Inc.*)

## Differential Diagnosis

- *Tinea corporis*: Usually itches and has a scaly red border; the fungus can be demonstrated with a potassium hydroxide scraping or culture (see Chapter 25).
- *Lichen planus, annular form:* Characterized by violaceous flat-topped papules with Wickham's striae. Mucous membrane lesions are also often seen.
- *Secondary syphilis:* Can be clinically similar but has a positive serology (see Chapter 22).
- *Other granulomatous diseases:* Can usually be distinguished by biopsy.

There is a subcutaneous form of granuloma annulare that is difficult to distinguish histologically from a rheumatoid nodule or a soft tissue tumor.

## Treatment

### Localized Form

Some cases respond to the application of a corticosteroid cream for 8 hours over night with an occlusive dressing such as Saran wrap. Intralesional corticosteroids are effective for cases with only a few lesions. Light liquid nitrogen therapy is sometimes beneficial.

### Generalized Form

Numerous remedies have been tried with only anecdotal benefit. Dapsone and hydroxychloroquine have also been used.

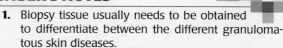

**SAUER'S NOTES**

1. Biopsy tissue usually needs to be obtained to differentiate between the different granulomatous skin diseases.
2. When trying to distinguish between granulomatous skin diseases, the biopsy must be deep enough to provide an adequate interpretation. A punch or ellipse biopsy rather than a shave biopsy needs to be done.
3. Culture for bacteria, acid-fast bacteria, and deep fungi should be done by submitting a portion of the harvested material in sterile saline for culture. If a viral etiology is considered, then a portion of tissue should be collected in viral culture media. This is important since organisms may be sparse in tissue even with appropriate staining and a superficial culture from a swab or skin scraping may be falsely negative.

## Suggested Readings

Bagwell C, Rosen T. Cutaneous sarcoid therapy updated. *J Am Acad Dermatol.* 2007;56:69–83.

English JC, Patel PJ, Greer KE. Sarcoidosis. *J Am Acad Dermatol.* 2001;44:725–743.

Hirsh BC, Johnson WC. Concepts of granulomatous inflammation. *Int J Dermatol.* 1984;23:90–100.

Iannuzzi, MC. Sarcoidosis. *N Engl J Med.* 2007;357:2153–2165.

Newman LS, Rose CS, Maier LA. Sarcoidosis. *N Engl J Med.* 1997;336:1224–1234.

Smith MD, Downie JB, DiCostanzo D. Granuloma annulare. *Int J Dermatol.* 1997;36:326–333.

Young RJ, Gilson RT, Yanase D. Cutaneous sarcoidosis. *Int J Dermatol.* 2001;40:249–253.

# CHAPTER 17

# Dermatologic Parasitology

*John C. Hall, MD*

Dermatologic parasitology is an extensive subject and includes the dermatoses caused by three main groups of organisms: protozoa, helminthes, and arthropods.

- The *protozoal dermatoses* are exemplified by the various forms of trypanosomiases and leishmaniases (see Chapter 45).
- *Helminthic dermatoses* include those due to roundworms (ground itch, creeping eruption, filariasis, and other rare tropical diseases) and those due to flatworms (schistosomiasis, swimmer's itch, and others) (see Chapter 45).
- *Arthropod dermatoses* are divided into those caused by two classes of organisms: the arachnids (spiders, scorpions, ticks, and mites) and the insects (lice, bugs, flies, moths, beetles, bees, and fleas). Lyme disease is caused by a spirochete that is transmitted by a tick and is discussed in Chapter 22. Rickettsial diseases are also tick borne (see Chapter 21).

In this chapter scabies, pediculosis, and bedbugs are discussed. Scabies are caused by mites, pediculosis is caused by lice, and bedbugs are caused by an insect that is usually found in mattresses and furniture. Fleabites, chigger bites, creeping eruption, swimmer's itch, and tropical dermatoses are discussed in Chapter 45.

## Scabies

Scabies (Figs. 17-1 and 17-2) is usually more prevalent in a populace ravaged by war, famine, or disease when personal hygiene becomes relatively unimportant. However, there are unexplained cyclic epidemics of this parasitic infestation. In the 1970s and 1980s, such a cycle plagued Americans. In normal times, scabies is seen in schoolchildren, elderly patients in nursing care centers, in poorer populations under crowded conditions, and in sexually active patients with multiple sex partners.

Animal scabies can occur in cats, dogs, foxes, cows, pigs, and other mammals. The disease is sarcoptic mange and is caused by *Sarcoptes scabiei* var *canis*. Direct contact with an infected animal causes a severe, generalized, polymorphous, pruritic eruption with absence of burrows and a negative wet mount for ova, parasites, or feces. This occurs 24 to 96 hours after exposure, is not associated with human-to-human transmission, and lasts only 14 to 21 days without further exposure. Treatment is accomplished by topical agents such as permethrin, malathion, or lindane for the pet and antipruritic therapy and topical or systemic corticosteroids for the temporary human host.

### Presentation and Characteristics

#### Primary Lesions

A burrow caused by the female of the mite *S. scabiei* (see Fig. 17-2) measures approximately 2 mm in length and can be hidden by the secondary eruption. Small vesicles may overlie the burrows. *Scabies incognito* is a form of the disease in which the burrows are not easily identified. It is seen most commonly in patients who are fastidiously clean and

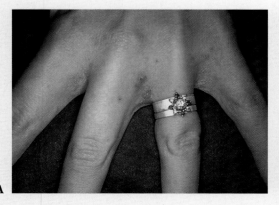 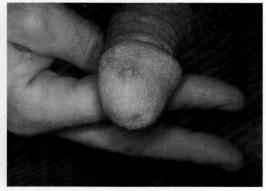

**FIGURE 17-1** ■ **(A)** Scabies on the hand. **(B)** Scabies on the penis. *(Courtesy of Hoechst-Roussel Pharmaceuticals.)*

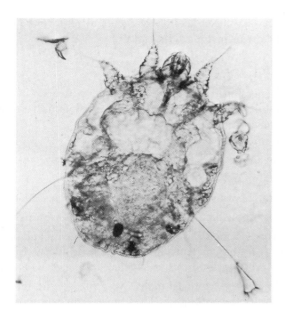

**FIGURE 17-2** ■ The female of the mite *Sarcoptes scabiei*. The small, oval, black body near the anal opening is a fecal pellet. Proximal to it is a vague, much larger, oval, pale-edged mass (an egg). *(Courtesy of Dr. H. Parlette.)*

bathe at least once a day. *Norwegian*, or *keratotic*, *scabies* occurs in immunosuppressed patients. Hundreds of organisms create a psoriasiform dermatitis.

### Secondary Lesions

Excoriations of the burrows may be the only visible pathologic process. These may be difficult to see, and magnification devices may be helpful. In severe, chronic cases, bacterial infection may be extensive and may take the form of impetigo, cellulitis, or furunculosis.

Residual nodular lesions may persist as an allergic reaction for many weeks or months after the organism is eliminated. They are often recalcitrant to therapy and topical, intralesional, and even systemic corticosteroids may be necessary. Excision may even be necessary. Nodular scabies is not contagious.

### Distribution

Most commonly, the excoriations are seen on the lower abdomen and the back, with extension to the pubic, genital, and axillary areas, the legs (ankles especially), the arms (flexor wrists especially), and the webs of the fingers.

---

**SAUER'S NOTES**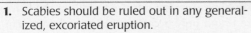

1. Scabies should be ruled out in any generalized, excoriated eruption.
2. The patient should always be asked if other members of the household itch.

---

### Subjective Complaints

Itching is intense, particularly at night when the patient is warm and in bed and the mite is more active. However, many skin diseases itch worse at night, presumably due to a lower itch threshold when relaxation occurs.

### Course

The mite can persist for months and years (7-year itch) in untreated persons.

### Contagiousness

Other members of the household or intimate contacts may or may not have the disease, depending on exposure and severity of the infestation.

### Laboratory Findings

The female scabies mite, ova, and fecal pellets may be seen in skin scrapings that are done with a no. 15 Bard-Parker blade. The scrapings are done at the site of burrows in the skin or in areas where itching is most severe. The scrapings are then examined under the low-power magnification of the microscope (see Fig. 17-2). Potassium hydroxide (KOH) (20% solution) can be used to clear the tissue. Another method of collection is to scrape the burrow through immersion oil and then transfer the scrapings to the microscopic slides. Skill is necessary to uncover the mite by curetting or scraping.

### Differential Diagnosis

■ *Pyoderma:* Rule out concurrent parasitic infestation; positive history of diabetes mellitus; only mild itching (see Chapter 21).
■ *Pediculosis pubis:* Lice and eggs on and around hairs; distribution different (see following section).
■ *Winter itch:* No burrows; seasonal incidence; elderly patient, usually; worse on legs and back (see Chapter 11).
■ *Dermatitis herpetiformis:* Vesicles; urticaria; excoriated papules; eosinophilia; no burrows; characteristic histopathologic appearance; direct immunofluorescence pattern (see Chapter 18).
■ *Neurotic excoriations:* Nervous person; patient admits picking at lesions; lesions present in areas where patient can easily reach; no burrows; characteristic stellate hypopigmented scars indicate a prolonged illness.
■ *Parasitophobia* (see Chapter 20): Usually the patient brings to the office pieces of skin and debris often carefully stored in a container (match box sign); showing the patient the debris under a microscope helps to convince him or her of the absence of parasites. This is a difficult problem to manage. Pimozide (Orap) or olanzapine (Zyprexa) can be used by a physician experienced in its use. Referral to a psychiatrist is ideal but seldom will the patient consent to this.

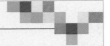
## Treatment

### Adults and Older Children

1. Inspect or question other members of the family or intimate contacts to rule out infestation in them. Any household members or intimate contacts must be treated at the same time as the patient to prevent "ping-pong" infestation. This is true even if itching is not present in contacts.
2. Instruct patient to bathe thoroughly and then apply a scabicide.
3. Permethrin (Elimite, Acticin) 5% cream 60.0 *or* gamma benzene hexachloride (Lindane, Kwell) 120.0 (not preferred due to toxicity)

   *Sig:* Apply to the entire body from the neck down. Repeat therapy in 1 week.
4. After 12 to 24 hours, the patient should bathe carefully and change to clean clothes and bedding.
5. Washing, dry cleaning, or ironing of clothes and bedding are sufficient to destroy the mite. Sterilization is unnecessary.
6. Itching may persist for a few days, even for 2 to 3 weeks or longer, in spite of the destruction of the mite. The itching may be worse for the first several days after treatment. For this apply b.i.d.:
   a. Crotamiton (Eurax) cream q.s. 60.0

      *Comment:* This cream has scabicidal power and antipruritic action combined.
   b. A topical corticosteroid ointment can be used or, if the pruritus persists, a 10- to 14-day course of systemic corticosteroids may have to be given.
7. If itching persists after 4 weeks, reexamine the patient carefully and repeat the KOH preparation to be sure reinfestation or inadequate treatment has not occurred. Ask if all people who are potential contacts have been treated. It takes a lot of reassurance to convince these itchy patients that they are not still infested with scabies. Repeated unnecessary topical therapy may only increase the itching because these topical agents can act as irritants. Overuse of gamma benzene hexachloride can cause seizures.
8. Oral ivermectin in a single dose is a therapy advocated by some authors. It is helpful in crusted scabies, which also may need keratolytic agents to remove the crusts before using topical therapy.

### Newborns and Infants

1. General instructions are as for older patients.
2. Lindane lotion used in newborns and infants has caused convulsions.
3. Elimite, Acticin, or Eurax cream 60.0

   *Sig:* Apply b.i.d. locally to affected areas only, *or*
4. Sulfur, ppt. 5%

   Water-washable cream base or Aquaphor q.s. 60.0

   *Sig:* Apply b.i.d. to affected areas for 3 consecutive days.

   This is a good choice of therapy in pregnant and breast-feeding patients due to its extreme safety. However, it is malodorous and stains clothing.
5. In patients younger than 1 year of age, the bite may occur above the neck. There have been rare reports of disease above the neck in adults. The immunocompromised patient is a candidate for this manifestation.

## Pediculosis

Lice infestation affects persons of all ages, but usually those in the lower income strata and military personnel in the field are affected most often because of lack of cleanliness and infrequent changes of clothing. It is also seen as a sexually transmitted disease. Three clinical entities are produced:

- infestation of the hair by the head louse *Pediculus humanus capitis,*
- infestation of the body by *Pediculus humanus corporis,* and
- infestation of the pubic area by the pubic louse *Pthirus pubis* (Fig. 17-3).

*P. pubis* infestation can also involve the hairy areas over the abdomen, chest, and eyelids. Because lice bite the skin and live on blood, it is impossible for them to live without human contact. The readily visible oval eggs or nits are attached to hairs or to clothing fibers by the female louse. After the eggs hatch, the newly born lice mature within 30 days. The female louse can live for another 30 days and deposit a few eggs daily.

### Presentation and Characteristics

#### Primary Lesions

The site of the bite is seldom seen because of the secondary changes produced by the resulting intense itching. In the scalp and pubic forms, the nits are found on the hairs, but the lice are found only occasionally. In the body form, the nits and lice can be found after careful searching in the seams of the clothing.

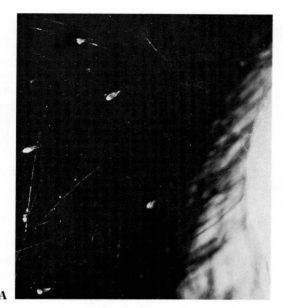
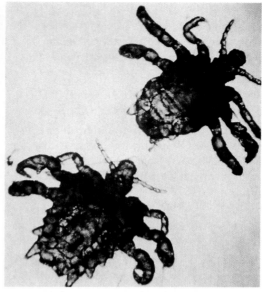

A                B

**FIGURE 17-3** Pediculosis. **(A)** Nits on the scalp hair behind the ear. *(Courtesy of Dr. L. Hyde.)* **(B)** Pubic louse, or *Phthirus pubis,* as seen with the 7.5× lens of a microscope. *(Courtesy of Dr. J. Boley.)*

### Secondary Lesions

In the scalp form, the skin is red and excoriated, with such severe secondary bacterial infection, in some cases, that the hairs become matted together in a crusty, foul-smelling "cap." Regional lymphadenopathy is common. A morbilliform rash on the body or a generalized papular "id" reaction can be seen in longstanding cases.

In the body form, linear excoriations and secondary infection mask the primary bites. These bites are seen mainly on the shoulders, the belt line, and the buttocks.

In the pubic form, secondary excoriations are again dominant and produce some matting of the hairs. This louse can also infest body, axillary, and eyelash hairs. An unusual eruption on the abdomen, the thighs, and the arms, called *maculae cerulea* because of the bluish-gray, pea-sized macules, can occur in chronic cases of pubic pediculosis.

### Differential Diagnosis

#### Pediculosis Capitis

- *Bacterial infection of the scalp:* Responds rapidly to correct antibacterial therapy (see Chapter 21), culture for bacteria is positive.
- *Seborrheic dermatitis or dandruff:* The scales of dandruff are readily detached from the hair, but oval nits are not so easily removed (see Chapter 13).

---

**SAUER'S NOTE**

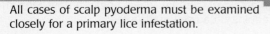

All cases of scalp pyoderma must be examined closely for a primary lice infestation.

---

Nits are easily seen when affected hairs are examined under low power on the microscope.

- *Hair casts (pseudonits):* Resemble nits but usually can be pulled off more easily; no eggs are seen on microscopic examination.

#### Pediculosis Corporis

- *Scabies:* May be small burrows; distribution of lesions different; no lice in clothes or nits on hairs (see beginning of this chapter).
- *Senile or winter itch:* History helpful; dry skin, aggravated by bathing; will not find lice in clothes or nits on hairs (see Chapter 11).

#### Pediculosis Pubis

- *Scabies:* No nits; burrows in pubic area and elsewhere (see beginning of this chapter).
- *Pyoderma:* Secondary to contact dermatitis from condoms, contraceptive jellies, new underwear, douches—history is important; acute onset, no nits (see Chapter 21).
- *Seborrheic dermatitis:* When in eyebrows and eyelashes, no nits are found. The scaling on the hair is less adherent than the nits in pediculosis (see Chapter 13).

### Treatment

#### Pediculosis Capitis

1. Shampoos or rinses
   a. Permethrin (Nix) cream rinse 60.0

   *Sig:* Use as a rinse for 10 minutes after shampooing. Only one application is recommended, but I usually recommend repeating in 3 days.

b. Lindane (Kwell) shampoo 60.0

*Sig:* Shampoo and comb hair thoroughly. Leave on the hair for 4 minutes. Repeat medicated shampoo in 3 days. Regular shampoo can be restarted in 24 hours.

c. Pyrethrins (RID) 60.0

*Sig:* Apply to scalp for 10 minutes and rinse off. Apply again in 7 days (nonprescription).

d. Step Two (formic acid) solution (obtainable without a prescription) can be used to help remove nits from the hair. Salicylic acid shampoo (T-Sal) may also help remove nits and may be left on overnight at least once.

e. Permethrin 5% (Elimite) cream 60.0

*Sig:* Leave on overnight under shower cap. May be the most effective topical treatment of all for recalcitrant cases.

f. A single oral dose of ivermectin (Stromectol), 200 μg/kg, repeated in 10 days may be the most effective oral agent in persistent cases. Some authors are concerned about the safety of this therapy.

g. Topical malathion (Ovide) is available in a scalp preparation and is quite safe.

2. For secondary scalp infection
   a. Trim hair as much as is possible and agreeable with the patient.
   b. Shampoo hair daily with a salicylic acid shampoo (T-Sal).
   c. Bactroban or Polysporin ointment 15.0

   *Sig:* Apply to scalp b.i.d.

3. Change and clean bedding and headwear after 24 hours of treatment. Storage of headwear for 30 days destroys the lice and nits.

4. Mayonnaise (not reduced fat) left overnight for 3 nights is effective and very safe.

### Pediculosis Corporis

1. Permethrin 5% (Elimite) cream overnight.
2. Have the clothing laundered or dry-cleaned. If this is impossible, dusting with 10% lindane powder kills the parasites. Care should be taken to prevent reinfestation. Storage of clothing in a plastic bag for 30 days kills both nits and lice.
3. Sulfur 5% to 10% in petrolatum overnight for 3 nights is effective and very safe. It is malodorous and stains bed clothes.

### Pediculosis Pubis

Treatment is the same as for the scalp form.

When the disease occurs on the eyelids, sulfacetamide ophthalmic ointment b.i.d. for 5 days is very safe and effective. Petrolatum can also be used in the same fashion.

# Bedbugs

Bedbugs (*Cimex lectularius*) usually present as nighttime papular urticaria. Not every patient has a reaction to the bite. Bedbugs are nocturnal and are attracted to the human host by carbon dioxide, which not all people emit in the same amount, and warmth. Personal cleanliness and good housekeeping are no protection. Bedbugs are visible with the naked eye as tiny reddish-brown insects about the size of a nonengorged tick. The mattress, or more rarely other furniture, is the usual location of the insects. They can also live in cracks in walls.

## Presentation and Characteristics

### Primary Lesions

Papular urticaria often seen in a row on exposed skin (**Fig. 17-4**). It often lasts 4 to 6 weeks after the infestation is eliminated.

### Secondary Lesions

Honey-colored oozing and crusting may be seen, indicating secondary infection. If continuously scratched, they can last indefinitely and mimic prurigo nodularis. Severe pruritus can result in bruising and bleeding.

## Differential Diagnosis

- *Urticaria:* More evanescent (1 to 2 days or less), scattered, and not in rows. Dermatographism may be present.
- *Scabies:* Has burrows and a positive KOH examination. Finger webs, flexor wrists, and genitalia often affected.

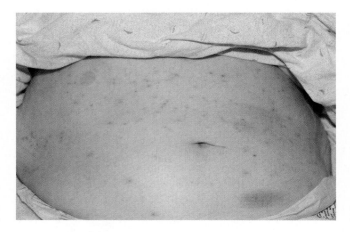

**FIGURE 17-4** ■ Grouped excoriated papules over the abdomen of an elderly female, which began 4 days after she began sleeping on a used mattress.

## Treatment

1. Symptomatic treatment consists of oral antihistamines, topical antipruritics, topical corticosteroids and, if severe, systemic corticosteroids.
2. The affected mattress, couch, stuffed chair, or other affected furniture is best discarded or fumigation carried out with specific instructions that bedbugs are suspected.

## Suggested Readings

Buntin DM, Rosen T, Lesher JL, et al. Sexually transmitted diseases: viruses and ectoparasites. *J Am Acad Dermatol.* 1991;25:527–534.

Centers for Disease Control and Prevention. Scabies in health-care facilities: Iowa. *Arch Dermatol.* 1988;124:837.

Goddard J. *Physician's Guide to Arthropods of Medical Importance.* 2nd ed. Boca Roton, Florida: CRC press LLC; 1996.

Ko CJ, Elston DM. Pediculosis. *J Am Acad Dermatol.* 2004;50:1–12.

Zhu YI, Stiller MJ. Arthropods and skin diseases. *Int J Dermatol.* 2002;41: 533–549.

# CHAPTER 18

# Bullous Dermatoses

*John C. Hall, MD*

To medical students and practitioners alike, the bullous skin diseases appear most dramatic. One of these diseases, pemphigus, is undoubtedly greatly responsible for the aura that surrounds the exhibition and discussion of an unfortunate patient with a bullous disease. Happy would be the instructor who could behold such student interest when a case of acne or hand dermatitis is being presented.

In almost all cases of bullous diseases, it is necessary to examine a fresh tissue biopsy specimen for deposits of immune reactants, immunoglobulins, and complement components at or near the basement membrane zone. Routine histologic examination of a formalin-fixed biopsy specimen is, of course, also usually indicated.

Four bullous diseases are discussed in this chapter: pemphigus vulgaris, dermatitis herpetiformis, bullous pemphigoid, and erythema multiforme bullosum. However, other bullous skin diseases do occur, and in this introduction they are differentiated from these four.

- *Bullous impetigo:* Bullous impetigo is differentiated from the other bullous diseases by its occurrence in infants and children, rapid development of the individual bullae, presence of impetigo lesions in siblings, bacterial culture positive for *Staphylococcus aureus,* and rapid response to antibiotic therapy (see Chapter 21). It can be a recurrent problem in HIV-positive patients in the groin area.
- *Contact dermatitis* due to poison ivy or similar plants: Bullae and vesicles are seen in a linear configuration. A history of pulling weeds, cleaning out fencerows, or burning brush is usually obtained, and a past history of poison ivy or related dermatitis is common. It is important to remember that this is a form of delayed hypersensitivity and the time between the exposure causing the eruption and the onset of symptoms can be anywhere from 1 to 2 days to 1 to 2 weeks. This delayed nature of the disease commonly leads to an erroneous diagnosis or a correct diagnosis with inability to establish when the exposure occurred and to therefore eliminate all traces of the plant oil from objects where it may be contacted again and result in another outbreak of the disease. The duration of disease is 10 to 21 days if untreated and is quite uncomfortable (see Chapter 8).

- *Drug eruption:* Elicit drug history (particularly of sulfonamides, nonsteroidal anti-inflammatory drugs [NSAIDs], and antiseizure medications). Fixed drug eruptions are not uncommonly bullous. Fixed drug eruptions are localized, very inflammatory, may blister, leave marked hyperpigmentation, and occur at the same site on drug rechallenge. The eruption usually clears upon discontinuing drugs but this can be delayed for 2 or more weeks. If the patient is not better within a few days of stopping the drug this does not mean that the drug is not the cause of the eruption. Bullae appear rapidly (see Chapter 8).

- *Epidermolysis bullosa* (see Chapter 40): This rare, chronic, hereditary skin disease is manifested by the formation of bullae, usually on the hands and the feet, following trauma. The full clinical and immunologic spectra of these diseases are protean in form of inheritance, severity of disease, and tendency to improve with age.
  - The simple form (epidermolysis bullosa simplex) of dominant inheritance can begin in infancy or adulthood with the formation of tense, slightly itchy bullae at sites of pressure that heal quickly without scarring. Forced marches or jogging can initiate this disease in patients who have the heredity factor. Such cases are usually treated erroneously as athlete's foot. The disease is worse in the summer or in climates with high humidity and may be present only at this time. This disease often improves with age.
  - The dystrophic form of recessive inheritance begins in infancy, and as time elapses, the bullae become hemorrhagic, heal slowly, and leave scars that can amputate digits. Death can result from secondary infection and metastatic squamous cell carcinomas. Mucous membrane lesions are more common in the dystrophic form than in the simple form. Treatment is supportive. Gene therapy may be a future modality but has been disappointing so far. Surgical dressings and skin substitutes (Apligraf) are an

important part of care. Various surgical dressings may be helpful. Mepitel is a dressing I have found especially useful. The blisters should be immediately drained to relieve pain and keep them from enlarging. Secondary infection should be watched for carefully and treated immediately.

■ A lethal, nonscarring form is also of recessive inheritance but is usually fatal within a few months (see Chapter 40).

■ *Epidermolysis bullosa acquisita:* An autoimmune response to collagen where skin lesions can appear similar to bullous pemphigoid, cicatricial pemphigoid, and recessive epidermolysis bullosa. Bulla, scarring, and esophageal disease all occur in this acquired illness. Direct immunofluorescence (DIF) is positive in a linear pattern positive for IgA in the epidermal basement membrane. Dapsone and systemic corticosteroids may be helpful. Trauma can induce blisters that result in scarring.

■ *Familial benign chronic pemphigus* (Hailey–Hailey disease): This is a rare, hereditary bullous eruption that is most common on the neck, groin, and in the axillae. It can be distinguished from pemphigus by its chronicity and benign nature and by its histologic picture. Some consider this disease to be a bullous variety of keratosis follicularis (Darier's disease). It is very painful and can be debilitating. It is caused by a mutation of the *ATP2C1* gene.

■ *Herpes gestationis* (see Chapter 48): This is a vesicular and bullous disease that occurs in relation to pregnancy. It usually develops during the second or the third trimester and commonly disappears after giving birth, only to return with subsequent pregnancies. The histologic features are believed significantly distinctive so this disease can be separated from dermatitis herpetiformis. Immunologic findings of C3 bound to the basement membrane of the epidermis and occasional immunoglobulin (IgG) deposition may be significant. Therapy with systemic corticosteroids is usually indicated.

■ *Porphyria:* The congenital erythropoietic type and the chronic hepatic type (porphyria cutanea tarda) commonly have bullae on the sun-exposed areas of the body (see the Dictionary–Index under *Porphyria*).

■ *Cicatricial pemphigoid:* This disabling but nonfatal bullous eruption of the mucous membranes most commonly involves the eyes. The skin and mucous membranes may be involved, usually in a localized pattern. As the result of scarring, which is characteristic of this disease and separates it from true pemphigus, eyesight is eventually lost. Over 50% of the cases have skin lesions. Histologically, the bullae are subepidermal and do not show acantholysis. There is quite a bit of immunologic similarity between this disease and bullous pemphigoid.

■ *Linear IgA bullous disease:* Most of the children and adults with this disease differ from classic dermatitis herpetiformis in the morphology and distribution of their lesions, have a poorer response to dapsone, and have linear IgA anti–basement membrane zone antibodies. Nontropical sprue is not a part of this illness.

■ *Incontinentia pigmenti:* The first stage of this rare disease of infants manifests itself with bullous lesions, primarily on the hands and feet (see Chapter 41). This stage may appear in utero and may not be seen clinically.

■ *Toxic epidermal necrolysis* (TEN): Most authors consider Stevens–Johnson syndrome a variant of TEN with less skin and more mucous membrane involvement but with the same clinical picture, histology, prognosis, and treatment. This rare disease is characterized by large bullae and a quite generalized Nikolsky's sign, in which large sheets of epidermis become detached from the underlying skin with gentle pressure from a finger. The mucous membranes are frequently involved. The patient is toxic. Adults are most commonly affected. Drugs are usually the causative factor, especially in adults. Most commonly implicated are sulfonamides, anticonvulsants, and NSAIDs. There may be a genetic predisposition to this bullous drug reaction. Therapy is supportive, and an appreciable number of cases are fatal. Intravenous immunoglobulins (IVIG) may be lifesaving. Cyclosporine is a preferred mode of therapy by some authors. High-dose systemic corticosteroids are controversial, with opinions ranging from contraindicated to lifesaving if given in very high doses very early in the course of the disease. Some authors would argue that only supportive measures have been shown to be of any benefit. Wound care is essential. Debridement should be avoided. Silver nitrate irrigation and soft gauze dressings (SofSorb gauze, which may be fitted on as a garment) are used in wound care. This is usually done in an intensive care unit because electrolyte and fluid balance is crucial. A central venous line helps greatly in managing these patients. The most crucial factor in survival is stopping any potential offending drug as quickly as possible. Acute graft-versus-host disease can be an identical disease process and should be treated in a similar manner. Mortality for this disease can be significant. A helpful prognostic scoring system is as follows:

Age >40
Underlying malignancy
Heart rate >120
>10% epidermal detachment
BUN >10 mmol/L
Serum glucose >14 mmol/L
Bicarbonate <20 mmol/L

| SCORTEN | Mortality |
|---------|-----------|
| 0–1 | 3.2% |
| 2 | 12.1% |
| 3 | 35.3% |
| 4 | 58.3% |
| 5 | >90% |

- *Staphylococcal scalded skin syndrome:* Clinically, this disorder is similar to TEN but has been separated from this disease because of the finding that phage group 2 *S. aureus* is the usual cause. In newborns, this formerly was known as Ritter von Ritterschein's disease. It also occurs in children and rarely in adults. The prognosis is very favorable. If suspected, antistaphylococcus drugs should be started intravenously immediately. The break in the skin is higher in the epidermis than in drug-induced TEN, and this can be rapidly ascertained with a skin biopsy.
- *Impetigo herpetiformis:* One of the rarest of skin diseases, this disease is characterized by groups of pustules mainly seen in the axillae and the groin, high fever, prostration, severe malaise, and, generally, a fatal outcome. It occurs most commonly in pregnant or postpartum women. It can be distinguished from pemphigus vegetans or dermatitis herpetiformis by the fact that these diseases do not produce such general, acute, toxic manifestations. Laboratory abnormalities include elevated white blood count, elevated sedimentation rate, and low calcium, phosphate, albumin, and vitamin D levels. Bacterial cultures of skin and blood are negative; high-dose (60 to 100 mg q.d.) prednisone and fluid and electrolyte replacement can be life saving (see Chapter 48).

In spite of high medical student and general practitioner interest in the bullous skin conditions, the diagnosis and the management of the three main bullous skin diseases, bullous pemphigoid, pemphigus vulgaris, and dermatitis herpetiformis, should be in the realm of the dermatologist. In this chapter, the salient features of these diseases are presented, with therapy briefly outlined.

# Bullous Pemphigoid

Bullous pemphigoid is a chronic bullous eruption most commonly occurring in elderly adults. Bullous pemphigoid can uncommonly occur in children and infants.

## Presentation and Characteristics

### Primary Lesions

Large tense blisters tend to mushroom out of normal skin and can grow to many centimeters before breaking. The disease less commonly can begin with large pruritic erythematous plaques.

### Secondary Lesions

When the blisters eventually break down they leave large superficial erosions that heal without scars. Oral lesions are extremely rare. The urticarial plaques may show excoriations and also heal without scarring.

### Course

When untreated, the disease lasts years before resolution.

### Causes

Bullous pemphigoid is an idiopathic autoimmune disease that shows antibody deposition at the basement membrane zone of IgG and C3, which recruits neutrophils and eosinophils with destruction of the basement membrane and results in a large subepidermal blister. Some drugs such as furosemide, penicillin, sulfasalazine, and ibuprofen can cause a blistering skin disease that mimics bullous pemphigoid but dissipates after the drug is discontinued.

### Laboratory Findings

DIF of IgG and C3 seen at the dermoepidermal junction and indirect immunofluorescence (IF) and circulation IgG may be present. Subepidermal blisters with invasion of neutrophils and eosinophils are seen. The urticarial plaques are more nonspecific histologically but still have positive DIF. Some studies have suggested an increased incidence of underlying systemic malignancy.

## Differential Diagnosis

- *Pemphigus:* See Table 18-1.
- *Dermatitis herpetiformis:* More pruritic; marked response to dapsone; rarely tense blisters; resolves with hyperpigmentation; characteristic DIF
- *Erythema multiforme:* Younger patients with "iris" or "bull's eye" configuration; disease of the palms and soles as well as mucous membrane disease; association with drugs or herpes simplex (in the milder form of the disease) often seen. DIF and IF are negative.

## Treatment

This can usually be done as an outpatient.

1. High-dose (50 to 100 mg) prednisone is required for early remission. Other immunosuppressive therapy is begun at the same time and is used on a more chronic basis as the patient is tapered off systemic corticosteroids.
2. Occasionally tetracycline (500 mg q.i.d.) and niacinamide (500 mg q.i.d.) are helpful alone or as a steroid-sparing regimen.
3. Dapsone (although with a much slower response than in dermatitis herpetiformis) 100 mg/d, can occasionally be helpful.

**TABLE 18-1 ■ Differences between Bullous Pemphigoid and Pemphigus Vulgaris**

|  | Bullous Pemphigoid | Pemphigus Vulgaris |
|---|---|---|
| Common age of onset | >70 yr; "old man's pemphigus" | 40–60 yr |
| Prognosis | Resolves over years | Usually fatal without therapy; lifelong |
| Clinical characteristics | Large blisters mushroom out of normal skin; can appear urticarial | Fragile blisters break to form confluent erosions; positive Nikolsky's sign |
| Location of blisters | Widespread on skin | Oral lesions common and may be localized to this location |
| Inheritance | None | Mediterranean; Jewish |
| Histopathology | Subepidermal blister; neutrophils; eosinophils | Intraepidermal blister |
| Direct immunofluorescence | Linear IgG, C3 at dermoepidermal junction in bullous and perilesional skin; binding site is proteins of basement membrane zone | IgG around cell surface of keratinocytes; binding site is desmoglein 3 |
| Indirect immunofluorescence | Variable | Present and used to follow disease |

4. Azathioprine (50 mg/d or b.i.d.) is a commonly used steroid-sparing agent.
5. Methotrexate (15 mg PO or IM) has been used successfully as a steroid-sparing agent.
6. IVIG has also had success as a single agent or steroid-sparing drug. It is very expensive and must be given intravenously for several days.

## Pemphigus Vulgaris

Pemphigus vulgaris is rare. These patients are miserable, odoriferous, and debilitated (Fig. 18-1). Before the advent of corticosteroid therapy, the disease was fatal.

### Presentation and Characteristics

#### Primary Lesions

The early lesions of pemphigus are small vesicles or bullae that appear on apparently normal skin. Redness of the base of the bullae is unusual. Without treatment, the bullae enlarge and spread and new ones balloon up on different areas of the skin or the mucous membranes. Rarely, mucous membrane lesions may be the main or only manifestation of the disease. Rupturing of the bullae leaves large eroded areas. Nikolsky's sign is positive; that is, a top layer of the skin adjacent to a bulla readily separates from the underlying skin after firm but gentle pressure.

#### Secondary Lesions

Bacterial infection with crusting is marked and accounts, in part, for the characteristic mousy odor. Lesions that heal spontaneously or under therapy do not leave scars.

#### Course

When untreated, pemphigus vulgaris can be rapidly fatal or assume a slow lingering course, with debility, painful mouth and body erosions, systemic bacterial infection, and toxemia.

Spontaneous temporary remissions do occur without therapy. The following clinical variations of pemphigus also exist:

■ *Pemphigus vegetans:* It is characterized by the development of large granulomatous masses in the intertriginous areas of the axillae and the groin. Secondary bacterial infection, although often present in all cases of pemphigus, is most marked in this form. Pemphigus vegetans is to be differentiated from a granulomatous ioderma or bromoderma (see Chapter 9) and from impetigo herpetiformis (see beginning of this chapter). This type of pemphigus can often be treated more conservatively such as with potent topical corticosteroids.

■ *Pemphigus foliaceus* (fogo selvagem): It appears as a scaly, moist, generalized exfoliative dermatitis. The characteristic mousy odor of pemphigus is dominant in this variant, which is also remarkable for its chronicity. The response to corticosteroid therapy is less favorable in the foliaceus form than in the other types (see also Chapter 45 for a Brazilian form). Complementary DNA cloning has shown the autoimmune target to be desmoglein 1. There is some evidence that this may be a disease borne by an insect vector in tropical areas near rivers.

■ *Pemphigus erythematosus:* It clinically resembles a mixture of pemphigus vulgaris, seborrheic dermatitis, and lupus erythematosus. The distribution of the red, greasy, crusted, and eroded lesions is on the butterfly area of the face, the sternal area, the scalp, and occasionally in the mouth. The course is more chronic than for pemphigus vulgaris, and remissions are common.

■ *Pemphigus herpetiformis:* It appears as grouped vesicles, bullae, or erythematous papules that are very pruritic. DIF of IgG in upper or entire epidermal cell surfaces and circulating IgG autoantibodies are present.

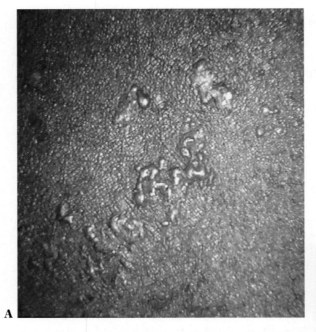

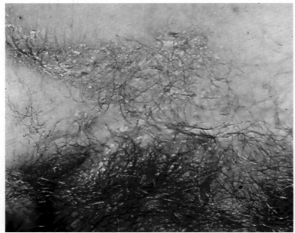

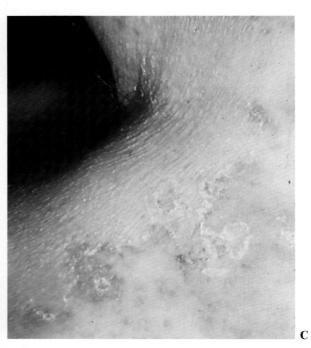

**FIGURE 18-1** ■ Hailey–Hailey on the back (**A**), suprapubic (**B**), and shoulder (**C**).

- *Paraneoplastic pemphigus:* It is an often fatal, severe, rare, polymorphous eruption with erosions, bullae, or targetoid lesions and severe mucous membrane disease. DIF shows IgG on all epidermal surfaces and often linear confluent deposits at the dermoepidermal junction; complement may also be on epidermal surfaces. Circulating IgG autoantibodies are present, and 75% of cases have circulating IgG to rat bladder epithelium. Non-Hodgkin's lymphoma is the most common underlying malignancy.

- *IgA pemphigus:* It shows flaccid, pruritc vesicles or pustules in an annular pattern with central crusting. It can show neutrophils with IgA DIF, either subcorneal or intraepidermal with less acantholysis. It is more common in females and usually less severe than pemphigus vulgaris with less morbidity and without mucous membrane disease. It responds to dapsone, or if there is sulfa allergy then methotrexate or retinoids may be helpful. Corticosteroids are usually not helpful, and there may be monoclonal antibodies present.

Some dermatologists believe that pemphigus foliaceus and pemphigus erythematosus may be distinct diseases from pemphigus vulgaris and pemphigus vegetans.

### Causes

The cause of pemphigus vulgaris is unknown, but autoimmunity is a factor. Some cases are associated with underlying malignancy (paraneoplastic pemphigus). Paraneoplastic pemphigus has unique immunofluorescent findings and is usually rapidly fatal. Human herpesvirus 8 has been isolated from the skin lesions of some patients. There is some suggestion that an increased lifetime exposure to penicillin may be associated with an increased incidence.

### Laboratory Findings

The histopathology of early cases is characteristic and serves to differentiate most cases of pemphigus vulgaris from dermatitis herpetiformis and the other bullous diseases. Acantholysis, or separation of intercellular contact between the keratinocytes, is characteristic. The bulla is intraepidermal. Cytologic smears (Tzanck test) for diagnosis of pemphigus vulgaris reveal numerous rounded acantholytic epidermal cells with large nuclei in a condensed cytoplasm. Antiepithelial autoantibodies against the intercellular substance are found by DIF and IF tests. Fresh tissue biopsy specimens taken from noninvolved skin best show immunoglobulins. IF tests are performed on serum. Complementary DNA cloning shows the autoimmune target to be desmoglein 3.

### Differential Diagnosis

See introduction to this chapter as well as the sections on dermatitis herpetiformis and erythema multiforme bullosum.

### Treatment

1. If possible, a dermatologist and internist should be called in to share the responsibility of the care.
2. Hospitalization is necessary for the patient with large areas of bullae and erosions. Mild cases of pemphigus can be managed in the office.
3. Prednisone, 10 mg #100

   *Sig:* 1 or 2 tablets q.i.d. until healing occurs, then reduce the dose slowly as warranted.

   *Comment:* Very high doses of prednisone may be needed to produce a remission in severe cases.
4. Local therapy is prescribed to make the patient more comfortable and to decrease the odor by reducing secondary infection. This can be accomplished by the following, which must be varied for individual cases:

   a. Potassium permanganate crystals

   *Sig:* Place 2 tsp of the crystals in the bathtub with approximately 10-in lukewarm water.

   *Comment:* To prevent the crystals from burning the skin they should be dissolved completely in a glass of water before adding to the tub. The solution should be made fresh daily. The tub stains can be removed by applying acetic acid or "hypo" solution.

   b. Talc

   *Sig:* Dispense in a powder can. Apply to bed sheets and to erosions twice a day (called a "powder bed").

   c. Polysporin, Bactroban, or other antibiotic ointment q.s.

   *Sig:* Apply to small infected areas b.i.d.

5. Supportive therapy should be used when necessary. This includes vitamins, iron, blood transfusions, and oral antibiotics. Dapsone and gold therapy can be used with benefit in some cases as a corticosteroid-sparing agent. Methotrexate, azathioprine, cyclosporine, and other immunosuppressive agents are also being used. IVIG may invoke long-term remission in some patients.
6. Nursing care of the highest caliber is a prerequisite for the severe case of pemphigus with generalized erosions and bullae. The nursing personnel should be told that this disease is not contagious or infectious. Surgical dressings such as Mepitel that are not adherent but quite protective may be of great benefit.
7. Mycophenolate mofetil may be an effective and safer immunosuppressive drug according to some authors.
8. Sun avoidance and sunscreen use may be beneficial, especially in pemphigus vulgaris and pemphigus foliaceus.
9. Plasmapheresis has been used with some success.
10. Immunoablative cytoxan has been used in paraneoplastic pemphigus and life-threatening recalcitrant disease.
11. Rituximab, IVIG, and cyclosporine are other immunosuppressive options.

## Dermatitis Herpetiformis (Duhring's Disease)

Dermatitis herpetiformis is a rare (11.2 per 100,000 in the United States), chronic, markedly pruritic, papular, vesicular, and bullous skin disease of unknown etiology (**Fig. 18-2**). It is probably an autoimmune disease and is activated via the alternate complement pathway. The patient describes the itching of a new blister as a burning itch that disappears when the blister top is scratched off. The severe scratching results in the formation of excoriations and papular hives, which may be the only visible pathology of the disease. Individual lesions heal, leaving an area of hyperpigmentation. The typical distribution of the blisters or excoriations is on the scalp, sacral area, buttocks, scapular area, forearms, elbows, and thighs. Large spared areas especially over the trunk are sometimes seen. In some cases, the resulting bullae may be indistinguishable from pemphigus or bullous pemphigoid.

The duration of dermatitis herpetiformis varies from months to as long as 40 years, with periods of remission scattered in-between. The illness is associated with nontropical sprue. Most patients with dermatitis herpetiformis have nontropical sprue, but it is usually asymptomatic. Some authors have found an association with underlying solid tumors in approximately 10% of patients.

Autoimmune thyroiditis, diabetes mellitus, and T-cell lymphomas are increased. Anemia and osteoporosis can develop from malabsorption.

Laboratory tests should include fixed tissue and fresh tissue biopsy. The DIF shows, in most cases, granular IgA in the dermal papillae of perilesional skin, along with the third component of complement (C3). The finding of endomysial

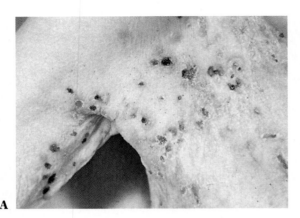

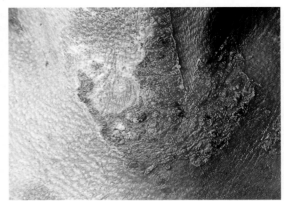

**FIGURE 18-2** ■ **(A)** Pemphigus vulgaris on anterior chest and right arm areas. **(B)** Pemphigus vulgaris on neck area. *(Courtesy of Roche Laboratories.)*

antibodies in the blood is highly specific for the disease. Antiendomysial antibodies are present in approximately 60% of patients. A blood cell count usually shows an eosinophilia.

### Differential Diagnosis

- *Pemphigus vulgaris:* Large, flaccid bullae; mouth involvement more common; debilitating course; biopsy specimen characteristic; eosinophilia is uncommon (see *Pemphigus*).
- *Erythema multiforme bullosum:* Bullae usually arise on a red, iris-like base; burning itch is absent; residual pigmentation is minor; course is shorter and palmar–plantar lesions are common (see Chapter 12).
- *Neurotic excoriations:* If this diagnosis is being considered, it is very important to rule out dermatitis herpetiformis. In a case of neurotic excoriations one usually does not find scalp lesions, blisters, or eosinophilia. Skin lesions are seen only where the patient can reach. If the patient is right handed then it is often worse on the left side of the body. The skin biopsy is helpful.
- *Scabies:* No vesicles (rarely can occur) or bullae; burrows and lesions are found in other members of the household (see Chapter 17). Potassium hydroxide scraping is diagnostic.
- *Subcorneal pustular dermatosis (Sneddon–Wilkinson disease):* Rare, chronic dermatosis characterized by an annular and serpiginous arrangement of pustules and vesiculopustules on the abdomen, groin, and axillae. Histopathologically, the pustule is found directly beneath the stratum corneum. Dapsone (avlosulfone) or sulfapyridine therapy is effective.

### Treatment

A dermatologist should be consulted to establish the diagnosis and to outline therapy, which consists of local and oral measures to control itching and a course of one of the following quite effective drugs: sulfapyridine (0.5 g q.i.d.) or dapsone (25 mg t.i.d.). Rapid response to these medicines should make the diagnosis suspect. These initial doses should be decreased or increased depending on the patient's response. These drugs can be toxic, and the patient must be under the close surveillance of the physician. The drugs should be avoided in the presence of a G6PD deficiency. Mild to moderate anemia is present in almost all patients on chronic dapsone therapy but is usually well tolerated. Dapsone can cause liver damage and pancytopenia. Cimetidine 800 mgms twice a day helps decrease dapsone toxicity. A diet that is gluten free is curative for both the skin and the bowel disease, but it must be maintained for a lifetime and is a very difficult diet to follow. It takes a committed physician and patient to maintain a gluten-free diet.

## Erythema Multiforme Bullosum

Erythema multiforme bullosum (Fig. 18-3) has a clinical picture and course distinct from that of erythema multiforme (Fig. 18-4; see Chapter 10). Many drugs can cause an erythema multiforme bullosum–like picture, but in these cases, the manifestation should be labeled a "drug eruption."

True erythema multiforme bullosum has no known cause. Clinically, one sees large vesicles and bullae usually overlying red, iris-like macules. The lesions most commonly appear on the arms, legs, and face, but can occur elsewhere, including, on occasion, the mouth. Erythema multiforme bullosum can last from days to months.

Slight malaise and fever may precede a new shower of bullae, but for the most part the patient's general health is unaffected. Itching may be mild or severe enough to interfere with sleep.

When the characteristic iris lesions are absent, it is difficult to differentiate this bullous eruption from early pemphigus vulgaris, dermatitis herpetiformis, and bullous pemphigoid. However, the histopathology and immunofluorescent studies are often helpful. DIF and IF studies are negative.

### Treatment

These patients should be referred to a dermatologist or an internist to substantiate the diagnosis and initiate therapy.

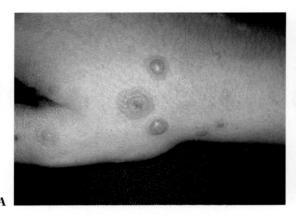
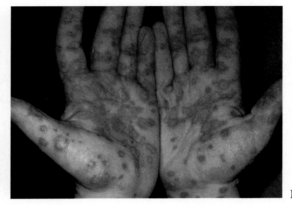

**FIGURE 18-3** ■ Erythema multiforme bullosum on the dorsum of the hand (**A**) and on the palms (**B**) 5 days later in the same patient. *(Courtesy of Roche Laboratories.)*

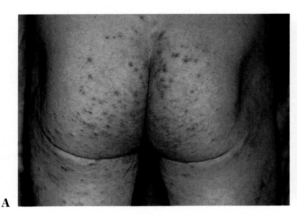
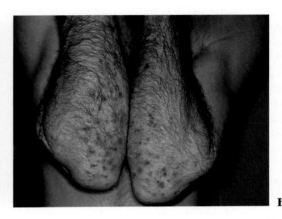

**FIGURE 18-4** ■ Dermatitis herpetiform on the buttocks (**A**) and elbows (**B**) of the same patient. *(Courtesy of Roche Laboratories.)*

Corticosteroids orally and by injection are the single most effective drugs in use today. For widespread cases requiring hospitalization, the local care is similar to that for pemphigus.

### SAUER'S NOTES

1. The bullous diseases must be differentiated by biopsy.
2. An intact blister with some edge of normal skin is ideal.
3. Part of the specimen should be sent in formaldehyde and part as fresh tissue or in Michael's solution for DIF.
4. Rapid accurate diagnosis is important since these diseases are not treated the same and early therapy is important in these sometimes life-threatening and always life-altering diseases.

## Suggested Readings

Ahmed AR, Kurgis BS, Rogers RS III. Cicatricial pemphigoid. *J Am Acad Dermatol.* 1991;24:987–1001.

Bastuji-Gavin S, Rzany B, Stern RS, et al. Clinical classification of cases of toxic epidermal necrolysis, Stevens–Johnson syndrome, and erythema multiforme. *Arch Dermatol.* 1993;129:92–96.

Diaz LA, Sampaio SA, Rivitti EA, et al. Endemic pemphigus foliaceus (fogo selvagem). *J Am Acad Dermatol.* 1989;20:657–669.

Jordon RE. *Atlas of Bullous Disease.* Philadelphia: WB Saunders; 2000.

Rogers RS III. Bullous pemphigoid: therapy and management. *J Geriatr Dermatol.* 1995;3:91–98.

Stanley JR. Therapy of pemphigus vulgaris. *Arch Dermatol.* 1999;135:76–78.

Zemstov A, Neldner KH. Successful treatment of dermatitis herpetiformis with tetracycline and nicotinamide in a patient unable to tolerate dapsone. *J Am Acad Dermatol.* 1993;28:505–506.

# CHAPTER 19

# Exfoliative Dermatitis

*John C. Hall, MD*

As the term implies, *exfoliative dermatitis* is a generalized scaling eruption of the skin. The causes are many. This diagnosis should never be made without additional qualifying etiologic terms.

This is a rare skin condition, but many general physicians, residents, and interns occasionally see these cases. Hospitalization serves two purposes, namely (1) to perform a diagnostic workup, because the cause, in many cases, is difficult to ascertain and (2) to administer intensive therapy under close supervision, especially in cases where the overall condition of the patient is poor. Exfoliative dermatitis can lead to sepsis, high-output congestive heart failure, and dehydration.

Classification of the cases of exfoliative dermatitis is facilitated by dividing them into primary and secondary forms.

## Primary Exfoliative Dermatitis

These cases develop in apparently healthy persons from no ascertainable cause.

### Presentation and Characteristics

#### Skin Lesions

Clinically, it may be impossible to differentiate this primary form from the one in which the cause is known or suspected.

---

**SAUER'S NOTES**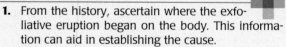

1. From the history, ascertain where the exfoliative eruption began on the body. This information can aid in establishing the cause.
2. Look at the edge of an advancing exfoliative dermatitis for the characteristic lesions of the primary disease, if present.
3. As the exfoliative dermatitis becomes more widespread, the characteristics of the original skin disease become less obvious or may completely disappear. History, therefore, can be critical in making the correct diagnosis.
4. The underlying cause may not be apparent upon first evaluation, and biopsy may show no definite diagnosis. With time, however, the underlying cause, such as CTCL, may become evident. This is why close follow-up with repeated skin biopsy attempts is important.

---

Various degrees of scaling and redness are seen, ranging from fine, generalized, granular scales with mild erythema to scaling in large plaques, with marked erythema (generalized erythroderma) and lichenification. Widespread lymphadenopathy is usually present. The nails become thick and lusterless, and the hair falls out in varying degrees.

#### Subjective Complaint

Itching, in most cases, is intense. The patient may be toxic and febrile.

#### Course

The prognosis for early cure of the disease is poor. The mortality rate is high in older patients because of generalized debility and secondary infection.

#### Causes

Various authors have studied the relationship of lymphomas with cases of exfoliative dermatitis. Some believe the incidence to be low, but others state that from 35% to 50% of these exfoliative cases, particularly those in patients older than the age of 40 years, are the result of lymphomas. However, years may pass before the lymphoma becomes obvious.

#### Laboratory Findings

There are no diagnostic changes, but the patient with a usual case has an elevated white blood cell count with eosinophilia. Biopsy of the skin is not diagnostic in the primary type, but may help to rule out a more specific diagnosis. Biopsy of an enlarged lymph node, in either the primary or the secondary form, reveals lipomelanotic reticulosis (dermatopathic lymphadenopathy) which is benign.

### Treatment

***Case Example:*** A 50-year-old man presents with a generalized, pruritic, scaly, erythematous eruption that he has had for 3 months.

***First Visit.***

1. A general medical workup is indicated.
2. A high-protein diet should be prescribed because these patients have an increased basal metabolic rate and catabolize protein.

3. Bathing instructions are variable. Some patients prefer a daily cool bath in a colloid solution for relief of itching (one box of soluble starch or 1 cup of oilated Aveeno to 10 in of bathwater). For most cases, however, generalized bathing dries the skin and intensifies the itching.

4. Provide heating blankets or extra blankets for the bed. These patients lose a lot of heat through their red skin and consequently feel chilly.

5. Locally, an ointment is most desired, but some patients prefer an oily liquid. Formulas for both are as follows:
   a. White petrolatum 240.0

   *or* a generic corticosteroid ointment, such as triamcinolone 0.025% or 0.1% ointment 240.0
   *Sig:* Apply locally b.i.d.
   Remember that on large areas of inflamed skin with a defective epidermal barrier, absorption will be dramatic and a systemic corticosteroid effect should be expected.

   b. Zinc oxide 40%

   Olive oil q.s. 240.0
   *Sig:* Apply locally with hands or a paintbrush b.i.d.
   *Comment*: Antipruritic chemicals can also be added to this.

6. Oral antihistamine, for example:

   Chlorpheniramine, 8 or 12 mg #100
   *Sig:* 1 tablet b.i.d. for itching. Warn the patient of possible drowsiness.
   *Or for more sedation* hydroxyzine 10, 25, or even 50 mg q 8 hours while awake.

**Subsequent Visits.**

1. Systemic corticosteroids: For resistant cases, the corticosteroids have consistently provided more relief than any other single form of therapy. Any of the preparations can be used. For example:

   Prednisone, 10 mg #100
   *Sig:* 4 tablets every morning for 1 week, and then 2 tablets every morning.
   *Comment:* Regulate dosage as indicated.

2. Systemic antibiotics may or may not be indicated.

## Secondary Exfoliative Dermatitis

Most patients with secondary exfoliative dermatitis have had a previous skin disease that became generalized because of overtreatment or for unknown reasons. There always remain a few cases of exfoliative dermatitis in which the cause is unknown but suspected.

### Presentation and Characteristics

#### Skin Lesions

The clinical picture of this secondary form is indistinguishable from the primary form unless some of the original dermatitis is present. As the exfoliation and erythroderma spread, the characteristics of a primary skin disease, such as psoriasis, become harder to ascertain (Fig. 19-1).

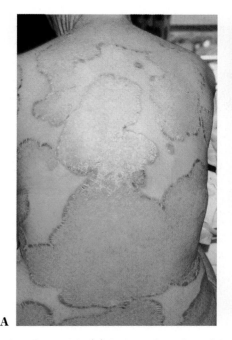
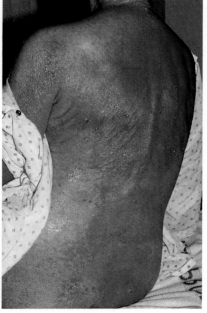

**A**    **B**

**FIGURE 19-1** ■ Exfoliative dermatitis. **(A)** Only at the edge of the large plaques is there a suggestion of psoriasis as the underlying diagnosis. **(B)** Exfoliative dermatitis due to a Dilantin drug eruption.

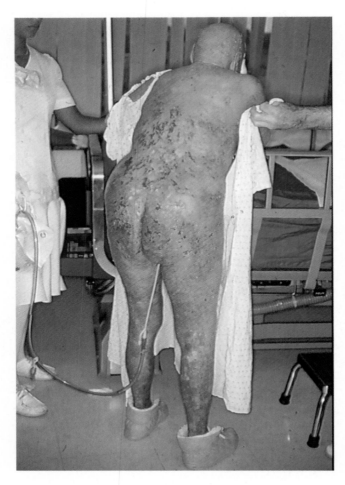

**FIGURE 19-2** ■ Exfoliative erythroderma in a patient with CTCL. A search for Sézary cells should be done.

## Course

The prognosis in the secondary form is better than that in the primary form, particularly if the original cause is definitely known and more specific therapy can be administered.

## Causes

The more common causes of secondary exfoliative dermatitis are as follows:

- Contact dermatitis (see Chapter 8)
- Drug eruption (see Chapter 8)
- Psoriasis (see Chapter 14)
- Atopic eczema (see Chapter 8)
- Pyoderma or other severe localized inflammation with a secondary id reaction (see Chapter 21)
- Inflammatory fungal disease (i.e., a kerion) with id reaction (see Chapter 25)
- Seborrheic dermatitis, especially in a newborn or an AIDS patient (see Chapter 13)
- T-cell lymphoma, especially cutaneous T-cell lymphoma (CTCL) (see Chapter 31). A useful rule is that 50% of all patients older than age 50 years who have an exfoliative dermatitis have a lymphoma. The Sézary syndrome form of lymphoma is a rare cause of exfoliative dermatitis. It is considered the leukemic form of CTCL. The patient is described as having a "lobster-like" appearance (Fig. 19-2).
- Internal cancer, leukemia, and other lymphomas.

## Treatment

The treatment of these cases consists of a combination of treatment for the primary form of exfoliative dermatitis plus the cautious institution of stronger therapy directed toward the original causative skin condition. This therapy should be reviewed in the section devoted to the specific disease (see the preceding text).

## Suggested Readings

Botella-Estrada R, Sanmartin O, Oliver V, et al. Erythroderma. *Arch Dermatol.* 1994;130:1503–1507.
Pal S, Haroon TS. Erythroderma: a clinico-etiologic study of 90 cases. *Int J Dermatol.* 1998;37:104–107.
Rym BM, Mourad M, Bechir Z, et al. Erythroderma in adults: a report of 80 cases. *Int J Dermatol.* 2005;44:731–735.
Sehgal VN, Srivastava G. Erythroderma/generalized exfoliative dermatitis in pediatric practice: an overview. *Int J Dermatol.* 2006;45:831–839.
Wilson DC, Jester JD, King LE Jr. Erythroderma and exfoliative dermatitis [review]. *Clin Dermatol.* 1993;11:67–72.194

# CHAPTER 20

# Psychodermatology

*John Koo, MD and Ellen De Coninck, MD*

*Psychodermatology* and *psychocutaneous medicine* are unfamiliar terms to many physicians. It is reported that up to 18% of dermatologists routinely prescribe psychotropic drugs. These terms describe a field of medicine that focuses on the interface between psychiatry and dermatology. In a surprisingly large proportion of dermatologic disorders, the understanding of the psychosocial and, sometimes, the occupational context is critical for optimal patient management. Examples range from common skin rashes, such as eczema or psoriasis, to flare-ups during emotional stress, to cases in which there is no real skin disorder, but the patient targets his or her skin to express an underlying psychopathologic condition. Neurotic excoriations, trichotillomania, and delusions of parasitosis are examples. Moreover, because skin disease is visible, patients commonly experience a significant negative impact on their psychological stability resulting from the disfigurement caused by their skin disorder. Patients with disfiguring skin disorders, such as alopecia areata, vitiligo, and psoriasis, frequently report problems with self-esteem, depression, and social anxiety.

The management of psychodermatologic disorders requires special skills. First, to understand what is going on and what the actual diagnosis is, a clinician must not only evaluate the skin manifestation based on the usual dermatologic differential diagnosis, but also evaluate the underlying psychopathology and the relevant social, familial, and occupational issues.

Once the diagnosis is made, optimal management often requires a dual approach to address both the dermatologic and the psychological aspects. Even in cases where the main problem is psychopathologic and the skin manifestations are entirely self-induced, the authors cannot overemphasize the importance of maintaining supportive dermatologic care to avoid secondary complications such as infection and to ensure that the patient does not feel "abandoned" by the nonpsychiatric physician. Such demonstrated support by the nonpsychiatric physician can enhance acceptance of a psychiatric consultation or referral by the patient, should there be a need for one. At the same time, it is important for the clinician to try to understand the nature of the underlying psychopathology so that the appropriate psychiatric management can be initiated. This ranges from providing appropriate psychotropic medication and encouraging the patient to attend stress management courses to making a formal referral to a psychiatrist (depending on the severity of the underlying psychopathology). Psychodermatology cases, just like those in any other field of medical practice, can range from mild to severe. In fact, when a clinician becomes aware of the mind–skin interaction and looks for psychological elements in patients, he or she finds that the large majority of these patients have easily treatable psychopathologies impacting their skin disease, such as situational stress or mild depression. Clinicians who are not fully aware of this field may only be reminded of the skin–mind interaction when they encounter the most difficult and most florid cases, such as delusions of parasitosis. It is the recommendation of the authors that clinicians become familiar with the entire range of psychodermatologic disorders so that their perception of this field is not warped by only being forced to deal with the most difficult and frustrating cases.

## Classification

Psychodermatologic disorders can be broadly classified into four categories: psychophysiologic disorders, primary psychiatric disorders, secondary psychiatric disorders, and miscellaneous cases. *Psychophysiologic disorder* refers to a situation where a real skin disorder, such as eczema or psoriasis, is worsened by emotional stress. *Primary psychiatric disorder* refers to cases such as trichotillomania where the primary problem is psychological. There is no primary skin disorder and all the manifestations are self-induced. *Secondary psychiatric disorder* refers to those cases where significant psychological problems, such as profoundly negative impact on self-esteem and body image, depression, humiliation, frustration, and social phobia, develop as a consequence of having a disfiguring skin disorder. The "miscellaneous" category refers to less well-defined situations where involvement of the central nervous system is suspected, such as cutaneous sensory syndrome. In this condition, a patient with no visible rash presents to a clinician with a purely sensory complaint, such as itching, burning, or stinging, but an extensive medical workup fails to reveal an underlying diagnosis. These patients usually respond better to psychotropic medications than to usual dermatologic therapeutics, such as topical steroids.

It is important to be able to distinguish between these broad categories for several reasons. First, the severity of the underlying psychopathologic condition tends to be different depending on the categories, with psychophysiologic disorders generally involving "milder" psychopathologies (such as situational stress) than the primary psychiatric disorders. Second, the approach to patients is frequently different among these categories. For example, with psychophysiologic cases, it is easy to talk to the patient about his or her situation, whereas in certain cases of primary psychiatric disorder, such as delusions of parasitosis or neurotic excoriation with underlying depression that is being denied by the patient, one must be extremely diplomatic, because these patients may not be ready to be confronted with the psychogenic aspect of their condition.

## Psychophysiologic Disorders

Psychophysiologic disorders are skin disorders that are known to be frequently precipitated or exacerbated by emotional stress. However, with each of these conditions, there are "stress responders" and "non–stress responders," depending on whether a patient's skin disease is or is not frequently and predictably exacerbated by stress.

The proportion of stress responders depends on the particular dermatologic diagnosis involved. In minor, treatment-responsive cases of eczema, psoriasis, or acne, the issue of stress may not be that important. However, when a clinician is faced with a more recalcitrant case, it is important to remember to ask the patient whether psychological, social, or occupational stress might be contributing to the activity of the skin disorder. Because of the propensity of so many chronic dermatoses to be exacerbated by emotional stress, and because emotional stress can initiate a vicious cycle referred to as the *itch–scratch cycle*, recalcitrant patients with chronic dermatoses may be difficult to "turn around" without addressing stress as an exacerbating factor.

With regard to psychological issues, patients often feel embarrassed discussing them, especially if they feel hurried. Once the clinician inquires, patients are frequently glad to share whatever psychosocial or occupational stress might be exacerbating or perpetuating the dermatitis. If the situation is relatively mild, simple encouragement by an authority figure (the physician) to join a stress management class, study relaxation techniques, or even use music or exercise as a stress reducer might suffice. If there is a specific psychosocial

or occupational issue that needs to be vented, referral to a therapist or counselor is appropriate.

If the stress or tension is of significant intensity to warrant considering the use of an antianxiety agent, there are three general types of agents available to meet these clinical needs. The first type, the benzodiazepines, can be used on an as-needed basis and can provide relatively quick relief from anxiety, "stress," and tension. The authors generally recommend relatively "newer" benzodiazepines, such as alprazolam (Xanax), available generically. The much older ones, such as diazepam (Valium) or chlordiazepoxide (Librium), are more often associated with possible cumulative side effects owing to their longer or unpredictable half-lives. Benzodiazepines should be reserved for short-term situations whenever possible because continued usage for more than several weeks can be associated with tolerance, dependence, and withdrawal.

On the other hand, if the "stress" proves to be a chronic predicament, a nonsedating and nonaddictive antianxiety agent such as buspirone (BuSpar) is safer for long-term use. Because of its slower onset of action, which may take up to 2 weeks or more, buspirone cannot be used on an as-needed basis. A common starting dose is 15 mg/d in divided doses, followed by 15 mg twice a day for 1 week, and up to 60 mgQD if required. The therapeutic range for most patients is between 15 and 30 mg/qd. It is not uncommon for a benzodiazepine to be started in conjunction with buspirone and then tapered after 2 or 4 weeks after the therapeutic effect of buspirone is achieved.

Antidepressants are the third type of agents used in the treatment of anxiety. The antidepressant agents paroxetine (Paxil) and venlafaxine (Effexor) are examples of selective serotonin reuptake inhibitors (SSRIs) that are useful not only in the treatment of depression but also in the treatment of chronic anxiety. It was found in an open-label study of paroxetine, imipramine, and a benzodiazepine that by the fourth week of treatment, paroxetine and imipramine were superior to the benzodiazepine for the relief of anxiety symptoms. Furthermore, the effectiveness of a venlafaxine extended-release preparation (Effexor XR) was demonstrated in a series of double-blind, randomized, placebo-controlled trials in the treatment of patients with generalized anxiety disorder.

If the intensity and the complexity of the anxiety disorder warrant a psychiatric referral, such a referral should be discussed with the patient in a most supportive and diplomatic way so as to maximize the chance of the patient accepting the referral as an adjunct to continuing dermatologic therapy.

## Primary Psychiatric Disorders

Primary psychiatric disorders are less commonly encountered than those in which stress exacerbates a common dermatosis. However, they tend to be more "florid" with a striking presentation.

### Delusions of Parasitosis

Delusions of parasitosis belong to a group of disorders called *monosymptomatic hypochondriachal psychosis* (MHP), where seemingly "normal" patients present with an encapsulated, somatic delusional ideation of a hypochondriachal nature. Because of the truly encapsulated nature of the delusional disorder, these cases are usually quite different from schizophrenia, which involves multiple functional defects, including auditory hallucinations, lack of social skills, and flat affect in addition to delusional ideation.

The most common form of MHP encountered by dermatologists is called *delusion of parasitosis*. In this type of MHP, patients firmly believe that their bodies are infested by some type of organism. They frequently present with elaborate ideation involving how these "organisms" mate, reproduce, move in the skin, and, sometimes, come out of the skin. Patients often present with the "matchbox" sign, in which bits of excoriated skin, debris, or unrelated insects or insect parts are brought in matchboxes or other containers as proof of infestation (Figs. 20-1 and 20-2). A family member or friend may come in with the patient to confirm the patient's delusion.

### Differential Diagnosis

The psychiatric differential diagnosis includes

- schizophrenia,
- psychotic depression,
- psychosis with florid mania,
- drug-induced and other forms of psychosis, and
- formication without delusions, in which the patient experiences crawling, biting, and stinging sensations without believing that they are due to organisms.

The other organic forms of psychosis include

- vitamin $B_{12}$ deficiency,
- withdrawal from cocaine, amphetamines, or alcohol,
- multiple sclerosis,
- cerebrovascular disease, and
- syphilis.

If any of these other underlying diagnoses are made, the separate diagnosis of delusions of parasitosis is not made. Once again, delusions of parasitosis are a separate psychiatric entity

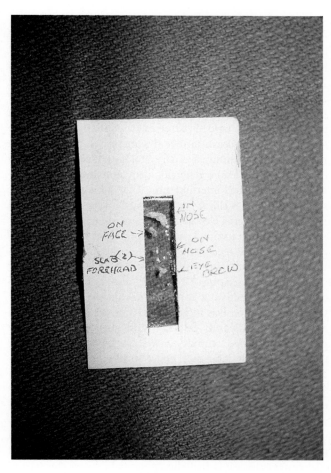

**FIGURE 20-2** ■ A carefully constructed specimen board of alleged parasites from another patient with delusions of parasitosis.

characterized by very encapsulated ideation, where none of the other psychiatric diagnoses are involved.

### Treatment

Currently, the treatment of choice for delusions of parasitosis is an antipsychotic medication called pimozide (ORAP). This antipsychotic medication with a chemical structure and potency similar to those of haloperidol (Haldol) has been known to be uniquely effective for this condition, especially in decreasing formication (crawling, stinging, and biting sensations). The dosage used is much lower than that used for chronic schizophrenics. Pimozide is generally started at the lowest possible dose of half a tablet (1 mg) and increased by 1 mg/wk. By the time the dosage of 4 to 6 mg (two to three tablets) is reached, most patients experience a great decrease in crawling and biting sensations, as well as the sensations of "organisms" moving in their skin. At the same time, patients generally become much less agitated. In younger patients, pimozide can often be continued at the lowest effective dose for several months, and then gradually tapered off without necessarily inviting recurrence of the symptoms. If the condition recurs, another course of therapy with pimozide can be instituted.

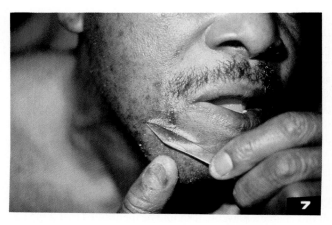

**FIGURE 20-1** ■ A man with delusions of parasitosis uses his knife to dig out a "parasite" to demonstrate it to the author (J.K.).

The main adverse effects of pimozide are its extrapyramidal side effects (EPS), just as with many other antipsychotic agents. The most common of these, namely stiffness and restlessness, can be effectively treated with benztropine (Cogentin) 2 mg up to four times per day. Diphenhydramine (Benadryl) 25 mg can also be substituted for benztropine. In elderly patients, long-term maintenance with a very small dose of pimozide (1 to 2 mg/d) is sometimes required. Although the long-term side effect of tardive dyskinesia is a possibility, the risk appears to be minimal in dermatology patients where a low dose (6 mg/qd or less) is generally adequate and where the medication is often used intermittently. If the patient has a cardiac rhythm disorder, is elderly, or if a dosage higher than 10 mg/qd is needed, then serial electrocardiograms are required.

A new generation of antipsychotic agents called *atypical antipsychotics* has recently been introduced into clinical practice. These atypical antipsychotics, which include risperidone (Risperdal), olanzapine (Zyprexa), and quetiapine (Seroquel), are as effective as conventional antipsychotics for the treatment of psychosis in general. These are better tolerated and cause significantly less EPS and tardive dyskinesia in placebo-controlled studies as well as in clinical practice. Given the much safer side effect profile, atypical antipsychotics may prove useful in the treatment of MHP, although studies comparing pimozide with the new atypical antipsychotics in the treatment of delusions of parasitosis have not yet been performed.

A word of caution when using atypical antipsychotics in patients with a history of seizures or with conditions such as Alzheimer's disease is that they potentially lower the seizure threshold. Early testing performed prior to market sales found that seizures occurred in 22 (0.9%) of 2,500 olanzapine-treated patients; 18 (0.8%) of 2,387 quetiapine-treated patients; and 9 (0.3%) of 2,607 risperidone-treated patients.

## Neurotic Excoriations/Factitial Dermatitis

*Neurotic excoriations* is used when individuals self-inflict excoriations (scratch marks) with the fingernails. Although *neurotic excoriations* and *factitial dermatitis* are sometimes used interchangeably, *factitial dermatitis* should be used more selectively to refer to situations where the patient uses something more elaborate than the fingernails, such as lit cigarette butts, chemicals, or sharp instruments, to damage his or her own skin. Factitial dermatitis tends to be bizarre in shape, depth, and distribution, unlike neurotic excoriations, which are "scooped out" with a butterfly distribution on the back with sparing of the interscapular region and worse on the left side in a right-handed person and vice versa. Factitial dermatitis patients do not admit to manipulating the skin but think the cause of their disease is some mysterious unknown etiology. Neurotic excoriations patients often admit to scratching but cannot control themselves. In both cases, scarring and infection are not uncommon complications. Although *neurotic excoriations* contains the word *neurotic*, clinicians need to recognize that this term is essentially dermatologic and does not imply any particular psychopathology in the patient. In fact,

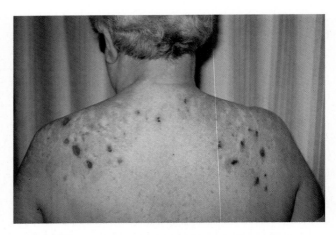

**FIGURE 20-3** ■ Multiple neurotic excoriations are present only in the areas easily accessed by the patient's hands on the back of this depressed woman.

the clinician needs to go a step further and determine what the underlying psychopathology is. The most common underlying psychopathologies encountered are major depressive episodes, anxiety, and obsessive–compulsive disorders. Rarely, patients excoriate their skin in response to a delusional ideation, in which case psychosis is the appropriate diagnosis. Patients with neurotic excoriations are usually suffering from depression or anxiety, whereas those with factitial dermatitis tend to be much "sicker" psychologically and they more frequently represent manifestations of underlying psychosis characterized by a delusional ideation (Fig. 20-3).

### Treatment

The management of anxiety is as discussed. However, if the patient proves to have underlying depression resulting in neurotic excoriations, one antidepressant that is frequently used by dermatologists is doxepin (Sinequan). Doxepin is a tricyclic antidepressant with one of the most powerful anti-itch and antihistamine effects, as well as sedative/tranquilizing effects. Because many people with depression who excoriate their skin tend to be agitated ("agitated depression"), the sedative and tranquilizing effects of doxepin frequently prove to be therapeutic in addition to its antidepressant effects. Moreover, the profound antipruritic effect is also an added benefit. Even though these patients create their own skin lesions, as they keep picking on their skin and not letting them heal, the itch–scratch cycle can become an issue, which can effectively be addressed with the antipruritic effect of doxepin (Fig. 20-4).

The use of doxepin requires all of the usual precautions regarding the use of older tricyclic antidepressants, including an absence of cardiac arrhythmias since doxepin can cause QT prolongation. A detailed description is beyond the scope of this chapter; however, it should be mentioned that if the patient is truly depressed, an antidepressant dosage of 100 mg/d or higher is usually required so that the patient is not undertreated. Elderly patients may respond to a lower dose.

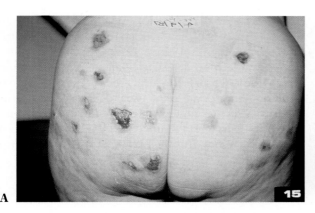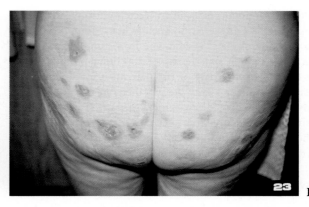

**FIGURE 20-4** ▪ **(A)** Pretreatment photograph of the buttocks of the patient depicted in Figure 20-3. **(B)** After 1 week of therapy with doxepin, the patient demonstrates significant improvement in excoriations owing to the antipruritic effect. However, the antidepressant effect of doxepin was not evidenced until later.

## Trichotillomania

*Trichotillomania*, according to the dermatologic usage of the word, refers to any patient who pulls out his or her own hair. The psychiatric definition of trichotillomania requires the presence of "impulsivity." However, using the less specific dermatologic definition, the clinician once again needs to ascertain the nature of the underlying psychopathology to select the most appropriate treatment. The most common underlying psychopathology is obsessive–compulsive behavior, whether or not it formally meets the DSM-IV criteria for obsessive–compulsive disorder. The other possible underlying psychiatric diagnosis includes depression with or without anxiety, as well as extremely rare cases of delusion, in which the patient pulls out his or her hair based on the delusional belief that something in the roots needs to be "dug out" for the hair to grow normally. This latter, rare, clinical condition is called *trichophobia*.

Trichotillomania is one of the rare conditions in which a pathologic examination of the skin can be diagnostic. There is a unique change in the hair root called *trichomalacia*, which is only seen in trichotillomania. Therefore, if the patient continues to deny pulling his or her own hair, a scalp biopsy can be helpful in determining the diagnosis.

### Treatment

As with other conditions, treatment is based on the nature of the underlying psychopathology. Because the most common underlying psychopathology is obsessive–compulsive tendency, medications such as fluoxetine (Prozac), paroxetine (Paxil), fluvoxamine (Luvox), sertraline (Zoloft), and clomipramine (Anafranil) in dosages appropriate for the treatment of obsessive–compulsive disorder can be helpful in pharmacologic management. It should be noted that when these medications are used in the treatment of obsessive–compulsive disorder, the dosage tends to be higher and the time to initial response is longer than when treating depression. For example, 20 mg/d of fluoxetine or paroxetine is often adequate for the treatment of depression.

In contrast, when treating obsessive–compulsive disorder, the required dosage may be in the 40- to 80-mg/d range. The initial treatment response time in obsessive–compulsive disorder may take 4 to 8 weeks with a maximal response time of up to 20 weeks. Once a therapeutic response is achieved, therapy should be continued for 6 months to 1 year. Many clinicians have found that a complete remission is unusual. The nonpharmacologic approach includes psychotherapy, which can be useful if there is a definable issue that can be discussed. The other treatment modality includes behavioral therapy conducted by a behaviorally oriented psychologist.

## Secondary Psychiatric Disorders

Although skin conditions are usually not life threatening, because they are visible, they can be life ruining. Patients frequently feel psychologically and socially devastated because of the disfigurement (Fig. 20-5). Moreover, it is difficult for patients with skin disorders to get jobs where appearance is important. It is also well documented that patients with

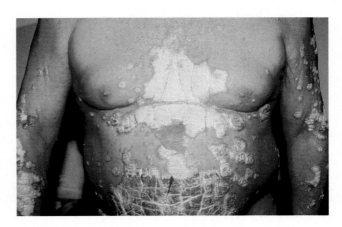

**FIGURE 20-5** ▪ The disfiguring effects of psoriasis are seen on the arms and torso of this patient with plaque psoriasis. This man experienced severe social, sexual, occupational, as well as psychological impact due to his psoriasis.

visible disfigurement, especially if the condition is perceived to be contagious, are generally treated worse than those with other obvious physical disabilities. Even though many patients adjust to their skin disease, if the clinician notes significant distress on the part of the patient, it is important to explore this issue and evaluate whether referral to a mental health professional or dermatologic support group might be of benefit. If the depression, social phobia, or any secondary psychopathology is of significant intensity, a referral to a psychiatrist might be warranted.

## Miscellaneous Cases

There are some cases that do not neatly fit into the above three categories. For example, there are patients with cutaneous sensory syndrome, who present to the clinician with nothing but a sensory complaint. There is no visible rash, and an extensive workup fails to reveal any underlying medical condition that can be associated with the chief complaint. The chief complaints can vary from itching, stinging, and biting sensations to other forms of cutaneous discomfort. It is well documented that itching can occur as a manifestation of central nervous system insult, such as multiple sclerosis, brain abscess, brain tumor, or sensory stroke. However, in many of these cases, it is not possible to demonstrate a focal neurologic deficit. In general, patients with chronic sensory disorders are frustrated because they often do not respond to the usual dermatologic treatment modalities such as topical steroids, emollients, and antibiotics. However, the authors' experience is that they frequently do respond to the empirical use of psychotropic medications.

### Treatment

If the primary complaint is pruritus, patients often respond to doxepin in doses that are significantly lower than those used for the treatment of depression. Often a dosage of less than 10 mg at bedtime to 50 to 75 mg during the day suffices (**Fig. 20-6**). If chronic pruritus can be suppressed this way and suppression is maintained with the lowest effective dose of doxepin for several months, the pruritus frequently does not return if the doxepin is gradually tapered.

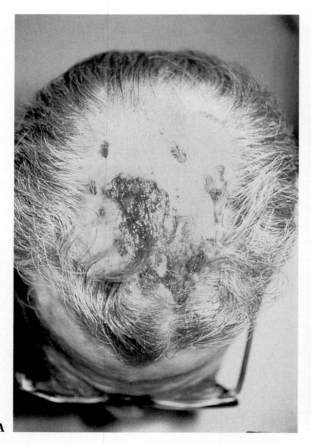 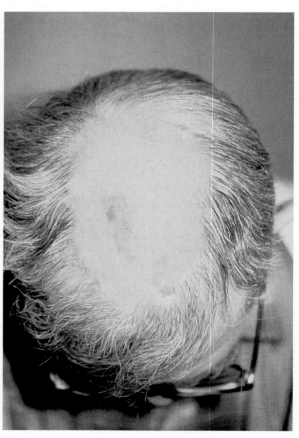

A     B

**FIGURE 20-6** ■ **(A)** For decades this older man experienced severe, intermittent attacks of scalp pruritus that failed conventional dermatologic therapy and for which no primary skin lesion or systemic organic etiology was ever identified. A mental status examination by the author (J.K.) was entirely negative for any diagnosable psychiatric disorder. **(B)** After 2 weeks of empirical treatment with 25 to 50 mg/d of doxepin, the patient experienced complete resolution of pruritus that recurred when doxepin was discontinued. This observation may illustrate a case of central nervous system–mediated pruritus.

If the primary sensory complaint relates to pain, including burning sensations, amitriptyline (Elavil), once again in a dosage lower than the antidepressant dosage, is frequently effective. If the patient cannot tolerate amitriptyline because older tricyclics are associated with more side effects than new ones, then desipramine (Norpramin) can be a good substitute. If the patient cannot tolerate any tricyclic antidepressants, the last option would be the newer, nontricyclic agents such as the SSRIs. SSRIs have the least documentation regarding their efficacy as analgesics, in contrast to tricyclics, which are better documented for their analgesic therapeutic effect.

It is important to tell the patient ahead of time that improvement occurs extremely slowly whether one is treating pruritus or dysesthesia. However, the authors' experience has been that, when treatment is conducted with a long-term view, it is generally possible to find the optimal agent and optimal dose to resolve the chronic sensory disorder, and then eventually taper the patient off the medication altogether.

## Suggested Readings

Fenollosa P, Pallares J, Cerver J, et al. Chronic pain in the spinal cord injured: statistical approach and pharmacological treatment. *Paraplegia.* 1993; 31:722–729.

Gaston L, Lassone M, Bernier-Buzzanga J, et al. Role of emotional factors in adults with atopic dermatitis. *Int J Dermatol.* 1987;17:82–86.

Ginsburg IH, Prystowsky JH, Kornfeld DS, et al. Role of emotional factors in adults with atopic dermatitis. *Int J Dermatol.* 1993;32:65–66.

Koblezer CS. *Psychocutaneous Disease.* Orlando, FL: Grune & Stratton; 1987: 77–78, 117.

Koo JY. Skin disorders. In: Kaplan HI, Saduch BJ, eds. *Comprehensive Textbook of Psychiatry.* 6th ed. Baltimore: Williams & Wilkins; 1995.

Koo JY, Pham CT. Psychodermatology: practical guidelines on pharmacotherapy. *Arch Dermatol.* 1992;128: 381–388.

Koo JYM. Psychotropic agents in dermatology. *Dermatol Clin.* 1993;11: 215–224.

Koo JYM. Psychodermatology: a practice manual for clinicians. *Curr Probl Dermatol.* 1995;6:204–232.

Medansky RS, Handler RM. Dermatopsychosomatics: classification, physiology and therapeutic approaches. *J Am Acad Dermatol.* 1981;5:125–136.

Rasmussen SA, Eisen JL. Treatment strategies for chronic and refractory obsessive–compulsive disorder. *J Clin Psychiatry.* 1997;58(suppl 13):9–13.

Stein DJ, Mullen L, Islam MN, et al. Compulsive and impulsive symptomatology in trichotillomania. *Psychopathology.* 1995;28:208–213.

Zanol K, Slaughter J, Hall R. An approach to the treatment of psychogenic parasitosis. *Int Dermatol.* 1998;37:56–63.

# CHAPTER 21

# Dermatologic Bacteriology

*John C. Hall, MD*

Bacteria exist on the skin as normal nonpathogenic resident flora or as pathogenic organisms. The pathogenic bacteria cause primary, secondary, and systemic infections. For clinical purposes it is justifiable to divide the problem of bacterial infection into three classifications (Table 21-1). Some of the diseases listed are of dubious bacterial etiology, but they appear bacterial, may have a bacterial component, can be treated with antibacterial agents, and are, therefore, included in this chapter.

With an alteration in immune capabilities in a person, bacteria and other infectious agents can have erratic behavior. Ordinary nonpathogens can act as pathogens, and pathogenic agents can act more aggressively.

## Primary Bacterial Infections (Pyodermas)

The most common causative agents of the primary skin infections are the coagulase-positive micrococci (staphylococci) and the β-hemolytic streptococci. Superficial or deep bacterial lesions can be produced by these organisms. In managing the pyodermas, certain general principles of treatment must be initiated.

- *Improve bathing habits:* More frequent bathing and the use of bactericidal soap, such as Dial, Cetaphil Antibacterial, or Lever 2000, are indicated. Any pustules or crusts should be removed during bathing to facilitate penetration of the local medications. In rare instances when these infections are recalcitrant to standard therapies, use half to one cup of bleach in a full tub of water to soak daily.
- *General isolation procedures:* Clothing and bedding should be changed frequently and cleaned. The patient should have a separate towel and washcloth.
- *Systemic drugs:* The patient should be questioned regarding ingestion of drugs that can cause lesions that mimic or cause pyodermas, such as iodides, bromides, testosterone, corticosteroids, progesterone, and lithium.
- *Diabetes:* In chronic skin infections, particularly recurrent boils, diabetes should be ruled out by history and laboratory examination.

- *Immunosuppressed patients:* A history of abnormal findings should alert the physician to the increasing number of patients now who are on chemotherapy for cancer, are posttransplant, or have the acquired immunodeficiency syndrome (AIDS).

**TABLE 21-1 ■ Classification of Bacterial Infection**

**Primary Bacterial Infections**
Impetigo
Ecthyma
Folliculitis
Superficial folliculitis
   Staphylococcus folliculitis
   Chronic noninfectious folliulitis
Folliculitis of the scalp
Superficial—acne necrotica miliaris
Deep scarring—folliculitis decalvans
Folliculitis of the beard
Stye
Furuncle
Carbuncle
Sweat gland inflammations
Erysipelas

**Secondary Bacterial Infections**
Cutaneous diseases with secondary infection
Infected ulcers
Infectious eczematoid dermatitis
Bacterial intertrigo

**Systemic Bacterial Infections**
Scarlet fever
Granuloma inguinale
Chancroid
Mycobacterial infections
Tuberculosis of the skin
Leprosy
Gonorrhea
Rickettsial diseases
Actinomycosis

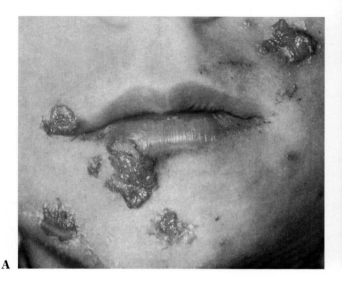

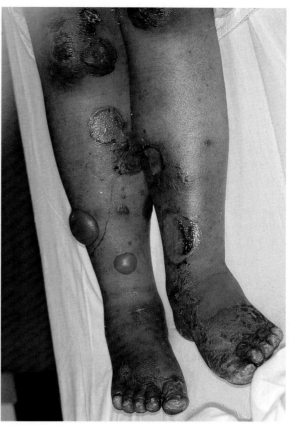

A                                                                                                          B

**FIGURE 21-1** ■ **(A)** Impetigo of the face. The honey-colored crusts are typical. *(Courtesy of Abner Kurtin, Folia Dermatologica, No. 2. Geigy Pharmaceuticals.)* **(B)** Bullous impetigo on the legs of a young child.

## Impetigo

Impetigo is a common superficial bacterial infection seen most often in children. It is the "infantigo" every parent respects.

### Primary Lesions

The lesions vary from small vesicles to large bullae that rapidly rupture and discharge a honey-colored serous liquid (Fig. 21-1). New lesions can develop in a matter of hours. The blisters are evanescent and often are not present but leave their oval or scalloped edges.

### Secondary Lesions

Crusts form from the discharge and appear to be lightly stuck on the skin surface. When removed, a superficial erosion remains, which may be the only evidence of the disease. In debilitated infants, the bullae may coalesce to form an exfoliative type of infection called *Ritter's disease* or *pemphigus neonatorum*.

### Distribution

The lesions occur most commonly on the face but may be anywhere.

### Contagiousness

It is not unusual to see brothers or sisters of the patient and, rarely, the parents similarly infected.

### Differential Diagnosis

- *Contact dermatitis* due to poison ivy or oak: Linear blisters and itches severely (see Chapter 8).
- *Tinea of smooth skin:* Fewer lesions; spreads slowly; central clearing; small vesicles in an annular configuration and elevated edge; fungi found on scraping; culture is positive (see Chapter 25).

---

**SAUER'S NOTES**

Body piercing has frequently been associated with localized staphylococcal infection and pseudomonas infection and rarely bacteremia and endocarditis. Tuberculosis, hepatitis C and B, and even HIV can be transmitted in this way. Noninfectious complications include keloids and allergic dermatitis. This fad should not be recommended, especially in the tongue, lips, navels, nipples, nose, or genitalia.

■ *Toxic epidermal necrolysis:* In infants and rarely in adults, massive bullae can develop rapidly, particularly with staphylococcal infection. The severe form of this infection is known as the *staphylococcal scalded skin syndrome,* which is a type of toxic epidermal necrolysis (see Chapter 18).

### Treatment

1. Outline the general principles of treatment. Emphasize the removal of the crusts once or twice a day during bathing with an antibacterial soap such as Lever 2000 or chlorhexidine (Hibiclens) skin cleanser.

2. Mupirocin (Bactroban) or gentamicin (Garamycin) ointment or Polysporin ointment q.s. 15.0

   *Sig:* Apply t.i.d. locally for 10 days. Treat all affected family members or other affected contacts.

3. Oral antibiotics such as a 10-day course of erythromycin, cephalexin, or clindamycin may be necessary.

4. Methicillin-resistant *Staphylococcus aureus* in the community-acquired form (CA-MRSA) now occurs in epidemic proportions. Fortunately it often is sensitive to sulfamethoxazole with trimethoprim (Septra or Bactrim), clindamycin, or tetracycline derivatives. Abscesses are common and when present must be treated aggressively by incision and drainage.

### Ecthyma

Ecthyma is another superficial bacterial infection, but it is seen less commonly and is deeper than impetigo. It is usually caused by β-hemolytic streptococci and occurs on the buttocks and the thighs of children (Fig. 21-2).

### Primary Lesion

A vesicle or vesiculopustule appears and rapidly changes into the secondary lesion.

---

### Secondary Lesion

This is a piled-up crust, 1 to 3 cm in diameter, overlying a superficial erosion or ulcer. In neglected cases, scarring can occur as a result of extension of the infection into the dermis.

### Distribution

Most commonly the disease is seen on the posterior aspect of the thighs and the buttocks, from where it can spread.

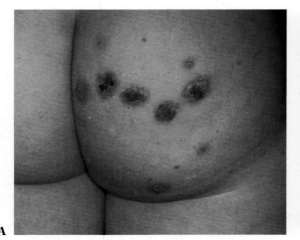

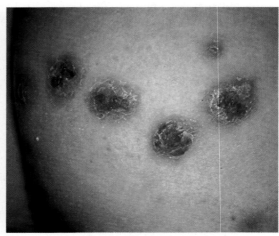

A                                                                      B

**FIGURE 21-2** ■ **(A)** Ecthyma on the buttocks of 13-year-old boy. **(B)** Closeup of lesions. (*Courtesy of Burroughs Wellcome Co.*)

Ecthyma commonly follows the scratching of chigger bites.

### Age Group

Children are the most common age group affected.

### Contagiousness

Ecthyma is rarely found in other members of the family.

### Differential Diagnosis

- *Psoriasis:* Less common in children; whitish, firmly attached scaly lesion, also on the scalp, knees, and/or elbows (see Chapter 14).
- *Impetigo:* Much smaller crusted lesions, not as deep (see preceding section).

### Treatment

1. The general principles of treatment are listed earlier in the chapter. The crusts must be removed daily. Response to therapy is slower than with impetigo, but the treatment is the same for both conditions.
2. *Systemic antibiotics:* If there is a low-grade fever and evidence of bacterial infection in other organs due to sepsis, one of the antibiotic syrups or tablets can be given orally for 10 days. This is commonly seen in children with extensive ecthyma. It is rarely seen with impetigo.

## Folliculitis

Folliculitis is a common pyogenic infection of the hair follicles, usually caused by coagulase-positive staphylococci (**Fig. 21-3**). Seldom does a patient consult the physician for a single outbreak of folliculitis. The physician is consulted because of recurrent and chronic pustular lesions. The patient realizes that the present acute episode clears with the help of nature, but seeks medicine and advice to prevent recurrences. For this reason, the general principles of treatment are listed.

The physician must pay particular attention to the drug history and the diabetes investigation. Some physicians believe that a focus of infection in the teeth, tonsils, gallbladder, or genitourinary tract should be ruled out when folliculitis is recurrent.

The folliculitis may invade only the superficial part of the hair follicle, or it may extend down to the hair bulb. Many variously named clinical entities based on the location and the chronicity of the lesions have been carried down through the years. A few of these entities bear presentation here, but most are defined in the Dictionary–Index.

### Superficial Folliculitis

The physician is rarely consulted for this minor problem, which is most commonly seen on the arms, scalp, face, and buttocks of children and adults with the acne–seborrhea complex. A history of excessive use of hair oils, bath oils, moisturizers, or suntan oils can often be obtained. The use of these oily agents should be avoided. Culture for *Staphylococcus* or *Streptococcus* may be negative and in these cases, the same therapeutic regiments that are usually used for acne should be used. Chronic noninfectious folliculitis is the term I use for this clinical picture.

### Folliculitis of the Scalp (Superficial Form)

A superficial form has the appellation *acne necrotica miliaris.* This is an annoying, pruritic, chronic, recurrent folliculitis of the scalp in adults. The scratching of the crusted lesions occupies the patient's evening hours.

**Treatment.**

1. Follow the general principles of treatment.
2. Selenium sulfide (Selsun, Head & Shoulders Intensive Treatment) suspension shampoo 120.0

   *Sig:* Shampoo twice a week as directed on the label.
3. Other shampoos such as T-Sal and sulfur washes, such as Ovace, Plexion, or a generic form of these used as a shampoo, can be tried.

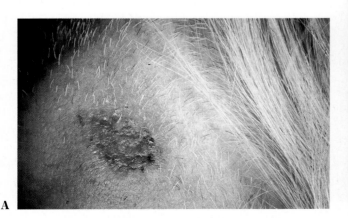
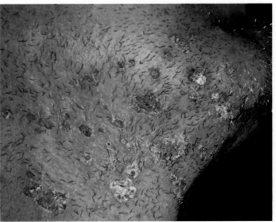

A                 B

**FIGURE 21-3** ■ **(A)** Folliculitis of the scalp. **(B)** Folliculitis of the beard area (*Courtesy of Burroughs Wellcome Co.*).

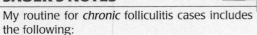

**SAUER'S NOTES**

My routine for *chronic* folliculitis cases includes the following:

1. Sulfur ppt. 5%
   Hydrocortisone 1%
   Bactroban cream q.s. 15.0
   *Sig:* Apply b.i.d. locally.
2. Long-term low-dose antibiotic therapy can be used, such as erythromycin, 250 mg, q.i.d. for 3 days then two or three times a day for months.
3. Lichenified papules of excoriated folliculitis respond to superficial liquid nitrogen applications or intralesional corticosteroid injections.

4. Antibiotic and corticosteroid cream mixture q.s. 15.0
   *Sig:* Apply to scalp h.s.

### Folliculitis of the Scalp (Deep Form)

The deep form of scalp folliculitis is called *folliculitis decalvans*. This is a chronic, slowly progressive folliculitis with an active border and scarred atrophic center. The end result, after years of progression, is patchy, scarred areas of alopecia, with eventual burning out of the inflammation. It is not a true infection and bacterial cultures are negative. Long-term tetracycline derivatives may be helpful.

### Differential Diagnosis.

- *Chronic discoid lupus erythematosus:* Redness, hypopigmentation, and hyperpigmentation; enlarged hair follicles with follicular plugs (see Chapter 37).
- *Alopecia cicatrisata* (pseudopelade of Brocq): Rare; no evidence of inflammation. Some authors think this is burnt out lichen planus of the scalp (see Chapter 32).
- *Tinea of the scalp:* It is important to culture the hair for fungi in any chronic infection of the scalp; *Trichophyton tonsurans* group can cause a subtle non-inflammatory clinical picture (black dot tinea in children, which is endemic in large urban areas in African-American children who braid their hair) (see Chapter 25).
- *Excoriated folliculitis:* Chronic thickened excoriated papules or nodules (can be called *prurigo nodularis*), usually seen on the posterior scalp, posterior neck, anus, and legs. When allowed to heal, whitish scars remain. The inflammation can last for years. Liquid nitrogen applied to the papules is effective, as are intralesional corticosteroids. Occasionally, these patients can be treated with a drug to decrease obsessive–compulsive behavior, such as a selective serotonin reuptake inhibitor. Common in dialysis patients and can be seen in hepatitis C and AIDS.
- *Lichen planopilaris:* Scarring lichen planus in the scalp, which is usually characteristic on biopsy.

It may have follicular plugging and is characterized by perifollicular cuffing of fine adheren scale and a purplish pink color. Topical or intralesional corticosteriods and antimalarials are often used with success.

**Treatment.** Results of treatment may be disappointing. Long-term antibiotics, especially tetracycline derivatives, may be helpful. Occasionally intralesional corticosteroids may be palliative.

### Folliculitis of the Beard

This is the familiar "barber's itch," which in the days before antibiotics was resistant to therapy. This bacterial infection of the hair follicles is spread rather rapidly by shaving.

### Differential Diagnosis.

- *Contact dermatitis* caused by shaving lotions: History of new lotion applied; general redness of the area with some vesicles (see Chapter 8).
- *Tinea of the beard:* Very slowly spreading infection; hairs broken off; usually a deeper, nodular type of inflammation (Majocchi's granuloma); culture of hair produces fungi (see Chapter 25).
- *Ingrown beard hairs* (pseudofolliculitis barbae): Hair circling back into the skin with resultant chronic inflammation; a hereditary trait, especially in African-Americans. Close shaving aggravates the condition. Local antibiotics rarely help, but locally applied depilatories may help. Other local therapy to consider is Retin-A gel and Benzashave (shaving cream with benzoyl peroxide). Permanent hair removal by electrolysis or laser can be helpful. Vaniqa applied twice a day after hair removal can be used to reduce the rate of regrowth of hair. Growing a beard or mustache eliminates the problem. Hairs may also become ingrown in axillae, pubic area, or legs, especially when closely shaved in places with curly hair.

**Treatment.**

1. Follow the general principles of treatment, stressing the use of Dial or other antibacterial soap for washing of the face.
2. Shaving instructions:
   a. Change the razor blade daily or sterilize the head of the electric razor by placing it in 70% alcohol for 1 hour.
   b. Apply the following salve very lightly to the face before shaving and again after shaving. *Do not shave closely.*
3. Antibiotic and hydrocortisone cream mixture q.s. 15.0
   *Sig:* Apply to the face before shaving, after shaving, and at bedtime.
   *Comment:* For stubborn cases, add sulfur 5% to the cream.
4. Oral therapy with erythromycin, 250 mg (can also use cephalexin on clindamycin)
   *Sig:* one capsule q.i.d. for 7 days, then one capsule b.i.d. for 7 days.

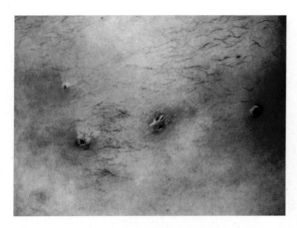

**FIGURE 21-4** ■ Multiple furuncles (boils) on the chest. *(Courtesy of Abner Kurtin, Folia Dermatologica, No. 2. Geigy Pharmaceuticals.)*

### Sty (Hordeolum)

A *sty* is a deep folliculitis of the stiff eyelid hairs. A single lesion is treated with hot packs of 1% boric acid solution and an ophthalmic antibiotic ointment. Recurrent lesions may be linked with the blepharitis of seborrheic dermatitis (dandruff) or rosacea. For this type, vytone or cleansing the eyelashes with Johnson's baby shampoo is indicated. If it is a chronic problem then tetracycline antibiotics short term or long term can be used.

### Furuncle

A furuncle, or boil (Fig. 21-4), is a more extensive infection of the hair follicle, usually due to *Staphylococcus*. A boil can occur in any person at any age, but certain predisposing factors account for most outbreaks. An important factor is the acne–seborrhea complex (oily skin and a history of acne and dandruff). Other factors include poor hygiene, diabetes, local skin trauma from friction of clothing, and maceration in obese persons. One boil usually does not bring the patient to the physician, but recurrent boils do.

**Differential Diagnosis.**

*Single Lesion*
 ■ *Primary chancre-type diseases:* See list in Dictionary–Index.

*Multiple Lesions*
 ■ *Drug eruption from iodides or bromides:* See Chapter 8.
 ■ *Hidradenitis suppurativa:* See later in this chapter.

### Treatment

*Case Example:* A young man has had recurrent boils for 6 months. He does not have diabetes, is not obese, is taking no drugs, and bathes daily. He now has a large boil on his buttocks.

1. Burow's solution hot packs.

 *Sig:* 1 packet of Domeboro powder to 1 quart of hot water. Apply hot wet packs for 30 minutes twice a day.

2. Incision and drainage: This should be done only on "ripe" lesions where a necrotic white area appears at the top of the nodule. Drains are not necessary unless the lesion has extended deep enough to form a fluctuant abscess. If near the rectum, consider a perirectal abscess as the diagnosis. This has a communicating tract with the rectum, which must be treated surgically. Referral to a general surgeon or proctologist is indicated.

3. Oral antistaphylococcal penicillin, such as dicloxacillin or cephalexin, should be prescribed for 5 to 10 days. (Bacteriologic culture and sensitivity studies are helpful in determining which antibiotic to use.) I often now use sulfamethoxazole/trimethoprim empirically to cover MRSA before culture results are known.

4. For recurrent form:
   a. Follow general principles of treatment by use of an antibacterial soap.
   b. Rule out focus of infection in teeth, tonsils, genitourinary tract, and so on.
   c. Begin oral therapy with erythromycin, 250 mg, which is very effective in breaking the cycle of recurrent cases.

    *Sig:* four capsules a day for 10 days.

Cultures should be done to determine sensitivity and antibiotic choices altered as indicated.

### Carbuncle

A carbuncle is an extensive infection of several adjoining hair follicles that drains with multiple openings onto the skin surface (Fig. 21-5). Fatal cases were not unusual in the preantibiotic days. A common location for a carbuncle is the posterior neck region. Large, ugly, criss-cross scars in this area in an older patient demonstrate the outdated treatment for this disease, namely, multiple bold incisions. Because a carbuncle is, in reality, a multiple furuncle, the same etiologic factors apply. Recurrences are uncommon.

**Treatment.** Treatment is the same as for a boil (see preceding section) but with greater emphasis on systemic antibiotic therapy.

## Sweat Gland Inflammations

Although not true infections, inflammations of the sweat gland are included here because of similar clinical appearance (Fig. 21-6) and similar treatment. Primary eccrine sweat gland or duct infections are very rare. However, prickly heat, a sweat-retention disease, frequently develops a secondary bacterial infection. Primary apocrine gland inflammation is rather common. Two types of inflammation exist:

 ■ *Apocrinitis* denotes inflammation of a single apocrine gland, usually in the axilla, and is commonly associated with a change in deodorant. It responds to the therapy listed for furuncles. In addition, a lotion containing an antibiotic aids in keeping the area dry, such as an erythromycin solution (A/T/S, Erymax, EryDerm, Erycette, T-Stat, Staticin).

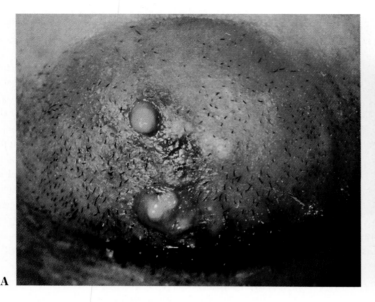
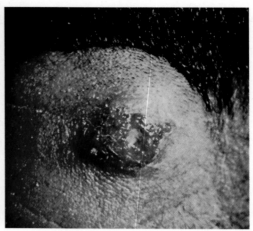

**FIGURE 21-5** ■ **(A)** Carbuncle on the chin. Notice the multiple openings. *(Courtesy of Abner Kurtin, Folia Dermatologica, No. 2. Geigy Pharmaceuticals.)* **(B)** Carbuncle on the back of the neck. *(Courtesy of J. Lamar Callaway, Folia Dermatologica, No. 4. Geigy Pharmaceuticals.)*

■ The second form of apocrine gland inflammation is *hidradenitis suppurativa*. This chronic, recurring inflammation is characterized by the development of multiple nodules, abscesses, draining sinuses, and eventual hypertrophic bands of scars. The most common location is in the axillae, but it can also occur in the groin, perianal, submammary, buttocks, and suprapubic regions. It does not occur before

puberty. Etiologically, there appears to be a hereditary tendency in these patients toward occlusion of the follicular orifice and subsequent retention of the secretory products. Two other diseases are related to hidradenitis suppurativa and may be present in the same patient: (1) a severe form of acne called *acne conglobata* and (2) *dissecting cellulitis of the scalp* (see Chapter 13).

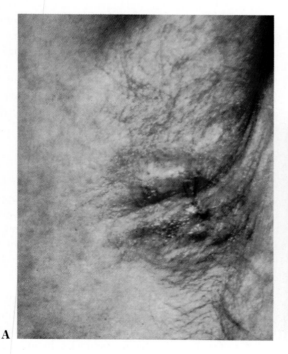
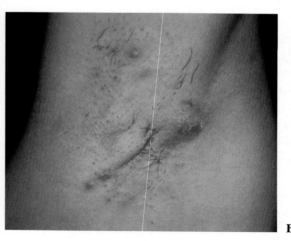

**FIGURE 21-6** ■ **(A)** Sweat gland inflammation of the axilla (hidradenitis suppurativa). *(Courtesy of Abner Kurtin, Folia Dermatologica, No. 2. Geigy Pharmaceuticals.)* **(B)** Hidradenitis suppurativa of the axilla of 6 years' duration. *(Courtesy of Burroughs Wellcome Co.)*

## Treatment

The management of these cases is difficult. In addition to the general principles mentioned previously, hot packs used locally and an oral antibiotic, especially tetracycline, should be given for several weeks.

Plastic surgery or a marsupialization operation is indicated in severe cases. When draining canals or sinuses are present, the marsupialization operation is curative and can be done in the office. After the bridge over the canal has been trimmed away, bleeding is controlled by electrosurgery. These areas can be treated with intralesional corticosteroid injections. Laser therapy has its advocates. Isotretinoin (Accutane) can be tried for 5 to 10 months (see Chapter 13). Do not give if there is a chance of pregnancy.

## Erysipelas

Erysipelas is an uncommon β-hemolytic streptococcal infection of the subcutaneous tissue that produces a characteristic type of cellulitis (**Fig. 21-7**), with fever and malaise. Recurrences are frequent.

### Primary Lesion

A red, warm, raised, brawny, sharply bordered plaque enlarges peripherally. Vesicles and bullae may form on the surface of the plaque. Multiple lesions of erysipelas are rare.

### Distribution

Most commonly lesions occur on the face and around the ears (following ear piercing), but no area is exempt. Some authors now think the legs are the most common site.

### Course

When treated with systemic antibiotics, response is rapid. Recurrences are common in the same location and may lead to lymphedema of that area, which eventually can become

irreversible. The lips, cheeks, and legs are particularly prone to this chronic change, which is called *elephantiasis nostras* or when the area develops a more warty appearance, elephantiasis nostra verrucosa.

### Subjective Complaints

Fever and general malaise can precede the development of the skin lesion and persist until therapy is instituted. Elderly patients may present with altered sensorium and somnolence. Pain at the site of the infection can be severe.

### Differential Diagnosis

- *Cellulitis:* Lacks a sharp border; recurrences are less common
- *Contact dermatitis:* Sharp border absent; fever and malaise absent; eruption predominantly vesicular and very pruritic rather than painful (see Chapter 8)

### Treatment

1. Institute bed rest and direct therapy toward reducing the fever. If the patient is hospitalized, semi-isolation procedures should be initiated. Blood cultures should be considered to rule out sepsis.
2. Give an appropriate systemic antibiotic, such as erythromycin or a penicillin derivative, for 10 days.
3. Apply local, cool, wet dressing, as necessary for comfort.

## Erythrasma

Erythrasma is an uncommon bacterial infection of the skin that clinically resembles regular tinea or tinea versicolor (**Fig. 21-8**). It affects the crural area, axillae, and webs of the toes with flat, hyperpigmented, fine, scaly patches without central clearing or an elevated edge as in tinea cruris. If the patient has not been using an antibacterial soap, these patches fluoresce a striking reddish orange coral color under Wood's light. The causative agent is a diphtheroid organism called *Corynebacterium minutussimum.*

The most effective treatment is erythromycin, 250 mg, q.i.d. for 5 to 7 days. Locally the erythromycin lotions are quite effective (e.g., Staticin, T-Stat, EryDerm, and A/T/S lotion [can obtain generically]). They are applied twice daily for 10 days.

## Secondary Bacterial Infections

Secondary infection develops as a complicating factor on a preexisting skin disease. The invasion of an injured skin surface with pathogenic streptococci or staphylococci is enhanced in skin conditions that are open, deep, oozing, and of long duration.

### Cutaneous Diseases with Secondary Infection

Failure in the treatment of many common skin diseases can be attributed to the physician's not recognizing the presence of the secondary bacterial infection.

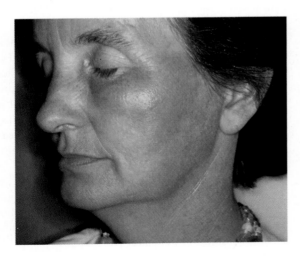

**FIGURE 21-7** ■ Erysipelas of the cheek. (*Courtesy of Burroughs Wellcome Co.*)

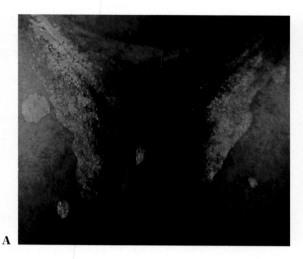
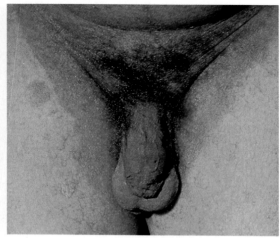

**FIGURE 21-8** ■ Erythrasma of the crural area with fluorescence under Wood's light (**A**) and in natural light (**B**). *(Courtesy of Burroughs Wellcome Co.)*

## Infected Ulcers

Infected ulcers (see Chapter 12) are deep skin infections owing to an injury or disease that invades the subcutaneous tissue and, upon healing, leaves scars. Ulcers can be divided into primary and secondary ulcers, but most become secondarily infected with bacteria.

### Primary Infected Ulcers

Primary ulcers from infection result from the following causes: gangrene owing to pathogenic streptococci, staphylococci, and *Clostridium* species; syphilis; chancroid; tuberculosis; diphtheria; fungi; leprosy; anthrax; cancer; and lymphomas.

### Secondary Infected Ulcers

Secondary ulcers can be related to the following diseases: vascular disorders (arteriosclerosis, thromboangiitis obliterans, Raynaud's phenomenon, phlebitis, thrombosis); neurologic disorders (spinal cord injury with bedsores or decubiti, central nervous system syphilis, spina bifida, poliomyelitis, syringomyelia); diabetes; trauma; ulcerative colitis; Crohn's disease; immunosuppression; allergic local anaphylaxis; and other conditions. Finally, there is a group of secondary ulcers called *phagedenic ulcers,* variously described under many different names. These arise in diseased skin or on the apparently normal skin of debilitated persons. These ulcers undermine the skin in large areas, are notoriously chronic, and are resistant to therapy.

### Treatment

1. For primary ulcers, specific therapy is indicated, if available. The response to therapy is usually quite rapid.
2. For secondary ulcers, appropriate therapy should be directed toward the primary disease. The response to therapy is usually quite slow. This is especially true for the decubitus ulcer of the immobile, incontinent person. These must be kept clean and the patient must be kept off the pressure site where the ulcer has developed as much as possible. Early in these ulcers, I use Johnson & Johnson self-healing pads for protection. It is cheap and can be left on and replaced indefinitely.
3. The basic rules of local therapy for ulcers can be illustrated best by outlining the management of a patient with a stasis leg ulcer (see Stasis (Venous) Dermatitis and Ulcers section in Chapter 12).
   a. Rest of the affected area: If rest in bed is not feasible, then an Ace elastic bandage, 4 in wide, should be worn. This bandage is applied over the local medication and before getting out of bed in the morning. A more permanent support is a modification of an Unna boot (Dome-Paste bandage, Gelocast, or an easy-to-apply and effective adhesive flexible bandage). This boot can be applied for 1 week or more at a time if secondary infection is under control.
   b. Elevation of the affected extremity: This should be carried out in bed and can be accomplished by placing two bricks, flat surface down, under both feet of the bed. (Arteriosclerotic leg ulcers should not be elevated.)
   c. Burow's solution wet packs

      *Sig:* one packet of Domeboro powder to 1 quart of warm water. Apply wet dressings of gauze or sheeting for 30 minutes t.i.d.

---

**SAUER'S NOTES**

1. Any type of skin lesion, such as hand dermatitis, poison weed dermatitis, atopic eczema, chigger bites, fungus infection, traumatic abrasion, and so on, can become secondarily infected.
2. The treatment is usually simple: An antibacterial agent is added to the local treatment one would ordinarily use for the dermatosis in question. For extensive secondary bacterial infection, the appropriate systemic antibiotic is indicated, based on bacterial culture and sensitivity studies.

d. If debridement is necessary, this can be accomplished by enzymes, such as Debrisan, Santyl (collagenase) ointment, Acuzyme, Panafil, or Elase ointment, applied twice a day and covered with gauze. Surgical debridement is often beneficial.

e. Gentian violet 1%

Distilled water q.s. 15.0

*Sig:* Apply to ulcer b.i.d. with applicator.

*Comment:* A liquid is usually better tolerated on ulcers than a salve. If the gentian violet solution becomes too drying, the following salve can be used alternately for short periods.

f. Bactroban or other antibiotic ointment q.s. 15.0

*Sig:* Apply to ulcer and surrounding skin b.i.d.

g. Long-term erythromycin or cephalexin therapy: 250 mg, one capsule q.i.d. for 14 or more days, then one capsule b.i.d. for weeks, is helpful for chronic pyogenic ulcers. Other systemic antibiotics may be used.

h. Low-dose oral corticosteroid therapy: prednisone, 10 mg

*Sig:* one or two tablets every morning for 3 to 4 weeks, then one tablet every other morning for months. When this is added to the above routine many indolent ulcers heal.

*Comment:* The best treatment for one ulcer does not necessarily work for another ulcer. Many other local medications are available and valuable.

4. Surgical management, such as excision and grafting, may be indicated.

5. Various surgical dressings may be beneficial, such as OpSite, Duoderm, Tegaderm, or Polymem; Johnson & Johnson makes an inexpensive surgical wound dressing.

6. Silver-impregnated topicals and negative pressure therapy are newer therapies.

7. Hyperbaric oxygenation may also be beneficial.

## Infectious Eczematoid Dermatitis

The term *infectious eczematoid dermatitis* or *auto eczematous dermatitis* is more often used incorrectly than correctly. Infectious eczematoid dermatitis is an uncommon disease characterized by the development of an acute eruption around an infected exudative primary site, such as a draining ear, mastitis, a boil, or a seeping ulcer (Fig. 21-9). Widespread

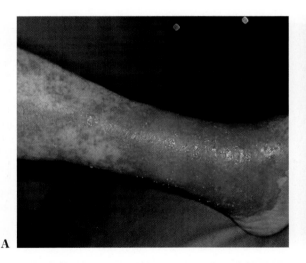
A

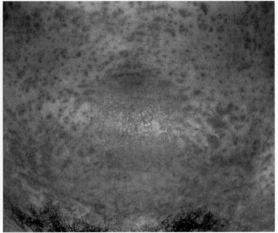
B

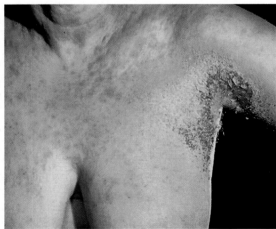
C

**FIGURE 21-9** ■ Bacterial infections of skin. *(Courtesy of Burroughs Wellcome Co.)* Infectious eczematoid dermatitis **(A)** from stasis dermatitis of the legs with a spread to the body **(B)**. **(C)** Infectious eczematoid dermatitis in the axilla.

**SAUER'S NOTES**

The primary factor in the management of an ulcer is to not let it happen. This is especially appropriate for decubitus ulcers. Frequent turning of the bedridden patient, air pressure mattresses, and devices to prevent rollover onto the back are helpful.

eczematous lesions can develop at a distant site from the primary infection, presumably owing to an immune phenomenon, and *autoeczemtous dermatitis* or so-called *id reaction*.

### Primary Lesions

Vesicles and pustules in circumscribed plaques spread peripherally from an infected central source. Central healing usually does not occur, as in ringworm infection.

### Secondary Lesions

Crusting, oozing, and scaling predominate in widespread cases.

### Distribution

Mild cases may be confined to a small area around the exudative primary infection, but widespread cases can cover the entire body, obscuring the initial cause.

### Course

The course depends on the extent of the eruption. Chronic cases respond poorly to therapy. Recurrences are common even after the primary source is healed.

### Subjective Complaints

Itching is usually present.

### Cause

Coagulase-positive staphylococci are frequently isolated.

### Differential Diagnosis

- *Contact dermatitis with secondary infection:* No history or finding of primary exudative infection; history of contact with poison ivy, new clothes, cosmetics, or dishwater; responds faster to therapy (see Chapter 8)
- *Nummular eczema:* No primary infected source; coin-shaped lesions on extremities; clinical differentiation of some cases difficult (see Chapter 8)
- *Seborrheic dermatitis:* No primary infected source; seborrhea–acne complex, with greasy, scaly eruption in hairy areas (see Chapter 13)
- *Eczematous psoriasis:* A recently described skin ailment with the appearance of diffuse severe nummular eczema, but with a response to therapy mimicking that of psoriasis

### Treatment

*Case Example:* An 8-year-old boy presents with draining otitis media and pustular, crusted dermatitis on the side of the face, neck, and scalp.

1. Treat the primary source—the ear infection, in this case.
2. Apply Burow's solution wet packs
   *Sig:* one packet of Domeboro powder to 1 quart of warm water. Apply wet sheeting or gauze to the area for 20 minutes t.i.d.
3. Apply antibiotic and corticosteroid cream, such as

   Bactroban ointment 15.0
   Triamcinolone 0.1% cream 15.0
   *Sig:* Apply t.i.d. locally, after the wet packs are removed. A patient with a widespread case might require hospitalization, daily mild soap baths, oral antibiotics, or corticosteroid systemic therapy.

## Bacterial Intertrigo

The presence of friction, heat, and moisture in areas where two opposing skin surfaces contact each other leads to a secondary bacterial, fungus, or yeast infection.

### Primary Lesion

Redness from friction and heat of opposing forces and maceration from an inability of the sweat to evaporate freely leads to an eroded patch of dermatitis.

### Secondary Lesion

The bacterial infection may become severe enough to result in fissures and cellulitis.

### Distribution

The inframammary region, axillae, umbilicus, pubic, crural, genital, and perianal areas as well as the areas between the toes may be involved.

### Course

In certain persons intertrigo tends to recur each summer.

### Causes

The factors of obesity, diabetes, and prolonged contact with urine, feces, and menstrual discharges predispose to the development of intertrigo. AIDS may present with recurrent bullous groin impetigo.

### Differential Diagnosis

- *Candidal intertrigo:* Scaling at the border of the erosion with an overhanging fringe of epidermis; presence of surrounding small satellite lesions; scraping and culture reveals *Candida albicans* (see Chapter 25)
- *Tinea:* Scaly or papulovesicular elevated border; scraping and culture are positive for fungi (see Chapter 25)

- *Seborrheic dermatitis:* Greasy red scaly areas, also seen on the scalp. Bacterial intertrigo may coexist with seborrheic dermatitis (see Chapter 13)

### Treatment

**Case Example.** A 6-month-old infant presents with red, pustular dermatitis in the diaper area, axillae, and folds of the neck.

1. Bathe the child once a day in lukewarm water with antibacterial soap. Dry affected areas thoroughly.
2. Double rinse diapers to remove all soap or use disposable diapers.
3. Change diapers as frequently as possible and apply a powder each time, such as

   Talc, unscented (Zeasorb) 45.0
4. Hydrocortisone 1%

   Bactroban ointment q.s. 15.0

   *Sig:* Apply to affected areas t.i.d. Continue local therapy for at least 1 week after dermatitis is apparently clear—"therapy plus." Allow only two refills of this salve to avoid atrophy of the skin.

## Systemic Bacterial Infections

### Scarlet Fever

Scarlet fever is a less common streptococcal infection characterized by a streptococci pyogenes culture (+) sore throat, high fever, and a scarlet rash. Less commonly, the skin can be the source of the streptoccoal infection. Decreased incidence in recent decades is probably related to different "phase"-type streptococci. The skin rash is caused by the production of an exotoxin. Pastia's sign is pink, red, or hemorrhagic transverse lines at the elbow, wrist, or inguinal areas 2 to 3 days after the fever. Pastia's sign occurs before the skin eruption begins and persists after the eruption is gone. The eruption develops after a day of rapidly rising fever, headache, sore throat, and various other symptoms. The rash begins first on the neck and the chest, and rapidly spreads over the entire body, except for the area around the mouth. Close examination of the pale scarlet eruption reveals it to be made up of diffuse pinhead-sized, or larger, macules. In untreated cases the rash reaches its peak on the fourth day, and scaling commences around the seventh day and continues for 1 or 2 weeks. "Strawberry tongue" is seen at the height of the eruption. Erythema nodosum can also occur.

The presence of petechiae on the body is a grave prognostic sign. Complications are numerous and common in untreated cases. Glomerulonephritis and rheumatic fever with consequent rheumatic heart disease may develop.

### Differential Diagnosis

- *Measles:* Early rash on face and forehead; larger macular rash; running eyes; photophobia; cough (see Chapter 23)

- *Drug eruption:* Lack of high fever and other constitutional signs; atropine and quinine can cause an eruption that is clinically similar to scarlet fever (see Chapter 8)

### Treatment

Penicillin or a similar systemic antibiotic is the therapy of choice. Complications should be watched for and should be treated early.

## Granuloma Inguinale

Before the use of antibiotics, particularly streptomycin and tetracycline, this disease was one of the most chronic and resistant afflictions of humans. Formerly, it was a rather common disease. Granuloma inguinale should be considered a venereal disease, although other factors may have to be present to initiate infection.

### Primary Lesion

An irregularly shaped, bright red, velvety appearing, flat ulcer with a rolled border is seen (Fig. 21-10).

### Secondary Lesions

Scarring may lead to complications similar to those seen with lymphogranuloma venereum. Squamous cell carcinoma can develop in old, chronic lesions.

### Distribution

Genital lesions are most common on the penis, scrotum, labia, cervix, or inguinal region.

### Course

Without therapy, the granuloma grows slowly and persists for years, causing marked scarring and mutilation. Under modern therapy, healing is rapid, but recurrences are not unusual.

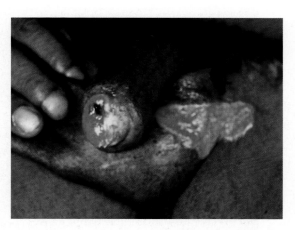

**FIGURE 21-10** ■ Granuloma inguinale of the penis and crural area. *(Courtesy of Derm-Arts Laboratories.)*

### Cause

Granuloma inguinale is due to *Calymmatobacterium granulomatis,* which can be cultured on special media.

### Laboratory Findings

Scrapings of the lesion reveal Donovan bodies, which are dark-staining, intracytoplasmic, cigar-shaped bacilli found in large macrophages. The material for the smear can be obtained best by snipping off a piece of the lesion with small scissors and rubbing the tissue on several slides. Wright or Giemsa stains can be used.

### Differential Diagnosis

- *Granuloma pyogenicum:* Small lesion; history of injury, usually; short duration; rarely on genitalia; bright red and bleeds easily; no Donovan bodies
- *Primary syphilis:* Short duration; inguinal adenopathy; serology may be positive; spirochetes (see Chapter 26)
- *Chancroid:* Short duration; lesion is small, not red and velvety; no Donovan bodies (see next section)
- *Squamous cell carcinoma:* More indurated lesion with nodule; may coexist with granuloma inguinale; biopsy specific

### Treatment

Tetracycline, 500 mg q.i.d., is continued until all the lesions are healed.

## Chancroid

Chancroid is a venereal disease with a very short incubation period of 1 to 5 days. It is caused by *Haemophilus ducreyi.*

### Primary Lesion

Small, superficial, or deep erosions occur with surrounding redness and edema (Fig. 21-11). This is referred to as a, "soft chancre" versus the "hard chancre" of syphilis with an indurated border. Multiple genital or distant lesions can be produced by autoinoculation.

### Secondary Lesions

Deep, destructive ulcers form in chronic cases, which may lead to gangrene. Marked regional adenopathy, usually unilateral, is common and eventually suppurates in untreated cases.

### Course

Without therapy most cases heal within 1 to 2 weeks. In rare cases, severe local destruction and draining lymph nodes (buboes) result. Early therapy is effective.

### Laboratory Findings

The organisms are arranged in "schools of fish" and can often be demonstrated in smears of clean lesions.

### Differential Diagnosis

- *Primary or secondary syphilis genital lesions:* Longer incubation period; more induration; *Treponema pallidum* found on darkfield examination; serology positive in late primary and secondary stage (see Chapter 26)
- *Herpes simplex progenitalis:* Recurrent multiple painful blisters or erosions; mild inguinal adenopathy; initial episode may have systemic symptoms (see Chapter 26)

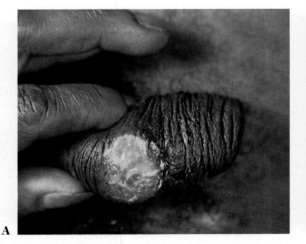

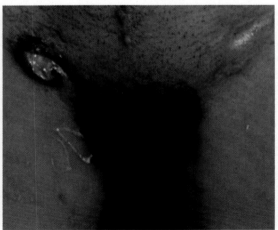

**FIGURE 21-11** ■ **(A)** Chancroid of the penis. **(B)** Chancroid buboes in the inguinal area. *(Courtesy of Derm-Arts Laboratories.)*

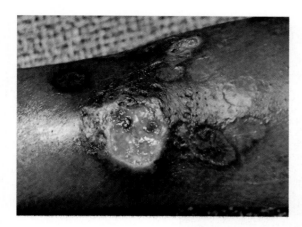

**FIGURE 21-12** ■ Tuberculosis ulcer of the leg. *(Courtesy of Derm-Arts Laboratories.)*

■ *Lymphogranuloma venereum:* Primary lesion rare; Frei test positive (see Chapter 26)
■ *Granuloma inguinale:* Chronic, red velvety plaque; Donovan bodies seen on tissue smear (see preceding section)

### Treatment

The therapy for chancroid is a sulfonamide such as sulfisoxazole, 1 g q.i.d. for 2 weeks, or erythromycin, 2 g/d for 10 to 15 days. Third-generation cephalosporins are also effective. A fluctuant bubo should never be incised but should be aspirated with a large needle.

## Tuberculosis

Skin tuberculosis (Fig. 21-12) is rare in the United States. However, a text on dermatology would not be complete without some mention of this infection. Although the incidence has been decreasing in the United States and leveled off worldwide since 1992, it is still a significant disease worldwide, and multidrug-resistant tuberculosis (MDR-TB), especially in AIDS patients, is a particularly difficult problem. AIDS and tuberculosis act as synergestic infections. An even more resistant form of tuberculosis is now reported called extensively drug-resistant tuberculosis (XDR-TB). The most common cutaneous tuberculosis infection, lupus vulgaris, is discussed. A classification of skin tuberculosis is given in Table 21-2.

### Presentation and Characteristics

*Lupus vulgaris* is a chronic, granulomatous disease characterized by the development of nodules, ulcers, and plaques arranged in any conceivable configuration. In severe, untreated cases, scarring in the center of active lesions or at the edge can lead to atrophy and contraction. This can result in mutilating changes.

### Distribution

Facial involvement is most common.

---

**TABLE 21-2** ■ **Classification of Cutaneous Tuberculosis**

**True Cutaneous Tuberculosis (Lesions Contain Tubercle Bacilli)**

1. *Primary tuberculosis* (no previous infection; tuberculin-negative in initial stages)
   a. Primary inoculation tuberculosis; Tuberculosis chancre (exogenous implantation into skin producing the primary complex)
   b. Miliary tuberculosis of the skin (hematogenous dispersion)
2. *Secondary tuberculosis* (lesions develop in a person already sensitive to tuberculin as a result of prior tuberculous lesion; tubercle bacilli are difficult or impossible to demonstrate)
   a. Lupus vulgaris (inoculation of tubercle bacilli into the skin from external or internal sources)
   b. Tuberculosis verrucosa cutis (inoculation of tubercle bacilli into the skin from external or internal sources)
   c. Scrofuloderma (extension to the skin from an underlying focus in the bones or glands)
   d. Tuberculosis cutis orificialis (mucous membrane lesions and extension onto the skin near mucocutaneous junctions)

**Tuberculids (Allergic Origin; No Tubercle Bacilli in Lesions)**

1. *Papular forms*
   a. Lupus miliaris disseminatus faciei (purely papular)
   b. Papulonecrotic tuberculid (papules with necrosis)
   c. Lichen scrofulosorum (follicular papules or lichenoid papules)
2. *Granulomatous, ulceronodular forms*
   a. Erythema induratum (nodules or plaques subsequently ulcerating; may be a nonspecific vasculitis)

---

### Course

The course is often slow and progressive, in spite of therapy.

### Laboratory Findings

The histopathology shows typical tubercle formation with epithelioid cells, giant cells, and a peripheral zone of lymphocytes. The causative organism, *Mycobacterium tuberculosis,* is not abundant in the lesions. The 48-hour tuberculin test is usually positive.

### Differential Diagnosis

Other granulomas, such as those associated with syphilis, leprosy, sarcoidosis, deep fungal disease, and neoplasm, are to be ruled out by appropriate studies (see Chapter 16).

### Treatment

Early localized lesions can be treated by surgical excision. For more widespread cases, long-term systemic therapy offers

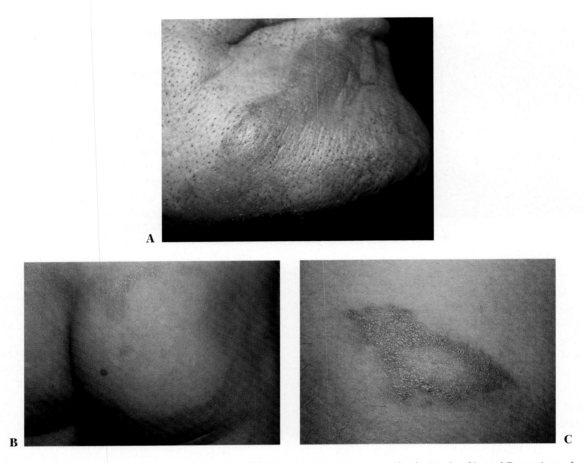

**FIGURE 21-13** ■ **(A)** Tuberculoid leprosy of the chin. **(B)** Tuberculoid leprosy on the buttocks. (A and B *courtesy of Drs. W. Schorr and F. Kerdel-Vegas.*) **(C)** Tuberculoid leprosy on the chest. *(Courtesy of Dr. M. Rico, Durham, NC.)*

high hopes for cure. Isoniazid is usually prescribed along with other antituberculous drugs, such as rifampin and ethambutol (Myambutol). MDR-TB is an increasing problem in AIDS patients.

## Leprosy

Leprosy, or Hansen's disease, is to be considered in the differential diagnosis of any skin granulomas. It is endemic in the southern part of the United States and all over the world in semitropical and tropical areas.

### Presentation and Characteristics

Two definite types of leprosy are recognized: tuberculoid (Fig. 21-13) and lepromatous (Fig. 21-14). In addition, there are cases, called *dimorphic leprosy* (Fig. 21-15) that cannot presently be classified in either of these two categories. These

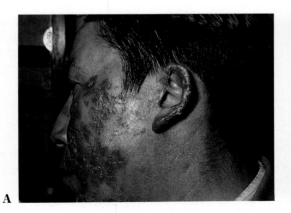

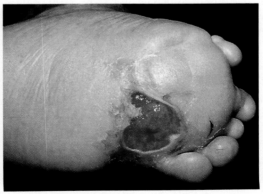

**FIGURE 21-14** ■ **(A)** Lepromatous leprosy. *(Courtesy of Dr. A. Gongalez-Ochoa, Mexico.)* **(B)** Lepromatous leprosy on the foot. *(Courtesy of Dr. M. Rico, Durham, NC.)*

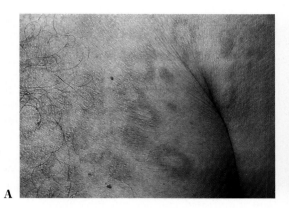 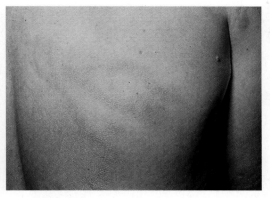

**FIGURE 21-15** ■ **(A)** Dimorphic leprosy on the chest. *(Courtesy of Dr. R. Caputo, Atlanta, GA.)* **(B)** Dimorphic leprosy on the back. *(Courtesy of Dr. M. Rico, Durham, NC.)*

patients eventually develop either lepromatous or tuberculoid leprosy.

*Tuberculoid leprosy* is generally benign in its course because of considerable resistance to the disease on the part of the host. This is manifested by a positive lepromin test, histology that is not diagnostic, cutaneous lesions that are frequently erythematous with elevated borders, and minimal effect of the disease on the general health of the patient.

*Lepromatous leprosy* is the malignant form, and represents minimal resistance to the disease, with a negative lepromin reaction, characteristic histologic appearance, infiltrated cutaneous lesions with ill-defined borders, and unless treated, progression to death, usually from secondary amyloidosis.

Early symptoms of the lepromatous type include reddish macules with an indefinite border, nasal obstruction, and nosebleeds. Erythema nodosum–like lesions commonly occur. The tuberculoid type of leprosy is often first diagnosed in what's called an indeterminant form. The indeterminant form presents as an area of skin with decreased sensation, polyneuritis, and skin lesions with a sharp border and central atrophy.

### Cause

The causative organism is *Mycobacterium leprae.*

### Contagiousness

The source of infection is believed to be from patients with the lepromatous form.

### Laboratory Findings

The bacilli are usually discovered in the lepromatous type but seldom in the tuberculoid type. Smears should be obtained from the exposed tissue by a small incision made into the dermis through an infiltrated lesion.

The lepromin reaction, a delayed reaction test similar to the tuberculin test, is of value in differentiating the lepromatous form from the tuberculoid form of leprosy, as previously mentioned. False-positive reactions do occur.

Biologic false-positive tests for syphilis are common in patients with the lepromatous type of leprosy.

### Differential Diagnosis

Consider any of the granulomatous diseases, such as

- *syphilis,*
- *tuberculosis,*
- *sarcoidosis,* and
- *deep fungal infections.*

See also Chapter 16.

### Treatment

Dapsone (diaminodiphenylsulfone), rifampin, and isoniazid are all effective.

## Other Mycobacterial Dermatoses

Mycobacteria are pathogenic (tuberculosis and leprosy) and saprophytic or environmental (atypical mycobacteria). *Mycobacterium marinum* is the most common saprophytic mycobacteria to cause disease in humans and can cause swimming pool granuloma, granulomas in fishermen, and granulomas in workers or people involved with fish tanks. Minocycline and combinations of either ethambutol, rifampin, clarithromycin, or levofloxacin have been used as treatments.

*Mycobacterium avium-intracellulare* is seen in patients with AIDS, but skin lesions are rare.

## Gonorrhea

Gonorrhea is considerably more prevalent than syphilis. Skin lesions with gonorrheal infection are rare. Untreated or inadequately treated infection due to *Neisseria gonorrhoeae* can involve the skin through metastatic spread (**Fig. 21-16**). Primary cutaneous infection with multiple erosions at the site of the purulent discharge is very rare.

Metastatic complications include a bacteremia, in which there is an intermittent high fever, arthralgia, and

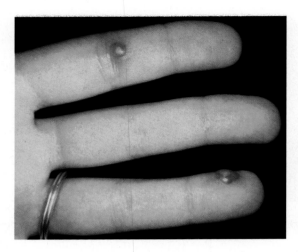

**FIGURE 21-16** ■ Gonococcal septicemia with hemor-rhagic vesicles. *(Courtesy of Derm-Arts Laboratories.)*

skin lesions. The skin lesions are characteristic hemorrhagic vesiculopustules, most commonly seen on the fingers. Arthalgias are common. Treatment with intravenous penicillin for 10 days at 5 to 10 million units per day is indicated.

The rarer septicemic form, with very high fever and meningitis or endocarditis, can have purpuric skin lesions similar to those seen in meningococcemia.

## Rickettsial Diseases

The most common rickettsial disease in the United States is Rocky Mountain spotted fever, which is spread by ticks of various types. The skin eruption occurs after 3 to 7 days of fever and other toxic signs. It is characterized by purpuric lesions on the extremities, mainly the wrists and the ankles, which then become generalized. The Weil–Felix test using *Proteus* OX19 and OX2 is positive. Tetracycline and chloramphenicol are effective treatment modalities.

The typhus group of rickettsial diseases includes epidemic or louse-borne typhus, Brill's disease, and endemic murine or flea-borne typhus. Less common forms include scrub typhus (tsutsugamushi disease), trench fever, and rickettsialpox, which are produced by a mite bite. The mite ordinarily lives on rodents. Approximately 10 days after the bite a primary lesion develops in the form of a papule that becomes vesicular. After a few days of fever and other toxic signs, a generalized eruption that resembles chickenpox appears. The disease subsides without therapy.

Ehrlichiosis is another rickettsial disease well known in dogs and now seen in humans. It is transmitted by a tick bite. The nonspecific symptoms are similar to those of Rocky Mountain spotted fever, but only 20% of the patients have a rash.

## Actinomycosis

Actinomycosis is a chronic, granulomatous, suppurative infection that characteristically causes the formation of a draining sinus. The most common location of the draining sinus is in the jaw region, but thoracic and abdominal sinuses can also occur.

### Primary Lesion

A red, firm, nontender tumor in the jaw area slowly extends locally to form a "lumpy jaw." It mimics a draining dental sinus from an infected tooth.

### Secondary Lesions

Discharging sinuses become infected with other bacteria and, if untreated, may develop into osteomyelitis.

### Course

General health is usually unaffected unless extension occurs into bone or deeper neck tissues. Recurrence is unusual if treatment is continued long enough.

### Cause

*Actinomyces israelii,* which is an anaerobic bacterium that lives as a normal inhabitant of the mouth, particularly in persons who have poor dental hygiene, is the causative agent. Injury to the jaw or a tooth extraction usually precedes the development of the infection. Infected cattle are not the source of human infection. The disease is twice as common in men as in women.

### Laboratory Findings

Pinpoint-sized "sulfur" granules, which are colonies of the organism, can be seen grossly and microscopically in the draining pus. A Gram stain of the pus shows masses of interlacing gram-positive fibers with or without club-shaped processes at the tips of these fibers. The organism can be cultured anaerobically on special media.

### Differential Diagnosis

- *Pyodermas*
- *Tuberculosis*
- *Draining dental abscess*
- *Neoplasm*

### Treatment

1. Penicillin, 2.4 million units intramuscularly, is given daily, until definite improvement is noted. Then oral penicillin in the same dosage should be continued for 3 weeks after the infection apparently has been cured. In severe cases, 10 million or more units of penicillin given intravenously, daily, may be necessary.
2. Incision and drainage is performed on the lumps in the sinuses.
3. Good oral hygiene is required.
4. In resistant cases, broad-spectrum antibiotics can be used alone or in combination with the penicillin.

## Suggested Readings

Aly R, Maibach H. *Atlas of the infections of the skin.* Philadelphia, PA: WB Saunders; 1998.

Daum SD. Skin and soft tissue infections caused by methicillin-resistant *Staphylococcus aureus. N Engl J Med.* 2007;357:380–390.

Drugs for sexually transmitted infections. *Med Lett Drugs Ther.* 1999;41: 85–90.

Epstein ME, Amodio-Groton M, Sadick NS. Antimicrobial agents for the dermatologist: I. β-Lactam antibiotics and related compounds. *J Am Acad Dermatol.* 1997;37(2):149–165.

Epstein ME, Amodio-Groton M, Sadick NS. Antimicrobial agents for the dermatologist: II. Macrolides, fluoroquinolones, rifamycins, tetracyclines, trimethoprim-sulfamethoxazole, and clindamycin. *J Am Acad Dermatol.* 1997;37(3):365–381.

Lesher JL. *An atlas of microbiology of the skin.* London: Parthenon Publishing Group; 2000.

Modlin RL, Rea TH. Leprosy: New insight into an ancient disease. *J Am Acad Dermatol.* 1987;17(1):1–13.

Moschella SL. An update on the diagnosis and treatment of leprosy. *J Am Acad Dermatol.* 2004;51:417–426.

Parish LC, Witkowksi JA, Crissey JT. *The decubitus ulcer in clinical practice.* New York: Springer; 1997.

Sanders CV. *Skin and infection: A color atlas and text.* Baltimore: Williams & Wilkins; 1995.

Sehgal VN, Wagh SA. Cutaneous tuberculosis. *Int J Dermatol.* 1990;29: 237–252.

Spach DH, Liles WC, Campbell GL, et al. Tick-borne diseases in the United States: Review article. *N Engl J Med.* 1993;329:936–947.

# CHAPTER 22

# Spirochetal Infections

*John C. Hall, MD*

Two spirochetal diseases are discussed in this chapter: syphilis and Lyme disease.

## Syphilis

When Gordon C. Sauer was stationed at the West Virginia State Rapid Treatment Center, from 1946 to 1948, the average for patient admittance was 30 a day. Approximately one third of these patients had infectious syphilis. In 1949, the center was closed because of the patient census. Today, the incidence of reported syphilis has risen again to alarming heights. Many patients with acquired immunodeficiency syndrome (AIDS) also have syphilis. Because of this resurgence, it is imperative that all physicians have a basic understanding of this polymorphous disease.

Cutaneous lesions of syphilis occur in all three stages of the disease. Under what circumstances will the present-day physician be called on to diagnose, evaluate, or manage a patient with syphilis?

1. The cutaneous manifestations, such as a penile lesion or a rash that could be secondary syphilis, may bring a patient into the office.
2. A positive blood test found on a premarital examination or as part of a routine physical examination may be the reason for a patient's visit to the dermatologist.
3. Syphilis may be seen in conjunction with AIDS. The problem becomes complicated because the serologic test for syphilis (STS) may not be positive in patients with AIDS and routine antibiotic dosage regimens may be ineffective.
4. Cardiac, central nervous system, or other organ disease may be a reason for a patient to consult a physician.

To manage these patients properly, a thorough knowledge of the natural untreated course of the disease is essential.

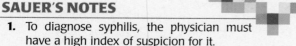

**SAUER'S NOTES**

1. To diagnose syphilis, the physician must have a high index of suspicion for it.
2. Syphilis is the great imitator and can mimic many other conditions.
3. Serologic tests for syphilis in AIDS may be falsely (−).

### Primary Syphilis

The first stage of acquired syphilis usually develops within 2 to 6 weeks (average 3 weeks) after exposure. The *primary chancre* most commonly occurs on the genitalia (Figs. 22-1 and 22-2), but extragenital chancres are not rare and are often misdiagnosed. Without treatment the chancre heals within 1 to 4 weeks but is dependent on the location, the amount of secondary infection, and host resistance.

The blood STS may be negative in the early days of the chancre but eventually becomes positive. The spirochete, *Treponema pallidum,* is readily found with darkfield examination. This test is of limited value since there are few people with the expertise to interpret the test reliably. A cerebrospinal fluid examination by darkfield during the primary stage reveals invasion of the spirochete in approximately 25% of cases.

Clinically, the chancre may vary in appearance from a single small erosion to multiple indurated ulcers of the genitalia. It is usually painless and with an indurated border ("hard chancre"). Primary syphilis commonly goes unnoticed in the female patient due to its intravaginal or rectal location. Men who have sex with men (MSM) may also have hidden rectal chancres. Bilateral or unilateral regional lymphadenopathy is common. Malaise and fever may also be present.

### Early Latent Stage

Latency, manifested by positive serologic findings and no other subjective or objective evidence of syphilis, may occur between the primary and secondary stages.

### Secondary Syphilis

*Early secondary lesions* may develop before the primary chancre has healed or after latency of a few weeks (Figs. 22-3 to 22-5). *Late secondary lesions* are more rare and usually are seen after the early secondary lesions have healed. Both types of secondary lesions contain the spirochete *T. pallidum,* which can be easily seen with the darkfield microscope. The STS is positive (an exception is in some patients with AIDS), and approximately 30% of the cases have abnormal cerebrospinal fluid findings.

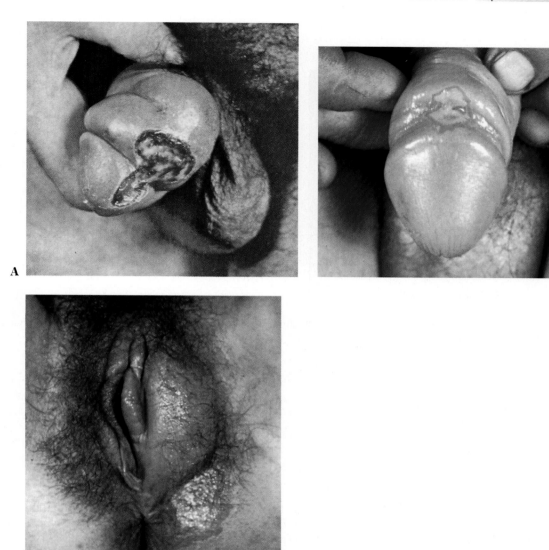

**FIGURE 22-1** ■ Primary syphilis with primary chancres of the genitalia. **(A)** Chancre of the penis is accompanied by marked edema of the penis. **(B)** Penile chancre. **(C)** Vulvar chancre with edema of the labia majora. *(Courtesy of J.E. Moore and The Upjohn Company.)*

Clinically, the early secondary rash can consist of macular, papular, pustular, squamous, or eroded lesions or combinations of any of these lesions. Papulosquamous is most common with oval lesions and fine dry adherent scale. This can easily be confused with pityriasis rosea. Palm and sole involvement is characteristic and there is no herald patch. Secondary syphilis can be generalized or localized to the palms and soles, genital area, or mucous membranes. A "moth-eaten" scalp alopecia may develop in the late secondary stage.

*Condylomata lata* is the name applied to the flat, moist, warty lesions teeming with spirochetes found in the groin and the axillae (Figs. 22-4 and 22-5). Mucous patches are white elevated verrucous skin lesions usually on the oral mucous membranes.

The late secondary lesions are nodular, squamous, and ulcerative and are distinguished from the tertiary lesions only by the time interval after the onset of the infection and by the finding of the spirochete in superficial smears of serum from the lesions. Annular and semiannular configurations of late secondary lesions are common.

Generalized lymphadenopathy, malaise, fever, and arthralgias occur in many patients with secondary syphilis.

*Early Latent Stage*

Following the secondary stage, many patients with untreated syphilis have only a positive STS. After 4 years of infection, the patient enters the late latent stage.

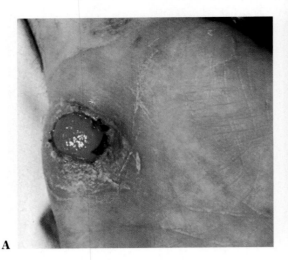
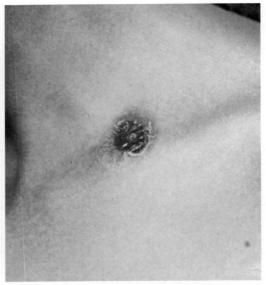

A                                                            B

**FIGURE 22-2** ■ Primary syphilis with extragenital chancres. **(A)** Chancre of the palm. **(B)** Chancre over the clavicle. *(Courtesy of The Upjohn Company.)*

### Late Latent Stage

This time span of 4 years arbitrarily divides the early infectious stages from the later noninfectious stages, which may or may not develop.

### Tertiary Syphilis

This late stage is manifested by subjective or objective involvement of any of the organs of the body, including the skin (Figs. 22-6 and 22-7; see also Fig. 3-1A). Tertiary changes may be precocious but most often develop 5 to 20 years after the onset of the primary stage. Clinically, the skin lesions are characterized by nodular and gummatous ulcerations. Solitary multiple annular and nodular lesions are common. Subjective complaints are rare unless considerable secondary bacterial infection is present in a gumma. Scarring is inevitable in the majority of the tertiary skin lesions. Larger texts should be consulted for the late changes seen in the central nervous system, the cardiovascular system, the bones, the eyes, and the viscera. Approximately 15% of the patients who acquire syphilis and receive no treatment will die of the disease.

### Late Latent Stage

Another latent period may occur after natural healing of some types of benign tertiary syphilis.

### Congenital Syphilis

Congenital syphilis is acquired in utero from an infectious mother (Fig. 22-8). The STS required of pregnant women by most states has lowered the incidence of this unfortunate disease. Stillbirths are not uncommon from mothers who are untreated. After the birth of a live infected child, the mortality rate depends on the duration of the infection, the natural host resistance, and the rapidity of initiating treatment. Early and late lesions are seen in these children, similar to those found in the adult cases of acquired syphilis. Blistering can occur.

### Laboratory Findings

#### Darkfield Examination

The etiologic agent, *T. pallidum*, can be found in the serum from the primary or secondary lesions. However, a darkfield microscope is necessary, and very few physicians' offices or laboratories have this instrument. A considerable amount of experience is necessary to distinguish *T. pallidum* from other *Treponema* species.

### Serologic Test for Syphilis

The STS is simple, readily available, and has several modifications. The rapid plasma reagin (RPR) test and the Venereal Disease Research Laboratories (VDRL) flocculation test are used most commonly. Treponemal tests such as the fluorescent treponemal antibody absorption (FTA-ABS) test and modifications are more difficult to perform in the laboratory and therefore are used primarily when the RPR and VDRL tests are "reactive."

When a report is received from the laboratory that the STS is positive (RPR or VDRL reactive), a second blood specimen should be submitted to obtain a quantitative report. In many laboratories this repeat test is not necessary, because a quantitative test is run routinely on all positive blood specimens. A dilution of 1:2 is only weakly positive and might be a biologic false-positive reaction. A test positive in a dilution of 1:32 is strongly positive. In evaluating the response of the STS to treatment, one must remember that a

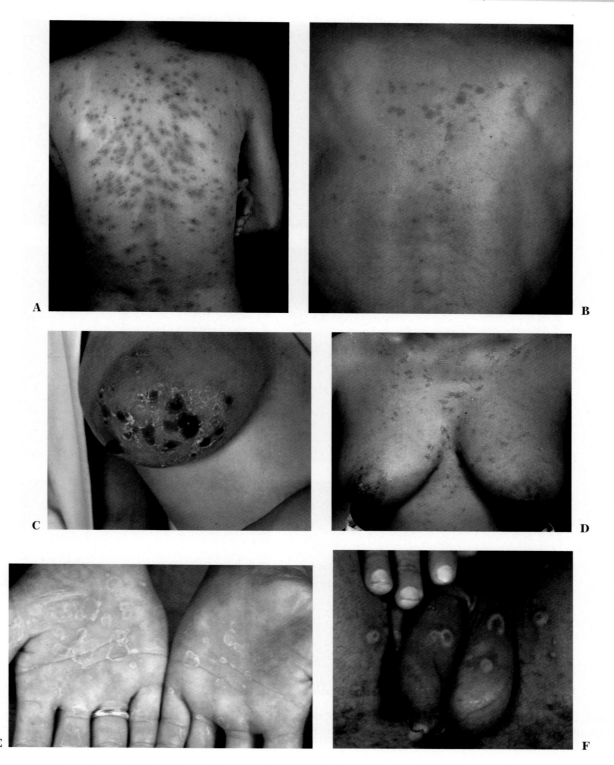

**FIGURE 22-3** ■ Secondary syphilis. **(A)** Secondary papulosquamous lesions on the back. **(B)** Papulosquamous lesions on the back. **(C)** Crusted lesions on the breast. **(D)** Papular lesions on the chest. *(Courtesy of K.U.M.C.)* **(E)** Papulosquamous lesions on the palms. **(F)** Late secondary annular lesions on the penis and scrotum.

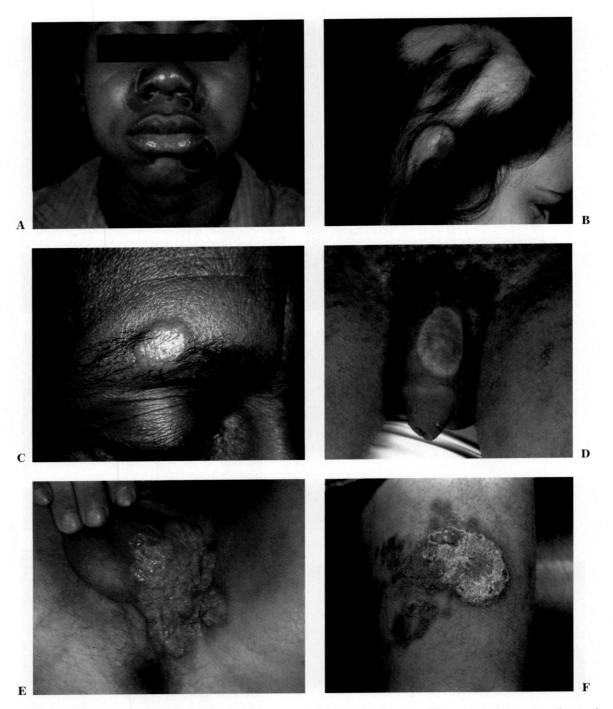

**FIGURE 22-4** ■ Late secondary syphilis. **(A)** Annular lesions. **(B)** Syphilitic alopecia. **(C)** A nodular lesion on the eyebrow. **(D)** An annular lesion on the penis. **(E)** *Condylomata lata* in the groin area. **(F)** Psoriatic-type lesion on the leg.

change in titer from 1:2 to 1:4 to 1:16 to 1:32 to 1:64, or downward in the same gradations in each instance is only a change in one tube. Thus, a change from 1:2 to 1:4 is of the same magnitude as a change from 1:32 to 1:64. Quantitative tests enable the physician to

- evaluate the efficacy of the treatment,
- discover a relapse before it becomes infectious,
- differentiate between a relapse and a reinfection,

- establish a reaction as a seroresistant type, and
- differentiate between true and biologic false-positive serologic reactions.

In most laboratories, it is now routine to do an FTA-ABS test on all patients with reactive RPR and VDRL tests. With rare exceptions, a positive FTA-ABS test means that the patient has or had syphilis and is not a biologic false-positive reactor. The STS may not be positive in patients with AIDS.

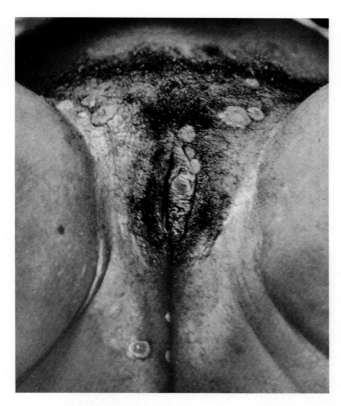

**FIGURE 22-5** ■ Secondary syphilis with *condylomata lata* of the vulva. *(Courtesy of J.E. Moore and The Upjohn Company.)*

## Tissue Examination

A direct fluorescent antibody test for *T. pallidum* can be performed on a lesion exudate or on biopsy tissue.

## Cerebrospinal Fluid Test

As has been stated, the cerebrospinal fluid is frequently positive in the primary and secondary stages of the disease. Invasion of the central nervous system is an early manifestation, even though the perceptible clinical effects are a late manifestation. The cerebrospinal fluid should be examined at least once during the course of the disease. However, in actual practice, primary or secondary disease is usually treated without a cerebrospinal fluid exam but with antibiotic doses that are sufficient to eliminate the treponeme from the cerebrospinal fluid. Cerebrospinal fluid examination is appropriate for all patients with syphilis who are at a high risk for human immunodeficiency virus (HIV) infection. The best routine is to perform a cerebrospinal fluid test before treatment is initiated and repeat the test as indicated. If the cerebrospinal fluid is negative in a patient who has had syphilis for 4 years, central nervous system syphilis will not occur, and future cerebrospinal fluid tests are not necessary. If the test is positive, repeat tests should be done every 6 months for 4 years. The following three tests are run on the cerebrospinal fluid:

- *Cell count:* The finding of four or more lymphocytes or polymorphonuclear leukocytes per cubic

millimeter is considered positive. The cell count is the most labile of the tests. It becomes increased early in the infection and responds fastest to therapy. Therefore, it is a good index of activity of the disease. The cell count must be done within an hour after the fluid is withdrawn.

- *Total protein:* Measured in milligrams per deciliter, it normally should be below 40.
- *Nontreponemal flocculation test:* Presently, the most common test performed is the qualitative and quantitative VDRL. This test is the last to turn positive and the slowest to return to negativity. In some cases, therapy causes a decrease in the titer, but slight positivity or "fastness" can remain for the lifetime of the patient.

## Differential Diagnosis

- *Primary syphilis:* From chancroid, herpes simplex, fusospirochetal balanitis, granuloma inguinale, and any of the *primary chancre-type diseases* (see Dictionary/Index).
- *Secondary syphilis:* From any of the papulosquamous diseases (especially pityriasis rosea), fungal diseases, drug eruption, and alopecia areata.
- *Tertiary skin syphilis:* From any of the granulomatous diseases, particularly tuberculosis, leprosy, sarcoidosis, deep mycoses, and lymphomas.
- *Congenital syphilis:* From atopic eczema, diseases with lymphadenopathy, hepatomegaly, and splenomegaly.

A true-positive syphilitic serology is to be differentiated from a biologic false-positive reaction. This serologic differentiation is accomplished best by using the FTA-ABS test, or one of its modifications, along with a good history and a thorough examination of the patient. Many patients with biologic false-positive reactions develop one of the collagen diseases at a later date.

## Treatment

*Case Example:* A 22-year-old married man presents with a sore 1 cm in diameter on his glans penis of 5 days' duration. Three weeks earlier he had an extramarital intercourse, and 10 days before this office visit he had marital intercourse. The patient knows his extramarital sexual contact only as "Jane," and he cannot remember the bar where he met her.

### First Visit.

1. Perform a darkfield examination of the penile lesion. Treatment can be started if *T. pallidum* is found. If you cannot perform a darkfield examination, refer the patient to the local health department or another facility that can perform a darkfield examination.
2. If a darkfield examination cannot be performed or is negative, obtain a blood specimen for an STS.

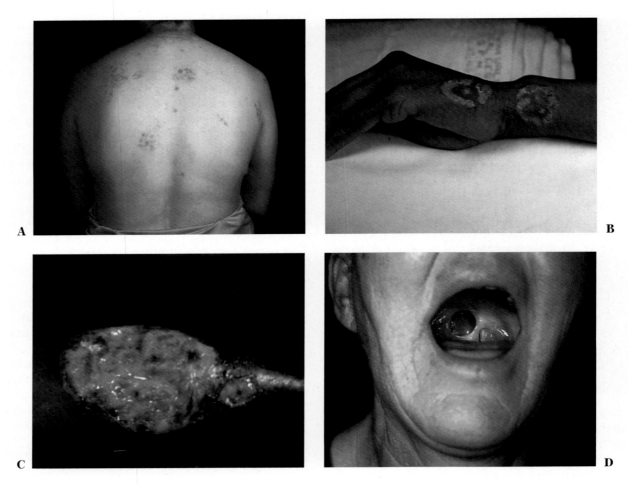

**FIGURE 22-6** ■ Tertiary syphilis. **(A)** Grouped papular lesions on the back. **(B)** Annular nodular lesions on the hand. **(C)** Gumma on the leg. **(D)** Perforation from an old gumma of the soft palate.

3. While waiting for the STS report, advise the patient to soak the site in saline solution for 15 minutes twice a day. The solution is made by placing 1/4 teaspoon of salt in a glass of water.
4. Advise the patient against sexual intercourse until the reports are completed.
5. Explain to the patient the seriousness of treating him for syphilis if he does not have it. The "syphilitic" label is one he should not want, if it is at all possible to avoid it and that allergic reactions to penicillin are not rare and can be serious.

***Second Visit.*** Three days later, the lesion is larger and the STS report is "nonreactive."

1. Obtain a blood specimen for a second STS.
2. Antibiotic ointment 15.0
   *Sig:* Apply t.i.d. locally after soaking in saline solution.
3. Explain again why you are delaying therapy until a definite diagnosis is made.

***Third Visit.*** Three days later, the sore is smaller, but the STS report is "reactive." The diagnosis is now known to be "primary syphilis."

1. The patient is reassured that present-day therapy is highly successful but that he must follow your instructions closely.
2. His wife should be brought in for examination and a blood test. If the blood test is negative, it should be repeated weekly for 1 month. However, some syphilologists believe that therapy is indicated for the marital partner in the presence of a negative STS if the husband has infectious syphilis and is being treated. A single injection of 2.4 million units of a long-acting type of penicillin is used. This prevents "ping-pong" syphilis, which is a cycle of reinfection from one marital partner to another.
3. The patient's contact should be found. The patient's findings, including his contact with an unidentified sexual partner, should be reported to the local health department. This is usually done automatically by the laboratory where the blood tests were done but this does not relieve the physician of the responsibility of reporting the patient to the health department. In some local health departments (author's experience), the health officials will give free treatment and follow-up of patient and contacts.

4. A cerebrospinal fluid specimen should be obtained. (The report was returned as normal for all three tests.)
5. Penicillin therapy should be initiated. Here, two factors are important:
   a. The dose must be adequate.
   b. The effective blood levels of medication must be maintained for a period of 10 to 14 days.

## Dosage

### Primary and Secondary Syphilis

1. Administer 2.4 million units of benzathine penicillin G, half in each buttock, in a single session.
2. Consult larger texts or relevant literature for other treatment modalities.

### Latent (Both Early and Late) Syphilis

1. If a spinal tap is not performed, administer 7.2 million units benzathine penicillin G divided into three weekly injections.
2. If cerebrospinal fluid examination is nonreactive, give 2.4 million units in a single dose.

### Neurosyphilis or Cardiovascular Syphilis

1. Administer 9 to 12 million units of a long-acting penicillin.
2. For other routines or complicated cases, consult larger texts for therapy and care.
3. HIV-infected patients with neurosyphilis should be treated for 10 days at least with aqueous crystalline penicillin G in a dosage of 2 to 4 million units IV every 4 hours.

### Benign Late Syphilis

Treatment is the same as for neurosyphilis.

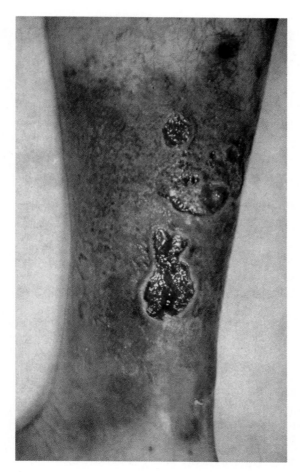

FIGURE 22-7 ■ Tertiary syphilis with a gumma of the leg. This resembles a stasis ulcer. *(Courtesy of J.E. Moore and The Upjohn Company.)*

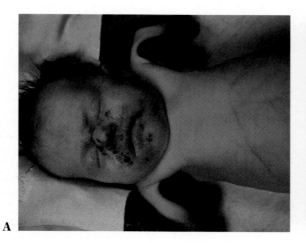
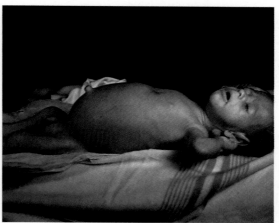

**A**   **B**

FIGURE 22-8 ■ Congenital syphilis. **(A)** Scaly and erosive lesions with a large liver (fatal). **(B)** Massively enlarged liver and spleen.

*Congenital Syphilis*

1. Early congenital syphilis
   a. *Younger than 6 months of age:* Aqueous procaine penicillin G, 10 daily IM doses totaling 100,000 to 200,000 units/kg.
   b. *Six months to 2 years of age:* As above, *or* benzathine penicillin G, 100,000 units/kg IM in one single dose.
2. Late congenital syphilis
   a. *Ages 2 to 11 years, or weighing less than 70 pounds:* Same as for 6 months to 2 years.
   b. *Twelve years or older, and weighing more than 70 pounds:* Same treatment as for adult-acquired syphilis, with comparable time and progression of infection.

## Lyme Disease

Originally described as Lyme arthritis, Lyme disease is caused by a spirochete that is transmitted by several species of *Ixodes* tick. Early removal of the tick (<24 hours) usually prevents disease transmission. The disease has been reported from most states and on every continent except Antarctica. Endemic areas include the northeastern United States and the upper Midwestern states. Clinical manifestations include erythema chronicum migrans (ECM) skin lesions, flu-like symptoms, and possible neurologic, cardiac, and rheumatologic involvement.

Late cutaneous manifestations of Lyme disease are borrelia lymphocytoma, acrodermatitis chronica atrophicans and, although controversial, possibly in some cases (especially in Europe) morphea (localized scleroderma).

### Presentation and Characteristics

#### Primary Lesion

The erythematous circular rash appears at the site of the tick bite and enlarges with central clearing, but multiple ECM eruptions can occur. The rash typically develops within 2 to 30 days after the bite. The bite area can become necrotic.

#### Secondary Lesion

Multiple ECM eruptions can develop.

#### Distribution

Usually ECM begins at the site of the tick bite.

#### Season

The disease occurs from late May through early fall.

#### Course

In untreated patients, the ECM lesions may last only 10 to 14 days, but they may persist for months, or they may come and go over a year's time. The bite papule and ECM fade rapidly after therapy is begun. Late-stage cutaneous lesions include acrodermatitis chronic atrophicans and borrelia lymphocytoma (see Chapter 38).

---

**SAUER'S NOTES: SYPHILIS**

1. Any patient treated for gonorrhea should have an STS 4 to 6 weeks later.
2. Persons with HIV infection acquired through sexual contact or IV drug abuse should be tested for syphilis.
3. Seventy-five percent of the persons who acquire syphilis suffer no serious manifestations of the disease.
4. Syphilis does not cause vesicular or bullous skin lesions, except in infants with congenital infection.

**PRIMARY STAGE**

1. Syphilis should be ruled in or out in the diagnosis of any penile or vulvar sores.
2. Multiple primary chancres are moderately common.

**SECONDARY STAGE**

1. The rash of secondary syphilis, except for the rare follicular form, does not usually itch.
2. Secondary syphilis should be ruled in or out in any patient with a generalized, nonpruritic rash especially when it is papulosquamous. A high index of suspicion is necessary.

**LATENT STAGE**

The diagnosis of "latent syphilis" cannot be made for a particular patient unless cerebrospinal fluid tests have been done and are negative for syphilis.

**TERTIARY STAGE**

1. Tertiary syphilis should be considered in any patient with a chronic granuloma of the skin, particularly if it has an annular or circular configuration.
2. Invasion of the central nervous system occurs in the primary and secondary stages of the disease. A cerebrospinal fluid test is indicated during these stages.
3. If the cerebrospinal fluid tests for syphilis are negative in a patient who has had syphilis for 4 years, central nervous system syphilis usually will not occur and future spinal punctures are not necessary.
4. Twenty percent of patients with late asymptomatic neurosyphilis have a negative STS.

**CONGENITAL SYPHILIS**

An STS should be done on every pregnant woman to prevent congenital syphilis of the newborn.

**SEROLOGY**

1. The STS may be negative in the early days of the primary chancre. The STS is always positive in the secondary stage. An exception to this rule is in patients with AIDS.
2. A quantitative STS should be done on all syphilitic patients to evaluate the response to treatment or the development of relapse or reinfection.
3. The finding of a low-titer STS in a patient not previously treated for syphilis calls for a careful evaluation to rule out a biologic false-positive reaction.

## Subjective Symptoms

Flu-like symptoms, with fever, chills, myalgias, and headache, appear with the rash but in the author's experience systemic symptoms are not commonly reported. Later, other organs may be affected.

## Cause

The spirochete *Borrelia burgdorferi* is transmitted by Ixodes species of ticks and possibly by the hard-bodied ticks. The white-tailed deer and white-footed mouse are preferred hosts of the tick.

## Diagnosis

A high index of suspicion, history of a tick bite (patient is not always aware of the bite), a previous "ringworm-type" rash, and, later, a positive Lyme disease antibody titer may be present (however these tests are not reliable).

Histologic findings are not specific and culture of the spirochete is often not practical. Polymerase chain reaction may be helpful on biopsy tissue in a qualified laboratory.

### Differential Diagnosis

Cutaneously, the ECM rash can resemble an allergic reaction or tinea. See *figurate erythemas* in the Dictionary/Index. Any patient who presents with fever, myalgia, cardiac, joint, or neurologic manifestations should have a broad differential diagnosis.

ECM is nonspecific and has many mimickers (Table 22-1). It is common in skin creases and under clothing straps and tends to be central in location. It may be multiple (90% single), is usually large (mean is 16 cm but can be 5 to 70 cm), and evolves over days to weeks (2 to 3 cm a day) with or without central clearing. It does not have a scale as in erythema annulare centrifugum and does not have a scaling, vesicular, or elevated border as in tinea corporis. It is not a generalized cutaneous condition as is erythema gyratum repens. It is asymptomatic but may have mild pain, pruritus, or mild systemic symptoms. These may occur days to weeks after the tick bite.

### Treatment

Because a diagnosis of Lyme disease is difficult, treatment may be indicated, especially in endemic areas, based on history and clinical findings alone. Early therapy for this disease is doxycycline, 100 mg, b.i.d. for 21 days, or amoxicillin, 500 mg, t.i.d. for 21 days. Early tick removal (< 24 hours) probably prevents disease transmission. Removing deer and mice habitats such as brush, leaves, stonewalls, and woodpiles may be helpful.

For late stages of the disease with cardiac or neurologic manifestations, treatment is ceftriaxone, 2 to 4 g/d IM or IV for 14 days. Because efficacy of therapy is difficult to evaluate, the literature is replete with other therapeutic regimens.

**TABLE 22-1 ▪ Mimics of Erythema Chronicum Migrans**

1. Tinea-clearing may occur in the center with a peripheral scale or crusts or vesicles. It is usually very pruritic, spreads over days to weeks, and may have satellite lesions.

2. Hypersensitivity to a tick bite is often itchy, the tick is often still attached, small (several centimeters), inflammatory papules rapidly develop without much evolution over days, and will occur at multiple sites of multiple bites.

3. Granuloma annulare—acral, especially over the dorsal hands, feet, knees, and elbows, dull red with central clearing and no scale, chronic over months to years with slow evolution, and asymptomatic.

4. Herald patch of pityriasis rosea—a collarette of scale just inside the pinkish plaque, will be followed usually within 5–7 days with an explosion of similar lesions that line up along Langer's lines.

5. Nummular eczema—extremely pruritic with oozing and crusting and does not remain single for long.

6. Cutaneous T-cell lymphoma—chronic rather than sudden in onset, eventually becomes multiple, often asymmetric.

Lyme vaccination is effective and should be considered in people at high risk in endemic areas. It takes 12 months to confer immunity.

*Lymephobia* is a term coined to describe a common psychological problem owing to the nonspecific nature of symptoms and the lack of specific tests. Well-meaning physicians can fall into the trap of long-term antibiotics for multiple vague systemic complaints.

Permethrin 5% applied to clothing is a helpful tick repellant.

## Suggested Readings

Abele DC, Anders KH. The many faces and phases of borreliosis: I. Lyme disease. *J Am Acad Dermatol.* 1990;23:167–186.

Abele DC, Anders KH. The many faces and phases of borreliosis: II. *J Am Acad Dermatol.* 1990;23:401–410.

Anonymous. Drugs for sexually transmitted infections. *Med Lett Drugs Ther.* 1999;41(1062):85–90.

Anonymous. Treatment of Lyme disease. *Med Lett Drugs Ther.* 2007;49:47–51.

Baum EW, Bernhardt M, Sams WM Jr. Secondary syphilis, still the great imitator. *JAMA.* 1983;249:3069–3070.

Bennet ML, Lynn AW, Klein LE. Congenital syphilis: subtle presentation of fulminant disease. *J Am Acad Dermatol.* 1997;36(2):351–354.

Burlington DB. *FDA Public Health Advisory: Assays for Antibodies to Borrelia burgdorferi: Limitations, Use, and Interpretation for Supporting a Clinical Diagnosis of Lyme Disease.* FDA; July 7, 1997.

Don PC, Rubinstein R, Christie S. Malignant syphilis (lues maligna) and concurrent infection with HIV. *Int J Dermatol.* 1995;34:403–407.

Trevisan G, Cinco M. Lyme disease. *Int J Dermatol.* 1990;29:1–8.

Stere AC, Taylor E, McHugh GL, et al. The overdiagnosis of Lyme disease. *JAMA.* 1993;269:1812–1816.

# CHAPTER 23

# Dermatologic Virology

*Anita Satyaprakash, MD, Parisa Ravanfar, MD, MBA, MS, and Stephen K. Tyring, MD, PhD*

Viral diseases of the skin are exceedingly common. The various clinical entities are distinct and because we have no specific antiviral drug for many diseases, the treatment varies for each entity. The following viral diseases are discussed here:

- Herpes simplex virus 1 and 2
- Varicella–zoster virus
- Human herpesvirus 6
- Human herpesvirus 7
- Human papillomaviruses
- Molluscum contagiosum virus
- Measles (rubeola)
- German measles (rubella)
- Erythema infectiosum
- Coxsackievirus infections
- Herpangina
- Hand, foot, and mouth disease
- Echovirus exanthema

## Herpes Simplex Virus 1

Herpes simplex virus 1 (HSV-1) is the usual cause of herpes labialis as well as the cause of up to 50% of first-episode genital herpes infections. Approximately 90% of people between 20 to 40 years of age have antibodies against HSV-1. The primary infection typically occurs early in life, with viral latency established in the neural ganglia. Reactivation can occur due to several different triggers, including immunosuppression, respiratory tract viral infection, or any febrile disease, physical trauma, psychological stress, or sun exposure. Transmission of HSV-1 occurs with viral shedding during the asymptomatic and symptomatic periods through direct contact with infected secretions (i.e., saliva).

### Presentation and Characteristics

True primary infection occurs when a patient is seronegative for HSV types 1 and 2 prior to the episode. Nonprimary initial episodes occur when the first symptomatic episode occurs later than the initial infection and tend to be less severe. Asymptomatic primary infection is the rule. During symptomatic episodes, 60% of patients experience prodromal symptoms such as burning, itching, or tingling. Systemic symptoms such as fever, chills, fatigue, and muscle aches may also accompany primary infection. The mouth and lips are the most common areas of primary infection (Figs. 23-1 and 23-2). Lesions start as papules on an erythematous base that become vesicular, progress to ulcers, then crust, and eventually heal, generally within 72 to 96 hours. Symptomatic primary episodes tend to be followed by less severe recurrences; however, some patients may never experience a second episode. Recurrent episodes often present as three to five vesicles at the vermilion border of the lip, which last at least 48 hours. Other locations include the palate, chin, and oral mucosa. Recurrent labial herpes affects approximately one third of the US population, with patients typically experiencing one to six episodes annually.

### Treatment

Oral acyclovir, famciclovir (the prodrug of penciclovir), and valacyclovir are effective for the treatment of herpes labialis. Different doses are recommended depending on whether the patient is presenting with his or her primary episode, a recurrent episode, or qualifies for suppressive therapy (Table 23-1). The use of suppressive therapy requires periodic reevaluation, generally within a year, in order to assess its necessity. Topical therapies that may be used are acyclovir 5% cream five times daily for 4 days and penciclovir 1% cream every 2 hours (while awake) for 4 days.

## Herpes Simplex Virus 2

Herpes simplex virus 2 (HSV-2) is one of the most widespread sexually transmitted diseases (STDs) in the world. It causes 70% of primary genital herpes and over 95% of recurrent genital herpes (Fig. 23-3). In the United States, the prevalence of genital herpes is 40 to 60 million, and the incidence is 500,000 to 1,000,000 cases per year, with approximately 22% of the general population being seropositive for HSV-2. Similar to HSV-1, HSV-2 causes primary, latent, and recurrent infections, and is transmitted during both asymptomatic and symptomatic phases, typically through sexual contact. Genital herpes infections caused by HSV-2 tend to be more severe than those caused by HSV-1, are more likely to have recurrent episodes, and have a greater frequency of subclinical viral shedding. HSV-2 can also cause neonatal herpes, with the highest risk occurring when the mother has primary genital herpes during delivery. In addition to cutaneous lesions, the infected neonate may develop multiorgan involvement, which carries a high mortality rate.

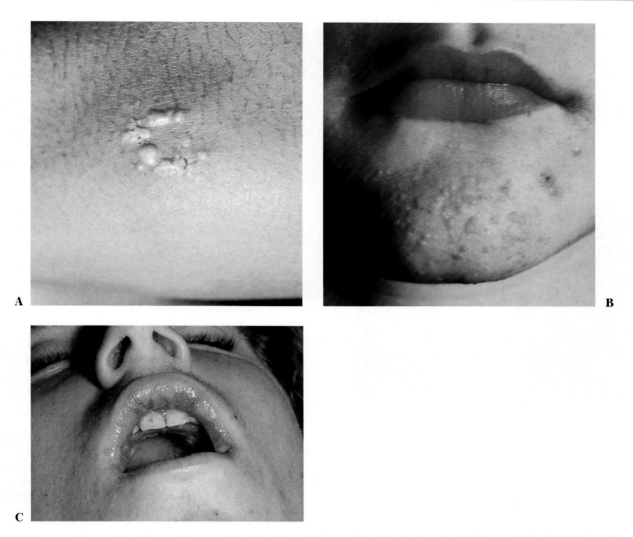

**FIGURE 23-1** ■ Herpes simplex on the arm (**A**), chin (**B**), and true primary infection on the lips and mouth (interoral) (**C**). *(Courtesy of Dermik Laboratories, Inc.)*

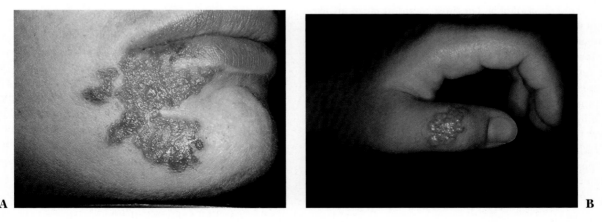

**FIGURE 23-2** ■ (**A**) Recurrent herpes simplex on the chin with secondary bacterial infection. (**B**) Recurrent herpes simplex on the thumb. *(Courtesy of Dermik Laboratories, Inc.)*

**TABLE 23-1 ■ Treatments for Herpes Labialis**

| First Clinical Episode of Herpes Labialis | Intermittent Episodic Therapy for Recurrent Herpes Labialis | Suppressive Therapy for Recurrent Herpes Labialis |
|---|---|---|
| Acyclovir 400 mg PO 5 times daily for 7–10 days | Acyclovir 400 mg PO 5 times daily for 5 days | Acyclovir 400 mg PO b.i.d. |
| Famciclovir 500 mg PO b.i.d. for 7 days | Famciclovir 1.5 g PO once | Famciclovir 500 mg PO b.i.d. |
| Valacyclovir 1 g PO b.i.d. for 1 day | Valacyclovir 1 g PO BID for 1 day | Valacyclovir 500 mg PO q.d. |

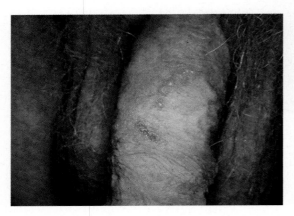

**FIGURE 23-3 ■** Recurrent herpes simplex on the penis. *(Courtesy of Dermik Laboratories, Inc.)*

## Presentation and Characteristics

Up to 90% of patients infected with HSV-2 become infected via asymptomatic viral shedding. Genital herpes infection is typically asymptomatic, because the lesions may be painless and inapparent. The first clinically recognized lesions of genital herpes may be either true primary or a first-episode, nonprimary. True primary genital herpes usually develops after 2 to 14 days of HSV exposure. There may be widespread vesicles and ulcers on the genitalia with inguinal adenopathy, and the patient may complain of discharge, dysuria, fever, lethargy, myalgias, and photophobia. The most common site of involvement in women is the cervix, although the classic painful clinical presentation is mostly that of vaginal and vulvar lesions.

More than half of patients with the first recognized signs and symptoms of genital herpes have a nonprimary first episode, which occurs when the initial infection is asymptomatic. This may occur weeks, months, or even years after initial HSV infection. A strong immune response may prevent the infection from becoming clinically recognizable. The initial immune response does attenuate the severity of first-episode nonprimary genital herpes. Lesions are often less extensive, and systemic symptoms are less common and severe compared to that of true primary genital herpes.

## Treatment

Because there is no cure for genital herpes, therapy is aimed at controlling the signs and symptoms of an outbreak. In 2006, the Centers for Disease Control and Prevention (CDC)

made therapeutic recommendations for individuals with a first clinical episode of genital herpes; for episodic development of genital herpes; and for suppressive therapy for recurrent genital herpes (Table 23-2). Pharmacologic therapies for genital herpes include

- acyclovir,
- valacyclovir,
- famciclovir,
- cidofovir,
- foscarnet (especially in immunocompromised HIV patients), and
- penciclovir.

## Varicella–Zoster Virus

Varicella–zoster virus (VZV) causes primary varicella (chickenpox) and herpes zoster (shingles), which is a reactivation of the primary varicella infection. Primary varicella is usually a self-limited disease in immunocompetent children. Prior to the availability of the varicella vaccine, there were more than 11,000 hospitalizations each year in the United States due to complications of varicella infection in children who were often otherwise healthy. Susceptible adults typically develop more extensive skin lesions, more frequent complications, and more severe constitutional symptoms, such as prolonged fever.

Following primary VZV infection, the virus resides in a latent state in the sensory ganglia. With aging or a weakened immune system, the VZV may reactivate as shingles, which is also known as herpes zoster. With the highest incidence of all neurologic diseases, herpes zoster occurs annually in more than 1,000,000 people in the United States and has a lifetime incidence of 20%. Since childhood varicella vaccination was introduced in the United States in 1995, the incidence of shingles has increased. This is presumably due to the lack of subclinical immune boosting that generally results from the wild-type virus in the environment.

## Presentation and Characteristics

Two weeks after exposure, primary varicella may start with 2 to 3 days of prodromal symptoms such as low-grade fever, chills, headache, malaise, nausea, and vomiting. The rash appears as crops of small red macules on the face and scalp, which then spreads to the trunk with sparing of the distal

**TABLE 23-2** ■ **Treatments for Genital Herpes**

| First Clinical Episode of Genital Herpes | Intermittent Episodic Therapy for Recurrent Genital Herpes | Suppressive Therapy for Recurrent Genital Herpes |
|---|---|---|
| Acyclovir 400 mg PO t.i.d. for 7–10 days | Acyclovir 400 mg PO t.i.d. for 5 days | Acyclovir 400 mg PO b.i.d. |
| Acyclovir 200 mg PO 5 times a day for 7–10 days | Acyclovir 800 mg PO t.i.d. for 2 days | Famciclovir 250 mg PO b.i.d. |
| Famciclovir 250 mg PO t.i.d. for 7–10 days | Acyclovir 800 mg PO b.i.d. for 5 days | Valacyclovir 500 mg PO q.d. (≤9 outbreaks/year) |
| Valacyclovir 1 g PO b.i.d. for 7–10 days | Famciclovir 125 mg PO b.i.d. for 5 days | |
| Famciclovir 1 g PO b.i.d. for 1 day | Valacyclovir 1 g PO q.d. (>9 outbreaks/year) | |
| | Valacyclovir 500 mg PO b.i.d. for 3 days | |
| | Valacyclovir 1 g PO q.d. for 5 days | |

upper and lower extremities. Over 12 hours, the macules progress to 1- to 3-mm papules, vesicles, and then pustules. Crusting occurs within a few days, and complete healing occurs in approximately 1 month. Lesions are generally found to be in different stages of healing in the same skin region.

More than 90% of patients with herpes zoster have a prodrome of intense pain in the involved single sensory ganglion (dermatome) preceding the zoster rash (Fig. 23-4). The appearance of the characteristic dermatomal rash (erythematous vesicles with subsequent crusting) is often accompanied by severe pain. Shingles is typically localized to a dermatome, does not significantly cross the midline of the body, and occurs at the site which was most severely affected during primary varicella infection. Although any dermatome can be

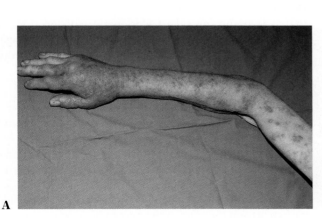
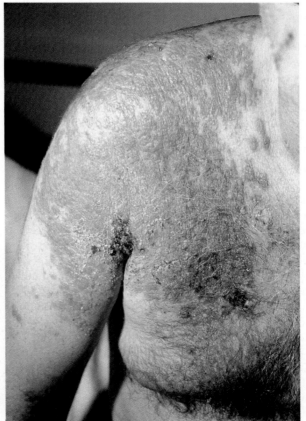

**FIGURE 23-4** ■ Herpes zoster in a lymphoma patient. (**A**) Right upper extremity. (**B**) Right chest.

affected, the most common regions of involvement are the ophthalmic (V1) and midthoracic to upper lumbar (T3 to L2) dermatomes. The rash heals within 2 to 4 weeks, but the pain associated with herpes zoster is its most distressing symptom. Pain that persists well after cutaneous healing is referred to as postherpetic neuralgia (PHN), a chronic neuropathic pain syndrome that can last for months or even years.

## Treatment

Primary varicella in immunocompetent children is self-limited and may be treated symptomatically. However, if the rash appears within 24 to 72 hours of medical attention, primary varicella in children may be treated with acyclovir 20 mg/kg q.i.d. up to 800 mg/dose for 5 to 7 days. Systemic antiviral treatment is recommended for primary varicella in adults and in immunocompromised patients. Although valacyclovir and famciclovir have anti-VZV activity, there are no clinical trials reporting their efficacy in primary varicella. Both antiviral agents, however, are used at the herpes zoster dose for therapy of primary VZV in adults. In patients who are at high risk of complications from varicella–zoster and are not eligible for vaccination due to age or immunodeficiency, varicella–zoster immune globulin can prevent or decrease the severity of disease if given as soon as possible, but no later than 96 hours after exposure to chickenpox.

Both oral and IV acyclovir have an important role in the treatment of herpes zoster. Oral acyclovir in immunocompetent patients leads to an accelerated healing of lesions and reduction in acute pain, but it has only modest effects on the incidence or duration of PHN. IV administration (10 mg/kg every 8 hours for 10 days) is indicated for the treatment of severe complications in immunocompetent patients and the treatment of zoster in severely immunosuppressed patients. Adverse effects with acyclovir are rare and include headache, nausea, diarrhea, and renal toxicity (especially in dehydrated elderly patients).

Valacyclovir, the orally administered prodrug of acyclovir, is effective in reducing time to crusting, the appearance of new zoster lesions, and time to 50% healing. The typical dose is 1 g t.i.d. for 7 days. Valacyclovir, when compared to acyclovir, decreased the median duration of pain from 60 to 40 days. It has a similar adverse event profile as acyclovir but without reports of nephropathy or neurotoxicity. Valacyclovir (1 g t.i.d. for 7 days) is safe and effective for the treatment of uncomplicated herpes zoster in most immunocompromised patients as well.

Famciclovir, the prodrug of penciclovir, is at least equal to acyclovir in promoting cutaneous healing and decreasing the duration of acute pain. The typical dose is 500 mg t.i.d. for 7 days. Its efficacy and safety are equivalent to that of valacyclovir. Like all antiviral agents, therapy should be started as soon as possible after the onset of the zoster rash, preferably within 72 hours. However, it has been reported that patients may also benefit if antiviral therapy is started after 72 hours of rash onset. The upper limit of time for initiation of antiviral therapy has not been determined.

### Vaccination

Varivax, a live, attenuated, varicella vaccine, was approved for use in the United States in 1995. It prevents chickenpox in 70% to 90% of vaccinees and prevents severe chickenpox in over 95% of vaccinees. Zostavax, a live, attenuated, varicella–zoster vaccine that is greater than 10 times the strength of Varivax, was approved in 2006 for use in individuals aged 60 and older for the prevention of herpes zoster. In patients who develop herpes zoster despite receiving the vaccination, the incidence of PHN is decreased by 39%.

## Human Herpesvirus 6

Human herpesvirus 6 (HHV-6) was first isolated in 1986 and has been found to be associated with roseola infantum (exanthem subitum). HHV-6 infects over 90% of the population by early childhood.

### Presentation and Characteristics

Primary infection with HHV-6 usually occurs by 2 years of age and is often accompanied by an indistinctive febrile illness. The characteristic rash is observed either during the illness or following defervescence in approximately 20% of patients experiencing primary HHV-6 infection. Some individuals may experience the classic roseola rash which starts on the trunk and may later spread to the arms, face, and neck. It is characteristically a faint pink maculopapular rash that rarely coalesces and blanches with pressure. Other skin manifestations associated with HHV-6 include exanthem subitum, "glove-and-socks" syndrome, hypersensitivity drug reactions, Gianotti–Crosti syndrome, pityriasis rosea, and lymphoproliferative malignancies.

### Treatment

Treatment is symptomatic. Antipyretics may be used to reduce fevers.

## Human Herpesvirus 7

Human herpesvirus 7 (HHV-7) is very similar to HHV-6 in that it is highly prevalent worldwide with greater than 90% of humans experiencing primary infection by the age of 10 years. The mode of transmission is most likely through salivary fluid.

### Presentation and Characteristics

HHV-7 has been thought to be the causative agent of pityriasis rosea and has also been associated with exanthem subitum in addition to HHV-6. Pityriasis rosea is a common, benign disease that often has a very characteristic pattern. In approximately 75% of the cases, a single, isolated oval scaly patch, referred to as the "herald patch," appears on the body, particularly on the trunk, upper arms, neck, or thighs. Additional pink scaly patches later occur on the body and on the arms and legs that are typically smaller than the herald patch. These patches often form a pattern over the back resembling a Christmas tree outline. The rash is self-limiting and disappears within 6 to 14 weeks. HHV-7 infection has also been linked to chronic fatigue syndrome, post-transplant skin eruptions, reactivation of HHV-6 infection, and febrile illness of infancy.

### Differential Diagnosis

> *Tinea corporis*
> *Eczema*
> *Drug eruption*
> *Syphilis*

### Treatment

The lesions are often pruritic and treatment is symptomatic.

## Human Papillomavirus

There are over 100 genotypes of human papillomavirus (HPV), which are DNA viruses of the family Papillomaviridae that infect the epithelial cells of skin and mucosa and cause warts, benign papillomas, or neoplasias. HPV infection in sexually active women is very common, with an incidence of 15% to 40%. Some HPV types, primarily 16 and 18, are considered high risk because they are the primary etiologic agents for cervical cancer and other anogenital cancers, as well as some upper aerodigestive tract and skin cancers. Vaccines to prevent infections from oncogenic human papilloma viruses are available.

### Presentation and Characteristics

Warts appear as hyperkeratotic papillomas with black specks, which are thrombosed capillaries, within the wart. These lesions can manifest on any body site, but specific HPV subtypes may have a tendency to affect a certain anatomic location. HPV-1 infection often causes palmar and plantar warts. HPV-2 causes common warts. HPV-3 and HPV-10 typically cause flat warts. HPV-6 and HPV-11 are the main causes of anogenital warts, or condyloma acuminatum, which are soft, flesh-colored, and flat, papular, or pedunculated lesions that occur on the genitals or surrounding skin. Cervical warts, or condyloma acuminata, may be difficult to visualize by examination without application of acetic acid, which can cause subclinical lesions to become white. However, this test has a high false-positive and false-negative rate.

### Treatment

Currently, there is no curative treatment for HPV infections. The 2006 CDC recommendations for therapy of HPV lesions include

- podofilox 0.5% solution or gel,
- imiquimod 5% cream,

- cryotherapy,
- podophyllin resin 10% to 25% tincture, and
- trichloroacetic acid (TCA) or bichloroacetic acid (BCA) 80% to 90%.

Imiquimod stimulates the host's immune response against infected cells and has the lowest recurrence rate following a complete response. This therapy can be used after any other therapy to reduce recurrences. Both podofilox and imiquimod are patient-applied therapies, while the other listed therapies must be applied or performed by a health-care provider. Alternative treatments include

- laser surgery,
- surgical excision,
- intralesional interferon,
- 5-fluorouracil,
- retinoids,
- bleomycin (intralesional and systemic),
- salicylic acid, and
- cidofovir (topical and intravenous).

Sinecatechin (Veregen), a 15% green-tea extract ointment, was recently approved by the FDA for the treatment of external anogenital warts.

### Vaccination

Gardasil is a quadrivalent vaccine that is effective against HPV types 6, 11, 16, and 18—the major types causing anogenital warts as well as cervical cancer. It was approved by the FDA for use in the United States in 2006 for females 9 to 26 years of age. Cervarix, a bivalent vaccine that is effective against HPV types 16 and 18, is currently used in Europe and is in the process of FDA approval.

## Molluscum Contagiosum Virus

Molluscum contagiosum (Fig. 23-5), caused by the molluscum contagiosum virus of the DNA poxvirus group, is a benign skin infection that affects children and young adults worldwide. Molluscum contagiosum commonly affects immunocompromised patients, and the prevalence of molluscum contagiosum infection among HIV-infected patients ranges from 5% to 18%. Because the infection is limited to the epidermis, most lesions regress spontaneously within 9 to 12 months, and molluscum contagiosum has not been reported to progress to malignancy.

The prevalence in the general population is unknown. The molluscum contagiosum virus has not been cultured. In the United States, it is estimated that the incidence of genital molluscum contagiosum is relatively low compared to other STDs (1 case per 42 to 60 cases of gonorrhea), and the age distribution of patients with genital molluscum contagiosum is similar to that of other STDs. Outbreaks of molluscum contagiosum may be spread between family members from casual contact. It is common in the pediatric age group usually as a non-STD.

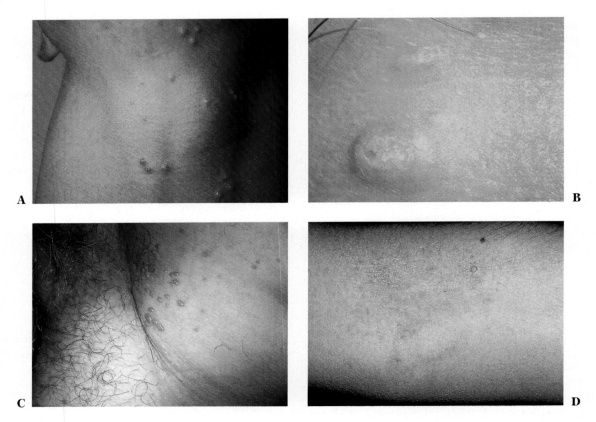

**FIGURE 23-5** ■ Molluscum contagiosum on the neck (**A**), in close-up (**B**) *(Drs. L. Calkins, A. Lemoine, and L. Hyde)*, of vulvar area (**C**), and with atopic eczema of cubital fossae (**D**). *(Courtesy of Glaxo Dermatology.)*

## Presentation and Characteristics

Molluscum contagiosum lesions present as small, smooth, umbilicated papules. In sexually active young adults, these lesions are spread through sexual contact and are found primarily on the lower abdomen, inner thighs, genitalia, and pubic areas. In children, the mode of transmission is nonsexual skin contact. Lesions are found primarily on the trunk and extremities and are often spread from one area to another on a patient's body via autoinoculation. The lesions are generally found in groups, but may also be widely disseminated.

## Treatment

Molluscum contagiosum lesions are self-limiting and generally resolve within 6 months in immunocompetent individuals. However, they may persist for up to 4 years. Therapeutic modalities are similar to those available for warts, and treatment is generally administered in order to control transmission and for cosmetic reasons. Effective therapies are:

- imiquimod,
- cryotherapy,
- cantharidin,
- electrosurgery, and
- curettage.

Less commonly used therapies are:

- topical cidofovir,
- lasers,
- podofilox,
- TCA, and
- retinoids.

## Measles (Rubeola)

Measles is a very common childhood disease. It is highly contagious and is spread by contact with infected individuals, through coughing or sneezing. The disease can be spread from 4 days prior to the onset of the rash to 4 days after onset. The incubation period averages 14 days before the appearance of the rash. The prodromal stage appears around the 9th day after exposure and consists of fever, conjunctivitis, rhinorrhea, and Koplik spots. The Koplik spots measure from 1 to 3 mm in diameter, are bluish-white on a red base, and occur bilaterally on the mucous membranes around the parotid duct and on the lower lip. With increasing fever and cough, the "morbilliform" rash appears first behind the ears and on the forehead and then spreads over the face, neck, trunk, and extremities. The fever begins to decrease as the rash develops. The rash is a faint, reddish, patchy eruption, and occasionally papular. The disease may resolve with scaling. Complications include secondary bacterial infection and encephalitis.

## Differential Diagnosis

- *German measles:* Postauricular lymphadenopathy; milder fever and rash; no Koplik spots (see following section).
- *Scarlet fever:* Circumoral pallor; rash brighter red and confluent (see Chapter 21).
- *Drug eruption:* History of new drugs; usually no fever (see Chapter 8).
- *Infectious mononucleosis:* Rash similar; characteristic hematology; high titer of heterophile antibodies.

## Treatment

Supportive therapy for the cough, bed rest, and protection from bright light are generally sufficient measures for treatment of the active disease. The availability of antibiotics has eliminated most of the bacterial complications. Corticosteroids are of value for the rare but serious complication of encephalitis.

## Vaccination

A live, attenuated measles vaccine is available and a routine childhood immunization in the United States.

# Rubella (German Measles)

Although German measles is a benign disease of children, it is severe if it develops in a pregnant woman during the first trimester because infection can cause serious birth defects in a small percentage of newborns.

The incubation period is approximately 18 days, and, as in measles, there may be a short prodromal stage of fever and malaise. The rash also resembles measles, because it occurs first on the face, then spreads. However, the redness is less intense and the rash disappears within 2 to 3 days. Enlargement of the cervical and the postauricular nodes is a characteristic finding. Serious complications are rare.

## Differential Diagnosis

- *Measles:* Koplik spots; the fever and the rash are more severe; no postauricular nodes.
- *Scarlet fever:* High fever; perioral pallor; rash may be similar (see Chapter 21).
- *Drug eruption:* Get new drug history; usually no fever (see Chapter 8).

## Treatment

Active treatment is generally unnecessary. Immune globulin given to an exposed pregnant woman in the first trimester of pregnancy may prevent the disease in the fetus. A live, attenuated rubella vaccine is available and is a routine childhood vaccination in the United States.

## Congenital Rubella Syndrome

Infants born to mothers who had rubella in the first trimester of pregnancy can have multiple systemic abnormalities. The skin lesions that may be seen include:

- thrombocytopenic purpura,
- hyperpigmentation of the navel, forehead, and cheeks,
- acne,
- seborrhea, and
- reticulated erythema of the face and extremities.

# Erythema Infectiosum

Also known as "fifth disease," erythema infectiosum occurs in epidemics and is believed to be caused by parvovirus B19. It affects children primarily, but in a large epidemic, many cases may be seen in adults.

## Presentation and Characteristics

The incubation period varies from 1 to 7 weeks. In children, the prodromal stage lasts from 2 to 4 days and is manifested by low-grade fever and occasionally, joint pains. When the red macular rash develops, it begins on the arms and the face and then spreads to the body. In children, the rash on the body is morbilliform, but on the face, the cheeks may appear to have been slapped, lending the colloquial term "slapped cheek disease." The rash is more red and confluent on the extensor surfaces of the extremities. A low-grade fever persists for a few days after the onset of the rash, which lasts for approximately 1 week. In adults, the rash on the face is less conspicuous, joint complaints are more common, and pruritus is present. Parvovirus infection may also result in the papular-purpuric gloves-and-socks syndrome (PPGSS), which occurs more often in adults and is characterized by petechiae and small purpuric papules on the hands and feet in a gloves-and-socks distribution. In the acropetechial variant of this syndrome, involvement may also be seen in the perioral and chin area and, less commonly, the buttocks, genital, and axillary regions.

## Differential Diagnosis

- *Drug eruption:* See Chapter 8.
- *Measles:* Coryza, eruption begins on face and behind ears.
- *Other morbilliform eruptions.*

## Treatment

Treatment is generally unnecessary.

# Coxsackievirus Infections

Coxsackieviruses are in the genus *Enterovirus*. Coxsackievirus infections are identified by type-specific antigens that appear in the blood 7 days or so after the onset of the disease.

## Differential Diagnosis

- measles,
- German measles,
- scarlet fever,
- infectious mononucleosis, and
- drug eruption.

## Treatment

Treatment is symptomatic. Antipyretics may be used to reduce the high fever.

## Herpangina

Herpangina is an acute febrile disease that occurs mainly in children in the summer months. The first complaints are fever, headache, sore throat, nausea, and stiff neck. Blisters are seen in the throat that are approximately 2 mm in size and surrounded by an intense erythema. These lesions may coalesce and some may ulcerate. The course of symptomatic infection is usually 7 to 10 days.

The cause of herpangina is primarily coxsackievirus A, but echovirus types have also been isolated from sporadic cases.

## Differential Diagnosis

- aphthous stomatitis,
- drug eruption,
- primary herpes gingivostomatitis, and
- hand–foot–mouth disease.

## Treatment

Treatment is symptomatic. Soothing mouthwashes and antipyretics may be used.

## Hand, Foot, and Mouth Disease

Hand, foot, and mouth disease (HFMD) is caused by viruses in the *Enterovirus* genus, most commonly Coxsackievirus A16 and Enterovirus 71. Other coxsackieviruses and other enteroviruses are also associated with HFMD. Infection is spread by direct contact with the virus, which is found in the nasal and pharyngeal secretions, saliva, vesicular fluid, and stool of infected individuals as well as by fomites. Individuals are most infectious the first week after the onset of symptoms. Generally, the infection begins with constitutional symptoms such as fever, malaise, anorexia, and pharyngitis. One to two days after onset of the fever, painful oral lesions develop on the tongue, gingival, and buccal mucosa that start as erythematous macules, progress to vesicles, and then eventually ulcerate. Concurrently, a rash also develops on the palms and soles, consisting of erythematous macules and papules as well as vesicles. These lesions may also be present on the buttocks and/or genitalia. HFMD most commonly occurs in children under the age of 10. Rare complications include meningitis and

### SAUER'S NOTES

1. Viral diseases are the most adaptable of all infections and the most difficult to treat.
2. There are few cutaneous viral diseases that cannot become a serious systemic disease in the proper setting.
3. Even the lowly human papilloma virus can lead to the most dreaded of all systemic diseases—metastatic cancer.
4. Tremendous progress in therapy and prevention of this group of skin disorders has been made, and recognition of this progress is mandatory in order for good medicine to continue to be practiced.

encephalitis; these complications are more likely in cases caused by Enterovirus 71.

## Treatment

Treatment is symptomatic. Mouthwashes, sprays, or analgesics can be used for mouth pain due to ulcers, and antipyretics may be used for fever.

## Echovirus Exanthem

Echoviruses are RNA viruses in the *Enterovirus* genus. Symptoms of infection include fever, nausea, vomiting, diarrhea, sore throat, and cough; rare complications include viral meningitis, encephalitis, myositis, pleurodynia, and myopericarditis. A viral exanthem, which may be maculopapular, morbilliform, macular, petechial, or papulopustular, occurs in one third of cases. Small erosions may develop on the buccal mucosa. Echoviruses 5, 9, and 25 are most commonly isolated from cases with skin lesions or exanthems. The duration of symptomatic infection is generally 1 to 2 weeks.

## Treatment

Treatment is symptomatic. Antipyretics may be used to reduce fever.

## Suggested Readings

Ahmed AM, Madkan V, Tyring SK. Human papillomaviruses and genital disease. *Dermatol Clin.* 2006;24:157–165.

Arduino PG, Porter SR. Herpes simplex virus type I infection: overview on relevant clinico-pathological features. *J Oral Pathol Med.* 2008;37:107–121.

Arora A, Mendoza N, Brantley J, et al. Double-blind study comparing 2 dosages of valacyclovir hydrochloride for the treatment of uncomplicated herpes zoster in immunocompromised patients 18 years of age and older. *J Infect Dis.* 2008;197:1289–1295.

Beutner KR. Antivirals in the treatment of pain. *J Geriatr Dermatol.* 1994; 6 (2 suppl):23A–28A.

Brown ST, Nalley JF, Kraus SJ. Molluscum contagiosum. *Sex Transm Dis.* 1981;8:227–334.

Brown TJ, Yen-Moore A, Tyring SK. An overview of sexually transmitted disease, Part I. *J Am Acad Dermatol.* 1999;41:511–529.

Cernik C, Gallina K, Brodell RT. The treatment of herpes simplex infections: an evidence-based review. *Arch Intern Med.* 2008;168:1137–1144.

Donohue JG, Choo PW, Manson JE, et al. The incidence of herpes zoster. *Arch Intern Med.* 1995;155:1605–1609.

Foti C, Bonamonte D, Conserva A, et al. Erythema infectiosum following generalized petechial eruption induced by human parvovirus B19. *New Microbiol.* 2006;29:45–48.

Tyring SK, ed. *Mucocutaneous Manifestations of Viral Diseases.* New York: Marcel Dekker; 2002.

Pereira FA. Herpes simplex: evolving concepts. *J Am Acad Dermatol.* 1996; 35:503–520.

Rivera A, Tyring SK. Therapy of cutaneous human Papillomavirus infections. *Dermatol Ther.* 2004;17:441–448.

Sexually transmitted diseases treatment guidelines, 2006. Centers for Disease Control and Prevention. *MMWR Recomm Rep.* 2006;55:1–100.

Spruance SL, Stewart JC, Rowe NH, et al. Treatment of recurrent herpes simplex labialis with oral acyclovir. *J Infect Dis.* 1990;161:185–190.

Ting PT, Dytoc MT. Therapy of external anogenital warts and molluscum contagiosum: a literature review. *Dermatol Ther.* 2004;17:68–101.

Tyring SK. Belanger R, Bezwoda W, et al. A randomized, double-blind trial of famciclovir versus acyclovir for the treatment of localized dermatomal herpes zoster in immunocompromised patients. *Cancer Invest.* 2001;19:13–22.

Tyring SK, Beutner KR, Tucker BA, et al. Antiviral therapy for herpes zoster: randomized, controlled clinical trial of valacyclovir and famciclovir therapy in immunocompetent patients 50 years and older. *Arch Fam Med.* 2000;9:863–869.

Tyring SK. Management of herpes zoster and postherpetic neuralgia. *J Am Acad Dermatol.* 2007;57(6 suppl):S136–S142.

Wu JJ, Huang DB, Pan KR, et al. Vaccines and immunotherapies for the prevention of infectious diseases having cutaneous manifestations. *J Am Acad Dermatol.* 2004;50:495–528.

Yeung-Yue KA, Brentjens MH, Lee PC, et al. Herpes simplex viruses 1 and 2. *Dermatol Clin.* 2002;20:249–266.

# CHAPTER 24

# Cutaneous Diseases Associated with Human Immunodeficiency Virus

*Crystal Thomas, MD, Antoanella Calame, MD, and Clay Cockerell, MD*

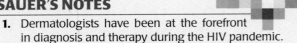

> ### SAUER'S NOTES
>
> 1. Dermatologists have been at the forefront in diagnosis and therapy during the HIV pandemic.
> 2. The skin can be used as a marker for early diagnosis and follow-up for disease regression or progression.
> 3. Morbidity and occasionally mortality from skin diseases underline the importance of dermatology in HIV.

Worldwide, there are an estimated 33 million individuals infected with human immunodeficiency virus (HIV) and up to 3 million cases diagnosed annually. Cutaneous diseases are frequently an initial manifestation of HIV, and knowledge of the most common presentations may aid in the diagnosis of immunodeficiency. Over the course of the disease, more than 90% of HIV-positive patients will present with one or more dermatologic disorders. The spectrum of HIV-associated cutaneous manifestations is broad and includes infectious diseases, inflammatory disorders, neoplastic conditions, and hypersensitivity reactions, some of which may be related to antiretroviral therapies. The following is an outline of the most commonly encountered skin disorders in the HIV-infected population and the array of cutaneous manifestations associated with each entity.

## Infectious Diseases

### Viral Infections

#### Acute Retroviral Syndrome

Acute HIV infection, also termed acute retroviral syndrome (ARS), is the period from primary infection with HIV to complete seroconversion and is often subclinical. When symptomatic, ARS resembles an acute, transient, nonspecific viral infection with fever, malaise, myalgias, headache, pharyngitis, and lymphadenopathy. It has been shown that early identification and treatment of patients with ARS may help preserve immune function. Cutaneous manifestations

may be seen in up to 75% of symptomatic patients with ARS and usually appear several days after the onset of symptoms. The most common presentation is a morbilliform eruption with erythematous macules and papules measuring up to 1 cm in diameter. The trunk is most commonly involved, followed by the face and extremities. Vesicles, pustules, urticarial lesions, alopecia, and desquamation of the palms and soles have also been reported. In addition, approximately 25% of patients with ARS exhibit painful erosions and shallow ulcerations of the mucous membranes, most commonly in the oral cavity.

### Molluscum Contagiosum

Molluscum contagiosum (MC) is a viral infection present in 5% to 20% of HIV-positive patients. The causative virus is a member of the family Poxviridae and is passed by direct skin-to-skin contact. In adults the lesions are often sexually transmitted and occur most commonly in the genital region, lower abdomen, and thighs as solitary or multiple, skin-colored, umbilicated papules or nodules measuring 1 to 10 mm in diameter. Severely immunocompromised patients, particularly those with CD4 cell counts below 200/mm³, may exhibit unusual morphologies and growth patterns such as giant (>1 cm) lesions, clusters of several hundred papules, and extensive facial involvement. Although most lesions are generally self-limited, MC in immunocompromised patients is characteristically difficult to treat and lesions rarely spontaneously regress. Treatment options include cryotherapy, electrocauterization, laser surgery, and topical tretinoin, intralesional interferon, or the antiviral agent cidofovir for refractory lesions.

### Human Papillomavirus

Human papillomavirus (HPV) is a double-stranded DNA virus of the Papovavirus class that induces hyperproliferative lesions of the skin and mucous membranes and is transmitted by direct skin-to-skin contact. More than 150 types of HPV have been identified, and several strains have been shown to play a role in oncogenesis, particularly HPV types 16 and 18. HPV infections can be subdivided clinically into three categories: cutaneous lesions (e.g., verruca vulgaris), anogenital/mucosal lesions (e.g., condyloma acuminata), and epidermodysplasia verruciformis (EDV). EDV is believed to be related to an autosomal recessive impairment of cell-mediated immunity. HIV is associated with an increased incidence of high-grade anogenital intraepithelial dysplasias and invasive squamous cell carcinomas (SCCs), and therefore, these patients should undergo frequent surveillance. Treatment modalities for cutaneous lesions include cryotherapy, podophyllin, salicylic acid, trichloroacetic acid, laser therapy, topical imiquimod, and surgical techniques.

### Herpes Simplex Virus

Herpes simplex virus (HSV) infections are seen in 2% to 27% of HIV-positive patients and demonstrate an increased incidence when CD4 cell counts decrease to $100/mm^3$ or less. HSV-1 typically causes oral lesions, while HSV-2 is generally localized to the anogenital region, although significant crossover infection is present. Transmission occurs through the exchange of bodily fluids, as well as direct contact with vesicular fluid of active herpetic lesions. In the early stages of HIV infection, the clinical presentation of HSV infections is similar to that seen in immunocompetent individuals (Fig. 24-1). However, with advanced immunosuppression, lesions of herpes simplex often are atypical and can generally be divided into three clinical forms: chronic ulcerative herpes simplex, generalized acute mucocutaneous herpes simplex, and systemic herpes simplex. Chronic ulcerative herpes simplex exhibits recalcitrant ulcerations, most often of the anogenital and perioral regions, that peripherally expand, deepen, and become confluent. Generalized acute muco-cutaneous herpes simplex is characterized by disseminated

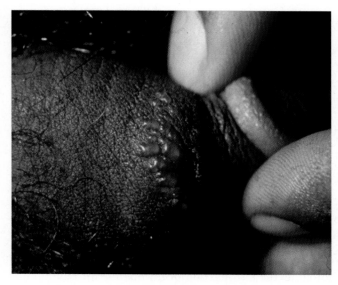

**FIGURE 24-1** ■ Grouped vesicles in a posterior auricular location in an AIDS patient. There is nothing characteristic about this as differing from an HIV(−) patient.

vesicular skin and mucous membrane lesions accompanied by high fever and other systemic symptoms. Systemic herpes simplex infection is relatively rare and most commonly involves the lungs, liver, adrenal glands, pericardium, and brain with an associated high mortality. Acyclovir remains the intravenous therapy of choice for severe local disease and disseminated cutaneous or systemic infections. However, acyclovir resistance has a prevalence of 6.4% and is encountered most commonly among AIDS patients in whom prolonged, low-dose administration is used for suppressive therapy. Foscarnet (vidarabine) has been shown to be effective against some acyclovir-resistant strains.

### Varicella–Zoster Virus

Varicella–zoster virus (VZV) infection, transmitted via aerosol droplets, initially manifests as varicella (chickenpox), whereas a reoccurrence of the disease is termed herpes zoster (shingles). When occurring in immunocompromised patients, VZV infection is often severe and can generally be categorized clinically as severe and persistent varicella, dermatomal zoster, recurrent zoster, chronic zoster, and disseminated zoster with or without precedent dermatomal lesions. Recurrent episodes of herpes zoster have an incidence of 10% to 23% in immunocompromised patients and serves as an indicator of progression of HIV-related immunosuppression. Chronic herpes zoster manifests as hyperkeratotic nodules, verrucous lesions, or ulcerations, most commonly affecting the buttock and lower extremities, with resolution requiring weeks to months. Disseminated zoster is defined as more than 20 lesions outside the originally affected dermatome, greater than 3 contiguous dermatomes involved, or systemic infections such as pneumonitis, hepatitis, or encephalitis. When HIV-positive individuals are exposed to VZV, varicella–zoster immune globulin (VZIG) should be given as soon as possible to prevent disease or alleviate its severity. If VZV infection occurs, acyclovir is the drug of choice, albeit administered at higher dosages than used for the treatment of HSV.

## Bacterial Infections

### Bacillary Angiomatosis

Bacillary angiomatosis is a rare cutaneous disease caused by the *Bartonella* species *B. henselae* and *B. quintana* and presents most commonly in HIV-positive patients, particularly those with CD4 cell counts of less than $200/mm^3$. Cutaneous lesions may manifest as tender violaceous papules resembling pyogenic granuloma, ulcerated or crusted nodules similar to Kaposi's sarcoma, subcutaneous nodules, or widespread erythematous plaques (Fig. 24-2). While cutaneous manifestations are most common, visceral involvement may also occur and most commonly presents as peliosis hepatis of the liver. Lymph node, soft tissue, and lytic bone lesions have also been described. Erythromycin and doxycycline have been shown to be effective in eradicating the infection. Some patients may experience a disseminated inflammatory reaction after antibiotic administration, which may be alleviated by the use of an anti-inflammatory agent.

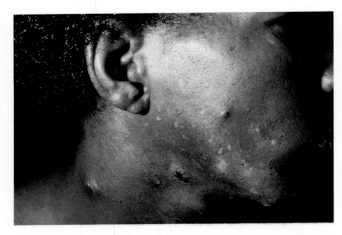

**FIGURE 24-2** ▪ Bacillary angiomatosis in an AIDS patient showing crusted, pyogenic granuloma like, papules on side of the face and neck.

## Syphilis

Syphilis is caused by the spirochete *Treponema pallidum* and has a higher prevalence among HIV-positive populations. *T. pallidum* is sexually transmitted and initially manifests as a nontender, clean-based ulceration, or chancre, which is the hallmark of primary syphilis. Within 4 to 10 weeks, secondary syphilis develops and presents as numerous erythematous macules and papules presenting diffusely on the face, trunk, and genital region. Mucous membrane and palmoplantar involvement may also be noted. Latent syphilis, the asymptomatic period following the resolution of secondary syphilis, may continue indefinitely. However, if untreated, one third of patients develop tertiary syphilis within 15 years. The cutaneous manifestations of tertiary disease include granulomas, psoriasiform plaques, and gummas (painless, indurated nodules which may ulcerate and become locally destructive). Unusual features may be seen in immunocompromised hosts and include extensive chancres, lues maligna (syphilis with vasculitis), and a rapid progression to neurosyphilis despite appropriate treatment. In general, the treatment of syphilis in HIV-positive patients is similar to those without HIV, that is, parenteral penicillin G. HIV-positive patients should be followed closely for clinical and serologic evidence of treatment failure and if confirmed, treated appropriately.

## Mycobacteria

Cutaneous mycobacterial disease, most commonly caused by *Mycobacterium tuberculosis*, often is a manifestation of systemic disease. Although relatively rare in developed countries, its incidence is increased among HIV-positive patients. There appears to be a synergistic effect with tuberculosis and HIV causing each condition to become more virulent. Multidrug resistant tuberculosis and extensively (extensively is sometimes used) drug resistant tuberculosis are major problems in the HIV population worldwide. Other mycobacterial species known to cause cutaneous infections include *M. kansasii*, *M. szulgai*, *M. marinum* and *M. avium-intracellulare*.

## Fungal Infections

### Dermatophytosis

The incidence of epidermal dermatophytosis in HIV-positive patients is similar to that of immunocompetent individuals. However, the severity and variability of presentation is typically increased in the setting of HIV infection. The most common dermatophytic pathogens seen in this patient population, *Tinea rubrum* and *Tinea mentagrophytes*, are also most commonly encountered in individuals not infected with HIV. Patients not receiving antiretroviral or antifungal therapy may develop chronic infections that can serve as portals of entry for superinfections, most commonly with *Staphylococcus aureus* or group A *Streptococcus*. Dermatophytosis occurring in HIV disease is most effectively treated with oral antifungal medications, such as terbinafine, itraconazole, or fluconazole. Topical antifungal preparations may serve as a useful adjunct to systemic therapy and may help to prevent recurrences.

### Candidiasis

The most common form of yeast infection in HIV-positive patients is oral candidiasis, most commonly caused by *Candida albicans*, documented in 43% to 93% of individuals with AIDS. Four clinical variants of oral candidiasis have been described in HIV-infected individuals: pseudomembranous candidiasis, erythematous (atrophic) candidiasis, hyperplastic candidiasis, and angular cheilitis. When possible, topical therapy, such as clotrimazole (available as a troche) or nystatin (available as an oral solution), is the preferred treatment due to the emergence of systemic antifungal-resistant organisms. If necessary, systemic medications may be utilized, such as fluconazole, ketoconazole, itraconazole, or amphotericin B.

### Cryptococcosis

Cryptococcosis, caused by *Cryptococcus neoformans*, is the most common life-threatening fungal infection in HIV-positive patients and is most commonly seen when the CD4 cell count is below $100/mm^3$. Infection with *C. neoformans* occurs via inhalation of organisms found in soil contaminated with excreta from birds. Cutaneous manifestations are seen in 10% to 20% of cases of disseminated cryptococcosis and may present 2 to 6 weeks prior to systemic symptoms. The most common findings of cutaneous cryptococcosis are umbilicated flesh-colored papules or nodules that resemble lesions of MC (**Fig. 24-3**). Lesions may also appear as pustules, ulcers, subcutaneous abscesses, cellulitis, panniculitis, palpable purpura, and plaques. The face is most commonly involved, although the lesions may be widespread. For nonmeningeal cryptococcosis, an induction phase with amphotericin B followed by the introduction of fluconazole for a minimum of 10 weeks is recommended. The addition of 5-flucytosine during the induction phase has been shown to reduce the risk of relapse.

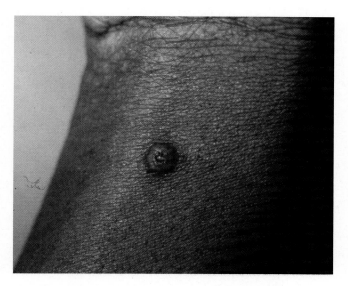

**FIGURE 24-3** ■ Umbilicated papule on the flexor wrist of disseminated cryptococcosis in an AIDS patient mimicking molluscum contagiosum.

## Histoplasmosis

Histoplasmosis, an AIDS-defining illness, is a granulomatous disease caused by the intracellular fungus, *Histoplasma capsulatum*, present in the soil within the vicinity of chicken coops, roosting places of birds, or bat caves. Disseminated disease is seen in 2% to 5% of HIV-positive individuals, particularly those with CD4 cell counts less than 150/mm³ who inhabit or have traveled to endemic regions of the United States, South America, and the Caribbean. Cutaneous manifestations, present in less than 10% of cases, most often occur on the face, followed by the extremities and trunk, as macules, papules, pustules, ulcers, subcutaneous nodules, or rosacea-like eruptions. Oropharyngeal plaques, nodules, and ulcers are also common when skin disease occurs. The treatment of choice in severe or disseminated histoplasmosis is amphotericin B. Maintenance or prophylactic therapy with itraconazole is recommended in patients with CD4 cell counts below 150/mm³.

## Coccidioidomycosis

Coccidioidomycosis is caused by *Coccidioides immitis*, a dimorphic fungus present in soil, endemic to the southwestern United States, northern Mexico, and scattered regions of Central and South America. Clinically significant infections occur more frequently in individuals with CD4 cell counts below 250/mm³. Cutaneous lesions are the most common presentation of disseminated coccidioidomycosis and predominantly manifest as papules and verrucous lesions. In some cases, lesions will expand and become confluent with the formation of ulcers, abscesses, or sinus tracts. The presence of skin lesions warrants a detailed investigation for other possible sites of dissemination. HIV-positive patients with disseminated disease should be treated initially with amphotericin B. Once clinically improved, patients may be switched to oral azole therapy, which should be continued indefinitely.

## Neoplastic Diseases

### Kaposi's Sarcoma

Kaposi's sarcoma (KS) is the most frequent neoplastic disorder occurring in HIV-positive patients and is seen most frequently in homosexual or bisexual men. Human herpesvirus type 8 (HHV-8) is present in all lesions. Initial lesions of KS occur on the face or trunk as unilateral, violaceous to yellowish-green macules or patches. With time, these lesions may progress to bilateral involvement and enlarge to form confluent plaques. A later stage of the disease is represented by nodules and tumors with areas of erosion or ulceration. KS may also involve the oral cavity, particularly the hard palate (Fig. 24-4) and serves as an indication of CD4 cell counts of less than 200/mm³. Extracutaneous KS commonly occurs in the lymph nodes, gastrointestinal tract, and lungs. Local treatment modalities include local radiation therapy, cryosurgery, laser surgery, excisional surgery, and electrocauterization. In patients with visceral involvement and life-threatening disease, chemotherapy, radiotherapy, and immunotherapy should be considered.

### Lymphomas

The incidence of lymphoma in HIV-positive patients is increased up to 200 times that of normal individuals and is the first AIDS-defining illness in 3% to 5% of patients. These are mainly non-Hodgkin lymphomas, predominantly of B-cell origin. Cutaneous lymphomas arising in HIV-positive patients may include mycosis fungoides (MF), CD30⁺ anaplastic large cell lymphoma or diffuse large B-cell lymphoma. An association with Epstein–Barr virus has been noted in many cutaneous B-cell lymphomas.

### Carcinomas and Melanoma

There is an increased incidence of nonmelanoma skin cancer including basal cell carcinoma, SCC, and Bowen's disease in HIV-positive patients, with rates approximately three to five times that of HIV-negative individuals. Epithelial neoplasms of

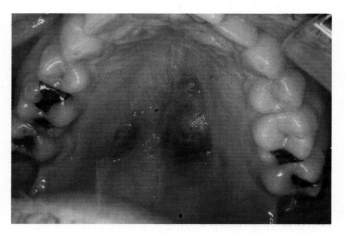

**FIGURE 24-4** ■ Asymmetric, purple, plaques of Kaposi's sarcoma on the hard palate in an AIDS patient.

oral and anogenital sites are especially increased in this patient population. In addition, neoplasms developing in a setting of immune suppression are often more aggressive, with higher rates of metastases. Adequate surgical margins providing early control of carcinomas have been shown to be important in reducing morbidity and mortality in HIV-infected patients.

Although no definitive data exist regarding the relationship between melanoma and HIV infection, the development of multiple primary melanomas and early nodular lesions has been reported in the literature. Currently it is uncertain whether this finding is secondary to increased surveillance, detection, and reporting, or an actual increase of melanoma in these patients. HIV-positive patients with melanoma have demonstrated a significantly decreased disease-free survival, with lower CD4 cell counts predictive of a poorer prognosis. Primary prevention, routine skin examinations, and early biopsy of suspicious lesions are essential in this patient population.

## Inflammatory Diseases

### Seborrheic Dermatitis

Seborrheic dermatitis, with a prevalence of approximately 85%, is one of the most common cutaneous diseases occurring in the HIV-positive patient population. The severity of the clinical presentation has been shown to correlate with the extent of immune suppression and lower CD4 cell counts. Clinically, seborrheic dermatitis presents as well-demarcated, erythematous, scaly patches and plaques of the scalp, eyebrows, nasolabial folds, ears, and intertriginous areas. Five features characteristic of AIDS-related seborrheic dermatitis include a greater degree of inflammation, more indurated plaques resembling psoriasis, involvement of atypical areas such as the trunk, groin, and extremities, "cradle cap" of the scalp producing a nonscarring alopecia, and hypo- or hyperpigmentation of affected areas. Recommended treatment consists of the use of topical corticosteroid and antifungal medications. Some refractory cases may require adjunctive therapies such as UVB phototherapy, coal tar, sulfur, salicylic acid shampoos, and pimecrolimus (Elidel) cream.

### Eosinophilic Folliculitis

HIV-associated eosinophilic folliculitis (EF) has an incidence of 9% and most commonly presents in patients with CD4 cell counts less than 250/mm$^3$. The etiology of the disease is currently uncertain. However, the folliculotropic nature of the inflammation has led to the hypothesis that an opportunistic infection, possibly secondary to bacteria, *Pityrosporum*, or *Demodex* mites, or a hypersensitivity response due to HIV-related immune dysregulation may be the cause. Patients with HIV-associated EF classically present with a persistent, erythematous, intensely pruritic, cutaneous eruption on the face, trunk, shoulders, upper arms, and neck (Fig. 24-5). Currently recommended treatment options include UVB phototherapy and topical or systemic corticosteroids.

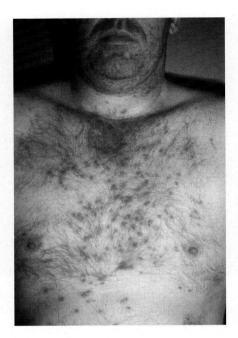

**FIGURE 24-5** ■ Inflammatory papules on the chest that were intensely pruritic and persistent which is typical of eosinophilic folliculitis in AIDS.

## Hypersensitivity Diseases

### Drug Reactions Associated with Highly Active Antiretroviral Therapy

The advent of highly active antiretroviral therapy (HAART) in the mid-1990s produced a dramatic decrease in the morbidity and mortality among patients infected with HIV. However, HAART administration has also been associated with adverse effects, many of which are dermatologic in nature. The drugs that comprise HAART regimens are categorized into four main groups based on their specific mechanism of action: nonnucleoside reverse transcriptase inhibitors (NNRTIs), nucleoside reverse transcriptase inhibitors (NRTIs), protease inhibitors (PIs), and fusion or entry inhibitors (FIs). Side effects associated with NNRTIs, which include nevirapine, delavirdine, and efavirenz, may manifest in several forms including urticaria, morbilliform eruptions, leukocytoclastic vasculitis, as well as Stevens–Johnson syndrome or "drug rash with eosinophilia and systemic symptoms" (DRESS). NRTIs, particularly zidovudine and abacavir, are known for nail and mucocutaneous hyperpigmentation (Fig. 24-6), a multisystem hypersensitivity reaction, and lipodystrophy. As a group, PIs are associated with an increased association with lipodystrophy, a morbilliform or urticarial hypersensitivity reaction, acute generalized eruptive pustulosis, generalized pruritus, xerosis, desquamative cheilitis, striae formation, and angiolipomatosis. Only one FI, enfuvirtide, is currently approved for use in HIV-positive patients, and its subcutaneous administration has been associated with injection site reactions in a significant proportion of patients.

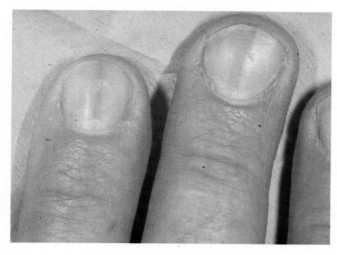

**FIGURE 24-6** ▪ Hyperpigmented streaks on fingernails which is seen in patients on NRTI medications for AIDS.

## Photosensitivity Reactions

Photoeruptions have become increasingly recognized in the setting of HIV disease and in general, can be classified into the following categories: chronic actinic dermatitis (CAD), lichenoid photoeruptions, photosensitive hyperpigmentation, porphyria cutanea tarda, and photosensitive granuloma annulare. Among these, CAD and lichenoid photoeruptions are the two categories most commonly witnessed in HIV-positive patients. CAD, which persists for months to years, demonstrates a marked male predominance and presents as erythematous or lichenified papules and plaques in a photodistributed pattern. An increased incidence of lichenoid photoeruptions is seen in African-American patients infected with HIV, particularly those with advanced disease and CD4 cell counts below 50/mm$^3$. The eruptions are usually chronic, lasting several months and, similar to lichen planus, are characterized by violaceous, flat-topped papules and plaques. Lesions are predominantly on the face, neck, and dorsa of the forearms and hands. The lack of mucosal involvement, with the exception of the lower lip, can aid in distinguishing these lesions from idiopathic lichen planus.

## Suggested Readings

Akgul B, Cooke JC, Storey A. HPV-associated skin disease. *J Pathol.* 2006;208(2):165–175.

Ampel NM, Dols CL, Galgiani JN. Coccidioidomycosis during human immunodeficiency virus infection: results of a prospective study in a coccidioidal endemic area. *Am J Med.* 1993;94(3):235–240.

Aquilina C, Viraben R, Roueire A. Acute generalized exanthematous pustulosis: a cutaneous adverse effect due to prophylactic antiviral therapy with protease inhibitor. *Arch Intern Med.* 1998;158(19):2160–2161.

Bourezane Y, Salard D, Hoen B, et al. DRESS (drug rash with eosinophilia and systemic symptoms) syndrome associated with nevirapine therapy. *Clin Infect Dis.* 1998;27(5):1321–1322.

Buchbinder SP, Katz MH, Hessol NA, et al. Herpes zoster and human immunodeficiency virus infection. *J Infect Dis.* 1992;166(5):1153–1156.

Cattelan AM, Trevenzoli M, Aversa SM. Recent advances in the treatment of AIDS-related Kaposi's sarcoma. *Am J Clin Dermatol.* 2002;3(7):451–462.

Chatis PA, Crumpacker CS. Resistance of herpesviruses to antiviral drugs. *Antimicrob Agents Chemother.* 1992;36(8):1589–1595.

Cockerell CJ. Cutaneous manifestations of HIV infection other than Kaposi's sarcoma: clinical and histologic aspects. *J Am Acad Dermatol.* 1990;22(6 pt 2):1260–1269.

Cockerell CJ. Seborrheic dermatitis-like and atopic dermatitis-like eruptions in HIV-infected patients. *Clin Dermatol.* 1991;9(1):49–51.

Cockerell CJ. Bacillary angiomatosis and related diseases caused by Rochalimaea. *J Am Acad Dermatol.* 1995;32(5 pt 1):783–790.

Coldiron BM, Bergstresser PR. Prevalence and clinical spectrum of skin disease in patients infected with human immunodeficiency virus. *Arch Dermatol.* 1989;125(3):357–361.

Cooley TP. Non-AIDS-defining cancer in HIV-infected people. *Hematol Oncol Clin North Am.* 2003;17(3):889–899.

Garcia-Silva J, Almagro M, Juega J, et al. Protease inhibitor-related paronychia, ingrown toenails, desquamative cheilitis and cutaneous xerosis. *AIDS.* 2000;14(9):1289–1291.

Golden MR, Marra CM, Holmes KK. Update on syphilis: resurgence of an old problem. *JAMA.* 2003;290(11):1510–1514.

Grayson W. The HIV-positive skin biopsy. *J Clin Pathol.* 2008;61(7):802–817.

Gregory N, DeLeo VA. Clinical manifestations of photosensitivity in patients with human immunodeficiency virus infection. *Arch Dermatol.* 1994;130(5):630–633.

Hetherington S, McGuirk S, Powell G, et al. Hypersensitivity reactions during therapy with the nucleoside reverse transcriptase inhibitor abacavir. *Clin Ther.* 2001;23(10):1603–1614.

Kahn JO, Walker BD. Acute human immunodeficiency virus type 1 infection. *N Engl J Med.* 1998;339(1):33–39.

Kaviarasan PK, Jaisankar TJ, Thappa DM, et al. Clinical variations in dermatophytosis in HIV infected patients. *Indian J Dermatol Venereol Leprol.* 2002;68(4):213–216.

Lapins J, Lindback S, Lidbrink P, et al. Mucocutaneous manifestations in 22 consecutive cases of primary HIV-1 infection. *Br J Dermatol.* 1996;134(2):257–261.

Nguyen P, Vin-Christian K, Ming ME, et al. Aggressive squamous cell carcinomas in persons infected with the human immunodeficiency virus. *Arch Dermatol.* 2002;138(6):758–763.

Noy A. Update on HIV lymphoma. *Curr Oncol Rep.* 2007;9(5):384–390.

Patel SM, Johnson S, Belknap SM, et al. Serious adverse cutaneous and hepatic toxicities associated with nevirapine use by non-HIV-infected individuals. *J Acquir Immune Defic Syndr.* 2004;35(2):120–125.

Phelan JA. Oral manifestations of human immunodeficiency virus infection. *Med Clin North Am.* 1997;81(2):511–531.

Rasokat H, Steigleder GK, Bendick C, et al. Malignant melanoma and HIV infection. *Z Hautkr.* 1989;64(7):581–582, 7.

Sadick NS, McNutt NS, Kaplan MH. Papulosquamous dermatoses of AIDS. *J Am Acad Dermatol.* 1990;22(6 pt 2):1270–1277.

Samaranayake LP, Holmstrup P. Oral candidiasis and human immunodeficiency virus infection. *J Oral Pathol Med.* 1989;18(10):554–564.

Schwartz JJ, Myskowski PL. Molluscum contagiosum in patients with human immunodeficiency virus infection. A review of twenty-seven patients. *J Am Acad Dermatol.* 1992;27(4):583–588.

Simpson-Dent S, Fearfield LA, Staughton RC. HIV associated eosinophilic folliculitis—differential diagnosis and management. *Sex Transm Infect.* 1999;75(5):291–293.

Vanhems P, Beaulieu R. Primary infection by type 1 human immunodeficiency virus: diagnosis and prognosis. *Postgrad Med J.* 1997;73(861):403–408.

Wheat J, Sarosi G, McKinsey D, et al. Practice guidelines for the management of patients with histoplasmosis. Infectious Diseases Society of America. *Clin Infect Dis.* 2000;30(4):688–695.

Wheat LJ, Kauffman CA. Histoplasmosis. *Infect Dis Clin North Am.* 2003;17(1):1–19, vii.

Wilkins K, Dolev JC, Turner R, et al. Approach to the treatment of cutaneous malignancy in HIV-infected patients. *Dermatol Ther.* 2005;18(1):77–86.

Wilks D, Boyd A, Clutterbuck D, et al. Clinical and pathological review of HIV-associated lymphoma in Edinburgh, United Kingdom. *Eur J Clin Microbiol Infect Dis.* 2001;20(9):603–608.

Zuger A, Louie E, Holzman RS, et al. Cryptococcal disease in patients with the acquired immunodeficiency syndrome. Diagnostic features and outcome of treatment. *Ann Intern Med.* 1986;104(2):234–240.

# CHAPTER 25

# Dermatologic Mycology

*John C. Hall, MD*

Fungi can be present as part of the normal flora of the skin or as abnormal inhabitants. Dermatologists are concerned with the abnormal inhabitants, or pathogenic fungi. However, so-called nonpathogenic fungi can proliferate and invade immunosuppressed persons.

Pathogenic fungi have a predilection for certain body areas; most commonly they infect the skin, but the lungs, the brain, and other organs can also be infected. Pathogenic fungi can invade the skin *superficially* and *deeply* and are thus divided into these two groups.

## Superficial Fungal Infections

The superficial fungi live on the dead horny layer of the skin and elaborate an enzyme that enables them to digest keratin, causing the superficial skin to scale and disintegrate, the nails to crumble, and the hairs to break off. The deeper reactions of vesicles, erythema, and infiltration are presumably due to the fungi liberating an exotoxin. Fungi are also capable of eliciting an allergic or id reaction.

When a skin scraping, a hair, or a culture growth is examined with the microscope in a wet preparation, the three structural elements of the fungi are seen: the spores, the hyphae, and the mycelia.

> *Spores* are the reproducing bodies of the fungi. Sexual and asexual forms occur. Spores are rarely seen in skin scrapings, but they are the identifying structures on microscopic examination of fungal cultures.
>
> *Hyphae* are threadlike, branching filaments that grow out from the fungus spore. The hyphae are the identifying filaments seen in skin scrapings in potassium hydroxide (KOH) solution.
>
> *Mycelia* are matted clumps of hyphae that grow on culture plates.

Culture media vary greatly in content, but modifications of Sabouraud's dextrose agar are used to grow the superficial fungi. Sabouraud's agar and corn meal agar are both used to identify the deep fungi. Hyphae and spores grow on the media, and identification of the species of fungi is established by the gross appearance of the mycelia, the color of the substrate, and the microscopic appearance of the spores and the hyphae when a sample of the growth is placed on a slide. Some media show a color change when pathogenic fungi are isolated.

## Classification

Superficial dermatophyte fungi are divided into three genera: *Microsporum*, *Epidermophyton*, and *Trichophyton*. Species of only two of these invade the hair: *Microsporum* and *Trichophyton*. As seen in a KOH preparation, *Microsporum* species cause an ectothrix infection of the hair shaft, whereas *Trichophyton* species cause either an ectothrix or an endothrix infection. The ectothrix fungi cause the formation of an external spore sheath around the hair, whereas the endothrix fungi do not. The filaments of mycelia penetrate the hair in both types of infection.

The species of fungi is correlated with the clinical diseases in Table 25-1.

## Clinical Classifications

Superficial fungal infections of the skin affect various sites of the body. The clinical lesions, the species of fungi, and the therapy vary for these different sites. Therefore, fungal diseases of the skin are classified, for clinical purposes, according to the location of the infection. These clinical types are as follows:

- Tinea of the feet (tinea pedis)
- Tinea of the hands (tinea manus)
- Tinea of the nails (onychomycosis)
- Tinea of the groin (tinea cruris)
- Tinea of the smooth skin (tinea corporis)
- Tinea of the scalp (tinea capitis)
- Tinea of the beard (tinea barbae)
- Dermatophytid (generalized allergic reaction)
- Tinea versicolor
- Tinea of the external ear.

1. Correct diagnosis of a fungal infection is necessary. An oral antifungal drug should not be prescribed for a patient if the diagnosis has not been confirmed. Systemic antifungal agents are of no value in treating atopic eczema, contact dermatitis, psoriasis, pityriasis rosea, and so on.

2. Except for tinea of the scalp and nails, true fungal infections are noticeably improved after only 1 to 2 weeks of oral antifungal therapy. If there is no improvement, the diagnosis of the dermatosis as a fungus disease is erroneous and the therapy should be stopped.

**TABLE 25-1 ■ Relationship of Fungi to Body Areas**

| Fungus | Feet and Hands | Nails | Groin | Smooth Skin | Scalp | Beard |
|---|---|---|---|---|---|---|
| **Microsporum species** | | | | | | |
| *M. audouini* | 0 | 0 | 0 | Uncommon | Uncommon | 0 |
| *M. canis* | 0 | 0 | 0 | Common | Uncommon | Rare |
| *M. gypseum* | 0 | 0 | 0 | Rare | Rare | 0 |
| **Epidermophyton species** | | | | | | |
| *E. floccosum* | Moderately common | Rare | Common | Moderately common | 0 | 0 |
| **Trychophyton species** | | | | | | |
| **Endothrix species** | | | | | | |
| *T. schoenleini* | 0 | Rare | 0 | Rare | (Favus) rare, especially tropics | 0 |
| *T. violaceum* | 0 | Rare | 0 | 0 | Rare | Rare |
| *T. tonsurans* | 0 | Rare | 0 | Rare | Common | 0 |
| **Ectothrix species** | | | | | | |
| *T. mentagrophytes* | Common | Moderately common | 0 | Common | Rare | Moderately common |
| *T. rubrum* | Common | Common | Moderately common | Common | 0 | Rare |

3. An adequate dosage is necessary, including (a) the correct daily dose for the particular type of fungal infection and (b) the correct duration of such dosage.

4. In general, systemic antifungal therapy should not be used to treat tinea of the feet. The recurrence rate after completion of therapy is very high.

5. Candidal infections should not be treated with oral griseofulvin. Very commonly, candidal intertrigo of the groin or candidal paronychias are erroneously treated with griseofulvin. Griseofulvin is of no value in these conditions. Because it is a penicillin-related drug, it can cause an allergic reaction in patients with a penicillin sensitivity.

6. Tinea versicolor does not respond to oral griseofulvin therapy.

7. So-called fungal infection of the ear does not respond to oral antifungal therapy. Most external ear diseases are not caused by a fungus.

---

**SAUER'S NOTES**

Since the discovery of specific systemic antifungal agents many physicians have believed that

1. These agents are indicated for every fungus infection.
2. Most skin diseases are due to a fungus, so they should treat the patient with an antifungal agent and make a diagnosis later.

Both of these assumptions are erroneous.

---

There is a predilection for certain sites of tinea in which the frequency varies with the age of the patient. This is outlined in **Table 25-2**.

## Tinea of the Feet (Tinea Pedis) (**Figs. 25-1 to 25-3**)

Tinea of the feet (athlete's foot, fungal infection of the feet, and ringworm of the feet) is a very common skin infection. Many persons have the disease and are not even aware of it. The clinical appearance varies.

*Primary Lesions*

*Acute form:* Blisters (vesicular tinea pedis) occur on the soles and the sides of feet or between the toes.

**TABLE 25-2 ■ Sites of Tinea in Relationship to Age Groups**

| Tinea Site | Children (0–16 yr) | Adults |
|---|---|---|
| Tinea capitis (scalp) | Common | Very rare |
| Tinea corporis (body) | Common | Fairly common |
| Tinea cruris (groin) | Rare | Common (esp. males) |
| Tinea pedis (feet) | Rare (mimics eczema) | Very common |
| Onychomycosis (nails) | Very rare | Very common |

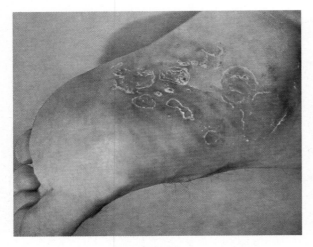

**FIGURE 25-1** ▪ Tinea of the foot. This dry, scaly form of fungus infection is usually due to *T. rubrum*. ▪ *(Courtesy of Smith Kline & French Laboratories.)*

*Chronic form:* Lesions are dry and scaly ("moccasin" tinea pedis).
*Interdigital form:* Macerated skin appears between the toes.

### Secondary Lesions

Bacterial infection may occur in the acute and interdigital form. Fissures are not uncommon in the interdigital form.

### Course

Recurrent acute infections can lead to a chronic infection. If the toenails become infected, a cure is highly improbable, because this focus is very difficult to eradicate and the fungus is ubiquitous and the patient's susceptibility (almost always lifelong) cannot be decreased.

The species of fungus influences the response to therapy. Most vesicular, acute fungal infections are due to *Trichophyton mentagrophytes* and respond readily to correct treatment. The chronic scaly type of infection is usually due to *Trichophyton rubrum* and is exceedingly difficult, if not impossible, to cure.

### Contagiousness

Experiments have shown that there is a susceptibility factor necessary for infection. Males are much more susceptible than are females.

### Laboratory Findings

KOH-ink preparations of scrapings and cultures on Sabouraud's media serve to demonstrate the presence of fungi and the specific type. A KOH preparation is a very simple office procedure and should be resorted to when the diagnosis is uncertain or the response to therapy is slow.

### Differential Diagnosis

*Contact dermatitis:* Due to shoes, socks, gloves, foot powder usually on dorsum of feet; history of new shoes or new foot powder; fungi not found.

*Atopic eczema:* Especially on dorsum of toes in children; quite chronic; usually worse in winter; very pruritic; atopic family history; fungi not found.

*Psoriasis:* Affects soles and palms; pustular, thickened, well-circumscribed lesions; psoriasis elsewhere on body; fungi not found.

*Pustular bacterid:* Pustular lesions only especially on palms and soles; chronic; resistant to local therapy; fungi not found. This condition may be associated with a focus of infection, as in tonsil, teeth, or gallbladder.

*Hyperhidrosis of feet:* Can be severe and cause white, eroded maceration of the soles, accompanied by a foul odor. No fungi found. Zeasorb AF powder is helpful, as is Drysol solution.

*Pitted keratolysis (keratolysis plantare sulcatum):* Produces circular areas of erosions with a punched-out appearance on the soles of the feet; associated with hyperhidrosis; filamentous, gram-positive, branching microorganisms are found on skin scrapings caused by corynebacterium, actinomyces, Kytococcus sedentarius (*Dermatococcus sedentarius*) or *Dermatophilus congolensis*. Topical or systemic erythromycin is usually beneficial.

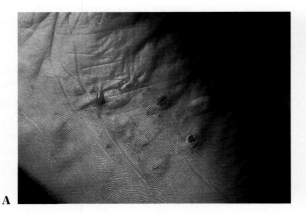
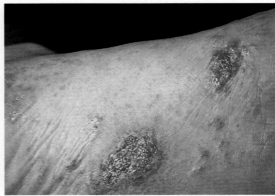

A    B

**FIGURE 25-2** ▪ **(A and B)** Acute vesicular tinea of the foot often due to *T. mentagrophytes. (Courtesy of Schering Corp.)*

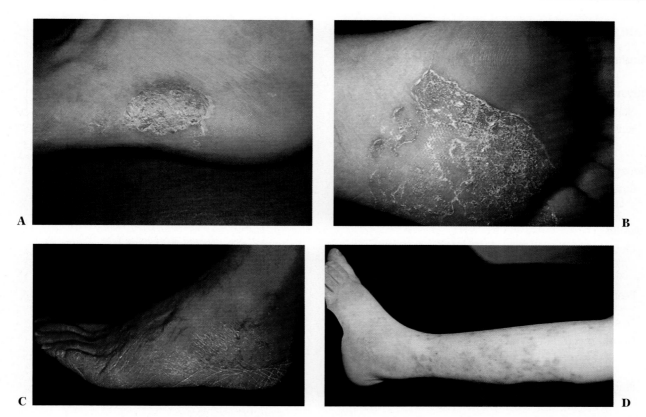

**FIGURE 25-3** ■ Tinea of the foot. *(Courtesy of Schering Corp.)* (**A**) Chronic tinea of side of foot. (**B**) Chronic tinea of sole due to *T. rubrum* (**C**) Chronic extensive tinea on patient on corticosteroids. (**D**) Chronic tinea extending up leg.

*Treatment*

***Case Example:*** *Acute Infection.* An acute vesicular, pustular fungal infection of 2 weeks duration is present on the soles of the feet and between the toes in a 16-year-old boy. This clinical picture is usually due to the organism *T. mentagrophytes.*

***First Visit***

1. The fear of the infectiousness of athlete's foot should be minimized but normal cleanliness emphasized, including the wearing of slippers over bare feet, wiping the feet last after a bath (not the groin last), and changing socks daily (white socks are not necessary).
2. Debridement. The physician or the patient should snip off the tops of the blister with small scissors. This enables the pus to drain out and allows the medication to reach the organisms. The edges of any blister should be kept trimmed, since the fungi spread under these edges. This debridement is followed by a foot soak.

---

**SAUER'S NOTES**

A favorite medication of mine for tinea of the feet and body is

| | |
|---|---|
| Sulfur, ppt. | 5% |
| Hydrocortisone | 1% |
| Antifungal cream q.s. | 30.0 |

---

3. Burow's solution soak

   *Sig:* One packet of Domeboro powder to 1 quart of warm water. Soak feet for 10 minutes b.i.d. Dry skin carefully afterward.

4. Antifungal cream 15.0

   Miconazole (Monistat-Derm, Micatin), clotrimazole (Lotrimin, Mycelex), econazole (Spectazole), ketoconazole (Nizoral), ciclopirox (Loprox), oxiconazole (Oxistat), naftifine (Naftin), terbenifine (Lamisil), butenafine (Mentax, Lotrimin AF is over the counter), econazole(Ertaczo), and tolnaftate (Tinactin) (see Table 25-3 for detailed list of antifungal agents).

   *Sig:* Apply b.i.d. locally to feet after soaking.
   *Sig:* Apply b.i.d. locally for long term.

5. Rest at home for 2 to 4 days may be advisable, if severe.
6. Place small pieces of cotton sheeting or cotton between the toes when wearing shoes.

   Five days later, the secondary infection and blisters should have decreased.

7. Oral terbenifine 250 mg once a day for 1 week is safe and very effective.

***Subsequent Visits***

1. The soaks may be continued for another 3 days or stopped if no marked redness or infection is present.

**TABLE 25-3 ■ Antifungal Agents**

| Antifungal Agents | Route of Administration | Organism Responsive | Side Effects |
|---|---|---|---|
| **Allylamines** | | | |
| Naftifine (Naftin) | Cream, gel | Dermatophytes | Rare |
| Terbinafine (Lamisil) | Cream, spray, oral | Dermatophytes, tinea versicolor | Oral, rarely liver toxicity |
| **Benzylamines** | | | |
| Butenafine HCL (Mentax, Lotrimin Ultra Cream) | Cream | Dermatophytes | Rare |
| **−Azoles** | | | |
| Clotrimazole (Mycelex, Lotrimin cream, solution Troches suppositories) | Cream | Dermatophytes, tinea versicolor, Candida | Rare |
| Econazole (Spectazole) | Cream | Dermatophytes, tinea versicolor, gram(+) bacteria | Rare |
| Fluconazole (Diflucan) | Oral | Dermatophytes, tinea versicolor, cryptococcosis, Candida | Rare |
| Itraconazole (Sporanox) | Oral (with food) | Dermatophytes, tinea versicolor, Candida, sporotrichosis, some deep fungi | Rare liver toxicity |
| Ketoconazole (Nizoral) | Cream shampoo, oral | Dermatophytes, some deep fungi, Candida, tinea versicolor | Liver toxicity when oral |
| Miconazole (Micatin, Monistat, Zeasorb AF) | Cream, powder spray, suppositories | Dermatophytes, tinea versicolor, Candida | Rare |
| Oxiconazole (Oxistat) | Cream | Dermatophytes, tinea versicolor, Candida | Rare |
| Sertaconazole (ertaczol) | Cream | Dermatophytes, tinea versicolor, Candida | Rare |
| **Polyenes** | | | |
| Amphotericin B (Fungizone, Abelcet) | Intravenous | Deep fungi sepsis, Candida sepsis | Common renal toxicity thrombophlebitis, hypokalemia |
| Nystatin (Mycostatin) | Cream, ointment, powder, oral (not absorbed), pastilles, with triamcinolone (Mycolog II cream, ointment) | Candida | Rare |
| **Miscellaneous** | | | |
| Flucytosine (Ancobon) | Oral, usually given with amphotericin B | Deep fungi sepsis, Candida sepsis | Liver, renal, bone marrow toxicity, gastrointestinal |
| Ciclopirox (Loprox, Penlac) Penlac Nail Lacquer | Gel, cream, shampoo, suspensions | Dermatophytes, Candida | Rare |
| Griseofulvin (Gris-Peg), Fulvicin, Grifulvin | Oral (evening with fatty meal) tablets, suspension | | Rare |

**TABLE 25-3** ■ *(Continued)*

| Antifungal Agents | Route of Administration | Organism Responsive | Side Effects |
|---|---|---|---|
| Selenium sulfide (Selsun, Head & Shoulders Intensive Treatment) | Shampoo (sometimes used as lotion) | Tinea versicolor | Irritation |
| Saturated solution of potassium iodide (SSKI) | Oral | Sporotrichosis | Gastrointestinal toxicity, bitter-taste, goiter if long-term |
| Tolnaftate (Tinactin) | Cream | Dermatophytes | Rare |
| Undecylenic acid (Desenex) | Cream | Dermatophytes | Rare |
| Capsofungin (Candidas) | Intravenous | Candidiasis sepsis, Aspergillosis sepsis | Common, fever, headache thrombophlebitis, rash |
| Micafungin (Mycoviral) | Intravenous | Candidiasis sepsis, esophagitis | Common, headaches, rash, fever, bone marrow thrombophlebitis |
| Vericonazole (Ufend) | Intravenous, oral | Candida sepsis, esophageal, Aspergillosis sepsis, Fusariesis sepsis | Visceral impairment, liver toxicity, fever, cardiac toxicity |

2. The previously described salve is continued or the following salves are substituted: A combination of an antifungal cream and a corticosteroid, as in Lotrisone cream, is beneficial. Antifungal solutions, such as Lotrimin or Mycelex or Loprox are quite effective. Apply a few drops on affected skin and rub in.

3. Antifungal powder q.s. 45.0.

Zeasorb AF, Micatin, Tinactin, and Desenex.

*Sig:* Supply in powder can. Apply small amount to feet over the salve and to the shoes in the morning.

***Case Example:*** *Chronic Infection.* A patient presents with chronic, scaly, thickened fungal infection of 4 years duration. In the past week, a few small tense blisters on the sole of the feet had developed. This type of clinical picture probably is due to the organism *T. rubrum.*

### First Visit

1. The patient is told that the acute flare-up (the blisters) can be cleared but that it will be difficult and time-consuming to cure the chronic infection. If the toenails are found to be infected, the prognosis for cure is even poorer (see Tinea of the Nails section).

2. The blisters are debrided and trimmed with manicure scissors.

3. Any of the antifungal creams,

*Sig:* Apply locally to soles b.i.d., or
Antifungal solution 10.0.
*Sig:* Rub in a few drops b.i.d.

### Subsequent Visits

1. Systemic antifungal therapy: This type of oral therapy is not recommended for chronic tinea of the feet. But the patient may have heard or read about the "pill for athlete's feet," so it would be wise for you to discuss this with the patient. If you mention that you cannot guarantee a cure, most patients will be content with keeping the chronic infection in an innocuous state with sporadic local therapy.

2. However, if the patient still wants to try oral therapy, then consider the systemic antifungal agents listed in the following section on Tinea of the Hands and in Table 25-3. Long-term pulse therapy is indicated.

## Tinea of the Hands (Tinea Manum)

A primary fungal infection of the hand or hands is quite rare. In spite of this fact, the diagnosis of "fungal infection of the hand" is commonly applied to cases that in reality are contact dermatitis, atopic eczema, pustular bacterid, or psoriasis. The best differential point is that tinea of the hand usually is seen only on one hand, not bilaterally. It mimics dry skin in the common chronic form and may have fingernail involvement (**Fig. 25-4A–E**).

### Primary Lesions

*Acute form:* Blisters on the palms and the fingers are seen at the edge of red areas.

*Chronic form:* Lesions are dry and scaly; usually there is a single patch, not separate patches.

### Secondary Lesions

Bacterial infection is rather unusual.

### Course

This gradually progressive disease spreads to fingernails. It usually is asymptomatic.

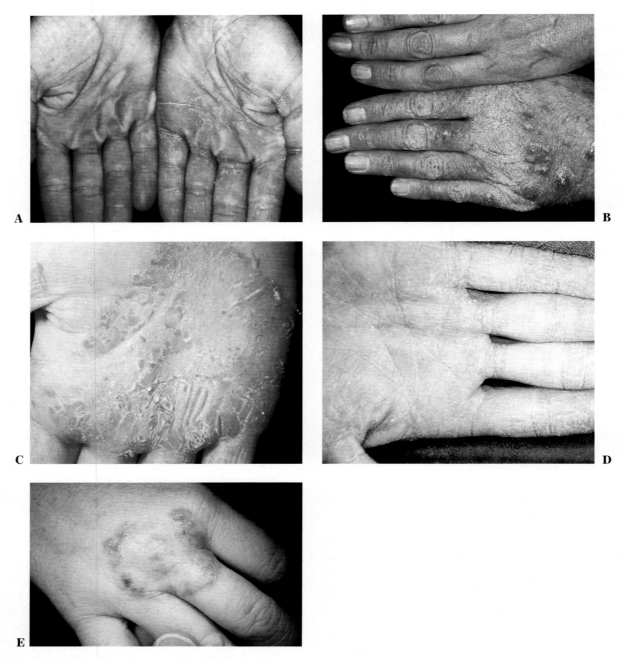

**FIGURE 25-4** ■ **(A)** Tinea of the left palm only, due to *T. mentagrophytes*. **(B)** Deep tinea of left hand, due to *T. mentagrophytes*. **(C)** Tinea of the palm, due to *T. rubrum*. **(D)** Tinea of the palm, of dry, scaly type, due to *T. rubrum*. **(E)** Tinea on the back of the hand.

*Laboratory Findings*

KOH or ink preparations reveal mycelia, or cultures on Sabouraud's media grow the fungus.

*Differential Diagnosis*

> *Contact dermatitis of hands:* Due to soap, detergents, and other irritants; usually bilateral, periodic, more vesicular, and less frequently chronic; fungi not found. Prefers backs of hands to palms.

*Atopic eczema:* History of atopy in patient or family; bilateral; periodic; fungi not found.

*Psoriasis:* See thick patch or patches in palms, usually bilateral; occasionally see psoriasis elsewhere; fungi not found. Psoriatic nail involvement may mimic onychomycosis of fingernails.

*Pustular bacterid:* Pustular lesions only; periodic and chronic; resistant to local therapy; fungi not found.

*Dyshidrosis of palms:* Recurrent; seasonal incidence; mainly vesicular on the sides of the fingers: not scaly; bilateral; may be related to atopic eczema; fungi not found.

## Treatment

**Case Example:** A man presents with scaly thickening of one palm of 8 years duration. His fingernails are not involved. Itching is noted slightly at times.

1. Antifungal creams, especially naftifine (Naftin), terbinafine (Lamisil) cream, or butenafine (Mentax) may control or occasionally cure the tinea of the hand.
2. Systemic therapy (Table 25-3). The following medicines are all expensive, especially because therapy must be continued, as for hand tinea, for several months. Appropriate monitoring of the patient during therapy is necessary. There are also drug interactions that can occur.
   a. Griseofulvin (Gris-Peg, 250 mg; Fulvicin P/G, 330 mg; Grisactin, 330 mg; Grifulvin, 330 mg).
      *Sig:* One tablet t.i.d after meals for at least 8 weeks, and probably for 4 to 6 months.
      *Comment:* Griseofulvin commonly causes headaches in the first few days of therapy. It is a penicillin derivative and cross reactions may occur.
   b. Ketoconazole (Nizoral), 200 mg (rarely 400 mg)
      *Sig:* One tablet once a day for 3 to 4 months.
      *Comment:* Hepatotoxicity has been rarely reported with ketoconazole therapy, also impotence.
   c. Itraconazole (Sporanox) capsule, 100 mg. 200 mg b.i.d. for 7 days, repeated once a month for 3 to 4 months. Monitoring for rare liver toxicity must be done. Drug interactions are numerous.
   d. Fluconazole (Diflucan) has not been approved for superficial dermatophyte therapy. It may be effective in doses of 200 mg per week for 1 to 3 months. Drug interactions are numerous.
   e. Terbinafine (Lamisil) 250 mg is author's choice
      *Sig:* One tablet each day for 1 week is cheap, safe and effective. It can be periodically repeated or topical agents used once control is achieved.

## Tinea of the Nails (Onychomycosis)

Tinea of the toenails is very common, but tinea of the fingernails (Fig. 25-5) is uncommon. Tinea of the toenails is almost inevitable in patients who have recurrent attacks of tinea of the feet. Once developed, the infected nail serves as a resistant focus for future skin infection.

### Primary Lesions

Distal and lateral detachment of the nail occurs with subsequent thickening, subungual white keratotic debris, and deformity.

### Secondary Lesions

Bacterial infection can result. Ingrown toenails are another undesirable consequence.

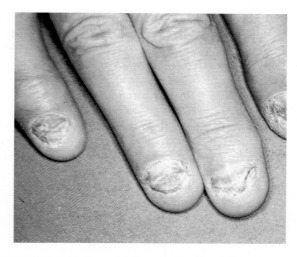

**FIGURE 25-5** ■ Tinea of fingernails, due to *T. rubrum*. *(Courtesy of Duke Laboratories, Inc.)*

### Distribution

The infection usually begins in the fifth toenail and may remain there or spread to involve the other nails.

### Course

*Tinea of the fingernails can rarely be cured.* Aside from the deformity, ingrown toenail (especially in diabetes mellitus and marked vascular or neurologic compromise to the feet) and an occasional mild flare-up of acute tinea, treatment is not necessary. Progression is slow and recurrence is the rule.

*Tinea of the fingernails* can be treated, but the treatment usually takes months.

### Etiology

This type of tinea is usually due to *T. rubrum* and, less likely, to *T. mentagrophytes*. Approximately 8% of cases are due to nondermatophyte molds especially scopulariopsis, scylidium (treatment by surgery only), fusarium, aspergillosis, and acremonium. These nondermatophyte molds are very difficult to treat. Approximately 1% are yeast, especially candida species.

### Laboratory Findings

These organisms can be found in a KOH preparation of a scraping and occasionally can be grown on culture media. The material should be gathered from the most proximal debris under the nail plate. It is often difficult to obtain a positive test. Author's favorite technique is obtaining the most proximally involved nail and sending it in a dry container for histopathology and PAS staining. I find it greatly decreases false-negative results and has virtually no false-positive results.

### Differential Diagnosis

*Nail injury:* A history of the injury must be obtained (Jogger's nails or pseudoonychomycosis), although tinea infection often starts in an injured nail; fungi are absent. If the second toe is longer then pseudoonychomycosis is more common in this digit. Otherwise, the great toe is most often affected.

*Psoriasis of fingernails:* Pitting, red areas occur under nail with resulting detachment; psoriasis is elsewhere, usually; no fungi are found. Appearance of "oil drop" on the nail. Arthritis may be present in fingers.

*Psoriasis of toenails:* This may be impossible to differentiate from tinea, because many psoriatic nails have some secondary fungal invasion and they are so similar clinically.

*Candidiasis of fingernails:* Common in people who frequently wash their hands; paronychial involvement common; *Candida* found (see later in this chapter).

*Green nails:* This fingernail infection yields *Candida albicans* and *Pseudomonas aeruginosa* most commonly. Clinically, there is a distal detachment of the nail plate, with underlying greenish black debris. For cure, complete debridement of the detached part of the nail is necessary, plus local or systemic antiyeast therapy.

### Treatment

**Case Example:** *Tinea of the Fingernails.* A young salesman presents with a fungal infection in three fingernails of his left hand of 9 months duration. The surrounding skin shows mild redness and scaling.

1. Griseofulvin therapy (see earlier and Table 25-3). Griseofulvin ultrafine type, 250 to 330 mg or equivalent.

   *Sig:* One tablet b.i.d. or t.i.d. for 9 months.

   *Comment:* Therapy is stopped when there is no clinical evidence of infection (crumbling, thickening of nail plate, or subungual debris) and no cultural or KOH or ink mount evidence of fungi.

2. Ketoconazole (Nizoral) therapy. If the patient and the physician are aware of the possibility of liver and other toxicity, then a 200-mg tablet once a day for 9 months might be curative. Close patient monitoring is necessary. Many drug interactions.

3. Itraconazole (Sporanox) therapy has been reported to be curative, 200 mg b.i.d. for 7 days, repeated monthly for 4 to 6 months. Available as a Pulse Pack. Many drug interactions.

4. Terbinafine (Lamisil) 250 mg. Author's experience is terbenifine 250 mg a day for 1 week. This is repeated every 3 months. It is safe, inexpensive ($4 for 30 pills at some discount pharmacies in the United States), and effective. This is referred to as pulse therapy and there are many other regiments recommended for this drug as well as other oral antifungals.

5. Loprox (ciclopirox) nail lacquer two times a week. It is expensive.

**Case Example:** *Tinea of the Toenails.* A 45-year-old woman presents with three infected toenails on the right foot and two on the left foot. These are causing mild pain when she wears certain tight-fitting shoes. Scaliness of soles of feet is also evident.

1. Griseofulvin or ketoconazole therapy. This oral therapy is not effective or indicated for tinea of the toenails. Apparently some dermatologists have cured cases after oral therapy was continued for several years or when oral therapy was combined with evulsion of the toenails. The only time such therapy for toenails is prescribed, in our practice, is when the patient understands the problem but still wants to attempt a cure or a cosmetic improvement. At least 12 months of griseofulvin therapy is necessary. Women respond to this therapy better than men.

2. Itraconazole (Sporanox) may be used. A dosage of 200 mg b.i.d. for 7 days, repeated monthly for 4 to 8 months, has been suggested. A Pulse Pack is available. Watch for drug interactions. Monitoring of the patient is necessary for rare liver toxicity. Very expensive.

3. Terbinafine (Lamisil) 250 mg a day for 1 week every 3 months for 1 year. Author's choice since inexpensive, safe, and effective.

4. Antifungal solution, 15 mL. For the patient who wants to "do something," applications two times a day for months might help some mild cases. One can combine this therapy with debridement of the nails. These solutions include Fungi-Nail, Fungoid, and Loprox (ciclpirox, also comes as a gel). Penlac (ciclopirox) nail lacquer is expensive but helpful if systemic therapy wants to be avoided. Unlike package insert, I use it only twice weekly with success.

5. Debriding of thick nails by patient, dermatologist, or podiatrist offers obvious relief from discomfort. This can be accomplished by the use of nail clippers, filing or a motor-driven drill (Dremel).

6. Surgical evulsion of the toenail is rarely curative. As stated previously, this surgical approach can be combined with oral systemic therapy with probable enhancement of the end result. Permanent removal of nail and nail matrix is advocated by some. Author's experience has been occasional regrowth of nail spicules due to incomplete matrix removal.

### Tinea of the Groin

Tinea of the groin is a common, itching, annoying fungal infection appearing usually in men and often concurrently with tinea of the feet. Home remedies often result in a contact dermatitis that adds "fuel to the fire."

### Primary Lesions

Bilateral, fan-shaped, red, scaly patches with a sharp, slightly raised border and central clearing occur. Small vesicles may be seen in the active border. No scrotal involvement.

### Secondary Lesions

Oozing, crusting, edema, and secondary bacterial infection. In chronic cases lichenification may be marked. Lichen simplex chronicus can develop.

*Distribution*

The infection affects the crural fold, thighs, perianal area, and buttocks.

*Course*

Factors that affect the course and recurrences are obesity, hot weather, sweating, and chafing garments.

*Etiology*

Tinea of the groin is commonly due to the fungi of tinea of the feet, *T. rubrum*, and *T. mentagrophytes*, and also to the fungus *Epidermophyton floccosum*.

*Contagiousness*

This is minimal, even between husband and wife.

*Laboratory Findings*

The organism is found in KOH preparations of scrapings and can be grown on culture. Material is taken from the active border.

*Differential Diagnosis*

*Candidiasis:* No sharp border; fine scales, oozing, redness, satellite pustule-like lesions at edges; more common in obese females; marked itching and burning; *Candida* found. History of oral antibiotics is common.

*Contact dermatitis:* Often coexistent but can be separate entity; new contactant history; no fungi found; no active border; very pruritic and can be vesicular.

*Prickly heat:* Pustular, papular; no active border, no fungi; may also be present with tinea.

*Lichen simplex chronicus:* Unilateral, usually; may have resulted from old chronic tinea; no fungi. Severe paroxysmal pruritis.

*Psoriasis:* Often unilateral; may or may not have raised border; psoriasis elsewhere; no fungi.

*Erythrasma:* Faint redness, fine scaling with no elevated border, also seen in axilla and webs of toes; coral reddish fluorescence under Wood's light; due to a diphtheroid organism called *Corynebacterium minutissimum*. Responds to topical erythromycin.

*Bowen's Disease or Extramammary Paget's Disease:* Consider these diagnoses if unilateral and recalcitrant to therapy; biopsy necessary to make these diagnoses.

*Treatment*

**Case Example:** Oozing, symmetrical, red dermatitis with sharp border occurring in crural area of young man.

1. Because the infection may come from chronic tinea of the feet, to prevent recurrences, advise the patient to dry the feet last and not the groin area last when taking a bath.

---

> **SAUER'S NOTES**
>
> An effective therapy for tinea of the groin is:
> Sulfur, ppt. 5%
> Hydrocortisone 1%
> Antifungal cream q.s. 15.0
> *Sig:* Apply b.i.d. locally, and continue for 7 days after apparently clear ("therapy-plus" routine).

2. Vinegar wet packs
   *Sig:* Half cup of white vinegar to 1 quart of warm water. Wet the sheeting or thin toweling and apply to area for 15 minutes twice a day.

3. Antifungal cream 15.0.
   *Sig:* Apply b.i.d. locally (Table 25-3).

4. Griseofulvin oral therapy
   Griseofulvin ultrafine types, 250 to 330 mg
   *Sig:* One tablet b.i.d. for 6 to 8 weeks for extensive case.

5. Ketoconazole, itraconazole, or terbinafine therapy may also be used.

6. Author uses terbifine 250 mg daily for seven days and then a topical for further control.

## Tinea of the Smooth Skin (Tinea Corporis)

The familiar ringworm of the skin is most common in children partially because of their intimacy with animals and other children. The lay public believes that *most* skin conditions are "ringworm," and many physicians erroneously agree with them (Fig. 25-6A–D).

*Primary Lesions*

Round, oval, or semicircular scaly patches have a slightly raised border that commonly is vesicular. Rarely, deep, ulcerated, granulomatous lesions (Majocchi's granuloma) are due to superficial dermatophyte fungi.

*Secondary Lesions*

Bacterial infection, particularly at the advancing border.

*Course*

Infection is short lived, if treated correctly. It seldom recurs unless treatment is inadequate.

*Etiology*

This disorder is most commonly due to *M. canis* from kittens and puppies and less commonly due to *E. floccosum* and *T. mentagrophytes* from groin and foot infections.

*Contagiousness*

It is very contagious.

*Laboratory Findings*

This is the same as for previously discussed fungal diseases.

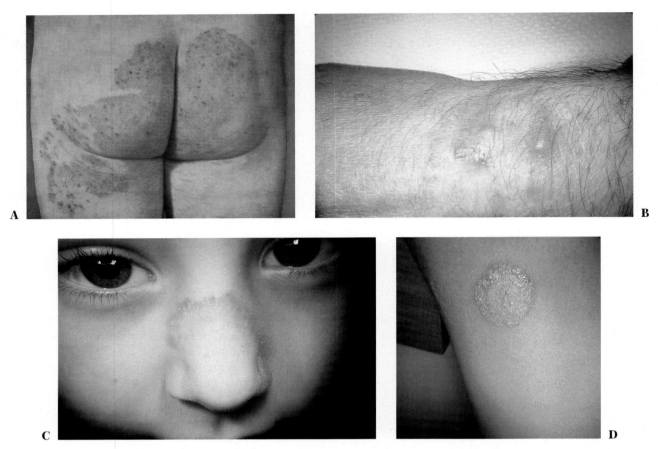

**FIGURE 25-6** ■ Tinea of the smooth skin. **(A)** This infection on the buttocks had spread from the crural region. *(Courtesy of Smith Kline & French Laboratories.)* **(B)** Majocchi granulomas on flexor wrist. **(C)** Tinea faciei on young girl caught from cat. **(D)** Tinea corporis on arm.

### Differential Diagnosis

*Pityriasis rosea*: History of herald patch; sudden shower of oval lesions; fungi not found.

*Impetigo*: Vesicular, honey-colored, crusted; most commonly on face; no fungi found.

*Contact dermatitis*: No sharp border or central healing; may be coexistent with ringworm worsened by overtreatment.

### Treatment

**Case Example:** A child has several 2 to 4 cm scaly lesions on his arms of 1 week's duration. He has a new kitten that he holds and plays with.

1. Examine the scalp, preferably with a Wood's light, to rule out scalp infection.
2. Advise the mother regarding moderate isolation procedures in relation to the family and others.
3. Antifungal salve q.s. 15.0.
   *Sig*: Apply b.i.d. locally (Table 25-3).

**Subsequent Visit of Resistant Case or a New Widespread Case: Griseofulvin Oral Therapy** Griseofulvin (ultrafine

types) can be given in tablet or oral suspension form. The usual dose for children is 165 mg b.i.d., but the pharmaceutical company's product information sheet should be consulted. Therapy should be maintained for 3 to 6 weeks or until lesions are gone. Occasionally, a higher dose is needed in deeper forms of infection. Terbenifine (author's choice) 250 mg daily for 2 weeks.

### Tinea of the Scalp (Tinea Capitis)

Tinea of the scalp (Fig. 25-7A–D) is the most common cause of patchy hair loss in children (Fig. 25-10). Endemic cases are with us always, but epidemics, usually due to the human type, were, until the discovery of griseofulvin, the real therapeutic problem. Griseofulvin orally finds its

---

**SAUER'S NOTES**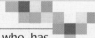

1. Examine the scalp in any child who has body ringworm.
2. Perform hair KOH mounts, cultures, or Wood's light examination of suspicious scalp areas.
3. Inquire about siblings having similar scalp lesions.

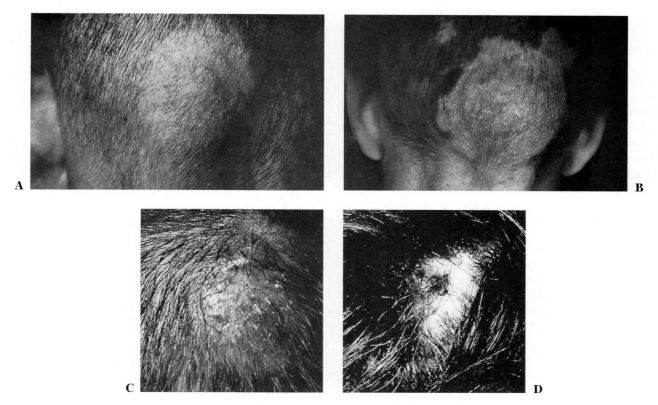

**FIGURE 25-7** ■ Tinea of the scalp. *(Courtesy of Ortho Pharmaceutical Corp.)* (**A**) Due to *M. audouini*. Note absence of visible inflammation. (**B**) Due to *T. tonsurans*. Wood's light examination revealed no fluorescence. (**C**) Due to *T. mentagrophytes*. Note inflammation., (**D**) Favus, due to *T. shoenleini*, of 11 years' duration.

greatest therapeutic usefulness and triumph in the management of tinea of the scalp. Before griseofulvin, children with the human type of scalp tinea had to be subjected to traumatic shampoos and salves for weeks or months, or they had to be epilated by x-ray. Often they were kept out of school for this entire period of therapy.

Ketoconazole, terbinafine (author's choice), or itraconazole systemic therapy is available for griseofulvin-resistant cases, if these truly occur in tinea of the scalp.

Tinea capitis infections can be divided into two clinical types: (1) *noninflammatory* and (2) *inflammatory*. The treatment, the cause, and the course vary for these two types.

### Noninflammatory Type

**Primary Lesions.** Grayish, scaly, round patches with broken-off hairs are seen, causing balding areas. The size of the areas varies.

**Secondary Lesions.** Bacterial infection and id reactions are rare. A noninflammatory patch can become inflamed spontaneously or as the result of strong local treatment. Scarring almost never occurs. "Black dot" hairs (short broken-off hairs) are seen with *Trichophyton tonsurans* on culture.

**Distribution.** The infection is most common in the posterior scalp region. Body ringworm from the scalp lesions is common, particularly on the neck and the shoulders.

**Course.** Incubation is usually 3 or more weeks after exposure. Parents often do not notice the infection for another 3 weeks to several months, particularly in girls. Spontaneous cures are rare in 2 to 6 months but after that time occur with greater frequency. Some cases last for years, if untreated. Recurrence of the infection after the cure of a previous episode is possible, because adequate immunity does not develop.

**Age Group.** Infection of the noninflammatory type is most common between the ages of 3 and 8 years and is rare after the age of puberty. This adult resistance to infection is attributed in part to the higher content of fungistatic fatty acids in the sebum after puberty.

*T. tonsurans* infection is seen mainly in African-American urban preadolescent children (often females who braid their hair). It is endemic in this population and may go unnoticed. Spontaneous cures at puberty, particularly for girls, do not always occur.

**Etiology.** The noninflammatory type of scalp ringworm is caused most frequently by *T. tonsurans* and occasionally by *Microsporum canis* and *Microsporum audouini*. *M. audouini* and *T. tonsurans* are anthropophilic fungi (human-to-human passage only), whereas *M. canis* is a zoophilic fungus (animals are the original source, mainly kittens and puppies).

***Contagiousness.*** This can be a part of a large urban epidemic.

***Laboratory Findings.*** *Wood's light examination of the scalp hair* is an important diagnostic test, but hairs infected with *T. tonsurans* do not fluoresce. The Wood's light is a specially filtered long-wavelength ultraviolet light. The hairs infected with *M. audouini* and *M. canis* fluoresce with a bright yellowish-green color. The bright fluorescence of fungus-infected hairs is not to be confused with the white or dull yellow color emitted by lint particles or sulfur-laden scales.

*Microscopic examination* of the infected hairs in 20% KOH solution shows an ectothrix arrangement of the spores when due to the *Microsporum* species and endothrix spores when due to *T. tonsurans*. Culture is necessary for species identification. The cultural characteristics of the various fungi can be found in many larger dermatologic or mycologic texts and are not presented here.

### Treatment
*Prophylactic*

1. Hair is washed with Loprox (ciclopirox) shampoo or Nizoral (ketaconazole) shampoo after every haircut by a barber, beautician, or parent.
2. Parents and teachers should be educated on methods of spread of disease, particularly during an epidemic.
3. Suggestions should be given for provision for individual storage of clothing, particularly caps, combs, barrettes and other hair styling products, in school and at home.

*Active*

1. Griseofulvin oral therapy. The ultrafine types of griseofulvin (Fulvicin U/F, Fulvicin P/G, Gris-Peg, Grifulvin V, and Grisactin) can be administered in tablet form or liquid suspension (not all brands available in liquid form). The usual dose for a child aged 4 to 8 years is 250 mg b.i.d., but some require a larger dose. The duration of therapy is usually 6 to 8 weeks. Both dose and duration have to be individualized and based on clinical, Wood's light, or culture response.
2. Ketoconazole, terfinafine, itriconazole, or fluconazole oral therapy. This type of therapy is usually not indicated or necessary, but regimens are effective and preferred by some.
3. Selenium sulfide (Selsun, Head & Shoulders Intensive Treatment) shampoo is sporicidal and may help decrease the spread of infection.
4. Manual epilation of hairs. Near the end of therapy, the remaining infected and fluorescent hairs can be plucked out, or the involved area can be shaved closely. This will eliminate the infected distal end of the growing hair.

***Primary Lesions.*** Pustular, scaly, round patches with broken-off hairs are found, resulting in bald areas.

***Secondary Lesions.*** Bacterial infection may occur. When the secondary reaction is marked, the area becomes swollen and tender. This inflammation is called a *kerion*. Minimal scarring sometimes remains.

***Distribution.*** Any scalp area is involved. Concurrent body ringworm infection is common.

***Course.*** Duration is much shorter than the noninflammatory type of infection. Spontaneous cures will result after 2 to 4 months in many cases, even if untreated, except for the *T. tonsurans* type.

***Etiology.*** The inflammatory type of scalp ringworm is most commonly caused by *T. tonsurans* and *M. canis* and rarely by *M. audouini*, *M. gypseum*, *T. mentagrophytes*, and *T. verrucosum*. *T. tonsurans*, *M. audouini*, and *T. mentagrophytes* are anthropophilic (coming from humans); *M. canis* and *T. verrucosum* are zoophilic (passed from infected animals); and *M. gypseum* is geophilic (coming from the soil).

***Contagiousness.*** Contagiousness is high in children. It is mainly endemic, except for cases due to *M. audouini*.

***Laboratory Findings.*** Microscopic examination of the infected hairs in 20% KOH solution shows an ectothrix arrangement of the spores, but *T. tonsurans* shows endothrix spores. The hairs infected with *M. canis* and *M. audouini* fluoresce with a bright yellowish-green color under the Wood's light.

***Differential Diagnosis*** See Table 25-4.

### Treatment

*Prophylactic* This is the same as for noninflammatory cases.

*Active*

1. Griseofulvin oral therapy (as under noninflammatory type).
2. If kerion is severe, with or without oral terbenifine or griseofulvin therapy:
   a. Burow's solution wet packs.
      *Sig:* One Domeboro packet to 1 pint of warm water. Apply soaked cloths for 15 minutes twice a day.
   b. Antibiotic therapy orally helps to eliminate secondary bacterial infection.
3. Some authors advocate a 1- to 2-week course of systemic corticosteroids to decrease inflammation.

### Tinea of the Beard (Tinea Barbae)

Fungal infection is a rare cause of dermatitis in the beard area (Fig. 25-8). Farmers occasionally contract it from infected cattle. Any presumed bacterial infection of the beard that

## Course

A large lesion develops over several months. Therapy is moderately effective on a long-term basis. Relapses are common.

## Cause

The fungus *Blastomyces dermtitidis* is believed to invade the lungs primarily and the skin is secondarily as a metastatic lesion. High native immunity prevents the development of more than one skin lesion. This immunity is low in the rare systemic form of blastomycosis in which multiple lesions occur in the skin, bones, and other organs.

## Laboratory Findings

The material for a 20% KOH solution mount is collected from the pustules at the border. Round, budding organisms can be found in this manner or in a histopathology specimen. A chest x-ray is indicated in every case.

## Treatment

- Surgical excision and plastic repair of early lesions is effective.
- Amphotericin B suppresses the chronic lesion more effectively than any other drug. It is administered by IV infusion daily in varying schedules, which are best described in larger texts or reviews. Albacet (liposomal amphotericin B) is a safer, expensive form of amphotericin B.
- Ketaonazole or intraconazole therapy on a long-term basis is also beneficial. Higher than normal dosages for a longer period of time are necessary for immunosuppressed patients.

## Coccidioidomycosis (San Juaquin Valley Fever)

There are three cutaneous types. The skin has a cutaneous form mainly in farmers and laboratory workers who become accidentally inoculated. There is a sporotrichoid form that mimics sporotrichosis with a chancre and nodules that spread up a lymphatic channel. The most severe and common form is a disseminated form from the lungs seen mainly in immunocompromised patients.

## Primary Lesion

In the disseminated form, nodules, papules or plaques appear on a dusky red indurated border.

## Secondary Lesion

Sinuses, ulcers, and cold abscesses may appear. Healing occurs with a scar. Erythema multiforme and erythema nodosum may occur as immune responses.

## Course

The severity of the disseminated form depends on the immune status of the patient and the amount of inoculum inhaled.

## Cause

*Coccidioides immitis* is a dimorphic fungus seen endemically in the United States (southwestern areas, "San Juaquin Valley Fever"), South and Central America, and Mexico. Blood types A and AB are more frequently pathogenic. It is common in Filipino immigrants to the United States.

## Laboratory Findings

Tissue examination shows brown yeast organisms called Medlar bodies within giant cells, pseudoepitheliomatous hyperplasia, and granulomas. Fungal culture on Sabouraud's agar shows aerial hyphae grossly and branched septate hypae with arthrospores microscopically.

## Treatment

Surgical excision or incision and drainage along with IV amphotericin B, or oral ketaconazole or itriconazole as second choices.

## Paracoccidioidomycosis (South American Blastomycosis)

Chronic disease is seen mainly in the lungs and lymph nodes with occasional spread to the skin and mucous membranes. It can be latent for decades, only to show up after immunosuppression. It is dimorphic and seen only in the yeast phase in humans. Primary infection is in the lung where it is often asymptomatic and not contagious. It may rarely be directly inoculated in the skin. Seen in AIDS patients who have traveled to an endemic area.

## Primary Lesion

Oral disease is seen commonly as granulomas (punctate vessels over a fungating base give a mulberry appearance) and crusts of the mouth, throat, larynx, and nasal cavities. Crusts, papules nodules, and verrucous plaques prefer a central facial location.

## Secondary Lesion

Hoarseness, dysphagia, destruction of the uvula, and perforation of the hard palate may occur. Disfiguring scars occur especially over the face.

## Course

Response to therapy is variable since most patients are immunocompromised. Pulmonary fibrosis, adrenal, and CNS disease are sequelae.

## Cause

*Paracoccidioides brasiliensis* is found in the soil mainly between latitudes 23 degrees to 34 degrees in Mexico, Latin America, and South America. The exact natural history is not completely understood.

### Laboratory Findings

Histologic examination of tissue reveals a mother cell with yeasts forming from the cell wall giving the look of a "pilot's wheel." Culture at 19°C to 28°C grows slowly, producing thin septate hyphae with chlamydospores. Serology is helpful in diagnosis.

### Treatment

Sulfamethoxazole/trimethoprim for at least 30 days by mouth. Amphotericin B for more severe disease with ketaconazole and intriconazole as second choices.

## Histoplasmosis

Mainly an asymptomatic lung infection. It can spread from the lung to the skin or rarely be primarily inoculated into the skin. AIDS is particularly a commonly associated underlying illness.

### Primary Lesion

Papules (mimicking molluscum contagiousum) and hemorrhagic necrotic areas.

### Secondary Lesion

Ulcers and scars.

### Course

Immunocomponent patients usually recover without treatment but in AIDS patients therapy must be given or CNS disease will ensue and become serious. Serology can be helpful. Culture on Sabouraud's agar reveals white colonies at 30°C, which microscopically show tuberculate macroconidia.

### Treatment

Amphotericin B in AIDS patients with concomitant azoles (itriconazole, fluconazole). The azoles are also often used as maintenance therapy.

## Candidiasis

Candidiasis (moniliasis) (Fig. 25-10A–H) is a fungal infection caused by *Candida albicans* that produces lesions in the mouth, the vagina, the skin, the nails, the lungs, or the gastrointestinal tract and occasionally results in sepsis. The latter condition is seen in patients who are on long-term, high-dose antibiotic therapy and in those who are immunosuppressed. Because *C. albicans* exists commonly as a harmless skin inhabitant, the laboratory findings of this organism are not adequate proof of its pathogenicity and etiologic role. *Candida* organisms commonly seed preexisting skin conditions. Concern here is with the *cutaneous* and the *mucocutaneous* candidal diseases. The following classification is helpful.

### Cutaneous Candidiasis

1. Localized diseases
   a. Candidal paronychia. This common candidal infection is characterized by the development of painful, red swellings of the skin around the nail plate. In chronic infections the nail becomes secondarily thickened and hardened. Candidal paronychia is commonly seen in housewives and those persons whose occupations predispose to frequent immersion of the hands in water. Terms such a "housewife's nail" or "barmaid's nail" relate to this water exposure.

      This nail involvement is to be differentiated from *superficial tinea of the nails* (the candidal infection usually does not cause the nail to lose its luster or to become crumbly, and debris does not accumulate beneath the nail, except in chronic mucocutaneous candidiasis) and from *bacterial paronychia* (this is more acute in onset and throbs with pain and may drain pus).
   b. Candidal intertrigo. This moderately common condition is characterized by red, eroded patches, with scaly, pustular or pustulovesicular lesions, with an indefinite border of satellite papules or pustules. The most common sites are axillae, inframammary areas, umbilicus, genital area, anal area, and webs of toes and fingers. Obesity, diabetes, and systemic antibiotics predispose to the development of this infection.

      Candidal intertrigo is to be differentiated from *superficial tinea infections*, which are not as red and eroded, and from *seborrheic dermatitis* or *psoriasis* which both may show signs of disease elsewhere.
2. Generalized mucocutaneous candidiasis. This rare infection involves the smooth skin, mucocutaneous orifices, and intertriginous areas. It follows in the wake of general debility, as seen in immunosuppressed patients, and was very resistant to treatment before the discovery of ketoconazole and, more recently, fluconazole and itraconazole. Thickened toenails and fingernails mimic onychomycosis. It can be associated with multiple endocrinopathies and thymoma.

### Mucous Membrane Candidiasis

#### Oral candidiasis (thrush and perlèche).

Thrush is characterized by creamy white flakes on a red, inflamed mucous membrane. The tongue may be smooth and atrophic, or the papillae may be hypertrophic, as in the condition labeled "hairy tongue." Therapy with Mycostatin pastilles (lozenges) or Mycelex troches is effective. Perlèche is seen as cracks or fissures at the corners of the mouth and is usually associated with candidal disease elsewhere, ill-fitting dental appliances, any alteration in a patient's bite that allows for collection of saliva at the corner of the mouth, and rarely a dietary deficiency (usually vitamin B complex or iron deficiency). Thrush is seen commonly in immunosuppressed patients.

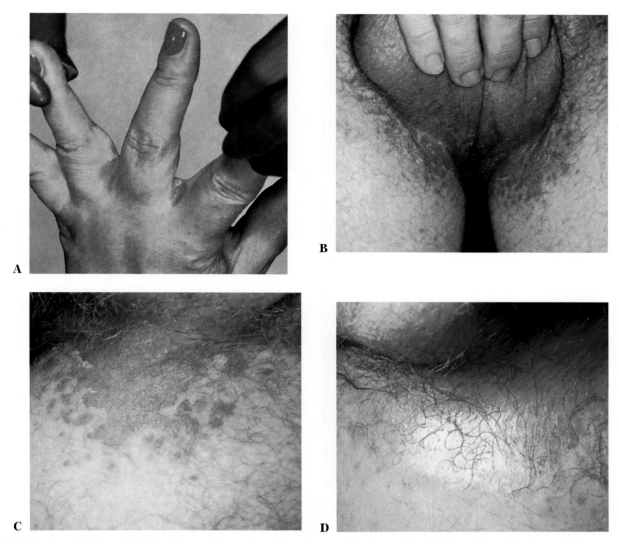

**FIGURE 25-10** ■ **(A)** Candidal intertrigo of the webs of the fingers. *(Courtesy of Smith Kline & French Laboratories.)* **(B, C, and D)** Candidal intertrigo of crural area and close-up showing satellite lesions without the sharp border as seen in tinea cruris.

Oral candidiasis is to be differentiated from allergic conditions, such as those due to toothpaste or mouthwash and leukoplakia.

***Candidal vulvovaginitis.*** The clinical picture is an oozing, red, sharply bordered skin infection surrounding an inflamed vagina that contains a buttermilk-like discharge. This type of candidal infection is frequently seen in pregnant women, diabetics, and those who have been on antibiotics systemically.

It is to be differentiated from an *allergic contact dermatitis, bacillary vaginosis, trichomonas infection* or *chlamydial vaginitis.*

***Laboratory Findings.*** Skin or mucous-membrane scrapings placed in 20% KOH solution and examined with the high-power microscope lens reveal small, oval, budding, thin-walled, yeast-like cells with occasional mycelia. Culture on Sabouraud's media produces creamy dull-white colonies in 4 to 5 days.

Further cultural studies on corn meal agar are necessary to identify the species as *C. albicans.*

***Treatment***

*Case 1* Candidal paronychia of two fingers is seen in a 37-year-old male bartender.

1. Advise the patient to avoid exposure of his hands to soap and water by wearing cotton gloves under rubber gloves, hiring a dishwasher, and so on.
2. Antifungal imidazole-type solution (Lotrimin or Mycelex solution 1%) 15.0

   *or* Fungi-nail 15.0

   *or* Mycolog II (generic) cream or ointment (nystatin and triamcinilone) 15.0

   *Sig:* Apply to base of nail q.i.d. especially after handwashing. Continue treatment for several weeks.

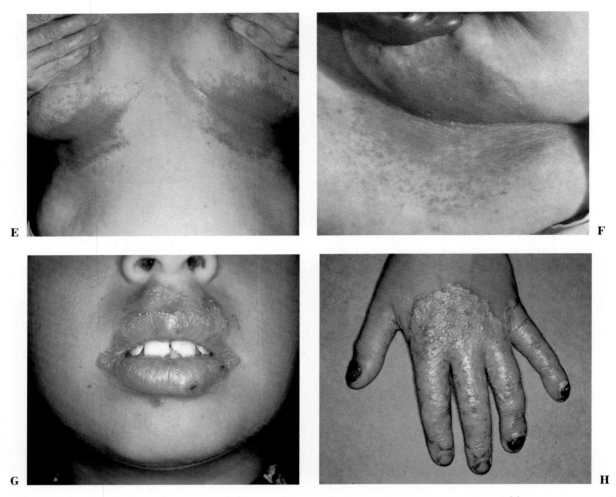

**FIGURE 25-10** ■ *(continued)* **(E)** Candida intertrigo under breasts. *(Courtesy of Herbert Laboratories.)* **(F)** Note the lack of a definite border to the eruption, which distinguishes it from a tinea infection. **(G)** Extensive candidiasis around the mouth. **(H)** Candida on the dorsum of the hand in a child with Addison's disease. *(Courtesy of Herbert Laboratories.)*

3. Consider, if severe, a brief course of fluconazole such as 200 mg a week for 1 month.

*Case 2* Candidal intertrigo of inframammary and crural region is seen in an elderly obese woman.

1. Advise the patient to wear pieces of cotton sheeting under breasts to keep the apposing tissues drier. Frequent bathing with thorough drying is helpful. Use of antibacterial soap should be avoided.

2. Sulfur, ppt. 5%

   Hydrocortisone 1%
   Mycostatin cream q.s. 30.0
   *Sig:* Apply locally t.i.d.

3. Powder can be used over cream:

   Mycostatin dusting powder q.s. 15.0
   *Sig:* Apply locally t.i.d.

*Case 3* Candidal vulvovaginitis is found in a woman who is 6 months pregnant.

1. Mycostatin vaginal tablets, 100,000 units #20

   *Sig:* Insert one tablet b.i.d. in vagina.

2. Monistat-Derm lotion, or

   Sulfur, ppt. 5%
   Hydrocortisone 1%
   Mycostatin cream q.s. 30.0
   *Sig:* Apply locally b.i.d. to vulvar skin.

3. Diflucan (fluconazole)

   150 mg tablet. Single dose p.o. Can repeat for resistant cases.

   Ketaconazole (Nizoral), itriconazole (Sporanox), or fluconazole (Difulcan) systemic therapy is rarely indicated for routine candidal infections. For *chronic* mucocutaneous candidiasis, ketoconazole and fluconazole can heal dramatically. Dosage information is provided in the package insert. The patient must be monitored carefully.

## Sporotrichosis

Sporotrichosis (Fig. 25-11A and B) is a granulomatous fungal infection of the skin and the subcutaneous tissues.

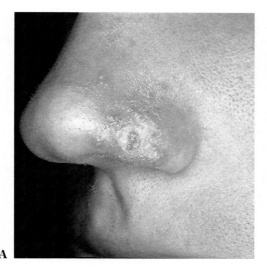
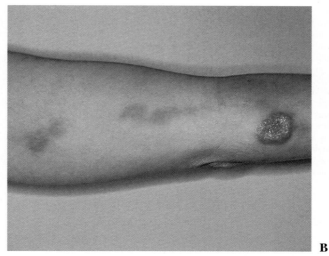

**FIGURE 25-11** ▪ **(A)** Sporotrichotic primary lesion on the nose. **(B)** Sporotrichotic chancre on arm with subcutaneous nodules. *(Courtesy of Stiefel Laboratories.)*

Characteristically, a primary chancre precedes more extensive skin involvement. Invasion of the internal viscera is rare.

### Primary Lesion

A sporotrichotic chancre develops at the site of skin inoculation, which is commonly the hand and less commonly the face or the feet. The chancre begins as a painless, movable, subcutaneous nodule that eventually softens and breaks down to form an ulcer.

### Secondary Lesions

Within a few weeks subcutaneous nodules arise along the course of the draining lymphatics and form a chain of tumors that develop into ulcers. This is the classic clinical picture, of which there are variations.

### Course

The development of the skin lesions is slow and rarely affects the general health.

### Etiology

The causative agent is *Sporothrix schenckii*, a fungus that grows on wood, sphagnum moss, and in the soil. It invades open wounds and is an occupational hazard of farmers (especially sphagnum moss), gardeners (especially roses), laborers, and miners.

### Laboratory Findings

Cultures of the purulent material from unopened lesions readily grow on Sabouraud's media. The organism is difficult to see, even with special stains or tissue examination from a biopsy.

### Differential Diagnosis

Any of the skin granulomas should be considered, such as *pyodermas, syphilis, tuberculosis, sarcoidosis*, and *leprosy*. An *ioderma* or *bromoderma* can cause a similar clinical picture.

### Treatment

1. Saturated solution of potassium iodide, 60.0 mL.

   *Sig:* On the first day, 10 drops t.i.d., p.c., added to milk or water; second day, 15 drops t.i.d.; third day, 20 drops t.i.d., and increase until 30 to 40 drops t.i.d. is given.

   *Comment:* The initial doses may be smaller and the increase more gradual if one is concerned about tolerance. Gastric irritation and ioderma should be watched for. There is a very bitter taste. This very specific treatment must be continued for 1 month after apparent cure.

2. Ketoconazole (Nizoral), 200 mg.

   *Sig:* Two tablets a day for 8 weeks.
   *Comment:* Some cases are not helped. The patient must be monitored closely.

3. Itraconazole (Sporanox), 100 mg.

   *Sig:* One tablet daily for 4 to 6 weeks.
   *Comment:* Patient should be monitored for rare liver toxicity.

## Suggested Readings

Baran R, Hay R, Haneke E. et al *Onychomycosis the current approach to diagnosis and therapy*. 2nd ed. Boca Raton, FL: Taylor and Francis; 2006.

Drake LA, Dinehart SM, Farmer ER, et al. Guidelines of care for superficial mycotic infections of the skin: Mucocutaneous candidiasis. *J Am Acad Dermatol*. 1996; 34:287.

Ellis D. Systemic antifungal agents for cutaneous fungal infections, *Aust Prescr*. 1996;19:72–75.

Gupta AK, Hofstader SLR, Adam P, et al. Tinea capitis: an overview with emphasis on management. *Pediatr Dermatol.* 1999;16(3):171–189.

Hart R, Bell-Syer SE, Crawford F, et al Systematic review of topcial treatments for fungal infections of the skin and nails of the feet. *BMJ.* 1999;319:79–82

Mooney MA, Thomas I, Sirois D. Oral candidosis. *Int J Dermatol.* 1995;34:759–765.

Odom R. Pathophysiology of dermatophyte infections. *J Am Acad Dermatol.* 1993;28:S2–S7.

Onychomycosis. *Int J Dermatol.* 1999;38(suppl 2).

Proceedings of the International Summit on Cutaneous Antifungal Therapy and Mycology Workshop, San Francisco, CA. *J Am Acad Dermatol Suppl* 1994;31:S1–S116.

Proceedings of a Symposium. Onychomycosis: Issues and Observations, Chicago, IL. *J Am Acad Dermatol Suppl.* 1995;35:3.

Radentz WH. Opportunistic fungal infections in immunocompromised hosts. *J Am Acad Dermatol.* 1989; 20:989–1003.

Rand S. Overview: The treatment of dermatophytosis. *J Am Acad Dermatol.* 2000;43(5 Suppl):S104–S112.

Sehgal VN, Jain S. Onychomycosis: clinical perspective. *Int J Dermatol.* 2000;39:241–249.

Smith EB. Topical antifungal drugs in the treatment of tinea pedis, tinea cruris, and tinea corporis. *J Am Acad Dermatol.* 1993;28:S24–S28.

Sugar AM, Lyman CA. *A Practical guide to medically important fungi and the diseases they cause.* Philadelphia, PA: Lippincott–Raven Publishers; 1997.

Suhonen RE, Ellis DH, Dawber RPR. *Fungal infections of the skin hair and nails.* London: Informa Health Care; 1999.

Systemic antifungal drugs. *Med Lett Drugs Ther.* 1997;39(1009):86–89.

# CHAPTER 26

# Sexually Transmitted Infections

*Clifton S. Hall, MD, Jason S. Reichenberg, MD, and Dayna Diven, MD*

Sexually transmitted infections (STIs) are a very common problem throughout the world. Those having sex with multiple partners are the most at risk, and men and women are more likely to have sex with multiple partners between ages 18 and 24, so it is not surprising that two thirds of all cases of STIs occur in people less than 25 years of age. All people who are sexually active are at risk, regardless of socioeconomic status. Carriers of STIs are often asymptomatic and spread their infections unknowingly.

There are at least 20 different types of STIs. Many STIs produce erosions and ulcers on the perineum and lymphadenopathy during one of the stages in their development (Table 26-1), which makes obtaining a detailed skin examination critical to their diagnosis. The types of STIs in this chapter have been grouped into these categories: viruses, bacteria, parasites, and fungi.

## Viruses

### Genital Herpes

Herpes simplex virus (HSV) subtypes 1 and 2 can result in oral or genital lesions. HSV-2 is the most common culprit for genital herpes, and is much more likely to cause recurrent outbreaks. HSV-1, which most commonly causes oral lesions, is associated with about 30% of HSV primary genital ulcers. Transmission via oral–genital sex is often implicated in these cases. The virus initially infects the contacted area, then travels to the sensory root ganglia, where it lies dormant. A recurrence occurs when the dormant virus in the ganglia travels back down the nerve to the skin.

*Skin Manifestations*

HSV lesions present as groups of discrete vesicles of clear fluid on an erythematous base that develop into erosions and then crust over time (Fig. 26-1). The lesions are painful because there is inflammation of the affected nerves. The lesions are neither suppurative nor indurated.

*Course*

After initial exposure, symptomatic "primary" herpes occurs after a 3- to 14-day incubation period. The vesicular lesions of primary herpes last 10 to 14 days, and new vesicles will continue to form over a 1- or 2-week period. There can be extensive bilateral inguinal lymphadenopathy. Overall, a

**TABLE 26-1 ■ STIs with Genital Ulcers**

| STI | Skin Lesion | Painful | Incubation | Inguinal Lymphadenopathy | Diagnosis | Organism |
|---|---|---|---|---|---|---|
| Herpes | Groups of vesicles, erosions, and ulcers on a red base | Yes | 3–14 d | Bilateral, tender, discrete, nonsuppurative, and nonindurated | Clinical, PCR, Tzanck, culture | HSV-2 > HSV-1 |
| LGV | Vesicle or shallow ulcer that heals rapidly | No | 3–20 d | Mostly unilateral, becomes violaceous and tender before fistula formation | PCR | *Chlamydia trachomatis* serovariants $L_1$, $L_2$, and $L_3$ |
| Granuloma inguinale | Papule that ulcerates with overhanging edges | No | 2–3 wk | Not typical | Giemsa stain of smear | *Calymmatobacterium granulomatis* |
| Primary syphilis | Ulcer with firm indurated border | No | 3 wk | Painless, regional, nonsuppurative, and rubbery | Serology, dark field microscopy | *Treponema pallidum* |
| Chancroid | Papule that becomes a friable, shallow, nonindurated ulcer | Yes | 1–5 d | Mostly unilateral, painful, and suppurative | Culture, rule out other causes of ulcers | *Haemophilus ducreyi* |

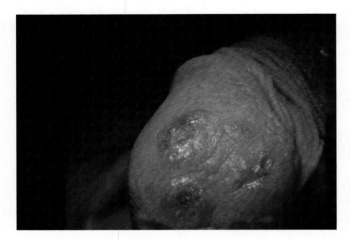

**FIGURE 26-1** ■ Genital herpes erosions and crusts.

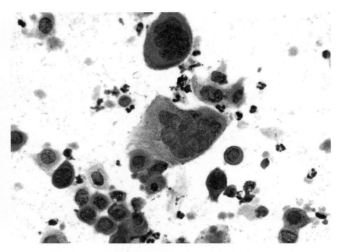

**FIGURE 26-2** ■ Positive Tzanck smear with Giemsa stain demonstrates giant multinucleated keratinocytes.

primary infection lasts about 3 weeks. Only a slight majority (57%) of primary HSV-2 infections are symptomatic. With so many asymptomatic primary infections, an outbreak of recurrent herpes may often be confused with a primary infection.

A recurrent episode of herpes will usually be preceded by a prodrome of burning, itching, or tingling in the affected area. Usually herpetic vesicles follow in less than 24 hours. The duration of recurrent herpes is much shorter than that of primary herpes. Recurrent outbreaks usually last about 1 week. Herpes can recur for years, but typically becomes less frequent over time.

### Contagiousness

Genital herpes is spread by direct physical contact. The virus is fragile and does not survive long outside of its host. Active vesicles and erosions have high viral titers and are the most contagious. Asymptomatic viral shedding and transmission is extremely common. As a result, patients who have asymptomatic primary or recurrent infections may unknowingly transmit the virus to others. Among monogamous couples, an uninfected partner will acquire the virus at a rate of 5% to 10% annually. Chronic suppression of the infected partner can halve this rate.

### Diagnosis

The diagnosis is based on the characteristic lesions and/or the history of recurrent vesicles and erosions in the perineal area. To confirm a diagnosis, the gold standard is a viral culture from a vesicle or moist erosion. Culturing dry, crusted lesions should be avoided as they are frequently negative. More rapid diagnostic methods such as direct fluorescent antibody test and polymerase chain reaction (PCR) assays are also available. The Tzanck smear is a rapid diagnostic test, where the base of a vesicle is gently scraped with a scalpel, smeared onto a glass slide, and stained with Wright or Giemsa stain. A positive Tzanck has large,

multinucleated keratinocytes (Fig. 26-2). A positive result, however, cannot distinguish between HSV-1, HSV-2, or varicella-zoster virus.

### Treatment

At this time, there is no cure for genital herpes. The goal of treatment is to decrease the frequency, duration, and severity of outbreaks. Treatment can also decrease, but not eliminate asymptomatic shedding. To decrease transmission of the virus, sex should be avoided when there are vesicles and moist erosions. Also, condoms should be used to decrease transmission during asymptomatic shedding. The antiviral medications currently available to treat herpes are acyclovir, famciclovir, and valacyclovir. These medications are relatively safe and are preferentially absorbed by infected cells. Valacyclovir and famciclovir offer the advantage of less frequent dosing.

Patients with a primary or initial genital herpes eruption should be treated to help avoid developing severe or prolonged symptoms. They should be treated for 7 to 10 days using any of the following: acyclovir 400 mg orally three times a day, acyclovir 200 mg orally five times a day, famciclovir 250 mg orally three times a day, or valacyclovir 1 g orally twice a day.

Patients with recurrent genital herpes can be treated either episodically or continually for suppressive therapy. Chronic suppressive therapy is generally used in patients with greater than six outbreaks a year or for those whose outbreaks are symptomatically severe. Suppressive therapy can reduce outbreaks by 70% to 80%. Twenty percent of suppressed patients have no visible outbreaks. As the frequency of recurrences decreases with time, a "drug holiday" can be tried every year to assess whether the patient still requires suppressive therapy. The recommended dosages for suppressive therapy are acyclovir 400 mg orally twice a day, famciclovir 250 mg orally twice a day, valacyclovir 500 mg orally once a day, or valacyclovir 1 g orally once a day.

Episodic treatment of recurrent genital herpes entails that the patient start treatment as soon as prodromal symptoms are noticed, in order to obtain maximum benefit. Once a skin eruption begins, only mild symptomatic improvement occurs. The dosage for episodic treatment is usually a 5-day course of acyclovir 400 mg three times a day or 800 mg twice a day; famciclovir 125 mg twice a day; or valacyclovir 1 g once a day. Shorter treatment durations include acyclovir 800 mg for 2 days, famciclovir 1,000 mg twice daily for 1 day, or valacyclovir 500 mg twice daily for 3 days.

## Venereal Warts (Condylomata Acuminata)

Venereal warts are the most common STI in the world. Half of all sexually active young adults in Europe and the United States have been infected. Venereal warts are caused by the human papillomavirus (HPV). HPV is a circular, double-stranded DNA virus. There are greater than 200 different types of HPV. The HPV types can be grouped as either low risk or high risk, depending on their risk for causing cervical cancer. Fortunately, the most common types, HPV-6 and HPV-11, are low risk. The most common high-risk types are 16, 18, 31, and 33.

### Skin Manifestations

Venereal warts, also known as condylomata acuminata, are multiple, painless, cauliflower-shaped, soft, lobulated papules located in moist anogenital regions (Fig. 26-3). In females, they are typically found on the vulva, cervix, perineum, or anus. In males, they are usually on the penis or perianal area. Warts are less common on the scrotum, unless the immune system is deficient. Bowenoid papulosis is a rare phenotype of venereal wart that is more often associated with the high-risk HPV types. These warts are less prominent flat papules that may have hyperpigmentation.

### Course

The incubation period can vary from several weeks to over a year. Most infections, particularly the low-risk visible warts of

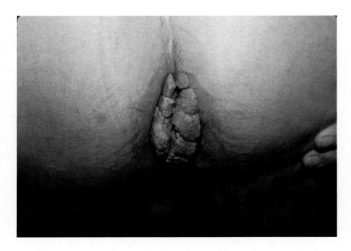

**FIGURE 26-3** ■ Large perianal condylomata acuminata.

HPV types 6 and 11, are transient, lasting 1 to 2 years on average. Most "recurrent" warts are actually areas that were subclinical at the time of treatment. High-risk HPV types can not only lead to cervical cancer but also increase the risk of developing cancers of the vulva, vagina, glans penis, and anus.

### Contagiousness

HPV spreads via direct skin-to-skin contact and fomites. Men are more at risk for genital warts if they have sex before they are 17, have greater than six sexual partners, have sex with prostitutes, or are not circumcised. Genital warts in children less than 2 years old do not necessarily signify abuse, since warts can spread during delivery, from autoinoculation, and from nonsexual contact.

### Diagnosis

Most venereal warts can be diagnosed clinically. Flat or sessile warts may occasionally warrant a biopsy for bowenoid papulosis given its higher association with cancer. PCR and in situ hybridization tests are also available and frequently used for cervical warts. These tests can differentiate between high- and low-risk HPV types.

### Treatment

There are a large number of treatment options for genital warts. These treatments can be grouped into those that physically destroy the wart, those that kill infected cells, and those that stimulate the immune system to destroy the wart.

Liquid nitrogen cryotherapy is the most commonly used in-office destructive method. It is quick, effective, and inexpensive. The warts and 2 mm of surrounding skin are frozen white once or twice with a liquid nitrogen dispenser or cotton swab.

Electrofulguration and electrocautery are slightly more effective than cryotherapy and work well for large warts. However, fewer physicians are using these methods because the smoke plume can theoretically cause warts in the respiratory tract. In response to this theory, many wear masks or use smoke evacuators. Other disadvantages of these modalities include the need for anesthesia and frequent scarring. Other in-office treatment options are trichloroacetic acid and podophyllin.

Imiquimod 5% cream is less effective (~50% efficacious) and often slow (sometimes taking 10 or more weeks of treatment); however, it has a low recurrence rate and can be done at home. The cream is applied three times a week at bedtime for up to 16 weeks. The cream causes mild to moderate irritation and has been reported to flare concomitant psoriasis.

5-Fluorouracil 5% cream twice a day can be effective and works well for intraurethral warts, but it can cause inflammation and painful scrotal erosions. Another effective option is podophyllotoxin 0.5% solution applied to the warts at home twice daily for 3 consecutive days per week for 1 to 4 weeks. It is contraindicated in pregnancy and can cause erythema and erosions in treated areas.

Gardasil, a quadrivalent vaccine against HPV types 6, 11, 16, and 18 is very effective at preventing warts caused by the four most common high- and low-risk HPV types. No therapeutic vaccine currently exists.

## Hepatitis B Virus

Hepatitis B virus (HBV) is an enveloped double-stranded DNA virus of the Hepadnaviridae family. It is unrelated to any other human virus. Chronic carriers are most commonly found in the Far East, where it is often spread from mother to child perinatally. In the United States, half of all cases arise from sexual contact.

### Skin Manifestations

HBV does not produce any genital lesions. Nevertheless, HBV can cause jaundice, urticaria, and vasculitis.

### Course

HBV has an average incubation time of 10 weeks before an acute infection becomes clinically apparent. Patients complain of fevers, anorexia, nausea, diarrhea, right upper quadrant pain, and general malaise. Few (<1%) acute infections go on to liver failure. About one fifth of acute infections develop a serum sickness–like infection 1 to 6 weeks before clinical liver disease. These patients typically have urticaria and arthralgias and occasionally vasculitis, arthritis, and glomerulonephritis. This sickness gradually resolves spontaneously. Polyarteritis nodosa develops in 7% to 8% of cases, usually within the first 6 months. A chronic liver infection develops in 10% of patients, a quarter of whom go on to develop cirrhosis and/or hepatocellular carcinoma.

### Contagiousness

The virus is found in body fluids such as blood, saliva, semen, and cervical fluid. The disease typically spreads via close physical contact, intravenous drug use, and perinatally.

### Diagnosis

The diagnosis of an HBV infection is typically made serologically. Acute infections are diagnosed by finding elevated liver tests and IgM antibodies against hepatitis B core antigen, which is almost always positive when jaundice is present. Chronic infections are diagnosed by finding HBV surface antigens in the blood. If antibodies to the surface antigen are present, the patient has eliminated the virus and does not have a chronic infection.

### Treatment

Acute infections generally require only supportive care, as most cases resolve on their own. Chronic infections are treated with $\alpha_{2b}$-interferon, lamivudine, or adefovir dipivoxil. HBV-associated polyarteritis nodosa is typically treated with systemic steroids, lamivudine, and rarely plasma exchange. A

vaccine is available to prevent infections, and it is recommended for health care workers and children.

## Hepatitis C Virus

Hepatitis C virus (HCV) is the most common cause of cirrhosis in the United States. It is a single-stranded RNA flavivirus. Other notable flaviviruses are yellow fever and dengue fever.

### Skin Manifestations

There are no acute genital lesions. The stigmata of liver cirrhosis such as jaundice, caput medusa, palmar erythema, and telangiectasias develop with chronic infections.

### Course

Most acute infections are asymptomatic; however, 55% to 85% of those infected develop a chronic infection that can lead to liver cirrhosis. Chronic HCV has also been associated with polyarteritis nodosa, sporadic porphyria cutanea tarda, lichen planus, necrolytic acral erythema, and cutaneous necrotizing vasculitis.

### Contagiousness

Sexual transmission of HCV is uncommon. A majority of cases in developed nations are acquired from intravenous illicit drug use, now that blood and blood products are screened for HCV.

### Diagnosis

Diagnosis is made via PCR for HCV RNA in the blood.

### Treatment

Chronic HCV infections are treated with a combination of interferon-$\alpha$ and ribavirin, which is effective half of the time. Eczema and pruritus are common side effects, which start 2 to 4 months after starting treatment. These side effects can be controlled with oral antihistamines, moisturizers, and topical steroids.

## HIV/AIDS

The human immunodeficiency virus (HIV) was first recognized in the United States in 1981, but it is thought to have been present in Africa for decades before the virus was discovered. HIV causes an immunodeficient state principally by depleting the body of CD4+ helper T cells. Acquired immunodeficiency syndrome (AIDS) is a term used to describe the later stages of HIV infection, in which the CD4 count has dropped below 200 cells/mL. Patients with AIDS usually present with an opportunistic infection (characteristic viral or fungal pneumonia), malignancy (Kaposi's sarcoma or one of several lymphomas), or chronic fatigue syndrome (encephalopathy, wasting). A great majority of HIV-infected individuals develop skin disorders related to their immunocompromised status.

### Skin Manifestations

Acute HIV infections are not associated with specific genital lesions. Most initial infections are asymptomatic, but some present with a mononucleosis-like illness 2 to 4 weeks after exposure. This illness consists of a nonspecific rash with discrete, erythematous macules and papules primarily on the trunk but occasionally involving the palms or soles. Systemic symptoms include fevers, pharyngitis, cervical lymphadenopathy, arthralgias, and oral/genital ulcers.

For patients with HIV, common skin findings include refractory psoriasis, severe seborrheic dermatitis, and dry skin. Once HIV has developed into AIDS, the examiner may see stigmata of disease such as the reddish-brown plaques of Kaposi's sarcoma, the whitish plaques of oral candidiasis, or cutaneous nodules caused by tuberculosis or disseminated fungal infections such as cryptococcus, histoplasmosis, or coccidioides.

### Course

After the initial infection, many years can pass before symptoms appear. The virus can directly cause muscle wasting, neurologic degeneration, diarrhea, and increase the risk of malignancies. The immunodeficient status leads to opportunistic infections and severe manifestations of common infections. Syphilis can be accelerated to tertiary syphilis, chancres can become uncharacteristically painful from coinfection, and syphilitic serologic tests can be falsely negative. Genital warts, HSV lesions, and molluscum contagiosum can be more widespread, larger, and more resistant to treatment. Also, patients are more likely to have candidiasis, tinea ("ringworm"), and staphylococcal infections.

### Contagiousness

HIV is spread through exposure to infected fluids, often via sexual contact. The probability of transmission per sexual act is actually low (0.0003 to 0.0015). Male-to-female transmission rates are much greater than female-to-male rates. Having a sore, such as a syphilitic chancre, can increase the risk of transmission. HIV can also be spread from blood transfusions (uncommon in the United States since the universal screening of all donated blood in the mid 1980s), sharing contaminated needles during intravenous drug use, and from mother to child either transplacentally, perinatally, or via breast-feeding.

### Diagnosis

The diagnosis is typically made by a highly sensitive serum enzyme immunoassay (EIA) that is confirmed by a Western blot test that is very specific for HIV-targeted antibodies. Since antibodies to HIV do not form for 2 to 4 weeks, early testing can lead to false negatives.

### Treatment

HIV is treated with a cocktail of antiviral proteases and reverse transcriptase inhibitors called HAART or highly active antiretroviral therapy. Most of the opportunistic infections and malignancies associated with HIV infection will also resolve with HAART therapy, with the notable exception of cytomegalovirus, herpes zoster, and *Mycobacterium avium intracellulare* infections, which may initially flare after HAART, or HPV and molluscum contagiosum, which may continue to worsen. Nevertheless, since HAART use has become widespread, extensive molluscum contagiosum cases in HIV patients are now rare.

## Molluscum Contagiosum

Molluscum contagiosum is a common infection in young children, but it can also be found among sexually active young adults and among immunocompromised patients. The infection is caused by a poxvirus.

### Skin Manifestations

The primary lesion is a small, firm, shiny, smooth-surfaced, dome-shaped, flesh-colored papule with a central umbilication (Fig. 26-4). Papules that are scratched or irritated can become crusted or pustular. Genital papules can occur in children as part of a more widespread infection. Abuse might be considered if the papules are limited only to the genitalia. Adults typically have fewer papules, which are usually found on the penile shaft, upper thighs, and lower abdomen.

### Course

Molluscum contagiosum frequently resolves within a year in healthy individuals but can take longer. Treatment might expedite the resolution.

### Contagiousness

The disease typically spreads from skin-to-skin contact that is amplified in wet environments such as bathtubs or swimming pools.

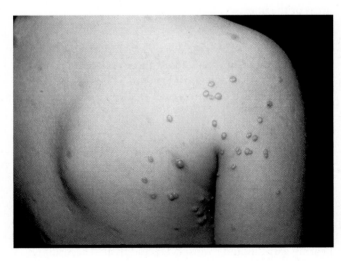

**FIGURE 26-4** ■ Molluscum contagiosum demonstrates classic umbilicated papules.

*Diagnosis*

The diagnosis is made clinically with identification of the distinctive umbilicated papules. Light cryotherapy can aid in making the diagnosis by making the umbilication more apparent. When necessary, a technique similar to a Tzanck smear will demonstrate characteristic "molluscum bodies." These bodies can also be seen on a skin biopsy.

*Treatment*

Many modalities can be used to physically destroy the papules. Commonly used treatments include cryotherapy with liquid nitrogen, topical imiquimod, and curettage. Chemical removal with topical cantharidin, KOH, or tretinoin can be used to avoid the pain of the latter treatments. Plucking out the core of the papules can also help.

## Parasites

### Pubic Lice

Pubic lice, also known as crabs or pediculosis pubis, is caused by the crab louse, *Pthirus pubis*. Lice have three pairs of legs and attach their eggs, called nits, to hair shafts. More than half of the time, pubic lice infest a second area, such as the eyelashes, eyebrows, axilla, or the scalp.

*Skin Manifestations*

Tiny crab lice and nits can be seen attached to the base of hairs. Pruritus may be present, as well as excoriations, crusts, and perifollicular erythema. Secondary bacterial infections can occur.

*Course*

The adult crab louse can live for 36 hours away from the host, and its eggs are viable for up to 10 days. Lice that survive shaving or treatment can find refuge in other hair-bearing areas of the body.

*Contagiousness*

Pubic lice more commonly infest those with ample amounts of pubic hair. Although considered an STI, pubic lice can be spread from infested fomites such as sheets and clothing.

*Diagnosis*

The infestation is clinically diagnosed by finding the crabs (**Fig. 26-5**) and nits.

*Treatment*

Treatment of only the pubic area with one round of treatment has a very high recurrence rate. Therefore, all hair-bearing areas should be inspected and treated accordingly. A second treatment, 1 week later, should be performed to kill newly hatched lice. Partners and close contacts should be

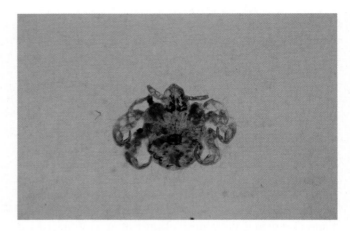

**FIGURE 26-5** ▪ Microscopic view of a pubic louse.

treated, and the presence of additional STIs should be considered. The most effective topical treatment is permethrin 5% cream left on overnight. If the eyelashes are involved, erythromycin ophthalmic ointment can be applied. An off-label but very effective option is ivermectin 200 μg/kg orally. Ivermectin should be considered if topical treatments have failed or if the eyelashes or the perianal areas are infested. Less effective treatments include lindane 1% shampoo and over-the-counter regular shampoo followed by permethrin 1% cream rinse/shampoo.

### Scabies

Scabies is caused by the human-specific parasitic mite *Sarcoptes scabiei* var *hominis*. It is found worldwide. The female burrows into the upper epidermis, lays her eggs, and lives for a month feeding and defecating within her burrow.

*Skin Manifestations*

Severe itching that worsens at night and after hot showers is typically the first manifestation of scabies. The most common lesions are small, erythematous, pruritic papules. Papules and indurated nodules can be found on the scrotum and shaft and glans of the penis (**Fig. 26-6**). The most pathognomonic sign is the linear burrow with fine scale. These burrows are most often seen in the interdigital web spaces and volar wrist. Other common infested areas include the elbows, axillae, central abdomen, buttocks, and anterior thighs.

*Course*

After an initial infestation, itching and cutaneous lesions may take 2 to 6 weeks to develop. As a result, many asymptomatic carriers exist. Subsequent infestations may become symptomatic in only 1 or 2 days, due to previous sensitization of the host to the mite antigens. Those who are immunosuppressed or who are unable to sense itching or scratch themselves adequately are at risk for developing crusted or Norwegian scabies. Crusted scabies is a massive

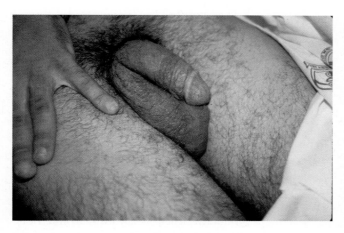

FIGURE 26-6 ■ Scabies-induced pruritic papules.

infestation of mites that frequently leads to a thickened, crusted epidermis.

### Contagiousness

The mite is spread by sexual and nonsexual close physical contact, often with children, and by fomites such as clothing.

### Diagnosis

The diagnosis can be made by scraping infested areas with mineral oil and finding mites, eggs, or scybala (fecal material) under the light microscope (**Figs. 26-7 and 26-8**). Most patients will have only a few mites, which can make it difficult to get a positive scraping. Mites are particularly hard to find in excessively clean, easily scratched, or partially treated areas.

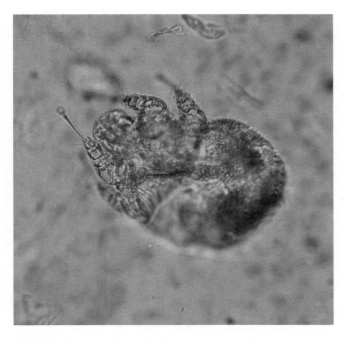

FIGURE 26-7 ■ Mineral oil smear demonstrating a scabies mite at 40×.

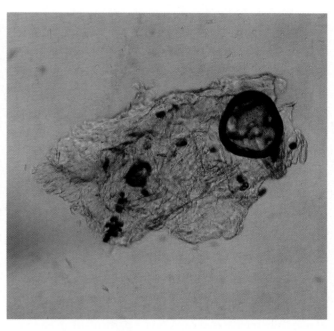

FIGURE 26-8 ■ Mineral oil smear of an epidermal scale containing brown scybala at 10×.

### Treatment

Permethrin 5% cream should be applied overnight from the neck down (head to toe if crusted scabies or an infant) with particular attention paid to covering the subungual, genital, and waistline areas completely. The treatment is repeated in 4 to 5 days. For crusted or treatment-resistant scabies, ivermectin is increasingly being used as it is very safe, convenient, and effective, despite being off-label. Nevertheless, ivermectin should be avoided in pregnant women, nursing mothers, and children less than 15 kg. Two doses of oral ivermectin at 200 to 400 $\mu$g/kg are needed: an initial dose and a dose 14 days later. It is common for itching and lesions to last 2 to 4 weeks following adequate treatment. To prevent reinfection, the entire household and close contacts should be treated because asymptomatic carriers are so common. Also, following each treatment, pajamas, bedding, and towels should be cleaned with hot water and a hot dryer or they can be stored in an airtight bag for 10 days.

### Trichomoniasis

One hundred and eighty million women worldwide are infected with the protozoan trophozoite *Trichomonas vaginalis*. A quarter of all sexually active women will acquire the disease, usually between the ages of 16 and 35.

### Skin Manifestations

There are typically no skin manifestations, but erythema can often be found in the vagina or on the cervix of symptomatic individuals. In severe cases, erosions and petechial hemorrhages may be seen. The association with a red, friable endocervix ("strawberry cervix") is well known, but is uncommonly found. Vaginal discharge is classically thin, yellow, and frothy, but in practice, these characteristics vary widely.

### Course

Trichomonas causes a chronic vaginitis that lasts for weeks to months and can worsen with menses or pregnancy. Clinically significant immunity never develops. Half of diagnosed women are asymptomatic, but most will go on to develop symptoms within 6 months. Common symptoms are discharge, itching, burning, dyspareunia, dysuria, and foul odor. Men typically are asymptomatic, but can complain of dysuria and scant discharge.

### Contagiousness

The disease is mostly linked to sexual contact. However, trichomonads can survive 1 to 2 hours on moist surfaces and for 24 hours in urine, semen, and water. As a result, a few nonsexually transmitted cases occur, particularly in environments where washcloths are shared.

### Diagnosis

Diagnosis is commonly made by performing wet mounts of vaginal discharge and finding trichomonads. Trichomonads can be identified by their jerky movements and five flagella. However, wet mounts are only 60% sensitive and are likely to be negative in asymptomatic, mildly symptomatic, and recently douched women. Culture is slow but is the gold standard for diagnosis. Direct fluorescent antibody staining and DNA and RNA probes are now available that are more sensitive than wet mounts and faster than culture. Even so, they are not commonly used.

### Treatment

Metronidazole is the most commonly used treatment, resulting in a cure in 95% of cases. Metronidazole is given either as a single 2,000 mg dose or as a seven-day regimen of 373 mg twice a day. Metronidazole should not be taken concomitantly with alcoholic beverages nor given to pregnant women in their first trimester.

## Bacteria

### Chlamydia

*Chlamydia trachomatis* causes the most common bacterial STI in the United States. A large majority (~80%) of infected females are asymptomatic carriers. Most men, on the other hand, are symptomatic. Serovariants B, D, E, F, G, H, I, J, and K frequently cause genital infections and will be discussed in this section. Serovariants $L_1$, $L_2$, and $L_3$ produce a clinically distinct variant known as lymphogranuloma venereum, which is discussed in the section following this one. Serovariants A, B, and C are associated with trachoma, a chronic follicular conjunctivitis that can lead to blindness.

### Skin Manifestations

Most infections are asymptomatic. Symptomatic infections can produce a white discharge from the penile urethra or from the vagina. Chlamydia is the most common cause of epididymitis in young men.

### Course

Urethritis in men usually develops after a 2- to 6-week incubation period. Symptomatic women may develop cervicitis or vaginitis. With decreasing rates of gonorrhea, chlamydial infections are the most common cause of pelvic inflammatory disease (PID) and of preventable infertility. PID can scar the reproductive tract, which leads to infertility. Infected males with the HLA-B27 genotype are most at risk for developing reactive arthritis (also known as Reiter's syndrome), which is the triad of arthritis, urethritis, and conjunctivitis. Reactive arthritis patients can develop small, scattered, thick, or pustular lesions on their genitals, palms, and soles. On the glans penis this is called balanitis circinata, and on the plantar feet this condition is called keratoderma blenorrhagicum. Painless oral erosions also occur. Reactive arthritis is a rare complication and typically develops 1 to 3 weeks after infection.

### Contagiousness

Chlamydial genital infections are typically transmitted via sexual contact. Chlamydia transmission rates are quite high, with approximately one third of exposed males developing urethritis. Reinfection is common.

### Diagnosis

As most of the clinical findings are nonspecific, laboratory testing is required to make the diagnosis. Nucleic acid amplification tests like PCR are gaining diagnostic popularity as they are more sensitive than cell cultures and can be used on self-collected vaginal swabs or urine samples.

### Treatment

Chlamydia is treated with azithromycin 1 g orally once or with doxycycline 100 mg orally twice a day for 7 days.

### Lymphogranuloma venereum

Lymphogranuloma venereum (LGV) is a rare STI caused by *C. trachomatis* serovariants $L_1$, $L_2$, and $L_3$. Most cases are found in Africa, India, Southeast Asia, and South America, but there are occasional outbreaks elsewhere.

### Skin Manifestations

At the primary site of infection, a 2 to 3 mm vesicle or shallow erosion appears on the glans penis, coronal sulcus, prepuce, or urethral meatus in men or on the vulva, vagina, or cervix in women. The lesion is painless and usually heals rapidly. Urethritis may also occur. Two weeks after the primary infection, the inguinal lymph nodes enlarge, typically unilaterally but occasionally bilaterally. The chain of enlarging inguinal nodes (buboes) fuse and the overlying skin becomes red and tender. A characteristic groove (the "groove sign") can be seen as lymph nodes both above and below the inguinal ligament become swollen. The firm buboes spontaneously ulcerate, drain pus, and then involute. An alternative site of infection is the rectum, where a proctitis with mucopurulent discharge can progress to rectal strictures. In the United States, the rectal presentation is more common and increasingly found among gay men.

### Course

There is a 3- to 20-day incubation period after exposure before a primary infection manifests itself. In addition to skin manifestations, infected individuals may complain of malaise, arthritis, conjunctivitis, fever, weight loss, and a poor appetite. Additional complications include hepatosplenomegaly, encephalitis, and chronic genital swelling (elephantiasis) secondary to scarring of the lymphatic system (**Fig. 26-9**). Untreated infections recur one fifth of the time.

### Contagiousness

The disease is chiefly spread through sexual contact. Men are more commonly symptomatic. Symptomatic women rarely have an observed primary lesion and have fewer buboes; they are more likely to present at a later stage with rectal strictures or genital elephantiasis.

### Diagnosis

A PCR test on lesional tissue can identify Chlamydia DNA. A complement fixation test can be used in conjunction with the PCR to identify serovariant-specific antibodies. These antibodies can only be detected 4 weeks after disease onset.

### Treatment

The first-line treatment is doxycycline 100 mg orally twice a day for 3 weeks, with erythromycin 500 mg orally four times

daily for 3 weeks as a second-line treatment. Large fluctuant buboes may need to be aspirated or drained to either prevent rupture or help clear the infection. All sexual contacts over the previous 30 days should be treated.

## Granuloma Inguinale

Granuloma inguinale, also known as donovanosis or granuloma venereum, is a rare, mildly contagious locally, destructive disease caused by the encapsulated gram-negative bacillus *Calymmatobacterium granulomatis*. The disease is principally found in tropical developing countries such as India, South Africa, and Papua New Guinea.

### Skin Manifestations

The first manifestation of the disease is a painless or mildly painful papule or nodule that slowly grows and erodes through the skin producing a clean, well-defined ulcer with overhanging edges. The ulcers are composed of beefy-red, friable hypertrophic granulation tissue. A majority of the lesions are found on the genitals with the prepuce, glans, and labia majora being the most common sites. However, the lesions can also be found perianally, in the inguinal folds, and occasionally at more distant locations. Lymphadenopathy is not a typical feature.

### Course

The incubation period is highly variable, but signs usually appear in 2 to 3 weeks. The disease progresses slowly and spreads by both peripheral extension and autoinoculation. Ulcers can lead to persistent draining sinuses and depigmented scars. Long-standing disease can occasionally scar the local lymphatic channels causing pseudoelephantiasis (swelling).

### Contagiousness

Sexual transmission is considered the most likely manner of transmission. The disease is only mildly contagious and likely needs to be inoculated through broken skin.

### Diagnosis

As no reliable serologic tests or cultures exist, clinical suspicion and smears of active lesions demonstrating Donovan bodies diagnose the disease. To make a smear, an ulcer is scraped and smeared onto a glass slide, air-dried, and then stained with either Wright or Giemsa stain. The diagnostic Donovan bodies are darkly staining clusters of encapsulated coccobacilli within the cytoplasm of mononuclear cells.

### Treatment

The first-line treatment is doxycycline 100 mg orally twice a day for a minimum of 3 weeks and until the lesions are completely healed. Alternative medications include erythromycin 500 mg four times daily, trimethoprim/sulfamethoxazole 160 mg/800 mg tablet twice daily, azithromycin 1 g every week, or ciprofloxacin 750 mg twice daily. Relapses are common.

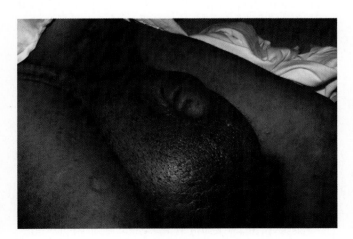

**FIGURE 26-9 ■** Lymphogranuloma venereum—induced genital elephantiasis.

## Gonorrhea

Gonorrhea, also known as GC or "the clap," is a common STI that has been with humans for millennia. Galen, the Roman physician, named it gonorrhea or "flowing seed" because of the disease's characteristic purulent urethral discharge. Gonorrhea is caused by the gram-negative diplococcus *Neisseria gonorrhoeae* and is most commonly found among young adults between the ages of 15 and 25. The incidence of the disease has been slowly decreasing over the last 20 years. Both gonorrhea and chlamydia infections can cause PID, the most common preventable cause of infertility.

### Skin Manifestations

The primary symptoms are dysuria and a purulent discharge from the male urethra or from the female cervix. Rarely, a gonococcal dermatitis may occur on the median raphe of the penis.

### Course

Symptoms of gonorrhea usually develop within 1 to 2 weeks. A majority of men develop symptoms, but only half of infected women do. Untreated symptomatic individuals often become asymptomatic carriers, a state which can last for months. Occasionally, gonorrhea disseminates hematogenously causing fevers, arthralgias, arthritis, and hemorrhagic vesiculopustules on the skin (Fig. 26-10). The vesiculopustules are tender, sparse, and usually on the palms, soles, or joints. The lesions start out as tiny erythematous macules before they become vesiculopustules ("blisters") on a deeply erythematous or hemorrhagic base. The macules can also become purpuric patches up to 2 cm in diameter. Disseminated disease in females often occurs during pregnancy or menstruation. Other complications of untreated gonorrhea infection include PID, sterility, epididymitis, proctitis, and rarely myocarditis or meningitis.

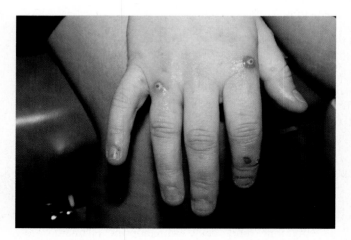

**FIGURE 26-10** ■ Disseminated gonorrhea with hemorrhagic vesiculopustules.

### Contagiousness

The disease is highly contagious, with a 20% to 50% transmission rate per episode of intercourse. Since a large reservoir of asymptomatic carriers exists, controlling the spread of the disease has been difficult. The disease can also be spread from the genitals to the oral cavity and rectal vaults. Nonsexual transmission is rare, so sexual abuse should be considered in all infected children.

### Diagnosis

A Gram-stained smear of urethral discharge is 95% sensitive and specific in symptomatic men. Endocervical smears are only half as sensitive. A positive smear demonstrates gram-negative diplococci within neutrophils. Cultures can also be obtained from the cervix or male urethra. Though more expensive, PCR tests are becoming widely popular as they are just as sensitive and specific as cultures, more rapid, and can be used on noninvasively obtained urine samples.

### Treatment

The first-line treatment of an uncomplicated infection is a single dose of a third-generation cephalosporin, such as cefixime 400 mg orally or ceftriaxone 125 mg intramuscularly. Other options include ciprofloxacin 500 mg orally or ofloxacin 400 mg orally. Since many patients are coinfected with Chlamydia, patients should be presumed to have chlamydia and treated accordingly, unless ruled out by laboratory testing. Disseminated infections should receive ceftriaxone 1 g each day until they have shown 1 to 2 days of clinical improvement. Then, they should use an oral antibiotic for 1 week after that. Partners over the previous 30 to 60 days should be treated.

## Syphilis

Epidemic syphilis, caused by the spirochete *Treponema pallidum*, subspecies *pallidum*, has been present for centuries, with early references in the works of Shakespeare and Voltaire. Some historians believe that it may have originated in the New World and traveled to Europe via Christopher Columbus's crew, where it became known as the Great Pox. In recent times, within the United States, the incidence of syphilis decreased dramatically throughout the 1990s, but since 2000 the incidence has slowly increased. Currently, most cases of syphilis in the United States are among men who have sex with men. Syphilis infections are divided into four stages: the initial infection called primary syphilis, the disseminated stage called secondary syphilis, the clinically asymptomatic stage called latent syphilis, and the late stage infection called tertiary syphilis.

### Skin Manifestations

The classic primary lesion is the chancre, a single, nonpainful ulcer with a firm indurated border, most commonly found on the genitals. The anus and lip are the next most

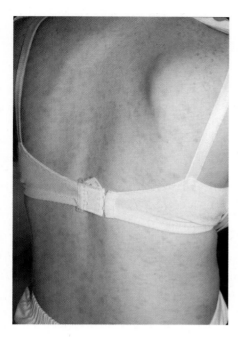

**FIGURE 26-11** ■ Secondary syphilis papulosquamous eruption.

common chancre sites. Half of all chancres are not "classical", in that they can be nonindurated, painful, or multiple in number. A week after a chancre appears, a painless, regional, nonsuppurative, rubbery lymphadenopathy can develop.

A secondary syphilis infection can mimic many diseases and has a large number of possible skin findings. The most common finding is a widespread, symmetric, nonpruritic, papulosquamous eruption (Fig. 26-11). The palms and soles are classically affected. Moist areas such as the anus, penis, labia, and inner thighs may grow wartlike condyloma lata, which are whitish or grayish flat papules (Fig. 26-12). Painful shallow erosions called mucous patches may affect the

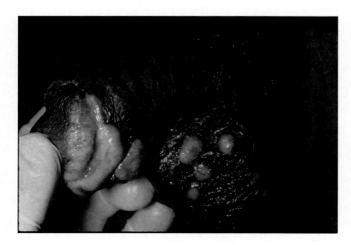

**FIGURE 26-12** ■ Moist, whitish, flat-topped, syphilitic papules of condylomata lata.

mucous membranes. A diffuse, nonscarring alopecia may affect the scalp and eyebrows. The classic moth-eaten patchy alopecia of syphilis is uncommon.

Tertiary syphilis's principal skin manifestation is the gumma. The gumma is a scarring, locally destructive plaque, nodule, or ulcer that is sometimes arciform in shape. Ulcerative gummas, particularly on the chest and calves, may appear "punched out." Gummas are not limited to the skin and can be found on the nasal septum, palate, bones, and internal organs.

### Course

The primary chancre develops after an average incubation of 3 weeks and lasts for 2 to 8 weeks. Secondary syphilis develops about 6 weeks after the primary chancre appears (the chancre may still be present at this time). Secondary syphilis is the result of a disseminated infection, and, as such, it typically has systemic symptoms such as headaches, low-grade fevers, generalized lymphadenopathy, malaise, loss of appetite, hepatosplenomegaly, pharyngitis, and myalgias. This stage, if left untreated, spontaneously resolves in 2 to 10 weeks. Latent syphilis follows. Tertiary syphilis appears an average of 3 to 10 years after secondary syphilis in about a quarter of untreated patients, but its onset may be accelerated in immunocompromised individuals. Besides gummas, tertiary syphilis can affect the neurologic and cardiovascular systems.

### Contagiousness

Syphilis is primarily transmitted via direct sexual contact with a primary or secondary syphilitic lesion. Much less commonly, it spreads via nongenital contact, intravenous drug use, or transplacentally. Fomite transmission is unlikely as *T. pallidum* is easily killed outside of its host environment.

### Diagnosis

Most cases of syphilis are diagnosed via clinical suspicion and positive serologic testing. Suspected patients are typically screened with the sensitive, but not specific, rapid plasma reagin (RPR) or Venereal Disease Research Laboratory (VDRL) tests. The RPR and VDRL tests can be negative early in a primary infection. Thus, if syphilis is suspected, these tests should be repeated weekly for a month to rule out syphilis. These tests can be falsely positive from many things including autoimmune diseases, hyperlipidemia, and pregnancy. As a result, a specific serologic test that targets treponemal antigens is used to confirm the infection. The fluorescent treponemal antibody-absorption test (FTA-ABS) and the microhemagglutination test for *T. pallidum* (MHA-TP) are two such tests. These specific tests, unlike the RPR and VDRL, remain positive after effective syphilis treatment. Syphilis can be diagnosed microscopically in experienced hands from primary and secondary syphilitic lesions, using dark field microscopy to visualize the corkscrew-shaped organisms.

Slow-release penicillin, penicillin G benzathine, is the treatment of choice for syphilis. Primary and secondary syphilis can be treated with a single intramuscular injection of 2.4 million units of benzathine penicillin G. For those allergic to penicillin, doxycycline 100 mg twice a day orally for 28 days, tetracycline 500 mg orally four times daily for 28 days, or ceftriaxone 125 mg daily intramuscularly for 10 days can be used. An acute febrile reaction with chills, myalgias, increased lesional inflammation, pharyngitis, and headaches, called the Jarisch–Herxheimer reaction, can occur within a day of starting penicillin or occasionally after other antibiotic treatments. To ensure clearance of the infection, RPR or VDRL titers should be drawn at 3, 6, 12, and 24 months post-treatment to document a fourfold titer decrease. Sexual partners of the patient should also be treated.

## Chancroid

Chancroid is an ulcerative STI caused by the gram-negative bacterium *Haemophilus ducreyi*. Chancroid is very common in developing countries such as India and in Africa, Southeast Asia, and the Caribbean. It is rare in industrialized nations, but outbreaks linked to prostitution do occur. Men are much more likely to be affected by the disease than women by a factor of 10 to 1.

### Skin Manifestations

The primary lesion is an erythematous papule that progresses to a pustule and then ruptures to form an ulcer. The ulcer has a purulent base and a well-demarcated, undermined, hyperemic edge (Fig. 26-13). It is painful, friable, nonindurated, and most commonly found around the prepuce. Other ulcer sites include the anus, vulva, and the cervix. "Kissing lesions" can be present from autoinoculation of opposing skin surfaces. Almost half of patients develop a painful, mostly unilateral, suppurative lymphadenitis (bubo) that may rupture and produce a chancrous-appearing lesion.

### Course

The primary lesion usually appears after a 1- to 5-day incubation period. The disease is rarely asymptomatic.

### Contagiousness

Chancroid is spread via sexual contact with females in the sex industry who have sex despite having a painful ulcer. Asymptomatic carriers are rare.

### Diagnosis

There is no perfect test to diagnose chancroid; even bacterial culture is only 80% sensitive. A probable diagnosis is often made by noting clinical presentation and ruling out other causes of genital ulcers such as syphilis, herpes, and LGV. Smears of chancroid ulcers may reveal the characteristic gram-negative rods in chains, but this finding is neither

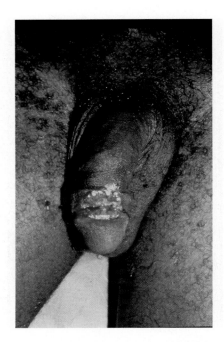

**FIGURE 26-13** ■ Chancroid ulcer demonstrating a purulent base with well-demarcated, undermined edges.

specific nor sensitive. The rods are only found on smears less than half the time. Culture is often unavailable as it requires a special medium. If a diagnosis of chancroid is made by culture, syphilis should still be ruled out as syphilis often coinfects chancroid ulcers.

### Treatment

A single 1-g oral dose of azithromycin is the first-line treatment. Other treatment options include erythromycin 500 mg orally four times daily for 7 days, ceftriaxone 250 mg intramuscularly once, and ciprofloxacin 500 mg orally twice daily for 3 days. Ciprofloxacin is not for pregnant or lactating women or for children. Sexual partners from the 10 days prior to symptom onset should be treated.

## Fungi

### Candidiasis

*Candida albicans* is a common inhabitant of the oropharynx, the gastrointestinal tract, and the female genitalia. *Candida* infections are normally overgrowths of normal flora, but they can also be acquired sexually. Vaginal candidiasis often occurs following changes in the vaginal pH, weakening of the immune system, or disruption of competing flora by antibiotics.

### Skin Manifestations

*Candida* can cause a vulvovaginitis in females and a balanitis in uncircumcised males. Itching is the most common finding. The vulva can be erythematous, swollen, and macerated. There can be a watery to thick cottage cheese–appearing

**SAUER'S NOTES**

The field of dermatology has long been considered the specialty most expert in the diagnosis of sexually transmitted diseases. In fact, the American Academy of Dermatology was formerly called "American Academy of Dermatology and Syphilology." As the cosmetic aspects of skin care have begun to replace the medical aspects, the expertise of the dermatologist has been waning. It is imperative that this trend be reversed for the sake of the specialty and more importantly for the sake of our patients.

vaginal discharge. The cervix can be hyperemic, swollen, and covered with small erosions and small vesicles.

*Course*

The lifetime prevalence of candidiasis is 75%, with 50% of women having more than one episode. Five percent of women develop recurrent vaginal candidiasis (greater than three episodes per year). Factors associated with recurrent candidiasis are sexual transmittance and poor perineal hygiene. Symptoms typically worsen a week before menses.

*Contagiousness*

Most infections are merely an overgrowth of endogenous *Candida*, but some cases can be caused by direct mucosal contact as in sexual intercourse.

*Diagnosis*

The diagnosis is made clinically with a KOH or Gram stain smear positive for yeast and pseudohyphae.

*Treatment*

Commonly, topical medications such as miconazole, nystatin, clotrimazole, and terconazole can be used as first-line agents. Terconazole may interfere with the effectiveness of condoms. They are used once daily for 1 to 7 days. Another treatment option is a single 150-mg oral dose of fluconazole. This can be repeated in 72 hours if symptoms persist. If the patient is immunosuppressed, diabetic, or possesses other predisposing factors, he or she may need a 5- to 10-day course of fluconazole. The antifungals griseofulvin, terbinafine, and naftifine are not effective treatment options.

## Suggested Readings

Bolognia JL, Jorizzo JL, Rapini RP. *Dermatology*. 2nd ed. Philadelphia: Elsevier Inc; 2008.

Centers for Disease Control Advance Data from Vital and Health Statistics. Sexual behavior and selected health measures: men and women 15–44 years of age, United States, 2002. Available at: http://www.cdc.gov/nchs/data/ad/ad362.pdf. Accessed August 2009.

James WD, Berger TG, Elston DM. *Andrews' Diseases of the Skin*. 10th ed. Philadelphia: Elsevier Inc; 2006.

Ryan KJ, Ray CG. *Sherris Medical Microbiology: An Introduction to Infectious Diseases*. 4th ed. New York: McGraw-Hill; 2004.

Sobel JD. Vulvovaginal candidosis. *Lancet*. 2007;369:1961–1971.

# CHAPTER 27

# Tumors of the Skin

*John C. Hall, MD*

## Classification

A patient comes into your office for care of a tumor on his skin. What kind is it? What is the best treatment? This complex process of diagnosing and managing skin tumors is not learned easily. As an aid to the establishment of the correct diagnosis, all skin tumors (excluding warts, which are caused by a virus) are classified

1. as to their histologic origin (Table 27-1),
2. according to the patient's age group (Table 27-2),
3. by location (Table 27-3), and
4. on the basis of clinical appearance (Table 27-4).

A complete histologic classification is found at the end of this chapter; only the more common tumors are classified and discussed here. This histologic classification is divided into epidermal tumors, mesodermal tumors, nevus cell tumors, lymphomas, and myeloses. In making a clinical diagnosis of any skin tumor, one should apply a histopathologic label if possible. Whether the label is correct or not depends on the clinical acumen of the physician and whether the tumor, or a part of it, has been examined microscopically.

An age group classification is helpful from a differential diagnostic viewpoint. Viral warts are considered in this classification because of the frequent necessity of differentiating them from other skin tumors.

The clinical appearance of any tumor is a most important diagnostic factor. Some tumors have a characteristic color and growth that is readily distinguishable from any other tumor, but a large number, unfortunately, have clinical characteristics common to several similar tumors or are nonspecific in appearance even to the most trained observer. A further hindrance to making a correct diagnosis is that the same histopathologic lesion may vary in clinical appearance. The following generalizing classification should be helpful, but, if in doubt, the lesion should be examined histologically.

---

**SAUER'S NOTES**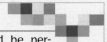

1. A histologic examination should be performed on every malignant skin tumor.
2. Similarly, a biopsy should be performed on any tumor when clinically a malignancy cannot be definitely ruled out.

---

## Seborrheic Keratoses

It is a rare elderly patient who does not have any seborrheic keratoses. These are the unattractive "moles" or "warts" that perturb the elderly patient, occasionally become irritated, but are benign (Fig. 27-1).

Dermatosis papulosa nigra is a form of seborrheic keratosis of African-Americans that occurs on the face, mainly in women. These small, black, multiple tumors can be removed, but there is a possibility of causing keloids or hypopigmentation. Stucco keratoses are numerous white 1- to 3-mm seborrheic keratoses mainly over the feet, ankles, and lower legs. A very large seborrheic keratosis is sometimes referred to as a *melanoacanthoma*.

### Presentation and Characteristics

#### Description

The size of the seborrheic keratoses varies up to 3 cm for the largest, but the average diameter is 1 cm. The color may be flesh-colored, tan, brown, or coal black. They are usually oval in shape, elevated, and have a greasy, warty sensation to the touch. White, brown, or black pinhead-sized keratotic areas called *pseudohorned cysts* are commonly seen within this tumor. They have the appearance of being superficial and "stuck on" the skin. Markings on the skin may be accentuated in superficial seborrheic keratoses. Pruritus is common and sudden appearance may occur. Numerous lesions coming on rapidly can be a marker of underlying cancer (sign of Leser–Trélat). They can suddenly appear at the site of inflamed skin (Myerson's phenomenon) and may dissipate as the inflammation is brought under control.

#### Distribution

The lesions appear on the face, neck, scalp, back, and upper chest, and less frequently on the arms, legs, and the lower part of the trunk. Mucous membranes, palms, and soles are spared.

#### Course

Lesions become darker and enlarge slowly. However, sometimes they can enlarge rapidly and this can be accompanied by bleeding and inflammation, which can be very frightening to the patient. Trauma from clothing occasionally results in infection and bleeding, and this prompts the patient to seek

## TABLE 27-1 ■ Histologic Classification of Tumors of the Skin

### Epidermal Tumors

### Tumors of the Surface Epidermis

1. *Benign tumors:* defined as neoplasms that probably arise from arrested embryonal cells

    a. Seborrheic keratosis
    b. Pedunculated fibroma (skin tag, fibroepithelial polyp, acrochordon)
    c. Cysts
        - Epidermal cyst
        - Trichilemmal (pilar or sebaceous cyst)
        - Milium
        - Dermoid cyst
        - Mucous cyst

2. Precancerous tumors

    a. Actinic keratosis and cutaneous horn
    b. Arsenical keratosis
    c. Leukoplakia
    d. Porokeratosis

3. *Carcinoma:* squamous cell carcinoma

### Tumors of the Epidermal Appendages

1. Basal cell carcinoma
2. Sebaceous gland hyperplasia
3. Numerous other types benign and malignant, usually classified by appendage of origin

### Mesodermal Tumors

### Tumors of Fibrous Tissue

1. Histiocytoma and dermatofibroma
2. Keloid

### Tumors of Vascular Tissue

1. Hemangiomas

### Nevus Cell Tumors

### Nevi

1. Junctional (active) nevus
2. Intradermal (resting) nevus
3. Dysplastic nevus syndrome (familial atypical mole–melanoma syndrome or sporadic atypical mole–melanoma syndrome)

### Malignant Melanoma

### Lymphoma and Myelosis

### Monomorphous Group

### Polymorphous Group

1. Mycosis fungoides (cutaneous T-cell lymphoma)

*Source:* Modified from Lever WF, Schaumberg-Lever G. *Histopathology of the skin.* 8th ed. Philadelphia: Lippincott; 1997.

## TABLE 27-2 ■ Age-Based Classification of Tumors of the Skin

| Age Group | Possible Tumor Types* |
|---|---|
| Children | 1. Warts (viral), very common<br>2. Nevi, junctional type, common<br>3. Molluscum contagiosum (viral)<br>4. Hemangiomas<br>5. Café-au-lait spot<br>6. Granuloma pyogenicum<br>7. Mongolian spot<br>8. Xanthogranulomas |
| Adults | 1. Warts (viral), plantar-type common<br>2. Nevi<br>3. Cysts<br>4. Pedunculated fibromas (skin tags, acrochordons)<br>5. Sebaceous gland hyperplasias<br>6. Histiocytomas (dermatofibromas, sclerosing hemangiomas)<br>7. Keloids<br>8. Lipomas<br>9. Granuloma pyogenicum |
| Older Adults** | 1. Seborrheic keratoses<br>2. Actinic keratoses<br>3. Capillary hemangiomas (cherry angiomas, senile angiomas)<br>4. Basal cell carcinomas<br>5. Squamous cell carcinomas<br>6. Leukoplakia |

*The most common tumors are listed first.
**In addition to tumors of adults.

medical care. Any inflammatory dermatitis around these lesions causes them to enlarge temporarily and become more evident, so much so that many patients suddenly note them for the first time. After the inflammation subsides the seborrheic keratosis may dissipate. Malignant degeneration of seborrheic keratoses does not occur.

*Cause*

Heredity is the biggest factor, along with old age.

### Differential Diagnosis

- *Actinic keratoses:* See Table 27-5 on page 286
- *Pigmented nevi:* Longer duration, smoother surface, softer to the touch; may not be able to differentiate clinically (see later in this chapter)
- *Flat warts:* In younger patients; acute onset, with rapid development of new lesions, colorless and flat topped without pseudohorned cysts; tiny black

**TABLE 27-3** ■ **Classification of Tumors Based on Location**

| Location | Possible Tumor Type | Location | Possible Tumor Type |
|---|---|---|---|
| Scalp | Seborrheic keratosis | | Trichilemmoma |
| | Epidermal cyst (pilar cyst) | | Trichofolliculoma |
| | Nevus | | Merkel cell carcinoma |
| | Actinic keratosis (bald males) | | Angiosarcoma (elderly men) |
| | Wart | | Nevus of Ota |
| | Trichilemmal cyst | | Warty dyskeratoma |
| | Basal cell carcinoma | | Atypical fibroxanthoma |
| | Squamous cell carcinoma | | Angiolymphoid hyperplasia with |
| | Nevus sebaceous | | eosinophilia |
| | Proliferating trichilemmal tumor | | Blue nevus |
| | Cylindroma | | Pedunculated fibroma |
| | Syringocystadenoma | Eyelids | Seborrheic keratosis |
| | papilliferum | | Milium |
| | Seborrheic keratosis | | Syringomas |
| Ear | Actinic keratoses | | Basal cell carcinoma |
| | Basal cell carcinoma | | Xanthoma |
| | Nevus | | Pedunculated fibroma |
| | Squamous cell carcinoma | Neck | Seborrheic keratosis |
| | Keloid | | Epidermal cyst |
| | Epidermal cyst | | Keloid |
| | Chondrodermatitis nodularis | Lip and mouth | Fordyce's disease |
| | helices | | Lentigo |
| | Venous lakes (varix) | | Venous lake (varix) |
| | Gouty tophus | | Mucous retention cyst |
| Face | Seborrheic keratosis | | Leukoplakia |
| | Sebaceous gland hyperplasia | | Pyogenic granuloma |
| | Actinic keratosis | | Squamous cell carcinoma |
| | Lentigo | | Granular cell tumor (tongue) |
| | Milium | | Giant cell epulis (gingivae) |
| | Nevi | | Verrucous carcinoma |
| | Basal cell carcinoma | | White sponge nevus |
| | Squamous cell carcinoma | | Acral lentiginous melanoma |
| | Lentigo maligna melanoma | | Pedunculated fibroma |
| | Flat wart | Axilla | Epidermal cyst |
| | Trichoepithelioma | | Molluscum contagiosum |
| | Dermatosis papulosa nigra | | Lentigo (multiple lentigo in the |
| | (African-American women) | | axillae neurofibromatosis called |
| | Fibrous papule of the nose | | Crowe's sign) |
| | Colloid milium | | Seborrheic keratosis |
| | Dilated pore of Winer | Chest and back | Angioma |
| | Keratoacanthoma | | Nevi |
| | Pyogenic granuloma | | Ephelides |
| | Spitz nevus | | Actinic keratosis |
| | Ephelides | | Lipoma |
| | Hemangioma | | Basal cell carcinoma |
| | Adenoma sebaceum | | Epidermal cyst |
| | Apocrine hydrocystoma | | Keloid |
| | Eccrine hydrocystoma | | |

*(continued)*

**TABLE 27-3** ■ *(continued)*

| Location | Possible Tumor Type | Location | Possible Tumor Type |
|---|---|---|---|
| | Lentigo | | Myxoid cyst (proximal nail fold) |
| | Café-au-lait spot | | Squamous cell carcinoma |
| | Squamous cell carcinoma | | Glomus tumor (nail bed) |
| | Melanoma | | Ganglion |
| | Hemangioma | | Common blue nevus |
| | Histiocytoma | | Acral lentigines melanoma |
| | Steatocystoma multiplex | | Giant cell tumor of tendon sheath |
| | Eruptive vellus hair cyst | | Pyogenic granuloma |
| | Blue nevus | | Acquired digital fibrokeratoma |
| | Nevus of Ito | | Recurrent infantile digital fibroma |
| | Becker's nevus | | Traumatic fibroma |
| | Pedunculated fibroma | | Xanthoma |
| *Groin and* | Seborrheic keratosis | | Dupuytren contracture |
| *crural areas* | Molluscum contagiosum | | Wart |
| | Wart | *Feet* | Nevi |
| | Bowen's disease | | Blue nevus |
| | Extramammary Paget disease | | Acral lentigines melanoma |
| | Wart | | Seborrheic keratosis |
| *Genitalia* | Molluscum contagiosum | | Verrucous carcinoma |
| | Squamous intraepithelial lesions | | Eccrine poroma |
| | Epidermal cyst | | Seborrheic keratosis |
| | Angiokeratoma (scrotum) | *Arms and legs* | Lentigo |
| | Pearly penile papules (around edge of glans) | | *Wart* |
| | | | *Histiocytoma* |
| | Squamous cell carcinoma | | *Actinic keratosis* |
| | Seborrheic keratosis | | *Squamous cell carcinoma* |
| | Erythroplasia of Queyrat | | *Melanoma* |
| | Bowen's disease | | *Lipoma* |
| | Median raphe cyst of penis | | *Xanthoma* |
| | Verrucous carcinoma | | *Clear cell acanthoma (legs)* |
| | Hidradenoma papilliferum (labia majora) | | *Kaposi's sarcoma (legs, classic type)* |
| | Wart | | |
| *Hands* | Seborrheic keratosis | | |
| | Actinic keratosis | | |
| | Lentigo | | |

thrombosed capillaries may be seen, usually smaller; may koebnerize (see Chapter 23)

■ *Malignant melanoma:* Less common, usually with rapid growth, indurated; histological examination with biopsy may be necessary (see later)

## Treatment

***Case Example:*** A 58-year-old woman requests the removal of a warty, tannish, slightly elevated 2 × 2 cm lesion of the right side of her forehead.

1. The lesion should be examined carefully. The diagnosis usually can be made clinically, but if there is any question, a scissor biopsy (see Chapter 2) can be performed. It would be ideal if all of these seborrheic keratoses could be examined histologically, but this is not economically feasible or necessary. If in doubt, always send for histologic examination.

2. An adequate form of therapy is curettement, with or without local anesthesia, followed by a light application of trichloroacetic acid, Monsel's solution, or aluminum

**TABLE 27-4 ■ Classification of Skin Tumors Based on Clinical Appearance**

| Appearance | Possible Tumor Type |
| --- | --- |
| Flat, skin-colored tumors | 1. Flat warts (viral) |
| | 2. Histiocytomas |
| | 3. Leukoplakia |
| Flat, pigmented tumors | 1. Nevi, usually junctional type |
| | 2. Lentigo |
| | 3. Café-au-lait spot |
| | 4. Histiocytomas |
| | 5. Mongolian spot |
| | 6. Melanoma (superficial spreading type) |
| Raised, skin-colored tumors | 1. Warts (viral) |
| | 2. Pedunculated fibromas (skin tags) |
| | 3. Nevi, usually intradermal type |
| | 4. Cysts |
| | 5. Lipomas |
| | 6. Keloids |
| | 7. Basal cell carcinomas |
| | 8. Squamous cell carcinoma |
| | 9. Molluscum contagiosum (viral) |
| | 10. Xanthogranuloma (yellowish, usually children) |
| Raised, brownish tumors | 1. Warts (viral) |
| | 2. Nevi, usually compound type |
| | 3. Actinic keratoses |
| | 4. Seborrheic keratoses |
| | 5. Pedunculated fibromas (skin tags) |
| | 6. Basal cell epitheliomas |
| | 7. Squamous cell carcinoma |
| | 8. Malignant melanoma |
| | 9. Granuloma pyogenicum |
| | 10. Keratoacanthomas |
| Raised, reddish tumors | 1. Hemangiomas |
| | 2. Actinic keratoses |
| | 3. Granuloma pyogenicum |
| | 4. Glomus tumors |
| | 5. Senile or cherry angiomas |
| Raised, blackish tumors | 1. Seborrheic keratoses |
| | 2. Nevi |
| | 3. Granuloma pyogenicum |
| | 4. Malignant melanomas |
| | 5. Blue nevi |
| | 6. Thrombosed angiomas or hemangiomas |

**SAUER'S NOTES**

1. For many benign lesions, it often is best cosmetically to err on the side of surgical undertreatment rather than overtreatment. You can always remove any remaining growth later, but you cannot put back what you took off.
2. Scarring should be kept to a minimum.
3. After any surgical procedure, I hand out a "Surgical Notes" sheet that indicates postoperative care. Skin surgery sites usually heal without any complication. However, there are always questions and concerns from the patient about aftercare.

chloride. The resulting fine atrophic scar will hardly be noticeable in several months.

3. Electrosurgery can be used, but this usually requires anesthesia and if the physician is not careful, it may scar.
4. If available, liquid nitrogen freezing therapy works well. It is the therapy of choice of most dermatologists. Do not freeze excessively.
5. Laser therapy has been used recently by some authors.
6. Surgical excision is an unnecessary and more expensive form of removal.

## Pedunculated Fibromas (Skin Tags, Acrochordons)

Multiple skin tags are common on the neck and the axillae of middle-aged, usually obese, men and women (Fig. 27-2). The indications for removal are twofold: cosmetic, as desired and requested by the patient, and to prevent the irritation and the secondary infection of the pedicle that frequently develops from trauma of a collar, necklace, or other article of clothing. These are often inherited and may be part of the metabolic syndrome.

### Presentation and Characteristics

#### Description

Pedunculated pinhead-sized to pea-sized soft tumors of normal skin color or light brown are seen. The base may be inflamed from injury, and the lesion may thrombose and turn black if twisted. This can cause alarm in the patient.

#### Distribution

The lesions occur on the neck, axillae, submammary or groin, or less frequently on any area.

#### Course

These fibromas grow very slowly. They may increase in size during pregnancy. Some become infected or thrombosed and drop off.

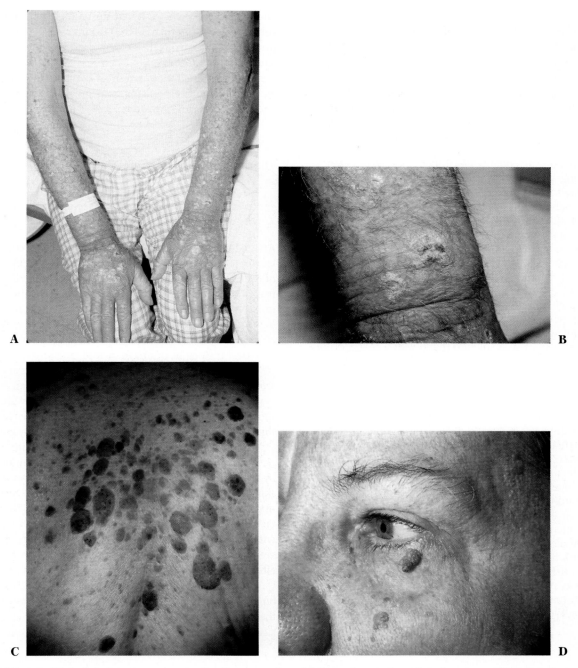

**FIGURE 27-1** ■ **(A)** Actinic keratoses in an oil refinery worker. **(B)** Hyperkeratotic actinic keratoses. **(C)** Seborrheic keratoses on the back. **(D)** Pedunculated seborrheic keratosis of the eyelid. *(Courtesy of Stiefel Laboratories, Inc.)*

## Differential Diagnosis

- *Filiform wart:* Digitate projections, more horny; also seen on the chin area (see Chapter 23)
- *Pedunculated seborrheic keratosis:* Larger lesion, darker color, warty, or velvety appearance (see preceding section)
- *Neurofibromatosis:* Lesions seen elsewhere; larger; can be pushed back into the skin; also café-au-lait spots; hereditary; single lesions do not indicate systemic disease (see Chapters 38 and 40)

## Treatment

***Case Example:*** A 42-year-old woman has 20 small pedunculated fibromas on her neck and axillae that she wants removed. This could be done by electrosurgery. Without anesthesia, gently grab the small tumor in a thumb forceps

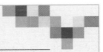

Minor surgery has been performed for the removal or biopsy of a skin lesion.

If liquid nitrogen was used to remove the growth, a blister or peeling at the growth site will develop in 24 hours; if electrosurgery, laser, or burning was used, a crust and scab will form; if a biopsy was made, there will be a crust or suture(s).

The treated sites heal better if they are covered with a dressing with polysporin ointment underneath during the day for 5 to 7 days and left uncovered at night and while bathing. Do not pick at the spot and try to avoid accidentally hitting the area.

You can wash over the area lightly.

A certain amount of redness and swelling around the surgery site is to be expected. Also you might have a small amount of drainage and crusting. A mild amount of redness and infection can be treated with polysporin ointment locally three times a day.

If more drainage or infection develops, apply a wet dressing with sheeting, or soak the area. Oral antibiotics can be given. Use a solution made with 1 teaspoon of salt to 1 pint of cool water or Domeboro compresses and apply for 20 minutes three times a day. Make a fresh solution every day.

If the infection becomes excessive, call the office or go to a hospital emergency department.

If the scab is knocked off prematurely, bleeding may occur. This can be stopped by applying firm pressure with gauze or cotton for 10 minutes by the clock, and then releasing pressure gradually.

Depending on the size of the surgery site, healing takes from 1 to 8 weeks. Some scarring or loss of pigment at the surgery site is possible. A few individuals have a tendency to form thick or keloidal scars, which is not predictable.

If a biopsy was done, you may receive a separate bill for the pathology study from the laboratory. Call the office in 7 days for this report.

Return to the office for further care or follow-up as directed.

and stretch the pedicle. Touch this pedicle with the electrosurgery needle and turn on the current for a split second. The tumor separates from the skin, and no bleeding occurs. The site heals in 4 to 7 days.

For very small lesions, a short spark with the electrosurgical needle suffices. Scissor excision with or without local anesthetic is commonly done.

## Cysts

The three common types are

- epidermal cyst,
- trichilemmal (pilar) or sebaceous cyst, and
- milium.

An *epidermal cyst* (Fig. 27-3A and B) has a wall composed of true epidermis and probably originates from an invagination of the epidermis into the dermis and subsequent detachment from the epidermis, or it can originate spontaneously. The most common locations for epidermal cysts are the face, ears, neck, back, and scalp, where tumors of varying size can be found. A central pore may be seen over the surface. There may be a history of drainage of foul smelling cheesy debris.

*Trichilemmal cysts*, formerly known as *wens* and *pilar* or *sebaceous cysts* (Fig. 27-3C), are less common than epidermal cysts, occur mainly on the scalp, usually are multiple, and show an autosomal-dominant inheritance. The sac wall is thick, smooth, and whitish and can be quite easily enucleated.

*Milia* (Fig. 27-3D) are very common, white, pinhead-sized, firm lesions that are seen on the face. They are formed by proliferation of epithelial buds following trauma to the skin (dermabrasion for acne scars), following certain dermatoses (pemphigus, epidermolysis bullosa, and acute contact dermatitis), or from no apparent cause. Occurrences with porphyria cutanea tarda, after 5-fluorouracil therapy, in areas of corticosteroid-induced atrophy, after burns, and after radiation therapy are other causes.

They can occur spontaneously at any age including newborns where they may dissipate. Treatment consists of opening the lesion with a No. 11 Bard Parker blade and expression with a comedone extractor. This is done for cosmetic reasons only.

TABLE 27-5 ■ **Differential Diagnosis of Keratoses**

| Parameter | Actinic or Senile Keratosis | Seborrheic Keratosis |
|---|---|---|
| Appearance | Flat, brownish, reddish, or tan scale firmly attached to the skin, poorly demarcated | Greasy, elevated, brown, black, flesh-colored, warty scale and can be easily scratched away at times, "stuck on," well demarcated |
| Location | Sun-exposed areas | Face, back |
| Complexion | Blue eyes, light hair, dry skin | Brown eyes, dark hair, oily skin |
| Symptoms | Some burning and stinging | Occasional itching |
| Precancerous | Yes | No |
| Cause | Sun | Inherited |

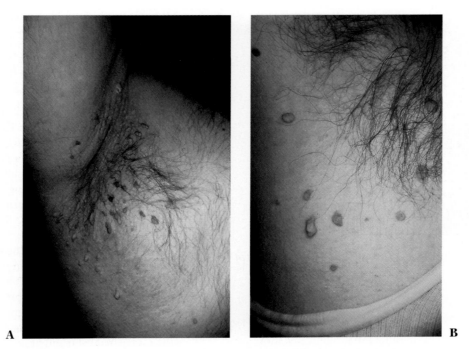

**FIGURE 27-2** ■ (**A, B**) Pedunculated fibromas in the axilla. *(Courtesy of Stiefel Laboratories, Inc.)*

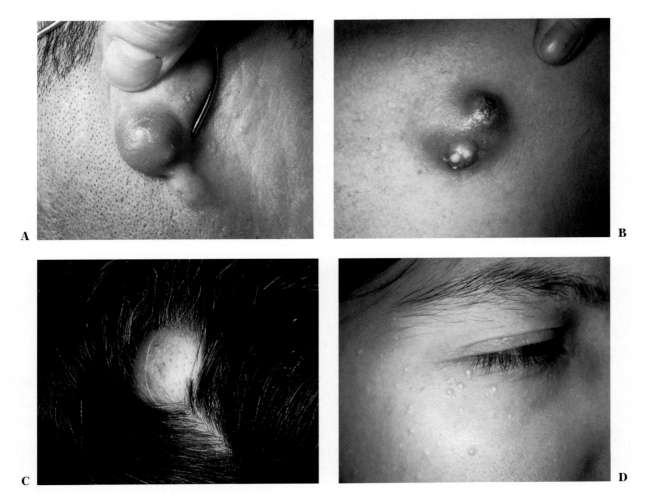

**FIGURE 27-3** ■ (**A**) Epidermal cyst of the earlobe. (**B**) Infected epidermal cyst on the shoulder. (**C**) Pilar or sebaceous cyst of the scalp. (**D**) Milia on the upper cheek of 21-year-old woman. *(Courtesy of Texas Pharmacal.)*

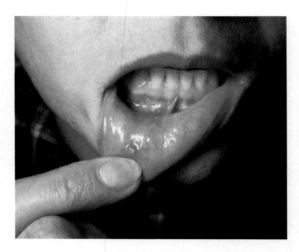

**FIGURE 27-4** ■ Mucous cyst on the lower lip. *(Courtesy of Texas Pharmacal.)*

### Differential Diagnosis of Epidermal and Trichilemmal Cysts

- *Lipoma:* Difficult to differentiate clinically; more firm, no central pore, lobulated; no cheesy material extrudes on incision; removal is by complete excision or by liposuction; clinically similar to hibernoma
- *Dermoid cyst:* Clinically similar; can also be found internally; usually a solitary skin tumor; histologically, contains hairs, eccrine glands, and sebaceous glands
- *Mucous cysts* (Fig. 27-4): Translucent pea-sized or smaller lesions on the lips, treated by cutting off the top of the lesion and carefully, lightly cauterizing the base with a silver nitrate stick or light electrosurgery; laser therapy can also be used
- *Synovial cysts (myxoid cysts) of the skin* (Fig. 27-5): Globoid, translucent, pea-sized swellings around the joints of fingers and toes that drain a syrupy clear liquid and are most common at the base of the nail on the proximal nail fold

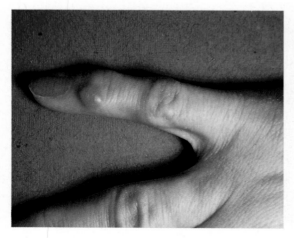

**FIGURE 27-5** ■ Synovial cyst on the finger. *(Courtesy of Texas Pharmacal.)*

### Treatment of Epidermal and Trichilemmal Cysts

Several methods can be used with success. The choice depends on the ability of the operator, the site, and the number of cysts. Cysts can regrow after even the best surgical care because of incomplete removal of the sac.

1. A single 3-cm cyst on the back should be removed by surgical excision and suturing. This can be done in two ways: either by incising the skin and skillfully removing the intact cyst sac with an ellipse excision or by cutting straight into the sac with a small incision, shelling out the evacuated lining by applying strong pressure to the sides of the incision, and suturing the skin. The latter procedure is simpler, requires a smaller incision, and is quite successful.
2. A patient with several cysts in the scalp can be treated in another simple way. A 3- to 4-mm incision can be made directly over and into the cyst. The cheesy, foul-smelling contents can be evacuated by pressure and the use of a small curette. The sac can then be popped out of the hole with very firm pressure, or the sac can be grasped with a small hemostat and pulled out of the opening. No suturing or only a single suture is necessary. The resulting scar is imperceptible after a short time.
3. If, during incision by any technique, a solid tumor is found instead of a cyst, the lesion should be excised completely and the material studied histologically. This diagnostic error is common because of the clinical similarity of cysts, lipomas, and other related tumors.

### Treatment of Milia

1. Simple incision of the small tumors with a scalpel or a Hagedorn needle and expression of the contents by a comedone extractor is sufficient.
2. Another procedure is to remove the top of the milia lightly with electrodesiccation.
3. An 11 Bard Parker blade can be used to open the top and then an acne stylette used to express the contents.

## Precancerous Tumors

Precancerous types of tumors include actinic keratoses, cutaneous horns, arsenical keratoses, and leukoplakia.

---

**SAUER'S NOTES**

1. Patients with actinic keratoses should be advised to return every 6 to 12 months for examination; this is especially important if they have extensive actinic damage.
2. All patients with actinic keratoses should be told to use a sunscreen lotion or cream to lessen the occurrence of future keratoses. Wear protective clothing and avoid sun exposure between 10:00 AM and 4:00 PM.

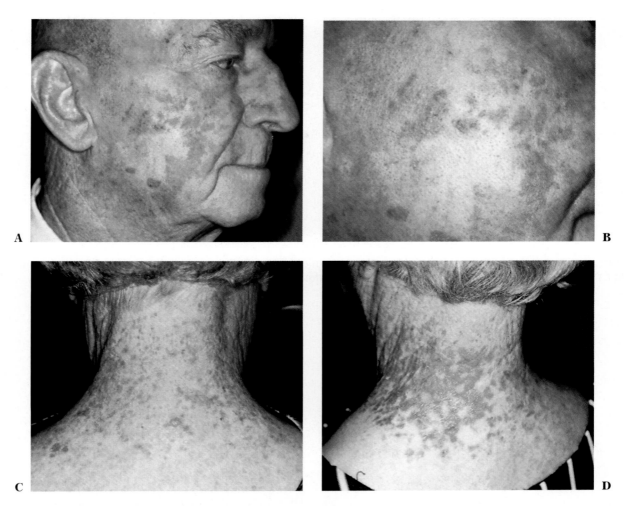

**FIGURE 27-6** ▪ Actinic keratoses. **(A)** Multiple actinic keratoses on the face of an 80-year-old, fair-complexioned farmer. **(B)** Close up. **(C)** Actinic keratoses of the back of the neck showing lesions before therapy. **(D)** Normal accentuation after therapy with 5-fluorouracil for 2 weeks. *(Courtesy of Dermik Laboratories, Inc., and Owen Laboratories, Inc.)*

## Actinic Keratosis

Actinic keratosis is a common skin lesion of light-complexioned older persons that occurs on the skin surfaces exposed to sunlight (**Fig. 27-6**). A small percentage of these lesions develop into squamous cell carcinomas (approximately 5% to 10%). Because of the popularity of sunbathing and the use of suntanning salons, these lesions (probably 5% to 10%) are also seen in persons in the 30- to 50-year-old age group.

### Description

Lesions are usually multiple, flat or slightly elevated, pink, brownish or tan colored, scaly and adherent, measuring up to 1.5 cm in diameter, and often arising on an ill-defined pink base (**Fig. 27-7**). There is a dark variant called a superficial pigmented actinic keratosis (SPAK). Individual lesions may become confluent. A *cutaneous horn* may be a proliferative, hyperkeratotic form of actinic keratosis that resembles a horn (**Fig. 27-8**). A cutaneous horn can also originate from a seborrheic keratosis, wart, squamous cell carcinoma, keratotic basal cell carcinoma, keratoacanthoma, and, most commonly, an actinic keratosis. If a biopsy is done, enough of the base of the lesion must be removed to obtain an accurate histologic diagnosis.

### Distribution

Areas of skin exposed to sunlight, such as the face, ears, neck, extensor forearms, lower legs distal to the knees, and dorsum of the hands, are involved.

### Course

The lesion begins as a faint red, slightly scaly patch that enlarges slowly, peripherally and deeply, over many years. Early actinic keratoses may come and go but do not dissipate completely. A sudden spurt of growth, increased thickness, or surrounding induration could indicate a change to a squamous cell carcinoma.

### Subjective Symptoms

Patients often complain that these lesions are sensitive or they burn and sting.

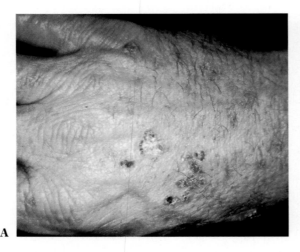
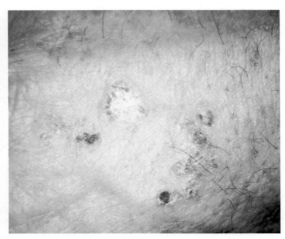

**FIGURE 27-7** ■ Actinic keratoses. **(A)** Lesions on the dorsum of hands. **(B)** Closeup in a 44-year-old, blue-eyed outdoor worker. *(Courtesy of Dermik Laboratories, Inc. and Owen Laboratories, Inc.)*

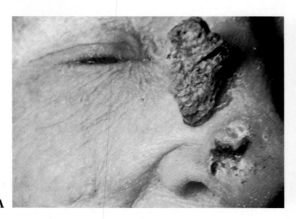
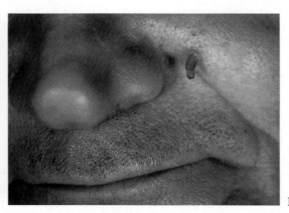

**FIGURE 27-8** ■ **(A)** A cutaneous horn with basal cell carcinomatous degeneration of the base. *(Courtesy of Texas Pharmacal).* **(B)** A cutaneous horn, on the cheek. *(Courtesy of Syntex Laboratories, Inc.)*

*Cause*

Heredity and sun exposure are the two main causative factors. The blue-eyed, thin-skinned, light-haired person with a family history of such lesions is the best subject for multiple actinic keratoses.

*Sex Incidence*

The disorder is most commonly seen in men.

*Differential Diagnosis*

- *Seborrheic keratosis:* See Table 27-5
- *Squamous cell carcinoma:* Any thickened lesion that has grown rapidly should undergo biopsy (see later in this chapter)
- *Arsenical keratosis:* Mainly on the palms and soles; history of arsenic ingestion
- *Porokeratosis:* Mainly on the legs in women; thread-like keratotic border (coronoid lamellae) that sharply demarcates tumor from surrounding skin

*Treatment*

***Case Example:*** A 60-year-old farmer has three small actinic keratoses on his face. The lesions should be examined carefully. If there is any evidence of induration or marked inflammation, the lesion should undergo biopsy (see Chapter 2). There are two methods of removal of these keratoses. For a single lesion, or only three or four lesions, a one-visit surgical treatment is usually preferable, especially if the lesion is relatively thick.

***Surgical Method.*** Liquid nitrogen, if available, applied very lightly to the lesion is an effective and rapid method of removal. This is the therapy of choice of dermatologists.

Curettement, followed by destruction of the base by acid or electrosurgery, is satisfactory. Local anesthesia is usually necessary. Firmly scrape the lesion with the dermal curette, which removes the mushy, scaly keratosis and exposes the more fibrous normal skin. Experience provides the necessary "feel" of abnormal versus normal tissue. Some of the bleeding can be controlled by pressure or use of either one of the two following procedures

1. application with a cotton-tipped applicator of a saturated solution of trichloroacetic acid, aluminum chloride solution, or Monsel solution cautiously to the bleeding site; or
2. electrocoagulation of the bleeding base.

Small lesions heal in 7 to 14 days. No bandage is required. Laser is also an acceptable form of therapy used by some dermatologists.

***Solareze Method.*** Apply a thin coat over the area of involvement twice a day for 3 months. Not as much irritation as fluorouracil and imiquimod.

***Fluorouracil Method.*** For the patient with multiple superficial actinic keratoses, fluorouracil therapy is effective and eliminates for some months or years the early damaged epidermal cells. Thus, this fluorouracil therapy is really a cancer-prevention routine.

Three preparations available are as follows:

1. Fluoroplex 1% solution, or cream 30.0 used as below for Efudex.
2. Efudex 2% solution or Efudex 5% cream 10.0

   *Sig:* Apply with fingers to area to be treated twice a day.
   *Comment:* It is wise to treat only a small area on the face at a time. Give instructions carefully and warn the patient that it is natural for the skin to get quite red and irritated and sore after 4 to 5 days. The most common method of therapy in the past was a thin coat twice a day for 2 weeks. Some patients must stop therapy sooner, and some need more time to get the desired effect.

   After completion of the course of therapy, the skin usually heals rapidly. A corticosteroid cream may be prescribed to hasten healing.

   Another form of administration of fluorouracil is the pulse method. Here the medication is applied twice a day for only 2 to 4 consecutive days of each week, for a total duration of 3 or 4 months of therapy or another example is each night Mon–Wed–Fri for approximately 3 months.

   This therapy may have to be repeated in several months or years. If some keratoses are too thick to be removed by this fluorouracil method, then the liquid nitrogen or surgical method, as described, is indicated for these lesions.
3. Carac (0.5%) Cream used as above for Efudex.

***Aldara (Imiquimod) Method.*** This can be used twice a day for 2 weeks or as a pulse therapy three times a week for 3 months. Unlike fluorouracil therapy, it does not cause a more severe reaction in the sun, but topical steroids probably should not be used to lessen the reaction because they may decrease the benefit.

***Retinoic Acid Preparations.*** These may treat early actinic keratoses but their main efficacy has been shown to be as a preventative in a thin coat at night. There are many preparations that can be applied as a thin coat each night. Irritation can be a problem, but with time the skin may become more tolerant. Tazorac (tazarotene) is a similar topical retinoid preparation that may be even more effective but irritation may be more severe.

### Treatment of a Cutaneous Horn

The same surgical technique as for actinic keratosis is used. To rule out cancer, most cutaneous horns should be sent with an intact base for histopathologic examination.

## Arsenical Keratosis

Prolonged ingestion of inorganic arsenic (e.g., Fowler's solution, Asiatic pills, well water that is high in arsenic) can result in the formation many years later of small, punctate keratotic lesions, mainly seen on the palms and the soles. Progression to a squamous cell carcinoma can occur but is unusual. These patients have an increased risk of underlying solid tumor malignancies.

### Treatment

Small arsenical keratoses can be removed by electrosurgery; larger lesions can be excised and skin grafted if necessary.

## Leukoplakia

Leukoplakia is an actinic keratosis of the mucous membrane (**Fig. 27-9**).

### Description

A flat, whitish plaque occurs localized to the mucous membranes of the lips, mouth, vulva, and vagina. Single or multiple lesions may be present.

### Course

Progression to squamous cell carcinoma occurs in 20% to 30% of chronic cases. Squamous cell cancer of the mucous membrane is more aggressive with 40% to 50% metastasis versus only 4% to 5% on the skin.

### Cause

Smoking, sunlight, ethanol ingestion, chewing tobacco, snuff, and chronic irritation are the important factors in the development of leukoplakia. Recurrent actinic cheilitis may precede leukoplakia of the lips. The vulvar form may develop from presenile or senile atrophy of this area.

### Differential Diagnosis

- *Lichen planus:* A lacy network of whitish lesions, mainly on the sides of the buccal cavity; when on lips, it may clinically resemble leukoplakia; lichen

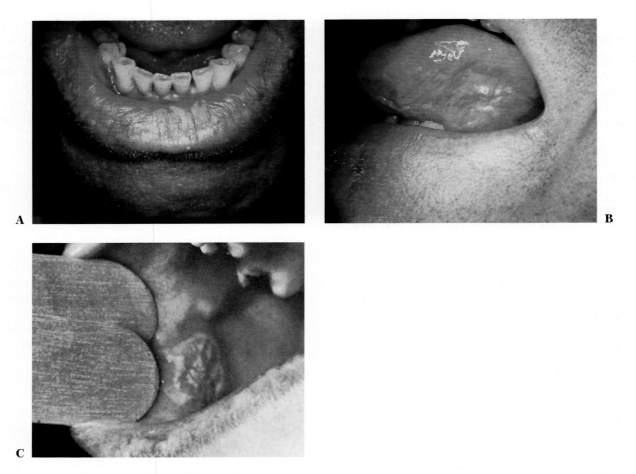

**FIGURE 27-9** ■ **(A)** Leukoplakia on the lower lip, mild. **(B)** Leukoplakia on the tongue, from chronic biting. (*Courtesy of Westwood Pharmaceuticals.*) **(C)** Biopsy-proven leukoplakia on the mucous membrane of the cheek. This was erroneously diagnosed, clinically, as lichen planus.

planus elsewhere on the body (see Chapter 15); biopsy is often indicated; ulcerative lichen planus in the oral mucous membranes may have an increased risk of squamous cell carcinoma

- *Pressure calluses* from teeth or dentures: Evidence of irritation; differentiation may be possible only by biopsy
- On the vulva, *lichen sclerosus et atrophicus* or *kraurosis vulvae:* No induration, as in leukoplakia of this area; can extend onto skin of the inguinal folds and perianal region; pruritus may or may not be present and can be severe with dyspareunia; biopsy is helpful; up to 5% of lichen sclerosis et atrophicus may develop a squamous cell cancer
- Oral lichen simplex chronicus (benign alveolar ridge keratosis) is felt by some authors to be a distinct clinicopathological entity which, unlike leukoplakia, is without cancer potential. It occurs more commonly in males on the attached ginigival mucosa especially retromolar and on the alveolar ridge. Histologically and clinically it mimics lichen simplex chronicus in the skin

*Treatment*

***Case Example:*** Small patch of leukoplakia is seen on the lower lip of man who smokes considerably.

1. The lesion should be examined carefully. Perform a biopsy on any questionable area that shows inflammation and induration. If a squamous cell carcinoma is present, the patient should receive surgical or radiation therapy by a physician who is an expert in this form of treatment.
2. Advise against use of tobacco products. The seriousness of continued smoking or other use of tobacco must be pointed out to the patient. Many early cases of leukoplakia disappear when smoking is stopped.
3. Eliminate any chronic irritation from teeth or dentures.
4. Protect the lips from sunlight with a sunscreen stick.
5. Electrosurgery, preceded by local anesthesia, is excellent for small, persistent areas of leukoplakia. The coagulating current is effective. Healing is usually rapid. Laser therapy or a surgical lip shave are used by some dermatologists.
6. Liquid nitrogen freezing is also effective.

7. If alcohol abuse is present, cessation is advisable.
8. Topical 5-FU or aldara can be used.

## Epitheliomas and Carcinomas

Basal Cell Carcinoma (see Chapter 28)

Squamous Cell Carcinoma (see Chapter 28)

## Histiocytoma and Dermatofibroma

Histiocytomas and dermatofibromas are common, usually single, flat, or only slightly elevated, tannish, reddish, or brownish nodules, less than 1 cm in size that occur mainly on the extremities (**Fig. 27-10**). These tumors have a characteristic clinical appearance and firm button-like feel that establishes the diagnosis. They often dimple when firm pressure is applied from both sides. They occur in adults and are usually asymptomatic and unchanging.

The histologic picture varies with the age of the lesion. The younger lesions are called *histiocytomas and are quite cellular,* the older ones *dermatofibromas and are more fibrous.* If the nodule contains many blood vessels, it is histologically labeled a *sclerosing hemangioma.* It is thought to possibly be a scar-like reaction to an insect bite.

### Differential Diagnosis

■ *Fibrosarcoma:* Active growth with invasion of subcutaneous fat; any questionable lesions should be excised and examined histologically

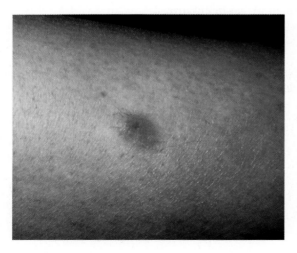

**FIGURE 27-10** ■ Histiocytoma, on the leg. *(Courtesy of Syntex Laboratories, Inc.)*

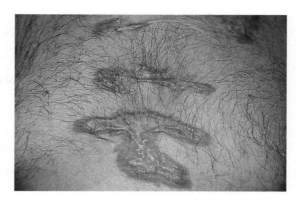

**FIGURE 27-11** ■ Keloids on the chest (common).

### Treatment

No treatment is indicated. If there is any doubt as to the diagnosis, surgical excision and histologic examination are indicated.

For the female patient who shaves her legs and hits this lesion, liquid nitrogen applied to the papule flattens it and excision with an ellipse or a punch eliminates it.

## Keloid

A keloid is a tumor resulting from an abnormal overgrowth of fibrous tissue following injury in certain predisposed persons (**Fig. 27-11**). Unusual configurations can occur, depending on the site, extent, and variety of the trauma. This tendency occurs so commonly in African-Americans that one should think twice before attempting a cosmetic procedure on a dark-skinned person or on any other person with a history of keloids. The back and the upper chest areas are especially prone to this proliferation. They may be tender and painful especially on the chest after coronary artery bypass surgery.

### Differential Diagnosis

■ *Hypertrophic scar:* Initially the same clinically and histologically as a keloid; flattens spontaneously in most cases after one or several years and does not extend beyond the original site of trauma

### Treatment

Therapy is unsatisfactory. Intralesional corticosteroids after cryospray or massaging with a corticosteroid ointment for 60 seconds daily after bath or shower can be tried. Occasionally,

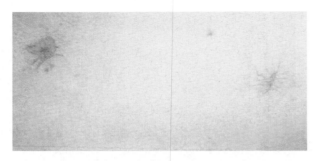

**FIGURE 27-12** ■ Two spider hemangiomas on the arm of a pregnant woman.

combined procedures using excision or laser and intralesional corticosteroid injections or interferon α-2b (Intron A) injections have been successful. Silicone sheeting therapy has its advocates. Excision should be done cautiously because recurrence of a larger tumor may occur. If removal is done, intralesional corticosteroids should be used to attempt to prevent a recurrence.

## Hemangiomas

### Spider Hemangioma

A spider hemangioma consists of a small pinpoint- to pinhead-sized central red arteriole with radiating smaller vessels like the spokes of a wheel or the legs of a spider (Fig. 27-12). On diascopy, they dissipate and rapidly refill from the center. These lesions develop for no apparent reason or may develop in association with pregnancy or, in chronic liver disease when very numerous on the upper trunk. The most common location is on the face. The reason for removal is cosmetic. In younger children, they may spontaneously disappear.

### Differential Diagnosis

- *Venous stars:* Small, bluish, telangiectatic veins, usually seen on the legs and the face but may appear anywhere on the body; these can be removed, if desired, by the same method as for spider hemangioma
- *Hereditary hemorrhagic telangiectasis* (Rendu–Osler–Weber disease): Small, red lesions on any organ of the body that can hemorrhage and are numerous on the lips and oral mucous membranes as well as far into the gastrointestinal tract; get family history

### Treatment

***Case Example:*** A spider hemangioma is present on the cheek of a young woman who is 6 months postpartum. This lesion developed during her pregnancy and has persisted unchanged.

Electrosurgery or laser is the treatment of choice. The fine epilating needle is used with either a very low coagulating sparking current or a low cutting current. The needle is stuck into the central vessel and the current turned on for 1 or 2 seconds until the vessel blanches. No anesthetic is necessary in most patients. The area forms a scab and heals in about 4 days, leaving an imperceptible scar. Rarely, a second treatment is necessary to eliminate the central vessel. If the radiating vessels are large and persistent, they can be treated in the same manner as the central vessel. For laser therapy, see Chapter 5.

### Venous Lake (Varix)

Another vascular lesion that occurs in older persons is a *venous lake.* Clinically, it is a soft, compressible, flat or slightly elevated, bluish-red, 3- to 6-mm lesion, usually located on the lips or the ears. The color decreases on diascopy. Lack of induration and rapid growth distinguish it from a melanoma. Lack of pulsation distinguishes a venous lake on the lower lip from a tortuous segment of the inferior labial artery.

Treatment is usually not desired, only reassurance concerning its nonmalignant nature.

### Angiokeratomas

Three forms of angiokeratoma are known:

- *Mibelli's form* occurs on the dorsa of the fingers, the toes, and the knees;
- *Fabry's form* occurs over the entire trunk in an extensive pattern; and
- the *Fordyce form* occurs on the scrotum.

The lesions are dark-red, pinhead-sized papules with a somewhat warty appearance. Treatment or further workup is not indicated for Mibelli form and the Fordyce form. The Fabry form (angiokeratoma corporis diffusum), however, is the cutaneous manifestation of a systemic phospholipid storage disease (fucosidosis) in which phospholipids are deposited in the skin, as well as in various internal organs. Death usually occurs in the fifth decade from the result of such deposits in the smooth muscles of the blood vessels, in the heart, and in the kidneys (see Chapter 38). Renal transplantation may be curative.

## Nevus Cell Tumors

Nevus cell tumors can be classified as melanocytic nevi or as malignant melanoma. Nevi, in turn are classified as

- Junctional or active nevus
- Intradermal or resting nevus
- Compound nevus (components of both junctional nevus manifested by color and intradermal nevus manifested by elevation)
- Dysplastic nevus syndrome (BK mole syndrome, FAMM [familial atypical malignant melanoma mole syndrome], SAMM [sporadic atypical malignant melanoma mole syndrome])

Nevi are discussed here, but malignant melanoma is discussed separately in Chapter 29.

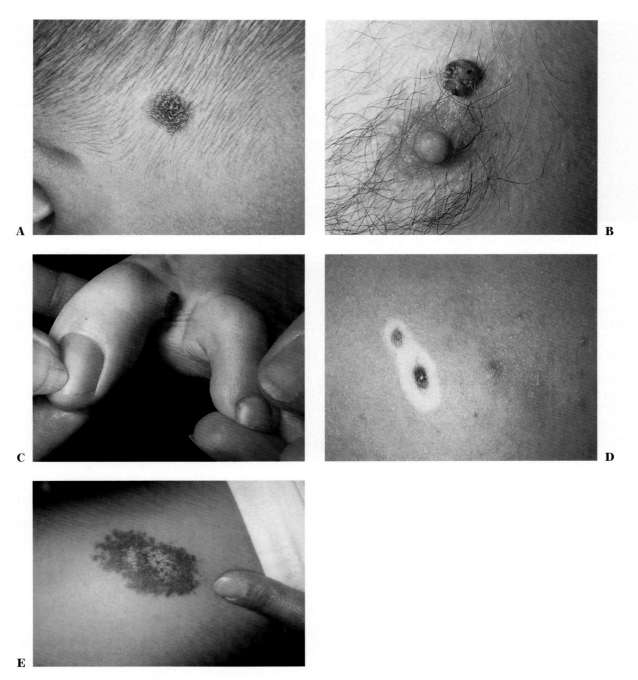

**FIGURE 27-13** ■ **(A)** Junctional nevus in the scalp of a 12-year-old child. **(B)** Compound nevus, on the chest above the nipple. **(C)** Junctional nevus on the web of the toe of an 8-year-old child. **(D)** Halo nevus, or leukoderma acquisitum centrifugum, on the back. **(E)** Giant pigmented nevus on the thigh. *(Courtesy of the Upjohn Company.)*

## Melanocytic Nevi

Nevi are pigmented or nonpigmented tumors of the skin that contain nevus cells (Fig. 27-13). Nevi are present on every adult, but some persons have more than others. There are two main questions concerning nevi or moles: When and how should they be removed? What is the relationship between nevi and malignant melanomas?

Histologically, it is possible to divide benign nevi into *junctional (active nevi)* and *intradermal (resting nevi)*.

Combinations of these two forms commonly exist and are labeled *compound nevi*.

In the dysplastic nevus syndrome (FAMM when a positive family history and SAMM when no family history), the nevi are more numerous and larger than ordinary (usually 5 to 15 mm in size), have an irregular border, and show a haphazard mixture of tan, brown, pink, and black. There is a propensity when this type of nevus is present, especially when familial, for these patients to develop a malignant melanoma.

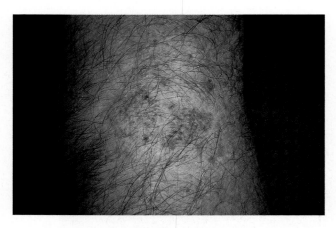

**FIGURE 27-14** ■ Speckled lentigines nevus on the forearm (nevus spilus).

Clinically, one never can be positive with which histopathologic type of nevus one is dealing, but certain criteria are helpful in establishing a differentiation between the forms.

### Description

Clinically, nevi can be pigmented or nonpigmented, flat or elevated, hairy or nonhairy, warty, papillomatous, or pedunculated. They can have a small or a wide base. The brown- or black-pigmented, flat or slightly elevated, nonhairy nevi are usually junctional nevi. The nonpigmented or pigmented, elevated, hairy nevi are more likely to be the intradermal nevi.

A nevus with a depigmented area surrounding it is called a *halo nevus, Sutton's nevus* or *leukoderma acquisitum centrifugum* (**Fig. 27-14**). The nevus in the center of the halo that histologically has an inflammatory infiltrate around it usually involutes in several months in contradistinction to the rarer noninflammatory halo nevus which may not involute. Excision of the halo nevus is usually not indicated unless the central nevus has the appearance of melanoma.

### Distribution

Nevi are very prevalent on the head and the neck but may be on any part of the body. The nevi on the palms, the soles, and the genitalia are usually junctional nevi.

### Course

A child is born with no, or relatively few, nevi, but with increasing age, particularly after puberty, nevi slowly become larger, can remain flat or become elevated, and may become hairy and darker. A change is also seen histologically with age. A junctional-type active nevus, although it may remain as such throughout the life of the person, more commonly changes slowly into an intradermal or resting nevus. Some nevi do not appear until adult or later life, but the precursor cells for the nevus were present at birth. A malignant melanoma can originate from a junctional nevus, compound

nevus, very rarely an intradermal nevus, and from dysplastic nevi, particularly in relationship to ultraviolet exposure. Most melanomas arise de novo. A benign junctional nevus in a child can histologically look like a malignant melanoma. Known as a *Spitz nevus (spindle cell nevus)*, this poses a difficult diagnostic and management problem. It is usually a dome-shaped reddish-brown tumor and rarely can occur in adults. It is histologically very difficult to distinguish from a melanoma. This a good to use a dermatopathologist as a first or second opinion and always consider a second opinion.

### Histogenesis

The origin of the nevus cell is disputed, but the most commonly accepted theory is that it originates from melanocytes.

### Differential Diagnosis

#### In Childhood

- *Warts:* Flat or common warts not on the hands or the feet may be difficult to differentiate clinically; should see warty growth with black "seeds" (the capillary loops), rather acute onset, and rapid growth (see Chapter 23)
- *Freckles:* On exposed areas of the body; many lesions; fade in winter; not raised
- *Blue nevus:* Flat or elevated, soft, dark bluish, steel-gray or black nodule
- *Granuloma pyogenicum:* Rapid onset of reddish or blackish vascular tumor, usually at the site of an injury and often with a history of bleeding
- *Molluscum contagiosum:* One, or usually more, crater-shaped, waxy tumors (see Chapter 23)
- *Urticaria pigmentosa:* Single, or multiple slightly elevated, yellowish to brown papules that urticate with trauma (Darier's sign) (see Chapter 41)

#### In Adulthood

- *Warts:* Usually rather obvious; black "seeds" (see Chapter 23).
- *Pedunculated fibromas:* On the neck and axillae (see Chapter 28)
- *Histiocytoma* (see Fig. 27-10): On the extremities; flat, button-like in consistency (see earlier in this chapter) that indents upon squeezing

Other epidermal and mesodermal tumors are differentiated histologically.

#### In Older Adults

- *Actinic or senile keratosis:* On exposed areas; scaly surrounding pink skin usually thin and dry; not a sharply demarcated lesion (see earlier in this chapter)
- *Seborrheic keratosis:* Greasy, waxy, warty tumor, "stuck on" the skin; white, brown or black dots (pseudohorned cysts); however, some are difficult to

differentiate clinically from nevus or malignant melanoma (see earlier in this chapter)

- *Lentigo:* Flat, tan or brown spot, usually on exposed skin surface, sometimes appears as a small splotchy, splash of flat black color (solar ink-spot lentigo)
- *Malignant melanoma:* Seen at the site of a junction nevus or can arise from skin that appears normal, shows a change in pigmentation either by spreading, becoming spotty, or turning darker; may bleed, form a crust, or ulcerate (see Chapter 29)
- *Basal cell and squamous cell carcinomas:* If there is any question of malignancy, a biopsy is indicated (see earlier in this chapter)

### Treatment

**Case Example 1:** A mother comes into your office with her 5-year-old son, who has an 8 × 8-mm flat, brown nevus on the forehead. She wants to know if this "mole" is dangerous and if it should be removed.

1. Examine the lesion carefully. This lesion shows no sign of recent growth or change in pigmentation. (If it did, it should be excised and examined histologically.)
2. Reassure the mother that this mole does not appear to be dangerous and that it would be unusual for it to become dangerous. If any change in the color or growth appears, the lesion should be examined again.
3. Tell the mother that it is best to leave the nevus alone at this time. The only treatment would be surgical excision, and you are quite sure that her boy would not sit still for this procedure unless he was given a general anesthetic. When the boy is 10 years of age or older, the lesion can be examined again and possibly removed at that time by a simpler method under local anesthesia.

**Case Example 2:** A 25-year-old woman desires a brown, raised, hairy nevus on her upper lip removed. There has been no recent change in the tumor.

1. Examine the lesion carefully for induration, scaling, ulceration, and bleeding. None of these signs are present. (If the diagnosis is not definite, a scissor biopsy may be performed safely and the base gently coagulated by electrosurgery or Monsel solution applied. Further treatment depends on the biopsy report.)
2. Tell the patient that you can perform a biopsy and remove the mole safely but that there will be a residual, very slightly depressed scar and that probably the hairs will have to be removed separately after the first surgery has healed.
3. Surgical excision with tissue examination is the best method of removal. However, hairy, raised, pigmented nevi have been removed by shave excision with biopsy for years with no proof that this form of removal has caused a malignant melanoma.

---

**SAUER'S NOTES**

### DO'S AND DONT'S REGARDING NEVI

1. Do not remove a nevus in a child by destructive methods. Remove only by surgical excision and submit nevus for histopathologic examination.
2. Do remember that in a child a benign junctional nevus may resemble a malignant melanoma histologically (Spitz nevus). Do not alarm the parents unnecessarily, because these nevi are no threat to life. A second pathology opinion can be helpful in equivocal cases.
3. Do not perform a radical deforming surgical procedure on a possible malignant melanoma until the biopsy report has been returned. Many of these tumors can turn out to be seborrheic keratoses, granuloma pyogenicum, and so on.

---

4. First, following local anesthesia, perform a shave biopsy. Then electrosurgery can be done with the coagulating or cutting current or with cautery or applying aluminum chloride or Monsel solution. The site should not be covered and will heal in 7 to 14 days, depending on the size. If the hairs regrow, they can be removed later by electrosurgical epilation or laser (see Chapter 6).

## Malignant Melanoma (see Chapter 29)

## Lymphomas (Table 27-6) (see Chapter 31)

## Complete Histologic Classification

A histologic classification of tumors of the skin is listed here. Those tumors discussed in the first part of this chapter are marked with an asterisk. The rarer tumors listed are defined or can be found in the Dictionary–Index. This classification is modified from Lever and Schaumberg–Lever (1997).

I. EPIDERMAL TUMORS
A. Tumors of the Surface Epidermis
 1. Benign tumors
  a. Linear epidermal nevus (Fig. 27-15): A rather common tumor usually present at birth, consisting of single or multiple lesions in various forms that give rise to several clinical designations, such as hard nevus, nevus verrucous, nevus unius lateris, and, when systematized (more generalized), ichthyosis hystrix. No nevus cells are present but there is verrucous overgrowth of epidermal tissue. There is epidermal nevus syndrome with multiple underlying abnormalities.
  *b. Seborrheic keratosis and dermatosis papulosa nigra
  *c. Fibroma

**TABLE 27-6 ■ WHO-EORTC classification**

Cutaneous T-cell lymphoma

  Indolent clinical behavior

    Mycosis fungoides

    Folliculotropic MF

    Pagetoid reticulosis

    Granulomatous slack skin

    Primary cutaneous anaplastic large cell lymphoma

    Lymphomatoid papulosis

    Subcutaneous panniculitis-like T-cell lymphoma

    Primary cutaneous CD4+ small/medium pleomorphic T-cell lymphoma

  Aggressive clinical behavior

    Sézary syndrome

    Primary cutaneous NK/T-cell lymphoma, nasal-type

    Primary cutaneous aggressive CD8+ T-cell lymphoma

    Primary cutaneous/T-cell lymphoma

    Primary cutaneous peripheral T-cell lymphoma, unspecified

Cutaneous B-cell lymphoma

  Indolent clinical behavior

    Primary cutaneous marginal zone B-cell lymphoma

    Primary cutaneous follicle center lymphoma

  Intermediate clinical behavior

    Primary cutaneous diffuse large B-cell lymphoma, leg type

    Primary cutaneous diffuse large B-cell lymphoma, other

    Primary cutaneous intravascular large B-cell lymphoma

*Source:* This research was originally published in *Blood*. Willemze R et al. WHO-EORTC classification for cutaneous lymphomas. *Blood*. 2005;105(10):3768–85.

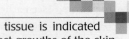

**SAUER'S NOTES**

A histologic examination of tissue is indicated for a definite diagnosis of most growths of the skin.

    d. Cysts
      *(1) Epidermal cyst
      *(2) Trichilemmal, pilar, or sebaceous cyst
      (3) Steatocystoma multiplex: A dominantly inherited condition with small, moderately firm, cystic nodules adherent to the overlying skin, which on incision yield an oily fluid.
      *(4) Milium
      *(5) Dermoid cyst
      *(6) Mucous retention cyst
    e. Clear cell acanthoma: A rare, usually single, slightly elevated, flat, pale red, scaling nodule less than 2 cm in diameter, nearly always located on the lower extremities.
    f. Warty dyskeratoma: A solitary warty lesion with a central keratotic plug, most commonly seen on the scalp, face, and neck. Histology is characteristic.
    g. Keratoacanthoma (see Chapter 28)

2. Precancerous tumors
  *a. Senile or actinic keratosis and cutaneous horn
  *b. Arsenical keratosis
  *c. Leukoplakia

3. Epiheliomas and carcinomas
  a. Basal cell cancer (see Chapter 28)
  b. Squamous cell cancer (see Chapter 28)
  c. Bowen's disease and erythroplasia of Queyrat: Bowen's disease is a single red scaly lesion with a sharp but irregular border that grows slowly by peripheral extension. Histologically, it is an intraepidermal squamous cell carcinoma (Fig. 27-16). Erythroplasia of Queyrat represents Bowen's disease of the mucous membranes and occurs on the glans penis and rarely on the vulva. The lesion has a bright red, velvety surface.

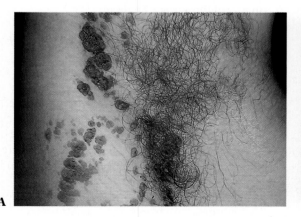
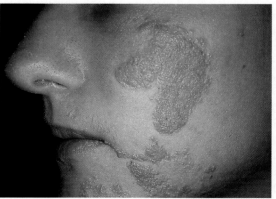

FIGURE 27-15 ■ (A) Linear epidermal nevus in the axilla. (B) Nevus unius lateris of the face. *(Courtesy of Owen/Galderma.)*

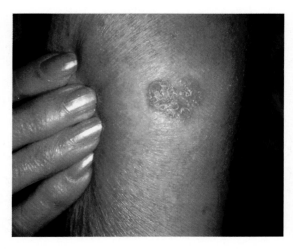

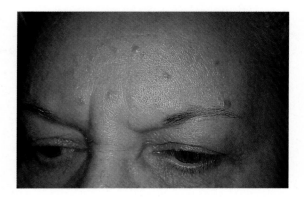

FIGURE 27-18 ■ Sebaceous gland hyperplasia (common).

FIGURE 27-16 ■ Bowen's disease, on the arm. *(Courtesy of Syntex Laboratories, Inc.)*

d. Paget's disease: A unilateral scaly red lesion resembling dermatitis, usually present on the female nipple, but the lesion can be extramammary. The early lesion on the nipple is an intraductal carcinoma that also involves the mammary ducts and deeper connective tissue. In the perirectal area, it can be associated with underlying bowel cancer.

B. Tumors of the Epidermal Appendages
  1. Nevoid tumors
    a. Organic nevi or hamartomas
      (1) Sebaceous nevi
        (a) Nevus sebaceous (Jadassohn) (Fig. 27-17): Seen on the scalp or face as a single lesion present from birth, slightly raised, firm, hairless, yellowish, with furrowed surface. Large examples may be associated with a "neurocutaneous syndrome" of epilepsy and mental retardation. Basal cell and squamous cell carcinomas can develop within these growths in approximately 10% of cases.

      (b) Adenoma sebaceum (Pringle's disease): Part of a triad of epilepsy, mental deficiency, and the skin lesions of adenoma sebaceum. This is called *tuberous sclerosis*. The skin lesions occur on the face and consist of yellowish brown, papular, nodular lesions with telangiectasias. Histopathology shows an angiofibroma (see Chapter 38).
      (c) Sebaceous hyperplasia (Fig. 27-18): Very common on the face in older persons and consists of one or several small, yellowish, translucent, slightly umbilicated nodules. It may be the most common tumor to be confused clinically with a basal cell cancer.
      (d) Fordyce's disease (see Chapter 34): A rather common condition of pinpoint-sized yellowish lesions of the vermilion border of the lips or the oral mucosa that represent ectopic sebaceous glands.
    b. Adenomas or organoid hamartomas
      (1) Sebaceous adenoma: A very rare solitary tumor of the face or the scalp, smooth, firm, elevated, often slightly pedunculated, and measuring less than 1 cm in diameter; may be associated with

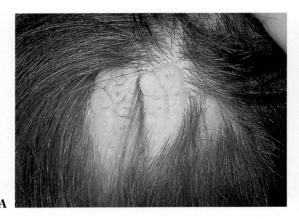

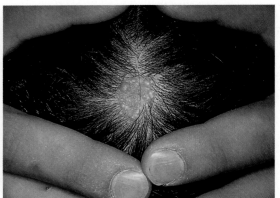

FIGURE 27-17 ■ **(A)** Nevus sebaceous of Jadassohn on the scalp. **(B)** Nevus sebaceous on the scalp. *(Courtesy of Owen/Galderma.)*

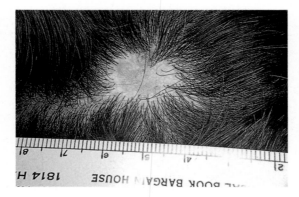

FIGURE 27-19 ■ Syringocystadenoma papilliferum. (*Courtesy of Owen/Galderma.*)

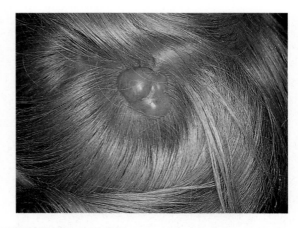

FIGURE 27-20 ■ Cylindroma of the scalp.

an adenocarcinoma of the bowel (Muir–Torre syndrome).

(2) Apocrine adenomas

(a) Syringocystadenoma papilliferum (Fig. 27-19): This adenoma of the apocrine ducts appears as a single verrucous plaque, usually seen on the scalp. Basal cell epitheliomatous change occasionally does occur and may arise in sebaceous nevi.

(b) Hidradenoma papilliferum: This adenoma of the apocrine glands occurs almost exclusively on the labia majora and the perineum of women as a single, intracutaneous, benign tumor covered by normal epidermis.

(3) Eccrine syringofibroadenoma (ESFA): Solitary or multiple nodules with the following subtypes:

(a) Solitary ESFA.

(b) Multiple ESFAs with hidrotic ectodermal dysplasia.

(c) Multiple ESFA.

(d) Nonfamilial linear ESFA.

(e) Reactive ESFA associated with inflammatory or neoplastic dermatoses usually seen on the lower extremities and easily confused with squamous cell carcinoma.

c. Benign epitheliomas or suborganoid hamartomas

(1) Apocrine epitheliomas

(a) Syringoma: This is characterized by the appearance of pinhead-sized soft, yellowish nodules at the age of puberty in women, developing around the eyelids, the chest, the abdomen, and the anterior aspects of the thighs.

(b) Cylindroma (Fig. 27-20): These appear as numerous smooth, rounded tumors of various sizes on the scalp in adults and resemble bunches of grapes or tomatoes. These tumors may cover the entire scalp like a turban and are then referred to as *turban*

*tumors.* It can be multiple and autosomal dominant with associated trichoepitheliomas and eccrine spiradenomas.

(2) Hair epitheliomas

(a) Trichoepithelioma (Fig. 27-21): Also known as epithelioma adenoides cysticum and multiple benign cystic epithelioma when multiple. This begins at the age of puberty, frequently on a hereditary basis, and is characterized by the presence of numerous pinhead- to pea-sized, rounded, yellowish or pink nodules on the face and occasionally on the upper trunk. This may also appear as a single lesion that can be confused with a basal cell cancer histologically.

(b) Calcifying epithelioma of Malherbe (Fig. 27-22) or pilomatrixoma: Hand, nodular, nondescript 0.5 to 1.0 cm tumors especially on the scalp and face. Malignant degeneration is very rare. There is a perforating form.

(c) Microcystic adnexal carcinoma: Relatively rare often extensive and invasive with perineural invasion. Up to 25% misdiagnosed

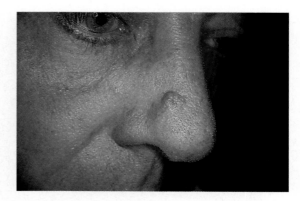

FIGURE 27-21 ■ Trichoepithelioma on the nose. (*Courtesy of Owen/Galderma.*)

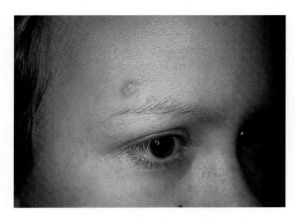

**FIGURE 27-22** ■ Rarer tumors of the skin. Calcifying epithelioma of Malherbe on the forehead. *(Courtesy of Owen/Galderma.)*

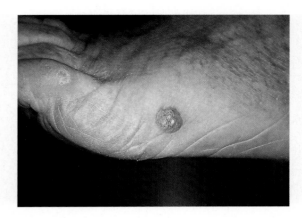

**FIGURE 27-24** ■ Eccrine poroma on the foot.

on initial biopsy. Slow growing and 5- to 10-year follow-up needed. Mohs, surgery may be the best therapy.

   (3) Eccrine epitheliomas

     (a) Eccrine spiradenoma (Fig. 27-23): A rare, usually solitary, intradermal, firm, tender nodule.

     (b) Clear cell hidradenoma: A rare, well-circumscribed, often encapsulated tumor of dermis and subcutaneous tissue.

     (c) Eccrine poroma (Fig. 27-24): This occurs as an asymptomatic solitary tumor on the soles and the palms. There is a rare malignant eccrine poroma.

**2.** Carcinomas of sebaceous glands and eccrine and apocrine sweat glands (rare)

C. Metastatic Carcinoma of the Skin

This occurs frequently from carcinoma of the breast and melanoma but rarely from other internal carcinomas. Metastatic carcinoid nodules may appear in the skin, as well as in lymph nodes and the liver. The primary tumor and the metastases produce excess 5-hydroxytryptamine (serotonin), which in turn produces attacks of flushing of the skin.

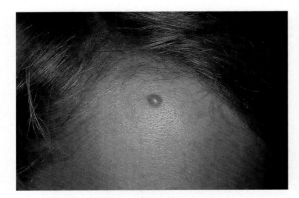

**FIGURE 27-23** ■ Eccrine spiradenoma of the forehead.

## II. MESODERMAL TUMORS

A. Tumors of Fibrous Tissue

   *1. Histiocytoma and dermatofibroma

   *2. Keloid

   *3. Fibrosarcomas

     a. True fibrosarcoma: A rare tumor that starts most commonly in the subcutaneous fat, grows rapidly, causes the overlying skin to appear purplish, and finally ulcerates.

     b. Dermatofibrosarcoma protuberans: A tumor that grows slowly in the corium and spreads by the development of adjoining reddish or bluish nodules that may coalesce to form a plaque that can eventually ulcerate. Margins are very difficult to evaluate making recurrence common. Mohs' surgery and positive CD34 immunohistochemical staining are helpful.

B. Tumors of Mucoid Tissue

   1. Myxoma: Clinically seen as fairly well circumscribed, rather soft intracutaneous tumors with normal overlying epidermis.

   2. Myxosarcoma: Subcutaneous tumors that eventually ulcerate the skin.

   3. Synovial cyst of the skin.

C. Tumors of Fatty Tissue

   1. Nevus lipomatosus superficialis: A rare, circumscribed nodular lesion, usually in the gluteal area.

   2. Lipoma: A rather common tumor that can be multiple or single, lobulated, of varying size, and in the subcutaneous tissue.

   3. Hibernoma: A form of lipoma composed of embryonic type of fat cells.

   4. Liposarcoma.

   5. Malignant hibernoma.

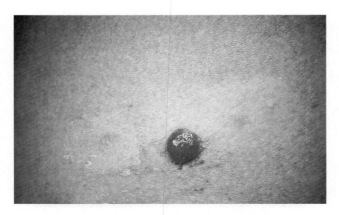

**FIGURE 27-25** ■ Pyogenic granuloma of 0.75 cm size on the back. *(Courtesy of Syntex Laboratories, Inc.)*

D. Tumors of Nerve Tissue and Mesodermal Nerve Sheath Cells
1. Neuroma: Rare, single, or multiple small reddish or brown nodules that are usually tender as well as painful.
2. Neurofibroma: Benign flesh-colored soft tumor that is frequently single, but when multiple it is associated with neurofibromatosis; when very large it is called a plexiform neuroma. Can have sarcomatous degeneration.
3. Neurofibromatosis: Also known as von Recklinghausen's disease, this hereditary disease classically consists of pigmented patches (café-au-lait spots), pedunculated skin tumors, and nerve tumors. All of these lesions may not be present in a particular case.
4. Neurilemoma.
5. Granular cell schwannoma (granular cell tumor) or myoblastoma: From neural sheath cells, this appears usually as a solitary tumor of the tongue, the skin, or the subcutaneous tissue. Also, multiple, nodular, or plaque-like.
6. Malignant granular cell schwannoma or myoblastoma.

E. Tumors of Vascular Tissue
*1. Hemangioma: See Chapter 30.
2. Granuloma pyogenicum (Fig. 27-25): This is a rather common (especially in pregnancy on the gums) end result of an injury to the skin that may or may not have been apparent. Vascular proliferation, with or without infection, produces a small red tumor that bleeds easily. It is to be differentiated from a malignant melanoma. Biopsy and mild electrocoagulation are curative.
3. Osler's disease: See Rendu–Osler–Weber disease in the Dictionary–Index.
4. Lymphangioma: A superficial form, lymphangioma circumscriptum, appears as a group of thin-walled vesicles on the skin surface, whereas the deeper variety, lymphangioma cavernosum, causes a poorly defined enlargement of the affected area, such as the lip or the tongue. Large lymphatic cisternae may underlie apparently superficial tumors.
5. Glomus tumor: A rather unusual small, deep-seated, red or purplish nodule that is tender and may produce severe paroxysmal pains. The solitary lesion is usually seen under a nail plate, on the fingertips, or elsewhere on the body and may erode underlying bone.
6. Hemangiopericytoma.
7. Kaposi's sarcoma (multiple idiopathic hemorrhagic sarcoma) (Fig. 27-26: Kaposi's sarcoma-associated herpes virus [HHV-8] is associated with all forms): Most commonly seen on the feet and the ankles as multiple bluish-red or dark brown nodules and plaques associated with visceral lesions. It is most prevalent in elderly men of Mediterranean or Jewish origin. Sarcomatous malignant degeneration can occur.
   a. Kaposi's sarcoma (KS) is also seen as part of the acquired immunodeficiency syndrome (see Chapter 24). In this complex, the sarcoma lesions are small, oval, red, or pink papules that occur on any area of the body. If HIV is not treated aggressively then KS can rapidly grow into tumors, spreading internally (especially to the gastrointestinal tract) and become fatal from bleeding or general debility.
   b. There is an endemic African form often associated with reticuloendothelial cancer.
   c. An immunosuppressive drug related form often seen in transplant patients that may dissipate after immunosuppression is decreased.

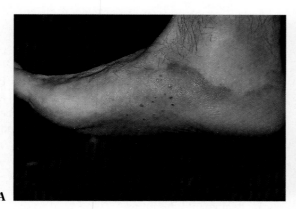
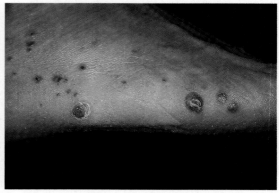

**A**    **B**

**FIGURE 27-26** ■ **(A)** Kaposi's sarcoma of the foot. **(B)** Kaposi's sarcoma of the foot. *(Courtesy of Owen/Galderma.)*

8. Hemangioendothelioma.
9. Postmastectomy lymphangiosarcoma (Stewart–Treves syndrome).
10. Glomangiomas: Large dilated vessels lined with glomus cells as in a glomus tumor but are larger tumors that mimic large venous malformations clinically. Considered by some authors better termed glomuvenous malformations to indicate they are not true tumors. The rare congenital plaque-type is extensively distributed, difficult to diagnose and progressive. Deep blue or purple, poorly compressible and usually on the face. They can be large, disfiguring, inherited in an autosomal dominant manner.

F. Tumors of Muscular Tissue
1. Leiomyoma: Solitary leiomyomas may be found on the extremities and on the scrotum, whereas multiple leiomyomas can occur on the back and elsewhere as pinhead- to pea-sized, brown or bluish, firm, elevated nodules. Both forms are painful and sensitive to pressure, particularly as they enlarge. They may have a butterfly shape.
2. Leiomyosarcoma: Very rare.
3. Multiple leiomyomas may be associated with uterine leiomyomas and renal cancer as a familial syndrome.

G. Tumors of Osseous Tissue
1. Osteoma cutis
   a. Primary: The primary form of osteoma cutis develops from embryonal cell rests; these may be single or multiple.
   b. Secondary: Secondary bone formation may occur as a form of tissue degeneration in tumors, in scar tissue (such as acne), in scleroderma lesions (see CREST syndrome), and in various granulomas.

H. Tumors of Cartilaginous Tissue
1. Nodular chondrodermatitis of the ear: A painful, benign, hyperkeratotic nodule, usually on the inner rim of the helix of the ear of elderly men. Trauma may be the inciting cause. Often awakens the patient at night when pressure is applied. Can be treated by excision or sometimes with intralesional corticosteroids.

III. NEVUS CELL TUMORS

A. Melanocytic Nevi
   *1. Junctional (active) nevus
   *2. Intradermal (resting) nevus
   *3. Dysplastic nevus syndrome
   4. Lentigines: These are to be differentiated from freckles (ephelides). A freckle histologically shows hyperpigmentation of the basal layer but no elongation of the rete pegs and no increase in the number of clear cells and dendritic cells. Juvenile lentigines (lentigo simplex) begin to appear in childhood and occur on all parts of the body. Senile lentigines, (solar lentigo)

also known as "liver spots," occur in elderly persons on the dorsa of the hands, the forearms, and the face and are related to sun exposure. Solar ink-spot lentigo is commonly seen on sun-exposed areas and has a characteristic black, splotchy, reticulated pattern. Lentigo maligna melanoma (Hutchinson's Freckle) is a dark brown or black macular, malignant lesion, usually on the face or arms of elderly persons that has a slow peripheral growth (see Chapter 29). Lentigines can be caused by ionizing radiation, a tanning bed, a sunlamp, PUVA therapy, and, most commonly, from sun exposure.

5. Mongolian spots: These are seen chiefly in Asian or African-American infants, usually around the buttocks. They disappear spontaneously during childhood. Related bluish patchy lesions are the nevus of Ota, seen on the side of the face (may have scleral pigment), and the nevus of Ito, located in the supraclavicular, scapular, and deltoid regions. Laser therapy may be beneficial.
*6. Blue nevus: Clinically, the blue nevus appears as a slate blue or bluish black, sharply circumscribed, flat or slightly elevated nodule, occurring on any area of the body. It originates from mesodermal cells. The common blue nevus is always benign. Cellular blue nevus is larger, especially on buttocks and can degenerate into malignant melanoma.

*B. Malignant Melanoma

IV. LYMPHOMAS (see Chapter 31)

A. Monomorphous Group
1. The non-Hodgkin's lymphomas are referred to as monomorphous lymphomas because, in contrast to Hodgkin's disease, they lack a significant admixture of inflammatory cells and are composed almost entirely of lymphoma cells largely derived from B or T lymphocytes.
2. Lymphomas may have specific skin lesions containing the lymphomatous infiltrate, or nonspecific lesions may be seen. These latter consist of macules, papules, tumors, purpuric lesions, blisters, eczematous lesions, exfoliative dermatitis, and secondarily infected excoriations.

**SAUER'S NOTES**

Sun tanning salons should be strongly discouraged. They are associated with increased risk of malignant melanoma, squamous cell cancer, and basal cell cancer. All aspects of photoaging are increased. Lupus erythematosus, various porphyrias, photo drug reactions, dermatomyositis, actinic keratoses, and solar urticaria are all caused by or worsened by sun tanning salon usage. The false tan or immediate pigment darkening of high-dose UVA given by most sun tanning salons does not protect from future sun burning as the sun-induced tan does.

B. Polymorphous Group
   1. Hodgkin's disease: Specific lesions are very rare, but nonspecific dermatoses are commonly seen.
   2. Mycosis fungoides
      a. Sézary's syndrome: This is a very rare form of exfoliative dermatitis (see Chapter 19) that occurs at an early leukemic stage of a CTCL. It is diagnosed by finding unusually large monocytoid cells (so-called Sézary cells) in the blood and in the skin. This cell is indistinguishable from the mycosis cell, both of which are derived from the T cell.

## V. Myelosis

A. Leukemia: Refers to circulating abnormal blood cells; may be seen along with lymphomas, but in skin almost always associated with myelosis, such as myeloid leukemia. Cutaneous lesions are quite uncommon but may be specific or nonspecific.

## VI. Pseudolymphoma Of Spiegler–Fendt

A benign, localized erythematous, nodular dermatosis usually on the face, with clinical and histologic features that make a distinction from lymphoma difficult. Some cases may eventually be diagnosed as a lymphoma.

## Suggested Reading

Barnhill RL. *Color Atlas and Synopsis of Pigmented Lesions*. New York: McGraw-Hill; 1995.

Drake LA, Ceilley RI, Cornelison RL, et al. Guidelines of care for actinic keratoses. *J Am Acad Dermatol*. 1995;32(1):95–98.

Drake LA, Ceilley RI, Cornelison RL, et al. Guidelines of care for nevi: II. Nonmelanocytic nevi, hamartomas, neoplasms, and potentially malignant lesions. *J Am Acad Dermatol*. 1995;32(1):104–108.

Drake LA, Salasche S, Ceilley RI, et al. Guidelines of care for cutaneous squamous cell carcinoma. *J Am Acad Dermatol*. 1993;28:628–631.

Lever WF, Schaumburg-Lever G. *Histopathology of the Skin*. 8th ed. Philadelphia, PA: JB Lippincott; 1997.

# CHAPTER 28

# Non-Melanoma Skin Cancer

*Victor J. Marks, MD and Nathan W. Hanson, MD*

## Background and Epidemiology

The term "non-melanoma skin cancer" (NMSC) refers to the types of skin cancers that are not melanomas and are grouped together because they tend to present and behave differently than melanomas. Generally speaking, this term also refers to two very common skin malignancies, basal cell carcinoma (BCC) and squamous cell carcinoma (SCC), which are derived from keratinocytes, the cells that make up the epidermal layer of the skin. BCC is the most common malignancy in mankind, representing about 7 out of 10 diagnosed skin cancers. SCC, the second most common skin malignancy, represents about 2 out of 10 newly diagnosed skin cancers. It is estimated that over 1 million new cases of non-melanoma cancer will be diagnosed in 2008 and that one in five or six Americans will develop skin cancer during their lifetime. Of particular concern is the alarming increase in NMSC cases in young adults, with a very significant increase in the age group from 20 to 40 years. Other rare skin cancers, such as Merkel cell carcinoma, adnexal tumors, some sarcomas, and others, fall into the heading of non-melanoma skin cancers, but will not be individually addressed in this chapter.

## Basal Cell Carcinoma

### Clinical

BCC generally presents quite innocuously as a red papule or small crusted area that tends to bleed and not heal. Most BCCs occur on sun-exposed areas, most commonly on the head and neck, but they may develop on any skin surface, including the extremities, trunk (particularly superficial BCC), genitalia, perineum, and around surgically created stomas. Often, they are mistaken by the patient for a nonhealing

acneiform papule or other benign entity, and they may develop a crusted appearance due to the friable and easily traumatized tissue associated with BCCs. Given their slow growth, it may be months before a patient seeks attention for the area of concern.

Clinically and histologically, there are many different variants of BCC that range from fairly slow growing and well-circumscribed nodular BCCs and superficial BCCs to relatively aggressive and clinically ill-defined variants known as morphea-form or sclerosing BCC. Other aggressive variants include infiltrative and micronodular BCC, which are mostly recognized by their histologic appearance. Nodular BCCs have a shiny, pearly appearance, and sometimes they have superficial blood vessels, called telangiectasias, running over their surface (Figs. 28-1 to 28-4). Some nodular BCCs are referred to as "rodent ulcers" due to the ragged central ulcer–like a rodent bite–within the nodule with smooth elevated borders. It is important to note that even small nodular BCCs often have a tiny central hemorrhagic crust. A sore that won't heal or a bleeding point recurring at the same site should alert the physician to the possibility of an underlying BCC even in the absence of classic morphology. Superficial BCCs have scaly, red, sometimes shiny appearances that are commonly mistaken for plaques of eczema and psoriasis. They are eventually recognized as BCCs due to their lack of response to treatment (Figs. 28-5 and 28-6). Morphea-form or sclerosing subtypes have clinical similarity to scars or scar-

> ### SAUER'S NOTES
> 1. Sun protection measures are the mainstay of prevention.
> 2. Early and sometimes repeated skin biopsies are the mainstay of diagnosis. If it is worth removing, then it is worth a biopsy.
> 3. Follow-up visits are the mainstay of adequate discovery and therapy for recurrences.

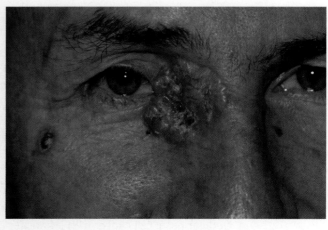

**FIGURE 28-1** ■ Basal cell cancer with telangiectasias and a pearly edge.

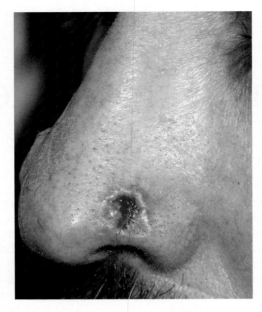

FIGURE 28-2 ■ Basal cell cancer with a central hemorrhagic crust.

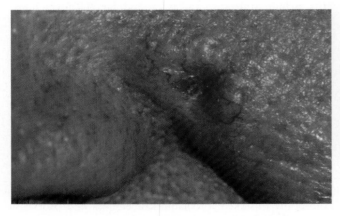

FIGURE 28-3 ■ Basal cell cancer at the nasolabial border with a central dell and translucent edge (often seen better with stretching of the skin) and telangiectasias.

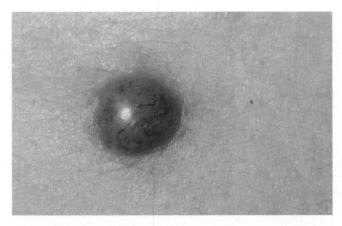

FIGURE 28-4 ■ Nodular basal cell cancer with a translucent, telangiectatic, domed appearance. It mimics an intradermal nevus.

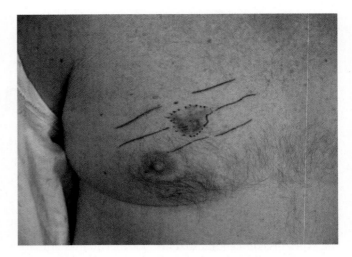

FIGURE 28-5 ■ Superficial basal cell cancer mimicking a dermatitis.

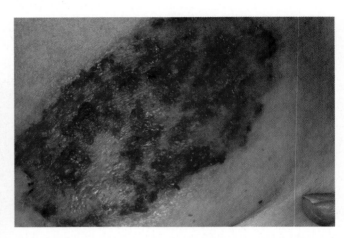

FIGURE 28-6 ■ Large eroded basal cell cancer with a thin pearly edge.

like plaques and have a tendency to grow rapidly and subtly and can, along with other aggressive subtypes, demonstrate perineural invasion histologically.

Although BCCs very rarely metastasize, and generally only in the setting of long-neglected tumors, they can be locally very destructive, invading neighboring skin, cartilage, bone, and other nearby structures (Figs. 28-7 to 28-10). The clinical differential diagnosis of BCC includes SCC, melanoma (especially when presented with pigmented variants of BCC or amelanotic melanomas), adnexal or follicular neoplasms, benign fibrous growths, scars, and other lesions.

## Pathogenesis

Unequivocally, ultraviolet (UV) radiation plays a significant and primary role in inducing BCCs. Those at most risk for development of BCC are patients with a history of chronic sun exposure, light-colored eyes, fair skin that burns easily and tans poorly, and light-colored hair. Darkly pigmented individuals develop BCC much less commonly. The most common site of presentation of BCC is on the head and

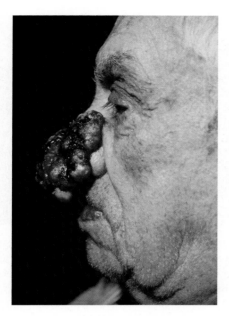

FIGURE 28-7 ▦ Large neglected basal cell cancer that mimics rhinophyma.

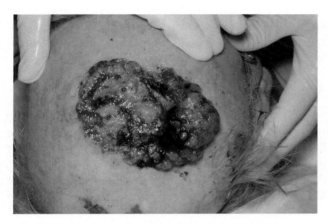

FIGURE 28-8 ▦ A neglected exophytic scalp basal cell cancer.

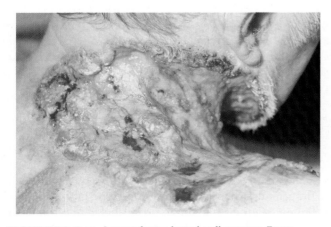

FIGURE 28-9 ▦ A very large basal cell cancer. Even though metastasis of these tumors is very uncommon, the size of this tumor would necessitate a consideration of metastatic disease.

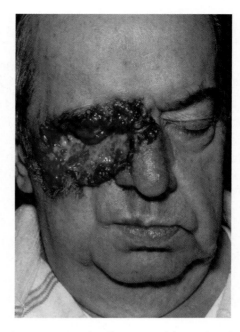

FIGURE 28-10 ▦ Basal cell cancer with eye involvement. Radiation therapy might be considered as palliative or potentially curative therapy.

neck, which are areas of the body that acquire the most exposure to UV light over an individual's lifetime. However, as noted previously, BCC may occur on any skin surface, even those with minimal sun exposure.

Two genodermatoses further confirm the primary role of UV light in BCC pathogenesis. Patients with a rare autosomal recessive genetic skin disorder known as xeroderma pigmentosum exhibit exquisite sensitivity to UV light and are over 1,000 times more likely than the general population to develop BCC and other skin cancers. These patients lack the enzymatic ability to repair DNA damage that occurs as a direct result of UV light. Their risk is significantly decreased if they practice vigilant sun protection, beginning in infancy and continuing throughout their lifetimes. The other group of patients have the autosomal dominant condition nevoid basal cell carcinoma syndrome. They have an allelic defect in a tumor suppressor gene, *PTCH*. They develop numerous BCCs in sun-exposed skin as their second, normal allele for the *PTCH* gene is damaged by UV light. Immunosuppression, regardless of the cause, seems to play a minor role in the development of BCC, but immunocompromised patients do carry a slightly increased risk for the development of BCC.

Other risk factors for the development of BCC include a history of x-ray exposure, either clinical or industrial, and other rare, inherited genetic disorders that predispose to the development of BCC specifically.

## Treatment

Treatment for BCC depends a great deal on the histologic subtype, size, and location of the tumor. A variety of modalities have been described, including, but not limited

**TABLE 28-1 ■ 5-Year Cure Rates for BCC with Various Treatment Modalities**

| Technique | Primary BCC, Percentage | Recurrent BCC, Percentage |
|---|---|---|
| MMS | 99.0 | 94.4 |
| Surgical excision | 89.9 | 82.6 |
| Radiotherapy | 91.3 | 90.2 |
| Cryosurgery | 92.5 | 87.0 |
| Electrodessication and curettage | 92.3 | 60.0 |

**TABLE 28-2 ■ Mohs Surgery 5-year Cure Rates for BCC and SCC**

| | |
|---|---|
| Primary BCC | 99% |
| Recurrent BCC | 94%–96% |
| Primary SCC | 97% |
| Recurrent SCC | 90% |

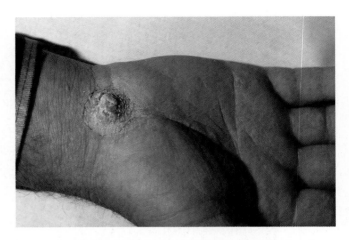

**FIGURE 28-11 ■** Squamous cell cancer on the palm that is quite symmetric indicating it may be of the keratoacanthoma type, especially if it grew quickly over weeks to months. Keratoacanthomas seldom metastasize.

to, excision, electrodessication and curettage, radiation therapy, cryosurgery, Mohs micrographic surgery (MMS), and topical therapies. The most reliable method is MMS because this modality offers complete histologic examination of the tumor margins, assuring 5-year cure rates of 99% for primary tumors (Tables 28-1 and 28-2), while sparing most of the normal tissue. This modality is often used for aggressive histologic subtypes, tumors in cosmetically sensitive areas such as the face, recurrent BCCs, large tumors, and tumors arising in irradiated skin. Other treatment regimens have varying 5-year cure rates, ranging from 70% to 80% for some topical therapies to 80% to 90% for curettage and excision. Regardless of the treatment, it is important to monitor the patient appropriately for recurrence.

## Prevention

BCC represents a UV light–induced malignancy, and as such, the most effective means of preventing BCC involves limiting sun exposure. Health care workers have an important role in educating the public about the role of UV light in skin cancer development and methods for sun protection and UV light avoidance. Appropriate use of broad-spectrum UVA and UVB sunscreen and sunblock will significantly reduce one's risk for development of BCC. Additionally, it is important to educate patients about wearing broad-brimmed hats and long-sleeved clothing, as well as avoiding the peak hours of UV transmissibility (~10:00 AM to 4:00 PM). Wearing light-colored, tightly woven, cotton blend, protective clothing provides a sun protective factor (SPF) range of 20 to 40, whereas an unblended, summer-weight, cotton shirt provides an SPF range of 6 to 10 and a wet t-shirt an SPF of only 3.

Epidemiologic studies have also demonstrated a direct correlation between the use of UV light tanning beds, regardless of wavelength, and the increased incidence of BCC. Young patients particularly benefit from early education and intervention because the damaging effect of cumulative UV exposure may not be evident for many years.

## Squamous Cell Carcinoma

SCC, on the other hand, is often a more rapidly growing malignancy. It generally starts as a scaly papule that can become indurated and "heaped up" with mounds of scale on its surface (Fig. 28-11). SCCs may or may not bleed, depending on the clinical nature of the lesion, but in the authors' opinion, they do not bleed as readily as equally sized BCCs. In general, "squames make squame"or, in other words, they produce scale while BCCs make crust from ulceration and bleeding.

The clinical appearance and location of these tumors varies based on etiology. Many SCCs arise from premalignant lesions, known as actinic keratoses, that clinically appear as red, scaly patches or papules on sun-exposed skin. Induration to the base of such precursor lesions often signals malignant degeneration. Some SCCs have the clinical appearance of a volcanolike lesion, with a central crater and sharply demarcated edges (Figs. 28-12 and 28-13). Bowen's disease or SCC in situ deserves special mention. It presents as a flat pink to red, often scaling plaque resembling eczema, psoriasis, or superficial BCC (Figs. 28-14 and 28-15) and can occur on sun-exposed or non–sun-exposed skin. SCC and SCC in situ on non–sun-exposed sites such as the genitalia can become quite impressive in size and distribution. Many genital tumors are related to infection with human papilloma virus (HPV), particularly types 16 and 18 (Fig. 28-16). Immunosuppressed patients are at particular risk for developing SCCs. Both UV light and viral infection are cofactors in the development of SCC in such patients,

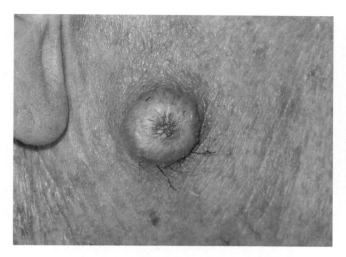

**FIGURE 28-12** ■ Preauricular squamous cell cancer, most likely of the keratoacanthoma type considering the marked symmetry of the lesion.

and tumors can number in the hundreds. Verrucous carcinoma, a type of well-differentiated SCC, clinically has a warty appearance and can be related to more common genital wart subtypes such as HPV-6 and HPV-11. It can occur in many locations but is most frequently described on the foot, hand, and genitalia. SCC sometimes occurs in areas of chronic scarring, such as burn scars, and in scarring skin diseases such as lichen sclerosus, epidermolysis bullosa, and chronic cutaneous lupus. Such "scar carcinomas" can be more aggressive than other variants of SCC and have a higher risk of metastasis.

Again, while SCCs usually occur in sun-exposed areas of the head, neck, ears, lips, and extremities, they can occur

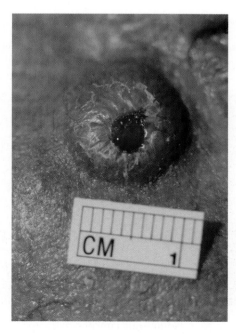

**FIGURE 28-13** ■ Squamous cell cancer with eye involvement.

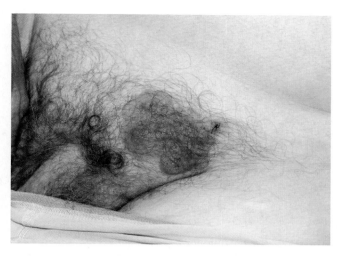

**FIGURE 28-14** ■ Squamous cell cancer in the groin that may well have begun as Bowen's disease. Dermatitis and extramammary Paget's disease, and condyloma acuminata are also diagnostic considerations.

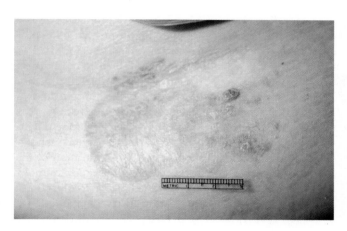

**FIGURE 28-15** ■ Superficial squamous cell cancer.

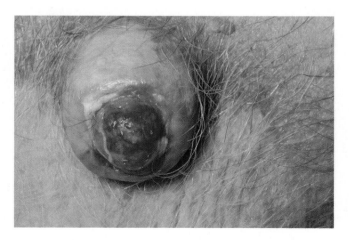

**FIGURE 28-16** ■ Squamous cell cancer of the penis. Condyloma acuminata of Lowenstein and Buschke (a human papilloma–induced neoplasm) may have preceded this malignancy considering its location.

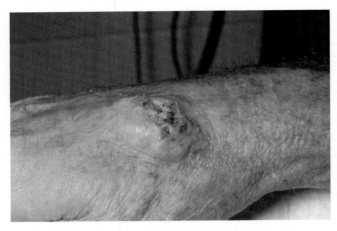

FIGURE 28-17 ■ Squamous cell cancer on the dorsal wrist. Excision with adequate margins is the treatment of choice. Up to 4% of these can metastasize, and lymph nodes of the upper extremity and axilla need careful palpation to see whether a nodal biopsy needs to be done.

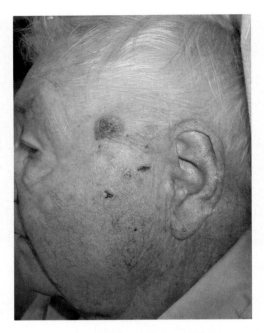

FIGURE 28-19 ■ Large flat squamous cell cancer on a sun-exposed area. History of radiation damage from acne therapy as a teenager is a historical fact of importance. Thyroid cancer is also more common in patients who have had x-ray therapy for acne.

in any location (Figs. 28-17 and 28-18). Histologically, SCCs can be quite variable as well, ranging from well-differentiated lesions that are well circumscribed and localized to those that are poorly differentiated, ill-defined, and deeply invasive. The occasional tumor requires special histopathologic staining to identify it as SCC or of keratinocyte derivation. Such poorly differentiated, highly aggressive SCCs may demonstrate unusual growth patterns such as perineural involvement. The risks of postsurgical recurrence and metastasis are higher in such tumors (Fig. 28-19). Location of the primary tumor can also affect metastatic risk. For example, lip, ear, and scalp SCCs are considered higher risk locations, and tumors arising in these locations carry a metastatic risk of 10% to 20% (Figs. 28-20 to 28-22). Tumor duration may

also affect metastatic risk. Long-standing, neglected SCC, regardless of the site, may metastasize. Metastasis usually occurs first to the regional lymph node basin, but SCC can metastasize to the lungs and other visceral organs. High-risk SCC (i.e., those that are large, neglected, poorly differentiated, neurotropic, or in higher risk anatomic sites) requires prompt attention.

## Pathogenesis

Similar to BCC, SCC is unequivocally linked pathogenically to UV light exposure. UV light induces covalent bonding

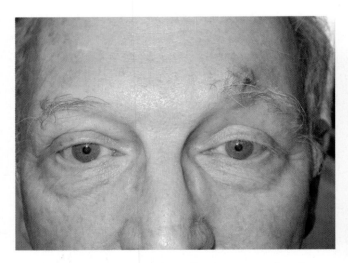

FIGURE 28-18 ■ Squamous cell cancer on a chronic sun-exposed site. Only a biopsy can distinguish a benign tumor from a basal cell cancer. Squamous cell cancers often have a nonspecific clinical appearance.

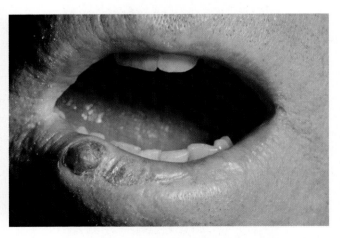

FIGURE 28-20 ■ Squamous cancer on the lip. This can be associated with tobacco abuse, alcohol abuse, and especially chronic sun exposure.

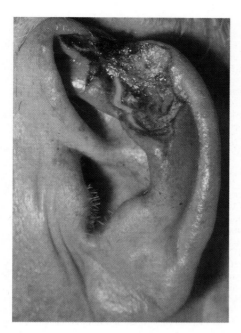

**FIGURE 28-21** ■ Squamous cell cancer with destruction of the ear making a benign diagnosis unlikely.

between nucleotide bases, called pyrimidine dimers, resulting in the loss of the function of tumor suppressing genes. Such genetic alterations have been demonstrated in chronically sun-exposed skin, in SCCs and in BCCs. As with BCC, patients at higher risk for SCC generally have light-colored eyes and hair, burn easily, and tan poorly. Often patients with SCC have a history of chronic sun exposure, and the cumulative effect of chronic sun exposure plays a definitive role in

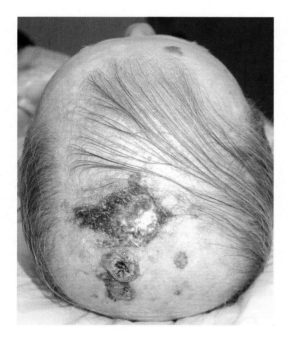

**FIGURE 28-22** ■ Extensive squamous cell cancer that will require extensive surgery, most likely with Mohs therapy and skin grafting.

the development of these skin cancers. In addition, as noted previously with BCC, there has been a substantial rise in the number of SCCs in younger patients.

Darkly pigmented patients are more likely to develop SCC rather than BCC. The development of SCC in races with darker pigment is usually related to an underlying, chronic, scarring condition or ulcer, occurs in less pigmented skin of the digits, or is related to immunosuppression or viral infection. It has been hypothesized that the underlying pathogenesis for tumors of chronic inflammation relates to the induction of mutations in highly proliferative tissue.

Other risk factors for the development of SCC include a history of x-ray exposure, exposure to arsenic, and rare, inherited, skin disorders that predispose one to increased risk of SCC such as xeroderma pigmentosum.

## Treatment

Treatment of SCC is similar to treatment of BCC, with the caveat that SCC has a much higher risk of metastasis than BCC and such knowledge must weigh into the therapeutic plan. For SCCs less than 1 cm in diameter, excision with 4 mm margins offers an 80% to 90% cure rate, depending on location and type of tumor. Tumors greater than 1 cm require broader margins, often approaching 10 mm, to reach such cure rates. For low-risk SCC less than 1 cm in diameter, curettage with or without electrodessication offers similar cure rates to excision. For SCC in situ, curettage and topical modalities, such as 5-fluorouracil and imiquimod, are viable options and offer acceptable cure rates. Recurrent tumors, large tumors, tumors with aggressive histologic subtypes, tumors involving the face and other critical structures, such as the ears, genitalia, and distal extremities (fingers/toes), and ill-defined tumors are best managed by MMS. This modality offers 5-year cure rates in the 95% range for primary tumors, and cure rates approaching 90% for recurrent SCC (Table 28-2). Radiation therapy has been shown to have acceptable cure rates. We reserve its use for those patients who are high surgical risks, when the patient refuses surgery, or for palliation when the lesions are deemed inoperable.

Physical examination of any patient with SCC should include palpation of the regional draining lymph nodes. Additionally, patients with histologically aggressive tumors, large tumors, and recurrent tumors may be considered for sentinel lymph node biopsy or other staging procedures such as computerized tomography of regional draining sites. Immunosuppressed patients with SCC should be considered high risk as well and require frequent clinical follow-up and appropriate, rapid treatment when tumors are diagnosed.

## Prevention

Appropriate sun-exposure precautions and sun avoidance are the keys to preventing SCC. The same precautions on sun exposure noted in the section on BCC should be followed. Immunosuppressed patients particularly need to be educated on strict sun protection with broad-spectrum UVA and UVB sunscreens/sunblocks, sun avoidance during peak UV hours, and regular dermatologic examination. These patients are at high risk for the development of aggressive and potentially life-threatening tumors and many die from metastasis of skin cancer. We recommend that immunosuppressed patients be examined and educated by a dermatologist as soon after their immunosuppression begins as is feasible. Rapid referral and timely treatment are important measures for any patient presenting with a lesion suspicious for SCC.

## Suggested Readings

Auerbach H. Geographic variation in incidence of skin cancer in the United States. *Public Health Rep.* 1961;76:345–348.

Brodland DG, Zitelli JA. Surgical margins for excision of primary cutaneous squamous cell carcinoma. *J Am Acad Dermatol.* 1992;27: 2241–2248.

Dinehart SM, Pollack SV. Metastases from squamous cell carcinoma of the skin and lip. *J Am Acad Dermatol.* 1989;21:242–248.

Gailani MR, Bale SJ, Leffell DJ, et al. Developmental defects in Gorlin syndrome related to putative tumor suppressor gene on chromosome 9. *Cell.* 1992;69:111–117.

Gailani MR, Stahle-Backadahl M, Leffell DJ, et al. The role of the human homologue of Drosophila patched in sporadic basal cell carcinomas. *Nat Genet.* 1996;13:78–81.

Gallagher RP, Hill GB, Bajdik CD, et al. Sunlight exposure, pigmentary factors and risk of non melanocytic skin cancer. I. Basal cell carcinoma. *Arch Dermatol.* 1995;131:157–163.

Karagas MR, Stannard VA, Mott LA, et al. Use of tanning devices and risk of basal cell and squamous cell skin cancers. *J Natl Cancer Inst.* 2002; 94(3): 224–226.

Knox JM, Freeman RG, Heaton CL. Curettage and electrodesiccation in the treatment of skin cancer. *South Med J.* 1962;55:1212–1215.

Kopf W, Bart RS, Schrager D, et al. Curettage-electrodesiccation treatment of basal cell carcinomas. *Arch Dermatol.* 1977;113:439–443.

Koutsky LA, Ault KA, Wheeler CM, et al. A controlled trial of a human papillomavirus type 16 vaccine. *N Engl J Med.* 2002;347:1645–1651.

Kraemer KH. Heritable diseases with increased sensitivity to cellular injury. In: Freedberg IM, Elsen AZ, Wolff K, et al., eds. *Fitzpatrick's Dermatology in General Medicine.* Vol 2. 5th ed. New York, NY: McGraw-Hill; 1999: 1848–1862.

Lang PG, Maize JC. Basal cell carcinoma. In: Rigel DS, Friedberg RJ, Dzubow LM, et al., eds. *Cancer of the Skin.* Philadelphia, PA: Elsevier-Saunders; 2005:101–132.

Marshall DR. The clinical and pathological effects of prolonged solar exposure. Part II. The association with basal cell carcinoma. *Aust NZ J Surg.* 1968;38:89–97.

Miller DL, Weinstock MA. Non-melanoma skin cancer in the United States: Incidence. *J Am Acad Dermatol.* 1994;30:774–780.

Mohs FE. Carcinoma of the skin. A summary of therapeutic results. In: *Chemosurgery: Microscopically Controlled Surgery for Skin Cancer.* Springfield, IL: Charles C Thomas; 1978:153.

Robins P. Chemosurgery: my 15 years of experience. *J Dermatol Surg Oncol.* 1981;7:779–789.

Rowe DE, Carroll RJ, Day CL Jr. Prognostic factors for local recurrence, metastasis, and survival rates in squamous cell carcinoma of the skin, ear, and lip: implications for treatment modality selection. *J Am Acad Dermatol.* 1992;26:976–990.

Sabin SR, Goldstein G, Rosenthal HG, et al. Aggressive squamous cell carcinoma originating as a marjolin's ulcer. *Dermatol Surg.* 2004;30: 229–230.

Sarasin A, Giglia-Maria G. p53 gene mutations in human skin cancers. *Exp Dermatol.* 2002;11:44–47.

Schwartz RA, Nychay SG, Lyons M, et al. Buschke-Lowenstein tumor: verrucous carcinoma of the anogenitalia. *Cutis.* 1991;47:263–266.

Setlow RB, Carrie WL. Pyrimidine dimmers in ultraviolet-irradiated DNAs. *J Mol Biol.* 1966;17:237–254.

Swanson NA, Taylor SB, Tromovitch TA. The evolution of Mohs surgery. *J Dermatol Surg Oncol.* 1982;8:650–654.

Tromovitch TA, Stegman SJ. Microscopic-controlled excision of cutaneous tumors. Chemosurgery fresh tissue technique. *Cancer.* 1978;41:653–658.

# CHAPTER 29

# Melanoma

*Robin S. Weiner, MD and Jaeyoung Yoon, MD, PhD*

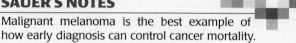

## SAUER'S NOTES

Malignant melanoma is the best example of how early diagnosis can control cancer mortality.

1. The incidence of melanoma continues to accelerate, but the death rate holds relatively steady.
2. This is not due to more aggressive therapy (surgical margins continue to shrink).
3. This is not because there are better therapies (therapy for metastatic disease remains woefully inadequate).
4. It is because the public and the medical community have increased their diagnostic acumen.
5. Until better therapy arrives, we must continue to press for early adequate skin exam by patient and physician alike.
6. You won't diagnose it if you don't look for it!

*Melanoma* (see malignant melanoma in Chapter 27) is defined as a malignant tumor arising from melanocytes, and although it may develop in a preexisting nevus, more than 50% of cases are believed to arise de novo without a preexisting lesion. Melanomas lacking pigment are termed *amelanotic melanomas.*

## Epidemiology

Cancer of the skin accounts for more than 50% of all cancers, and the majority of skin cancer deaths are attributable to melanoma. The American Cancer Society estimates that in 2008 there were 62,480 new cases of melanoma in this country, with 8,420 deaths from this disease. Incidence rates for melanoma have increased steadily over the past several decades, currently rising at a rate of approximately 3% per year. Melanoma has historically affected a younger population than most cancers, with half the patients under age 57.

## Risk Factors

Several risk factors have been identified for the development of melanoma:

- *Ultraviolet irradiation,* with intermittent intense exposure and sunburn posing a greater risk than cumulative lifetime exposure and increasing latitude correlating with decreased incidence of melanoma.
- *Atypical or dysplastic nevi,* especially in families with the so-called dysplastic nevus syndrome.
- *Increased numbers of benign nevi,* with those having greater than 50 nevi being at higher risk of developing melanoma.
- *Large congenital nevi,* defined as greater than 20 cm.
- *Phenotypic features,* including pale or light skin, blonde or red hair, blue or green eyes, a tendency toward freckling, and poor tanning ability.
- *Family history of melanoma.*
- *Host immunosuppression,* which includes transplant patients and patients on chronic immunosuppression for autoimmune diseases.
- *Genetic predisposition,* including defects in the *CDKN2A* gene and/or the *CDK4* gene, and genodermatoses such as xeroderma pigmentosum.

## Types of Primary Melanoma

*Superficial spreading melanoma* (Fig. 29-1) represents the most common clinical subtype, accounting for approximately 70% of cutaneous melanomas. These tumors typically experience a slow horizontal growth phase followed by a rapid vertical growth phase, which may be evident by the development of a papule or nodule. Sites of predilection include the backs of men and the backs and legs of women, although they can occur at any site.

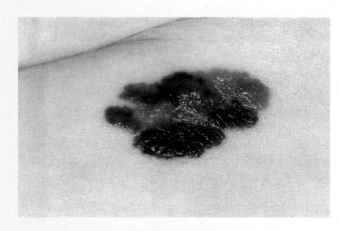

**FIGURE 29-1** ■ Superficial spreading melanoma.

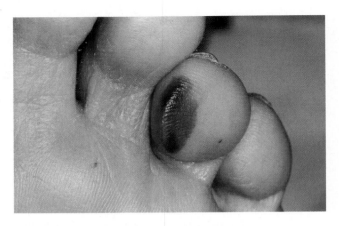

**FIGURE 29-2** ■ Acral lentiginous melanoma.

*Nodular melanoma* accounts for approximately 15% of cutaneous melanomas and has a short radial (horizontal) growth phase, accounting for its rapid invasion. It quickly enters the vertical growth phase. It is seen more frequently in men, and sites of predilection include the trunk, head, and neck. It typically appears as a dark blue-black papule or nodule that develops rapidly and may include a history of ulceration or bleeding. Amelanotic melanoma is often a variant of this subtype.

*Acral lentiginous melanoma* (Fig. 29-2) represents approximately 10% of cutaneous melanomas but is the most common type found in darker complected individuals. Most frequent sites include the palms, soles, or beneath the nail plate. Lesions frequently present as brown to black macules with irregular borders and variations in color, although papules and nodules may be present. This subtype typically has a poor prognosis, which may be related to delayed diagnosis. Therefore, early biopsy of suspected lesions is critical.

*Lentigo maligna melanoma* is a rare clinical subtype, comprising approximately 5% of cutaneous melanomas. This lesion arises from a lentigo maligna (melanoma in situ of sun-exposed skin) and involves dermal invasion. Tumors typically occur in the elderly and arise on sun-damaged skin, including the forearms and the face. These lesions present as large, irregularly shaped macules or patches with variations of tan, brown, or black pigment, and they may eventually develop a papular or nodular component.

## Diagnosis

Early identification and treatment of melanomas are essential as prognosis depends on the stage of disease at diagnosis. Pertinent data should be gathered from the medical history, including personal or family history of melanoma, any change in existing skin lesions including changes in size, shape, or pigmentation, as well as any history of bleeding or ulceration.

Physical examination should include evaluation of all skin, including scalp and mucous membranes, using the American Cancer Society's ABCD mnemonic to identify suspicious lesions. *A* is for asymmetry, *B* for irregular borders, *C* for irregular color, and *D* for diameter, with size greater than 6 mm typically considered suspicious. It has recently been suggested that the mnemonic be lengthened to include *E* for evolving. Dermatoscopy, also known as *epiluminescence microscopy*, is a noninvasive tool used for magnification and may contribute to diagnosis.

Once identified, suspicious lesions should be evaluated with full-thickness biopsy to allow assessment of lesion thickness. Excisional biopsy should be performed when possible to evaluate the entire lesion; prognosis and treatment are determined by tumor thickness. When excisional biopsy is impractical, such as when the lesion is large, or clinical suspicion is low, punch biopsy technique or deep shave may be used and should include the most suspicious area of the growth.

## Staging and Prognosis

The American Joint Committee on Cancer's *Cancer Staging Manual* was revised in 2002 and established the TNM staging system for melanoma given in Table 29-1. Stages I and II represent local disease, stage III represents regional involvement, and stage IV represents distant metastases (Table 29-2).

Important prognostic factors include tumor thickness and ulceration, as well as clinical variables such as anatomic site, sex, and age of the patient. Increased tumor thickness correlates with poorer prognosis and is the most important determinant. Presence of ulceration microscopically is the second most important determinant. Tumor thickness is known as *Breslow's depth*, which is defined as the distance from the

**TABLE 29-1** ■ **TNM Staging System for Melanoma**

|     |     |
| --- | --- |
|     | Primary tumor cannot be assessed |
| T0 | No evidence of primary tumor |
| Tis | Melanoma in situ |
| T1 | Melanoma, <1.0 mm in thickness |
| T2 | Melanoma 1.01−2.0 mm in thickness |
| T3 | Melanoma 2.01−4.0 mm in thickness |
| T4 | Melanoma >4.0 mm in thickness |
| NX | Regional lymph nodes cannot be assessed |
| N0 | No regional lymph node metastasis |
| N1 | Metastasis in one lymph node |
| N2 | Metastasis in 2−3 regional nodes or intralymphatic regional metastasis without nodal metastases |
| N3 | Metastasis in 4 or more regional nodes, matted metastatic nodes, or in-transit metastasis or satellite(s) *with* metastasis in regional node(s) |
| MX | Distant metastasis cannot be assessed |
| M0 | No distant metastasis |
| M1 | Distant metastasis |

**TABLE 29-2 ■ Clinical Stage Grouping (AJCC)**

| Stage 0 | Tis | N0 | M0 |
|---|---|---|---|
| Stage IA | T1a | N0 | M0 |
| Stage IB | T1b | N0 | M0 |
| | T2a | N0 | M0 |
| Stage IIA | T2b | N0 | M0 |
| | T3a | N0 | M0 |
| Stage IIB | T3b | N0 | M0 |
| | T4a | N0 | M0 |
| Stage IIC | T4b | N0 | M0 |
| Stage III | Any T | N1, N2, or N3 | M0 |
| Stage IV | Any T | Any N | M1 |

*Note:* a, no ulceration; b, ulceration

top of the granular cell layer to the deepest point of tumor invasion. Clark's level of invasion may also be described:

- Level 1 involves only the epidermis
- Level 2 invades the papillary dermis
- Level 3 fills the papillary dermis
- Level 4 invades the reticular dermis
- Level 5 involves the subcutaneous fat

According to Surveillance, Epidemiology and End Results data from 1988 to 2001, approximately 83% of melanomas are diagnosed at a localized stage. These tumors (stage I and II) have a 5-year survival rate of 97% with appropriate treatment. Melanomas with regional involvement at the time of diagnosis (stage III) have a 5-year survival rate of 60%, and those with distant metastases (stage IV) have a 5-year survival rate of 16%.

## Treatment

Once the diagnosis of melanoma is confirmed, complete excision of the tumor site is performed with margins determined based on Breslow's tumor thickness. Although there is some controversy regarding recommendations for tumors 1 to 2 mm in depth, the American Academy of Dermatology task force recommends the following:

- 0.5-cm margins for in situ melanoma
- 1-cm margins for tumor thickness less than 2 mm
- 2-cm margins for tumors with a thickness greater than 2 mm

Lymphatic mapping and sentinel lymph node biopsy can be performed as a staging tool and provides prognostic information. The therapeutic value of this procedure awaits further analysis. It is hoped that intense research into chemotherapy, immunotherapy, and cancer vaccinations will improve survival rates; however, the prognosis for advanced melanoma remains grim.

## Suggested Readings

Balch CM, Houghton AN, Sober AJ, et al. *Cutaneous Melanoma.* 4th ed. St. Louis, MO: Quality Medical Pub.; 2003.

Hearing VJ, Leong SPL. *From Melanocytes to Malignant Melanoma.* Totowa, NJ: Humana Press; 2005.

Kroon BBR, Morton, DL, Thompson, JF. *Textbook of Melanoma.* London: Martin Dunitz; 2004.

Massi G, LeBoit PE. *Histological Diagnosis of Nevi and Melanoma.* Darmstadt: Steinkopff; 2004.

Rigel DS, Friedman RJ, Kopf AW, et al. ABCDE–an evolving concept in the early detection of melanoma. *Arch Dermatol.* 2005;141(8):1032–1034.

Riker AI, Glass F, Perez I, et al. Cutaneous melanoma: methods of biopsy and definitive surgical excision. *Dermatol Ther.* 2005;18(5):387–393.

Schaffer JV, Rigel DS, Kopf AW, et al. Cutaneous melanoma—past, present, and future. *J Am Acad Dermatol.* 2004;51(1 suppl):S65–S69.

Scottish Intercollegiate Guidelines Network. *Cutaneous Melanoma: A National Clinical Guideline/Scottish Intercollegiate Guidelines Network.* Edinburgh, Scotland: SIGN; 2003.

# CHAPTER 30

# Vascular Tumors

*Margaret S. Lee, MD, PhD and Marilyn G. Liang, MD*

## Classification

Vascular tumors can be characterized by the following methods:

- Clinical and demographic characteristics of the patient (e.g., age, immune status)
- Gross clinical characteristics of the tumor (size, shape, color, distribution, evolution over time)
- Histology
- Radiologic studies to assess blood flow, circumscription, and depth of involvement (Doppler ultrasound, computed tomography [CT], magnetic resonance imaging [MRI])

In most cases, the tumors can be diagnosed using just the first two categories of information.

In this chapter, we will discuss the most common and most concerning vascular tumors: infantile hemangioma (IH), congenital hemangiomas, pyogenic granuloma (PG), kaposiform hemangioendothelioma (KHE), tufted angioma (TA), Kaposi's sarcoma (KS), and angiosarcoma.

## Tumors versus Malformations

Before we discuss tumors in detail, it is important to differentiate between *tumors* and *malformations*. This distinction is relatively new in the study of vascular anomalies. In the past, vascular lesions were not well understood and all were called *hemangiomas* or some derivative thereof using the suffix *-oma*. Mulliken and Glowacki proposed a new classification system for vascular anomalies in 1982 (revised formally in 1996 by the International Society for the Study of Vascular Anomalies) based on histologic and pathophysiologic features. *Tumors* are cellular masses with postnatal endothelial proliferative potential. *Malformations* are products of abnormal vasculogenesis during fetal development. They enlarge over time predominantly through distention of congenitally malformed vessels rather than true endothelial cell proliferation as in an infantile hemangioma.

## Benign Tumors

### Infantile Hemangioma

The most common vascular tumor is the benign infantile hemangioma (IH). These tumors are unique in that they eventually involute over years without treatment, sometimes leaving no trace on the skin surface.

*Presentation and Characteristics*

**Demographics.** Two percent of all newborns present with an IH. The prevalence of IH is about 10% of all Caucasian children. Less than 2% of black and Asian infants are affected. There is a clear female preponderance, in a ratio of about 3–5:1. IH are much more common in premature infants, twin/multiple gestations, infants of older mothers, and infants whose mothers underwent chorionic villus sampling.

**Description.** Most lesions are present at birth or appear within the first week of life, often as a precursor lesion that looks like telangiectasias or a "bruise like" macule. The final size of IH ranges tremendously, from spotty macules and papules a few millimeters in diameter to extensive plaques encompassing several developmental regions. IH can be described as superficial, deep, or mixed. Superficial IH are well-demarcated papules or plaques raised above the skin surface, with a bright red color during the proliferative and early plateau phases (Fig. 30-1). Deep IH are visible through the skin surface as a bluish-purple nodule and often seem softer and more compressible than superficial plaques (Fig. 30-2). Mixed superficial and deep IH combine a bright red superficial lesion overlying a deep component. Reticular IH are thinner, more discontinuous superficial lesions than the typical superficial plaque-type IH (Fig. 30-3).

**Distribution.** IH are most commonly found on the head and neck (up to 85%). However, they can present on any part

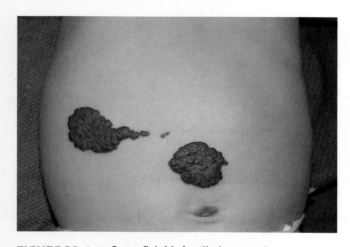

**FIGURE 30-1** ■ Superficial infantile hemangioma.

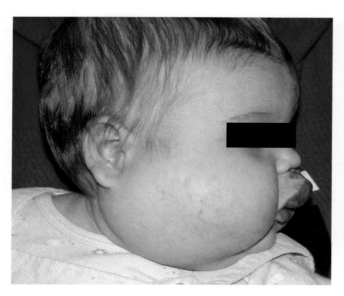

**FIGURE 30-2** ■ Deep infantile hemangioma. Also note mixed superficial and deep infantile hemangioma on the lip.

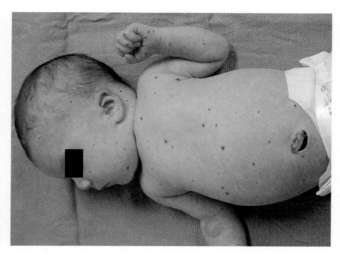

**FIGURE 30-4** ■ Multifocal infantile hemangioma.

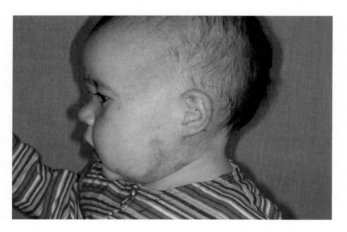

**FIGURE 30-3** ■ Reticular infantile hemangioma.

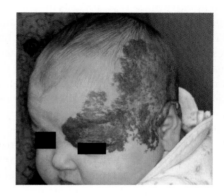

**FIGURE 30-5** ■ Regional infantile hemangioma.

of the body. A patient may have several lesions at the same time. IH can be described as focal, multifocal, or regional:

- Focal—a solitary lesion
- Multifocal—multiple lesions involving different anatomical regions (Fig. 30-4)
- Regional—a lesion encompassing a large surface area but limited to one anatomical or developmental region (also termed segmental) (Fig. 30-5)

***Course.*** A third of IH are present at birth, and the rest become apparent within the first few weeks of life. The clinical course of IH includes a proliferative, plateau, and involution phase. Superficial IH quickly become bright red over the first month of life. Deep IH may not become evident until 2 to 4 months of life. IH become softer and grayer or paler in color as they plateau in size, then involute (Fig. 30-6). At the end of involution, the lesions, if visible at all, range from scattered telangiectasias to pale, fibrofatty, baggy outpouchings or

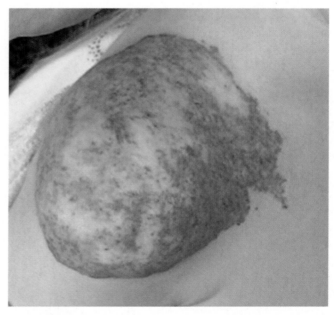

**FIGURE 30-6** ■ Involuting infantile hemangioma.

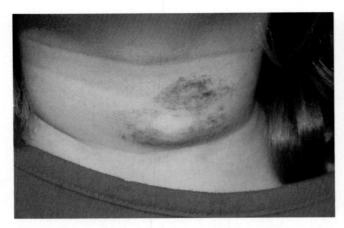

**FIGURE 30-7** ■ Residual fibrofatty infantile hemangioma.

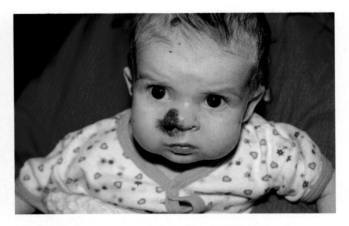

**FIGURE 30-9** ■ Nasal deformation risk in infantile hemangioma.

soft, irregular plaques (Fig. 30-7). Reticulate IH involute very nicely, leaving behind only telangiectasias.

The proliferative phase typically lasts for 6 to 10 months, although very small IH may not proliferate much and can involute away within the first year or two of life. The plateau phase varies from 1 to 4 months. Involution time tends to be proportionate to the size of the lesion; larger and thicker lesions require more time to involute. A general rule of thumb in counseling parents is that 50% of all IH stop involuting by the time a child is 5 years old. IH may continue to involute until age 10.

The most common complication is ulceration. This can occur due to rapid tumor proliferation, friction/trauma, or infection. Hence, the most common sites for ulceration are intertriginous sites, especially the perineum (Fig. 30-8). Other complications include impingement upon vital structures, such as the airway or visual axis, and deformation of anatomical structures such as the nose (Fig. 30-9) and lips. IH in the "beard" distribution correlate with risk of airway involvement and respiratory distress; the larger the IH in this location, the greater the risk of airway obstruction (Fig. 30-10). If an IH is large enough (e.g., in the liver), it can overburden the circulatory system, causing high-output cardiac overload.

***Cause.*** We do not yet fully understand what causes some children to be born with IH. Recent evidence supports the existence of an IH endothelial stem cell that drives the tremendous proliferative potential of these tumors. The source of these stem cells is unknown. One possibility is that they are derived from the embolization of placental cells to the developing fetus; support for this phenomenon lies in the increased incidence of IH in babies whose mothers underwent chorionic villus sampling during pregnancy. In the fetal or postnatal tissue environment, these stem cells may proliferate due to an angiogenic milieu as compared to that in placental tissues.

*Histology*

On hematoxylin and eosin (H&E) preparations, proliferating IH are composed of a dense collection of endothelial cells and pericytes forming many capillary vascular channels

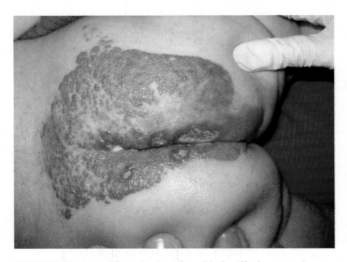

**FIGURE 30-8** ■ Ulcerated perineal infantile hemangioma.

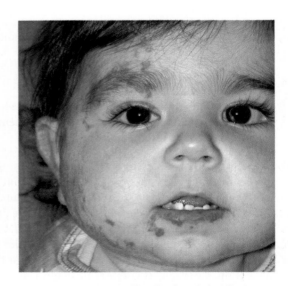

**FIGURE 30-10** ■ "Beard" distribution infantile hemangioma with airway obstruction.

arranged in lobules. These lobules are fed and drained by larger vessels. Naturally, larger tumors have larger feeding arteries and draining veins. IH are characterized by positive erythrocyte type glucose transporter-1 (GLUT-1) staining, which is also expressed by placental endothelial cells. Sometimes normal appendageal structures, such as hair follicles and nerves, may be found within the capillary lobules. During involution there is a steady increase in fibrofatty tissue replacing the endothelial and stromal cells and vascular channels. Persistence of some of the afferent and efferent vessels probably correlates with grossly visible remnant telangiectasias.

### Radiologic Studies

Imaging is usually not needed to diagnose or assess an IH. Doppler ultrasound can be very helpful in differentiating a bluish, deep IH from a venous malformation based on blood flow characteristics. IH are fast flow lesions whereas venous malformations and other tumors are slow flow lesions. Standard ultrasound can be used to screen for spinal dysraphism occurring with a sacral IH or for liver IH in a patient with multifocal cutaneous hemangiomas. MRI is necessary when vital structures are compromised or to identify intracranial abnormalities associated with regional facial IH.

### Associations to Consider

**PHACES Association (Posterior fossa malformations, Hemangioma, Arterial anomalies, Coarctation of the aorta and Cardiac anomalies, Eye anomalies, Sternal clefting).** This condition is much more common in females than in males. Patients with an IH encompassing one or more developmental regions on the head and neck should have a workup for the above defects. It is not necessary to have more than one or two of the additional associations to carry a diagnosis of PHACES (Fig. 30-11).

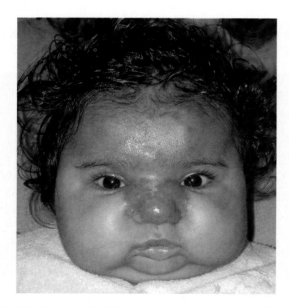

**FIGURE 30-11** ■ PHACES association: facial infantile hemangioma and absent corpus callosum.

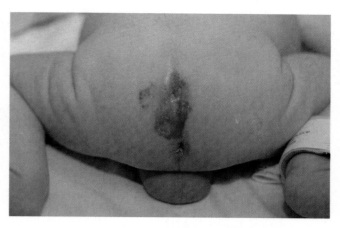

**FIGURE 30-12** ■ Sacral infantile hemangioma associated with tethered cord.

**Reticular Infantile Hemangioma of Perineum and/or Limb.** These IH can be associated with chronic ulceration and ventral-caudal anomalies such as omphalocele or genital anatomical defects such as fistulae or ambiguous genitalia. Renal anomalies, imperforate anus, and high-output cardiac overload has also been described.

**Tethered Cord or Other Spinal Abnormalities.** An IH, reticular or plaque type, overlying the lower spine should be investigated radiologically to rule out tethered cord (Fig. 30-12), occult spinal dysraphism, lipomeningocele, or, very rarely, extension of IH into the spine.

**Multifocal with Visceral Infantile Hemangiomas.** Patients who present with five or more superficial IH scattered over the body should be evaluated for visceral IH, anemia, and congestive heart failure. One should perform ultrasonography or MRI of the liver to rule out liver lesions, the most common visceral site of involvement. Large liver IH can cause profound hypothyroidism because IH produce type 3 iodothyronine deiodinase. This deiodinase inactivates thyroxine and triiodothyronine. The deiodinase has also been found in cutaneous IH, but there are no reports of clinical hypothyroidism associated with cutaneous IH. Hepatomegaly from liver IH can potentially lead to cardiac output overload and death. In other cases, the mass effect from large liver IH can cause abdominal compartment syndrome, leading to respiratory and renal failure.

### Differential Diagnosis

IH are relatively easy to diagnose clinically by the first month of life. If there is ambiguity for any reason (e.g., deep IH), a simple and important feature to keep in mind is that IH are fast-flow lesions. Doppler investigation detects an arterial signal in fast-flow lesions.
Precursor lesion DDx:

- *Ecchymosis/birth trauma*: Observation will easily clarify the difference since true ecchymoses will resolve within a week.
- Kaposiform hemangioendothelioma
- Tufted angioma

Superficial hemangiomas DDx:

- *Capillary malformation (CM)*: A very early superficial IH might theoretically be macular and confused with a CM. However, observation will show relatively rapid evolution from patch to papule or plaque. Usually an IH changes rapidly enough that a diagnosis of capillary malformation is not considered. CM are slow-flow lesions.

Deep hemangioma DDx:

- *Cyst or cyst-like lesions (e.g., dermoid cyst, pilomatrixoma)*: Ultrasonography is indicated if there is insufficient or inconsistent information supporting a clinical diagnosis of IH.
- *Congenital hemangiomas*: These are fully formed at birth and either involute much more rapidly than IH or do not involute.
- *Soft tissue sarcomas (fibrosarcoma, rhabdomyosarcoma)*: These are less vascularized than IH and do not exhibit a fast-flow signal via Doppler ultrasonography. MRI and CT imaging also appear distinct from IH. A tumor that appears later than four months of age, displays an unusual proliferation pattern, or lacks fast-flow Doppler signal should be biopsied or excised to rule out a malignancy.

### Treatment

Most IH do not require any intervention other than bland emollients to reduce risk of frictional breakdown and ulceration. Treatment depends on the body location and complications.

- Intralesional corticosteroid
- Systemic corticosteroid
- Vincristine
- Propranolol
- Interferon (IFN)-$\alpha$
- Laser
- Local treatment for ulceration (emollients, antibiotics with wound care, topical corticosteroids, laser, becaplermin)
- Excision

Many involuting hemangiomas on the face are treated before a child is 2 or 3 years old, which is the age most children begin to form lasting memories and a sense of self. Most patients are treated before starting kindergarten, when children become more conscious of social relationships and physical differences.

### Congenital Hemangiomas

Congenital hemangiomas are distinct from infantile hemangiomas (IH) even though many IH are also visible at birth. Congenital hemangiomas have no postnatal proliferation, and the gross clinical appearance is quite different from that of IH. RICH stands for *rapidly involuting congenital hemangioma* and NICH stands for *non-involuting congenital hemangioma*.

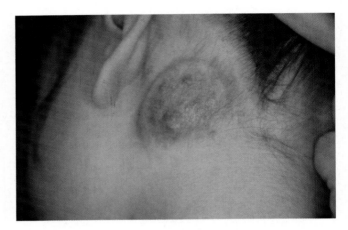

**FIGURE 30-13** ■ Non-involuting congenital hemangioma with characteristic halo.

*Presentation and Characteristics*

**Demographics.** Unlike IH, RICH and NICH occur equally in males and females.

**Description.** RICH and NICH can be indistinguishable from one another in appearance, especially at birth or during infancy. A pale halo on the skin around a congenital hemangioma is characteristic (Fig. 30-13). While most RICH and NICH are smooth, domed or slightly flat-topped tumors similar to IH (Fig. 30-14), they are often more blue-gray in color than IH. Many congenital hemangiomas exhibit large telangiectasias or coarse hairs. As a RICH involutes, it may become depressed or atrophic (Fig. 30-15).

**Distribution.** Both RICH and NICH tend to be found on the head and neck or extremities. Lesions on the torso are uncommon.

**Course.** As the name implies, RICH rapidly decreases in size over the first 6 to 14 months of life. There may be a residual fibrofatty lesion, as in IH, or even a partial regression leaving an NICH-like plaque. NICH do not change significantly with time.

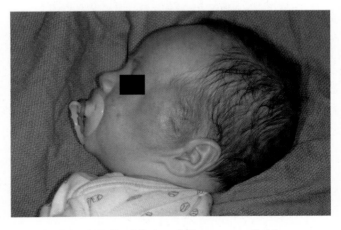

**FIGURE 30-14** ■ Rapidly involuting congenital hemangioma before involution.

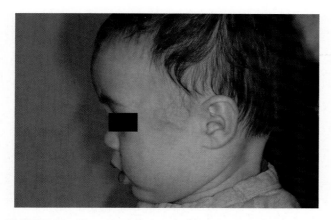

**FIGURE 30-15** ■ Rapidly involuting congenital hemangioma after involution (same patient as in Fig. 30-14).

**Cause.** As for IH, the root cause of congenital hemangiomas is unknown.

### Histology

On H&E staining, RICH displays a moderately prominent endothelium with rare hobnailing, interlobular fibrous tissue with zonation, and are typically GLUT-1 negative. As they involute, they may develop thrombi, infarctions, calcification, cysts, aneurysms, and extramedullary hematopoiesis. NICH tend to have endothelial hobnailing, dense fibrous tissue between lobules, no zonation, and are always GLUT-1 negative.

### Radiologic Studies

RICH are often detected during routine prenatal ultrasonography as uniformly hypoechoic masses. On MRI, they are characterized by high flow. There are large flow voids mixed with areas that are much less homogeneous than IH, as they may include AV fistulae, arterial aneurysms, thrombi, cysts, and calcifications. Ultrasonography of NICH often reveals arteriovenous fistulae. MRI and angiography of NICH is very similar to that of IH; uniform hyperintensity is seen on T2 imaging and with gadolinium injection.

### Differential Diagnosis

RICH and NICH are the main entities serving as differential diagnoses for each other in a neonate. Clinical behavior over time is a principal means of differentiating the two.

### Treatment

Many RICH are left to involute on their own. However, if there is risk of significant ulceration or bleeding, they may be excised. NICH may be excised, often after embolization of the largest vessels. Neither lesion recurs after excision.

## Pyogenic Granuloma

Pyogenic granuloma (PG) is one of the persisting misnomers in dermatologic nomenclature. It is neither pyogenic (generating pus) nor a granuloma (inflammatory collection of immune cells). It is a highly vascular tumor common in infants

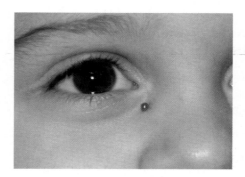

**FIGURE 30-16** ■ Pyogenic granuloma.

and children, often following minor trauma. Another name for PG used by pathologists is *lobular capillary hemangioma*.

### Presentation and Characteristics

**Demographics.** The male to female ratio is 3:2. Half of cases occur in children younger than 5 years of age; the mean age is 6.7 years. Adults with PG are most often pregnant women.

**Description.** Most PG are rounded, exophytic, or pedunculated red papules that are extremely friable and therefore likely to bleed with the slightest contact. Those that are not friable have a thicker surface that may or may not be lobulated (Fig. 30-16).

**Distribution.** The most common locations for PG are acral sites, such as the face and fingers. They may also appear on the gingiva and intraoral mucous membranes. PG are also known to arise within capillary malformations.

**Course.** PGs frequently come to the attention of a physician promptly due to the tendency to bleed as they enlarge over time, which can be rapid. At times a pedunculated lesion may disrupt and fall off at the stalk. Spontaneous regression is possible, but rare.

**Cause.** The cause of PG is unknown. Preceding trauma was associated in 7% of cases in one series.

### Histology

On H&E staining, PG are seen as a domed papule with a feeder vessel giving rise to many capillary vascular spaces and fibrotic stroma. The loose proliferation of vessels simulates granulation tissue. A collarette of epithelium encircles the base of the papule. There is often an area of ulceration from which the lesion bleeds easily.

### Radiologic Studies

These lesions are too small and superficial to be studied radiologically.

### Differential Diagnosis

- Spitz nevus
- Bacillary angiomatosis (multiple lesions, immunosuppression)

- Well-differentiated angiosarcoma
- Nodular Kaposi's sarcoma
- Squamous cell carcinoma
- Amelanotic melanoma
- Peripheral giant cell granuloma
- Peripheral ossifying granuloma
- Oral verrucous carcinoma

### Treatment

- Direct pressure usually stops bleeding before medical attention
- Electrodessication, surgical excision, curettage, chemical cauterization
- Sclerotherapy with 1% sodium tetradecyl sulfate
- $CO_2$ laser, pulsed dye laser
- Imiquimod

## Kaposiform Hemangioendothelioma

Kaposiform hemangioendothelioma (KHE) and tufted angioma (TA) are important entities because they are associated with the potentially fatal Kasabach-Merritt phenomenon (KMP), a consumptive coagulopathy with a mortality rate of 10% to 37%. It is not known why KHE and TA are associated with KMP while other vascular tumors are not. KHE is typically associated with KMP; TA is less often so. Some consider KHE a low-grade malignant neoplasm because the clinical course can be aggressive and deadly due to complications.

### Presentation and Characteristics

**Demographics.** KHE are more common in males than in females. They are usually congenital lesions but later onset or later diagnosis in childhood has been observed.

**Description.** KHE skin lesions are classically very violaceous or brawny-colored indurated, highly infiltrative plaques, sometimes with overlying papules or nodules. Lesions are poorly defined at the borders, unlike IHs (**Fig. 30-17**). Skin is less commonly involved than internal organs. KHE can extend through soft tissue, muscle, and bone.

**Distribution.** The most common location for KHE overall is head and neck, mediastinum, and retroperitoneum. On the skin it is typical to see a neck/shoulder/arm or hip/ buttock/ thigh distribution. There is no known metastatic potential but lesions can be locally very aggressive and infiltrative.

**Course.** KHE rarely involutes. In cases where the lesion responds to therapy, there is almost always residual tumor that remains. The residua are more fibrotic than the primary lesion.

**Cause.** Pathophysiology is not yet understood.

### Histology

On H&E staining, one can see infiltrating lobules of monomorphous spindled cells arranged in fascicles separated

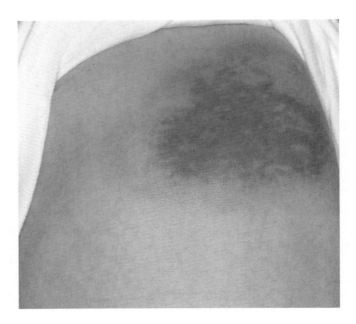

**FIGURE 30-17** ■ Kaposiform hemangioendothelioma.

by fibrous septae, and slit like vascular spaces. Lymphatic channels can also be seen. Microthrombi can be seen at the periphery of the lesion. There may be nests of epithelioid cells. KHE stains positively for the lymphatic marker D2-40.

### Radiologic Studies

These diffusely enhancing lesions are seen on MRI to be highly infiltrative, potentially involving skin, muscle, viscera and bone.

### Differential Diagnosis

- Tufted angioma (TA)
- Kaposi's sarcoma (KS)
- Spindle-cell hemangioma

### Treatment

There is no definitive therapy for KHE. Corticosteroids, vincristine, IFN, and excision are most commonly used.

## Tufted Angioma

TA are notable for their association with KMP, although less commonly than for KHE. It is also known as *angioblastoma of Nakagawa*. TA may be on a spectrum of KHE-like lesions, as some vascular lesions have features of both KHE and TA. The incidence of KMP in these two lesions supports the possibility of a pathophysiologic and histologic overlap.

### Presentation and Characteristics

**Demographics.** TA may be congenital or acquired (usually before 5 years of age).

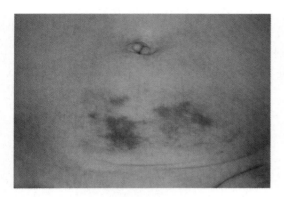

FIGURE 30-18 ■ Tufted angioma.

***Description.*** TA tend to be ruddier lesions than KHE but often cannot be distinguished from them without a biopsy. They may be pink, red, brown, or a combination thereof. Lesion morphology can vary widely, from macules to papules to plaques. Some lesions display hypertrichosis, hyperhidrosis, or small red papules overlying a plaque (**Fig. 30-18**). They can be tender to palpation. Occasionally TA can present as a dermal tumor with a blanching halo, mimicking a rapidly involuting congenital hemangioma (RICH). TA lesions are less well defined than IH.

***Distribution.*** TA are more common on the limbs but can be found anywhere on the body.

***Course.*** TA may increase in size and change shape slowly over time. Some spontaneously regress by the age of 2 years. However, most persist and remain painful to varying degrees.

***Cause.*** Cause is unknown.

### Histology

On H&E staining, one sees "tufts of cannonball-like aggregates" of hypertrophied endothelial cells in the middle and lower dermis. They may extend deeply into subcutaneous fat. Surrounding dermis may be fibrotic. These endothelial cells have scant cytoplasm. Vascular spaces are slit like. There may be lymphatic channels interspersed among the "cannonballs." The epidermis may be unaffected, or there may be some degree of acanthosis and papillomatosis. Lymphatic marker D2-40 staining is positive.

### Radiologic Studies

MRI can be used to assess depth of involvement in larger lesions. Sometimes TA can extend into muscle and fascia.

### Differential Diagnosis

- Kaposiform hemangioendothelioma
- Kaposi's sarcoma
- Infantile hemangioma

### Treatment

No therapy has proven uniformly effective for TA. For small lesions, observation for spontaneous involution is reasonable. Intralesional and systemic corticosteroids, intralesional and systemic IFN- α-2, laser, and other antiangiogenic agents have been tried. Excision and laser have been used with varying results. Non-steroidal anti-inflammatory drugs (NSAIDs) can be used for pain.

### Kasabach–Merritt Phenomenon

Kasabach-Merritt phenomenon (KMP) deserves further mention due to its high morbidity/mortality potential. It was first described in 1940 by Kasabach and Merritt as a consumptive thrombocytopenia occurring in association with a violaceous, indurated skin lesion called a hemangioma at the time. We now know that KMP occurs in the context of KHE and TA but not IH.

### Presentation and Characteristics

***Demographics.*** Males may be affected slightly more often than females. There is no racial predilection. Mortality is estimated to be between 10% and 40% and occurs in the context of aggressive visceral disease, profound thrombocytopenia, and infection or treatment complications.

***Description.*** Profound thrombocytopenia observed in a patient with a vascular anomaly should immediately raise concern for KMP. Thrombosis and platelet trapping occurs within the vascular spaces of KHE and TA. The lesion becomes engorged and increasingly violaceous as the condition progresses (**Fig. 30-19**). Ulceration and hemorrhage may occur. There is consumption of coagulation factors such as fibrinogen, with formation of D-dimers. Laboratory studies to evaluate/confirm KMP are complete blood count to assess for thrombocytopenia and anemia, decreased fibrinogen level, increased fibrin split products, and elevated D-dimers. Platelet counts fall to below 10,000/mm$^3$.

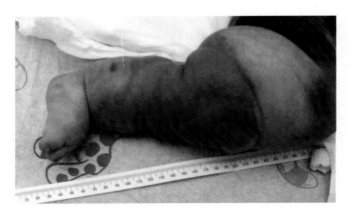

FIGURE 30-19 ■ Kasabach–Merritt phenomenon associated with kaposiform hemangioendothelioma.

***Course.*** KMP manifests early, at birth or within the first few months of life. Onset in utero and in adulthood are also reported. Platelet count tends to fall rapidly.

***Cause.*** The initial trigger for KMP is unknown. We do not know why some lesions develop KMP while others do not, or why some cases are more severe than others. However, there is some correlation of KMP with larger-sized tumors.

### Treatment

There is no uniformly effective medical therapy for KHE and TA in which KMP arises so management can be challenging. Surgical excision of these infiltrative and poorly defined lesions is often not feasible, but does correct KMP if it is an option. A typical progression of therapy is a trial of high-dose corticosteroids, then vincristine. Platelet transfusion does not correct the problem and therefore is reserved for hemorrhage due to the thrombocytopenia and just before surgical procedures. IFN-$\alpha$-2b and radiation have been tried in the past, but tend to have a poor risk/benefit ratio. Drawing from general DIC management, in some patients a combination of anticoagulants such as the antiplatelet drug ticlopidine and aspirin have been helpful.

## Malignant Tumors

### Kaposi's Sarcoma

Kaposi's sarcoma (KS) is a spindle-cell tumor derived from endothelial cells. It is uncertain if it is a malignancy or a benign vascular tumor with multiple sites of origin. This tumor became a recognizable sign of the AIDS epidemic in the 1970s and 1980s before effective antiretroviral therapy was developed. Now its appearance is much less common in the HIV/AIDS population overall but remains a sign of inadequate therapy or noncompliance. There are four subtypes of KS: classic/sporadic, immunocompromised, AIDS-related, and endemic (African).

### Presentation and Characteristics

**Demographics.**
*Classic:* This subtype typically presents in elderly men of Mediterranean and Eastern European descent. The male to female ratio is 10-15:1.

*Immunocompromised:* This subtype is most commonly seen in the organ transplant population, with an equal male to female ratio. The incidence of KS is 100-fold more common in transplant patients than other populations at risk. Patients at risk for classic KS who are immunocompromised have an even higher risk of disease.

*AIDS-related:* In the United States, KS is primarily seen in homosexual men, bisexual men, and the female partners of bisexual men. In Africa, KS is common in heterosexual patients as well as in the homosexual population. Nonsexual transmission occurs among intravenous drug abusers and those who received unscreened blood transfusions.

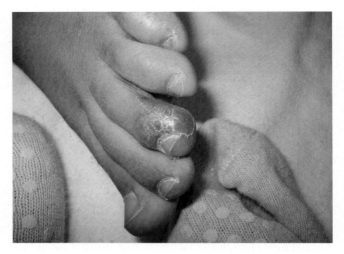

**FIGURE 30-20** ■ AIDS-related macular Kaposi's sarcoma.

*Endemic (African):* Heterosexual HIV-seronegative men and women are affected equally, with children less often so. HIV-negative children are more likely to develop a lymphadenopathic subtype that, if generalized with visceral involvement, is uniformly fatal by 3 years of age.

**Description.** KS skin lesions are classically dusky or violaceous, red-purple lesions. In darker-skinned patients, they may appear brown or bruise like, and early lesions may not be appreciated as KS without a high index of suspicion (Fig. 30-20). They evolve from a patch stage to a plaque stage, and in very advanced/aggressive cases, to nodules (Fig. 30-21). They have poorly defined borders. It is common to form more than one lesion. They occur not only in mucocutaneous locations but also in lymph nodes and viscera, potentially impairing organ function.

**Distribution.** Lesions are more common on the lower extremities and the head and neck, including oral mucosa, but they can form anywhere on the body. It is typical to

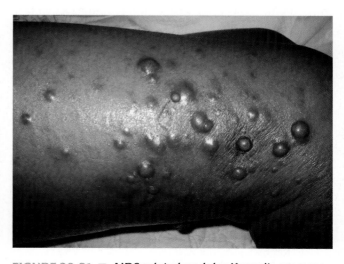

**FIGURE 30-21** ■ AIDS-related nodular Kaposi's sarcoma.

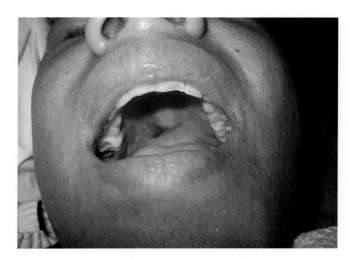

FIGURE 30-22 ■ AIDS-related mucosal Kaposi's sarcoma.

form linear lesions along skin lines in a bilateral, more or less symmetrical distribution. The most common mucous membranes affected are the palate, gingiva and conjunctivae (Fig. 30-22).

*Course.* Classic and endemic KS is an indolent disease. AIDS-associated KS, however, is much more aggressive. Nodular KS lesions are typically seen in this latter subtype in resistant strains of HIV or in patients not compliant to HAART. Involvement of lymph nodes leads to lymphedema.

*Cause.* There is an association between human herpes virus 8 (HHV-8) and low CD4 count. Restoration of NK cytotoxic effect and CD4 counts above 200 to 300/mL is associated with regression or indolence.

### Histology

KS is the classic lesion with slit like vascular spaces. Spindle cells, endothelial cells, extravasated erythrocytes, and hemosiderin-laden macrophages abound. Nuclear pleomorphism and many mitoses are seen. Iron, HHV-8, and CD34 or other vascular immunohistochemical stains are positive.

### Radiologic Studies

CT or MRI should be employed in AIDS-related KS to assess for lymphatic and visceral involvement, especially hepatosplenic disease. Endoscopy, CT, and angiography may be used to assess gastrointestinal involvement. In pulmonary KS, chest radiographs show perihilar and lower lobe involvement, and sometimes pleural effusions.

### Differential Diagnosis

- Bacillary angiomatosis
- Ecchymosis (early macular lesions)
- Angiokeratoma
- Pyogenic granuloma

- Pseudokaposiform angiomatosis in arteriovenous malformations
- Reactive angioendotheliomatosis

### Treatment

Therapy naturally depends in part on the subtype of KS. For AIDS-related KS, effective HAART is required and may even be sufficient for regression of lesions. Other medical therapy includes anti-HHV-8 agents (such as foscarnet and ganciclovir), antiangiogenesis agents (such as SU-5416, a VEGF inhibitor), and cytokine inhibitors. Chemotherapy using vincristine, vinblastine, and bleomycin is used for symptomatic visceral disease or rapidly progressive, severe, and widespread mucocutaneous disease. Antiangiogenic agents such as thalidomide have shown efficacy and may be combined with cytotoxic chemotherapy agents. Topical retinoids may be helpful for facial lesions.

Radiation therapy may be used for focal disease causing bleeding, pain, or functional impairment (e.g., oral mucosal involvement impeding speech or swallowing) or cosmetically distressful lesions. Patients with very widespread skin disease may be treated with extended-field electron beam radiation therapy.

Surgical excision may be required for visceral obstruction, lymphedema, and severe bleeding. Laser photocoagulation is appropriate for smaller focal lesions and palliation. Cryotherapy may be used for small, superficial lesions such as those on the face.

## Angiosarcoma

Angiosarcoma is an uncommon but aggressive vascular tumor with a high morbidity/mortality profile. Prompt workup and intervention is very important, but early diagnosis is often difficult. Stewart-Treves syndrome is angiosarcoma arising in areas of chronic lymphedema, whether congenital or secondary lymphedema due to disease or surgical complications.

### Presentation and Characteristics

*Demographics.* Cutaneous disease is more common in males, with a male to female ratio of 2:1. Bone and soft tissue disease is also more common in males. Caucasians are affected more than other races. Head and neck cutaneous disease is classically seen in elderly patients. Soft tissue angiosarcoma has a peak incidence in the seventh decade of life, but it can occur even in children. Bone angiosarcoma tends to occur in adults aged 20 and older. Immunosuppressed patients such as those with AIDS are at higher risk.

Stewart-Treves syndrome is most commonly seen in patients following radical mastectomy for breast cancer. While it classically follows chronic lymphedema of many years' duration, it can occur as soon as 1 year after mastectomy, with a median interval of about 11 years. There is no known racial predilection for Stewart-Treves. Patients with Stewart-Treves syndrome are middle-aged to elderly.

***Description.*** There are four variants of cutaneous angiosarcoma recognized

- Angiosarcoma of the scalp and face (or head and neck, also known as Wilson-Jones angiosarcoma) is the most common form
- Stewart-Treves syndrome
- Radiation-induced angiosarcoma
- Epithelioid angiosarcoma, a rare, highly aggressive variant leading to death less than 5 years after presentation

Lesions are usually obvious red or purple vascular papules and plaques (Fig. 30-23). They may be multifocal, arising as multiple lesions or forming satellites around a central focus with eventual coalescence of tumor cells. Early lesions may be macular and dusky, mimicking ecchymoses or radiation dermatitis, thus evading prompt diagnosis. Subcutaneous masses and necrotic, oozing, or bleeding lesions are also reported. In the setting of chronic lymphedema with chronic skin infections and poor wound healing, it can also be difficult to identify as tumor. Rapid and steady progression in tumor size is a clue to diagnosis. Metastasis to nodes occurs in 45% of cases.

***Distribution.*** Skin and soft tissues are most commonly affected, but angiosarcoma can occur anywhere. Lesions are most commonly found on the head and neck.

***Course.*** This is an aggressive tumor with high potential for local recurrence and metastasis regardless of the time of intervention and even with the most aggressive surgical treatment. The most common cause of death in Stewart–Treves syndrome is metastasis to the chest wall and lungs.

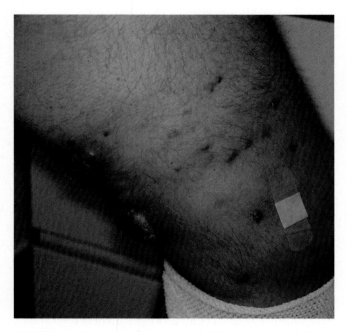

**FIGURE 30-23** ■ Angiosarcoma arising in a lymphedematous lower extremity. *(Courtesy John B. Mulliken, MD.)*

This is because the most common site of Stewart-Treves is the chest wall, following mastectomy for breast cancer. Metastasis also occurs to the liver and bones.

***Cause.*** While it is not known what molecular stimuli specifically trigger angiosarcoma, a high index of suspicion should be maintained in the following clinical scenarios:

- Primary lymphedema (e.g., congenital Milroy's disease, idiopathic disease)
- Postsurgical lymphedema in any body site
- Secondary lymphedema due to filariasis, trauma, or other obstructive chronic lymphedema
- Elderly patients with new head and neck vascular lesion(s)
- History of exposure to radiation or chemical carcinogens, even foreign materials such as shrapnel, implanted plastic grafts, surgical sponges, and bone wax

Local and systemic immunodeficiency has been considered as an underlying cause of malignant transformation in vascular cells. Local immunodeficiency has been demonstrated in lymphedematous tissues. Radiation may or may not play a direct role in the specific pathophysiology of angiosarcoma.

*Histology*

Vascular spaces are lined by and later invaded by atypical neoplastic endothelial cells. Higher-grade lesions are more cellular and display more mitoses. Low-grade tumors can be confused with more benign vascular lesions such as hemangioendotheliomas. High-grade, aggressive tumors display sheets of anaplastic cells that can be confused with melanomas and carcinomas.

Immunohistochemical staining is positive for CD34, vimentin, factor VIII–related antigen, and cytokeratins.

*Radiologic Studies*

MRI or CT scans are used for delineating the extent of involvement into deeper tissues, involvement of cervical lymph nodes, and response to therapy in head and neck angiosarcoma. Chest CT is used for assessment of lung, pleural, and mediastinal metastases. MRI with contrast is recommended for assessing extent of involvement in most soft tissues.

*Differential Diagnosis*

- Cellulitis
- Ecchymosis
- Stasis changes due to lymphedema
- Pyogenic granuloma
- Kaposi's sarcoma
- Metastasis from other neoplasms (e.g., breast carcinoma)
- Amelanotic melanoma
- Leiomyosarcoma
- Fibrosarcoma
- Liposarcoma

## Treatment

Prompt surgical excision is the primary and only proven intervention. Wide local excision (at least 5 cm) is performed, but is often insufficient. Large lesions require amputation of limbs and/or wide regional resection of affected areas, if possible. Adjuvant chemotherapy or radiotherapy generally does not confer added survival but surgery followed by radiotherapy helps with local disease control, and in focal cutaneous angiosarcoma may in fact prolong survival.

Chemotherapy and/or radiation therapy alone may be attempted if a patient refuses or is a poor candidate for surgical intervention, but this is typically unsuccessful. Surgical intervention is impractical if there is extension into vital structures, if the lesion is very extensive, or for multifocal lesions.

Doxorubicin and actinomycin D are the most commonly used chemotherapeutic agents. Paclitaxel is showing promise as a single agent for head and neck angiosarcoma, even following previous chemotherapy or radiotherapy.

Immunotherapy has been used to some effect in pleural effusions caused by metastatic angiosarcoma.

## Suggested Readings

Antman K, Chang Y. Kaposi's sarcoma. *N Engl J Med*. 2000; 342(14): 1027–1038.

Drolet BA, Esterly NB, Frieden IJ. Hemangiomas in children. *N Engl J Med*. 1999;341(3):173–181.

Hemangioma Investigator Group, Haggstrom AN et al. Prospective study of infantile hemangiomas: demographic, prenatal, and perinatal characteristics. *J Pediatr*. 2007;150(3):291–294.

Huang SA, Tu HM, Harney JW, et al. Severe hypothyroidism caused by Type 3 iodothyronine deiodinase in infantile hemangiomas. *N Engl J Med*. 2000;343(3):185–189.

Mendenhall WM, Mendenhall CM, Werning JW, et al. Cutaneous angiosarcoma. *Am J Clin Oncol*. 2006;29(5):524–528.

Metry DW, Garzon MC, Drolet BA, et al. PHACE syndrome: current knowledge, future directions. *Pediatr Dermatol*. 2009;26(4):381–398.

Mulliken JB, Fishman SJ, Burrows PE. Vascular anomalies. *Curr Probl Surg*. 2000;37(8):517–584.

Sarkar M, Mulliken JB, Kozakewich HP, et al. Thrombocytopenic coagulopathy (Kasabach–Merritt phenomenon) is associated with Kaposiform hemangioendothelioma and not with common infantile hemangioma. *Plast Reconstr Surg*. 1997;100(6):1377–1386.

# CHAPTER 31

# Cutaneous T-cell Lymphoma

*Stephen J. Nervi, MD, W. Clark Lambert, MD, PhD, and Robert A. Schwartz, MD, MPH*

## Introduction

The diagnosis of cutaneous lymphoma mandates consideration of a large and diverse group of malignant B-cell or T-cell lymphocytes in various stages of differentiation. In this chapter we focus on skin, the primary site of cutaneous lymphoma. Historically, primary cutaneous lymphomas were thought to be of T-cell origin; cutaneous B-cell lymphomas (CBCLs) were assumed to be secondary, or a dissemination of a nodal B-cell lymphoma. With the advent of immunohistochemical and molecular genetic modalities, it has become clear that B-cell cutaneous lymphomas are, in fact, a distinct and important group of primary cutaneous lymphomas. The majority are low-grade malignancies that have a good prognosis and slow course. This chapter will focus on primary cutaneous T-cell lymphomas (CTCLs).

CTCLs are the largest group of cutaneous lymphomas, accounting for 65% to 80% of all cases. They are classified by the World Health Organization (WHO)/European Organization for Research and Treatment of Cancer (EORTC) classification (WHO–EORTC classification) as follows:

- Mycosis fungoides (MF)
  - MF variants: Pagetoid reticulosis (localized), follicular, syringotropic, granulomatous, and granulomatous slack skin (GSS) syndrome
- Sézary syndrome (SS)

### SAUER'S NOTES

1. Cutaneous lymphoma is the wolf in sheep's clothing for the dermatologist. Any skin disease that does not respond to normal therapeutic intervention as would be expected, suddenly worsens in intensity or distribution, is unusually chronic, or appears to be following an unexpected course, should be suspect for lymphoma. Protean clinical manifestations of this group of diseases are the rule.

2. Can you ever biopsy the skin too frequently? I think it is very unlikely that the patient, the patient's family, the patient's referring physician, or the patient's attorney will be critical of a biopsy done to confirm benign disease. For better or worse, a biopsy not done and a malignancy missed are a recipe for problems.

- CD30$^+$ T-cell lymphoproliferative disorders of the skin
  - Lymphomatoid papulosis
  - Primary cutaneous anaplastic large cell lymphoma
- Subcutaneous panniculitis-like T-cell lymphoma (SPTL)
- Primary cutaneous peripheral T-cell lymphoma (PTL), unspecified
  - PTL subtypes:
    - Primary cutaneous aggressive epidermotropic CD8$^+$ T-cell lymphoma
    - Cutaneous gamma/delta-positive T-cell lymphoma (CGD-TCL)
    - Primary cutaneous CD4$^+$ small/medium-sized pleomorphic T-cell lymphoma
- Extranodal NK/T-cell lymphoma, nasal type
  - Variant—Hydroa vacciniforme-like lymphoma
- Adult T-cell leukemia/lymphoma (ATLL)
- Angioimmunoblastic T-cell lymphoma

CTCL, most commonly evident as MF, is usually a clonal expansion of T-helper cells, less often of T suppressor/killer cells or NK cells, manifesting as a widespread and long-standing cutaneous eruption. MF is characterized by the relatively predictable and often gradual evolution of patches into plaques and tumors composed of skin-targeting malignant T cells. This progression may be gradual and the patient may outlive the disease.

Pagetoid reticulosis is a noteworthy variant of MF characterized by the presence of localized discrete cutaneous patches or plaques with an intraepidermal proliferation of neoplastic T cells. The term pagetoid reticulosis should be restricted to the localized type (Woringer–Kolopp type) and should not be used to describe the disseminated form (Ketron–Goodman type). Generalized cases should probably be classified as aggressive epidermotropic CD8$^+$ CTCL, CGD-TCL, or tumor-stage MF.

GSS syndrome is a rare subtype of CTCL characterized by the development of folds of loose or "slack" skin in the major skin folds and, histologically, by an infiltrate of clonal T cells, with exceptionally large multinucleated giant cells sometimes showing inclusion of fragmented elastic fibers.

SS has been defined historically by the triad of erythroderma, generalized lymphadenopathy, and the presence of neoplastic T cells (Sézary cells) in skin, lymph nodes, and peripheral blood, respectively. Others assert that the definition of SS should include one or more of the following:

- An absolute Sézary cell count of least 1000/$\mu$L
- Demonstration of immunophenotypical abnormalities (an expanded CD4$^+$ T-cell population resulting in a CD4/CD8 ratio of more than 10:1; loss of any or all of the T-cell antigens CD2, CD3, CD4, CD5; or loss of both CD4 and CD5)
- Demonstration of a T-cell clone in the peripheral blood by molecular or cytogenetic methods

ATLL is an aggressive T-cell neoplasm associated with human T-cell leukemia virus 1 (HTLV-1). While an indolent form involving the skin may occur, cutaneous findings are usually a manifestation of widely disseminated disease.

SPTL is a type of T-cell lymphoma characterized by the presence of primarily subcutaneous infiltrates of neoplastic T cells and macrophages, predominantly affecting the legs and often complicated by a hemophagocytic syndrome. There are at least two groups of SPTL with different histologies, phenotypes, and prognoses. Cases with an alpha/beta-positive T-cell phenotype are usually CD8$^+$, are restricted to the subcutaneous tissue (with no dermal or epidermal involvement), and tend to run an indolent course. The SPTL designation is only used for patients with an alpha/beta-positive T-cell phenotype, whereas those with a gamma/delta T-cell phenotype are now categorized as having CGD-TCL.

Extranodal NK/T-cell lymphoma is an Epstein–Barr virus (EBV)–associated lymphoma usually with an NK cell, or, less commonly, a cytotoxic T-cell phenotype. The nasal cavity or nasopharynx is the most common site of involvement, and the skin is the second most common site. Cutaneous involvement may be primary or secondary; however, because both primary and secondary involvement are clinically aggressive and require the same type of treatment, distinction between the two cutaneous forms is largely academic.

Primary cutaneous PTL, type unspecified, encompasses those CTCLs that do not fit into any of the subtypes of CTCLs. These include the provisional entities described later, because primary cutaneous aggressive epidermotropic CD8$^+$ cytotoxic T-cell lymphoma, CGD-TCL, and primary cutaneous small/medium CD4$^+$ T-cell lymphoma are sufficiently characteristic that they can be separated as provisional entities:

- Primary cutaneous aggressive epidermotropic CD8$^+$ cytotoxic T-cell lymphoma, a provisional entity, is characterized by a proliferation of epidermotropic CD8$^+$ cytotoxic T cells and aggressive clinical behavior.
- CGD-TCL is composed of a clonal proliferation of mature, activated gamma/delta T cells with a cytotoxic phenotype. It may be a primary or secondary cutaneous lymphoma.

- Primary cutaneous CD4$^+$ small/medium-sized pleomorphic T-cell lymphoma is the diagnosis used when a predominance of small- to medium-sized CD4$^+$ pleomorphic T cells are present without a history of patches and plaques typical of MF.

## Pathophysiology

The primary pathophysiologic mechanisms for the development of CTCL (i.e., MF) have not been elucidated. Genetic, genotraumatic, immunologic, and environmental etiologies have all been considered. Chronic exposure to various irritants has been considered in the pathogenesis of CTCL, but evidence thus far is not conclusive. A persistent antigen that over time leads to an accumulation of mutations in oncogenes, suppressor genes, and signal-transducing genes has been suggested. One of us has proposed the thymus-bypass hypothesis that aberrant differentiation, in which T cells differentiate in the skin (rather than thymus), may be a cause.

## Epidemiology

In the United States, the incidence of CTCL is approximately five cases per million people per year. It is assumed that there is a similar worldwide incidence with some possible increases among workers using machine cutting oils. Areas where HTLV-1 is endemic, such as certain Caribbean Islands, parts of South America, Central Africa, and southwest Japan have a higher incidence of ATLL. In Jamaica and selected other Caribbean Islands, childhood-infective dermatitis is viewed a marker of HTLV-1 infection. CTCL is more common in men than women with an approximate ratio of 2:1. Most patients with CTCL are middle aged or elderly. Peak incidence is during the 5th decade, although it may rarely occur in children. Children with CTCL usually have a mild course and excellent prognosis, though extension to tumor stage and death may occur. There also does not seem to be a male predominance in children with one series observing a female predominance. As CTCL in its incipient stage may present as a chronic, poorly defined dermatitis, the average duration from onset to diagnosis of CTCL is 4 to 6 years. Most cases are treated with myriad topical agents preceding biopsy that obscure histologic diagnosis.

## History and Staging

### Classic MF

MF is divided into three stages: patch, plaque, and tumor (**Figs. 31-1 to 31-3**). The patch stage may persist for many years and is characterized by a nonspecific dermatitis usually consisting of patches most commonly centrally located on the lower trunk and buttocks. Sometimes, these patches have a thin, wrinkled quality, often with reticulated pigmentation. In this stage, pruritus is usually minimal or absent. Classic MF is usually preceded by a nonspecific indolent inflammatory process, manifesting as atopic dermatitis, nonspecific chronic dermatitis, or parapsoriasis (most commonly

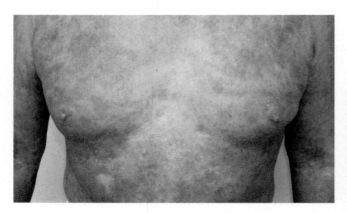

FIGURE 31-1 ■ Plaque-stage CTCL on the anterior trunk.

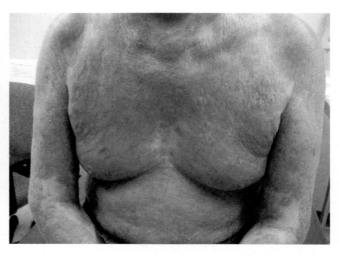

FIGURE 31-3 ■ Mycosis fungoides with partially confluent erythematous plaques.

large-plaque parapsoriasis), which may progress over years to decades to early plaque-stage MF. Some authorities regard large-plaque parapsoriasis as patch-stage MF. In many cases, the disease does not progress beyond this stage, and the diagnosis of MF is never confirmed. In other cases, the disease appears from the beginning as rather well-defined superficial plaques that range from 2 cm to more than 20 cm in diameter.

While well-developed plaques that are clinically diagnostic for MF are usually intensely pruritic, less characteristic ones typically are not, and the development of pruritus in such lesions is a sign of progression toward MF. Many cases remain at these stages for many years or decades without further progression.

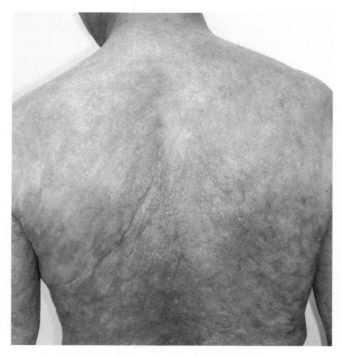

FIGURE 31-2 ■ Patch-stage CTCL with cigarette paper wrinkling atrophy and hyperpigmentation. Some areas are already forming plaques over the left lower back.

### Stages IA and IIA

The stage of disease determines the prognosis for most cases of CTCL, particularly MF and SS. Stage IA consists of patches and/or plaques affecting less than 10% of the total body surface without erythroderma, lymph node, or visceral involvement. Stage IB is defined by involvement of 10% or more of the total body surface.

### Stages IIA and IIB

CTCL is stage IIA if there are clinically enlarged lymph nodes that histologically do not show evidence of CTCL tumor cells. If skin tumors of CTCL are present with no visceral involvement or erythroderma, the disease is in stage IIB, regardless of lymph node involvement. Either process usually takes years or even decades to develop. Tumors once formed are prone to ulceration.

### Stages III, IVA, and IVB

The disease is classified as stage III if erythroderma is present but neither circulating lymphoma cells nor, histologically proven involvement of lymph nodes or viscera is present, regardless of whether lymphadenopathy is noted. If lymph nodes are histologically involved with the lymphomatous process, the disease is in stage IVA. Visceral involvement with histologically proven lymphoma denotes stage IVB.

### D'emblee MF

MF usually progresses sequentially through its stages. However, rarely the development of apparent MF tumors may occur without preceding patches or plaques. Most, if not all, such cases may represent primary cutaneous CD30+ pleomorphic, medium or large cell T-cell lymphomas.

### Transformation of MF

MF in any stage may suddenly accelerate or become much more aggressive, progressing rapidly to more advanced stages. This is associated with the histologic appearance of

**TABLE 31-1 ■ Staging of CTCL**

| | Skin Lesions | | | | | Histological Lymphoma | |
|---|---|---|---|---|---|---|---|
| Stage | Patches <10% | Plaques ≥10% | Tumors | Lymphadenopathy | Erythroderma | Lymph Nodes | Viscera |
| IA | + | − | − | − | − | − | − |
| IB | + or − | + | − | − | − | − | − |
| IIA | + or − | + or − | + or − | + | − | − | − |
| IIB | + or − | + or − | + | + or − | − | − | − |
| III | + or − | + or − | + or − | + or − | + | − | − |
| IVA | + or − | + or − | + or − | + or − | + or − | + | − |
| IVB | + or − | + or − | + or − | + or − | + or − | + or − | + |

large atypical cells. Often, these are CD30$^+$, and the process is termed large cell transformation.

### Pagetoid Reticulosis, Localized (Woringer–Kolopp) Type

Patients with this slowly progressive subtype are usually first seen with a solitary psoriasiform or hyperkeratotic patch or plaque most commonly located on the extremities. Extracutaneous dissemination or disease-related deaths rarely occur. In contrast, multilesional pagetoid reticulosis (Ketron–Goodman disease) has a clinical course similar to MF and is regarded as a variant of MF. Some cases may actually represent primary cutaneous epidermotropic CD8$^+$ (cytotoxic) T-cell lymphoma.

These definitions are depicted in Table 31-1. Table 31-2 lists the TNMB (tumor, node, metastasis, blood) stage definitions. Table 31-3 shows a comparison of the two systems.

### Variants of MF

■ Folliculotropic MF (FMF) presents commonly with alopecia, follicular cysts, or comedo-like lesions and is usually associated with follicular mucinosis and strong epidermotropism. This variant may also be called alopecia mucinosa when mucin is present. However, the benign form of alopecia mucinosa, not associated with MF, must be distinguished from MF associated with mucinosis. The most relevant feature, with and without associated follicular mucinosis, is the deep follicular and perifollicular localization of the neoplastic infiltrates, which makes them less accessible to skin-targeted therapies.

■ Hypopigmented MF tends to occur in young people of Indian, Latin American, or sub-Saharan African-American heritage. It manifests as irregular but fairly well-demarcated hypopigmented or white patches. They are either asymptomatic or slightly pruritic and may appear with or without other more characteristic MF lesions.

■ MF may demonstrate a granulomatous reaction pattern.

■ Bullous MF may present with flaccid or tense bullae arising on normal skin, an erythematous base, or

**TABLE 31-2 ■ TNMB Staging of CTCL**

| Stage Class | Stage | Definition |
|---|---|---|
| T (Tumor) | T$_1$ | Patches/plaques involving <10% of body surface |
| | T$_2$ | Patches/plaques involving ≥10% of body surface |
| | T$_3$ | Tumor(s) present on skin |
| | T$_4$ | Erythroderma |
| N (Nodes) | N$_0$ | No enlarged lymph node present |
| | N$_1$ | Enlarged lymph nodes, histologically uninvolved |
| | N$_2$ | No enlarged lymph node; one or more nodes histologically involved* |
| | N$_3$ | Enlarged lymph nodes, histologically involved |
| M (Metastasis to viscera) | M$_0$ | No visceral lesion present |
| | M$_1$ | Visceral involvement |
| B (Blood involvement) | B$_0$ | Circulating atypical lymphocytes (Sézary cells) ≤5% of lymphocytes |
| | B$_1$ | Circulating atypical lymphocytes ≥5% of lymphocytes (Sézary syndrome) |

*Uncommon finding, usually not considered/investigated.

**TABLE 31-3** ■ **Comparison of Staging Systems for CTCL**

| Clinical Stage | TNM (B) Stage | | | |
|---|---|---|---|---|
| IA | $T_1N_0M_0$ | | | |
| IB | $T_2N_0M_0$ | | | |
| IIA | $T_1N_1M_0$ | $T_2N_1M_0$ | | |
| IIB | $T_3N_0M_0$ | $T_3N_1M_0$ | | |
| III | $T_4N_0M_0$ | $T_4N_1M_0$ | | |
| IVA | $T_1N_2M_0$ | $T_2N_2M_0$ | $T_3N_2M_0$ | $T_4N_2M_0$ |
| | $T_1N_3M_0$ | $T_2N_3M_0$ | $T_3N_3M_0$ | $T_4N_3M_0$ |
| IVB | $T_1N_0M_1$ | $T_2N_0M_1$ | $T_3N_0M_1$ | $T_4N_0M_1$ |
| | $T_1N_1M_1$ | $T_2N_1M_1$ | $T_3N_1M_1$ | $T_4N_1M_1$ |
| | $T_1N_2M_1$ | $T_2N_2M_1$ | $T_3N_2M_1$ | $T_4N_2M_1$ |
| | $T_1N_3M_1$ | $T_2N_3M_1$ | $T_3N_3M_1$ | $T_4N_3M_1$ |

within typical patch- or plaque-stage lesions of MF. It most commonly is found on the trunk and extremities. Rarely, it may clinically resemble pemphigus foliaceous, pemphigus vulgaris, or erythema multiforme.

■ Pustular MF is most often found on the palms but may occur anywhere.

■ Hyperpigmented MF is a diffuse macular hyperpigmentation accompanied by typical MF, or, more rarely, as the sole manifestation of the disease. These lesions may resemble ashy dermatosis or postinflammatory hyperpigmentation.

■ Unilesional MF shows histologic changes that are identical to those that occur with multiple disseminated lesions of MF. The prognosis is excellent following treatment including excision or radiotherapy, although it may recur.

■ In addition to hair follicles (folliculotropism), MF cells may be seen in eccrine glands. Rarely, this may be the only manifestation of MF, designated as syringotropic MF (syringolymphoid hyperplasia). Both the eccrine duct and the eccrine gland may be affected and may mimic eccrine carcinoma. Lesions manifest as flesh colored, brown or red papules, patches, and/or scaly plaques. Hair loss without mucinous degeneration in the affected areas is common. All reported cases have occurred in men.

■ Pagetoid reticulosis (Woringer–Kolopp disease) arises preferentially on acral skin as a single, slowly growing psoriasiform plaque. Dissemination or extracutaneous manifestation does not occur. The classic histologic finding is the pagetoid spread of haloed lymphoid cells in the epidermis.

■ Poikilodermic MF, often evident as poikiloderma vasculare atrophicans, represents a combination of atrophic, dry, reticulated dyspigmented skin with telangiectasia developing in cases of otherwise typical MF. It can involve the entire body surface.

On occasion, it may be the only presenting manifestation of the disease.

■ Other variants of MF include hyperkeratotic/verrucous and vegetating/papillomatous MF, typically arising in the cervical neck, axillae, perineum, and sometimes on the breasts near the areolae, resembling acanthosis nigricans or multiple seborrheic keratosis.

■ Persistent pigmented purpura or lichenoid processes also may be manifestations of MF.

■ Mucosal involvement by MF is rare and may occur as part of a more generalized involvement in cases with extensive disease, particularly those that have undergone large cell transformation. It is a poor prognostic sign.

■ GSS syndrome, as described above, affects intertriginous skin, particularly axilla and groin.

Physical

■ Initially, MF has a predilection for central sun-protected areas such as the proximal lower extremities and buttocks. In tumor-stage MF, the usual presentation is a combination of patches, plaques, and tumors. The tumors are prone to ulceration. However, if only tumors are present, without preceding or concurrent patches or plaques, a diagnosis of MF is highly unlikely and another type of CTCL or CBCL should be considered.

■ SS occurs almost exclusively in adults. It is characterized by erythroderma, often associated with marked pruritus and exfoliative dermatitis, edema, and lichenification. Lymphadenopathy, alopecia, onychodystrophy, and palmoplantar hyperkeratosis are also associated.

■ GSS syndrome shows circumscribed areas of pendulous loose or slack skin with a predilection for the axillae and groin. An association with Hodgkin's lymphoma may exist. Most patients experience an indolent course of disease.

- Acute ATLL manifests with skin lesions in about 50% of cases. It is also characterized by the presence of leukemia, lymphadenopathy, organomegaly, and hypercalcemia. Skin lesions most commonly include nodules or tumors (33%), generalized papules (22%), or plaques (19%).
- SPTL is a rare form of CTCL. Patients usually present with single or multiple nodules and/or plaques, mainly involving the legs. Ulceration is rare, but constitutional symptoms may be present. Visceral or lymph node involvement is rare. SPTL may be preceded for years or decades by a seemingly benign panniculitis suggestive of chronic erythema nodosum or scalp alopecia.
- Primary cutaneous PTL, unspecified, is a heterogeneous group of diseases for which the common characteristic is a lack of typical physical features of MF.
- Cutaneous gamma/delta T-cell lymphoma lies within the PTL subset. It is usually aggressive and manifests with disseminated plaques or ulceronecrotic nodules or tumors, particularly on the extremities.
- Primary cutaneous aggressive epidermotropic CD8$^+$ cytotoxic T-cell lymphoma (provisional) manifests localized or disseminated eruptive papules, nodules, and tumors that show central ulceration and necrosis or superficial, hyperkeratotic patches and plaques.
- Primary cutaneous CD4$^+$ small/medium-sized pleomorphic T-cell lymphoma tends to be first apparent as a solitary plaque or tumor, generally on the head/neck, or upper trunk, although it may less commonly appear as one or several papules, nodules, or tumors.
- Extranodal NK/T-cell lymphoma, nasal type, usually appears as a midfacial destructive tumor or multiple plaques or tumors, often with ulceration. It preferentially occurs on the trunk and extremities. This was formerly termed lethal midline granuloma and was considered a destructive form of vasculitis. Constitutional symptoms may be present. Extranodal NK/T-cell lymphoma, nasal type, has a variant that resembles hydroa vacciniforme. It occurs in children, mainly in Latin America and Asia, and has a papulovesicular eruption that typically occurs on sun-exposed areas.

## Differential Diagnosis

Differential diagnosis includes atopic dermatitis, psoriasis, granulomatous disease, metastatic solid tumors, leukemia cutis, contact dermatitis, dermatophytosis, erythroderma, lichen planus, pemphigus foliaceous, and psoriasis.

## Lab Studies

- CTCL is a clinical and histologic diagnosis. The use of a molecular assay such as southern blot or PCR may aid in identifying a dominant lymphocyte clone in skin biopsy specimens and decipher the T-cell subtype.
- The neoplastic MF cells have a mature CD3$^+$, CD4$^+$, CD45RO$^+$, CD8$^-$ memory T-cell phenotype. Rarely, MF may have a CD4$^-$, CD8$^+$ mature T-cell phenotype. An aberrant phenotype, such as a loss of pan–T-cell antigens (e.g., CD2, CD3, CD5) is not unusual and is diagnostically helpful.

## Histologic Findings

The histopathology is nonspecific in early CTCL/MF. Thus, the condition is often misdiagnosed as a chronic inflammatory disorder. Early patches of MF show a superficial lichenoid lymphohistiocytic infiltrate. Scattered atypical lymphocytes with indented (cerebriform) and occasionally hyperchromatic nuclei are present. They are mostly confined to the epidermis. They usually are located in the basal layer of the epidermis either as single, often-haloed cells or in a linear configuration, especially at the tips of the rete ridges.

In MF plaques, the histologic changes are more clearly diagnostic. Epidermotropism is generally more pronounced. The presence of intraepidermal collections of atypical cells (Figs. 31-4 and 31-5) (Pautrier's microabscesses) is a highly characteristic feature observed in only a minority of patients. In the tumor stage, the infiltrates become more

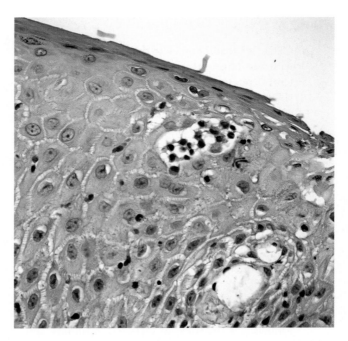

**FIGURE 31-4** ■ Five or more atypical cells surrounded by a clear space in the epidermis. This is a Pautrier's microabscess in a CTCL patient.

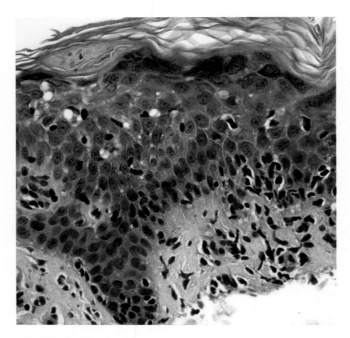

**FIGURE 31-5** ■ Atypical clusters of cells in the dermis and dermal–epidermal junction in CTCL.

diffuse and epidermotropism is less apparent. The tumor cells increase in number and size, demonstrating variable proportions of small, medium, and large cerebriform blast cells with prominent nuclei and intermediate forms. Transformation to a diffuse large cell lymphoma of either CD30⁻ or CD30+ phenotype may occur, which is a harbinger for a poor prognosis.

## Medical Care

■ CTCL/MF that is limited to the skin is often managed with skin-targeted therapies such as topical corticosteroids, photochemotherapy (e.g., psoralen plus UV-A [PUVA]), topical application of cytotoxic agents such as nitrogen mustard (mechlorethamine) and carmustine (BCNU), or radiotherapy, including total skin electron beam irradiation. Electron beam irradiation can only be used a very limited number of times because of bone marrow toxicity. Thus, it should be applied selectively bexarotene is also sometimes used for limited disease. Methotrexate (MTX) has been used, but some concern exists relating to large cell transformation. Tazarotene, long-term low-dose oral etoposide, and imiquimod may be of some value in the treatment of early CTCL. Patients with early stages of CTCL/MF should be treated relatively aggressively to avoid progression of the disease.

■ Biologic agents such as interferon-α and other cytokines (e.g., interleukin-2 [IL-2]), retinoids, and receptor-targeted cytotoxic fusion proteins (e.g., DAB389I-2; denileukin diftitox) are being used increasingly. Other agents include the IL-2 fusion toxin (Ontak), IL-12, pentostatin (a potent adenosine deaminase inhibitor), histone deacetylase inhibitors (e.g., depsipeptide), NF-κB inhibitors, cytokine receptor antagonists, immunomodulatory therapies, and allogeneic stem cell therapy. Combination therapy with bexarotene and PUVA should be considered for patients with treatment-resistant CTCL refractory to monotherapy. However, the precise use of these new treatments is yet to be established. Various regimens may be palliative but may not have an impact on prolonging overall survival.

■ Multiagent chemotherapy is used when lymph node or systemic involvement is present or in cases with widespread tumor-stage MF that is refractory to skin-targeted therapies.

■ Perifollicular disease in FMF is often less responsive to skin-targeted therapies than classic plaque-stage MF. In these cases, total skin electron beam irradiation is superior. However, because sustained complete remissions are rarely achieved with electron beam therapy, PUVA combined with retinoids or interferon-α may be used. Cysts and comedones found in follicular CTCL may benefit from isotretinoin therapy.

■ Extracorporeal photopheresis, either alone or in combination with other treatment modalities (e.g., interferon-α), is useful for SS and erythrodermic MF, with overall response rates of 30% to 80% and complete response rates of 14% to 25%. Beneficial results have also been described with interferon-α, either alone or in combination with PUVA therapy, prolonged treatment with a combination of low-dose chlorambucil (2 to 4 mg/d) and prednisone (10 to 20 mg/d), or with MTX (5 to 25 mg/wk), but complete responses are rare. Skin-directed therapies such as PUVA or potent topical steroids are good adjuvant therapies. Beneficial effects of bexarotene and alemtuzumab (anti-CD52) have been noted, but the long-term effects of these therapies remain to be established.

## Prognosis

■ As previously noted, the prognosis for CBCLs is generally good to excellent. The prognosis for CTCL/MF is dependent on stage and, in particular, the type and extent of skin lesions and the presence of visceral or lymph node involvement. Patients with limited patch/plaque-stage MF have similar life expectancies to age-, sex-, and race-matched control populations. For example, 10-year disease-specific survival rates were 97% to 98% for patients with limited patch/plaque disease (covering < 10% of the skin surface), 83% for patients with generalized patch/plaque disease (covering >10% of the skin surface), 42% for patients with tumor-stage disease, and approximately 20% for patients with histologically documented lymph node involvement. Patients with effaced lymph nodes, visceral involvement, and transformation to large T-cell lymphoma have an aggressive clinical course and usually die of systemic involvement or infections. Blood eosinophilia may also serve as a poor prognostic indicator.

■ The prognosis associated with FMF is worse than that for classic patch- and plaque-stage MF and corresponds more closely with tumor-stage disease (stage IIB). FMF has a 5-year survival rate of approximately 70% to 80%.

■ In SS, the prognosis is poor, with a median survival of 2 to 4 years. The 5-year survival rate has been reported to be 24%, with most patients dying of infection from immunosuppression.

■ In patients with ATLL, the clinical subtype is the main prognostic factor. Survival in persons with acute or lymphomatous variants is poor, ranging from 2 weeks to over 1 year. Chronic and smoldering forms have a more protracted clinical course and a longer survival, but transformation into an acute phase with an aggressive course can develop.

■ SPTL (with a CD8$^+$, alpha/beta$^+$ T-cell phenotype) tends to have a protracted clinical course with recurrent subcutaneous nodules but without extracutaneous spread. The 5-year survival rate of such patients may be greater than 80%.

■ Unilesional pagetoid reticulosis (Woringer–Kolopp disease) has an excellent prognosis due to its slow progression.

■ Primary cutaneous PTL, type unspecified, is also associated with a poor prognosis, with 5-year survival rates of less than 20%.

■ Primary cutaneous CD4$^+$ small/medium pleomorphic T-cell lymphoma (provisional entity) is associated with a more favorable prognosis, with an estimated 5-year survival of approximately 60% to 80%. Patients with solitary or localized skin lesions usually have an excellent prognosis.

■ Primary cutaneous aggressive epidermotropic CD8$^+$ cytotoxic T-cell lymphoma often has an aggressive clinical course, and patients have a median survival of 32 months.

■ CGD-TCL patients tend to have aggressive disease recalcitrant to both multiagent chemotherapy and radiation, with a median survival in one study of 15 months. Subcutaneous fat involvement is a poor prognostic indicator.

■ Nasal type NK/T-cell lymphoma manifesting in the skin is highly aggressive, and patients have a median survival of less than 1 year. The most important factor predicting a poor outcome is the presence of extracutaneous involvement at baseline or initial presentation. CD30$^+$ and CD56$^+$ tumor cells may indicate a better prognosis, possibly identifying examples of cutaneous anaplastic large cell lymphoma with coexpression of CD56.

## Suggested Readings

Barrionuevo C, Anderson VM, Zevallos-Giampietri E, et al. Hydroa-like cutaneous T-cell lymphoma: a clinicopathologic and molecular genetic study of 16 pediatric cases from Peru. *Appl Immunohistochem Mol Morphol.* 2002;10(1):7–14.

Bekkenk MW, Jansen PM, Meijer CJ, et al. CD56+ hematological neoplasms presenting in the skin: a retrospective analysis of 23 new cases and 130 cases from the literature. *Ann Oncol.* 2004;15(7):1097–1108.

Bekkenk MW, Vermeer MH, Jansen PM, et al. Peripheral T-cell lymphomas unspecified presenting in the skin: analysis of prognostic factors in a group of 82 patients. *Blood.* 2003;102(6):2213–2219.

Beljaards RC, Meijer CJ, Van der Putte SC, et al. Primary cutaneous T-cell lymphoma: clinicopathological features and prognostic parameters of 35 cases other than mycosis fungoides and CD30-positive large cell lymphoma. *J Pathol.* 1994;172(1):53–60.

Berthelot C, Rivera A, Duvic M. Skin directed therapy for mycosis fungoides: a review. *J Drugs Dermatol.* 2008;7(7):655–666.

Berti E, Tomasini D, Vermeer MH, et al. Primary cutaneous CD8-positive epidermotropic cytotoxic T cell lymphomas. A distinct clinicopathological entity with an aggressive clinical behavior. *Am J Pathol.* 1999;155(2):483–492.

Burg G, Kempf W. Etiology and pathogenesis of cutaneous lymphomas. In: Burg G, Kempf W, eds. *Cutaneous Lymphomas.* London: Taylor & Francis; 2005.

Burg G, Kempf W. Therapy of cutaneous lymphomas. In: Burg G, Kempf W, eds. *Cutaneous Lymphomas.* London: Taylor & Francis; 2005:475–528.

Burg G, Kempf W, Cozzio A, et al. WHO/EORTC classification of cutaneous lymphomas 2005: histological and molecular aspects. *J Cutan Pathol.* 2005;32(10):647–674.

Burg G, Kempf W, Cozzio A, et al. Cutaneous malignant lymphomas: update 2006. *J Dtsch Dermatol Ges.* 2006;4(11):914–933.

Burg G, Kempf W, Drummer R. Cutaneous lymphoma, leukemia, and related disorders. In: Schwartz RA, ed. *Skin Cancer Recognition and Management.* 2nd ed. Oxford: Blackwell; 238–266.

Chan JK, Sin VC, Wong KF, et al. Nonnasal lymphoma expressing the natural killer cell marker CD56: a clinicopathologic study of 49 cases of an uncommon aggressive neoplasm. *Blood.* 1997;89(12):4501–4513.

Clarijs M, Poot F, Laka A, et al. Granulomatous slack skin: treatment with extensive surgery and review of the literature. *Dermatology.* 2003;206(4):393–397.

Dummer R, Asagoe K, Cozzio A, et al. Recent advances in cutaneous lymphomas. *J Dermatol Sci.* 2007;48(3):157–167.

El Shabrawi-Caelen L, Cerroni L, Kerl H. The clinicopathologic spectrum of cytotoxic lymphomas of the skin. *Semin Cutan Med Surg.* 2000;19(2):118–123.

Foss F. Overview of cutaneous T-cell lymphoma: prognostic factors and novel therapeutic approaches. *Leuk Lymphoma.* 2003;44(suppl 3):S55–S61.

Haghighi B, Smoller BR, LeBoit PE, et al. Pagetoid reticulosis (Woringer–Kolopp disease): an immunophenotypic, molecular, and clinicopathologic study. *Mod Pathol.* 2000;13(5):502–510.

Jaffe ES, Krenacs L, Raffeld M. Classification of cytotoxic T-cell and natural killer cell lymphomas. *Semin Hematol.* 2003;40(3):175–184.

Jones GW, Hoppe RT, Glatstein E. Electron beam treatment for cutaneous T-cell lymphoma. *Hematol Oncol Clin North Am.* 1995;9(5):1057–1076.

Knobler E. Current management strategies for cutaneous T-cell lymphoma. *Clin Dermatol.* 2004;22(3):197–208.

La Grenade L, Janniger CK, Schwartz RA. Tropical dermatitis with special emphasis on infective dermatitis as a marker of HTLV-1 infection. *Cutis.* 1996;58:115–118.

Lambert WC, Gianotti B, Van Vloten WA, et al. Basic Mechanism of Physiologic and Aberrant Lymphoproliferation in the Skin. New York: Plenum Press, (Nato ASI Series B. Life Sciences. No. 265) 1994:657.

Lambert WC, Cohen PJ, Schwartz RA. Surgical management of mycosis fungoides. *J Med.* 1997;28(3–4):211–222.

Lambert WC, Schwartz RA. Dermatitic precursors of mycosis fungoides. In: Schwartz RA, ed. *Skin Cancer Recognition and Management.* 2nd ed. Oxford: Blackwell; 2008:227–237.

Leverkus M, Rose C, Brocker EB, et al. Follicular cutaneous T-cell lymphoma: beneficial effect of isotretinoin for persisting cysts and comedones. *Br J Dermatol.* 2005;152(1):193–194.

Lundin J, Hagberg H, Repp R, et al. Phase 2 study of alemtuzumab (anti-CD52 monoclonal antibody) in patients with advanced mycosis fungoides/Sezary syndrome. *Blood.* 2003;101(11):4267–4272.

Mao X, Lillington D, Scarisbrick JJ, et al. Molecular cytogenetic analysis of cutaneous T-cell lymphomas: identification of common genetic alterations in Sézary syndrome and mycosis fungoides. *Br J Dermatol.* 2002;147(3):464–475.

Marzano AV, Berti E, Paulli M, et al. Cytophagic histiocytic panniculitis and subcutaneous panniculitis-like T-cell lymphoma: report of 7 cases. *Arch Dermatol.* 2000;136(7):889–896.

Massone C, Chott A, Metze D, et al. Subcutaneous, blastic natural killer (NK), NK/T-cell, and other cytotoxic lymphomas of the skin: a morphologic, immunophenotypic, and molecular study of 50 patients. *Am J Surg Pathol.* 2004;28(6):719–735.

Miyamoto T, Yoshino T, Takehisa T, et al. Cutaneous presentation of nasal/nasal type T/NK cell lymphoma: clinicopathological findings of four cases. *Br J Dermatol.* 1998;139(3):481–487.

Mraz-Gernhard S, Natkunam Y, Hoppe RT, et al. Natural killer/natural killer-like T-cell lymphoma, CD56+, presenting in the skin: an increasingly recognized entity with an aggressive course. *J Clin Oncol.* 2001;19(8):2179–2188.

Natkunam Y, Smoller BR, Zehnder JL, et al. Aggressive cutaneous NK and NK-like T-cell lymphomas: clinicopathologic, immunohistochemical, and molecular analyses of 12 cases. *Am J Surg Pathol.* 1999;23(5): 571–581.

Pimpinelli N, Olsen EA, Santucci M, et al. Defining early mycosis fungoides. *J Am Acad Dermatol.* 2005;53(6):1053–1063.

Russell-Jones R. Diagnosing erythrodermic cutaneous T-cell lymphoma. *Br J Dermatol.* 2005;153(1):1–5.

Santucci M, Biggeri A, Feller AC, et al. Efficacy of histologic criteria for diagnosing early mycosis fungoides: an EORTC cutaneous lymphoma study group investigation. European Organization for Research and Treatment of Cancer. *Am J Surg Pathol.* 2000;24(1):40–50.

Santucci M, Pimpinelli N, Massi D, et al. Cytotoxic/natural killer cell cutaneous lymphomas. Report of EORTC Cutaneous Lymphoma Task Force Workshop. *Cancer.* 2003;97(3):610–627.

Schwartz RA, Lambert WC. *Cutaneous T-cell lymphoma. eMedicine Dematology 2009.* Available at http://emedicine.medscape.com/article/1098342-overview.

Senff NJ, Noordijk EM, Kim YH, et al. European Organization for Research and Treatment of Cancer and International Society for Cutaneous Lymphoma consensus recommendations for the management of cutaneous B-cell lymphomas. *Blood.* 2008;112(5):1600–1609.

Setoyama M, Katahira Y, Kanzaki T. Clinicopathologic analysis of 124 cases of adult T-cell leukemia/lymphoma with cutaneous manifestations: the smouldering type with skin manifestations has a poorer prognosis than previously thought. *J Dermatol.* 1999;26(12):785–790.

Shimoyama M. Diagnostic criteria and classification of clinical subtypes of adult T-cell leukaemia–lymphoma. A report from the Lymphoma Study Group (1984–87). *Br J Haematol.* 1991;79(3):428–437.

Smoller BR, Santucci M, Wood GS, et al. Histopathology and genetics of cutaneous T-cell lymphoma. *Hematol Oncol Clin North Am.* 2003;17(6): 1277–1311.

van Doorn R, Scheffer E, Willemze R. Follicular mycosis fungoides, a distinct disease entity with or without associated follicular mucinosis: a clinicopathologic and follow-up study of 51 patients. *Arch Dermatol.* 2002;138(2):191–198.

Vonderheid EC, Bernengo MG, Burg G, et al. Update on erythrodermic cutaneous T-cell lymphoma: report of the International Society for Cutaneous Lymphomas. *J Am Acad Dermatol.* 2002;46(1):95–106.

Vural F, Saydam G, Cagirgan S, et al. Primary cutaneous B-cell lymphoma: report of eight cases and review of the literature. *Int J Dermatol.* 2008;47(7):675–680.

Willemze R, Jaffe ES, Burg G, et al. WHO–EORTC classification for cutaneous lymphomas. *Blood.* 2005;105(10):3768–3785.

Willemze R, Jansen PM, Cerroni, BE, et al. Subcutaneous panniculitis-like T-cell lymphoma: definition, classification, and prognostic factors: an EORTC Cutaneous Lymphoma Group Study of 83 cases. *Blood.* 2008; 111:838–845.

Yi SR, Schwartz RA. Human T-lymphotropic virus type I-associated dermatitis: Human T-lymphotropic virus type I-associated infective dermatitis: a comprehensive review. J Am Acad Dermatol (in press).

# CHAPTER 32

# Diseases Affecting the Hair

*Thelda M. Kestenbaum, MD*

Hair is an extremely important part of an individual's appearance and sense of identity. Loss of hair on the scalp or an excessive amount of unwanted hair on other body parts causes great psychologic distress. Our perception of femininity and masculinity is greatly affected by hair quantity, hair distribution, and hair styling.

## Hair Physiology

There are three types of hairs: lanugo, vellus, and terminal hairs. Lanugo hairs are long, unmedullated hairs seen in utero and are shed during the end of pregnancy and the first several months postpartum. Vellus (or intermediate hairs) are short, nonpigmented hairs produced by follicles that penetrate only into the papillary dermis. Terminal hairs are produced by follicles that penetrate into the reticular dermis and are usually medullated (have a medulla), and are wider than the inner root sheath of the follicle that produces them. Hairs on the scalp and beard area are examples of terminal hairs. In the inherited types of balding some terminal hairs are lost and vellus hairs are seen instead.

Hair growth is not a continuous process. There is an anagen (growth) phase (about 85% to 95% of scalp hairs), a catagen (regressive) phase (about 1% of scalp hairs), and a telogen (resting) phase (about 10% to 15% of scalp hairs). The length of the anagen phase determines the length of the hair. Human scalp hair anagen phase is usually between 2 and 6 years, and the hair on the scalp grows about 1 cm/month. Therefore, some people can never have very long hair on the scalp even if they never cut their hair. Growth phases of hair on other body parts are much shorter than on the scalp. It is normal to lose between 50 and 100 scalp hairs per day. Plucking the resting hairs from follicles that have already entered anagen can advance the onset of the next anagen phase. Shaving the hair has no effect on the hair cycle. The telogen phase is the period between the completion of follicular regression (catagen) and the onset of the next anagen phase. On the human scalp, telogen phase lasts about 2 to 4 months, whereas catagen phase on the human scalp lasts 2 to 4 weeks.

With aging or with the inherited type of hair loss there is a shortening of the anagen phase and a lengthening of time between telogen and a new anagen phase. Hair cycles are influenced by multiple factors such as the season and a change in hormonal status as seen in pregnancy. Seasonal changes in hair shedding are usually not noticeable but are important when conducting studies on treatment of hair loss. During pregnancy there is an increase in the proportion of follicles in anagen, and postpartum there is an increase in the proportion of hairs in telogen, which results in a marked increase in shedding usually 3 months (1 to 5 months) postpartum. This problem rectifies itself usually within a year or less.

Hairs vary in diameter and number in different racial groups. The diameter of Asian hair is the widest and is round in cross section. Caucasian hair is round to oval in cross section. Black hair is more elliptical or flattened in cross section; black hair follicles are spiral in shape. The volume of the hair papilla determines the size of the hair shaft.

Hair amount varies among races with Caucasians (especially those of southern European extraction) generally being hairier than other racial groups. The number of scalp hairs is 10% greater in blonds and 10% less in redheads compared to Caucasian brunettes. Blacks have significantly fewer hair follicles and more fragile hair than Caucasians.

*Graying* of the hair is a normal process of aging and develops in Caucasians about a decade earlier than in blacks. Graying earlier than 20 years of age is considered premature in Caucasians, and graying earlier than 30 years of age is considered premature in blacks. By 50 years of age, the average Caucasian is 50% gray. In Caucasians, the age of onset of graying varies from 24 to 44 years; in blacks from 34 to 54 years; and in Asians in the 30s. Premature graying has been associated with pernicious anemia as well as thyroid disease (usually hyperthyroidism, may be seen with hypothyroidism), and a host of unusual inherited syndromes. A frontal white patch of hair may be inherited as an autosomal dominant trait (piebaldism). People with alopecia areata may note regrowing hairs that are light in color. People who are said to have "turned gray overnight" probably are those with "salt and pepper" hair that developed a diffuse form of alopecia areata in which the dark hairs were lost preferentially to the gray hairs.

Many people color their hair. The most common chemical used to dye the hair is paraphenylenediamine, which is sometimes the cause of a contact dermatitis.

## Hirsutism and Hypertrichosis

Hirsutism is the excessive growth of terminal hair in a male sexual pattern in a female or a child. Hypertrichosis is the hair growth that is abnormal for the age, gender, or race of an

**TABLE 32-1 ■ Drugs That Can Cause Hirsutism and Hypertrichosis**

| | Drug |
|---|---|
| **Hirsutism** | Androgens |
| | Danazol |
| | Progesterone |
| **Hypertrichosis** | Acetazolamide |
| | Corticosteroids |
| | Cyclosporine |
| | Diazoxide |
| | Interferon |
| | Latanoprost |
| | Minoxidil |
| | Penicillamine |
| | Phenytoin |
| | Psoralens |
| | Streptomycin |

individual or for a particular area of the body. Medications can cause either of these problems (Table 32-1).

## Hirsutism

The prevalence of hirsutism in women overall is said to vary from 5% to 15%. The most common diagnosis associated with hirsutism is polycystic ovary syndrome (PCOS). Overall, about 5% to 15% of cases of hirsutism are idiopathic, but about 50% of cases of mild hirsutism are idiopathic.

Asian and Scandinavian women are generally less hairy than Caucasian women of Mediterranean ancestry, so sometimes it is difficult to judge when the hair growth in women is abnormal. Also, menopausal women who are not on hormone replacement may note some hirsutism. Androgen excess and drug-induced hirsutism need to be ruled out. Laboratory tests should be guided by the history and physical examination. Certainly, other signs of virilization such as severe acne would lead one to do a more aggressive hormonal evaluation. In mild hirsutism, when menses are regular and there are no features to suggest other causes, holding off on further laboratory testing is reasonable.

If hirsutism is moderate or severe or there are features suggestive of a secondary cause, then androgen levels and ultrasonographic examination of the ovaries, adrenals, or both may be in order. Pelvic ultrasonography may be useful in establishing the diagnosis of PCOS. Plasma-free testosterone is 50% more sensitive than total testosterone for detecting androgen excess and is the best single indicator of hyperandrogenism. The most reliable method of establishing free testosterone is by computing it from the levels of total testosterone and the sex hormone binding globulin (SHBG). Finding a reputable laboratory for establishing this information is imperative.

In females with androgen excess, 1.5% to 2.5% have nonclassic congenital adrenal hyperplasia and 0.2% have androgen-secreting tumors (half of these tumors are malignant). Other causes of androgen excess include Cushing's syndrome, hyperprolactinemia, acromegaly, and thyroid dysfunction. About 8% of hirsute women have idiopathic hyperandrogenism.

Sometimes a serum testosterone and 17-α-hydroxyprogesterone may be sufficient, but women with irregular menses and hirsutism should be screened for thyroid dysfunction and prolactin disorders. A dehydroepiandrosterone sulfate (DHEAS) test is useful for screening for adrenal tumors but is not reliable for screening late-onset congenital adrenal hyperplasia. The presence of striae, central obesity, and peripheral weakness make the diagnosis of Cushing's syndrome possible where a 24-h urine free cortisol test would be indicated.

Normally 78% of the testosterone in women is bound to SHBG, only 1% to 2% is free (which is the bioactive portion), and 20% is bound to albumin. SHBG may be reduced in amount by obesity, hypothyroidism, and hyperinsulinemia, thereby increasing free testosterone levels and therefore possibly leading to hirsutism.

An early-morning follicular phase 17-α-progesterone level is one of the better tests to screen for congenital adrenal hyperplasia. There are some rare enzyme deficiencies that can lead to congenital adrenal hyperplasia that might be better treated by an endocrinologist.

PCOS has a prevalence of 5% to 10% in all women and is the most common diagnosis associated with hirsutism. Stein and Leventhal were the first to describe this syndrome of amenorrhea, obesity, and hirsutism in association with sclerocystic ovaries. PCOS may be better described as chronic anovulation and hyperandrogenism with the exclusion of androgen-secreting tumors, nonclassic adrenal hyperplasia, and hyperprolactinemia. Currently, PCOS is said to be characterized by the presence of two or more of the following: chronic oligo-ovulation or anovulation, androgen excess, and polycystic ovaries. Usually these women have hirsutism, irregular menses, acne, and alopecia.

Insulin resistance with compensatory hyperinsulinemia is a prominent feature in many but not all cases of PCOS. Prevalence of type 2 diabetes is 10 times the rate of normal women. In women with PCOS the prevalence of metabolic syndrome is two to three times the rate in normal women and it may be that the prevalence of fatal myocardial infarction (if oligomenorrhea is severe) may be double the rate of normal women. Commonly found laboratory abnormalities in PCOS include an elevated total testosterone (about twice the normal), an elevated luteinizing hormone (LH) level (at least twice the value for follicle stimulating hormone (FSH)), a slight elevation in prolactin, and a slight elevation in DHEAS. The PSA (prostate-specific antigen) test may or may not be helpful in distinguishing women with PCOS from those with idiopathic hirsutism.

Treatment of hirsutism involves finding the cause and obtaining the help of an endocrinologist in some cases. Oral spironolactone (Aldactone) may be helpful in PCOS and idiopathic hirsutism. Spironolactone interferes with androgen biosynthesis, blocks the action of androgens at the receptor level, and decreases the 5-α-reductase levels in the follicle. Six months' treatment of spironolactone at 100 to 200 mg/day is at least worth a trial. It is important that this should not be given to women who are not using adequate contraception since it is teratogenic (it is a pregnancy category D drug). Oral contraceptives, flutamide (not approved by the FDA), finasteride, and cyproterone acetate (this is an ingredient in the contraceptive pill called Dianette, which is not available in the United States) are some other treatments that are available. The use of the antihyperglycemic metformin does reduce markers of insulin resistance in PCOS, and this may help treat hirsutism. Eflornithine hydrochloride (Vaniqa) cream is an irreversible inhibitor of ornithine decarboxylase that slows (but does not remove hair) hair growth and has been approved by the FDA for treatment of facial hirsutism. Maximal effect is seen by 8–24 weeks of use with marked improvement in 32% of users (compared to 8% marked improvement in the placebo group). This drug is used systemically for treatment of African trypanosomiasis, and its side effect of hair loss has been utilized in the development of it as a cream for treatment of facial hirsutism. Removal of hair as discussed under treatment of hypertrichosis may be a helpful adjunct to treatments mentioned here.

## Hypertrichosis

Hypertrichosis is the hair growth that is abnormal for the age, gender, or race of an individual or for a particular area of the body. It may result from the conversion of vellus hairs to terminal hairs, more hairs being in a prolonged anagen (growth) phase (and therefore a decrease in the number of hairs in the telogen phase) or an increase in hair follicle density.

It may be helpful to divide hypertrichosis into *congenital or acquired* and then into *generalized and localized* types.

Congenital generalized hypertrichosis and congenital hypertrichosis lanuginosa both are very rare inherited disorders; "dog-faced" or "monkey-faced" people in circus sideshows may have had the former diagnosis. Congenital hypertrichosis may be a feature of numerous inherited syndromes such as mucopolysaccharidoses, leprechaunism, and Cornelia de Lange syndrome. Of particular note is that fetuses exposed to hydantoin (Dilantin) *during the first 9 weeks* of gestation may have hypertrichosis as part of the fetal hydantoin syndrome. Hypertrichosis may also be seen in fetal alcohol syndrome.

Congenital localized hypertrichosis over the vertebral column (faun tail) may be a marker of an underlying spinal abnormality. Magnetic resonance imaging is strongly recommended in such cases since the underlying problems may require early surgical intervention to prevent neurologic damage. Congenital hypertrichosis of the ears may be seen in the babies of diabetic mothers or in babies with XYY syndrome. Hairy elbows may be present at birth or acquired, and may or may not be associated with other abnormalities.

Acquired hypertrichosis may be generalized or localized. Generalized acquired hypertrichosis may be seen as acquired hypertrichosis lanuginosa (malignant down), which is a rare, but striking, marker of an internal malignancy (usually lung or colon cancer but a multiplicity of underlying tumors have been associated). Multiple normal hair follicles revert to lanugo hair usually starting on the face and progressing caudally. Generalized acquired hypertrichosis may occur in diverse conditions, including porphyrias, dermatomyositis, anorexia nervosa, mercury intoxication (acrodynia), insulin-resistant diabetes, hypothyroidism, posten cephalitis, multiple sclerosis, head injuries, and POEMS syndrome (*P*olyneuropathy, *O*rganomegaly, *E*ndocrinopathy, *M*onoclonal gammopathy *S*kin changes: hyperpigmentation, hypertrichosis, skin thickening, edema, digital clubbing, cutaneous angiomas, among other possible signs). Multiple drugs can cause hypertrichosis (see Table 32-1). Some cause generalized and some localized hypertrichosis. A newer drug in this latter category is one for treatment of glaucoma called latanoprost which is a prostaglandin $F_{2\alpha}$ analogue that causes hypertrichosis and hyperpigmentation of the eyelashes in most (77%) patients using it. (Unfortunately, latanoprost was not helpful for treatment of eyebrow alopecia areata.)

Localized acquired hypertrichosis on the pinnae may be an inherited trait (especially in men from India), or it may be seen with diabetes or with acquired immunodeficiency syndrome (AIDS). Localized hypertrichosis may develop under orthopaedic casts, or in areas that are chronically traumatized such as lichen simplex chronicus (neurodermatitis), areas in which habitual self-inflicted biting occurs (dermatophagia), over thrombophlebitis or over areas of osteomyelitis.

Treatment of hypertrichosis may include shaving, depilatories, bleaching, plucking, waxing (a sort of plucking of multiple hairs simultaneously), laser, and electrolysis. Electrolysis may require more than one treatment and should be carried out by someone trained in the procedure and who uses sterile needles so as to prevent transmission of bloodborne disease. Shaving, contrary to popular belief, does not increase the amount of hair that regrows. Chemical depilatories and bleaching agents are available over the counter and frequently prove effective, but they may irritate the skin of some users. Waxing and plucking have the advantage of removing the unwanted hair for longer periods without retreatment than does shaving or chemical removal. Electrolysis can cause scarring and is expensive. Laser (usually 694 to 1064 nm wavelengths) may be helpful in selected cases but may cause scarring. Light-skinned women with dark hair are the best candidates for laser.

## Alopecia (Hair Loss)

Alopecia of the scalp is of considerable concern to men and women. It is helpful in differentiating among the many causes of alopecia to examine the hair and scalp and observe whether the scalp is scarred or nonscarred and whether the hair loss is diffuse (the most common type) or

**TABLE 32-2 ■ Nonscarring and Scarring Hair Loss**

*Nonscarring Hair Loss*

Diffuse
  Androgenic* (female pattern; male pattern)
  Telogen effluvium
    Illness
    Postpartum
    Sudden weight loss
    Medication
    Toxins
  Endocrinopathy (hypothyroidism; hyperthyroidism)
  Alopecia areata
  Loose anagen syndrome

Patchy
  Tinea capitis
  Alopecia areata
  Trichotillomania
  Syphilis
  Traumatic (traction)
  Loose anagen syndrome

*Scarring Hair Loss*

Tinea†
Trauma (traction)
Tumors (malignant or benign)
Skin diseases (such as sarcoid; scleroderma)
Lymphocytic
  Central centrifugal cicatricial alopecia (CCCA)‡
  Discoid lupus§
  Lichen planopilaris
    Frontal fibrosing alopecia
  Pseudopelade of Brocq

Neutrophilic
  Folliculitis decalvans
  Dissecting cellulitis

Mixed
  Acne keloidalis
  Acne necrotica
  Erosive pustular dermatosis

---

*It is usually nonscarring; perhaps scarring can result in some cases.
†Usually nonscarring.
‡Formerly called "hot comb alopecia" or "follicular degeneration syndrome." CCCA may include pseudopelade, folliculitis decalvans, and some cases of acne keloidalis and dissecting cellulitis.
§May be seen in SLE; SLE patients may also have diffuse nonscarring hair loss.

---

patchy (Table 32-2). Establishing whether the hair is coming out by the roots or breaking off will help guide the physician how to proceed with the workup. If the hair loss is scarring, a scalp biopsy early on will probably prove helpful. If the hair is breaking off, fungal infection, trauma, or hair shaft defects are more likely causes. Loss of up to one-half of the scalp hair may occur before the hair loss is clinically obvious on casual inspection.

**SAUER'S NOTES**

1. Believe the complaint of diffuse hair loss in a patient who clinically appears to have a normal amount of scalp hair because one has to lose almost half the hair before it is clinically apparent.
2. It is normal to lose 50 to 100 scalp hairs per day.
3. In a patient with normal nutrition there are no vitamin supplements that make the hair grow faster or thicker.
4. Shaving does not increase the number of hairs; plucking can advance the onset of the next anagen (growth) phase.

## Nonscarring Diffuse Alopecia

This accounts for the vast majority of people presenting with hair loss. Among the more common causes are androgenetic (androgenic, male pattern or female pattern), telogen effluvium, diffuse alopecia areata, and tinea capitis. A detailed history, past medical history, review of systems, medication history, family history, and social history are helpful, and appropriate laboratory testing can then be obtained (Table 32-3). A gradual onset over more than a year is more likely to point to androgenetic hair loss.

*Androgenetic (androgenic, pattern hair loss, female pattern hair loss, male pattern hair loss, diffuse hormonal alopecia, common baldness)* is the most common cause of diffuse nonscarring hair loss in men and women. Some forms may be scarring but this is still being sorted out (see Scarring Alopecia section). Most laypeople can diagnose this in men but it is much more difficult to diagnose in women. It is an inherited hair loss induced by androgens in men and in some women who are genetically predisposed. Prevalence is over 50% of men and probably a similar number of women by menopause. Caucasians are more likely to have this than other racial groups. In men, androgenetic hair loss is both

**TABLE 32-3 ■ Laboratory Studies to Evaluate Nonscarring Alopecia**

Baseline
  Complete blood cell count
  Ferritin
  VDRL with dilutions
  Thyroid screening
  Microscopic examination of hair
  Fungal culture

Other
  Scalp biopsy
  Antinuclear antibody
  Hormones (e.g., dehydroepiandrosterone sulfate, testosterone, androstenedione)
  Borate and thallium levels
  Heavy metal screens

genetic and androgen dependent and can be inherited from either or both parents. In women with androgenetic hair loss (better termed female pattern hair loss), probably only a subset of them that have PCOS are truly the female counterparts of male pattern baldness. Clinically, both men and women with androgenetic hair loss have notable loss of hair on the top of the scalp (vertex, frontal, bitemporal, or mid-scalp). Men have a more severe amount of hair loss than do women, generally speaking. It used to be thought that in women with female pattern hair loss the frontal hairline was retained (unlike in men) and this could help distinguish it from telogen effluvium in which there is often a temporal recession. Olsen has pointed out that many women with female pattern hair loss have a frontal accentuation of hair loss, which may encroach on the frontal hairline in a "Christmas tree"-like pattern (with the base of the tree being the frontal hairline). The inheritance of androgenetic hair loss in men is probably autosomal dominant with variable penetrance and expression. This may not be true for androgenetic hair loss in women (female pattern hair loss), which is a more heterogeneous group. It can be stated that women with female pattern hair loss who are less than 50 years of age have a positive family history in their mothers and male relatives in over 50% of cases. It is probably polygenic in inheritance. Severe female pattern hair loss in women may be a marker of insulin resistance and these women are perhaps more likely to have a paternal history of alopecia than women with a milder version of this problem. Female pattern hair loss is the preferred term and its onset may be early (teens to 3rd decade) or late (5th decade) with or without androgen excess. It is best to classify it in this way especially when reporting clinical trials of treatment. Most women with female pattern hair loss do not have androgen excess, and androgen excess alone does not cause female pattern hair loss.

A workup to exclude other causes of hair loss such as medications, telogen effluvium, diffuse alopecia areata, and loose anagen syndrome is important (see Table 32-3). A detailed history and physical examination should help dictate how extensive the workup should be.

Treatment of the inherited types of alopecia includes minoxidil (Rogaine, 2% or 5%) for men or for women with the exclusion of women of childbearing years who are not using adequate contraception. Only 2% minoxidil concentration is approved for use in women but probably 5% is slightly more effective. Minoxidil 5% now comes in a new foam as well as the solution form. The foam does not contain propylene glycol and so may be less irritating and less likely to cause a contact dermatitis. Minoxidil (Rogaine) is a vasodilator in hypertension, and this may be just one of the mechanisms that makes it useful for treatment of alopecia. Side effects of topical minoxidil include contact or irritant dermatitis (in less than 8%) and facial hypertrichosis in women using it (in at least 3% to 5% of those using the 2% concentration). Frequently changing the pillow cases (at least every other day) will prevent the build up of the medication in the fabric of the pillow case and decrease the risk of growth of facial hair. The absorption of even 5% minoxidil is well below that necessary to change pulse rate, which is the most sensitive indicator of systemic minoxidil effects. The drug must be used indefinitely to maintain hair growth.

For young men with male pattern alopecia the use of finasteride (Propecia) 1 mg/d is an additional treatment option. Finasteride is a type II, 5-$\alpha$-reductase inhibitor. The enzyme 5-$\alpha$-reductase catalyzes conversion of testosterone to the more potent dihydrotestosterone. Finasteride is used in a higher dose of 5 mg (Proscar) for treatment of benign prostatic hypertrophy (BPH). In a study using finasteride in postmenopausal women with female pattern hair loss, it was not helpful for treatment, but was helpful in premenopausal women using it at a 2.5-mg dose along with oral contraceptives. In another report, it was helpful at the 5-mg dosage. Perhaps in women whose alopecia improves with finasteride they have an abnormal activity of the 5-$\alpha$-reductase enzyme. Finasteride should not be used in pregnant or lactating women. It can lower serum dihydrotestosterone and therefore has a potential risk of causing genital abnormalities in male fetuses exposed in utero (it is a pregnancy category X drug). Women who are pregnant or nursing should not even handle finasteride pills (especially crushed or broken pills) to avoid teratogenic problems. Four percent of men aged 18 to 41 years taking finasteride may have decreased libido, erectile dysfunction, or a decreased volume of ejaculate. The drug must be taken indefinitely to maintain hair growth.

Dutasteride (Avodart) inhibits both type I and type II 5-$\alpha$-reductase isoenzymes, and it is 3 times more potent than finasteride at inhibiting type II 5-$\alpha$-reductase and more than 100 times as potent at inhibiting type I 5-$\alpha$-reductase. It was approved in 2002 by the FDA for treatment of BPH at a dosage of 0.5 mg daily under the trade name Avodart. In a study in men who were given 2.5 mg dutasteride, it was superior to 5 mg of finasteride for treatment of alopecia. One woman who had failed treatment of female pattern alopecia with finasteride was given dutasteride at 0.5 mg/d along with an oral contraceptive and had significant improvement after 6 months of treatment. The FDA has not approved use of dutasteride for men or women with hair loss. Teratogenicity is a real issue especially since the half-life is very long (half-life is 5 weeks for dutasteride and 6 to 8 h for finasteride), and men taking it for BPH should *not* donate their blood for at least 6 months after stopping the drug. Drug interactions are a potential problem with dutasteride, which is not seen with finasteride. Dutasteride is processed by CYP3A4 enzymes, so it may affect the clearance of other potent CYP3A4 inhibitors such as ritonavir, ketoconazole, verapamil, diltiazem, cimetidine, ciprofloxacin, and troleandomycin.

Although the only FDA-approved treatment for women with female pattern hair loss is 2% minoxidil, other antiandrogens such as finasteride, spironolactone, cyproterone acetate, and flutamide may prove helpful for some women with androgen excess.

I am not advocating that these medications be used, but of these medications, spironolactone (Aldactone) is the most easily available and probably the safest (but remember it is a pregnancy category D drug). Flutamide has been associated (rarely) with hepatic deaths. None should be used in pregnant or lactating women.

*Telogen effluvium* is another important cause of diffuse nonscarring hair loss. It is the shedding of an abnormal number of hairs in the telogen (resting) phase. A telogen effluvium may be triggered by childbirth, surgical procedures with general anesthesia, major illness, high fevers, medications (Table 32-4), rapid marked weight loss, possibly smoking, toxin exposure (such as heavy metal, thallium, or borate intoxication), and virtually any major insult to the body that causes the ratio of telogen to anagen hairs to increase. Within 2 or 3 months of the triggering event, the person notices an abnormally large number of hairs coming out. It is usually reversible in 4 to 6 months. Some people with telogen effluvium may have a shortening of the anagen phase, which leads to shorter hairs in addition. Multiple medications can cause hair loss by inducing a telogen effluvium, but some medications such as chemotherapy agents cause an anagen effluvium because they interfere with mitosis. Anagen effluvium starts usually within 7 to 14 days after starting the medication. Since about 90% of scalp hairs are in anagen, there is an extremely marked hair loss with chemotherapy. Both hypothyroidism and perhaps low ferritin (<40 and some say <70) may trigger a telogen effluvium. There is a chronic telogen effluvium of unclear cause described primarily in middle aged women that affects the entire scalp, starts abruptly, often causes some temporal recession, and fluctuates over a prolonged time. Doing several hair pulls, which involves pulling firmly about 20 hairs between your fingers and extracting more than 2 hairs per pull, suggest a telogen effluvium. Inspecting the hair root under the microscope to make sure it is a telogen hair and not an abnormal anagen hair is important to clinch the diagnosis (and rule out loose anagen syndrome). Of course, if a patient has vigorously shampooed and/or brushed their hair prior to seeing you, the hair pull may not demonstrate an increased number of easily extractable telogen hairs. On the other hand, if a patient only shampoos and or brushes their hair very infrequently, their hair pull test may be falsely elevated with excessively large numbers of telogen hairs.

*Loose anagen syndrome* is a disorder usually presenting in young blonde girls (but can present in adults) that is sporadic or inherited (as autosomal dominant with variable expression and incomplete penetrance) characterized by easily (and painlessly) plucked dystrophic scalp hairs. The plucked hairs have misshapen, irregular, shrunken roots that may have a "mousetail"-like or "loose-sock"-like appearance microscopically. Normal anagen hairs are not pulled out with a firm or gentle pull, but anagen hairs in this syndrome are very easily extracted. In this condition there is a weak adhesion between the hair shaft cuticle and the inner root sheath cuticle. This may present clinically as a diffuse or as a patchy hair loss. It may be associated with other entities such as alopecia areata, Noonan's syndrome, and AIDS. The condition may improve with age.

Usually *alopecia areata* presents as a patchy hair loss, but sometimes it may present as a diffuse, and sometimes very severely diffuse, hair loss that has a fairly abrupt onset. Because pigmented hairs are lost preferentially to gray or white hairs, some people who say they "turned gray overnight" may have had salt and pepper hair and developed alopecia areata in which large numbers of their pigmented hairs were lost very rapidly (see alopecia areata discussion under Patchy Hair Loss section.).

### Patchy Nonscarring Alopecia

Patchy nonscarring alopecia is usually caused by *tinea capitis* (especially in children), *alopecia areata*, *trichotillomania*, or *syphilis*. *Trauma* from cosmetic procedures and *loose anagen syndrome* may be the causes as well. Certainly a fungal culture and a blood serology to rule out syphilis are important in the proper evaluation of patchy nonscarring hair loss (Table 32-2).

*Tinea capitis* may be diagnosed with a KOH examination of the hair and or fungal culture of the hair. It should always be suspected in children with patchy hair loss on the scalp. Oral antifungals are needed to eradicate this problem. Oral griseofulvin is still the "gold standard" of treatment for

---

**TABLE 32-4 ■ Some Drugs That Can Cause Alopecia**

| | |
|---|---|
| Allopurinol | Interferon |
| Amiodarone | Isoniazid |
| Amphetamine | Itraconazole |
| Anabolic steroid | Levodopa |
| Angiotensin-converting enzyme inhibitors | Lithium |
| Anticoagulants | Minoxidil (temporary) |
| Anticonvulsants | Monoamine oxidase inhibitor |
| Antifungals (in high dose) | Nicotinic acid |
| Antimalarials | Nitrofurantoin |
| Antithyroid | NSAIF |
| Benzimidazole | Oral contraceptive |
| β-Blockers | Progesterone |
| Bromocriptine | Retinoids |
| Captopril | Salicylates |
| Chemotherapeutic drugs | SSRIs (some)* |
| Cholesterol-lowering agents | Sulfasalazine |
| Chloramphenicol | Tacrolimus |
| Cimetidine | Terfenadine |
| Colchicine | Testosterone |
| Corticosteroids | Tricyclic antidepressants |
| Gentamicin | Venlafexime |
| Gold | Vitamin A |
| Immunoglobulin | |

*SSRIs (paroxetine, sertraline, fluoxetine).

children, but oral terbinafine (Lamisil) or oral itraconazole (Sporanox) may also be used.

*Alopecia areata* has a 0.1% to 0.2% prevalence in the general population and a lifetime incidence of 1.7%. It may account for 1% to 3% of new patient visits to a dermatologist. It is a nonscarring, usually patchy, but sometimes diffuse, hair loss of unclear cause that probably is autoimmune. It has typically an abrupt, asymptomatic onset. Usually the scalp is involved but any hair-bearing area of the body may be affected. At the margin of the bald spots there may be broken off hairs that are thicker distally and thinner proximally near the scalp like the top part of an exclamation point (!) and are very characteristic of this problem. Dermoscopy of the scalp shows numerous diffuse, round or polycylic yellow dots (hyperkeratotic plugs in hair follicles), black dots (cadaverized hairs), micro-exclamation hairs, and dystrophic and regrowing hairs. Remember too that black dots may indicate fungal infection. Regrowth may be with fine, white colored hair but with time the normal hair color returns. In adults, regrowth is often complete in 6 to 12 months. Factors that bode a bad prognosis are young age at onset, extensive early hair loss (especially if there is severe marginal hair loss called ophiasis), and associated atopy. If all the scalp hair is lost, the term alopecia totalis is used; if all the scalp and body hair is lost, the term alopecia universalis is used. These two extensive types of alopecia areata have an extremely poor prognosis. Nail pitting, longitudinal ridging, koilonychia, onycholysis, onychomadesis, and a host of other nail dystrophies may be associated in 10% to 66% of patients with alopecia areata and precede, accompany, or follow the hair disorder. An association of alopecia areata may be seen with multiple thyroid abnormalities including goiter, myxedema, and Hashimoto's thyroiditis. Patients are also more likely to have vitiligo, lupus, rheumatoid arthritis, pernicious anemia, inflammatory bowel disease, myasthenia gravis, lichen planus, or HIV infection. Patients with Down's syndrome, Turner's syndrome, and autoimmune polyglandular syndrome (APS-1) have an increased likelihood of developing alopecia areata.

Treatments of alopecia areata are primarily topical corticosteroids, topical anthralin (short contact), intralesional corticosteroids, systemic cortiosteroids (not usually warranted), ultraviolet light therapy, topical minoxidil, and topical sensitizers (such as squaric acid dibutylester, dinitrochlorobenzene, and diphencyprone).

A hodgepodge of miscellaneous therapies have been used including cryotherapy, aromatherapy, and hypnotherapy. Oral sulfasalazine and pulsed infrared diode laser are among newer agents that may be helpful. Interestingly, some of the newer biologics may help alopecia areata, such as alefacept, and some others (such as infliximab, adalimumab, and efalizumab) may induce alopecia areata. Keep in mind that none of these treatments are formally approved by the FDA, and none are resoundingly effective. In fact, in a recent review of controlled trials of therapy for alopecia areata, there was a lack of efficacy or no controlled trials available on many of the treatment modalities reported. Choosing fairly innocuous second-line or adjunctive agents may be prudent. Keep in mind that in most cases with mild to moderate hair loss, regrowth is spontaneous. The National Alopecia Areata Foundation (PO Box 150760, 14 Mitchell Blvd, San Rafael, CA 94903; Tel: 415-472-3780; http://www.naaf.org) provides support group information and a newsletter that patients may find helpful. Certainly, patients with severe, longstanding hair loss need help with choosing hair pieces, and this organization can help them.

*Trichotillomania* (hair pulling) is much more common than once thought and may well have a prevalence of at least 1% (based on one survey). In some surveys of students in college the prevalence may be 3.4% in female and 1.5% in male students. These latter figures on prevalence do not fit rigid criteria for *DSM-IV (Diagnostic and Statistical Manual of Mental Disorders)*. It may be that this disorder is heterogeneous with some patients probably fitting the criteria for obsessive–compulsive disorder (OCD). Most patients are reluctant to admit to hair pulling because they are ashamed of the problem or afraid they will be viewed as "crazy" by their physician, friends, or close family members.

The *DSM-IV* diagnostic criteria for trichotillomania includes (1) recurrent pulling out of one's hair resulting in noticeable hair loss, (2) an increasing sense of tension immediately before pulling out the hair or when attempting to resist the behavior, (3) pleasure, gratification, or relief when pulling out the hair, (4) the disturbance not better accounted for by another mental disorder and not due to a general medical condition (e.g., a dermatologic condition), and (5) the disturbance that provokes clinically marked distress and/or impairment in occupation, social, or other areas of functioning.

Chronic hair pulling has been associated with depression, anxiety, psychosis, and dysthymia. In some young children, it may be a transient problem. It also has been described with Sydenham's chorea. Certainly hair pulling may be seen with major mental retardation, schizophrenia, and in borderline personality disorder. In those patients in which OCD is suspected, behavioral therapy, oral clomipramine, or oral selective serotonin reuptake inhibitors (SSRIs) (gradually going to the highest recommended dosage for at least 12 weeks) may prove helpful. Cognitive behavioral therapy in particular should be tried. Providing a warm nonjudgmental environment for these patients is invaluable for helping them. The problem tends to be chronic with exacerbations and remissions. If medication is used it should be used probably for at least a year and may have to be utilized again if relapse occurs. Educational material can be provided at http://www.trich.org (Trichotillomania Learning Center, 207 McPherson Street, suite H, Santa Cruz, CA 95060; Tel: 831-457-1004), which may give these patients further support in dealing with this problem. Another web site that offers an interactive cognitive behavioral therapy program is http://www.StopPulling.com.

*Secondary syphilis* may cause a patchy or "moth-eaten" alopecia (typically) or it can cause a diffuse nonscarring alopecia. Treatment is discussed in Chapter 22.

*Traumatic* hair loss can result from chemical or physical trauma to the hair from hair grooming procedures such as permanents, relaxers, dyes, hot combs, or pulling the hair in tight braids. Usually this results in hair breakage rather than the hair coming out by the roots as it does in these other causes of patchy nonscarring hair loss. An underappreciated "traction folliculitis" may cause reversible or irreversible hair loss. It is often related to stretching the scalp hair with braids or ponytails or chemical or heat hair straighteners or relaxers. *Loose anagen syndrome* can cause diffuse or a patchy hair loss and has been discussed (see discussion on diffuse nonscarring hair loss).

## Scarring Alopecia (Cicatricial Alopecia)

The clinical diagnosis of a scarring hair loss should point the physician toward performing a scalp skin biopsy and a fungal culture. Certainly, diagnoses such as metastatic or benign tumors of the scalp, discoid lupus, sarcoid, lichen planopilaris (LPP), or scleroderma can be rapidly diagnosed with a biopsy. There is a larger, murkier group of scarring (cicatricial) alopecias that are undergoing constant renaming as our understanding of (or attempts at understanding) these disorders evolves. Overall, scarring hair loss accounts for the minority (about 3.2% to 7.3%) of all hair loss. An excellent discussion by Tan sorts primary cicatricial alopecia into lymphocytic and neutrophilic types. Lymphocytic types are four times as common as neutrophilic types and more common in middle-aged women, whereas neutrophilic types are more common in middle-aged men (see Table 32-2).

*Lymphocytic cicatricial alopecias* include *central centrifugal cicatricial alopecia* (CCCA) (formerly called "hot comb alopecia" or more recently "follicular degeneration syndrome"), *discoid lupus erythematosus*, *LPP* (and its variant *frontal fibrosing alopecia* [*FFA*]), and *pseudopelade of Brocq*. CCCA probably accounts for most scarring hair loss (certainly in blacks). Discoid lupus is discussed elsewhere in this text. *CCCA* is usually seen in black women and begins in the crown early on and may be confused with female pattern alopecia (and perhaps it is a scarring variant). Typically, it is thought that the inherited types of hair loss are nonscarring but perhaps this is not entirely true. It is slowly progressive. Certainly, ruling out traumatic alopecia is important. It was formerly called "hot comb alopecia" and its causation attributed to hot comb use. Later on it was appreciated that there were women (as well as some men) who did not use hot combs and had a similar picture and the histology showed premature degeneration of the inner root sheath in many hair follicles. This histologic change is not pathognomonic, however, for just one disease.

LPP presents typically in women as a patchy hair loss with perifollicular erythema, follicular spines, and scarring. About half of these patients develop other skin, mucous membrane, or nail changes of lichen planus. Treatments usually include (topical and intralesional) steroids and antimalarials. Topical tacrolimus and oral tetracycline (500 mg po b.i.d.) are some newer possible treatments. Other treatments that have been tried include minoxidil, dapsone, oral griseofulvin, retinoids, cyclosporine, and methotrexate. Some cases resolve spontaneously; others last for years. The average duration is 18 months.

FFA, a variant of LPP, is usually seen in women in their 60s as a recession of the frontal and temporal hairline with perifollicular erythema within the marginal hairline that is asymptomatic. There may be loss of eyebrows as well. Histology is that of LPP and the treatment is the same as for LPP.

*Pseudopelade of Brocq* is usually in women and presents as a noninflammatory, intermittently progressive, scarring alopecia of unknown cause that starts on the crown and spreads in a pseudopod-like fashion at irregular intervals and has been described as resembling "footprints in the snow" on the affected scalp.

Some people have used the term pseudopelade as an all-encompassing term for an end stage of various types of cicatricial alopecia of unclear cause, but that is probably better not done since it may be confusing. A "tufted folliculitis" may result as the end stage of multiple types of scarring alopecias. It has the clinical appearance of "doll's hair," which is numerous hair shafts exiting out of one aperture in multiple plugs. It is not diagnostic of any one disease, like the term pseudopelade is not.

*Neutrophilic cicatricial alopecias* include *folliculitis decalvans* and *dissecting cellulitis* (perifolliculitis capitis abscedens et suffodiens). There is a cicatricial alopecia group in which the inflammatory infiltrate is mixed and this includes acne keloidalis (folliculitis keloidalis), acne (folliculitis) necrotica, and erosive pustular dermatosis.

*Folliculitis decalvans* is a scarring folliculitis in which *Staphylococcus aureus* and sometimes other bacteria are frequently cultured, but response to antibiotics is not always that robust. In addition to giving the appropriate antibacterial agent based on culture and sensitivity, sometimes rifampin at 300 mg twice daily in combination is helpful. Besides being a good medication to eradicate staphylococci, it is effective against gram-negative as well as gram-positive organisms. It is capable of killing bacteria that are engulfed by phagocytic cells (maybe one of the reasons it works so well in granulomatous diseases such as tuberculosis and leprosy). Rifampin does have numerous drug interactions, and it will stain bodily fluids such as tears, saliva, perspiration, and urine a bright red color. Clindamycin at 300 mg/d can be used with rifampicin if other, safer antibiotics such as doxycycline are not effective, but one should be aware of the risk of *Clostridium difficile*–induced diarrhea with clindamycin. Topical fusidic acid, oral zinc sulfate (400 mg daily), steroids (topical and systemic), and intramuscular immunoglobulin may be other considerations for therapy. It has been postulated that the condition is characterized by an altered immunologic response to a variety of organisms, but an altered inflammatory foreign body response may play a role as well. Whether or not it is a subtype of CCCA is yet to be determined.

*Dissecting cellulitis (perifolliculitis capitis abscedens et suffodiens)* is more common in young black men and begins as inflammatory boggy, nodules that drain purulent material. Patients may be more likely to also have hidradenitis suppurativa and acne conglobata (often called the follicular occlusion triad). The cause is unknown and it tends to be a chronic problem. Usually it is not symptomatic but the disfiguring scarring and sometimes foul-smelling discharge are very problematic. Bacterial and fungal cultures should be performed. Treatment leaves a lot to be desired and has included various oral antibiotics (sometimes with the addition of rifampicin [600 mg/d] to cephalexin or to ciprofloxacin), and oral zinc sulphate 400 mg t.i.d. Oral isotretinoin is used in resistant cases for 4 to 5 months sometimes after oral antibiotics. Surgery, laser, and even radiation have been used in recalcitrant cases (I would be dubious about using radiation).

There are three scarring types of hair loss in which a mixed inflammatory infiltrate is seen histologically and these are: acne keloidalis, acne necrotica, and erosive pustulosis. *Acne keloidalis* is more common in young black men. It starts as smooth papules and pustules on the occipital scalp and posterior neck that evolve into keloid-like plaques. It may be asymptomatic or may have associated mild burning or itching. In mild cases a topical antibiotic maybe helpful, but usually an oral antibiotic such as tetracycline (500 mg to 1 g total dose per day), doxycycline (100 to 200 mg/d), minocycline (100 mg/d), or erythromycin (500 mg/d to 1 g/d) may prove helpful. *Acne necrotica* is usually presents as papules or necrotic pustules that are on the scalp and perhaps the face, neck, and chest as well that may lead to varioliform scars. It can be scarring or nonscarring. Oral antibiotics, intralesional or topical steroids, and even oral isotretinoin (Accutane) may be helpful for treatment. *Erosive pustular dermatosis* is a disease with pustular, necrotic, infundibular folliculitis with crusting that usually appears in older Caucasian women and later on has features of folliculitis decalvans.

Another manner of categorizing scarring hair loss was proffered by Sperling as CCCA (which encompasses pseudopelade, folliculitis decalvans, acne keloidalis, and dissecting folliculitis), LPP (with FFA as a subcategory), and lupus. The exact overlap and exclusivity of these diseases is constantly evolving. Scarring hair loss of unclear type is an appropriate label for some cases not fulfilling criteria for one of the entities described.

## Miscellaneous Hair Diseases

*Trichorrhexis nodosa* is the most common hair shaft disorder and most commonly is acquired secondary to damage from hair grooming procedures, although it may be associated with hypothyroidism and with other rarer syndromes such as argininosuccinic aciduria or Menkes' syndrome. Severe scratching or other trauma, as seen with lichen simplex chronicus, trichotillomania, or obsessive hair combing may lead to this hair shaft abnormality. Clinically, it presents as tiny white specks on the hair shaft that may superficially look like nits from head lice. When viewed microscopically, these specks resemble the bristles of two broom ends interlocked

and are the site of fractures. This condition is more likely to occur proximally in black hair and more distally in Caucasian or Asian hair. The resulting breakage may lead to the clinical complaint of the hair not growing very long.

*Uncombable hair syndrome* (spun glass hair) is an interesting hair shaft abnormality in which the hair shafts in cross section are triangular and on electron microscopy there are longitudinal grooves. The onset is usually around 3 years of age when the hair seems particularly wild and unruly. Typically, the hair is of a silver blond color and the problem may be generalized (usually) or localized. Spontaneous improvement may occur in childhood. Oral biotin may prove helpful. This same triangular hair shaft abnormality has been described in loose anagen syndrome and after spironolactone therapy.

*Acquired progressive kinking of the hair* is an odd entity that usually arises in the teens or early adult years in young Caucasian men. Gradually the hair becomes kinky, dry, and more unmanageable. The hair shaft is said to be elliptical with partial twists at irregular intervals. The anagen (growth) phase is said to be diminished. Oral retinoids or local radiation may induce a clinically similar problem.

Interestingly, a seemingly converse clinical picture has been described in African-American patients with AIDS who develop softer, silkier hair that replaces previously normal kinky hair. In addition, the color is said to become ashen and the hair becomes sparse.

*Trichoptilosis* (split ends) is the longitudinal splitting of the distal hair shaft and is a result of weathering and is made more striking by overuse of various cosmetic hair styling and grooming procedures. Hair pulling and scratching may be causative. Various unusual inherited hair shaft defects are more prone to trichoptilosis.

*Bubble hair* is the result of excessive heat from hair dryers (and perhaps other chemical treatments of the hair) leading to distinctive "bubbles" within the hair shaft. These hairs may appear brittle and broken off. Interestingly, with thallium intoxication a bubble-like inclusion can be seen within the hair shaft. Typically, thallium intoxication leads to massive hair loss.

*Pseudofolliculitis barbae* is a problem typically seen in the beard area of black men caused by close shaving in curly or kinky hair that may cause the newly emerging hair shaft to grow back into the skin surface or pierce the follicular wall, causing inflammation. Clinically it presents as papulopustules that may lead to hyperpigmentation and scarring. Hair plucking and electrolysis can induce the same type of problem. The best treatment is to avoid shaving or at least avoid close shaving. Topical tretinoin (Retin-A) and/or topical Vaniqa (used for treatment of hypertrichosis) may prove helpful. This can also occur in patients with curly or kinky hair that is shaved closely in the axillae, legs, and pubic areas. One author has suggested the terms pseudofolliculits axillae, pseudofolliculits corporis, and pseudofolliculitis pubis.

*Green hair* may result from the deposition of copper on light-colored hair from tap water used to shampoo or from water in a swimming pool. Pretreating the hair with some types of conditioners may help prevent the discoloration. Shampooing with a penicillamine-containing mixture may reduce the green color. Copper intoxication from ingestion of tap water can cause a diffuse alopecia.

*Trichomegaly* is the development of abnormally long eyelashes and can be seen in patients with AIDS, with underlying malignancy (such as adenocarcinoma), with kala azar, with various unusual syndromes in which it is just one feature (such as dwarfism or Cornelia-de-Lange syndrome), or with certain medications (alpha interferon, or latanoprost [which is an analogue of prostaglandin $F_{2\alpha}$ used topically for treatment of chronic open-angle glaucoma], and, perhaps, also with cyclosporine).

## Suggested Readings

Abramowicz M. Propecia and Rogaine extra strength for alopecia. *Med Lett.* 1998;40:25–27.

Barrett S. Commercial hair analysis: science or scam? *JAMA.* 1985;254:1041–1045.

Bernard J, ed. Ethnic hair and skin: what is the state of the science. *J Am Acad Dermatol.* 2003;48(6).

Blazek C, Megahed M. Lichen planopilaris: successful treatment with tacrolimus. *Hautarzt* 2008;59(11):874–877.

Brooke RCC, Griffiths CEM. folliculitis decalvans. *Clin Exp Dermatol.* 2001;26:120–122.

Bui K, Polisetty S, Gilchrist H, et al. Successful treatment of alopecia universalis with alefacept: a case report an review of the literature. *Cutis.* 2008;81:431–434.

Dawber R. *Diseases of the Hair and Scalp.* 3rd ed. Oxford, UK: Blackwell Science; 1997.

Dawber R and Van Neste D. *Hair and Scalp Disorders: Common Presenting Signs, Differential Diagnosis and Treatment.* Philadelphia, PA: JP Lippincott; 1995.

Delamere FM, Sladden MM, Dobbins HM, et al. Interventions for alopecia areata. *Cochrane Database Syst Rev.* 2008;(2): doi: 10.1002/14651858. CD004413.pub2.

Fox GN, Stausmire JM. Traction folliculitis: an underreported entity. *Cutis.* 2007;79:26–30.

Georgala S, Korfitis C. Dissecting cellulitis of the scalp treated with rifampicin and isotretinoin: case reports. *Cutis.* 2008;82:195–198.

Headington JT. Telogen effluvium: new concepts and review. *Arch Dermatol.* 1993;129:356–363.

Hordinsky MK. Alopecias. In: Bolognia J, Rapini RP, Jorizzo JL, eds. *Dermatology.* New York: Mosby Publishers; 2003:1033–1050.

Jackson J, Caro J, Caro J, et al. The effect of eflornithine 13.9% cream on the bother and discomfort due to hirsutism. *Int J Dermatol.* 2007;46:976–981.

Kossard S, Lee MS, Wilkinson B. Postmenopausal frontal fibrosing alopecia: a frontal variant of lichen planopilaris. *J Am Acad Dermatol.* 1997;36:59–66.

Leung AKC, Robson WLM. Hirsutism. *Int J Dermatol.* 1993;32:773–777.

Matilainen V, Laakso M, Hirsso P, et al. Hair loss, insulin resistance, and heredity in middle-aged women. A population based study. *J Cardiovasc Risk.* 2003;10:227.

Nuss MA, Carlisle D, Hall M, et al. Trichotillomania: a review and case report. *Cutis.* 2003;72:191–196.

Olsen EA. Female pattern hair loss. *J Am Acad Dermatol.* 2001;45(3):S70–S80.

Olsen EA. *Disorders of Hair Growth: Diagnosis and Treatment.* 2nd ed. New York: McGraw-Hill; 2003.

Rogers NE, Avram MR. Medical treatments for male and female pattern hair loss. *J Am Acad Dermatol.* 2008;59:547–566.

Rosenfield RL. Hirsutism. *N Engl J Med.* 2005;353(24):2578–2588.

Ross EK, Tan E, Shapiro J. Update on primary cicatricial alopecias. *J Am Acad Dermatol.* 2005;53(1):1–37.

Rushton DH, Ramsey ID, James KC, et al. Biochemical and trichological characterization of diffuse alopecia in women. *Br J Dermatol.* 1990;123:137–197.

Sawaya M. Clinical updates in hair. *Dermatol Clin.* 1997;15:37–43.

Schmidt S, Fischer TW, Chren MM, et al. Strategies of coping and quality of life in women with alopecia. *Br J Dermatol.* 2001;144(5):1038–1043.

Shapiro J. Hair loss in women. *N Engl J Med.* 2007;357(16):1620–1630.

Sommer S, Render C, Burd R, et al. Ruby laser treatment for hirsutism: clinical response and patient tolerance. *Br J Dermatol.* 1998;138:1009–1014.

Sperling LC. A new look at scarring alopecia. *Arch Dermatol.* 2000;136:235–242.

Sperling LC. Alopecias. In: Bolognia JL, ed. *Dermatology.* 2nd ed. Spain: Mosby (Elsevier Limited); 2008:987–1005.

Sperling LC, Sau P. The follicular degeneration syndrome in black patients: hot comb alopecia revisited and revised. *Arch Dermatol.* 1992;128:68–74.

Tan E, Martinka M, Ball N, et al. Primary cicatricial alopecias: clinicopathology of 112 cases. *J Am Acad Dermatol.* 2004;50:25–32.

Trueb RM. Association between smoking and hair loss: another opportunity for health education against smoking? *Dermatology.* 2003;206(3):189–191.

Wendelin DS, Pope DN, and Mallory S. Hypertrichosis. *J Am Acad Dermatol.* 2003;48:161–179.

Whiting DA. Update on hair disorders. *Dermatol Clin.* 1996;14(4).

Whiting DA. Male pattern hair loss: current understanding. *Int J Dermatol.* 1998;37:561–566.

Whiting, DA, Howsden FL. *Color Atlas of Differential Diagnosis of Hair Loss.* Cedar Grove, NJ: Canfield Publishing; 1996.

# CHAPTER 33

# Diseases Affecting the Nail Unit

*Brad Merritt, MD and Richard K. Scher, MD*

The nail unit is an essential component of the integumentary system that can be affected by primary diseases, dermatologic disorders with nail involvement, and systemic illnesses that alter the appearance of the nails. Primary nail disorders, as in the case of subungual melanoma and subungual squamous cell carcinoma, can be life threatening. Secondary nail changes can be a sign of underlying life-threatening diseases such as severe renal, hepatic, and cardiovascular disease. The nail unit's most important functions are to protect the distal digit and to improve dexterity in manipulating small objects. By providing counterpressure, the nail plate enhances the transmission of delicate sensations. Perhaps more important from an evolutionary standpoint, the nail unit facilitates scratching and grooming. Disorders of the nail unit can be physically and psychologically distressing to patients, because nails often serve socially as a cosmetic enhancement. This chapter reviews common and serious nail disorders, including those caused by infectious, traumatic, neoplastic, congenital, and primary dermatologic disorders.

A complete history and physical examination should be included in any evaluation of a patient with a nail disorder. A medication history is important and systemic diseases should be noted, as these factors often affect the appearance of the nail unit. The family history can give clues to hereditary nail abnormalities as can be found in the nail-patella syndrome (osteo-onychodysplasia), ectodermal dysplasia, pachyonychia congenita, and Darier's disease (keratosis follicularis). An occupational history can provide insight into possible allergic or irritant exposures. Treatments of the nail, including prior medical/surgical modalities, home remedies, and manicures/pedicures, are important to note because they can be factors contributing to persistent nail disease. All 20 nails should be examined. A magnifying glass can be employed to enhance fine details. A dermatoscope can be helpful when evaluating the nail folds for signs of connective tissue disease and the nail plate for melanonychia striata. A complete skin examination, including the oral mucosa, is also important. Subtle lesions can give clues as to the cause of nail disorders. Laboratory tests useful in the evaluation of nail disease include biopsy of the nail plate, cuticle, bed, or matrix, fungal cultures, bacterial cultures, and potassium hydroxide preparations. Imaging modalities including plain film and magnetic resonance imaging (MRI) can be helpful in determining the extent of disease

and evaluating possible involvement of bone underlying the nail apparatus.

## Anatomy of the Nail Unit

The nail unit is a specialized appendage of the skin, composed of unique structures not found elsewhere in the body. The nail unit consists of the nail plate, proximal and lateral nail folds, cuticle, nail matrix, nail bed, and the hyponychium (Fig. 33-1). What most people commonly consider the nail refers to the nail plate, which is the clear, hard portion of the nail made of keratin. The nail plate is divided into two sections: the dorsal plate that is created by the proximal nail matrix and the ventral plate that is created by the distal nail matrix with some contribution from the nail bed. The nail matrix is composed of a group of germative cells located proximal to the nail plate. The nail matrix contains a layer of actively dividing keratinocytes that mature and, after death, contribute to the formation of the nail plate. The nail plate is bordered by the proximal nail fold and two lateral nail folds. The lunula is the most distal portion of the matrix, visible as a white, half-moon–shaped area under the nail plate bordered by the proximal nail fold. The nail plate rests on the highly vascular nail bed. The hyponychium is the section of the skin located under the free edge of the nail plate between the nail bed and the distal nail groove.

Fingernails grow constantly at a rate of 0.1 mm/d or 3 mm/mo. At this rate, a fingernail can be totally replaced in 4 to 6 months. Toenails, however, grow at about half this rate and can take 8 to 12 months to be totally replaced. Certain disease states including psoriasis, minor trauma, pityriasis rubra pilaris, the brittle nail syndrome, hyperpituitarism, and hyperthyroidism can cause nails to grow at a faster rate than normal. Slower nail growth has been noted in patients with malnutrition, acute infections, peripheral neuropathy, onychomycosis, and hypothyroidism as well as in smokers. The rate of nail growth can also be affected by a variety of medications.

## Onychomycosis

Onychomycosis refers to fungal infection of the nail. Onychomycosis is the most common nail disorder and accounts for up to half of all nail problems encountered in clinical practice. The prevalence of onychomycosis increases with age. Other risk factors for developing onychomycosis include

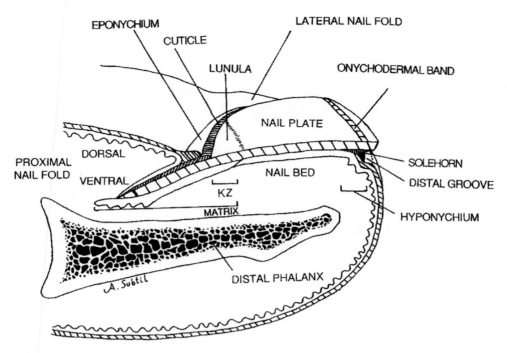

**FIGURE 33-1** ■ Anatomy of the nail unit. KZ, keratogenous zone. *(Reprinted from Hordinsky MK, Sawaya ME, Scher ME. Histology of the normal nail unit. In: Atlas of Hair and Nails. 1st ed. Philadelphia: Churchill Livingstone; 2000:19. Copyright 2000, with permission from Elsevier.)*

smoking, peripheral arterial disease, recurrent trauma, diabetes mellitus, family history, and immunosuppression including HIV infection. Fungal infections of the nail may be caused by dermatophytes (tinea unguium), nondermatophyte molds, or yeast. More than 90% of cases of onychomycosis are caused by the dermatophytes *Trichophyton rubrum* and *Trichophyton mentagrophytes*. Onychomycosis has been classified into five major types:

- distal and lateral subungual onychomycosis,
- superficial white onychomycosis,
- proximal subungual onychomycosis,
- endonyx onychomycosis, and
- total dystrophic onychomycosis.

Clinical signs of onychomycosis include

- thickening of the nail bed and nail plate,
- subungual debris,
- onycholysis (separation of the nail plate from the nail bed),
- nail discoloration (white/yellow or orange/brown patches or streaks),
- ridging of the nail, and
- nail pitting.

## Diagnosis

Before treating patients with clinical evidence of onychomycosis, the diagnosis should be confirmed by (1) direct microscopy of nail debris using a preparation of potassium hydroxide (KOH) with or without dimethyl sulfoxide or chlorazol black, or (2) fungal culture, or (3) histologic examination of the nail plate with periodic acid–Schiff (PAS) stain. Collection of an appropriate specimen is crucial to avoid a false-negative or false-positive result. In general, it is best to obtain a sample from the most proximal, central area of involved nail. Direct microscopy allows for rapid diagnosis but does not provide information for speciation. Fungal culture, while the least sensitive test, can be important for identifying the causative organism, especially in treatment-resistant cases. Histologic examination with PAS is the most sensitive test for onychomycosis and has the highest negative predictive value. It is also the most expensive and should be reserved for cases when direct microscopy is unavailable or negative but clinical suspicion is high.

## Presentation and Characteristics

Distal and lateral subungual onychomycosis is the most common form of onychomycosis (**Fig. 33-2**). The first sites of fungal invasion are the hyponychium or the lateral nail fold. Onycholysis occurs when subungual keratotic debris separates the nail plate from the nail bed. Paronychia can also occur. The nail bed is the ideal site for obtaining a specimen for microscopic examination. The most common organisms associated with distal and lateral subungual onychomycosis are the dermatophytes *T. rubrum* and *T. mentagrophytes*. *Candida albicans* and *Candida parapsilosis* are less frequently responsible, while the nondermatophyte molds, including *Scopulariopsis brevicaulis*, *Aspergillus* species, *Acremonium* species, and *Fusarium oxysporum*, are the least common causative organisms.

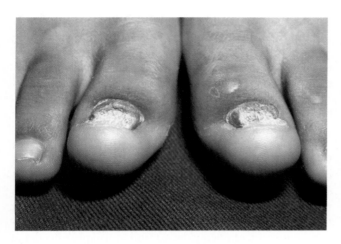

**FIGURE 33-2** ■ Distal and lateral subungual onychomycosis.

Superficial onychomycosis can be divided into white superficial onychomycosis and black superficial onychomycosis. White superficial onychomycosis is the most common of the two and is also known as leukonychia trichophytica and leukonychia mycotica. The first, second, and third toenails are more likely to be affected, and the exposed dorsal surface of the nail plate is the site of fungal invasion. Clinically, white superficial onychomycosis presents on the nail plate as white, opaque islands with distinct edges. Untreated lesions can develop a yellow color. Because of the superficial nature of the infection, organisms can often be scraped from the nail plate surface. White superficial onychomycosis is most often caused by the dermatophyte *T. mentagrophytes var. interdigitale* but can also be caused by *T. rubrum* as well as by molds including *Aspergillus*, *Acremonium*, and *Fusarium* spp. White superficial onychomycosis caused by *T. rubrum* often leads to more extensive nail involvement and is seen in otherwise healthy children and in patients infected with HIV. White superficial onychomycosis secondary to molds can be clinically indistinguishable from disease caused by dermatophytes, but can also lead to deeper, more extensive involvement of the nail. Black superficial onychomycosis presents with black, opaque plaques on the nails secondary to invading fungi that are pigmented. This variant occurs with *Scytalydium dimidiatum* and *T. rubrum*.

Endonyx onychomycosis is a fungal infection of the nail in which both the superficial and deep layers of the nail plate are affected without resulting in nail bed inflammatory changes. Tunnels formed by and filled with invading fungi may be present. Clinically, this appears as a milky-white discoloration of the nail plate that is not accompanied by subungual hyperkeratosis or onycholysis. There is lamellar splitting of the nail plate. Endonyx onychomycosis is caused by *Trichophyton soudanense* and *Trichophyton violaceum*.

Proximal subungual onychomycosis is a relatively uncommon subtype that occurs secondary to fungal invasion at the proximal nail fold through the cuticle. Clinically, it is a whitish discoloration of the proximal nail plate along with proximal subungual hyperkeratosis and onycholysis. The distal end of the nail plate appears normal in early infection. Proximal subungual onychomycosis can be seen with or without paronychia. In patients without paronychia, proximal subungual onychomycosis is usually caused by *T. rubrum*. In patients with paronychia, proximal subungual onychomycosis is usually secondary to *C. albicans*. Proximal subungual onychomycosis can also be caused by *Aspergillus*, *Fusarium*, and *Scopulariopsis* spp. Proximal white subungual onychomycosis with rapid progression is a variant most often associated with immunocompromised conditions, especially HIV infection. *T. rubrum* is the most common pathogen. Because of the association with HIV, clinicians should consider laboratory testing to investigate the patient's immune status when a diagnosis of proximal white subungual onychomycosis is made.

Total dystrophic onychomycosis can be primary or secondary. Secondary total dystrophic onychomycosis usually occurs because of extensive fungal infection involving the entire nail plate from distal and lateral subungual onychomycosis or proximal subungual onychomycosis. The entire nail plate is extensively thickened and can easily collapse. Primary total dystrophic onychomycosis is seen in patients with chronic mucocutaneous candidiasis and is caused by infection of all portions of the nail unit by *Candida*.

## Differential Diagnosis

A variety of diseases of the nail can mimic onychomycosis and must be considered in the differential diagnosis. Only 40% to 50% of abnormal appearing toenails are actually due to onychomycosis. Possible simulators of onychomycosis include psoriasis, chronic onycholysis, lichen planus, alopecia areata, chronic paronychia, hemorrhage/trauma, onychogryphosis, aging, median canaliform dystrophy, pincer nail deformity, yellow nail syndrome, subungual malignant melanoma, and subungual squamous cell carcinoma. Any of these disease states can coexist with onychomycosis, and proof of dermatophyte infection in the nail (Fig. 33-3) does not exclude a separate, concurrent disease of the nail unit.

## Treatment

Therapy for onychomycosis depends on the pattern of infection, pathogen, and degree of involvement. Treatments include oral and topical medications, as well as periodic clipping and filing of infected portions of the nail plate. White superficial onychomycosis involving less than the distal two thirds of the nail plate and moderate distal and lateral subungual onychomycosis can be treated effectively with the topical fungicidal lacquers ciclopirox and amorolfine. These lacquers have a broad range of antifungal activity against dermatophytes, as well as *C. albicans*. Additionally, ciclopirox has antibacterial and anti-inflammatory actions. Lacquers are less effective than oral treatments, but can be useful in patients with onychomycosis who cannot tolerate oral antifungals because of liver or kidney disease, or those taking multiple systemic medications where drug interactions may be a concern.

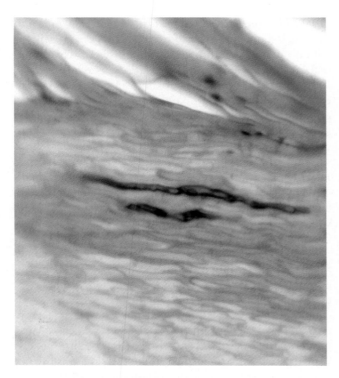

**FIGURE 33-3** ■ High-power microscopic view of a dermatophyte in the nail plate (PAS stain; original magnification 400×). *(Courtesy of Dr. George W. Niedt.)*

The first-line treatment for onychomycosis is oral terbinafine, an allylamine fungicidal medication. A meta-analysis of randomized clinical trials found terbinafine to be superior to placebo, itraconazole, fluconazole, and griseofulvin in achieving mycological cure in patients with onychomycosis. Terbinafine also demonstrates the lowest post-treatment recurrence rates. Typical dosing for terbinafine is 250 mg daily for 12 weeks for toenails and 6 weeks for fingernails. While previously considered cost-prohibitive by many patients, the cost of treatment with terbinafine has been significantly reduced with the advent of $4 generic plans that are now available at many pharmacies.

Other systemic medications used to treat onychomycosis include the azole antifungals itraconazole and fluconazole. Itraconazole can be given as 100 mg twice daily for 12 weeks for toenails or 6 weeks for fingernails. Alternatively, itraconazole can be pulsed at 200 mg twice daily for 1 week per month for 3 months for toenails and 2 months for fingernails, lowering the risk for hepatotoxicity. Various pulse therapies have also been advocated for oral terbinafine therapy but are generally less effective than continuous therapy. Fluconazole can be dosed from 150 to 300 mg once per week until the nails are clear but has a low clearance rate. Griseofulvin is a fungistatic medicine that must be taken until the entire nail is replaced. For this reason, as well as inferior efficacy compared to newer treatments and potential interactions with warfarin and oral contraceptives, griseofulvin is no longer used frequently for onychomycosis. Ketoconazole is also used infrequently for onychomycosis because of possible hepatotoxicity. Hepatotoxicity has been reported with itraconazole, fluconazole, and terbinafine, in decreasing order of frequency. Monitoring of liver enzymes is advised during continuous therapy. Systemic treatments for onychomycosis are generally well tolerated, with gastrointestinal side effects and headaches occurring most commonly. Combining oral and topical treatments may allow for shorter courses with higher cure rates.

Factors indicating a likely poor response to treatment with oral therapy include lateral nail disease, proximal nail disease, involvement of the entire nail unit, longitudinal streaks of fungal infection in the nail plate, presence of a dermatophytoma (a mass of fungi between the nail plate and the nail bed), and extensive onycholysis. If a dermatophytoma is present, removing the portion of nail plate overlying it and removing the concentration of fungi can help to achieve a cure. *Candida* onychomycosis can be more difficult to treat. Terbinafine is slightly less effective than itraconazole in achieving cure in onychomycosis secondary to *Candida* spp.

Onychomycosis is difficult to cure permanently. Many patients have recurrent infections. Factors associated with recurrent disease include persistent predisposing conditions such as peripheral vascular disease, diabetes mellitus, recurrent trauma, older age, as well as insufficient treatment from early termination or an insufficient dose of medication. Several measures have been suggested to avoid recurrence of onychomycosis. These include wearing footwear when walking in areas of high concentrations of dermatophytes (e.g., communal areas by pools, spas), avoiding shoes that may have dermatophytes present, drying feet (and interdigital spaces) after a bath or shower, using socks made of absorbent material (highly wicking socks), treating concurrent tinea pedis, using powder such as Zeasorb AF (very absorbent and has miconazole) to shake into shoes or socks, and prophylactic use of topical antifungal agents.

## Paronychia

Paronychia is defined as acute or chronic inflammation of the nail fold, typically with an associated infection. Acute paronychia is usually preceded by trauma that facilitates bacterial inoculation of the nail fold. It affects the digit with rapid development of erythema, tenderness, and in more advanced disease, purulent discharge. Untreated, acute paronychia can lead to a subungual abscess and nail dystrophy. The most commonly associated organism is *Staphylococcus aureus*, but *Streptococcus pyogenes*, *Pseudomonas pyocyanea*, *Proteus vulgaris*, and anaerobic bacteria have also been cultured from acute paronychia. Herpes simplex virus can cause recurrent acute paronychia in the form of herpetic whitlow. Pemphigus vulgaris is also associated with acute paronychia.

Chronic paronychia is defined as inflammation of the nail fold present for at least 6 weeks that develops from repeated exposure to moisture, irritants, and allergens. Patients present with erythema, swelling, and tenderness of the nail folds. Nail plate thickening, ridging, and discoloration can occur. Chronic paronychia most commonly affects patients with repeated exposure to a moist environment, including cooks, dishwashers, laundry workers, and nurses. *Candida* is often present, but its role in the pathogenesis is unclear. Chronic paronychia has been associated with isotretinoin (Accutane), protease inhibitors, and the epidermal growth factor inhibitors.

## Diagnosis

Squamous cell carcinoma, subungual melanoma, and metastatic carcinoma can simulate paronychia and are important to exclude. In patients with acute paronychia that responds poorly to conventional treatment, cultures can be beneficial in identifying the causative organism. The prevalence of skin infections secondary to methicillin-resistant *S. aureus* is increasing, and culture may be necessary to rule out this pathogen. If vesicles are present, herpetic whitlow should be suspected and a Tzanck smear and/or HSV culture or less often PCR should be performed. Biopsy should be considered in treatment of refractory cases or if there is any suspicion of a neoplastic process.

## Treatment

Mild acute paronychia responds well to warm compresses and topical antibacterial treatment. More severe and persistent disease often requires oral antibiotics or incision and drainage. Surgical drainage effectively treats acute paronychia and is indicated if an abscess has formed. Herpetic whitlow can be treated with acyclovir, valacyclovir, or famciclovir. Incision and drainage should be avoided if the presence of HSV is confirmed.

Chronic paronychia is best treated by avoidance of moisture and irritants. Patients should be advised to avoid manipulation of the cuticle, which is important in preventing entry of microorganisms. Topical antifungal treatment is also recommended because of the presence of *Candida*. Topical corticosteroids are the treatment of choice, however, especially if inflammation is prominent. A randomized trial found greater improvement of chronic paronychia treated with topical steroids compared to topical antifungal therapy.

## Nail Psoriasis

Nail involvement in psoriasis is common, occurring in up to half of all patients with psoriasis. Psoriatic nail changes are especially common in patients with psoriatic arthritis. Most patients with nail involvement have classic skin lesions as well, but nail disease can occur in the absence of cutaneous psoriasis. Clinical features of nail psoriasis include

- pitting,
- discoloration,
- onycholysis,
- subungual hyperkeratosis,
- nail plate crumbling and grooving, and
- splinter hemorrhages.

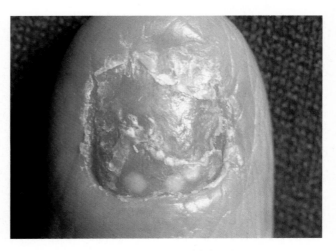

**FIGURE 33-4** ■ Pustular nail psoriasis.

Nail changes in psoriasis are variable, ranging from a few pits to total nail dystrophy. Nail pits are the most common finding and are formed by small psoriatic lesions in the proximal nail matrix. Oil drop or salmon-colored spots are yellow-red discolorations of the nail bed. They are caused by inclusion of neutrophilic exudates between the nail plate and the nail bed. Psoriasis can affect all of the components of the nail unit, and biopsy from affected areas including the proximal nail fold, nail plate, nail bed, and matrix may be appropriate to establish the diagnosis.

Pustular psoriasis of the nails (also known as acrodermatitis continua of Hallopeau) is a variant of nail psoriasis in which the characteristic clinical features include periungual or subungual pustules (Fig. 33-4). Pustular psoriasis of the nails can be difficult to distinguish from other nail disorders. In an evaluation of 38 patients with pustular psoriasis of the nails, all of whom had been evaluated by a prior physician, 35 (92%) had not been correctly diagnosed. The diagnosis of pustular psoriasis of the nails should be considered in patients with recurrent subungual and periungual pustules, recurrent painful onycholysis, and in patients with painful dystrophic and crusted nails. Nail bed biopsy can be useful in confirming the diagnosis of pustular psoriasis of the nails.

## Diagnosis

Nail psoriasis almost always occurs along with classic cutaneous lesions, in which case, diagnosis is straightforward. In patients without skin involvement, the diagnosis can be difficult unless a characteristic cluster of nail changes is present. Nail pits can be seen as a normal variant as well as in diseases such as chronic eczema, alopecia areata, and lichen planus. The pits in nail psoriasis are typically deeper and less regular than in other nail conditions. Onycholysis is a nonspecific nail change that can also be seen in nail infections, chronic dermatitis, repetitive trauma, and as a side effect of medications. Onycholysis increases the risk for infection, which should be excluded. Oil spots have been described as the most specific isolated change in psoriatic nails. The majority of patients with psoriatic arthritis have nail changes, so concomitant arthritis can be a clue to the diagnosis. Biopsy of the nail plate, bed, or matrix may be necessary for confirmation of the diagnosis.

## Treatment

Treatment of nail psoriasis requires patience, as correction of abnormal findings can require up to 6 months for fingernails and longer for toenails. The mainstay of psoriatic nail treatment is injected steroid, usually triamcinolone acetonide 2.5 mg/ml, directly into the nail matrix. Topical therapies for nail psoriasis include

- corticosteroids,
- vitamin D analogs,
- 5-fluorouracil, and
- topical psoralen plus ultraviolet A (PUVA).

Systemic therapies used to treat skin psoriasis, including cyclosporine, acitretin, and methotrexate, have also been effective in treating psoriatic nail disease. For the treatment of pustular psoriasis of the nail, systemic retinoids have been recommended for severe relapses and topical calcipotriol for maintenance therapy in patients with multiple nail involvement. For patients with one or two affected nails, topical calcipotriol alone is suggested.

## Subungual Hematoma

Subungual hematoma is a common problem encountered by clinicians. A sudden, strong, external force or repeated minor trauma to the digit can cause bleeding of the vascular nail bed. The collection of blood under the nail plate causes a bluish or violaceous discoloration (Fig. 33-5). Repeated minor trauma often leads to subungual hematoma that simulates melanonychia striata. Increased pressure in the space between the nail bed and the nail plate can cause intense pain, and larger hematomas can lead to shedding of the nail plate and permanent nail dystrophy.

## Diagnosis

The most important distinction to make when evaluating discoloration under the nail plate is differentiating subungual hematoma from subungual melanoma. Information obtained by taking a history can help clarify the diagnosis. A rapidly developing lesion that occurs after trauma is more likely to be a subungual hematoma, but it should be remembered that patients with subungual melanoma also occasionally report a history of trauma, and bleeding can be the first sign of a subungual melanoma. Distinguishing pigment secondary to blood from pigment of melanocytic origin can sometimes be accomplished using dermoscopy, but only a biopsy can render a final diagnosis.

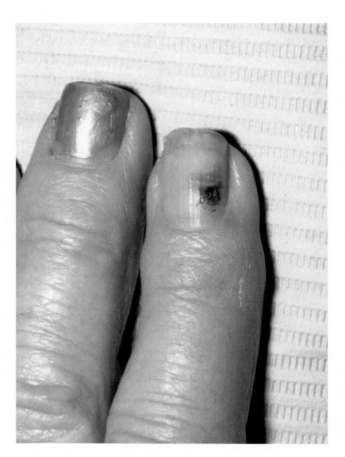

**FIGURE 33-5** ■ Subungual hematoma.

## Treatment

Treatment for subungual hematoma includes nail trephination or, in cases with more severe injury, nail removal with exploration for nail bed lacerations that may require repair. These techniques facilitate evacuation of the collection of blood from under the nail plate, thus relieving pressure and associated pain. Most recent articles suggest that in patients without significant injury to the digit, trephination is the preferred treatment, regardless of the size of the hematoma. A number of instruments have been used for nail trephination, including a heated paper clip, heated needle, scalpel blade, cautery device, 2-mm punch biopsy, and carbon dioxide laser. The use of an extrafine insulin syringe needle for the evacuation of subungual hematomas has also been reported. To avoid secondary nail dystrophy resulting from the subungual hematoma, it is recommended that evacuation not be delayed longer than 6 to 12 h after injury.

## Pincer Nail

The pincer nail deformity is defined as a transverse overcurvature of the nail plate that leads to progressive pinching of the nail bed. The lateral edges of the nail plate can break through the skin, resulting in the formation of granulation

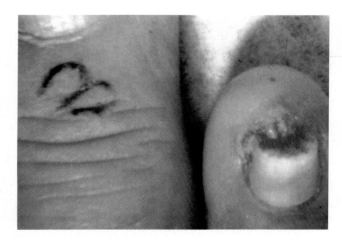

FIGURE 33-6 ■ Pincer nail.

tissue and paronychia (Fig. 33-6). Any nail can be involved, but the great toenails are most commonly affected. Pincer nail can lead to inflammation, pain, difficulty with footwear, and an undesirable cosmetic appearance. Pincer nail can be both familial and acquired. In the hereditary form, involvement is usually symmetric, whereas acquired pincer nail generally does not show symmetric involvement.

Pincer nail can be divided into three clinical types. The most common form is the trumpet nail deformity that occurs when the curvature increases from the proximal to distal portion. The second clinical type of pincer nail is the tile-shaped nail, which displays an even, transverse overcurvature with the lateral nail plate edges remaining parallel. The third form of pincer nail is the plicated nail, which shows a less drastic overcurvature with one or both lateral nail plate edges forming a vertical sheet pressing into the lateral nail groove.

### Diagnosis

Pincer nail deformity is usually diagnosed easily by the characteristic clinical appearance. It is important to determine the underlying cause, however, as there are a variety of treatable causes of acquired pincer nail. The most common cause is deviation of the phalanges of the feet secondary to poorly fitting shoes. Diseases associated with acquired pincer nail deformity include psoriasis, onychomycosis, subungual exostosis, epidermal cyst, or myxoid cyst. Pincer nails have also been reported in association with metastasis of colon carcinoma, placement of an arteriovenous fistula for hemodialysis, and the use of β-blockers. Pincer nail deformity can also be seen in association with osteoarthritis. Imaging with plain film or MRI can help identify the presence of osteophytes or hyperostosis, which unless treated, can lead to recurrence.

### Treatment

Pincer nail can be treated nonsurgically by placement of a brace on the nail plate that is fixed to the lateral edges. The brace is gradually adjusted, resulting in flattening of the nail plate. Recurrences are common with this method. Nail avulsion has also been shown to be an ineffective long-term treatment that can actually exacerbate the overcurvature of the nail plate. Several surgical treatments are effective in correcting pincer nail deformity. These include widening and flattening of the nail bed, tunneled dermal graft placement for flattening of the matrix, and selective destruction of the lateral matrix horns by phenol, electrocautery, or $CO_2$ laser. Improvement is more likely to be permanent when bony defects that contribute to the nail deformity are removed. Destruction of the entire nail matrix by phenol or surgical ablation may be required in recurrent cases.

## Onychocryptosis (Ingrown Nails)

Onychocryptosis occurs when the lateral edge of the nail plate grows into the nail fold, resulting in inflammation and soft tissue hypertrophy that can become secondarily infected. The great toenail is most often affected (Fig. 33-7). This condition can be extremely painful and restrict mobility. Onychocryptosis has been classified based on the extent of disease. Stage I is typified by pain with mild nail fold erythema and swelling without drainage. Stage II is characterized by swelling, purulent drainage, and ulceration of the nail fold. Stage III is characterized by chronic inflammation with granulation tissue and extensive nail fold hypertrophy.

### Diagnosis

In patients presenting with onychocryptosis, it is important to explore all potential etiologies. Onychocryptosis is usually caused by poorly fitting shoes or improper trimming of the nail. Other causes include onychomycosis that results in a thickened and dystrophic nail, arthritis, hyperhidrosis, obesity, injury to the nail, and medications. Isotretinoin is one of the more commonly reported causative medications, while the epidermal growth factor inhibitors have recently been found to cause onychocryptosis.

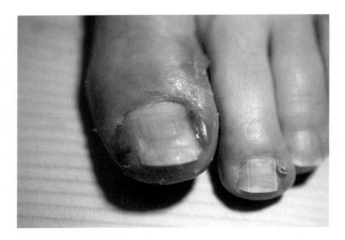

FIGURE 33-7 ■ Onychocryptosis.

## Treatment

Treatment of onychocryptosis depends on the extent of involvement. Early disease can be treated conservatively by separating the nail plate from the nail fold using a piece of cotton, a wedge of fabric treated with antiseptic solution, or a plastic tube splint. These stay in place until the nail plate grows beyond the lateral nail fold. In more advanced disease, the portion of nail plate pressing on the nail fold should be removed and if secondary infection is suspected, antibiotics should be added. For stage III onychocryptosis, avulsion of the lateral nail plate plus ablation of the corresponding lateral nail matrix using phenol, sodium hydroxide, or $CO_2$ laser is the preferred treatment. A Cochrane review found simple nail avulsion combined with the use of phenol for matrix ablation to be more effective at preventing symptomatic recurrence but more likely to be complicated by postoperative infection compared to surgical excision without phenol. In cases where the lateral nail fold is hypertrophied, excision of extra lateral nail fold tissue reduces pain and the risk of recurrence.

## Racket Nail

Racket nail is a short, broad, flat nail named after its similarity in shape to a tennis racket. The nail shape usually results from an underlying, shortened distal phalanx of the thumb. Other digits may be involved as well. Women are more often affected. Racket nails may be inherited in an autosomal dominant manner. One or both hands can be involved. Racket nails can be a source of cosmetic concern to patients, but do not otherwise affect function of the digit. Most cases of racket nail are congenital, but an acquired case has been reported in association with tertiary hyperparathyroidism.

## Habit-Tic Deformity

Habit-tic deformity presents as evenly spaced, parallel transverse grooves with a central depression of the nail plate (Fig. 33-8). The lunula is enlarged and the cuticle is often disrupted. The thumbnail is most commonly affected, but other nails can also be involved. This deformity is caused by repeated trauma to the nail matrix at the proximal nail fold secondary to picking from a conscious or unconscious habit. Body dysmorphic disorder, obsessive–compulsive disorder, and other psychiatric illnesses that involve a loss of impulse control can include ritualistic nail picking. A case of the habit-tic deformity has been reported to respond to treatment with fluoxetine (Prozac).

## Median Canaliform Dystrophy

Median canaliform dystrophy, also known as dystrophia unguium mediana canaliformis, is a nail plate defect in which a median (central) ridge develops, with short transverse ridges running from both sides of the central split. This has been described as an "inverted fir tree configuration." The thumbnails are most commonly affected. Median canaliform dystrophy can be hereditary. In most cases, an inciting cause cannot be identified and the nails normalize over a period of months to years. Although the pathogenesis of this disorder is not known, it is speculated that localized dyskeratinization of the nail matrix may be responsible. Self-inflicted damage to the middle part of the posterior nail fold has also been hypothesized to be the cause of median canaliform dystrophy. There are three case reports of patients who developed median canaliform dystrophy after treatment with isotretinoin for acne. In all cases, the nail changes reverted to normal after discontinuation of the drug.

## Trachyonychia

Trachyonychia or "rough nails" can be associated with a variety of dermatoses including

- lichen planus,
- psoriasis,
- alopecia areata,
- atopic dermatitis, and
- ichthyosis vulgaris.

Trachyonychia has also been associated with immunoglobulin A deficiency. Trachyonychia is described as having a sandpaper appearance, with a rough, lusterless nail plate (Fig. 33-9). The presence of numerous small, superficial pits in the nail plate in less severe cases can cause the nail to appear shiny. One or more nails can be affected. When all 20 nails are affected, the condition is often termed twenty-nail dystrophy. The peak incidence is between 2 and 12 years of age. Identification of a specific cause may require nail matrix biopsy. Trachyonychia associated with lichen planus in children usually resolves over time without treatment.

## Treatment

Local treatment of trachyonychia is best accomplished with intralesional triamcinolone acetonide into the proximal nail folds. A case report has demonstrated a beneficial effect of topical 5-fluorouracil cream in the treatment of psoriatic trachyonychia. Emollients or nail sticks with 50% urea may be beneficial.

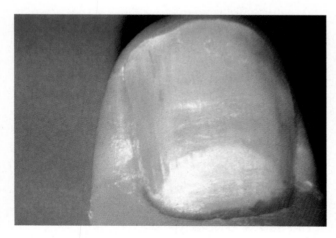

**FIGURE 33-8** ■ Habit-tic deformity.

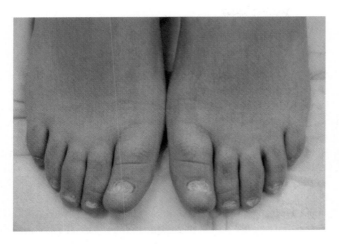

**FIGURE 33-9 ■** Trachyonychia.

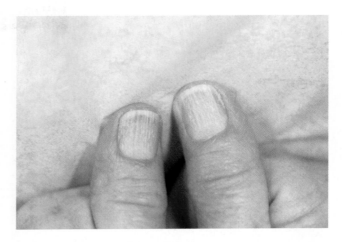

**FIGURE 33-10 ■** Brittle nails.

## Brittle Nails

Brittle nail syndrome is characterized by dry, easily damaged nail plates with onychorrhexis (longitudinal ridging), onychoschizia (horizontal layering), and excessive cracking and/or splitting (**Fig. 33-10**). A grading system based on the degree of lamellar and longitudinal splitting has been proposed. Dehydration of the nail plate is believed to be the main cause of brittle nails, leading to loss of flexibility and inelasticity of the nail plate. This can occur in patients exposed to organic solvents, acetone, alkaline liquids, and frequent handwashing. Psoriasis, lichen planus, and alopecia areata can be associated with brittle nails. Several systemic diseases are associated with brittle nails, including

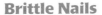

- tuberculosis,
- endocrinopathies,
- iron deficiency anemia,
- hemochromatosis,
- osteoporosis,
- glucagonoma, and
- vitamin deficiencies.

### Treatment

Treatment of brittle nails should first address underlying dermatologic or systemic disease. Determining the moisture content of the nail plate can also dictate treatment. There appears to be an optimal humidity for nail strength, and brittle nails can be divided into cases in which the plate is hard and brittle and those in which the plate is soft and brittle. Hard and brittle nails result from dehydration that may be exacerbated by low-humidity environments. In these cases, the goal of treatment is nail plate rehydration, accomplished by the addition of daily emollients, a humidifier, and nighttime nail soaks in water followed by application of urea or lactic acid creams. After soaking, the nail plate can also be massaged with mineral oil to prevent drying. Soft and brittle nails result from excess moisture, a condition that may worsen in high humidity. Treatment in these cases should focus on

minimizing exposure to moisture by the use of cotton gloves under vinyl gloves for wet work and avoidance of irritants.

Oral biotin, a B-complex vitamin, has proven effective in the treatment of brittle nails. The recommended dose is 2.5 mg/d, taken for 3 to 6 months. The average time before clinical improvement is 2 months. Silicon has also shown efficacy in improving brittle nails.

## Longitudinal Melanonychia (Melanonychia Striata)

Longitudinal melanonychia refers to a tan, brown, or black longitudinal band or streak affecting a nail (**Fig. 33-11**). One or multiple nails can be involved. When multiple bands are present, the inciting cause is most likely non-neoplastic. Causes of multiple bands of longitudinal melanonychia include

- dermatologic disorders (Laugier–Hunziker syndrome, lichen planus, lichen stratus),
- drugs (antimalarials, ketoconazole, minocycline, zidovudine, many chemotherapeutic agents),
- bacterial and fungal infections,
- racial variation (African American, Hispanic, Indian, Japanese), and
- a variety of systemic diseases (Addison's disease, hyperbilirubinemia, hyperthyroidism, malnutrition, Peutz–Jeghers syndrome, porphyria, and others).

A variety of causes can be responsible for isolated longitudinal melanonychia. Pigment may be present from exogenous sources, such as dirt, tobacco, or tar, and can usually be scratched off the nail plate. These sources typically do not present as a longitudinal streak. Nail plate infection with gram-negative bacteria such as *Klebsiella* and *Proteus* spp. can cause longitudinal melanonychia. When a greenish discoloration is present, infection with *Pseudomonas aeruginosa* is likely. Bacterial infection causing a pigmented streak usually presents at the junction of the lateral and proximal nail folds. The border of this streak is usually variable. Fungal infections of the nail plate can also cause hyperpigmented

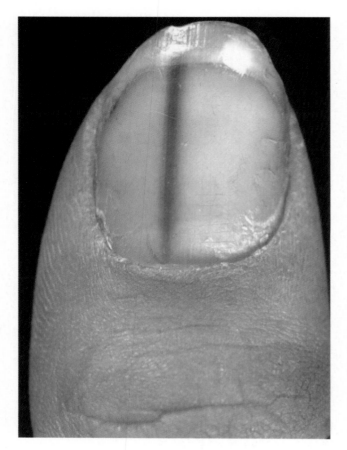

**FIGURE 33-11** ■ Longitudinal melanonychia.

streaks. These streaks are usually wider distally than proximally. Subungual hematomas caused by repeated minor trauma, usually from shoe friction, can cause an elliptical streak similar to longitudinal melanonychia. Local irradiation has also been reported to cause longitudinal melanonychia. A variety of melanocytic lesions, including acquired and congenital melanocytic nevi, benign and atypical melanocytic hyperplasias, and melanoma, can cause longitudinal melanonychia. Nail unit melanoma should always be in the differential diagnosis of isolated longitudinal melanonychia and can only be confirmed or excluded by biopsy.

## Diagnosis

Situations in which longitudinal melanonychia should trigger suspicion for ungual melanoma include longitudinal melanonychia that

- begins in a single digit of a person during the fourth to sixth decade of life or later,
- develops abruptly in a previously normal nail plate,
- becomes suddenly darker or wider than 5 mm,
- occurs in the thumb, index finger, or great toe,
- occurs in a person without a history of digital trauma,
- occurs singly in the digit of a dark-skinned patient,
- demonstrates blurred lateral borders,

- occurs in a person with a history or increased risk of melanoma, or
- is accompanied by nail dystrophy.

Dermoscopy is being used increasingly as a tool to aid in the decision to biopsy longitudinal melanonychia. Melanomas are more likely to be associated with irregular longitudinal lines varying in color, spacing, thickness, and parallelism. End-on nail plate dermoscopy can be used to determine the site of pigment origin in the matrix. Dorsal plate pigment corresponds to the proximal matrix and ventral plate pigment corresponds to the distal matrix. When malignancy is suspected, biopsy of the site of origin in the matrix is critical for an accurate diagnosis. Lesions with midline bands thinner than 3 mm can be biopsied using the punch technique in the matrix. Larger midline lesions can be biopsied by the shave technique. Lateral lesions can be biopsied by a longitudinal excision.

Longitudinal melanonychia in children is evaluated on a case-by-case basis and biopsy should be performed when appropriate. Among 85 cases of longitudinal melanonychia in children over a period of 35 years, no more than 5.9% displayed histologic evidence of malignancy. Although detection of a subungual melanoma in a child with longitudinal melanonychia is rare, the risk of nail dystrophy and anesthesia are outweighed by importance of an accurate diagnosis of a potentially malignant lesion.

## Treatment

Treatment of longitudinal melanonychia depends on the underlying cause.

# Tumors of the Nail Unit

## Subungual Melanoma

The nail apparatus is an uncommon site for melanoma, with an incidence between 0.7% and 3.5% of all melanomas. Timely diagnosis is critical, however, because the prognosis for melanoma involving the nail is significantly worse than cutaneous melanoma of the same thickness and stage. The prognosis is worse because subungual melanoma is diagnosed later (mean Breslow depth of 4.7 mm), it is felt to be more aggressive than cutaneous melanoma, and it has earlier metastasis leading to higher mortality. Patients most commonly present with subungual melanoma between the fifth and seventh decades. Amelanotic melanoma makes up a much higher percentage of melanomas affecting the nail compared to other sites, which further complicates the diagnosis. The most important factors contributing to prognosis include Breslow depth of invasion of the melanoma, presence of tumor ulceration, and presence of bone invasion.

### Diagnosis

Subungual melanoma can be misdiagnosed as onychomycosis, pyogenic granuloma, subungual hematoma, benign nevus, and paronychia. This can cause delay in potentially lifesaving treatment. Two important signs of subungual

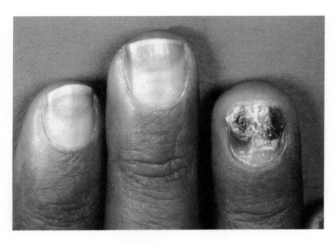

**FIGURE 33-12** ■ Subungual melanoma.

melanoma are longitudinal melanonychia (discussed before) and Hutchinson's sign (Fig. 33-12). Hutchinson's sign refers to the spread of pigment from the nail bed, matrix, and nail plate onto the adjacent cuticle and proximal and/or lateral nail folds. Pseudo-Hutchinson's sign refers to periungual pigmentation unrelated to melanoma that can be found in Laugier–Hunziker syndrome, as a side effect of certain medications, in the presence of nail infection, as a normal variant, and with a variety of systemic diseases.

The ABCDEF acronym for clinical detection of subungual melanoma is a useful screening method that was developed after a review of the world literature:

- A stands for African Americans, Asians, and Native Americans, the races most commonly affected by subungual melanoma.
- B stands for the diagnostic sign of a brown- to black-pigmented nail band with blurred borders and a breadth of 3 mm or more.
- C stands for a recent, sudden, or rapid change in the size of the nail band or lack of change despite treatment.
- D stands for the digit most commonly affected by subungual melanoma, the thumb, followed by the hallux or index finger. A single digit affected by a pigmented band should raise the suspicion of subungual melanoma more than a situation where multiple digits are affected by pigmented bands.
- E stands for extension of pigment onto the proximal and/or lateral nail fold (Hutchinson's sign).
- F stands for a family or personal history of the dysplastic nevus syndrome or previous melanoma, which would indicate an increased overall risk for subungual melanoma.

Final diagnosis of subungual melanoma requires a biopsy.

## Treatment

Treatment of subungual melanoma depends on the extent of disease and the presence or absence of systemic metastases.

Wide local excision is the only treatment proven to reduce mortality. For invasive tumors, most authors advocate distal amputation, but some suggest that digit sparing may be possible for in situ lesions and thinner invasive lesions. Sentinel lymph node mapping provides information regarding prognosis but has not shown any survival benefit and lymph node dissection itself carries morbidity.

## Subungual Squamous Cell Carcinoma

Subungual squamous cell carcinoma is rare. It is often associated with predisposing factors including prior radiation therapy (especially in physicians and dentists), infection with human papillomavirus, tar exposure, and trauma. The incidence of subungual squamous cell carcinoma is highest in men between 50 and 69 years of age. Most reported cases of subungual squamous cell carcinoma occur on the fingers, but cases have been described occurring on the toes as well. Usually one digit is affected, the most common site being the thumb (Fig. 33-13).

### Diagnosis

Definitive diagnosis of subungual squamous cell carcinoma requires a biopsy. Delay in diagnosis is common as the tumor can be confused with onychomycosis, verruca vulgaris, or

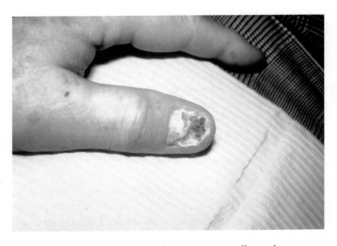

**FIGURE 33-13** ■ Subungual squamous cell carcinoma.

paronychia. Subungual squamous cell carcinoma involves the bone in 20% to 55% of cases. Squamous cell carcinoma of the nail unit is considered to have a good prognosis when compared with squamous cell carcinomas of other cutaneous sites. Lymph node and visceral metastasis are uncommon.

### Treatment

Smaller invasive tumors and in situ lesions are effectively treated with Mohs micrographic surgery. If there is bone involvement, amputation of the affected digit is recommended. Radiation therapy has been employed successfully in the treatment of unresectable subungual squamous cell carcinoma.

### Subungual Metastases

A comprehensive review of 133 patients diagnosed with subungual metastases shows that the three most common sites of primary malignancy are the lung (41% of cases), kidney (11% of cases), and breast (9% of cases). The appearance of these lesions takes a variety of forms, with some cases masquerading as pyogenic granuloma, acute paronychia, erysipelas, and herpes zoster. Subungual metastases are usually painful. Anatomic sites of presentation include both the hands and feet. One or multiple digits can be affected. An x-ray of the affected digit should be performed to evaluate bone involvement, which is a common complication of subungual metastases. A review of 39 patients with subungual metastases showed that in 44% of the cases the metastatic lesion was the initial expression of an undiagnosed malignancy or presented in the same month that the tumor was discovered.

### Digital Myxoid Cyst

Digital myxoid cyst is also known as a digital mucoid cyst, digital mucous cyst, myxoid pseudocyst, and synovial cyst. The variety of terms for this disorder reflects the controversial origin of the cyst development. It usually presents as an asymptomatic, single, soft to rubbery nodule on the dorsal surface of a finger, located between the proximal nail fold and distal interphalangeal joint, lateral to the midline. The material encased in the cyst has been described as viscous or gelatinous. The surface of the cyst is usually smooth, but verrucous variants have also been reported. Most cases occur in patients between the ages of 40 and 70. Women are more often affected than men. The most commonly affected anatomic sites are the middle and index fingers, but myxoid cysts are also sometimes found on the toes. Because of their location, cysts can exert pressure on the nail matrix, resulting in a linear nail plate dystrophy and a groove in the nail. Occasionally, these cysts can have a connection with the nearby distal interphalangeal joint.

### Treatment

When surgically excised, care must be taken to remove any communicating tracts between the cyst and joint to prevent recurrence. Other treatment options include cryotherapy, carbon dioxide laser vaporization, and injection of sclerosing solutions. Treatment by aspiration of the cyst contents

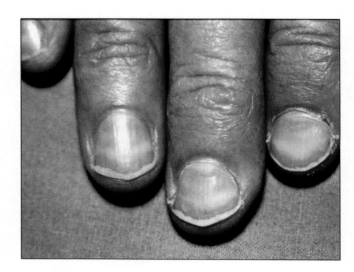

**FIGURE 33-14** ■ Muehrcke lines.

and injection of intralesional steroids can have high recurrence rates.

## Nail Manifestations of Systemic Disease

The nails can provide important clues in the diagnosis of systemic disease. Many morphologic changes can occur that point to an underlying renal, hepatic, pulmonary, and cardiac disease. Clubbing can suggest pulmonary infection, chronic pulmonary disease, and lung cancer. Koilonychia usually signifies underlying iron deficiency anemia. Transverse depressions in all nails are called Beau lines and indicate recent illness causing cessation of nail growth. Mees lines are transverse white bands that can be associated with arsenic poisoning, congestive heart failure (CHF), and Hodgkin's disease. Muehrcke lines are pairs of white lines extending across the nail that disappear with pressure (Fig. 33-14). They are classically associated with hypoalbuminemia. Terry nails are described as white nails with sparing of the tip of the nail plate. They are found most commonly in hepatic disease. Renal disease can be associated with nails with a half-white proximal portion and half-brown distal portion called half-and-half nails (Fig. 33-15). Yellow nail syndrome consists of

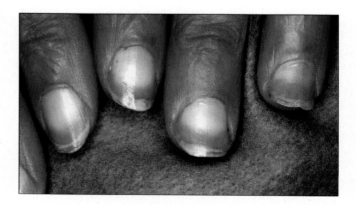

**FIGURE 33-15** ■ Half-and-half nails.

thickened yellow nails with absent lunula, pleural effusions, and lymphedema. Increased nail fold capillaries are best seen by dermoscopy and are indicative of connective tissue disease like lupus erythematosus, dermatomyositis, rheumatoid arthritis, or scleroderma. Diffuse pigmentation of the nails suggests medication side effects. Changes in the color of the lunula can be seen in Wilson's disease, CHF, connective tissue disease, and medication side effects.

## Suggested Readings

Baran R, Dawber RPR. *Baran and Dawber's Diseases of the Nails and Their Management.* 3rd ed. Malden, MA: Blackwell Science; 2001.

Baran R, Hay RJ, Garduno JI. Review of antifungal therapy and the severity index for assessing onychomycosis: part I. *J Dermatol Treat.* 2008;19: 72–81.

Baran R, Hay RJ, Tosti A, et al. A new classification of onychomycosis. *Br J Dermatol.* 1998;139:567–571.

Batrick N, Hashemi K, Freij R. Treatment of uncomplicated subungual hematoma. *Emerg Med J.* 2003;20:65.

Cohen PR. Metastatic tumors to the nail unit: subungual metastases. *Dermatol Surg.* 2001;27:280–293.

de Berker D. Management of nail psoriasis. *Clin Exp Dermatol.* 2000;25: 357–362.

Faergemann J, Baran R. Epidemiology, clinical presentation and diagnosis of onychomycosis. *Br J Dermatol.* 2003;149(suppl 65):1–4.

Farber EM, Nall L. Nail psoriasis. *Cutis.* 1992;50:174–178.

Fawcett RS, Linford S, Stulberg DL. Nail abnormalities: clues to systemic disease. *Am Fam Physician.* 2004;69:1417–1424.

Finch JJ, Warshaw EM. Toenail onychomycosis: current and future treatment options. *Dermatol Ther.* 2007;20:31–46.

Gupta AK. Types of onychomycosis. *Cutis.* 2001;68(2 suppl):4–7.

Gupta AK. Ciclopirox nail lacquer: a brush with onychomycosis. *Cutis.* 2001;68:13–16.

Gupta AK, Baran R, Summerbell R. Onychomycosis: strategies to improve efficacy and reduce recurrence. *J Eur Acad Dermatol Venereol.* 2002;16: 579–586.

Haneke E, Baran R. Longitudinal melanonychia. *Dermatol Surg.* 2001;27: 580–584.

Hay R. Literature review. Onychomycosis. *J Eur Acad Dermatol Venereol.* 2005;19(suppl 1):1–7.

Helms A, Brodell RT. Surgical pearl: prompt treatment of subungual hematoma by decompression. *J Am Acad Dermatol.* 2000;42:508–509.

Hordinsky MK, Sawaya ME, Scher RK. *Atlas of Hair and Nails.* 1st ed. Philadelphia: Churchill Livingstone; 2000.

Jellinek NJ. Primary malignant tumors of the nail unit. *Adv Dermatol.* 2005; 21:33–64.

Jellinek N. Nail matrix biopsy of longitudinal melanonychia: diagnostic algorithm including the matrix shave biopsy. *J Am Acad Dermatol.* 2007;56:803–810.

Jiaravuthisan MM, Sasseville D, Vender RB, et al. Psoriasis of the nail: anatomy, pathology, clinical presentation, and a review of the literature on therapy. *J Am Acad Dermatol.* 2007;57:1–27.

Levit EK, Kagen MH, Scher RK, et al. The ABC rule for clinical detection of subungual melanoma. *J Am Acad Dermatol.* 2000;42:269–274.

Lilly KK, Koshnick RL, Grill JP, et al. Cost-effectiveness of diagnostic tests for toenail onychomycosis: a repeated-measure, single-blinded, cross-sectional evaluation of 7 diagnostic tests. *J Am Acad Dermatol.* 2006; 55:620–626.

Peterson SR, Layton EG, Joseph AK. Squamous cell carcinoma of the nail unit with evidence of bony involvement: a multidisciplinary approach to resection and reconstruction. *Dermatol Surg.* 2004;30: 218–221.

Rich P, Scher RK. *An Atlas of Disease of the Nail.* 1st ed. New York: Parthenon Publishing Group; 2003.

Rigopoulos D, Larios G, Gregoriou S, et al. Acute and chronic paronychia. *Am Fam Physician.* 2008;77:339–346.

Rounding C, Bloomfield S. Surgical treatments for ingrowing toenails. *Cochrane Database Syst Rev.* 2005;2:CD001541.

Scher RK, Daniel, III, CR. Nails: Therapy, Diagnosis, Surgery. 3rd edition, WB Saunders, Philadelphia. 2005.

Scher RK, Tavakkol A, Sigurgeirsson B, et al. Onychomycosis: diagnosis and definition of cure. *J Am Acad Dermatol.* 2007;56:939–944.

Sonnex TS. Digital myxoid cysts: a review. *Cutis.* 1986;37:89–94.

Thai KE, Young R, Sinclair RD. Nail apparatus melanoma. *Australas J Dermatol* 2001;42:71–81:quiz 2–3.

Usman A, Silvers DN, Scher RK. Longitudinal melanonychia in children. *J Am Acad Dermatol.* 2001;44:547–548.

Uyttendaele H, Geyer A, Scher RK. Brittle nails: pathogenesis and treatment. *J Drugs Dermatol.* 2003;2:48–49.

# CHAPTER 34

# Diseases of the Mucous Membranes

*John C. Hall, MD*

The mucous membranes of the body adjoin the skin at the oral cavity, nose, conjunctiva, penis, vulva, and anus. Histologically, these membranes differ from the skin in that the horny layer and the hair follicles are absent. Disorders of the mucous membranes are usually associated with existing skin diseases or internal diseases. Only the most common diseases of the mucous membranes are discussed herein. At the end of the chapter is a listing of the uncommon conditions of these areas.

## Geographic Tongue

Geographic tongue is an extremely common condition of the tongue that usually occurs without symptoms. When these lesions are noticed for the first time by the individual, they may initiate fears of cancer.

### Presentation and Characteristics

#### Clinical Appearance

Irregularly shaped (maplike or geographic) pale red patches are seen on the tongue (Fig. 34-1). Close examination reveals that the filiform papillae are flatter or denuded in these areas. The patches slowly migrate over the tongue surface and heal without scarring.

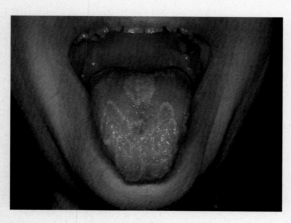

**FIGURE 34-1** ■ Geographic tongue. *(Courtesy of Neutrogena Corp.)*

#### Course

The disorder may come and go but may be constantly present in some persons.

#### Cause

The cause is unknown, but the lesions seem to be more extensive during a systemic illness. It has been suggested by some authors that geographic tongue is a form of psoriasis.

#### Subjective Symptoms

Some patients complain of burning and tenderness, especially when eating sour or salty foods.

### Differential Diagnosis

- *Syphilis,* secondary mucous membrane lesions: similar clinically, but acute in onset; usually more inflammatory; other cutaneous signs of syphilis; dark field examination and serology positive (see Chapters 22 and 26); does not come and go as rapidly.

### Treatment

1. Reassure patient that these are not cancerous lesions.
2. There is no effective or necessary therapy. However, if patient complains of burning and tenderness, prescribe triamcinolone (Kenalog) in Orabase 15.0

   *Sig:* Apply locally q.i.d. half hour p.c. and h.s.

## Gingival Enlargement

Excessive growth of periodontal tissue with raising and blunting of the gingival margins.

### Presentation and Characteristics

#### Clinical Appearance

If inflammation is present, the gingiva appears shiny, red, smooth, soft, and friable, with easy bleeding. If noninflammatory, it is firm with loss of stippling and contains a reddish-purple hue.

### Course

Improvement is common if the underlying cause is treated.

### Cause

Systemic diseases include primary amyloidosis, sarcoidosis, acromegaly, Kaposi's sarcoma, Wegener's granulomatosis, leukemia, aplastic anemia, lymphomas, Crohn's disease, scurvy, and neurofibromatosis.

Drug causes include phenytoin, calcium channel blockers, and cyclosporine. Less common drugs include lithium, tacrolimus, sertraline, birth control pills, ketaconazole, erythromycin, and other antisiezure medicines in addition to phenytoin. Poor dental hygiene with chronic gingivitis may be causative. It can be congenital, idiopathic, or physiologic in pregnancy or puberty.

### Symptoms

Pain, tenderness, halitosis, poor speech, difficult mastication and unsightly appearance are all reasons to initiate therapy.

### Treatment

Therapy is focused on the treatment of the underlying cause as well as aggressive oral hygiene. Surgical reduction is the last approach to be considered.

## Aphthous Stomatitis

Canker sores are extremely common, painful, superficial ulcerations of the mucous membranes of the mouth (Fig. 34-2).

### Presentation and Characteristics

### Course

One or more lesions develop at the same time and heal without scarring in 5 to 10 days. They can recur at irregular intervals. It is the most common oral inflammatory disease (affects 20% of population). It usually begins in adolescence and peaks in incidence in the third to fourth decade, after which the disease becomes less severe and less frequent.

### Clinical Appearance

Lesions are usually located on nonkeratinized mucosa (buccal, labial sulci, lateral and ventral tongue, soft palate, oropharynx).

There are three subtypes: (1) minor lesions (80%) are less than 5 mm to 1 cm, especially buccal and labial, and heal spontaneously in 7 to 10 days without a scar, (2) major (10%) are 5 to 10 mm deep, heal in weeks to months and often scar; other names are Sutton's ulcers or periadenitis mucosa necrotica recurrens, and (3) herpetiform (10%) occur on dorsal tongue, palate, or other keratinized mucosa, are small (1 to 3 mm) and grouped on coalescent ulcers, and heal in 1 to 4 weeks.

### Cause

The cause is unknown, but certain foods, especially chocolate, nuts, and fruits, can precipitate the lesions or may even be causative. Trauma from biting or dental procedures can initiate lesions (pathergy). Some cases in women recur in relation to menstruation. A viral cause has not been proved. A pleomorphic, transitional L-form of an $\alpha$-hemolytic *Streptococcus* sp (*Streptococcus sanguis*) has also been implicated as causative. Stress, nutritional deficiency, smoking cessation, and allergy may be triggers. Numerous underlying illnesses include Behçet's disease, human immunodeficiency virus (HIV), inflammatory bowel disease, cyclic neutropenia, FAPA (fever, aphthous stomatitis, pharyngitis, adenitis), and MAGIC (mouth and genital ulcers with inflamed cartilage and gluten-sensitive enteropathy). The disease can also be a sign of deficiencies of iron, zinc, folate, and B vitamins 1, 2, 6, and 12.

### Differential Diagnosis

- *Syphilis,* secondary lesions: clinically similar; less painful; other signs of syphilis; dark field examination and serology positive (see Chapters 22 and 26)

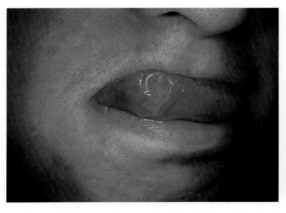
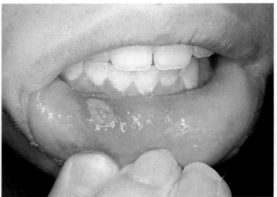

**FIGURE 34-2** ■ **(A)** Recurrent aphthous ulcer of the tongue. **(B)** Aphthous ulcer in patient with cyclic neutropenia. *(Courtesy of Neutrogena Corp.)*

■ *Herpes simplex virus:* usually a single lesion of grouped vesicles that erode. The first episode can be much more severe and widespread. Recurrence is usually at or near the original site and seldom intraoral. Can culture virus or see viral effect on biopsy (see Chapter 23)

## Treatment

Most persons who get these lesions learn that very little can be done for them and that the ulcers heal in a few days.

1. Toothpaste swish therapy: Brush the teeth and swish the toothpaste around in the mouth after each meal and at bedtime. If done soon after the onset of ulcers, extension of the lesions can be prevented and early healing can be helpful in many cases.
2. Triamcinolone in Orabase (prescription needed) applied locally after meals relieves some of the pain.
3. Tetracycline therapy: An oral suspension in a dosage of 250 mg per teaspoonful (or the powdery contents of a 250-mg capsule in a teaspoon of water) kept in the mouth for 2 minutes and then swallowed, four times a day, is beneficial. This mixture can be applied with a piece of cotton soaked in this solution.
4. Systemic corticosteroids may occasionally be used for severe ulcers.
5. A few reports in the literature have suggested limited benefit from the helicobacter elimination antibiotic regiment.

## Behçet's Disease

Behçet's disease is a triad of ulcers of oral and genital mucous membranes and uveitis. The "silk route disease" is so named because of its increased prevalence in the Middle East, Asia, and the Mediterranean (especially Turkey).

## Presentation and Characteristics

### O'Duffy Criteria for Behçet's Disease

Aphthous stomatitis
Genital ulcers
Uveitis
Cutaneous pustular vasculitis
Synovitis
Meningoencephalitis

---

**SAUER'S NOTES**

1. I wish to emphasize the value of the toothpaste swish therapy for aphthous stomatitis. It is especially valuable if begun soon after lesions appear.
2. The toothpaste swish also aids healing of self-inflicted tongue-bite sores.

---

At least three criteria, one being recurrent aphthous ulcers.
Incomplete form
At least two criteria, one being recurrent aphthous ulcers.

Must exclude inflammatory bowel disease, systemic lupus erythematosus, Reiter's disease, and herpes simplex virus infection.

*International 1990 Study Group for Diagnosis of Behçet's Syndrome*
Oral aphthae at least three times a year, plus two of the following:

Recurrent genital ulcers
Uveitis or retinal vasculitis
Papulopustular vasculitis or erythema nodosum
Pathergy—oblique insertion of 20-gauge needle showing perivascular neutrophils
Leukocytoclastic vasculitis at 24 to 48 hours

## Course

Behçet's disease can affect all ages, with no symptoms for weeks, months, or years and cycles of disease lasting days, weeks, or months. Oral aphthae can be the only sign of the disease for years (6 to 7 years on average). Blindness can occur in the 50% to 90% of Behçet's patients with eye disease. The disease affects the gastrointestinal tract (ulcers throughout the gastrointestinal tract), the neurologic system (vasculitis), the cardiopulmonary system (vasculitis), and the renal system. The oral and genital ulcers can be very debilitating.

## Cause

The cause is unknown, but it is hypothesized that exogenous trigger factors induce vasculitis in genetically predisposed individuals. Infectious triggers that may play a roll are herpes simplex virus or streptococci. There may be an immunologic or cytokine imbalance.

## Treatment

1. Topical and systemic corticosteroids are the mainstay of therapy
2. Nonsteroidal anti-inflammatory drugs, colchicines, and dapsone
3. Immunosuppressives and cytotoxic agents
4. Other therapies tried include tacrolimus, thalidomide, interferon-γ, etanercept, and infliximab

## Herpes Simplex

Herpes simplex virus infection can occur as a group of umbilicated vesicles on the mucous membranes of the lips, the conjunctiva, the penis, and the labia. Frequently recurring episodes of this disease can be quite disabling (see Chapter 23). Recurrent intraoral herpes simplex is uncommon, but the primary outbreak can have extensive intraoral mucous membrane involvement.

## Fordyce's Disease

This is a physiologic variant of oral sebaceous glands in which more than the normal number exist. When they are suddenly noticed, the person becomes concerned as to the diagnosis. The lesions are asymptomatic and yellowish-orange, and there are 1- to 2-mm papules on the lips and labia minora. No treatment is necessary; they are benign.

## Other Mucosal Lesions and Conditions

Mucosal lesions can also be caused by the following:

- *Physical causes:* Sucking of lips, pressure sores, burns, actinic or sunlight cheilitis, factitial disorders, tobacco, and other chemicals. Contact dermatitis almost never occurs due to constant bathing of the mucous membranes with saliva.
- *Infectious diseases* (from viruses, bacteria, spirochetes, fungi, and animal parasites): Gangrenous bacterial infections are called *noma*. *Ludwig's angina* is an acute cellulitis of the floor of the mouth caused by bacteria, abscesses, and sinuses and may be due to dental infection. *Trench mouth*, or *Plaut–Vincent's disease*, is an acute ulcerative infection of the mucous membranes caused by a combination of a spirochete and a fusiform bacillus.
- *Systemic diseases*: These include lesions seen with hematologic diseases (e.g., leukemia, agranulocytosis from drugs or other causes, thrombocytopenia, pernicious anemia, cyclic or periodic neutropenia), immunocompromised conditions (such as the acquired immunodeficiency syndrome, organ transplants, lymphomas), collagen diseases (such as lupus erythematosus, scleroderma), pigmentary diseases (e.g., Addison's disease, Peutz–Jeghers syndrome), and autoimmune diseases, which cross over in several categories but include pemphigus and benign mucosal pemphigoid.
- *Drugs:* Phenytoin sodium causes a hyperplastic gingivitis; bismuth orally and intramuscularly causes a bluish-black line at the edge of the dental gum (see Fig. 8-12B); certain drugs cause hemorrhage and secondary infection of the mucous membranes.
- *Metabolic diseases:* Mucosal lesions are seen in primary systemic amyloidosis, lipoidosis, reticuloendothelioses, diabetes, and other disorders.
- *Tumors, local or systemic:* These include leukoplakia, squamous cell carcinoma, epulis, and cysts.

## Rarer Conditions of Oral Mucous Membranes

- *Halitosis:* Halitosis, or fetor oris, is a disagreeable odor of the breath.

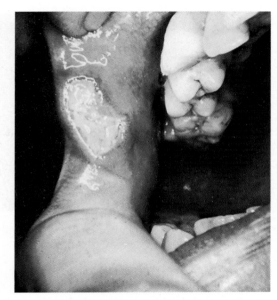

**FIGURE 34-3** ■ Periadenitis mucosa necrotica recurrens.

- *Periadenitis mucosa necrotica recurrens* (**Fig. 34-3**): Also known as Sutton's disease, this is a painful, recurrent, ulcerating disease of the mucous membranes of the oral cavity. The single or multiple deep ulcers exceed 10 mm and heal with scarring. Systemic corticosteroids may be indicated. It is considered by some to be a very severe type of aphthous ulcer.
- *Hand–foot–mouth disease:* This is a common vesicular eruption of the hands, feet, and mouth. Usually affecting children, it lasts up to 2 weeks. Most cases are caused by Coxsackievirus A16.
- *Koplik's spots:* Bright red, pinpoint-sized lesions on the mucous membranes of the cheek are seen in patients before the appearance of the rash of measles.
- *Erythema multiforme* (**Fig. 34-4**): This causes "bull's eye" lesions on the skin and erosions of the mucous membranes that may be severe. The commonest causes are herpes simplex and drug allergies.
- *Burning tongue* (glossodynia): This rather common complaint, particularly among middle-aged women, is usually accompanied by no visible pathology. The cause is unknown, and therapy is of little value, but the many diseases and local factors that cause painful tongue must be ruled out from a diagnostic viewpoint. The entire mouth can also burn. Tricyclic antidepressants have been used with some success.
- *Black tongue* (hairy tongue, lingua nigra; (**Fig. 34-5**): Overgrowth of the papillae of the tongue, apparently caused by an imbalance of bacterial flora, is due to the use of antibiotics and other agents. Black tongue without papillae hypertrophy can be seen with tobacco abuse, crack cocaine smoking, lansoprazole, chewing bismuth, methyldopa, minocycline, and hydroxychloroquine.

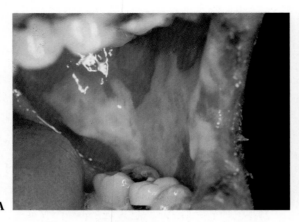
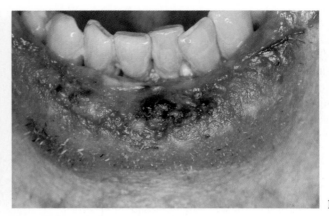

A                                                                              B

FIGURE 34-4 ■ Erythema multiforme of the left buccal mucosa (**A**) and on the lower lip (**B**).

■ *Hairy leukoplakia of the tongue:* This is a slightly raised, poorly demarcated lesion with a corrugated or "hairy" surface that appears on the sides of the tongue. It is seen mainly in immunosuppressed homosexual men infected with HIV. Human papillomavirus and Epstein–Barr virus have been identified in biopsy specimens (see Chapter 24). It is benign and no therapy is necessary.

■ *Moeller's glossitis:* This painful, persistent, red eruption on the sides and the tip of the tongue persists for weeks or months, subsides, and then recurs. The cause is unknown.

■ *Furrowed tongue* (grooved tongue, scrotal tongue): The tongue is usually larger than normal, containing deep longitudinal and lateral grooves of congenital origin due to syphilis or as part of Melkersson–Rosenthal syndrome (see Dictionary–Index).

■ *Glossitis rhomboidea mediana* (Fig. 34-6): This rare disorder, characterized by a smooth reddish lesion, usually occurs in the center of the tongue. This term is poor because there is no inflammation and the reddish plaque may not always be in the center.

■ *Sjögren's syndrome:* This rare entity is characterized by dryness of all of the mucous membranes and of the skin in middle-aged women. *Keratoconjunctivitis sicca* is used to describe the severe dryness of the eyes seen in this syndrome. The primary form of this syndrome is in many cases associated with a cutaneous vasculitis. The secondary type of Sjögren's syndrome is associated with rheumatic and collagen diseases. Evoxac is an oral medication that may help with the dry mouth. Sucking on hard lemon candy and artificial saliva can be tried.

■ *Cheilitis glandularis:* This chronic disorder of the lips is manifested by swelling and secondary inflammation caused by hypertrophy of the mucous glands and their ducts. There is up to a 35% risk of deterioration to squamous cell carcinoma. Surgical intervention has usually been the mainstay of therapy. Topical calcineurin inhibitors such as tacrolimus (Protopic) have been used with some success.

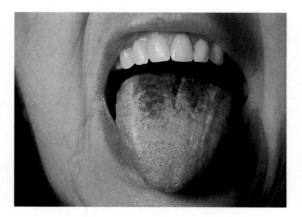

FIGURE 34-5 ■ Black tongue. *(Courtesy of Neutrogena Corp.)*

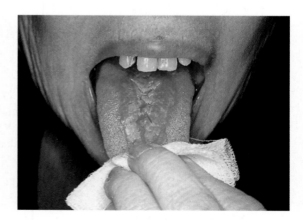

FIGURE 34-6 ■ Glossitis rhomboidea mediana. *(Courtesy of Neutrogena Corp.)*

## Rarer Conditions of Genital Mucous Membranes

- *Fusospirochetal balanitis:* This uncommon infection of the penis is characterized by superficial erosions. It must be differentiated from syphilis by a dark field examination and blood serology.
- *Balanitis xerotica obliterans* (see *Atrophies of the Skin* in the Dictionary–Index): This whitish atrophic lesion on the penis is to be differentiated from leukoplakia. The female counterpart is lichen sclerosus et atrophicus.
- *Lichen sclerosus et atrophicus:* This is a rare atrophy of the skin, usually of the genital and perirectal mucous membranes. In children (Fig. 34-7), it is the most common chronic genital dermatitis. The prognosis is better in younger patients. In older patients there is a slight increase in the incidence of squamous cell cancer (approximately 5%). (See *Atrophies of the Skin* in the Dictionary–Index.)

## Suggested Readings

Axell T. The oral mucosa as a mirror of general health or disease. *Scand J Dent Res.* 1992;100:9–16.

Daley TD. Common acanthotic and keratotic lesions of the oral mucosa: a review. *J Can Dent Assoc.* 1990;56:407–409.

Eisen D. The clinical features, malignant potential, and systemic associations of oral lichen planus: a study of 723 patients. *J Am Acad Dermatol.* 2002;46(2):2007–2014.

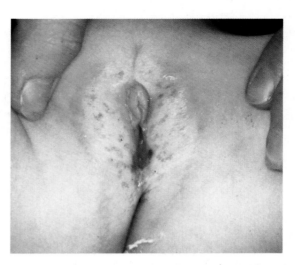

**FIGURE 34-7** ■ Lichen sclerosis et atrophicus of the labia in a patient aged 3 years.

Eisen D, Lynch DP. *The Mouth: Diagnosis and Treatment.* St. Louis: Mosby; 1998.

Eversole LR. Immunopathology of oral mucosal ulcerative, desquamative and bullous disease: selected review of the literature. *Oral Surg Oral Med Oral Pathol.* 1994;77:555–571.

Novick NL. Diseases of the mucous membrane. *Clin Dermatol.* 1987;5: 123–136.

Van der Waal I. *Diseases of the Salivary Glands: Including Dry Mouth and Sjögren's Syndrome Diagnosis and Treatment.* New York: Springer, 1997.

# CHAPTER 35

# Skin Diseases in Ethnic Skin

*Cheryl M. Burgess, MD and Beverly A. Johnson, MD*

## Learning Objectives/Goals

- Recognize diversity among skin types.
- Describe the changing demographics among ethnic populations in the United States.
- Recognize the market growth of ethnic consumers of dermatologic services.
- Recognize differences between white skin and ethnic skin.
- Identify skin types using established classification systems.
- Assess therapeutic considerations and identify potential for adverse effects in ethnic skin.
- Select treatment plans with respect to the potential for tissue response in ethnic skin.
- Identify the most common cosmetic concerns in ethnic skin.

## Chapter Overview

Dermatologists must take adequate steps for maintaining the necessary knowledge and instruction to provide all patients with thorough and comprehensive services. Therefore, additional knowledge and training must be considered to deliver the greatest efficacy with the lowest risk of adverse events when using state-of-the-art products and procedures in ethnic skin. This is especially true in light of daily advances in dermatologic services and growing diversity of skin types in the ethnic patient population. Clinicians must be fully prepared to recognize common problems in ethnic skin, identify appropriate treatments, and take steps to limit risk for any adverse events within this patient population.

### Terminology

Throughout the burgeoning research on ethnic skin, it has been difficult to provide consistent terminology in the medical literature that conveys appropriate categorization and accurate description of skin types. To address this challenge, the following conventions are used throughout this chapter: The term "white skin" refers to skin having a Fitzpatrick classification of I, II, or III. The term "Caucasian" is avoided because this term refers to a larger group of skin types, beyond people with white skin. The term "ethnic skin" refers to skin that has a Fitzpatrick classification of IV, V, and VI, which applies to skin types in people of black, Latino, and

Asian ethnic groups. The term "blacks" is used in place of "African Americans" because the latter term refers to only a subgroup of a much larger category of people with pigmented skin. These conventions have been selected to provide consistency, accuracy, and clarity in the following discussion. These conventions should not be substituted for careful clinical descriptions.

## Introduction and Background

### Demographic Trends and the Growth of Dermatologic Services in Ethnic Consumers

#### Diversity of Skin Types

The buzz phrase, "Skin of Color," has often been thought to refer primarily to black skin. However, in the United States, individuals with pigmented skin come from a variety of racial and ethnic groups. These groups are summarized in Table 35-1. The diversity of ethnic and racial groups yields a broad spectrum of pigmented skin types that is continuously changing. For example, the 1990 US Census Bureau listed 6 races with 23 racial subtypes. Only 10 years later, the same 6 race categories included at least 67 subtypes. The largest ethnic populations—black, Hispanic, and Asian—are expected to make up almost half of the total US population by the year 2050; the predictions are 25% Hispanic, 14% black, 8% Asian, and 1% other. Trends in the

---

**TABLE 35-1 ■ Racial and Ethnic Groups in the United States**

- African-American black persons (including Caribbean-American black persons)
- Asian and Pacific Islanders (including those of Filipino, Chinese, Japanese, Korean, Vietnamese, Thai, Malaysian, Laotian, Hmong)
- Latino or Hispanic (including those of Mexican, Cuban, Puerto Rican, Central American, Spanish descent)
- People traditionally categorized as Caucasoid (including a majority of Indians, Pakistanis, and those of Middle Eastern origin)
- Native Americans
- Alaskans
- Aleuts

growth of diversity must drive the practice of dermatology to new levels of knowledge and awareness, so that clinicians are prepared to meet the challenges of today's patient populations and provide the highest level of care to the largest possible number of patients.

## Categorizing Pigmented Skin Types

### Fitzpatrick Skin Phototype Classification System

In the United States, individuals with pigmented skin come from a large collection of racial and ethnic groups. The diversity of racial and ethnic groups yields a broad spectrum of pigmented skin types that defy easy categorization. Throughout the years, the fields of dermatology and cosmetics have struggled to characterize pigmented skin types adequately. After its development in the 1970s, the Fitzpatrick Skin Phototype classification became a surrogate classification system for this purpose.

The Fitzpatrick Skin Phototype classification system was originally developed to categorize the skin's response to UV radiation. Over time, dermatologists became accustomed to using the system to classify both UV sensitivity and skin color. However, the system has limited utility for accurately communicating patient information for either research or clinical purposes and is of almost no value for helping clinicians treat ethnic skin effectively and safely. Patients with ethnic skin would benefit more from a classification system based on the propensity of the skin to scar and/or become hyperpigmented—a unique characteristic of pigmented skin. Several classification systems have been developed or proposed to meet these obvious needs. However, none have risen to an industry standard.

### Roberts Skin Type Classification System

The recently introduced Roberts Skin Type classification system (Table 35-2) may provide the most comprehensive information to meet the needs of clinicians. This system uses a four-part serial profile to characterize the skin's likely response to insult, injury, and inflammation through a quantitative and qualitative assessment that includes a review of ancestral and clinical history, visual examination, test site reactions, and physical examination of the patient's skin. Skin is categorized using a numeric descriptor that provides information on the phototype, hyperpigmentation, photoaging, and scarring characteristics. The Roberts classification system can provide a means to help facilitate study designs and communicate data in the medical literature.

**TABLE 35-2 ■ The Roberts Classification System**

| Name (units) | Fitzpatrick Scale (FZ) | Roberts Hyperpigmentation Scale (H) | Glogau Scale (G) | Roberts Scarring Scale (S) |
|---|---|---|---|---|
| Scale | Measures skin phototypes | Propensity for pigmentation | Describes photoaging | Describes scar morphology |
| Categories | $FZ_1$ White skin. Always burns, never tans | $H_0$ Hypopigmentation | $G_1$ No wrinkles, early photoaging | $S_0$ Atrophy |
| | $FZ_2$ White skin. Always burns, minimal tan | $H_1$ Minimal and transient ($<1$ year) hyperpigmentation | $G_2$ Wrinkles with motion, early to moderate photoaging | $S_1$ None |
| | $FZ_3$ White skin. Burns minimally, tans moderately and gradually | $H_2$ Minimal and permanent ($>1$ year) hyperpigmentation | $G_3$ Wrinkles at rest, advanced photoaging | $S_2$ Macule |
| | $FZ_4$ Light brown skin. Burns minimally, tans well | $H_3$ Moderate and transient ($<1$ year) hyperpigmentation | $G_4$ Only wrinkles, severe photoaging | $S_3$ Plaque within scarred boundaries |
| | $FZ_5$ Brown skin. Rarely burns, tans deeply | $H_4$ Severe and transient ($>1$ year) hyperpigmentation | | $S_4$ Keloid |
| | $FZ_6$ Dark brown/black skin | $H_5$ Severe and transient ($<1$ year) hyperpigmentation | | $S_5$ Keloid nodule |
| | | $H_6$ Severe and permanent ($>1$ year) hyperpigmentation | | |

Note: Reprinted with permission from Roberts WE. The Roberts skin type classification system. *J Drugs Dermatol.* 2008;7(5):452–456.

**TABLE 35-3 ■ Characteristics of Darker Complexions**

- Black skin has larger, more dispersed melanosomes
- The minimal erythema dose of black skin is 30-fold greater than that of white skin
- The skin becomes darker in response to injury
- Thicker, more compact stratum corneum
- Thicker collagen bundles in the dermis
- Blacks have increased apocrine and sebaceous glands associated with increased follicular responses
- Increased transepidermal water loss

Note: Stephens TJ, Oresajo C. Ethnic sensitive skin: a review. *Cosmet Toiletries*. 1994;109(February):75–80.

Draelos ZD. Is all skin alike? *Cosmet Dermatol*. 2002;15(9):81–83.

## Distinguishing Characteristics of Black Skin

### Structure and Function

There are several distinguishing characteristics of black skin (Table 35-3). For example, in the skin of blacks, the stratum corneum layer counts are significantly higher and more compact, with thicker collagen bundles present in the dermis. The most evident difference between ethnic skin and white skin is epidermal melanin content. While no differences exist in the number of melanocytes, variations do exist in the number, size, packaging, and distribution of melanosomes. In the skin of blacks, melanosomes are larger and more dispersed. Moreover, the epidermal melanin unit in ethnic skin contains more melanin overall and may undergo slower degradation. These differences in melanin and melanosomes provide superior UV protection in ethnic skin.

In fact, the minimal erythema dose in black skin is 30-fold greater than that of white skin. In addition, black skin has increased apocrine and sebaceous glands that are associated with increased follicular responses. Transdermal water loss is also increased in the skin of blacks.

Because of these differences in skin structure and function, ethnic people suffer less photodamage than whites do. In fact, one study of adults living in Tucson, Arizona, found that the epidermis of black participants was largely spared the gross photodamage observed in white participants. Most of the white women, aged 45 to 50 years, had wrinkles in the area of the lateral epicanthus (this is also known as crow's feet) and on the corners of the mouth, while none of the black women of comparable age had obvious crow's feet wrinkles or perioral rhytides. The skin of blacks was also felt firmer, and the histology of the dermal elastic fibers in black skin was similar to the appearance of these fibers in sun-protected white skin.

## Common Dermatologic Concerns in Ethnic Skin

### Pseudofolliculitis Barbae and Acne Keloidalis Nuchae

These chronic inflammatory disorders are among the most common dermatologic concerns in ethnic skin (Table 35-4). It is observed primarily in individuals with tightly curled hair, and found most commonly in black men, followed by Hispanic men. It is also found in women of all races due to shaving in the bikini region where natural folds of the crural area in friction from underwear promote epidermal reentry of even straight hair (Fig. 35-1).

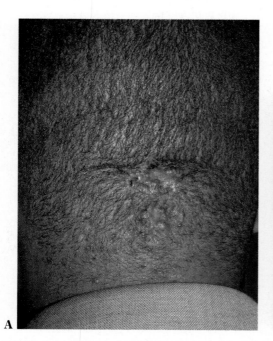

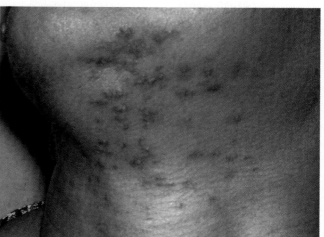

A B

**FIGURE 35-1 ■ (A)** Acne keloidalis nuchae. **(B)** Pseudofolliculitis barbae.

## TABLE 35-4 ■ Most Common Dermatologic Concerns in Ethnic Skin

- Pseudofolliculitis barbae and acne keloidalis nuchae
- Acne vulgaris and acne rosacea
- Seborrheic dermatitis
- Scarring alopecia
- Scalp folliculitis

All treatments should target elimination or reduction of the foreign body reaction surrounding an ingrown hair. Cessation of shaving is the first choice of treatment but is typically insufficient to break the cycle of ingrown hairs because many men must have a clean-shaven face, and discontinuation of shaving can continue to cause problems in approximately 10% to 20% of affected individuals. Shaving with single-blade razors can result in the extrafollicular reentry of the hair follicle. New or multiple blade systems can lead to transfollicular penetration. Plucking hairs can also lead to transfollicular penetration. An inflammatory response associated with these processes can lead to papules and pustules, which has the propensity to leave hyperpigmented macules and keloids.

### Treatment

To minimize pseudofolliculitis barbae, it is necessary to discontinue close shaves. This can be achieved by the use of a correct shaving tool with proper training of the patient. Single-bladed razors or The Bump Fighter Razor is an effective shaving tool for this purpose. Treatment can also be accomplished with fairly good success by the AM/PM alternation of a topical steroid and a topical retinoid. Treatment may also consist of depilatories, adjunctive topicals, electrolysis, chemical peels, and laser hair removal therapy. Ingrown hair follicles may be prevented by the use of retinoids, glycolic acid or salicylic acid preparations, topical anti-inflammatory agents, or the use of a soft toothbrush to lift the hair follicles above the skin.

### Seborrheic Dermatitis

Seborrheic dermatitis occurs in all types of skin and is commonly found in areas of the scalp and along the hairline; in and behind the ears; along the side of the nostrils, eyebrows, or T-zone of the face; midchest; and in the beard and mustache of men. Contrary to what the references have said regarding black skin, applying pomades and oils and lotions to these areas only exacerbates the condition. Seborrheic dermatitis may cause hypo- or hyperpigmented changes in skin color in affected areas of black skin (Fig. 35-2).

### Treatment

Treatment for seborrheic dermatitis includes topical medications and dandruff shampoos containing selenium sulfide, coal tar, sulfur, salicylic acid pyrithione zinc, ketoconazole, and mild steroids. When dandruff shampoos are recom-

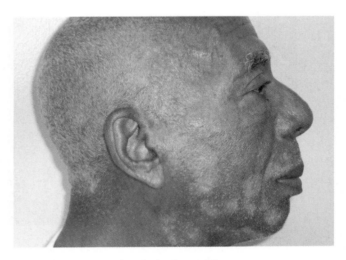

**FIGURE 35-2** ■ Seborrheic dermatitis.

mended, patients must routinely shampoo their scalp for a minimum of 5 minutes once or twice a week.

Frequent shampooing can lead to dry brittle hair and subsequent breakage; therefore, dandruff shampoos are not commonly used or recommended. Topical preparations with active ingredients containing ketoconazole or corticosteroids can be used as an alternative to the daily use of dandruff shampoos. Topical preparations are applied directly to the scalp several times a week until the condition is brought under control. The use of topical preparations limits the need to shampoo the scalp on a daily basis. With proper treatment, skin discoloration typically returns to normal.

### Scarring Alopecia

#### General Information

Scarring alopecia is a condition that commonly occurs in black women and some Hispanic women and is typically the result of some unique biologic attribute. For men and women of all ages, hair loss can be devastating and can cause serious psychologic and financial consequences. The spectrum of hair loss is broad. Causes of hair loss vary from

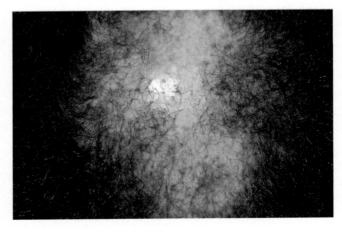

**FIGURE 35-3** ■ Scarring alopecia.

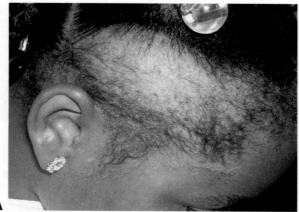

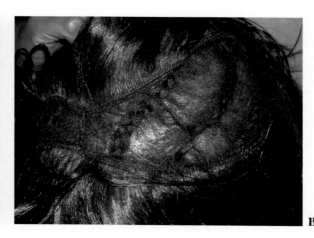

**FIGURE 35-4** ■ **(A)** Traction alopecia. **(B)** Hair tracks.

controllable to uncontrollable circumstances such as genetic predisposition to disease for unknown reasons. In addition, it is important to acknowledge and accommodate cultural differences that can serve as a barrier to the patient's acceptance of a recommended treatment protocol. Accurate diagnosis requires taking a comprehensive history of the patient, including influences from social and economic influences. For example, take into consideration weekly or twice-monthly hair shampooing, the use of braids or twists, as well as home remedies. Black patients may also have a presumed preference for oily vehicles and medications to treat dermatitis of the scalp (**Fig. 35-3**).

Common causes of alopecia may be due to (1) scarring alopecia (traction alopecia, discoid lupus erythematosus [DLE], chronic tinea capitis, central centrifugal cicatricial alopecia [CCCA]); (2) nonscarring alopecia (alopecia areata, tinea capitis); or (3) grooming alopecia.

### Traction Alopecia

Traction alopecia is a common cause of hair loss due to pulling forces exerted on the scalp hair. This excessive tension leads to breakage in the outermost hairs. The two types of traction alopecia are marginal and nonmarginal. Traction alopecia is unintentionally induced by various hairstyling practices (use of braids, hair rollers, weaves, twists, locks, or cornrows). When tensile forces are chronically present, an irritant type of folliculitis develops. Follicular scarring and permanent alopecia may result. Hair loss is reversible in the initial stages, but with prolonged traction, alopecia can be permanent. Therefore, the key is early prevention (**Fig. 35-4**).

### Discoid Lupus Erythematosus

DLE is a chronic skin disease that produces atrophic lesions of sores with inflammation and scarring on the face, ears, and scalp, and to a lesser degree, on other areas of the body. When lesions occur in hairy areas such as the beard or scalp, permanent scarring and hair loss can occur. The exact cause of DLE is unknown, but the condition is thought to be an autoimmune disease. This condition tends to run in families

and occurs about three times more often in females. In some patients with DLE, sunlight and cigarette smoking may trigger the lesions (**Fig. 35-5**).

### Treatment

Treating DLE lesions with topical corticosteroids often reduces the severity of the involved areas and slows their progression. A cortisone injection into the lesions is typically more effective than the topical form of cortisone. Alternatively, calcineurin inhibitors such as pimecrolimus cream or tacrolimus ointment may be used. Additionally, imiquimod has been identified as a successful treatment. Patients whose condition is sensitive to sunlight should use a UVA/UVB blocking sunscreen daily and wear a hat while outdoors. Follow-up with the doctor is important and necessary every 6 to 12 months to check for internal organ involvement and to minimize scarring.

### Grooming Alopecia

Hair breakage can occur in natural hairstyles because of friction that develops from dry hair grooming through narrow

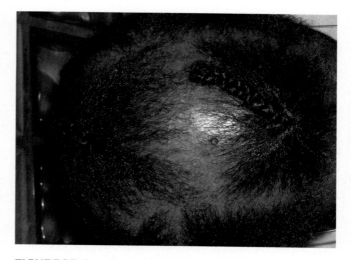

**FIGURE 35-5** ■ Traction alopecia due to braids.

combs or brushes. Hair breakage can also be caused by chronic use of chemical treatments. Hair processing solutions that contain sodium hydroxide (lye) or potassium hydroxide (non-lye) contribute to hair breakage by breaking disulfide bonds. Non-lye hair relaxers were developed for safe use at home by novices. However, contrary to popular belief, lye- and non-lye relaxers are equally damaging to hair. Therefore, most dermatologists and hair stylists prefer the use of lye relaxers. This is because the shorter processing time reduces the chemical contact exposure to the hair, which limits the degree of breakage.

Ammonium thioglycolate, ammonium sulfate, and ammonium bisulfate are known as perm salts that weaken the internal structures of the bonds, but stop short of breaking up disulfide bonds. Although these solutions are milder, they remove natural oils and moisture. Furthermore, after using ammonium thioglycolate, a mild alkaline solution is necessary to fix the perm.

Other products and practices that can contribute to hair breakage include hot comb and pomade use combined with blow-drying, the use of hot iron curling, hair rollers, hair dyes, and the use of various hairstyles, such as ponytails, extensions, and microbraids.

### Scalp Folliculitis

Individuals with scalp folliculitis often develop uncomfortable and embarrassing symptoms such as intense itching, tenderness, persistent bumps, sores, pus discharge, and even bleeding of the scalp. In some cases, these symptoms subside and the scalp returns to its normal condition. However, these symptoms often progress, leading to the loss of individual hair follicles, with permanent hair loss and scarring in later stages. Early intervention is crucial to successful treatment and can lead to the slowing or reversal of hair loss in many individuals (Figs. 35-6 and 35-7).

The etiology of scalp folliculitis is unclear. However, clinical observations suggest that variants of scalp folliculitis develop most often in black men and women. It is believed that the condition refers to folliculitis occurs more

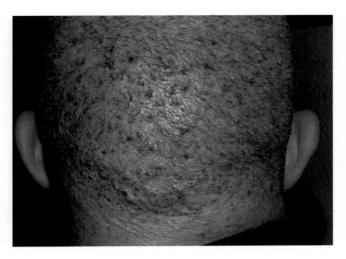

**FIGURE 35-7** ■ Scalp folliculitis.

often in women than in men, although the apparent prevalence of this condition in women may only be a reflection of women's tendency to seek medical attention more often than men, in the case of hair loss. Dermatologists have speculated that the condition is associated with hair care products and grooming practices used by blacks. Pressing of the hair, pomades, chemical relaxers, permanent wave agents, braiding, and other physically aggressive combing techniques are examples of possible causes suggested by this theory. However, dermatologists remain puzzled about the specific role of hair care products and grooming practices. For example, women and men with no prior use of these products or hair grooming practices develop scalp folliculitis. Other causes have also been proposed. For example, a family trait or genetic cause has been suggested by some experts, and a weakened immune system or hormonal change has also been suggested. Like many other skin conditions, a single cause may not be responsible for developing the condition; it may be multifactorial.

Throughout the years, dermatologists have explored a variety of treatments for scalp folliculitis with little or no success. Treatments have included the use of such medications as antibiotics, steroids, and oral retinoids. The prognosis (outcome) based on these treatments is not good. Either the condition persists through the treatment, or the condition briefly dissipates, only to stubbornly resurface shortly after halting the treatment.

### Treatment

Burgess et al. found that a combination of rifampicin 300 mg and cephalexin 500 mg given twice daily for 2 weeks led to nearly 100% improvement of symptoms in a majority of patients. Moreover, hair regrowth occurred in almost half of the patients treated. However, if the patient has experienced a long-standing, chronic condition, treatment may be less successful, because permanent damage to the hair follicle prevents regrowth of hair in the affected areas.

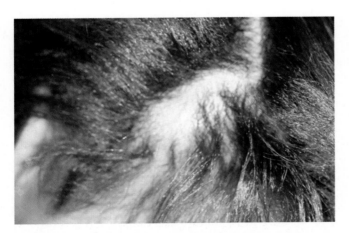

**FIGURE 35-6** ■ Scarring alopecia from discoid lupus erythematosus.

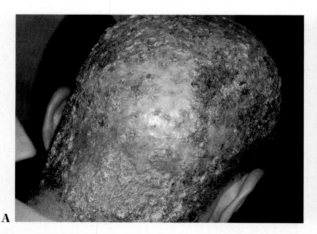
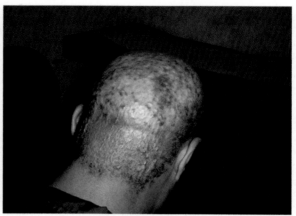

**FIGURE 35-8** ■ **(A)** Dissecting cellulitis and folliculitis. **(B)** After oral antibiotic treatment.

### Central Centrifugal Cicatricial Alopecia

CCCA can be divided into two categories: primary and secondary. Primary cicatricial alopecias are caused by an intrinsic process that specifically targets the hair follicle, leading to its destruction and replacement by fibrous tissue. Primary cicatricial alopecias are further classified as lymphocytic or neutrophilic according to the type of predominant inflammatory infiltrate. CCCA is a lymphocytic primary cicatricial alopecia.

CCCA begins with a patch of hair loss on the vertex of the scalp that expands centrifugally over the course of months to years. Affected areas of the scalp have a shiny appearance and can develop into large affected areas in late stages, while tenderness, pruritus, burning, and a "pins and needles" sensation are common associated symptoms. Histopathologically, CCCA is characterized by perifollicular lymphocytic inflammation and premature desquamation of the inner root sheath. Lamellar fibroplasia and follicular fibrosis are also seen. Biopsies taken of end-stage lesional scalp reveal diffuse scarring with a marked reduction or absence of hair follicles. Although the prevalence has not been studied, CCCA is one of the leading causes of hair loss in black women.

The cause of CCCA is poorly understood. Although thermal and chemical straightening of the hair has been implicated, conclusive evidence for this association is lacking. In particular, the term CCCA encompasses the previously described entity, hot comb alopecia, which refers to a scarring alopecia that is associated with the long-term use of heat and oil ("hot combing") to straighten the hair. However, CCCA has also been rarely reported in men who do not straighten the hair. Therefore, the etiology of CCCA is likely a combination of genetic and environmental factors.

## Common Dermatologic Diseases in Ethnic Skin

### Pityriasis Alba

Pityriasis Alba is a variation of atopic eczema that occurs in ethnic children. The round, light patches are covered with fine scale, but are otherwise asymptomatic. The condition can occur on any part of the body, but is usually first noticed on the face and upper arms, and can also involve the trunk. It is more noticeable in the summer months when the normal skin darkens and the affected skin looks paler by contrast. The loss of color is temporary and is not related to vitiligo. Treatment with topical immunomodulators is preferable to topical corticosteroids (which can further depigment the skin). Patients should be educated on sun protection and reassurance that the condition will not evolve into vitiligo. If the disease is widespread, topical PUVA is effective (Fig. 35-8).

### Dry or "Ashy" Skin

When dry or "ashy" skin develops in individuals with darker skin tones, the skin takes on a noticeable grayish or ashen hue that is easily observed. When dry skin occurs on the scalp, the ashiness may be mistaken for seborrhea. Treatment should include the use of moisturizers and avoidance of long hot baths or showers, or bath gels containing alcohol. To improve the condition of the scalp, patients should avoid the use of some of the antiseborrheic shampoos that can increase the dryness of the scalp and exacerbate the situation. Patients with dry ashy skin suffer more during cold weather seasons when dry air causes dry

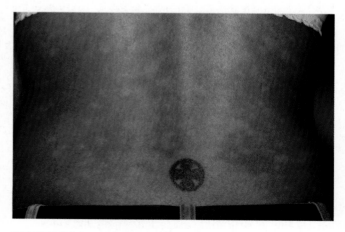

**FIGURE 35-9** ■ Pityriasis alba.

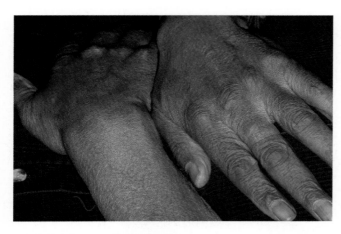

**FIGURE 35-10** ■ Dry ashy skin.

skin to worsen. Treatment can include humidifiers, and moisturizers applied immediately after showering while the skin is still damp. Moisturizing twice daily may be necessary for extremely dry skin (Fig. 35-9).

### Acne Vulgaris and Acne Rosacea

The morphology of acne lesions is the same in pigmented and white skin. However, there are several differences in the occurrence of acne between black and white individuals. Acne in blacks is often due to cultural preferences. For example, products such as pomades are typically applied to the hair for controlling hair and treating dryness, but can also cause comedonal acne on the forehead, hairline, and temples. The most significant difference in the acne of blacks is dramatic inflammation and subsequent development of postinflammatory hyperpigmentation (Fig. 35-10).

### Treatment

When treating ethnic patients, it is important to recognize that many topical products are poorly tolerated by black and Hispanic patients, especially women. In addition, clinicians should be careful to avoid hyperpigmentation or hypopigmentation that can be caused by the acne treatment, such as benzoyl peroxide, azelaic acid, and retinoids. The use of test spots with dermabrasion and chemical peeling treatments is strongly recommended before attempting dermal grafting, substation, punch grafting, and punch elevation.

Occasionally, dermatologists will want to use acne treatments that hypopigment the skin when dark macules are present. In such cases, it is important to blend the complexion. In addition, reports have suggested that among blacks, the incidence of "sensitive skin" and rosacea is more common than previously thought. Blacks have reported skin sensitivities as high as 50% in undocumented observations. Even though the prevalence of sensitivity might not be as high as reported by ethnic patients, dermatologists should have an increased awareness of potential irritation from acne products.

**TABLE 35-5** ■ **Unusual Variants of Diseases in Ethnic Skin**

- Inverse pityriasis rosea
- Pitted keratosis
- Hypopigmented cutaneous T-cell lymphoma
- Ichthyosiform sarcoidosis

## Unusual Variants of Disease in Ethnic Skin

With few exceptions, skin disease incidence is the same in all people, regardless of skin color. However, dermatologists should be aware of certain diseases with a higher incidence in ethnic skin (Table 35-5). For black skin, these diseases include inverse pityriasis rosea, hypopigmented cutaneous T-cell lymphoma (CTCL), pitted keratosis, and ichthyosiform sarcoidosis.

### Inverse Pityriasis Rosea

Inverse pityriasis rosea is a papulosquamous eruption that occurs on ethnic skin. More frequently, the eruption is mostly papular with prominent scales and occurs in distal regions such as on the legs, feet, arms, wrists, and neck, sparing the trunk. Prolonged dyspigmentation can cause suffering in ethnic patients with this disease (Fig. 35-11).

### Hypopigmented Cutaneous T-cell Lymphoma

Hypopigmented CTCL has a high prevalence in black patients. In a retrospective study at Howard University Hospital, 12.1% of skin cancers in black patients were due to CTCL. The disease is aggressive in black patients, and late-stage disease at the time of diagnosis contributes to a poor prognosis. These patients have a history of generalized eczematoid or psoriasiform dermatitis, which does not respond to routine therapy for those conditions. The hypopigmented variant can also be mistaken for pityriasis alba or postinflammatory hypopigmentation. Skin biopsy should include immunophenotyping studies for definitive diagnosis. Repeated histologic evaluation is usually necessary when patients with "eczema" are not improving with therapy. The hypopigmented form is more common in ethnic patients and is often seen in adolescents and children with CTCL (Fig. 35-12).

### Ichthyosiform Sarcoidosis

Black patients with cutaneous sarcoidosis are the only patients who seem to express ichthyosiform sarcoidosis. The skin lesions are clinically identical to those found in acquired ichthyosis or ichthyosis vulgaris and must be biopsied to determine the correct diagnosis. Noncaseating granulomas are observed even when the skin lesions precede the systemic disease. The skin findings are usually on the distal extremities and may precede the development of systemic disease.

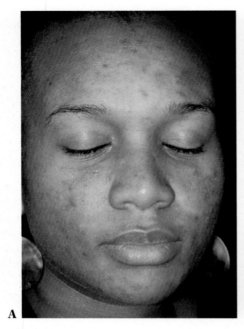
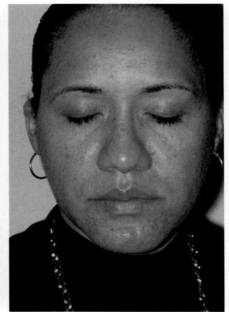

A                                                          B

**FIGURE 35-11** ■ **(A)** Acne. **(B)** Rosacea.

# Common Cosmetic Concerns in Ethnic Skin

## Keloid/Hypertrophic Scars

### *Growth of Cosmetic Products and Procedures in Ethnic Populations*

Growing diversity of skin types and shifting trends in US demographics are driving the increased growth of the ethnic patient population. However, products and procedures that target the ethnic market are also bringing more ethnic patients into the clinic. According to recent surveys, 11.7 million cosmetic procedures were performed in 2007, an overall increase of 8% in surgical procedures. As the total number of cosmetic procedures continues to increase, dermatologists can expect greater numbers of health-care consumers from specialized ethnic populations. For example, of the total 11.7 million cosmetic procedures performed in 2007, 2.48 million (22%) procedures were performed in ethnic groups. Hispanics accounted for 9%; blacks accounted for 6%; Asians, 5%; and other non-Caucasians, 2%. This represents an increase of more than 65% in ethnic groups since 2004. Therefore, it is especially important for the dermatologist to incorporate safe and effective, ethnic-specific treatment procedures.

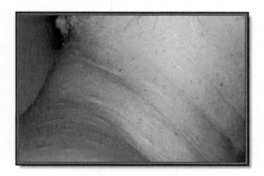

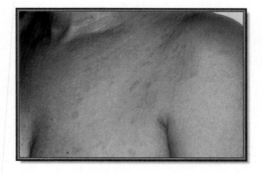

### *Keloids in Ethnic Populations*

Keloids are among the most common cosmetic concerns in ethnic skin (Table 35-6). These scars are benign, sometimes painful and/or pruritic, proliferative growths of dermal collagen that typically occur in ethnic skin because of excessive tissue response to trauma. These growths typically occur 3 to 18 times more often than in white skin. Patients with a Fitzgerald Phototype of IV–VI are at greater risk for keloid formation and keloid recurrence after treatment. A higher incidence occurs in younger females due to ear piercing. Keloids have also developed from tattoos. People aged 65 years or older seldom experience keloids; however, the incidence is increasing as more individuals experience coronary artery bypass surgery and midchest operations. Treatment success is variable and the first rule of keloid therapy is prevention. Success rates are low and the rate of recurrence is high—for example, 50% to 80% of lesions recur after excision therapy. Patients should be aware of familial keloid

**FIGURE 35-12** ■ Inverse pityriasis rosea.

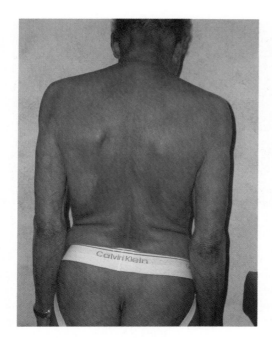

FIGURE 35-13 ■ Hypopigmented cutaneous T-cell lymphoma.

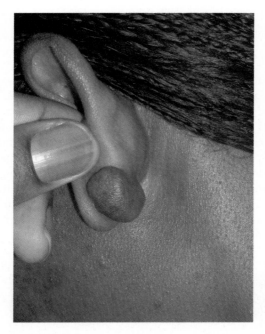

FIGURE 35-14 ■ Earlobe keloid scar.

history, especially in blacks. Therapy is more complex for large, nonpedunculated earlobe keloids, or keloids with wide bases (**Figs. 35-13 to 35-16**).

### Treatment

For many years, injection with triamcinolone acetonide (10 to 40 mg/mL) was the standard of care for treating keloids. Patients should be told in advance that injected areas might

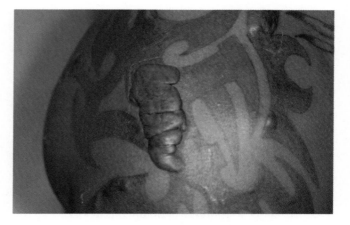

FIGURE 35-15 ■ Keloids caused by tattoos.

become hypopigmented for 6 to 12 months. Pain can be minimized by using topical anesthetic preparations prior to injection. With the exception of treating midsternal keloids, the current gold standard of treatment is primary excision followed by adjuvant therapy. Excision can be followed up with corticosteroid injection, radiation therapy, and pressure gradient garments. Other primary therapies include lasers and silicone gel-sheeting.

### Dermatosis Papulosa Nigra

Dermatosis papulosis nigra (DPN) presents as small (1 to 3 mm in diameter), discrete, rounded, brownish black skin growths on the face, and develops most often, on a person's cheeks, neck, upper chest, and back. Lesions begin to appear in the mid-20s as flesh colored to black papules and/or plaques on the face, neck, and upper torso. The condition is chronic, with new lesions continually developing as the person ages. The exact reason for the growth of these lesions remains unknown. However, researchers are confident that the appearance of DPNs has a hereditary tendency, which leads to DPNs observed on the skin of family members and relatives. DPN occurs more often in females, and overall, affects one in three blacks. Although most dermatologists believe that these growths are unique to black

---

**TABLE 35-6 ■ Common Cosmetic Concerns in Ethnic Skin**

- Dyschromia (postinflammatory hyperpigmentation/hypopigmentation, melasma, vitiligo)
- Scarring (hypertrophic scars, keloid scars) (surgical vs. nonsurgical) and discoloration
- Dermatosis papulosa nigra
- Seborrheic keratosis and acrochordons
- Striae distensae
- Accentuated facial lines of expression (especially glabellar frown lines)
- Lipoatrophy (deep nasolabial folds, skin laxity and cheek festooning)

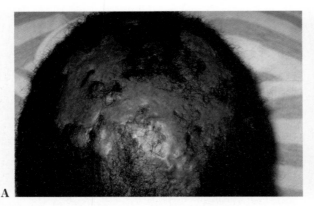

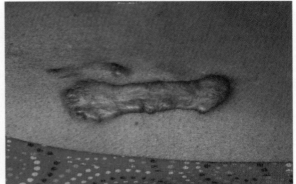

FIGURE 35-16 ■ **(A and B)** Spontaneous keloids.

skin, some dermatologists think these same growths occur on the skin of Asians.

*Treatment*

**Treatment of Dermatosis Papulosa Nigra/Seborrheic Keratoses/Acrochordons.** Some patients choose to treat DPNs for cosmetic reasons or as a medical necessity. For example, medical reasons for removing these lesions might include chronic irritations about the neck, caused by chains or collars rubbing on the lesions, or interference with the line of vision, caused by lesions that occur on the eyelids. More commonly, however, these lesions are removed for cosmetic reasons, as the DPNs are histologically and biologically benign. Effective cosmetic therapy is available to treat DPN/seborrheic keratoses/acrochordons. Treatment of these "skin tags" can effectively reduce the appearance of age by 10 years. Low-voltage electrodesiccation is an effective treatment for more common smaller, flat macules. Electrodesiccation causes very little pain, since the procedure is normally done under local anesthesia using a topical anesthetic cream. In about a week's time, the individual lesions begin to drop off the skin, leaving a normal skin appearance. Advise the patient not to pick the treated areas. Pedunculated lesions respond well to scissor excision of papules; use local anesthesia

to alleviate pain. If a person has hundreds of DPNs, several treatment sessions may be required to completely remove all of the lesions. Although cryosurgery is commonly used to destroy DPNs/seborrheic keratoses, the method has a high incidence of causing hyperpigmentation and hypopigmentation, and therefore, should be considered the last treatment option. Cryosurgery requires significant caution; risks should be minimized by using only short bursts of nitrogen since the risk for discoloration increases with the length of freezing. Trichloroacetic acid (50%) can be used for large seborrheic keratotic plaques.

## Dyschromia

Oftentimes, black patients will indicate that they want to be treated for a scar. However, in many cases, the purported scars are in fact postinflammatory hyperpigmentation (**Fig. 35-17**). It is important to discuss the significant differences between true scarring and postinflammatory hyperpigmentation since there are differences in the specific therapies and relative difficulty between treating true scarring and postinflammatory hyperpigmentation. In addition, problems involving misdiagnosis may occur with pityriasis alba, tinea versicolor, seborrheic dermatitis, and trichrome vitiligo (**Figs. 35-18 and 35-19**).

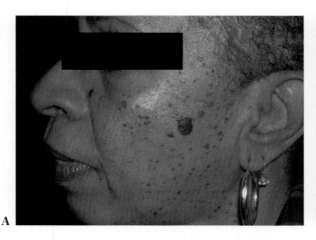

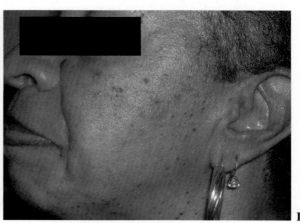

FIGURE 35-17 ■ Dermatosis papulosa nigra. **(A)** Before treatment. **(B)** After electrodesiccation treatment.

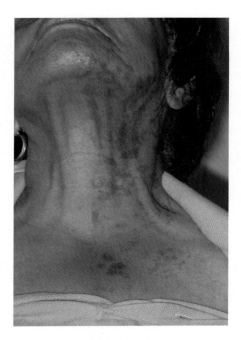

FIGURE 35-18 ■ Postinflammatory hyperpigmentation.

Pigmentary disorders are especially prevalent and distressing for blacks, Latinos, Asians, and Middle Easterners. Postinflammatory hyperpigmentation is caused by various inflammatory skin disorders, such as eczema, allergic contact or irritant contact dermatitis, acne, or other causes. In fact, ethnic patients are commonly more distressed by the resulting dark areas than the initial culprit—the acute acne lesion. Dermal incontinence of pigment also occurs in melasma and hereditary dyschromias. Postinflammatory hypopigmentation can develop from laser hair removal (**Figs. 35-20 and 35-21**). Unprotected sun exposure is also a significant source of additional skin discoloration because it prolongs melanin production in active melanocytes in various inflammatory conditions. Sun protection is typically required during procedures to blend skin discoloration. Chemical (organic) sun protection includes Parsol 1789 (avobenzone), ecamsule (Mexoryl), oxybenzone, and octinoxate. These are preferred because physical (inorganic) sun protection such as titanium dioxide, zinc oxide, and mineral makeup can leave a chalky or ashy residue on brown skin. Other options for sun protection include clothing, hats, and umbrellas.

### Treatment

Hyperpigmentation can be evaluated to provide a general idea of the prognosis and length of treatment. The evaluation can consist of both qualitative diagnosis and quantitative analysis (**Table 35-7**). A positive Wood's lamp examination reveals superficial (epidermal) incontinence of pigment, whereas a negative Wood's lamp examination reveals a deep (dermal) incontinence of pigment. Although not commonly used, quantitative analysis can be performed with a colorimeter.

Although disorders of hyperpigmentation may be difficult to treat, several therapeutic agents have been used over the years and others are in development (see **Table 35-7**). Epidermal incontinence of pigment can be seen in postinflammatory hyperpigmentation. Product ingredients of lightening agents containing hydroquinone 4% to 6%, mequinol, kojic acid, azelaic acid, licorice (glabridin), citric acid, retinol, soy, arbutin, *N*-acetylglucosamine, nicotinamide, and mulberry are used once to twice daily.

Topical agents are generally classified as phenolic or nonphenolic compounds. The goal of these therapeutic agents is to inhibit key regulatory steps of hyperactive melanocytes by regulating (1) melanin synthesis via transcription inhibition of tyrosinase or TRP-1, (2) the uptake and distribution of melanosomes in keratinocytes, and (3) melanosome degradation and cell turnover. Hydroquinone has been the standard for many years but has occasionally been mired in controversy pertaining to safety. Lightening agents are also used for pretreatment of areas that will undergo cosmetic procedures. The agents are typically applied in advance as a cautionary measure to minimize any hyperpigmentation that may result from procedures.

### Hydroquinone

The most commonly used ingredient in bleaching preparations to treat hyperpigmentation is hydroquinone. The concentration of hydroquinone can range from 2% (over-the-counter)

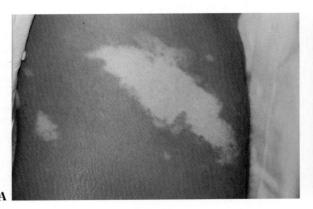
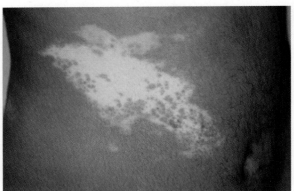

FIGURE 35-19 ■ **(A)** Vitiligo. **(B)** Stimulation of pigment with psoralen + UVA light treatment.

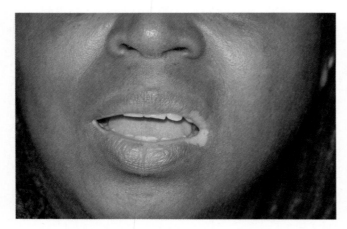

FIGURE 35-20 ■ Postinflammatory hypopigmentation caused by laser hair removal device.

to 4% to 8% prescription formulations. Currently, the Food and Drug Administration (FDA) is monitoring the use of hydroquinone products in the United States since they have been outlawed in several countries in Africa and Asia. The FDA is concerned about ochronosis or persistent darkening of the skin with chronic use of hydroquinone-containing products, in addition to the potential of hydroquinone to cause cancer in lab mice. Although the concern is noteworthy, the countries where hydroquinone has been outlawed have routinely overused large quantities of hydroquinone-containing products to lighten the entire body. Those who use the ingredient in excess are at risk for systemic absorption. There is little concern among dermatologists in the United States partly due to the standard use of smaller quantities or application to dark spots only and because it is not being routinely used to lighten the entire body. Therefore in the United States, there is not significant systemic absorption from topical hydroquinone bleaching, and if systemic levels are detected, it is primarily from natural sources of hydroquinone as seen with consumption of coffee, tea, red wine, wheat germ, pears, and berries and/or exposure to cigarette and wood smoke. The

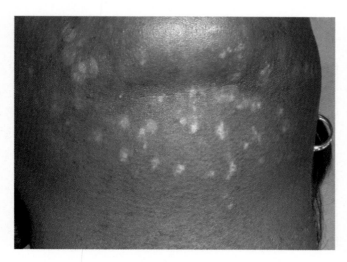

FIGURE 35-21 ■ Hypopigmentation.

**TABLE 35-7 ■ Hyperpigmentation Evaluation**

**Qualitative Diagnosis**

■ +Wood's lamp examination

Superficial (epidermal) incontinence of pigment

■ −Wood's lamp examination

Deep (dermal) incontinence of pigment

**Quantitative Analysis**

Colorimeter

■ Delta L, a and b

  ■ L (98.4) white-black

  ■ a (0.2) red-green

  ■ b (1.2) yellow-blue

Note: Wolff K, Goldsmith LA, Katz SI, et al. *Fitzpatrick's Dermatology in General Medicine*. 7th ed. New York: McGraw-Hill Publishing; 2008.

Shriver MD, Parra EJ. Comparison of narrow-band reflectance spectroscopy and tristimulus colorimetry for measurements of skin and hair color in persons of different biological ancestry. *Am J Phys Anthropol*. 2000;112(1):17–27.

American Academy of Dermatology reports no incidences of cancers associated with hydroquinone in the United States and supports the need for further clinical science information on the safety of hydroquinone.

## Summary

Although differences in the structure of ethnic skin can be beneficial, some of these differences can have the opposite effect. For example, the photoprotection afforded by differences in melanosome and melanin characteristics also causes frequent hyperpigmentation in ethnic skin and may be responsible for divergent responses observed in burn injuries.

**SAUER'S NOTES**

Members of ethnic groups will soon comprise a majority of the international and domestic population. As the importance of ethnic markets continues to increase, dermatologists and cosmetic surgeons will require more expertise in the treatment of ethnic skin. Ethnic consumers are increasingly seeking out products and procedures to provide dermatologic and cosmetic solutions in these patients. However, when treating ethnic patients, issues specific to ethnic skin such as skin sensitivity, hyperpigmentation, and keloid scarring require special consideration by clinicians. As with patients of all skin colors, a comprehensive approach to assessment and treatment is absolutely necessary. With proper training and technique, clinicians can provide successful outcomes with little risk of adverse events to patients with pigmented skin.

Indeed, individuals with darker skin experience more frequent postinflammatory hyperpigmentation compared to patients with lighter complexions. Moreover, surveys found that uneven skin tone was a chief complaint in more than one third of black women, while pigment disorders rated the third most commonly treated dermatoses. In a survey of 100 ethnic women, complaints about dark spots reached 86%, while 49% of women complained of sensitive or very sensitive skin.

## Suggested Readings

Callender VD, McMichael AJ, Cohen GF. Medical and surgical therapies for alopecias in black women. *Dermatol Ther.* 2004;17(2):164–176.

Kelly AP. Pseudofolliculitis barbae and acne keloidalis nuchae. *Dermatol Clin.* 2003;21(4):645–653.

Kelly AP. Medical and surgical therapies for keloids. *Dermatol Ther.* 2004;17(2):212–218.

Olsen EA, Bergfeld WF, Cotsarelis G, et al. Summary of North American Hair Research Society (NAHRS)-sponsored Workshop on Cicatricial Alopecia, Duke University Medical Center, February 10 and 11, 2001. *J Am Acad Dermatol.* 2003;48(1):103–110.

Olsen EA, Callender V, Sperling L, et al. Central scalp alopecia photographic scale in African American women. *Dermatol Ther.* 2008;21(4):264–267.

Ross EK, Tan E, Shapiro J. Update on primary cicatricial alopecias. *J Am Acad Dermatol.* 2005;53(1):1–37; quiz 38–40.

Sperling LC. Scarring alopecia and the dermatopathologist. *J Cutan Pathol.* 2001;28(7):333–342.

Tan E, Martinka M, Ball N, et al. Primary cicatricial alopecias: clinicopathology of 112 cases. *J Am Acad Dermatol.* 2004;50(1):25–32.

Taylor SC, Burgess CM, Callender VD, et al. Postinflammatory hyperpigmentation: evolving combination treatment strategies. *Cutis.* 2006; 78(2 suppl 2):6–19.

# CHAPTER 36

# Pigmentary Dermatoses

*John C. Hall, MD*

There are two variants of pigmentation of the skin: hyperpigmentation and hypopigmentation. The predominant skin pigment discussed in this chapter is melanin, but other pigments can be present in the skin. A complete classification of pigmentary disorders appears at the end of this chapter.

The melanin-forming cells and their relationship to the tyrosine–tyrosinase enzyme system are discussed in Chapter 1. The common clinical example of abnormal hyperpigmentation is *chloasma*, but secondary melanoderma can result from many causes. The most common form of hypopigmentation is *vitiligo*, but secondary leukoderma does occur.

## Chloasma (Melasma)

### Presentation and Characteristics

#### Clinical Lesions

An irregular hyperpigmentation of the skin that varies in shades of brown is seen. It is well demarcated and located most often on the face in sun-exposed areas (Fig. 36-1).

#### Distribution

The lesions usually occur on the sides of the face, forehead, and sides of the neck.

#### Course

The disorder is slowly progressive, but remissions do occur. It is more obvious in the summer.

#### Cause

The cause is unknown, but some cases appear during pregnancy (called "mask of pregnancy") or with chronic illness.

---

**SAUER'S NOTES**

1. Skin pigmentation is the most socially significant skin marker, and care must be taken not to underestimate its importance to the patient even if it is not harmful to the patient's medical well-being.
2. Change in skin pigmentation can be an important marker for underlying illness.
3. The safest and most beneficial therapy may be camouflage, that is, Lydea O'Leary Covermark or Dermablend.

---

There is an increased incidence of chloasma in women taking contraceptives, postmenopausal hormone replacement, or fertility hormones. The melanocyte-stimulating hormone of the pituitary may be excessive and affect the tyrosine–tyrosinase enzyme system.

### Differential Diagnosis

The causes of *secondary melanoderma* should be ruled out (see end of this chapter).

### Treatment

1. The patient should not be promised great therapeutic results. Most cases associated with pregnancy slowly fade or disappear completely after delivery. The pigmentation may be prolonged if the patient elects to breast-feed.
2. For a mild case in an unconcerned patient, cosmetic coverage can be adequate. Dermablend or Lydia O'Leary Covermark are two useful products.
3. Sunlight intensifies the pigmentation, so a sunscreen should be added to the routine each morning year-round.
4. Hydroquinone preparations (any of the following):
   Melanex solution 3%
   Lustra cream 4%
   Eldopaque Forte cream (tinted)
   Solaquin Forte cream (nontinted)
   Eldoquin Forte
   Lustra AF (sunscreen)
   Lustra-Ultra (sunscreen, retinol) 4% Hydroquinone Cream is an inexpensive generic preparation.

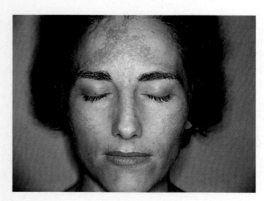

**FIGURE 36-1** ■ Chloasma of the face. *(Neutrogena Skin Care Institute.)*

Tri-Luma (fluocinolone, tretinoin)

EpiQuin (microsponge)

Glyquin (glycolic acid)

*Comment:* Tri-Luma contains a retinoid, a class VI corticosteroid, and hydroquinone. This product should show a response within 8 weeks and some authors restrict its use to this time period and then have a rest period because it contains a corticosteroid. They then switch to a sunscreen and hydroquinone combination. There are many variants of these topicals, all with hydroquinone and some with sunscreens, glycolic acid, and retinoids. They all tend to be expensive with the exception of over-the-counter hydroquinone. Insurance considers these products cosmetic and seldom defrays the cost.

*Sig:* Apply locally b.i.d. Stop if irritation develops.

*Comment:* The treatment with any of these hydroquinone preparations should be continued for at least 2 to 3 months. Response to therapy is slow. When they are stopped, the disease tends to recur. Prolonged use over many months to years can cause increased pigmentation owing to an acquired ochronosis. This resolves on discontinuing the hydroquinone.

5. Retinoic acid (Retin-A cream [0.025%, 0.05%, 0.1%] or gel, Renova [0.02%]) applied at night can slowly decrease the pigmentation, if tolerated.

6. Kojic acid is advocated by some authors.

7. Surgical procedures used by experienced physicians include microdermabrasion, laser, and chemical peels. Beware of the danger of hypopigmentation.

## Vitiligo

### Presentation and Characteristics

#### Clinical Lesions

Irregular areas of depigmented skin are seen with a hyperpigmented border (**Fig. 36-2**). There is a segmental variety that has pigment loss in a dermatomal (especially trigeminal) distribution.

#### Distribution

It is estimated to affect 1% to 2% of the population. It is a more severe cosmetic problem in darker skinned patients. Most commonly, the lesions occur on the face and the dorsum of hands and feet, but they can occur on all body areas.

#### Course

The disease is slowly progressive, but remissions and changes are frequent. It is more obvious during the summer because of the tanning of adjacent normal skin.

#### Cause

The cause is unknown, but believed by some to be an autoimmune disease. Heredity is a factor in some cases. Autoimmune diseases, especially thyroiditis and pernicious anemia, can be associated with vitiligo.

### Differential Diagnosis

Causes of *secondary hypopigmentation* need to be ruled out (see end of this chapter and **Fig. 36-3**).

### Treatment

***Case Example:*** A young woman with large depigmented patches on her face and dorsum of hands asks if something can be done for her "white spots." Her sister has a few lesions.

- *Cosmetics:* The use of the following covering or staining preparations is recommended: pancake-type cosmetics, such as Covermark, by Lydia O'Leary; Vitadye (Elder); dihydroxyacetone containing self-tanning creams, gels, and foams; walnut-juice stain; or potassium permanganate solution in appropriate dilution. Many patients with vitiligo become quite proficient in the application of these agents. A sunscreen used on the surrounding skin makes the contrast of light and dark skin less apparent.

- *Corticosteroid cream therapy:* This is effective for early mild cases of vitiligo, especially when one is mainly

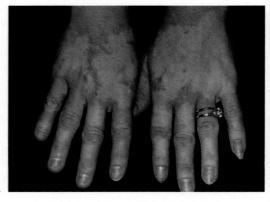
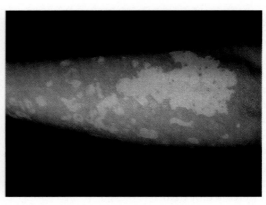

A                                                                                          B

**FIGURE 36-2** ■ **(A)** Vitiligo of the hands in a white patient. **(B)** Vitiligo of the forearm in a black patient. *(Neutrogena Skin Care Institute.)*

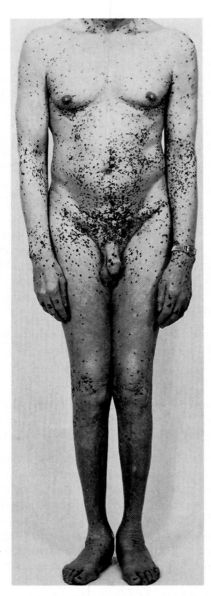

**FIGURE 36-3** ■ Secondary hypopigmentation. A marked example of loss of pigment that occurred in an African-American man following healing of an exfoliative dermatitis. Corticosteroids were used in the therapy.

concerned with face and hand lesions. Betamethasone valerate (Valisone) cream 0.1% can be prescribed for use on the hands for 4 months or so and for use on the face for only 3 months. It should not be used on the eyelids or as full-body therapy. Even class I topical corticosteroids can be used for a while if appropriate precautions are observed.

■ *Protopic 0.1% ointment* used twice a day avoids topical corticosteroid side effects and may be quite beneficial. Concern over induction of cutaneous lymphoma has been hypothesized but not proven and discredited by many.

■ *Sun avoidance:* Sun tanning should be avoided because this accentuates the normal pigmentation and

makes the nonpigmented vitiligo more noticeable. The white areas of vitiligo are more susceptible to sunburn. If the patient desires a more specific treatment, the following can be suggested with certain reservations.

■ *Psoralen derivatives:* For many years, Egyptians along the Nile River chewed certain plants to cause the disappearance of the white spots of vitiligo. Extraction of the chemicals from these plants revealed the psoralen derivatives to be the active agents, and one of these, 8-methoxypsoralen, was found to be the most effective. This chemical is available as Oxsoralen in 10-mg capsules and also as a topical liquid form. The oral form is to be ingested 2 hours before exposure to measured sun radiation. The package insert should be consulted. Our results with this long-term therapy have been disappointing.

■ Trisoralen is a synthetic psoralen in 5-mg tablets. The recommended dosage is 2 tablets taken 2 hours before measured sun exposure for a long-term course. Detailed instructions accompany the package. Some dermatologists believe this therapy to be more effective than Oxsoralen.

■ A short 2-week course of Oxsoralen capsules (20 mg/d) has been advocated for the purpose of acquiring a better and quicker suntan. The value of such a course has been questioned. The sun exposure must be gradual. Oral psoralens plus self-administered UVA or UVB in "tanning booths" can produce severe burns, which may be fatal.

■ *Psoralens and ultraviolet light (PUVA) therapy:* The combination of topical or oral psoralen therapy with UVA radiation has been somewhat successful in repigmenting vitiligo. The psoralen can be given orally, topically, or as a bath. Precautions concerning photoaging and skin cancer apply. Narrowband UVB has less short-term side effects with no photoprotective goggles needed, less cost, less phototoxicity, less skin cancer, and less photoaging than PUVA or broadband UVB.

■ *Depigmentation therapy:* In the hands of experts, monobenzyl ether of hydroquinone (Benoquin) can be used to remove skin pigment to even out the patient's skin color. Beware of this therapy since pigment loss is permanent. Author has never attempted this therapy.

■ *Skin grafting:* Autologous minigrafting and other similar surgical procedures have been used with success by some.

■ *Surgical therapy:* Various grafting procedures are valuable in recalcitrant disease. Epidermal or full-thickness autographs have been advocated by some authors.

■ Narrowband UVB therapy has been advocated and may be safer than PUVA or broadband UVB

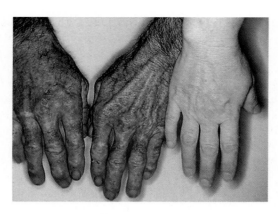

**FIGURE 36-4** ■ Porphyria cutanea tarda hyperpigmentation. *(Neutrogena Skin Care Institute.)*

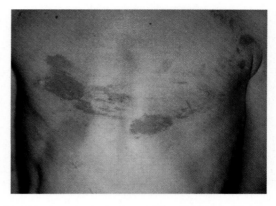

**FIGURE 36-5** ■ Berlock dermatitis: photosensitivity reaction from mother's perfume, age 7 years. *(Neutrogena Skin Care Institute.)*

## Classification of Pigmentary Disorders

### Melanin Hyperpigmentation or Melanoderma

1. Chloasma (melasma) (Fig. 36-1)
2. Incontinentia pigmenti
3. Secondary to skin diseases
   a. Chronic discoid lupus erythematosus
   b. Tinea versicolor
   c. Stasis dermatitis
   d. Lichen planus
   e. Fixed drug eruption
   f. Many cases of dermatitis in African Americans and other dark-skinned individuals (Fig. 36-3)
   g. Scleroderma
   h. Porphyria cutanea tarda (**Fig. 36-4**)
   i. Dermatitis herpetiformis
4. Secondary to external agents
   a. X-radiation
   b. Ultraviolet light
   c. Sunlight
   d. Tars
   e. Photosensitizing chemicals, as in cosmetics, causing development of clinical entities labeled as Riehl's melanosis, poikiloderma of Civatte on the sides of the neck due to chronic sun exposure, berloque dermatitis due to applying certain colognes or perfumes to the skin (**Fig. 36-5**), and others
5. Secondary to internal disorders
   a. Addison's disease (Fig. 38-6)
   b. Chronic liver disease
   c. Pregnancy
   d. Hyperthyroidism
   e. Internal carcinoma causing a malignant form of acanthosis nigricans
   f. Hormonal influence on benign acanthosis nigricans
   g. Intestinal polyposis causing mucous membrane pigmentation (Peutz–Jeghers syndrome)
   h. Albright's syndrome
   i. Schilder's disease
   j. Fanconi's syndrome (in HIV-positive patients)

6. Secondary to drugs such as adrenocorticotropic hormone, estrogens, progesterone, melanocyte-stimulating hormone, minocycline, nonsteroidal anti-inflammatory drugs, amiodarone, psychotropic drugs, antimalarials, tetracyclines, heavy metals, zidovudine, and fluoroquinolones

### Nonmelanin Pigmentations

1. Argyria owing to silver salt deposits
2. Arsenical pigmentation caused by ingestion of inorganic arsenic, as in Fowler's solution and Asiatic pills
3. Pigmentation from heavy metals such as bismuth, gold, and mercury
4. Tattoos
5. Black dermographism, the common bluish black or green stain seen under watches and rings in certain persons from the deposit of the metallic particles reacting with chemicals already on the skin or the granules in talc
6. Hemosiderin granules in hemochromatosis, stasis dermatitis, or pigmented purpuric eruptions (see Chapter 12)
7. Bile pigments from jaundice
8. Yellow pigments following atabrine and chlorpromazine ingestion
9. Carotene coloring in carotenemia and lycopene coloring in lycopenia
10. Homogentisic acid polymer deposit in ochronosis
11. Minocycline hyperpigmentation (characteristic histopathology) diffuse and also localized at scar sites (and rarely teeth)
12. Hyperpigmentation of Ito or OtaA

### Hypopigmentation

1. Albinism
2. Vitiligo
3. Nevus achromicus (nevus depigmentosus)
4. Vogt–Koyanagi–Harada syndrome
5. Whitaker syndrome
6. Chediak–Higashi syndrome

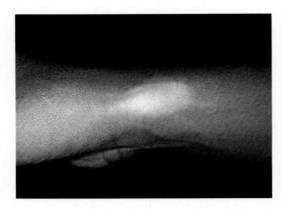

**FIGURE 36-6** ■ Leukoderma on the wrist from intralesional corticosteroid injections in a black patient. *(Neutrogena Skin Care Institute.)*

7. Hypomelanosis of Ito
8. Leukoderma or acquired hypopigmentation (Fig. 36-6)
   a. Secondary to skin diseases such as tinea versicolor, chronic discoid lupus erythematosus, localized scleroderma (may show perifollicular pigment retention), psoriasis, secondary syphilis, or pinta (Fig. 36-3)
   b. Secondary to chemicals such as mercury compounds, monobenzyl ether of hydroquinone, and cortisone-type drugs given intralesionally, especially in people of color (Fig. 36-6)
   c. Secondary to internal diseases, such as hormonal diseases, and in Vogt–Koyanagi syndrome
   d. Associated with pigmented nevi (halo nevus or leukoderma acquisitum centrifugum)
   e. Hypopigmented patch-stage mycosis fungoides
   f. Indeterminate leprosy with anesthesia
   g. Pinta
   h. Imatinib treatment for chronic myelogenous leukemia
   i. Idiopathic guttate hypomelanosis
9. Nevus anemicus
10. Waardenburg's syndrome
11. Ash-leaf macule of tuberous sclerosis

## Suggested Readings

Boersma BR, Westerhof W, Bos JD. Repigmentation in vitiligo vulgaris by autologous minigrafting: results in nineteen patients. *J Am Acad Dermatol.* 1995;33(6):990–995.

Drake LA, Dinehart SM, Farmer ER, et al. Guidelines of care for vitiligo. *J Am Acad Dermatol.* 1996;35:620–626.

Fulk CS. Primary disorders of hyperpigmentation. *J Am Acad Dermatol.* 1984; 10:1–16.

Grimes PE. New insights and new therapies in vitiligo. *JAMA.* 2005;293: 730–735.

Kovacs SO. Vitiligo. *J Am Acad Dermatol.* 1998;38(5):647–666.

Levine N. *Pigmentation and Pigmentary Disorders.* Boca Raton, FL: CRC Press; 1994.

Lio PA. Little white spots: an approach to hypopigmented macules. *Arch Dis Child.* 2008;93:98–102.

Nordlund JJ, Boissy R, Hearing VJ, et al. *The Pigmentary System: Physiology and Pathophysiology.* New York: Oxford University Press; 1998.

Taieb A, Picardo M. Clinical practice. Vitiligo. *N Engl J Med.* 2009;360(2): 160–169.

Victor FC, Gelber J, Rao B. Melasma: a review. *J Cutan Med Surg.* 2004;8: 97–102. [Epub 2004 May 4.]

# CHAPTER 37

# Collagen–Vascular Diseases

*Aaron Loyd, MD, Gary Goldenberg, MD, and Joseph L. Jorizzo, MD*

The collagen vascular diseases are a group of autoimmune diseases including lupus erythematosus (LE), scleroderma, dermatomyositis (DM), rheumatoid arthritis, Sjögren's syndrome, and many others. LE, scleroderma, and DM are discussed in detail herein. These diseases are characterized by autoimmune phenomena, including circulating autoantibodies (aAbs). There is a great deal of overlap of clinical and laboratory findings among these disorders. Cutaneous manifestations may be the presenting or dominant feature of collagent vascular disease. Nevertheless, systemic multiorgan disease needs to be excluded in each case.

A thorough laboratory evaluation is required. Much has been written about antinuclear antibody (ANA) testing. This assay identifies aAbs present in serum to autoantigens present in nuclei of mammalian cells. ANA testing is reported as a titer, and most commercial kits report ANA titers of 1:40 or 1:80 as abnormal. However, titers less than 1:160 are not diagnostic. Approximately 5% of otherwise healthy young individuals have an ANA titer of 1:160 or higher. The prevalence of this false-positive ANA increases with age. Therefore, it is important not to label patients with LE or another autoimmune disease simply based on one laboratory test. Additionally, ANA positivity is seen in multiple other autoimmune diseases and is not specific for LE.

After securing a diagnosis, much important work remains. A thorough medical history, including medicinal and social history, should be obtained. Paraneoplastic phenomena should

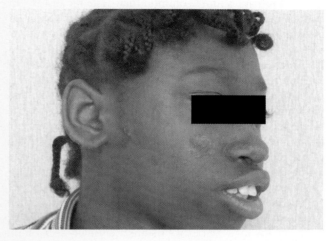

**FIGURE 37-1** ■ CCLE with discoid lesions—erythematous, hyperpigmented plaques with scarring characteristic of CCLE with discoid lesions.

also be considered, especially in the setting of DM. Finally, understanding the systemic effects of each disease is crucial for initial screening tests as well as appropriate referral.

## Lupus Erythematosus

Chronic cutaneous lupus erythematosus (CCLE), subacute cutaneous lupus erythematosus (SCLE) (Figs. 37-1 and 37-2), and

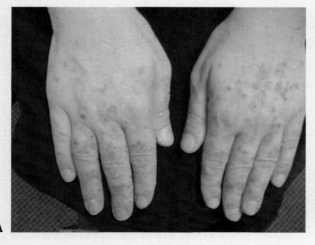
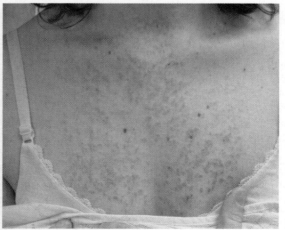

**FIGURE 37-2** ■ SCLE. **(A)** Erythematous papules and plaques on dorsal hands; typical distribution spares the knuckles. **(B)** Erythematous papules and plaques in a typical sun-exposed distribution of the V on the chest.

acute cutaneous lupus erythematosus (ACLE) are the most common variants encountered by dermatologists.

It has been estimated that cutaneous variants of LE are two to three times more common than systemic disease. LE is much more common in women than in men; the female to male ratio is at least 6:1. Young, fertile women are most commonly affected, and pregnancy issues should be addressed. LE is more common in blacks than in whites, and blacks have a higher frequency of systemic disease.

Drug-induced lupus has been reported with multiple medications, including hydrochlorothiazide, calcium channel blockers, isoniazid, phenytoin, angiotensin-converting enzyme inhibitors (captopril), tetracyclines (minocycline), and many others including over-the-counter nonsteroidal anti-inflammatory drugs. Antihistone aAbs is a serologic marker that occurs in patients with drug-induced LE.

Neonatal LE (NLE) is seen in newborns whose mothers have anti-Ro aAbs. Nearly 100% of patients with NLE also have anti-Ro aAbs. SCLE-like lesions are usually seen on the face of newborns. Congenital heart block is an important complication and is usually present at birth. Therefore, screening for heart disease should be performed in all patients with NLE. Children with this complication have a 20% mortality rate and two thirds require pacemakers.

Diagnosis of LE and its subtypes depends on a constellation of findings that include history, physical examination, histopathologic correlation, and laboratory evaluation that focuses on published American College of Rheumatology criteria (**Table 37-1**). See **Table 37-2** for a comparison of CCLE, SCLE, and ACLE. The treatment approach is outlined in **Table 37-3**.

## Scleroderma

Localized scleroderma (morphea), systemic (diffuse) sclerosis, and CREST syndrome (*c*alcinosis cutis, *R*aynaud's phenomenon, *e*sophageal dysfunction, sclerodactyly, *t*elangiectasias) are variants included under the general heading of scleroderma (**Fig. 37-3**).

Systemic sclerosis (SSc) is a systemic disease that affects the skin, lungs, heart, gastrointestinal (GI) tract, and other organ systems. It is upto 15 times more common in women, and the age of onset is between 30 and 50 years. Ten-year survival of patients with SSc is under 70%. Pathogenesis of SSc is unknown, but endothelial cell damage is suspected as the key pathogenic abnormality.

aAbs are often detected in nonlocalized forms of sclerosis. ANA may be used as a screen, while Scl 70 antibodies

**TABLE 37-1 ■ Systemic Lupus Erythematosus Criteria (4 of 11 needed for diagnosis of systemic disease)**

ANA positive

Arthritis

Butterfly rash

Discoid rash

Hematology disorder

Immunology disorder

Neurologic disorder

Oral or nasopharyngeal ulcers

Photosensitivity

Renal disorder

Serositis

differentiate SSc from the centromere antibody-associated CREST syndrome. Cutaneous and systemic findings of SSc and other variants of scleroderma are summarized in Table 37-4.

## Dermatomyositis

DM is an autoimmune proximal extensor inflammatory myopathy with specific cutaneous manifestations (**Fig. 37-4**). Polymyositis is an inflammatory myopathy without any skin involvement. DM sine myositis presents with the characteristic skin eruption of DM without muscle involvement.

Cutaneous disease is characteristic (**Table 37-5**) and can either precede or follow muscle disease. Adult and juvenile variants exist. Differential diagnosis of skin disease includes systemic lupus erythematosus (SLE), psoriasis, allergic contact dermatitis, phototoxic drug eruption, cutaneous T-cell lymphoma, atopic dermatitis, and scleroderma.

The pathogenesis of DM is unclear, but it is believed to be an autoimmune disease triggered by outside factors in genetically predisposed individuals. Photoirradiation

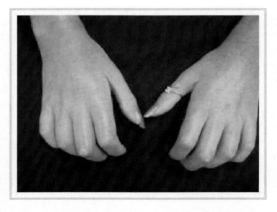

**FIGURE 37-3 ■** Systemic sclerosis. This patient demonstrates typical loss of wrinkles on the hands with waxy, shiny, bound down skin.

**TABLE 37-2** ■ **Comparison of Three Most Common Types of LE Encountered by Dermatologists**

| LE Subtype | CCLE | SCLE | ACLE |
|---|---|---|---|
| Distribution | Face, scalp, ears, extensor arms | V of the neck, upper back, shoulders, extensor arms, less commonly face | "Butterfly" malar distribution on face, V of neck, arms, hands (sparing knuckles) |
| Clinical features | *Early lesions:* sharply demarcated erythematous papules and plaques with prominent scale, follicular plugging, and early scarring; *late lesions:* atrophic plaques with central scarring, telangiectasia, and hypopigmentation; photosensitivity | Erythematous papules and scaly, hyperkeratotic, annular/polycyclic plaques; photosensitivity; nonscarring | Poorly marginated erythematous macules, fine scaling, poikiloderma, edema; photosensitivity; nonscarring |
| Course | Chronic with disease progression without treatment; 5%–10% eventually meet ACR criteria for SLE | 50% meet ACR criteria for SLE | Acute onset, usually with systemic signs and symptoms |
| Histopathology | Vacuolar change; dyskeratotic keratinocytes; follicular plugging; basement membrane thickening; superficial and deep perivascular and perifollicular lymphohistiocytic infiltrate; increased dermal mucin | Vacuolar change; dyskeratotic keratinocytes, epidermal atrophy; superficial and mid perivascular lymphohistiocytic infiltrate; increased dermal Mucin | Vacuolar change; dyskeratotic keratinocytes; superficial perivascular lymphohistiocytic infiltrate; dermal edema |
| Laboratory findings | Positive ANA (5%) | Positive ANA, anti-Ro aAb (>90%) | Positive ANA (99%); double-stranded DNA (60%); anemia (normocytic); leukopenia; thrombocytopenia; elevated ESR; proteinuria; cellular casts |
| Differential diagnosis | Polymorphous light eruption; psoriasis; sarcoidosis; lichen planus; granuloma faciale | Annular erythemas; atopic dermatitis; psoriasis; dermatophyte infection; secondary syphilis | Sunburn; rosacea; DM; phototoxic drug eruption; seborrheic dermatitis |

*Abbreviations:* LE, lupus erythematosus; CCLE, chronic cutaneous lupus erythematosus; SCLE, subacute cutaneous lupus erythematosus; ACLE, acute cutaneous lupus erythematosus; ACR, American College of Radiology; SLE, systemic lupus erythematosus; ANA, antinuclear antibody; ESR, erythrocyte sedimentation rate; DM, dermatomyositis.

**TABLE 37-3** ■ **Therapeutic Options for LE**

| | | | |
|---|---|---|---|
| Mild local disease | Sunscreens (high SPF with UVA blocker | Systemic disease | Prednisone |
| | Topical or intralesional corticosteroids | | Azathioprine |
| | Topical immunomodulators (e.g., tacrolimus) | | Mycophenolate mofetil |
| | Hydroxychloroquine (may add quinacrine) | | Cyclophosphamide |
| Extensive cutaneous disease | Oral retinoids | | Cyclosporine |
| | Dapsone/sulfapyridine | | Interferon |
| | Clofazimine | | IVIG |
| | Methotrexate | | Newer biologic therapies |
| | Thalidomide | | Extracorporeal immunomodulation |
| | Azathioprine | | Androgen therapy |
| | | | Stem cell transplantation |

*Abbreviations:* SPF, sun protective factor; UVA, ultraviolet A; IVIG, intravenous immunoglobulin.

**TABLE 37-4** ■ **Clinical Features of Scleroderma Variants**

| Scleroderma Subtype | Systemic Sclerosis | CREST Syndrome | Morphea |
|---|---|---|---|
| Cutaneous findings | Sclerodactyly (induration of fingers, waxy, shiny, hardened, bound down skin, loss of wrinkling), Raynaud's phenomenon (coldness, triphasic color changes, i.e., pallor, cyanosis, rubor), diffuse and salt-and-pepper hyperpigmentation, cutaneous ulcers ("rat bite necrosis"), trunk involvement | Telangiectasias, Raynaud's phenomenon, calcinosis cutis (especially over bony prominences), cutaneous ulcers ("rat bite" necrosis), sclerodactyly | *Plaque type:* erythematous, edematous plaque that becomes sclerotic and scar-like with hypopigmentation and hyperpigmentation; *deep (profunda) morphea:* deep tissue sclerosis; *en coupe de saber:* linear morphea affecting the forehead and scalp; *Parry–Romberg syndrome:* hyperpigmentation and soft tissue atrophy affecting the entire distribution of the trigeminal nerve leading to facial asymmetry |
| Systemic findings | *Esophagus:* reflux disease, dysmotility, dysphagia; *GI tract:* decreased peristalsis leading to constipation, diarrhea, bloating, malabsorption; *heart:* constrictive pericarditis, conduction abnormalities; *lungs:* diffuse pulmonary fibrosis; *kidneys:* uremia, renal hypertension | *Esophagus:* reflux disease, dysmotility, dysphagia; *GI tract:* telangiectasias | None |
| Histopathology | Diffuse dermal sclerosis, mild vacuolar change, excessive collagen deposition, decreased adnexal structures, mild perivascular infiltrate with plasma cells | Same (For sclerodactyly) | Same |
| Laboratory findings | Positive ANA (90%–95%), anti–Scl 70 aAb (DNA topoisomerase I; 60%) | Positive ANA, anticentromere aAb (80%) | Possibly a positive ANA (especially linear morphea), anti–fibrillin-1 aAb |
| Differential diagnosis | Eosinophilic fasciitis, scleromyxedema, scleredema, L-tryptophan syndrome, nephrogenic fibrosing dermopathy, toxic oil syndrome, graft-versus-host disease, drug reaction (bleomycin) | Pathognomonic if all features are present | Toxic oil syndrome, drug reaction (bleomycin), silicosis, chemical exposure (vinyl chloride, organic solvents, pesticides and epoxy resin), graft-versus-host disease |
| Treatment | *Skin sclerosis:* physical therapy, prednisone (controversial), methotrexate, D-penicillamine; *Raynaud's phenomenon:* calcium channel blockers, Viagra; *calcinosis cutis:* excision; *renal disease:* ACE inhibitors; *esophageal disease:* proton pump inhibitors; *pulmonary disease:* cyclophosphamide | *Calcinosis cutis:* excision; *Raynaud's phenomenon:* calcium channel blockers, Viagra; *esophageal disease:* proton pump inhibitors; *skin sclerosis:* physical therapy, methotrexate, D-penicillamine | *Mild disease:* topical/intralesional corticosteroids, topical immunomodulators (e.g., tacrolimus), with keratolytics; *severe disease:* hydroxychloroquine, methotrexate, D-penicillamine, cyclosporine, phototherapy, physical therapy |

*Abbreviations:* ANA, antinuclear antibody; ACE, angiotensin-converting enzyme.

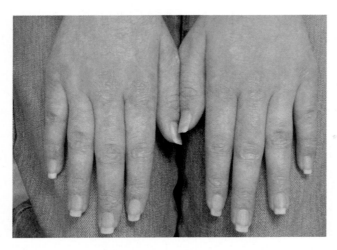

**FIGURE 37-4** ■ Gottron's papules on the dorsal hands of a patient with juvenile DM.

plays an important trigger role in cutaneous DM. Average age of onset of adult disease is 52 years and juvenile disease is 8 years. Adult DM is more common in women; the male to female ratio is 1:6. Juvenile DM is slightly more common in boys.

The inflammatory myopathy affects proximal muscle groups, especially the triceps and quadriceps. Patients present with proximal muscle weakness, muscle tenderness, and fatigue. Muscle workup should include creatine phosphokinase and aldolase levels, magnetic resonance imaging, electromyography, and triceps muscle biopsy. Pulmonary fibrosis can be seen in 15% to 30% of patients and is more common in patients with anti–transfer-RNA syndrome (which may include Jo-1 antibodies).

Internal malignancy is estimated to occur in 10% to 50% of patients with adult DM. Ovarian, breast, lung, and gastric cancers have been described. The risk of malignancy may return to normal after 2 years. Juvenile DM is not associated with increased malignancy risk.

**TABLE 37-5** ■ **Cutaneous Manifestations of Dermatomyositis**

| | |
|---|---|
| Gottron's papules (see Fig. 37-4) | Violaceous papules overlying dorsal interphalangeal and metacarpophalangeal joints |
| Gottron's sign | Confluent violaceous erythema overlying dorsal interphalangeal and metacarpophalangeal joints |
| Periorbital heliotrope rash | Confluent violaceous erythema and edema of the eyelids and periorbital tissue |
| Poikiloderma | Violaceous erythema with hypopigmentation, hyperpigmentation, and atrophy in sun-exposed distribution and over extensor surfaces |

**TABLE 37-6** ■ **Therapeutic Options for Treatment of Dermatomyositis**

| | |
|---|---|
| Cutaneous lesions | Sunscreens (high SPF with UVA blocker) |
| | Topical corticosteroids |
| | Topical immunomodulators (e.g., tacrolimus) |
| | Hydroxychloroquine |
| | Low-dose methotrexate |
| | Mycophenolate mofetil |
| | Retinoids |
| Systemic disease | Oral prednisone |
| | Low-dose methotrexate |
| | Cyclosporine |
| | Cyclophosphamide |
| | Chlorambucil |
| | Newer biologic therapies |
| | IVIG |

*Abbreviations:* SPF, sun protective factor; UVA, ultraviolet A; IVIG, intravenous immunoglobulin.

Histopathology reveals vacuolar change, sparse lymphocytic infiltrate, epidermal atrophy, and basement membrane degeneration. aAbs to Jo-1 and Mi-2 are found in 30% of patients with polymyositis and 10% of patients with DM, respectively. ANA positivity is seen in 60% to 80% of patients. Treatment is outlined in Table 37-6.

## Suggested Readings

Chung L, Lin J, Furst DE, et al. Systemic and localized scleroderma. *Clin Dermatol.* 2006;24:374–392.

Connolly MK. Systemic sclerosis (scleroderma) and related disorders. In: Bolognia JL, Jorizzo JL, Rapini RP, eds. *Dermatology.* 2nd ed. St. Louis: Mosby; 2008:585–596.

Doria A, Briani C. Lupus: improving long-term prognosis. *Lupus.* 2008; 17(3):166–170.

Gáti T, Pajor A, Géher P, et al. Systemic lupus erythematosus and pregnancy. *Orv Hetil.* 2008;149(16):723–731.

Hochberg MC, Boyd RE, Ahearn JM, et al. Systemic lupus erythematosus: a review of clinico-laboratory features and immunogenetic markers in 150 patients with emphasis on demographic subsets. *Medicine.* 1985; 64:285–295.

Iorizzo LJ 3rd, Jorizzo JL. The treatment and prognosis of dermatomyositis: an updated review. *J Am Acad Dermatol.* 2008;59(1):99–112.

Jacobe HT, Sontheimer RD. Autoantibodies encountered in patients with autoimmune connective tissue diseases. In: Bolognia JL, Jorizzo JL, Rapini RP, eds. *Dermatology.* 2nd ed. St. Louis: Mosby; 2008:549–560.

Jorizzo JL, Carroll CL, Sangueza OP. Dermatomyositis. In: Bolognia JL, Jorizzo JL, Rapini RP, eds. *Dermatology.* 2nd ed. St. Louis: Mosby; 2008:575–584.

Simard JF, Costenbader KH. What can epidemiology tell us about systemic lupus erythematosus? *Int J Clin Pract.* 2007;61(7):1170–1180.

Sontheimer RD. Skin manifestations of systemic autoimmune connective tissue disease: diagnostics and therapeutics. *Best Pract Res Clin Rheumatol.* 2004;18:429–462.

# CHAPTER 38

# The Skin and Internal Disease

*Sarah Asch, MS, Pascal Ferzli, MD, and Warren R. Heymann, MD*

A practicing dermatologist must be cognizant of the potential cutaneous manifestations of systemic diseases. Although certain skin findings are pathognomonic for particular maladies, more often than not cutaneous eruptions must be interpreted in the context of the complete clinical picture. Occasionally, a cutaneous finding may guide the clinician toward a previously undiagnosed systemic disease. It is the interplay between the skin and internal medicine that underscores the value of a cutaneous evaluation as a routine part of a complete physical examination.

Cutaneous findings can be classified as specific and nonspecific. *Specific changes* demonstrate the same pathologic process as internal disease and can, therefore, be diagnostic of the disease. *Nonspecific changes* do not demonstrate the primary disease process (Figs. 38-1 and 38-2). These changes can be helpful in establishing the diagnosis only if interpreted within the context of the clinical data. The following cases are a few selected examples of the many systemic diseases with skin involvement. Table 38-1 lists some internal diseases and their dermatologic manifestations.

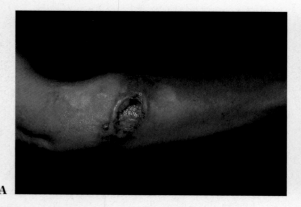
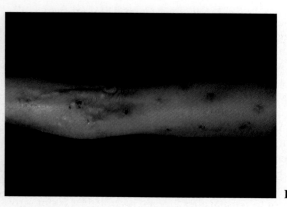

**FIGURE 38-1** ■ Nonspecific skin changes indicating an underlying psychologic disease state. **(A)** Delusional excoriation on the arm ("have to get the hairs out"). **(B)** Neurotic excoriations on the arm.

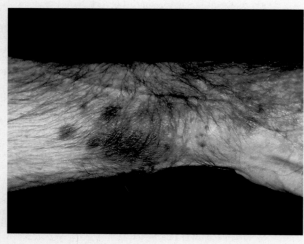
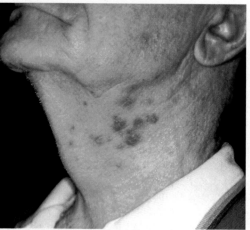

**FIGURE 38-2** ■ Nonspecific skin changes resulting from an internal disease. Purpura of the arm **(A)** and folliculitis of the neck **(B)** in a patient with myelogenous leukemia. *(Courtesy of Syntext Laboratories, Inc.)*

**TABLE 38-1** ■ **Internal Malignancies with Cutaneous Manifestations**

| Disorder | Cutaneous Findings | Associated Malignancies |
|---|---|---|
| Acanthosis nigricans | Velvety hyperpigmentation of flexures and, less commonly, mucosal surfaces and palms (tripe palms) | Adenocarcinoma of genitourinary or gastrointestinal tract. Most commonly associated with adenocarcinoma of the stomach (55.5%)* |
| Acquired ichthyosis | Adult onset hyperkeratosis indistinguishable from ichthyosis vulgaris | Hodgkin's lymphoma, mycosis fungoides, multiple myeloma, leiomyosarcoma |
| Acrokeratosis paraneoplastica (Bazex syndrome) | Acral psoriasiform plaques with nail dystrophy | Carcinomas of upper digestive and respiratory tracts. Also described in association with transitional cell bladder carcinoma† |
| Carcinoid syndrome | Deeply erythematous or violaceous flushing of upper body associated with pruritus, diaphoresis, lacrimation, and facial edema | Foregut, midgut, and bronchial neuroendocrine tumors |
| Cushing's syndrome | Generalized hyperpigmentation, including areolae, palmar creases, and scars; hirsutism; central obesity; moon facies, striae | Ectopic ACTH production by small cell lung cancer, bronchial carcinoid tumors and cancers of the thyroid, pancreas, and adrenals |
| Dermatomyositis | Heliotrope dermatitis, proximal nail fold telangiectasias, Gottron's papules, cutaneous necrosis | Ovarian, gastrointestinal, and nasopharyngeal carcinomas; adenocarcinomas of the lung and prostate; hematologic malignancies |
| Erythema gyratum repens | Migratory figurate erythema with "wood grain" pattern | Malignancies of the lung, breast, female reproductive tract, gastrointestinal tract, and prostate |
| Hypertrichosis lanuginosa acquisita | Excessive growth of vellus hairs on neck and face, but can involve any body surface | Most commonly observed with colorectal, breast, and lung cancers |
| Necrolytic migratory erythema | Acral and intertriginous papulosquamous dermatitis with occasional vesiculation | Pancreatic $\alpha$-cell tumor presents with glucagonoma syndrome |
| Paget's disease | (1) Unilateral eczematous nipple plaque (2) Eczematous plaque of the anorectal, genital, and axillary regions (extramammary Paget's disease) | (1) Associated with ductal adenocarcinoma (2) Regional associations are (a) anorectal—adenocarcinoma of the anus and colorectum, (b) vulvar—epithelial, eccrine, and apocrine neoplasms, and (c) male genitourinary reproductive tract malignancies |
| Paraneoplastic pemphigus | Diffuse mucocutaneous involvement with blisters, erosions, lichenoid, and erythema multiforme–like lesions. Head and neck skin is usually spared. Extensive oral erosions are notable. | Hematologic malignancies |
| Porphyria cutanea tarda | Vesicles and bullae with subsequent scarring, skin fragility on the dorsal hands, milia formation, and hypertrichosis on sun-exposed surfaces | Hepatocellular carcinoma, hematologic malignancies, myelodysplastic syndromes |
| Sweet's syndrome—atypical bullous pyoderma gangrenosum overlap | Indurated erythematous to violaceous plaques with or without bulla formation and ulceration | Hematologic malignancies, myeloproliferative disorders |
| Sign of Leser–Trélat | Eruptive multiple seborrheic keratoses | Adenocarcinomas of the lung and gastrointestinal tract |

*From Rigel DS, Jacobs MI. Malignant acanthosis nigricans: a review. *J Dermatol Surg Oncol*. 1980;6(11):923–927.

†From Arregui MA, Raton JA, Landa N, et al. Bazex's syndrome (acrokeratosis paraneoplastica)—first case report of association with a bladder carcinoma. *Clin Exp Dermatol*. 1993;18(5):445–448.

*Abbreviations:* ACTH, Adrenocorticotropic hormone.

## Cardiology

### Kawasaki's Syndrome

Kawasaki's syndrome, also known as *mucocutaneous lymph node syndrome,* is a self-limited acute vasculitis of childhood. It has a propensity for coronary artery involvement with aneurysms, angina pectoris, or myocardial infarction in up to 18% to 23% of untreated cases. With proper treatment, the percentage of coronary artery aneurysms decreases to 4% to 8%. Usually young children under the age of 5 are affected, with cases reported in infants and teenagers as well. There is a slight female preponderance. The diagnosis of Kawasaki's syndrome is based on a constellation of clinical findings including fever lasting at least 5 days, nonsuppurative cervical adenopathy, bilateral nonpurulent conjunctival injection, reddening and fissuring of the lips, "strawberry tongue," and several cutaneous findings. The skin changes begin with erythema of the palms and soles that may spread to the trunk. Then the syndrome progresses with the presence of an indurative edema and desquamation starting on the tips of the fingers and toes and around nails. A polymorphous rash that can vary from morbilliform to scarlatiniform may also be present.

### LEOPARD Syndrome

Multiple lentigines syndrome is an autosomal dominant disorder with abnormalities of various clinical expressions. LEOPARD is an acronym for the following abnormalities that may be present in an individual patient with this syndrome:

- *L*entigines: multiple lentigines are present at birth and may cover the entire body, including the palms and soles but sparing the lips and oral mucosa. The pigment can be seen in the iris and retina as well
- *E*lectrocardiogram conduction defects
- *O*cular hypertelorism
- *P*ulmonary stenosis
- *A*bnormalities of genitalia
- *R*etardation of growth
- *D*eafness (sensorineural)

### Pseudoxanthoma Elasticum

Pseudoxanthoma elasticum is a genetic connective tissue disease characterized by progressive mineralization of elastic fibers with cutaneous, cardiovascular, and ophthalmologic complications. The disease manifests as angioid streaks of the retina, retinal and gastrointestinal hemorrhages, hypertension, and occlusive vascular disease secondary to progressive calcification and fragmentation of the elastic fibers in the eye and blood vessels. Characteristic yellowish papules that appear like a "plucked chicken" are seen in the flexural areas of the neck as well as periumbilical areas. These lesions can also be seen in the oral, vaginal, and rectal mucosa.

## Endocrinology

### Diabetes Mellitus

Cutaneous manifestations associated with diabetes mellitus may correlate with metabolic derangements or may present as chronic degenerative changes with no apparent correlation to the degree of hyperglycemia. Metabolic changes in patients with poorly controlled diabetes tend to lead to a higher risk for the development of cutaneous infections by bacterial, fungal, and yeast pathogens. Diabetic dermopathy (atrophic, circumscribed, brownish plaques on the pretibial surfaces; Fig. 38-3) or bullous diabeticorum (spontaneous development of bullae on the extremities) can be seen as a result of chronic degenerative changes. Peripheral neuropathy, further compounded by

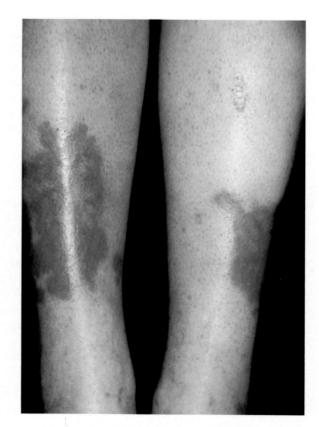

**FIGURE 38-3** ■ Necrobiosis lipoidica diabeticorum on the anterior tibial area of the legs. *(Courtesy of Smith Kline & French Laboratories.)*

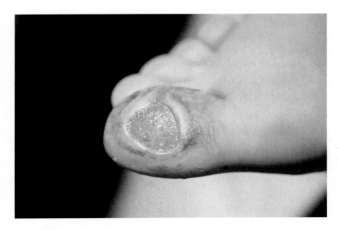

**FIGURE 38-4** ■ Mal perforans ulcer on the great toe of a diabetic man.

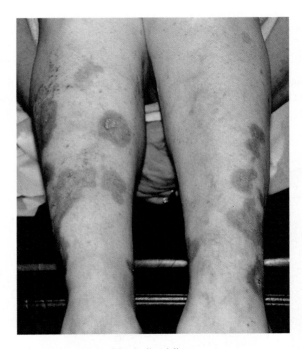

**FIGURE 38-5** ■ Necrobiosis lipoidica.

vascular compromise, may eventuate in neuropathic foot ulcers (Fig. 38-4).

Necrobiosis lipoidica (NL) is seen in less than 1% of diabetics, but the majority of patients with NL have diabetes mellitus (Fig. 38-5). NL begins as sharply circumscribed, dusky-red nodules or papules located most commonly on the anterior and lateral surfaces of the lower extremities. The lesions expand to form atrophic, waxy, yellowish, telangiectatic plaques with active brawny borders. The plaques occasionally ulcerate. New NL lesions may appear at the site of surgery or trauma (Koebner phenomenon).

## Disorders of the Hypothalamic–Pituitary–Adrenal Axis

Cushing's syndrome of glucocorticoid excess is caused by either endogenous overproduction of corticosteroids by the

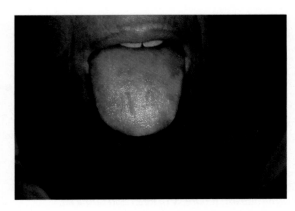

**FIGURE 38-6** ■ Hyperpigmentation of skin and tongue in a white woman with Addison's disease.

adrenal glands or by iatrogenically administered steroids, whereas Cushing's disease is caused by an adrenocorticotropic hormone–secreting anterior pituitary or nonpituitary neoplasm. The most profound cutaneous manifestations of Cushing's syndrome (and disease) include epidermal atrophy, striae, plethoric moon facies, buffalo hump, supraclavicular fat pads, and central obesity. There is a marked susceptibility to cutaneous fungal infections. The following findings may be observed in Cushing's syndrome:

- Addisonian hyperpigmentation
- Precocious puberty
- Virilization
- Pattern alopecia in females

Patients with Addison's disease, or primary adrenocortical insufficiency, suffer from a deficiency of glucocorticoids as well as mineralocorticoids. There is a hyperpigmentation of sun-exposed surfaces, flexural areas, pressure points, scars, and palmar creases (Fig. 38-6). Women may experience loss of axillary and pubic hair.

### Multiple Mucosal Neuroma Syndrome

Multiple mucosal neuroma syndrome is also known as *multiple endocrine neoplasia IIB*. In this autosomal dominant disorder, medullary thyroid carcinoma (MTC) and pheochromocytoma are associated with oral, nasal, upper gastrointestinal tract, and conjunctival neuromas. The skin lesions typically range from soft to firm intradermal nodules that tend to precede the MTC. However, MTC may occur in early childhood prior to the development of neuromas. Additional skin findings include "blubbery" lips, lentigines, café-au-lait macules, and localized intense unilateral pruritus on the back (notalgia paresthetica).

### Thyroid Disease

The activity of the thyroid gland is intimately reflected by changes in the skin and its appendages. In hyperthyroidism, the skin is thin, warm, moist, and flushed secondary to vasodilation of the dermal vasculature. Erythema and hyperhidrosis of the palms and soles may be present. Adnexal changes include rapidly growing, fine, soft hair with

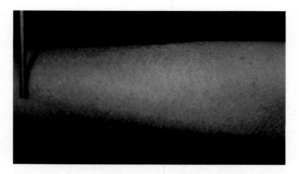

FIGURE 38-7 ■ Year-round dry skin associated with hypothyroidism. *(Courtesy of Reed and Carnick.)*

attendant nonscarring alopecia and soft nails with distal onycholysis. Graves' disease is associated with ophthalmopathy (proptosis, exophthalmos, and lid lag), thyroid dermopathy (pretibial myxedema), and acropachy.

In hypothyroidism, the skin is cold, dry, and pale secondary to vasoconstriction of the cutaneous vessels (Fig. 38-7). There is a generalized thinning and hyperkeratosis of the epidermis. Fine wrinkling and a yellow discoloration of the skin are also sometimes present. The hair is coarse, dry, brittle, and slow growing. Patchy or diffuse alopecia may be seen. Loss of the outer third of the eyebrow (madarosis) is a characteristic finding. Myxedema may be generalized in its distribution. Hypothyroid facies typically is expressionless, with thickening of the lips, broadening of the nose, drooping of the upper eyelids, and overall puffiness.

## Gastroenterology

### Dermatitis Herpetiformis

Also known as Duhring's disease, dermatitis herpetiformis manifests as vesicles on the buttocks, elbows, and knees. Dermatitis herpetiformis is associated with celiac sprue (gluten-sensitive enteropathy). Celiac sprue is often subclinical but can be confirmed by jejunal biopsy. Dermatitis herpetiformis should be considered in the differential diagnosis of children presenting with recalcitrant eczema or individuals with recalcitrant pruritus and ill-defined dermatoses.

### Inflammatory Bowel Disease

Ulcerative colitis is most commonly associated with pyoderma gangrenosum, a destructive neutrophilic dermatosis (Fig. 38-8). In pyoderma gangrenosum, a painful violaceous

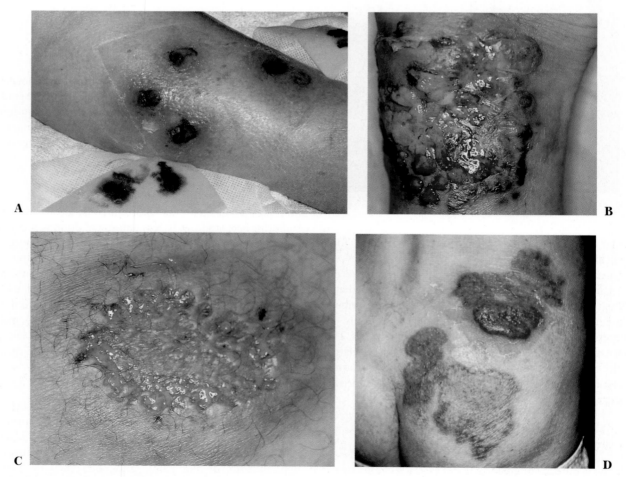

FIGURE 38-8 ■ Pyoderma gangrenosum associated with ulcerative colitis. *(Part D courtesy of Schering Corp.)*

nodule or pustule breaks down to form an enlarging ulcer with a raised, undetermined border and a boggy, necrotic base. Pyoderma gangrenosum has also been observed with Crohn's disease as well as hematologic malignancies, monoclonal gammopathies, and various arthritides.

### Peutz–Jeghers Syndrome

Peutz–Jeghers syndrome is an autosomal dominant disorder characterized by hamartomatous gastrointestinal polyposis and mucocutaneous pigmentation. Patients may present with abdominal pain, rectal bleeding, rectal prolapse, or intussusception. There is an increased risk of gastrointestinal tumors, ovarian and breast malignancies in females, and Sertoli cell tumors in males. Lentigines may be present at birth or develop in early childhood. Discrete brown, blue, or blue-brown macules are almost always located on the lips and oral mucosa, most commonly on buccal surfaces. Lentigines may also appear on the nail beds, hands, and feet, especially on palmar and plantar areas. With age, the cutaneous lesions may fade and even disappear, but the buccal mucosal lesions tend to persist into adulthood.

## Hematology–Oncology

Although cutaneous manifestations of systemic neoplastic disorders are diverse and often nonspecific, a practitioner must be vigilant for warning signs that warrant further investigation. For example, a patient presenting to a dermatologist with generalized pruritus may trigger a workup for underlying malignancy. Criteria of association pioneered by Curth and later expanded by Hill (Table 38-2) are applied to determine whether any given malignancy and dermatologic

---

**TABLE 38-2 ■ Criteria for Establishing Relationship between Dermatosis and Internal Malignancy. (Curth's Criteria with Modifications Noted.)**

- Both conditions develop at about the same time.
- Both conditions follow a parallel course.
- In certain syndromes, the course and onset of the dermatosis do not depend on the course and onset of the malignancy (and vice versa) because the two conditions are part of a genetic syndrome and they are coordinated with one another. Modified: Now classified as genodermatoses with malignant potential.
- A specific tumor occurs in connection with a certain dermatosis.*
- The dermatosis is usually uncommon.*
- The two conditions are strongly associated.*

*These criteria are not essential for a mucocutaneous condition to be considered a paraneoplastic syndrome.

From Cohen PR. Cutaneous paraneoplastic syndromes. *Am Fam Physician.* 1994;50(6):1273–1282.

---

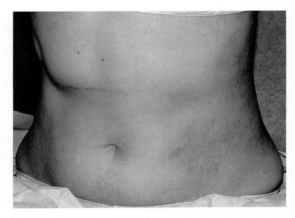

**FIGURE 38-9 ■** Acquired ichthyosis, which can be a sign of lymphoproliferative disorders.

condition are correlated. Examples of these associations include the following: Acquired ichthyosis (Fig. 38-9), which clinically appears as severely dry skin, is most often associated with lymphoproliferative disorders and other malignancies, including

- Hodgkin's disease
- Mycosis fungoides
- Multiple myeloma
- Kaposi's sarcoma
- Leiomyosarcomas
- Breast, cervical, and lung cancers

Erythroderma is a diffuse erythema of the skin, usually accompanied by induration and scaling. When scaling is diffuse, the condition is diagnosed as an exfoliative erythroderma. Erythrodermas are seen more commonly with hematologic malignancies, especially leukemia, lymphoma, and Sézary syndrome.

Acanthosis nigricans (AN) presents as hyperpigmented, velvety skin in flexural areas (Fig. 38-10). "Benign" forms are generally seen in obese patients or associated with endocrinopathies such as hyperandrogenism and insulin resistance as well as diabetes mellitus and the polycystic ovarian syndrome. AN is also observed in a number of

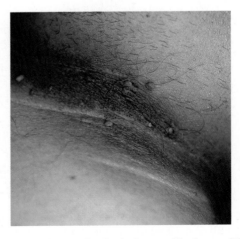

**FIGURE 38-10 ■** Acanthosis nigricans of the base of the neck.

genetic disorders. Occasionally, AN is induced by systemically administered corticosteroids, somatotropin, nicotinic acid, and insulin. AN in metabolic disturbances appears to be related to insulin and insulin-like growth factor (IGF) and their interaction with corresponding keratinocytic receptors (IGFR-1), and it is likely to be a reflection of insulin resistance.

"Malignant" AN is suspected in thin, older individuals with extensive involvement of the mucocutaneous integument. These gray-brown, symmetric, velvety, papillomatous plaques involve the axillae, neck, groin, antecubital fossae, vermilion border of the lip, and eyelids. Mucosal AN presents with verrucous pigmented plaques on the oral mucosa and conjunctivae and is especially suggestive of a neoplastic process. Association with rugated, velvety plaques of palmar surfaces (tripe palms) is observed. This variant of AN is most often associated with lung, ovarian, breast, gastric, bladder, and endometrial carcinomas.

Necrolytic migratory erythema (NME) is an integral part of a paraneoplastic syndrome observed in the context of glucagonoma (a neuroendocrine pancreatic tumor).

Although no longer considered pathognomonic of glucagonoma, NME accompanied by the new onset of diabetes, weight loss, glossitis, and angular cheilitis may be observed in a majority of patients with a glucagonoma. NME frequently presents as an annular psoriasiform eruption in an acral distribution affecting the central face, extremities, and groin. The lesions tend to have a waxing and waning course, healing without scarring. The NME course does not reflect the activity of the underlying tumor.

The classical paraneoplastic rheumatologic syndrome is dermatomyositis. Although the presentation of malignancy-associated rheumatologic disturbances is very similar to that of nonparaneoplastic rheumatologic diseases, there are certain laboratory and clinical findings that may suggest malignancy in otherwise typical cases. Rapid onset, cutaneous necrosis, extensive vasculitis, and a history of malignancy are all likely predictors of a concurrent neoplasm. Rheumatic symptoms and primary tumors may follow parallel clinical courses. Dermatologic manifestations of some lymphoproliferative disorders are shown in Fig. 38-11.

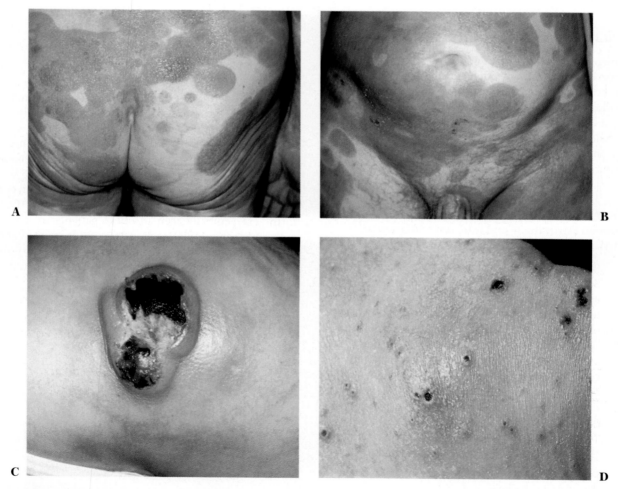

A   B

C   D

**FIGURE 38-11** ■ Dermatoses associated with lymphomas. Mycosis fungoides in plaque stage of the buttocks **(A)** and abdomen **(B)** of a 79-year-old man. **(C)** Mycosis fungoides in tumor stage on the thigh. **(D)** Nonspecific pyoderma with lymphocytic leukemia.

# Infectious Diseases

## Hepatitis C

Hepatitis C is associated with a variety of skin conditions that may often be the first indication of the patient's underlying infection. The more common manifestations include generalized pruritus, mixed cryoglobulinemia, necrolytic acral erythema, porphyria cutanea tarda (PCT), and lichen planus.

Generalized pruritus is a presenting symptom that raises flags for many underlying diseases. In the case of hepatitis C, it is seen in about 20% of patients and can be associated with nonspecific lesions such as prurigo nodules or excoriations.

Mixed cryoglobulinemia (types II and III) is a disorder of monoclonal or polyclonal immunoglobulins that reversibly precipitate at low temperatures. Hepatitis C infection is thought to cause an immune dysregulation that leads to the development of cryoglobulinemia. The classic presentation is a triad of purpura, arthralgias, and weakness. Palpable purpura appears in crops on the lower extremities, lasting 3 to 10 days, and is thought to be secondary to deposition of immune complexes in the vessels. Livedo reticularis, a netlike pattern of reddish-blue discoloration with central pallor, ischemic ulcers, acrocyanosis, and hemorrhagic bullae are also seen with mixed cryoglobulinemia.

Necrolytic acral erythema is a rarely seen, but pathognomonic, complication of hepatitis C infection. Well-circumscribed, annular, hyperkeratotic, violaceous plaques with raised scaly borders or vesiculobullous lesions appear on acral surfaces. Patients report burning and pruritus associated with the lesions.

Porphyria cutanea tarda is a photosensitivity disorder and can be familial. It can occur in association with renal disease (see later in the chapter), but may also be found in association with hepatitis C. Lesions occur in a photodistributed pattern and are characterized by tense bullae, erosions, and skin fragility and often heal with scarring and milia formation.

Lichen planus, predominantly the oral disease, may also be seen in association with hepatitis C. Oral and genital mucosal lesions begin as white, lacy papules and may become erosive. Cutaneous lichen planus is characterized by pruritic, purple, polygonal papules with an overlying reticulate pattern of white lines called Wickham's striae. These lesions are typically distributed over the flexor surfaces of the wrists and forearms, dorsal hands, the anterior aspect of the lower legs, the presacral area, and the neck, although cutaneous lesions are less commonly associated with hepatitis C than the oral form. The association of lichen planus with hepatitis C appears to be more common in patients from southern Europe and Japan.

## Human Immunodeficiency Virus

Untreated human immunodeficiency virus (HIV) infection may be associated with a host of dermatologic disorders ranging from mucocutaneous infections, papulosquamous diseases, and malignancies. With the advent of increased routine HIV screening and the institution of HAART (highly active antiretroviral therapy), the incidence of

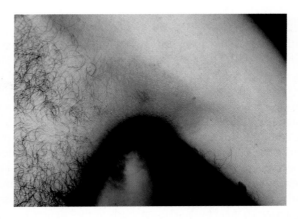

**FIGURE 38-12** ■ Erythema chronicum migrans of the axilla.

dermatologic diseases associated with terminal HIV infection has decreased significantly. A full discussion of cutaneous diseases associated with HIV is presented in Chapter 24.

## Lyme Disease

Lyme borreliosis is a spirochetal, multisystem illness borne by *Ixodes* sp (ticks). It is prevalent in the Northeastern, North Central, and Pacific coastal regions in the United States. *Borrelia burgdorferi* is the most commonly isolated causative organism in the United States, whereas in European countries, *B. afzelii* and *B. garinii* predominate. Erythema chronicum migrans (ECM) is the principal cutaneous hallmark of new-onset Lyme disease (Fig. 38-12). Early lesions display homogenous erythema at the site of the tick bite that subsequently spreads centrifugally. In North America, this lesion is less likely to show central clearing. However, in Europe the center of the lesion may fade or clear completely, leaving an annular, expanding erythema. ECM may present with a single or, less often, multiple lesions. Although ECM is by far the most common Lyme-associated dermatosis in the United States and Europe, other cutaneous disorders borrelial lymphocytoma (BL) and acrodermatitis chronica atrophicans (ACA) are observed more frequently in Europe. BL, also known as *lymphadenosis benigna cutis,* is usually noted at or near the tick bite site. Typically, BL presents as a solitary bluish-red nodule with regional lymphadenopathy. Sites of predilection include the earlobe, nipple and areola, scrotum, and nose. Patients with BL may present with or without preceding or concomitant ECM. Late Lyme disease may be associated with ACA, a chronic acral dermatitis that develops 6 months to 10 years after the initial arthropod assault. The onset is insidious, with waxing and waning edema and a reddish-blue discoloration of distal extremities, reminiscent of venous insufficiency. With time, the epidermis and dermis become atrophic and translucent. Late findings include fibrotic bands and nodule formation.

Of note, a Lyme disease mimic known as southern–tick-associated rash illness (STARI) is an emerging entity in the United States. While the etiology is still under investigation, physicians need to be aware of this clinical presentation when diagnosing and testing suspected cases, especially in areas that are not endemic for Lyme disease.

## Syphilis

With its incidence on the rise and its increasing prevalence coincident with HIV infection, syphilis has reemerged as an important treponemal disease. Syphilis (lues) is caused by the spirochete *Treponema pallidum*. The mode of acquisition (sexual versus vertical) and stage determine cutaneous and systemic manifestations. Cutaneous manifestations of syphilis are addressed in detail in Chapter 22. Briefly, lesions of primary syphilis present as a syphilitic chancre—a firm, painless, eroded plaque at the site of treponemal entry. Often syphilitic chancres are unrecognized as such because of their perianal, anal, intravaginal, or oral locations. Untreated, the classic hunterian chancre heals spontaneously. If the chancre is coinfected with other sexually transmitted agents, the presentation may be atypical.

Roughly one third of patients with untreated primary syphilis progress to secondary syphilis. More than 80% of these patients develop generalized cutaneous eruptions—syphilids that vary widely in their presentations including macular, maculopapular, papular, annular, and, less frequently, nodular and pustular lesions (Fig. 38-13). Condyloma lata are pathognomonic, patchy alopecia is rare, and mucous membrane lesions may be seen. Mucous patches are especially common on the tongue and lips. These lesions are highly infectious.

Nearly one third of untreated patients develop tertiary syphilis, which also presents with polymorphous lesions. Gummas are painless, pink to dusky-red nodules that can affect any organ system. These lesions may ulcerate and cause local tissue destruction. In tertiary syphilis, gummas are often seen in the skin and can also involve visceral organs and skeletal structures. Neurosyphilis and cardiovascular syphilis each affect 25% of patients with tertiary syphilis.

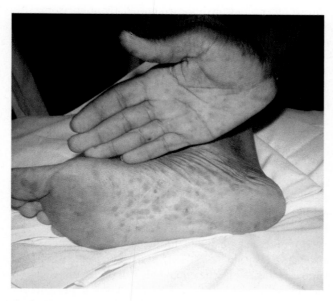

**FIGURE 38-13** ■ Ham-colored, scaly papules of the palm in secondary syphilis.

Presenting signs and symptoms of cerebrovascular syphilis range from the Argyll Robertson pupil that accommodates and converges but does not react to light, to blindness, deafness, and dementia. Tabes dorsalis is the degeneration of the posterior columns of the spinal cord leading to lancinating pain, ataxia, urinary incontinence, and loss of proprioception with resultant joint deterioration (Charcot's joints). Cardiovascular syphilis leads to a spectrum of manifestations: uncomplicated aortitis, aortic aneurysm (usually affecting the ascending aorta), aortic valvulitis with aortic insufficiency, coronary artery ostial stenosis, and myocarditis. Interestingly, early atherosclerosis in individuals with no known risk factors has been associated with tertiary syphilis.

Congenital syphilis tends to present soon after birth. However, a delay in presentation of up to 2 years may occur. Early manifestations are remarkably similar to syphilids in adults. In neonates, pemphigus syphiliticus with vesiculobullous lesions of the palms and soles, as well as other areas, has been described. Classically, syphilitic rhinitis (snuffles) is one of the more frequent specific signs of congenital syphilis. Mucosanguineous discharge with attendant nasal obstruction is present early in the disease; saddle nose deformity with septal perforation and perioral rhagades are stigmata of late congenital syphilis. Hutchinson's triad of congenital syphilis consists of Hutchinson's teeth (notched incisors), interstitial keratitis, and sensorineural deafness. Other important signs include bone lesions (saddle nose deformity, epiphysitis with resultant pain on motion—Parrot's pseudoparalysis), Higoumenakis's sign (unilateral clavicular thickening lateral to the patient's dexterity), neurosyphilis (seizures, hydrocephalus, cranial nerve palsies, tabes dorsalis), lymphadenopathy, and hepatosplenomegaly.

# Nephrology

## Acquired Perforating Disease

Acquired perforating disease (APD) of end-stage renal disease (ESRD) presents as a clinical aggregate of three primary perforating disorders:

- Kyrle's disease
- Reactive perforating collagenosis
- Perforating folliculitis

APD has also been associated with patients on dialysis. As with primary perforating disorders, an alteration in connective tissue (collagen or elastin) and transepithelial elimination have been implicated in the pathophysiology of APD. The lesions appear clinically as dome-shaped papules with keratotic plugs on the trunk and extensor extremities. Severe pruritus may accompany cutaneous eruption of APD. Koebnerization is frequently observed.

## Calcinosis Cutis and Calciphylaxis

Abnormal calcium and phosphate metabolism with subsequent secondary hyperparathyroidism predisposes patients with renal disease to metastatic calcifications. Calcinosis cutis frequently affects periarticular soft tissues. Discrete, mobile, skin-colored subcutaneous nodules are tender when present on the digits. Pasty or chalky contents occasionally extrude from these lesions. Calciphylaxis is a systemic vascular disease with mural calcification of small- and medium-sized arteries. Typical lesions are exquisitely tender, poorly defined, deep subcutaneous nodules and plaques with overlying livedoid purpura of proximal thighs and buttocks. Stellate ulcerations may be accompanied by marked cutaneous necrosis. Calciphylaxis is associated with a high mortality rate.

## Chronic Renal Failure and Dialysis

Several cutaneous changes are particularly prevalent in patients on dialysis. Generalized pruritus without a primary cutaneous eruption could be a sign of various underlying disorders, including uremia or chronic renal failure. Dialysis seems to be an important trigger of pruritus. Uremic frost is exceedingly rare in the present day but can be seen as white, crystalline precipitation on the skin. Pallor of the proximal nail bed, known as Lindsay's nail (half-and-half nail), may be observed in azotemic patients.

## Henoch–Schönlein Purpura

Henoch–Schönlein purpura is an immunoglobulin (Ig) A–mediated systemic leukocytoclastic vasculitis of small vessels that typically affects the skin, joints, gastrointestinal tract, and kidneys (see Chapter 12). Clinically, pediatric patients present with the classic tetrad of abdominal pain, polyarthritis, nephritis, and a purpuric eruption. Palpable purpura, typically of the lower legs and buttocks, occurs in almost every case and is the presenting sign in more than 50% of cases. Petechiae and ecchymoses may also be present. Urticarial and erythematous maculopapular lesions preceding the purpura have been described. A characteristic finding in children is painful edema of the face, scalp, ears, periorbital region, extremities, and genitalia. Scrotal edema and bruising is observed in up to one third of male patients. Rare cases of penile edema and purpura involving the glans penis have been reported.

## Fabry's Disease

Fabry's disease is an X-linked recessive defect in the activity of a lysosomal enzyme, $\alpha$-galactosidase A, causing accumulation of glycosphingolipids in tissues. The glycosphingolipid deposits primarily affect the vascular endothelium, which leads to cardiovascular, cerebral, and renal manifestations. Cutaneous findings give rise to vascular lesions known as angiokeratoma corporis diffusum universale. Angiokeratomas are of the utmost diagnostic importance as they appear in childhood and may be one of the earliest signs of the disease. These are nonblanchable, punctate, red to blue-black keratotic papules with slight hyperkeratosis in the larger lesions. Angiokeratomas, with time, increase in size and number. Lesions are mostly located between the umbilicus and the knees and are usually symmetrically distributed. Acroparesthesias and hypohidrosis with resultant heat intolerance have been described. Enzyme replacement therapy has revolutionized the treatment of Fabry's disease. It has recently been shown to decrease both organ dysfunction and cutaneous manifestations.

## Nephrogenic Systemic Fibrosis

First described in 1997, nephrogenic systemic fibrosis (NSF), formerly nephrogenic sclerosing (fibrosing) dermopathy, has been recognized in patients with renal insufficiency, with nearly 150 cases identified between 1997 and 2004. Patients may or may not require hemodialysis. NSF occurs equally in males and females without ethnic predilection. Gadolinium exposure from contrast agents used for imaging is the presumptive cause of NSF. Clinically, patients initially present with erythematous papules as well as a peau d'orange appearance of distal extremities. These primary lesions coalesce into woody, sclerodermoid, red-brawny plaques with an edge that advances proximally. Dependent areas are more severely involved. There is accompanying pruritus, burning, and lancinating pain. A marked decrease in the affected joints' range of motion may progress to joint contractures, thereby incapacitating patients. Systemic involvement with extensive calcifications and fibrosis of vital structures has been reported. The disease course closely parallels that of renal function.

## Porphyria Cutanea Tarda

PCT in renal disease patients is most often of the sporadic type. Clinical and laboratory findings are analogous to those of the inherited form of PCT, with photodistributed tense bullae that tend to rupture and heal with scars and milia. Hypertrichosis and hyperpigmentation are common. Pseudoporphyria, a bullous dermatosis clinically similar to PCT, has been described in patients on chronic hemodialysis or those taking one of several medications that have been reported to cause the condition. Patients with pseudoporphyria lack abnormal porphyrin levels and do not exhibit either hypertrichosis or sclerodermoid changes.

# Pulmonary

## Atopic Dermatitis

Asthma, penicillin allergy, urticaria, marked reaction to insect bites, multiple food allergies, allergic rhinitis, and conjunctivitis have all been associated with atopic dermatitis (see Chapter 10). These disorders may occur concomitantly or independently, and most patients develop only one or two components of an atopic diathesis. Several genetically inherited cutaneous disorders include atopic dermatitis as an integral part of the syndrome. Netherton's syndrome is an autosomal recessive genodermatosis characterized by pathognomonic erythematous patches with a double-edge scale termed *ichthyosis linearis circumflexa,* a "ball-and-socket" hair deformity (trichorrhexis invaginata), and atopic dermatitis. Other diseases associated with atopic dermatitis include ichthyosis vulgaris and the Wiskott–Aldrich syndrome. Recently, chronic atopic dermatitis has been implicated in increased susceptibility to CD30+ cutaneous lymphoma. However, the causal relationship between the two entities remains under scrutiny.

## Sarcoidosis

Sarcoidosis is a granulomatous process affecting various organ systems (see Chapter 16). The most characteristic cutaneous sarcoidal lesion is lupus pernio. Lesions of lupus pernio consist of chronic, reddish-brown to violaceous, indurated papules and plaques with a predilection for the nose, ears, and lips (**Fig. 38-14**). Sarcoidal skin plaques are also located on the limbs, back, and buttocks. These plaques may have central atrophy or a hypopigmented appearance. Erythema nodosum is the most common nonspecific cutaneous manifestation of sarcoidosis. Erythema nodosum is a hypersensitivity reaction to various agents, appearing clinically as tender, erythematous, subcutaneous nodules predominantly on the anterior shins. Lofgren's syndrome presents with erythema nodosum, fever, hilar adenopathy, and polyarthralgia. Lupus pernio is more frequent in African-American patients; erythema nodosum is commonly found in European and Latin-American patients. Heerfordt's syndrome is a manifestation of acute sarcoidosis and presents with fever, uveitis, parotitis, and Bell's palsy. Although rare in the general population, this syndrome has been most often reported in young Japanese patients, with females outnumbering males. Koebnerization of sarcoidal lesions is observed. Uncommon manifestations such as leonine facies, psoriasiform or lichenoid plaques, and pyoderma gangrenosum have been reported. Other nonspecific skin findings include scarring and nonscarring alopecia, hypopigmented patches, erythroderma, erythema multiforme, acquired ichthyosis, and dystrophic calcifications.

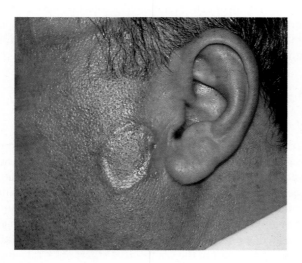

**FIGURE 38-14** ■ A granulomatous plaque in a man with sarcoidosis.

# Neurology

## Neurofibromatosis

Neurofibromatosis (NF) is an autosomal dominant genodermatosis (see Chapter 40). There are two subtypes of NF: Recklinghausen's disease (NF-1) and bilateral acoustic neurofibromatosis (NF-2). Both types involve congenital and acquired hamartomatous tumors of the central nervous system (CNS), skin, bone, endocrine glands, and eyes. Café-au-lait macules develop shortly after birth and may be found anywhere on the body. These hyperpigmented lesions can be found in normal individuals, but the presence of six or more macules 1.5 cm or greater in adults ($\geq$0.5 cm in children) is highly suggestive of NF. Intertriginous freckling (Crowe's sign) and pigmented hamartomas of the iris (Lisch nodules) are virtually diagnostic of NF. The principal dermatologic manifestations of this disease are cutaneous, subcutaneous, or plexiform neurofibromas (**Fig. 38-15**). These vary in size and shape and range from a few to as many as 9,000. Less common features include total or partial limb enlargement (elephantiasis neuromatosa), multiple lipomas, or a cutaneous sclerosing perineuroma. Segmental involvement with either NF subtype may represent a postzygotic mutation.

## Sturge–Weber Syndrome

In this neurocutaneous syndrome, a capillary malformation (port-wine stain, or nevus flammeus) involves the unilateral or, less commonly, the bilateral distribution of the ophthalmic division of the trigeminal nerve. Typically, the cutaneous involvement precedes the cerebral involvement, which appears later in childhood as a contralateral spastic hemiparesis, unilateral seizures, hemisensory defects, mental retardation, glaucoma, and homonymous hemianopia. Although plain skull x-rays reveal the classic "tram-track" calcifications, these do not appear until later in life. Therefore, either MRI/MRA (magnetic resonance imaging/angiography) or PET (positron emission tomography) scans are better modalities to screen for leptomeningeal angiomatosis and brain involvement.

## Tuberous Sclerosis

Tuberous sclerosis is a highly penetrant, genetically heterogeneous, autosomal dominant genodermatosis characterized by the triad of multiple hamartomas, seizures, and developmental difficulties. Hamartomas can involve any organ system, especially the skin, CNS, renal system, and cardiovascular system. Facial angiofibromas (adenoma sebaceum) (**Fig. 38-16**), Koenen tumors (**Fig. 38-17**), and fibrous plaques are the major cutaneous findings.

Angiofibromas are pink to red papules appearing after 4 years of age and localizing to the nasolabial folds, cheeks, and chin. Fibrous forehead plaques may present as early as the first weeks of life. The Koenen tumor is an ungual angiofibroma. A later finding appearing during childhood or adolescence is the shagreen patch, a connective tissue hamartoma.

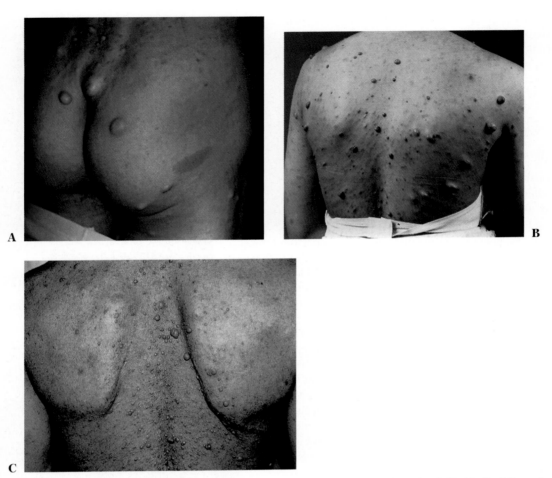

**FIGURE 38-15** ■ Neurofibromatosis of the buttocks **(A)**, with café-au-lait lesions on the back **(B, C)**. *(Part B courtesy of KUMC; Reed and Carnick.)*

It is characteristically found in the lumbosacral region and appears as a skin-colored, slightly elevated plaque with the texture and appearance of an orange peel. Hypomelanotic macules have been found in up to 90% of patients with tuberous sclerosis. These lesions, typically located on the trunk and limbs, appear before any other skin findings. Their configurations vary from guttate leukodermatous "confetti" macules to lance ovate ash-leaf macules. One or two hypopigmented macules may be seen in normal individuals; when three or more are present, the diagnosis of tuberous sclerosis must be considered. Although the most common

**FIGURE 38-16** ■ Angiofibromas (adenoma sebaceum) on the face of a patient with tuberous sclerosis.

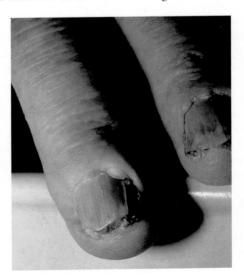

**FIGURE 38-17** ■ Periungual fibromas (Koenen tumor) associated with tuberous sclerosis.

renal lesion in tuberous sclerosis is the angiomyolipoma, tuberous sclerosis is associated with an increased risk of renal cancer, specifically clear cell carcinoma. Patients must be radiologically monitored as these tumors are likely to be multifocal, bilateral, and present at a younger age than the general population (30 vs. 60 years of age).

## Rheumatology (see Chapter 37)

### Dermatomyositis

Dermatomyositis is a complex autoimmune disease of adults and children that causes progressive muscular inflammation and weakness. Myositis preferentially involves the shoulder and hip girdles, manifesting as difficulty with such activities as combing hair or getting up from a chair. Interstitial lung disease may be a presenting sign of dermatomyositis, with 65% of newly diagnosed patients affected by it. In approximately 15% of patients, dermatomyositis may be complicated by associated malignancies, including cancers of the lung, ovary, and hematopoietic systems.

The cutaneous manifestations are pathognomonic. The most specific skin finding is Gottron's papules, which are erythematous papules of distant interphalangeal joints, elbows, and knees. The heliotrope rash, a subtle, erythematous or violaceous blush on the eyelids and periorbital region, is seen in approximately 60% of cases. Erythema may develop on sun-exposed areas, and chronic changes may include poikilodermatous lesions on the trunk and proximal extremities. Periungual telangiectasias and cuticular thromboses may also be observed. Of note, myositis and cutaneous manifestations often have divergent courses in terms of onset, progress, and severity. "Amyopathic" dermatomyositis displays classic cutaneous findings without an associated myopathy. These patients may also be at risk for associated malignancies.

### Lupus Erythematosus

Systemic lupus erythematosus (SLE) is an autoimmune connective tissue disease characterized by multiorgan involvement and the presence of autoantibodies to nuclear antigens (see Chapter 37). The stringent diagnostic criteria for SLE were originally set forth by the American College of Rheumatology in 1982 and revised in 1997. The butterfly rash is the sine qua non of an acute SLE eruption (**Fig. 38-18**). The shape of the eruption indeed resembles a butterfly with open wings, with erythematous to violaceous edematous plaques over the malar cheeks and dorsal nose. The nasolabial folds are typically spared. As with all SLE cutaneous manifestations, the malar rash typically appears after sun exposure. Other sites of predilection are the V of the chest, extensor extremities, mid-upper back, and shoulders (**Fig. 38-19**). On rare occasions, the atrophic, hyperpigmented scarring lesions of chronic cutaneous lupus erythematosus (discoid lupus erythematosus) may develop; the annular or papulosquamous lesions of subacute cutaneous lupus erythematosus have a more frequent association with systemic disease than discoid lupus erythematosus.

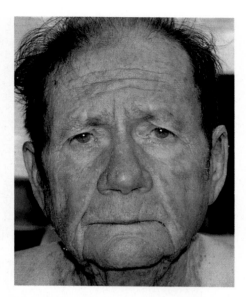

FIGURE 38-18 ■ Butterfly appearance in patient with SCLE.

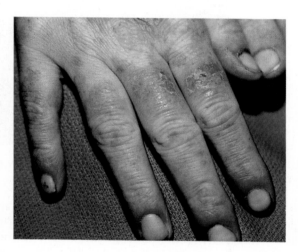

FIGURE 38-19 ■ Sparing of the knuckles in systemic lupus erythematosus (the opposite of dermatomyositis).

Mucous membranes may also be affected, with lesions on either the palatal or buccal mucosa. The former is involved with honeycombed plaques, hyperemia, and punched-out ulcerations, whereas lichen planus–like lesions appears on the latter. Discoid lesions may be observed on the palatal and buccal mucosa. Panniculitis (lupus profundus), alopecia, livedo reticularis, and periungual telangiectasias are other cutaneous features that may be seen in SLE.

### Scleroderma

Systemic scleroderma is a chronic disease of unknown origin that affects the connective tissue and the vasculature. The disease is characterized by fibrosis and obliteration of the vessels in the skin, lungs, heart, gastrointestinal tract, and kidneys (**Fig. 38-20**). Morphea (localized scleroderma) is only rarely associated with systemic disease. These cases tend to be when such lesions are multiple and diffuse.

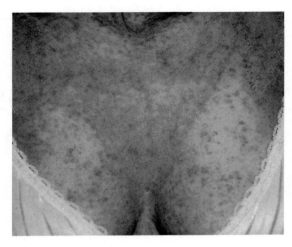

**FIGURE 38-20** ■ Hypopigmentation with perifollicular pigment retention and skin tightening of scleroderma.

There are two forms of systemic scleroderma: progressive and limited. Limited systemic scleroderma or CREST syndrome (*c*alcinosis, *R*aynaud's phenomenon, *e*sophageal dysmotility, *s*clerodactyly, *t*elangiectasias) predominantly affects the hands and may start as Raynaud's phenomenon or nonpitting edema of the hands and fingers (Fig. 38-21). Flexion contractures and sclerodactyly may eventually supervene. Progressive systemic scleroderma may also

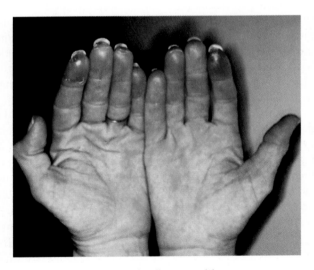

**FIGURE 38-21** ■ Raynaud's disease with gangrene.

present with Raynaud's phenomenon and, as the name implies, evolve to affect viscera and the skin. The disease slowly extends to involve upper extremities, face, trunk, and possibly the lower extremities. It begins as a painless edema that leads to tightening of the skin. In the final or atrophic stage, the skin becomes taut, smooth, and discolored, being tightly bound to underlying bony structures, with a resultant decrease in range of motion. The face takes on a masklike quality with microstomia with radial furrowing around the mouth, a beaked nose, and an unnaturally youthful countenance. Matlike telangiectasias of the face and upper trunk, alopecia, and anhidrosis are also seen.

## Suggested Readings

Abdelmalek NF, Gerber TL, Menter A. Cardiocutaneous syndromes and associations. *J Am Acad Dermatol.* 2002;46:161–183.

Bratton RL, Whiteside JW, Hovan MJ, et al. Diagnosis and treatment of Lyme disease. *Mayo Clin Proc.* 2008;83(5):566–571.

Brewster UC. Dermatological disease in patients with CKD. *Am J Kidney Dis.* 2008;51(2):331–344.

Cahill J, Sinclair R. Cutaneous manifestations of systemic disease. *Aust Fam Physician.* 2005;34(5):335–340.

Callen J. *Dermatological Signs of Internal Disease.* 3rd ed. Philadelphia: WB Saunders; 2003.

Centers for Disease Control and Prevention (CDC). Lyme disease—United States, 2003–2005. *MMWR Morb Mortal Wkly Rep.* 2007;56(23): 573–576.

Holman JD, Dyer JA. Genodermatoses with malignant potential. *Curr Opin Pediatr.* 2007;19(4):446–454.

Ianuzzi MC, Rybicki BA, Teirstein AS. Sarcoidosis. *N Engl J Med.* 2007;357(21):2153–2165.

Kent ME, Romanelli F. Reexamining syphilis: an update on epidemiology, clinical manifestations, and management. *Ann Pharmacother.* 2008; 42(2):226–236.

Kirsner RS, Federman DG. Cutaneous clues to systemic disease. *Postgrad Med.* 1997;101:137, 144–147.

Kleyn CE, Lai-Cheong JE, Bell HK. Cutaneous manifestations of internal malignancy: diagnosis and management. *Am J Clin Dermatol.* 2006;7(2):71–84.

Lebwohl M. *Atlas of the Skin and Systemic Disease.* New York: Churchill Livingstone; 2003.

Mannis MJ, Mascal MS, Huntley AC. *Eye and Skin Disease.* Philadelphia: Lippincott–Raven; 1996.

Ostezan LB, Callen JP. Cutaneous manifestations of selected rheumatologic diseases. *Am Fam Physician.* 1996;53:1625–1633.

Pipkin CA, Lio PA. Cutaneous manifestations of internal malignancies: an overview. *Dermatol Clin.* 2008;26(1):1–15, vii.

Tabor CA, Parlette EC. Cutaneous manifestations of diabetes. Signs of poor glycemic control or new-onset disease. *Postgrad Med.* 2006;119(3): 38–44.

Wohlrab J, Wohlrab D, Meiss F. Skin diseases in diabetes mellitus. *J Dtsch Dermatol Ges.* 2007;5(1):37–53.

Yell JA, Mbuagbaw J, Burge SM. Cutaneous manifestations of systemic lupus erythematosus. *Br J Dermatol.* 1996;135(3):355–362.

# Dermatologic Reactions to Ultraviolet Radiation and Visible Light

*Laurie L. Kohen, MD and Henry W. Lim, MD*

## The Ultraviolet Spectrum

By convention, ultraviolet (UV) radiation is divided into UVA, UVB, and UVC. UVA ranges from 320 to 400 nm. UVB spans from 290 to 320 nm, and UVC includes wavelengths measuring from 200 to 290 nm. UVC radiation emitted by the sun is absorbed by the atmosphere. Therefore, it does not reach the earth's surface and has no medical relevance. Sixty-five percent of UV radiation reaches the earth's surface between 10:00 AM and 2:00 PM when the sun is most directly overhead. UV radiation in noonday sun consists of 95% UVA and 5% UVB. This is the reason that, for optimal photoprotection, broad-spectrum sunscreens that absorb in both the UVA and UVB ranges are recommended. The type of UV light and chromophores in the skin, such as nucleic acids, melanin, and aromatic amino acids, determine the depth of penetration of UV radiation. UVA, being of a longer wavelength, penetrates deeper than UVB. Twenty to thirty percent of UVA radiation reaches the deep dermis, whereas only 10% of UVB reaches the superficial dermis. UVA, but not UVB radiation, can penetrate window glass.

## Sunburn and Tanning: Acute Effects of UV Radiation

Skin type plays an important role in the clinical outcome of sun exposure. Fitzpatrick's classification of skin types is widely used (Table 39-1). Sensitivity to UV is best assessed by the determination of minimal erythema dose (MED), which is defined as the smallest dose of radiation causing perceptible erythema covering the entire irradiated area. For individuals with skin type I, the MED for broadband UVB (MED-B) is between 20 and 40 mJ/cm$^2$ and for broadband UVA (MED-A), it is 20 to 40 J/cm$^2$, illustrating the 1,000-fold less efficiency of UVA radiation in causing erythema.

### Presentation and Characteristics

UVA-induced erythema is typically apparent by the end of the irradiation period and fades gradually in the next 24 to 72 hours. UVA is much more effective at inducing pigmentary alteration than causing erythema. Exposure to UVA radiation results in three types of pigmentation changes: immediate pigment darkening (IPD), persistent pigment darkening (PPD), and delayed tanning. IPD occurs immediately after exposure and fades within 10 to 20 minutes; it presents as a bluish-gray discoloration of the skin. The mechanism of IPD is oxidation of preexisting melanin in the epidermis; there is no neomelanogenesis. PPD occurs by the same mechanism and follows IPD if the UVA dose is sufficiently high. It lasts from 2 to 24 hours. Delayed tanning is due to the formation of new melanin in the epidermis; it may blend with IPD and PPD and lasts for days.

UVB-induced erythema consists of an immediate and a delayed phase; the former starts in 2 to 6 hours and peaks in 24 to 36 hours. There is no apparent IPD/PPD seen with UVB, just a delayed tanning reaction that is always preceded by erythema. UVB-induced delayed tanning peaks at 72 hours and fades rapidly. Similar to UVA-induced delayed tanning, neomelanogenesis also takes place.

**TABLE 39-1 ■ Fitzpatrick Skin Types**

| Skin Type | Characteristics |
| --- | --- |
| I | Never tan, always burn |
| II | Occasionally tan, usually burn |
| III | Usually tan, occasionally burn |
| IV | Easily tan, rarely burn |
| V | Brown skin |
| VI | Black skin |

Sunburn reactions present as erythema, edema, vesiculation, and pain, followed by scaling, desquamation, and hyperpigmentation. Acute reactions, when severe, may be accompanied by weakness, fatigue, and pruritus.

## Treatment

- *Photoprotection:* Photoprotection consists of minimizing sun exposure between 10 AM and 4 PM, the use of photoprotective clothing, wide-brimmed hats, and sunglasses, and the application of broad-spectrum sunscreens. Sunscreens with a sun protection factor (SPF) of 15 or greater should be applied 20 minutes before sun exposure and reapplied every 2 hours, especially after sweating or swimming. Sunscreens should be applied generously: 1 oz (30 mL) is needed to cover the entire body surface. Broad-spectrum sunscreens, which protect against both UVB and UVA radiation, are recommended. Commonly used sunscreen ingredients in the United States are listed in Table 39-2.
- *Nonsteroidal anti-inflammatory agents and corticosteroids:* These should be taken within 4 to 6 hours after sun exposure. Topical corticosteroids and cool compresses are helpful in reducing the inflammation. Oral prednisone (1 mg/kg) may be used for 5 to 7 days in severe cases.

**TABLE 39-2 ■ Commonly Used Sunscreen Ingredients in the United States**

| UVB Filters | UVA Filters |
|---|---|
| PABA derivatives | Benzophenones |
| Cinnamates | Avobenzone (Parsol 1789) |
| Salicylates | Anthranilate |
| Octocrylene | Titanium dioxide |
| | Zinc oxide |
| | Ecamsule (Mexoryl SX) |

*Abbreviation:* PABA, *para*-aminobenzoic acid

## Photoaging: Chronic Effects of UV Radiation

### Presentation and Characteristics

Photoaging accounts for 90% of age-associated cosmetic problems. The effects of photoaging can be broken down into the following categories:

- Pigmentation changes
- Texture changes
- Vascular changes
- Papillary changes

Pigmentation changes result from UV damage to the epidermis; the other changes result from dermal pathology. Both UVA and UVB radiation contribute to the process of photoaging.

The prototypical pigmentary change seen in older adults is a solar lentigo. Solar lentigines, or "age spots," appear in chronically sun-exposed areas, usually starting at around 40 years of age. They are macules with well-demarcated borders and vary in color from yellowish brown to dark brown. The mechanism of occurrence is thought to be an increase in melanin content within the keratinocytes and possibly reactive hyperplasia of melanocytes. Areas near the lentigines may be hypopigmented, giving the skin an overall mottled appearance.

The leathery texture and deep wrinkling of the skin from photoaging is called *solar elastosis* and is very characteristic of severe chronic sun damage. This typically occurs on the face and neck and gives the skin a yellowish hue. The pathologic hallmark is deposition in the papillary dermis of amorphous elastotic material that does not form functional elastic fibers. This altered connective tissue does not demonstrate the resilient properties of normal elastic tissue. There is also epidermal acanthosis seen on histology. Furthermore, collagen destruction, induced by downstream effects of oxidative and direct DNA damage from UV radiation, plays a role in the loss of the skin's tensile strength.

Blood vessel damage occurs with photoaging as well. Thinning of vessel walls and a decrease in vessel number are observed. Connective tissue support of the vasculature is diminished. Thus, fragility of vessels is demonstrated by the development of ecchymoses after minimal trauma. Telangiectasias are also seen in chronically sun-exposed regions.

A common example of a papillary change seen in photoaging is a seborrheic keratosis. This "wisdom spot" results from disrupted keratinocyte maturation imposed by accumulated UV radiation. Seborrheic keratoses appear "stuck on" to the skin and are more frequent on sun-exposed skin of the face, trunk, and extremities. They are completely benign growths and pose no risk of malignant transformation.

### Treatment

- *Topical retinoids:* These can cause slight reversal of photoaged skin. They increase collagen levels, which effaces wrinkles. Retinoids also stimulate epidermal hyperplasia, which manifests clinically as smoother skin with fewer fine lines. Deeper wrinkles caused by chronologic aging persist. Retinoids also lighten pigmentary changes associated with photodamage. Side effects include peeling, erythema, and dryness. Topical retinoids are not recommended during pregnancy.

- *Photorejuvenation:* This entails stimulation of dermal collagen synthesis by exposure to laser, intense pulse (visible) light, radiofrequency, or photodynamic therapy. This is a rapidly evolving area with numerous methods and equipment on the market. More studies are needed for many of the methods used.
- *Resurfacing:* This can occur at a superficial, medium, or deep level. Techniques employed include microdermabrasion, chemical peels, and, less commonly, laser resurfacing. Efficacy depends on the depth of wound infliction. The mechanism of wrinkle reduction is stimulation of wound healing with new collagen formation. Re-epithelization occurs from stem cells located in adnexal appendages. Side effects of resurfacing include permanent pigmentary changes and scarring.

## Photocarcinogenesis

### Actinic Keratoses

*Presentation and Characteristics*

Actinic keratoses (AKs) are premalignant lesions that predominately form on the chronically sun-exposed areas of skin type I and II (Table 39-1) patients. They occasionally appear in type III and IV individuals as well. Clinically, they present as discrete, rough, hyperkeratotic areas with a scale. They may be brown, yellowish-brown, flesh-colored, or red. When the lower lip is involved, the term *actinic cheilitis* is used (Fig. 39-1). Texture is the key to diagnosis. Histologically, an AK is an abnormal proliferation of cells confined to the epidermis with some evidence of cellular atypia. It has been estimated that over 10 years, 10.2% of AKs would evolve into invasive squamous cell carcinoma, thus necessitating the treatment of lesions that do not spontaneously remit. AKs are considered to be precursors of squamous cell carcinoma; hence, they should be treated appropriately.

*Treatment*

- *Cryotherapy:* This is the treatment of choice for most superficial lesions. For AK lesions that appear indurated, painful, or with a thick crust, surgical

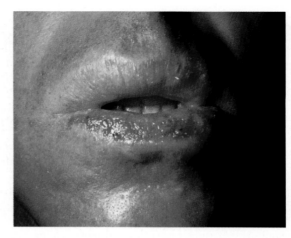

**FIGURE 39-1** ■ Actinic cheilitis, presenting as rough, keratotic patches on the lower lip.

removal may be required and a specimen should be sent for pathologic examination to rule out squamous cell carcinoma.

- *Topical agents:* 5-Fluorouracil, imiquimod cream, and diclofenac sodium gel are useful for patients with multiple or recurrent lesions.
- *Photodynamic therapy:* This modality utilizes 5-aminolevulinic acid (which gets converted into protoporphyrin) and blue light, or methyl aminolevulinate and red light. It has been shown to successfully eliminate AKs.

### Non-melanoma Skin Cancer

Basal cell carcinomas (BCCs) comprise 80% of non-melanoma skin cancers (NMSCs) diagnosed; squamous cell carcinomas (SCCs) comprise 20%. SCCs demonstrate a more linear correlation to the amount of UV exposure than do BCCs. Among whites, the incidence of NMSCs and melanomas has been increasing annually for several decades.

### Squamous Cell Carcinoma

***Presentation and Characteristics.*** The in situ form of SCC is known as Bowen's disease. Clinically, it appears as a well-demarcated, red, scaly patch, usually in sun-exposed areas. It is more likely to be found on the lower extremity of women and the scalp and ears of men. Treatment options include electrodessication and curettage, cryosurgery, and surgical excision.

Risk factors for development of SCCs include fair skin, light-colored iris, intermittent burns during childhood, ionizing radiation, immunosuppression, chronic inflammation, environmental carcinogens, certain genodermatoses, proximity to the equator, and cumulative exposure to UV radiation—specifically UVB radiation. UVB induces DNA damage and mutates tumor suppressor genes, such as *p53*. UVA also damages DNA and is thought to enhance the carcinogenic potential of UVB radiation.

SCCs are typically distributed on the scalp, dorsal hands, and pinna. SCCs have a greater potential for metastasis than

BCC's. The risk of metastasis depends on a multitude of factors including location of the primary lesion, immune status, size of tumor, degree of differentiation on histopathologic examination, and depth of invasion. A 12.5-year study done in Australia has shown that the use of broad-spectrum sunscreens could significantly decrease the development of SCCs.

**Treatment.** Treatment entails electrodessication and curettage, surgical excision, or Mohs micrographic surgery.

### Basal Cell Carcinoma

**Presentation and Characteristics.** BCCs are the single most common malignant neoplasm. They occur most often after the age of 40. Although sun exposure is an important cause of BCCs, other factors, such as ethnicity and skin type, play a role in its etiology. Cummulative, rather than intermittent, sun exposure is the more prominent factor in the development of BCCs. BCCs can appear in areas protected from the sun, such as behind the ear. Approximately 25% to 30% of BCCs occur on the nose.

Clinically, BCCs appear as pink or white pearly papules with areas of telangiectasia. As lesions progress, they may develop central ulceration and look as if they have been gnawed upon (i.e., the classic "rat bite" description). There are five histologic patterns of BCCs: nodular, superficial, micronodular, infiltrative, and morpheaform. Microscopically, BCCs are nests of basophilic cells originating from basal keratinocytes and hair follicles. Peripheral palisading is a hallmark histologic feature.

Risk factors include poor ability to tan, fair skin, immunosuppression, old age, and exposure to UV radiation. There are also genodermatoses associated with the development of BCCs, such as Gorlin's syndrome. Just as with SCCs, UVB radiation is thought to be more effective than UVA in photocarcinogenesis. DNA mutations involving the Sonic hedgehog pathway are thought to play a role.

BCCs grow by direct extension; therefore, the incidence of metastasis is low. Diagnosis is made only from biopsy.

**Treatment.** Treatment options include electrodessication and curettage, surgical excision, Mohs micrographic surgery, or radiation therapy for elderly patients who cannot tolerate surgical procedures. Photodynamic therapy has been used with success, especially for superficial tumors.

### Melanoma

**Presentation and Characteristics.** Melanoma demonstrates a less clear-cut relationship with sun exposure. Unlike BCCs, melanoma does not typically appear on skin that has received the most cumulative UV radiation. In fact, in individuals with skin of color, while the incidence of melanoma is low, when it occurs, palms and soles are common sites. Furthermore, melanoma has a peak incidence in younger patients, who have acquired less lifetime sun exposure than their elderly counterparts. Melanoma occurs more frequently in people who work indoors, as opposed to outdoors. One proposed

explanation for why indoor workers have a higher incidence of melanoma is that melanoma may be related to intense, intermittent sun exposure of untanned skin. This also supports the distribution pattern of melanoma seen on the trunk in men and lower extremities in women.

A helpful guideline to distinguish melanomas from benign nevi (moles) is the ABCDE rule. Melanoma tends to be *a*symmetrical, with *b*order irregularity, *c*olor variegation, and a *d*iameter greater than 6 mm. Lesions that are *e*volving must also be evaluated. This is, of course, just a clinical tool and does not help in the diagnosis of all melanomas. Moles that look different from the other moles on the patient are another clinical clue that should be considered.

There are four major clinical histopathologic subtypes:

- Superficial spreading
- Lentigo maligna
- Nodular
- Acral lentiginous

They differ with respect to the pattern of sun exposure and location. A more detailed discussion of these subtypes is beyond the scope of this chapter. Other risk factors for melanoma include the following:

- A first-degree relative with melanoma
- The presence of atypical or dysplastic nevi
- Fair skin and light eyes
- A history of severe childhood sunburns
- A history of NMSC
- Immunosuppression

One gene that has been linked to melanoma in certain families is *p16*. Its protein products code for cell cycle arrest. Mutations of *p16* would theoretically allow damaged DNA to replicate, leading to oncogenesis.

**Diagnosis.** The diagnosis of melanoma is made by biopsy. Under the microscope, melanomas appear as clusters of large and atypical melanocytes with visible mitotic figures proliferating above the epidermis. The pathology report includes the Breslow's depth (full tumor thickness) and the presence or absence of ulceration. The depth of the lesion is

---

**SAUER'S NOTES**

1. Chronic sun exposure, or repeated sunburn, is associated with the development of AKs, BCCs, and SCCs. The association of melanomas and sun exposure is less clear.
2. Treatment
   a. *Actinic keratoses:* cryotherapy, topical 5-fluorouracil, imiquimod cream, diclofenac sodium gel, photodynamic therapy.
   b. *BCCs, SCCs:* electrodessication and curettage, surgical excision, Mohs micrographic surgery, photodynamic therapy (for BCC only).
   c. *Melanomas:* wide local excision, α-interferon.

the strongest histologic factor influencing prognosis. Thus, superficial shave biopsies are not appropriate in cases of suspected melanoma because they have the potential to obscure an accurate report of tumor depth. Wide local excision is the only acceptable treatment, and surgical margins are determined by Breslow's depth and the diameter of the lesion. α-Interferon is considered for adjuvant therapy in certain cases. Melanomas, especially the deeper ones, are frequently lethal. They are responsible for 75% of skin cancer deaths.

## Photodermatoses

Although the aforementioned acute and chronic effects of UV radiation occur in exposed skin of all individuals, there are some abnormal reactions to sunlight that only manifest in the predisposed. These reactions are known as *photodermatoses*. The more commonly encountered ones (Table 39-3) are discussed below. Photoprotection is an integral part of the management of all photodermatoses.

### Immunologically Mediated Dermatoses

*Polymorphous Light Eruption*

***Presentation and Characteristics.*** Polymorphous light eruption (PMLE) is the most common photodermatosis in humans. It affects patients of all backgrounds and races and occurs more often in women than men. Its peak onset is during the third and fourth decades of life. In temperate climates, it flares during the spring and summer, after exposure to a certain threshold of UV radiation. Association with lupus erythematous and thyroid disease has been reported.

**TABLE 39-3 ■ Commonly Encountered Photodermatoses**

**Immunologically mediated photodermatoses**
Polymorphous light eruption
Chronic actinic dermatitis
Solar urticaria

**Endogenous photodermatoses**
Porphyria cutanea tarda
Erythropoietic protoporphyria

**Exogenous photodermatoses**
Phototoxicity
Photoallergy

**Photoaggravated dermatoses**
Lupus erythematosus
Dermatomyositis
Atopic dermatitis
Seborrheic dermatitis

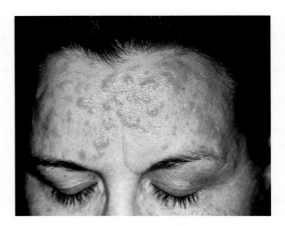

**FIGURE 39-2 ■** Polymorphous light eruption. Note erythematous papules on the forehead.

Patients are usually susceptible to broadband UVA and UVB radiation, with either able to elicit the symptoms. In most patients, however, the minimal dose of UV needed to induce redness in the skin is normal. There is recent evidence to indicate that patients with PMLE are less susceptible to UV-induced immunosuppression. Therefore, PMLE is a delayed type of hypersensitivity response to a photo-induced antigen. Clinically, PMLE presents minutes to hours after exposure to UV radiation and can persist from 1 day to weeks. Initial symptoms include mild burning and pruritus. Grouped erythematous papules appear in a symmetrical distribution on sun-exposed skin—notably, the forehead, upper chest, dorsum of hands, and forearms (**Fig. 39-2**). There are several different clinical manifestations, such as papules, plaques, nodules, and, rarely, vesicles. In individuals with skin of color, pinhead-sized papules are the most common presentation. General malaise, headache, fever, and nausea may infrequently accompany the cutaneous findings. Histologically, PMLE appears as a nonspecific, dermal, lymphocytic, perivascular infiltrate. Diagnosis is made by history and clinical findings in the context of a negative rheumatologic (lupus erythematosus, dermatomyositis) serology workup. Biopsy is not typically helpful, and phototesting is often unnecessary.

***Treatment.***

- *Desensitization:* This is attained by narrowband UVB phototherapy, two to three times per week for 15 treatments, usually done in the spring. 8-Methoxypsoralen and UVA (PUVA) therapy is also effective.
- *Antimalarials:* They have been shown to provide moderate protection during the spring and summer. Most commonly, hydroxychloroquine, 200 mg twice a day, is used.

Once the outbreak has occurred, the symptoms are best treated with topical or oral corticosteroids.

*Chronic Actinic Dermatitis*

***Description.*** Chronic actinic dermatitis is a chronic photodermatosis that occurs more commonly among older men.

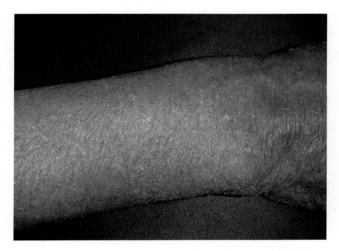

**FIGURE 39-3** ■ Chronic actinic dermatitis. Note hyperpigmentation and lichenification on the dorsum of the hand with sparing of a photoprotective area above the wrist.

It is most severe during the summer months. Clinically, it presents with lichenified papules or plaques on sun-exposed areas (**Fig. 39-3**). The lesions are usually pruritic. Histologically, there is mild epidermal spongiosis, perivascular lymphocytic infiltrate, and not infrequently, there are atypical mononuclear cells in the dermis and epidermis. Therefore, histologic changes of chronic actinic dermatitis may resemble those of cutaneous T-cell lymphoma. Diagnosis is confirmed by phototesting; there is an abnormal response to UVB and/or UVA and/or visible radiation.

***Treatment.***

- ■ *Corticosteroids and tacrolimus:* Symptom relief is accomplished with the use of topical and oral corticosteroids. Topical tacrolimus has been used with success in some patients.
- ■ *Others:* Management of refractory cases includes low-dose PUVA, mycophenolate mofetil, cyclosporine, and azathioprine.

### Solar Urticaria

***Presentation and Characteristics.*** Solar urticaria occurs slightly more often in females and is associated with atopic dermatitis in 21% to 48% of patients. Patients typically present in their 20s and 30s. The pathogenic mechanism is thought to involve mast cell degranulation in response to a yet-unidentified photosensitized allergen.

Patients present with urticaria minutes after exposure to the instigating wavelength (**Fig. 39-4**). Like all urticarias, lesions disappear within hours. The wheals may be pruritic and occasionally burn. In rare instances, patients may also experience a systemic anaphylactic reaction. Biopsy of the lesion shows mild dermal edema with a perivascular infiltrate consisting of neutrophils and eosinophils. Upon phototesting with the activating wavelengths, urticaria is induced within a few minutes after the exposure.

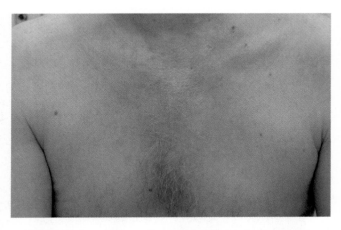

**FIGURE 39-4** ■ Solar urticaria. This patient developed urticaria on the chest within minutes of exposure to sunlight.

***Treatment.***

- ■ *Antihistamines*
- ■ *Desensitization:* This is done with incrementally increasing doses of UVA or PUVA.
- ■ *Plasmapheresis:* For refractory cases.

## Endogenous Photodermatoses: The Cutaneous Porphyrias

The porphyrias are a group of disorders caused by congenital defects of enzymes in the heme biosynthesis pathway. Plasma porphyrin determination is an excellent screening test, since it is elevated in all types of cutaneous porphyrias. This section discusses the two most common porphyrias that exhibit skin involvement most prominently.

### Porphyria Cutanea Tarda

***Presentation and Characteristics.*** Porphyria cutanea tarda (PCT) is the most common cutaneous porphyria. There are two forms: an inherited autosomal dominant form (20% of patients) and an acquired form (80% of patients). Men present with PCT slightly more commonly than women. Men with PCT are more likely to use alcohol and women are more likely to be exposed to estrogen replacement. Most patients present after their 40s, although childhood onset has been infrequently reported. There is a strong association of PCT with hepatitis C as well as with hemochromatosis. Association of PCT with HIV (human immunodeficiency virus) infection has been well reported. Therefore, HIV testing should be offered to all newly diagnosed patients with acquired PCT.

PCT is caused by a defect in hepatic uroporphyrinogen decarboxylase activity, which creates an excess of uroporphyrinogen, 7-, 6-, 5-, and 4-carboxyl porphyrinogens. All porphyrinogens are spontaneously oxidized to the corresponding porphyrins. These porphyrins are phototoxic when exposed to visible light (Soret band, 400 to 410 nm).

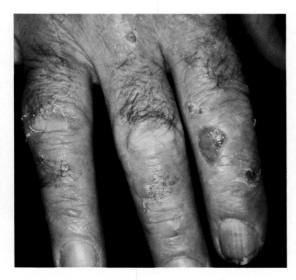

**FIGURE 39-5** ■ PCT, presenting with vesicles and postinflammatory hyperpigmentation on the dorsum of the hand.

Clinically, PCT manifests with skin fragility, blisters, erosions, crusting, and milia on sun-exposed areas (**Fig. 39-5**). Mottled hyper- and hypopigmentation and hypertrichosis on the periorbital areas are frequently observed. Scarring alopecia and sclerodermoid lesions are uncommon presentations. The latter can occur in both sun-exposed and sun-protected areas.

Histologically, a subepidermal blister with cell-poor dermal infiltrate is seen. Diagnosis is confirmed by the characteristic porphyrin profile. There are elevated levels of uroporphyrin, 7-, 6-, 5-, and 4-carboxyl porphyrins in urine and plasma and elevated isocoproporphyrin in the stool.

***Treatment.***

- *Photoprotection:* Because the action spectrum is in the visible light range, photoprotection with physical agents (nonmicronized titanium dioxide or zinc oxide, clothing, etc.) is required.
- *Phlebotomy:* This is done to decrease the iron load. It is the most effective treatment for patients. One unit of blood is usually removed weekly for 10 to 15 treatments. Alcohol, other hepatic toxins, and iron should be avoided. Interferon-$\alpha$ may be beneficial in the treatment of PCT in those patients with concomitant hepatitis C virus infection.
- *Antimalarials:* Low-dose (weekly or twice a week) chloroquine or hydroxychloroquine also produces a therapeutic response. Its mechanism of action is to form a porphyrin—antimalarial complex that can be excreted renally.

### Erythropoietic Protoporphyria

***Presentation and Characteristics.*** Unlike PCT, erythropoietic protoporphyria (EPP) presents in children, usually by age 2. It is inherited in an autosomal dominant fashion with variable penetrance. The enzyme deficient in EPP is ferrochelatase, which converts protoporphyrin into heme by insertion of iron. Elevated levels of phototoxic protoporphyrin in erythrocytes, plasma, and stool are seen in EPP. Because protoporphyrin is lipophilic, urine porphyrin level is normal in EPP.

Clinically, children with EPP usually cry or scream in pain minutes after exposure to sunlight. Sometimes this is misdiagnosed as psychoneurosis. The burning sensation lasts for hours and is followed by erythema, induration, and purpura. Vesicles are rarely seen. With repeated attacks, shallow erosions on the forehead and nasal bridge and waxy thickening of the skin of knuckles may be apparent. In rare instances, hepatic failure may occur. Histologically, thickening of the dermal–epidermal junction and blood vessel walls of superficial capillaries is observed.

***Treatment.***

- *Photoprotection:* Same as PCT, see previous section.
- *Oral $\beta$-carotene:* This is used to quench the reactive oxygen species. Lumitene, an over-the-counter preparation, at 30 to 300 mg/d, is usually recommended.
- *PUVA or narrowband UVB:* These are utilized to induce tolerance.

## Exogenous Photodermatoses

### Phototoxicity and Photoallergy

***Presentation and Characteristics.*** Exogenous agents can be categorized by whether they cause a phototoxic or photoallergic cutaneous reaction. *Phototoxic responses* occur when UV radiation activates a drug or chemical that subsequently produces tissue injury. It occurs in 100% of individuals provided they are exposed to sufficient doses of a phototoxic agent and the radiation. *Photoallergy* is a delayed-type hypersensitivity reaction, consisting of a sensitization phase on first exposure. Subsequent exposures precipitate a photoallergic response. Commonly encountered photosensitizers are listed in Table 39-4.

**TABLE 39-4** ■ **Common Exogenous Photosensitizers**

| Common Phototoxic Agents | Common Photoallergic Agents |
| --- | --- |
| Antiarrhythmics | Sunscreen filters |
| Diuretics | Fragrances |
| NSAIDs | Antibacterials |
| Phenothiazines | |
| Psoralens | |
| Quinolones | |
| Tetracyclines | |
| Thiazides | |
| Sulfonamides | |
| Sulfonylureas | |

*Abbreviation:* NSAIDs, nonsteroidal anti-inflammatory drugs

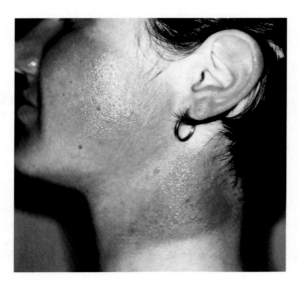

**FIGURE 39-6** ■ Phototoxicity secondary to demeclocycline.

Clinically, phototoxic eruptions consist of erythema, edema, stinging, and burning in sun-exposed areas (**Fig. 39-6**). Relatively sun-protected areas such as the submental, retroauricular areas and eyelids are usually spared. Occasionally, vesicles, bullae, and onycholysis may be observed. Symptoms resolve with hyperpigmentation over the course of days to weeks. Histologically, phototoxic reactions present with lymphocytic and neutrophilic dermal infiltrates and occasional necrotic keratinocytes.

UVA is the most common action spectrum for systemic, drug-induced phototoxicity. Exposure to furanocoumarin-producing plants causes a topical phototoxic reaction called *phytophotodermatitis*. Common plants evoking this condition include celery, parsnip, lime, and parsley.

Photoallergic reactions present with pruritus and eczematous dermatitis. Bullae and vesicles are rarely seen. The histologic changes are similar to those of contact dermatitis, namely, lymphohistiocytic dermal infiltrates and spongiosis. Currently, the most common cause of photoallergic reactions is sunscreen filters. However, it should be noted that considering the large number of individuals exposed to sunscreens, the incidence of photoallergy to sunscreen agents is very low.

Taking a careful history, paying special attention to medication and recent chemical exposures, is crucial for diagnosis. Photoallergy can be confirmed by photopatch testing.

***Treatment.*** Treatment includes avoidance of the offending agents along with appropriate photoprotection; symptomatic treatment, including topical or systemic corticosteroids, may be necessary in severe cases.

## Photoaggravated Dermatoses

Exacerbation of cutaneous lesions in lupus erythematosus following sun exposure is frequently seen, especially in subacute lupus erythematosus and in tumid lupus erythematosus. Patients with dermatomyositis also frequently complain of photosensitivity. Photoexacerbation of atopic dermatitis and, less commonly, seborrheic dermatitis has been well reported.

### Treatment

In addition to treatment of the primary disease, photoprotection is the appropriate management for these conditions.

## Suggested Readings

Frank J, Poblete-Gutierrez P. Porphyria. In: Bolognia JL, Jorizzo JL, Rapini RP, eds. *Dermatology.* London: Mosby; 2008:641–651.

Lim HW, ed. The diagnosis and treatment of photodermatitis. *Dermatol Ther.* 2003;16:1–72.

Lim HW, Hawk J. Photodermatoses. In: Bolognia JL, Jorizzo JL, Rapini RP, eds. *Dermatology.* 2nd ed. London: Mosby; 2008:1333–1351.

Moyal D, Fourtanier A. Acute and chronic effects of UV on skin: what are they and how to study them? In: Rigel DS, Weiss RA, Lim HW, et al., eds. *Photoaging.* New York: Marcel Dekker; 2004:15–33.

Wright DR, Khoo LSW, Lim HW. Acute and chronic effects of ultraviolet radiation, including photocarcinogenesis. In: Taylor S, Kelly P, eds. *Dermatology for Skin of Color.* New York: McGraw-Hill; 2009.

# CHAPTER 40

# Genodermatoses

*Amy Y. Jan, MD, PhD and Virginia P. Sybert, MD*

## Introduction

The inherited skin disorders are individually rare, but in the aggregate comprise a significant proportion of dermatologic practice. Some are of minimal medical significance; others are life threatening, life shortening, or debilitating. For some, treatment is available. For others, there is no management beyond diagnosis. For a growing number of conditions, both the causal mutations and the specific perturbations in cellular function are known.

Genetic skin disorders are unique in that the diagnosis automatically invokes the issues of recurrent risk to relatives and prenatal diagnosis. These are topics not usually in the domain of the dermatologist. Identification of a genodermatosis may require referral for medical genetics evaluation and counseling. The availability and applicability of molecular (DNA) testing changes daily. Medical genetics centers are most likely to be aware of these resources. Online resources include:

- GENE CLINICS
  http://www.geneclinics.org
  This web site includes a listing of laboratories offering molecular testing for research and/or clinical purposes and for many disorders, a review that is clinically focused with molecular information as well, along with support group information.

- OMIM
  http://www.ncbi.nlm.nih.gov/omim/
  A catalog web site of Mendelian disorders in man with references, clinical synopses, and hyperlinks to other databases.

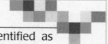

## SAUER'S NOTES

The genodermatoses need to be identified as soon as possible for three important reasons:

1. Genetic counseling can help avoid the tragic passing on of a genetic defect to future generations.
2. Prenatal diagnosis is becoming a more available option and can lead to optimal management of a genodermatosis at the earliest possible time.
3. Referral to an appropriate center for an exact diagnosis, specific recommendations, and research can be of great value.

Many common skin disorders also have a significant genetic component. The risk for psoriasis, atopic dermatitis, vitiligo, alopecia areata, or systemic lupus erythematosus is much higher among close relatives of affected individuals than for the general population. Even acne and onychomycosis enjoy genetic contribution. These disorders are discussed in Chapters 13 and 33, respectively, and will not be further addressed here. This chapter will deal with only a handful of the many inherited skin disorders.

## Disorders of Keratinization

### Ichthyoses

The ichthyoses (Table 40-1; Figs. 40-1 to 40-4) share in common a thickened stratum corneum, which results in scaly skin. The distribution and severity of scaling, the presence of erythroderma, the mode of inheritance, and associated abnormalities differ among them. The degree to which life is impaired ranges from minimal to lethal. The genetic alterations responsible for some of these conditions are known. Treatment remains general and nonspecific. Use of keratolytics ($\alpha$-hydroxy acids such as lactic acid, glycolic acid, and urea-based emollients) can be helpful. The oral retinoids are effective and should be considered in the more severe forms of ichthyoses. Their long-term use is limited by significant side effects including dryness of the mucous membranes, alterations in serum lipids, musculoskeletal pain, bony alterations, and teratogenicity.

### Palmar–Plantar Keratodermas

Palmar–plantar keratodermas (PPK) (Figs. 40-5 and 40-6) are conditions in which thickening of the stratum corneum and scaling, with or without erythroderma, are limited primarily to the palms and soles. They are distinguished, as are the more generalized ichthyoses, by mode of inheritance and associated findings. One autosomal dominant form (Howell-Evans) is associated with esophageal carcinoma. Papillon–Lefèvre is an autosomal recessive PPK caused by mutations in the cathepsin C gene and is associated with gingivitis and premature tooth loss. Unna–Thost disease or nonepidermolytic hyperkeratosis results from mutations in *KRT9* or *KRT1*. PPK with epidermolytic hyperkeratosis, Voener, can also be caused by mutations in *KRT1* and by mutations in *KRT16*.

**TABLE 40-1 ▪ Ichthyoses**

| Disorder | Inheritance | Basic Defect | Major Dermatologic Findings | Associated Features | Miscellaneous |
|---|---|---|---|---|---|
| Ichthyosis vulgaris | AD | Unknown | Mild-to-moderate white scales<br><br>Spares flexures and neck; involves face<br><br>Keratosis pilaris<br><br>Atopic dermatitis (50%) | None | Improves with age and warm weather |
| X-linked ichthyosis (sterol sulfatase deficiency) | XLR | Mutation/deletion of steroid sulfatase gene | Moderate-to-severe white-brown scale Spares face; involves neck | Corneal opacities Possible increased risk of testicular malignancy | Pregnancies with affected males have low to absent estriol levels; failure of spontaneous initiation of labor is common |
| Bullous congenital ichthyosiform erythroderma (epidermolytic hyperkeratosis) | AD | Mutations in K1 or K10 (suprabasal keratins) | Red skin with blisters and scale evident at birth<br><br>Marked hyperkeratosis<br><br>Face usually least affected<br><br>Inter- and intrafamilial variability | Secondary skin infection, bacterial and fungal common | Skin is tender; skin fragility improves with age |
| Lamellar ichthyosis/nonbullous congenital ichthyosiform erythroderma/congenital autosomal recessive ichthyosis | AR | Heterogenous. Some caused by mutations in transglutaminase 1 (*TGM1*), 12-R lipoxygenase (*ALOX12B*), lipoxygenase-3 (*ALOXE3*), ATP-binding cassette transporter 2 (*ABCA2*) | LI: mild erythroderma; brown, adherent plate-like scale<br><br>NCIE: Erythroderma; fine, white scale<br><br>Many cases with overlap in phenotype | Secondary tinea infection common | Collodion membrane common at birth<br><br>Ectropion/ecla-bium common |
| Harlequin fetus | AR | Unknown; probably heterogenous | Severe, armor plate-like hyperkeratosis In survivors, phenotype becomes similar to BCIE | Among survivors, mental retardation has been noted in a few | Rare spontaneous survival; handful of survivors treated with oral retinoids |
| Conradi Hunermann | XLD AR | XLD: mutation in gene encoding delta(8)-delta(7) sterol isomerase emopamil-binding protein<br><br>AR: mutations in *PEX7* gene | Feathery scale on erythrodermic base<br><br>Follicular atrophoderma | Seizures; MR<br><br>Chondrodysplasia punctata<br><br>Cataracts | Asymmetry typical in XLD form |

*(continued)*

**TABLE 40-1** ▪ *(continued)*

| Disorder | Inheritance | Basic Defect | Major Dermatologic Findings | Associated Features | Miscellaneous |
|---|---|---|---|---|---|
| Sjögren–Larsson syndrome | AR | Fatty aldehyde dehydrogenase deficiency | Mild-to-moderate fine, adherent scale<br><br>Pruritus | Progressive spastic paraparesis<br><br>Mild retardation<br><br>Glistening white dots on retina | |
| Netherton syndrome | AR | Mutations in *SPINK5* gene | Variable erythroderma and scale<br><br>Classic pattern of ichthyosis linearis circumflexa | Trichorrhexis invaginata (bamboo hair) | Failure to thrive<br><br>Food allergies |
| Collodion baby | AR if isolated<br><br>Otherwise, depends on underlying disorder | Heterogenous | Plastic wrap-like membrane peels within few weeks after birth, revealing underlying skin, which may range from minimally xerotic to lamellar ichthyosis | This is a feature of many disorders including lamellar ichthyosis, hypohidrotic ectodermal dysplasia, Gaucher disease and lamellar exfoliation of the newborn | |

*Abbreviations:* AD, autosomal dominant; AR, autosomal recessive; BCIE, bullous congenital ichthyosiform erythroderma; XLR, X-linked recessive; K, keratin; MR, mental retardation.

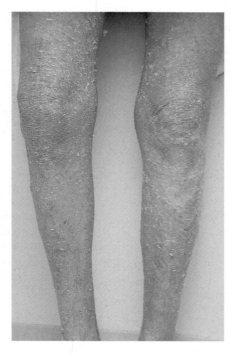

**FIGURE 40-1** ▪ X-linked ichthyosis. *(Reprinted from Sybert VP. Genetic Skin Disorders. New York: Oxford University Press; 1997.)*

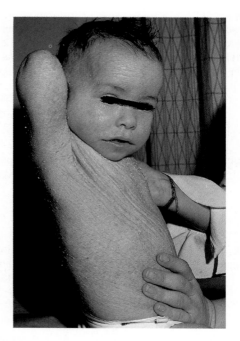

**FIGURE 40-2** ▪ A young girl with nonbullous congenital ichthyosiform erythroderma. *(Reprinted from Sybert VP. Genetic Skin Disorders. New York: Oxford University Press; 1997.)*

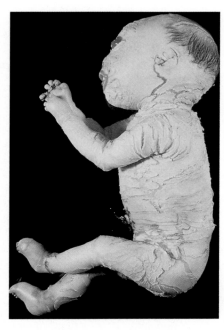

**FIGURE 40-3** ■ A newborn with Harlequin ichthyosis. *(Reprinted from Sybert VP. Genetic Skin Disorders. New York: Oxford University Press; 1997.)*

## Disorders of Adhesion

The epidermolysis bullosa syndromes (Table 40-2; Figs. 40-7 to 40-9) are mechanobullous disorders that share in common fragility of the skin. They are distinguished, one from the next, by the histologic level of blister formation, mode of inheritance, and associated cutaneous features. Most present at birth or soon thereafter. Scarring is primarily limited to the dystrophic forms, where the separation of the skin occurs below the basement membrane of the dermis. Extensive involvement in the newborn period can occur in epidermolysis bullosa simplex Dowling–Meara (EBS-DM), recessive epidermolysis bullosa dystrophica

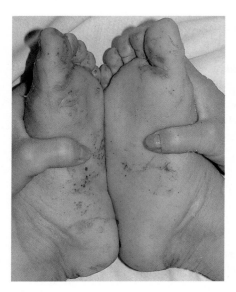

**FIGURE 40-5** ■ Palmar–plantar hyperkeratosis. The hands and soles are thickened, with erythroderma evident at the margins. A young girl shares the same condition as her father. *(Reprinted from Sybert VP. Genetic Skin Disorders. New York: Oxford University Press; 1997.)*

(REBD), and in junctional epidermolysis bullosa (JEB). Neonatal or infant death due to sepsis or intestinal protein loss and inanition is common in the most severe forms. Respiratory mucosa is often involved in the Herlitz form of JEB. Accurate diagnosis requires electron microscopy and/or immunofluorescence studies. Treatment consists of protection of skin surfaces and avoidance of trauma, lancing of small blisters to prevent lateral spread by the pressure of blister fluid, topical antibiotics, and nonadherent dressings. More severe forms may require a team approach to management of complications.

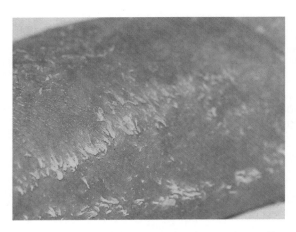

**FIGURE 40-4** ■ The feathery scale of X-LD Conradi Hunermann disease. *(Reprinted from Sybert VP. Genetic Skin Disorders. New York: Oxford University Press; 1997.)*

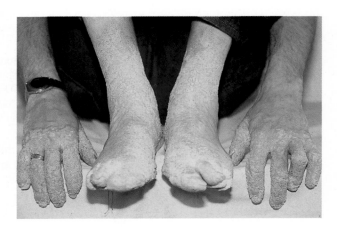

**FIGURE 40-6** ■ Palmar–plantar hyperkeratosis with severe palm/sole involvement and extension onto the wrists and shins. Some of these patients have involvement of the elbows, knees, and gluteal cleft. *(Reprinted from Sybert VP. Genetic Skin Disorders. New York: Oxford University Press; 1997.)*

**TABLE 40-2 ■ Epidermolysis Bullosa**

| Disorder | Mode of Inheritance | Basic Defect Mutations In | Major Dermatologic Findings | Associated Features | Electron Microscopy |
|---|---|---|---|---|---|
| EBS-WC (Weber–Cockayne) (localized) | AD | Basal keratins (*KRT 5*) (*KRT 14*) | Blisters primarily limited to hands and feet. Onset can be at birth but usually thereafter. Occasionally delayed until adolescence. Palmar–plantar hyperkeratosis may occur | None | Level of split within basal keratinocyte |
| EBS-K (Koebner) (generalized) | AD | Basal keratins (*KRT 5*) (*KRT 14*) | Blisters soon after birth, generalized. May have oral involvement/nail involvement | None | Level of split within basal keratinocyte |
| EBS-DM (Dowling–Meara) (herpetiform) | AD | Basal keratins (*KRT 5*) (*KRT 14*) | Marked blistering at birth. With time clustering of small blisters in rosettes may occur. Oral involvement common. Nails often dystrophic. Progressive palmar–plantar hyperkeratosis common. Dyspigmentation common | Can result in neonatal/ infant death. Blistering tends to diminish with age | Clumping of tonofilaments within basal cells with cytolysis |
| EBS with muscular dystrophy | AR/AD | Plectin (*PLEC1*) | Relatively severe simplex disease, may be mistaken for junctional EB | Muscular dystrophy of various types has been described | Split at hemidesmosomal attachment plate |
| EBS with mottled hyperpig- mentation | AD | Basal keratin (*KRT 5*) | Blisters similar to EBS-K. Development of hyper/hypopigmented spots | None | Level of split within basal keratinocyte |
| JEB-Herlitz (gravis) (letalis) | AR | Various components of laminin (*LAMA3*) (*LAMC2*) (*LAMB3*) | Widespread severe. GI, respiratory, and GU mucosa often involved. Usually lethal | | Level of split within lamina lucida, decrease/absence of hemidesmosomes |
| JEB-miti (GABEB) | AR | Type 17 collagen; Laminin (*BPAG2/ COL17A1*) (*LAMB3*) | More mild, gradual atopic appearance of healed skin | None | Similar to JEB-H. May have relatively more hemidesm- osomes |
| JEB with PA | AR | Integrins (*ITGB4*) (*ITGB6*) | Similar to JEB-L, usually lethal | Pyloric atresia, intestinal malabsorption | Same as JEB-H |

*(continued)*

**TABLE 40-2** ■ *(continued)*

| Disorder | Mode of Inheritance | Basic Defect Mutations In | Major Dermatologic Findings | Associated Features | Electron Microscopy |
|---|---|---|---|---|---|
| EBD-CT (Cockayne–Touraine) | AD | Type 7 collagen (*COL7A1*) | Blistering and scarring limited and localized to areas of greatest trauma. Mild oral involvement. Milia | None | Split below basement membrane Decrease in anchoring fibrils |
| EBD-HS (Hallopeau–Siemens) | AR | Type 7 collagen (*COL7A1*) | Widespread, severe blistering, progressive scarring. Pseudo-amputation of digits. Development of cutaneous malignancy common in adult life. Oral mucosa involved. Milia | FTT. Anemia, GI involvement is progressive | Same as EBD-CT. Absence of anchoring fibrils |

## Disorders of Pigmentation

There are many molecules that contribute to skin color. This discussion is limited to alterations in melanin, the major contributor to color in the skin. Perturbations in pigment production can be due to alterations or defects anywhere along the pathway from the differentiation and migration of neural crest derivatives, through the enzymatic production of melanin, to the packaging and transport of melanosomes.

### Hypopigmentation

Waardenburg syndromes I through III and piebaldism (**Fig. 40-10**) share in common white patches of skin, a white forelock, premature graying of the hair, and autosomal dominant inheritance. All are due to a failure of migration and invasion of melanocytes into the epidermis, resulting in lack of melanocytes in the depigmented areas. Individuals with Waardenburg syndrome may also have deafness and heterochromia irides. Those with Waardenburg syndromes I, III, and rarely IV, have dystrophia canthorum. Waardenburg III is associated with limb abnormalities. Hirschsprung disease occurs in Waardenburg syndrome type IV and rarely in piebaldism. Waardenburg I and III are due to mutations in PAX3. Mutations in MITF, SNAI2, or SOX 10 have been found in some cases of Waardenburg II, while mutations in EDNRB, EDN3, or SOX 10 have been identified in Waardenburg IV, confirming genetic heterogeneity within this group. Piebaldism, which is caused by mutations in the C-kit protooncogene, is usually characterized only by skin changes, although deafness has been reported in some patients.

The oculocutaneous albinisms (OCAs) are a group of autosomal recessive disorders that are distinguished from each other by the degree of pigment production. Affected individuals have pink skin, transillumination of the irises, white to light yellow hair, and often visual disturbances, foveal hypoplasia, and nystagmus. Many mutations in the

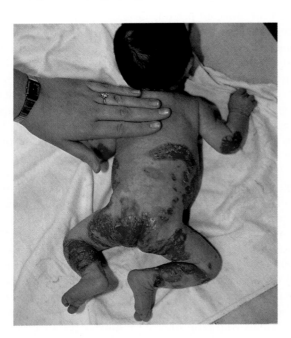

**FIGURE 40-7** ■ A newborn with junctional epidermolysis bullosa-Herlitz.

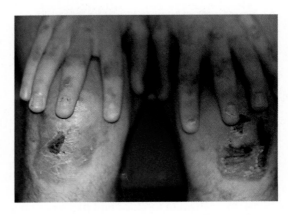

**FIGURE 40-8** ■ Scarring in a patient with DEBD.

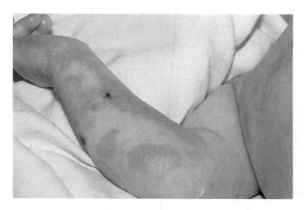

**FIGURE 40-9** ■ Extensive superficial blistering in a patient with EBS-Dowling–Meara.

tyrosinase gene have been identified in both OCA1A (the most severe form classically known as "tyrosinase-negative" with complete lack of tyrosinase activity) and OCA1B (with partial tyrosinase activity) forms of OCA, and many affected individuals are compound heterozygotes for mutations at this locus. In addition, mutations in other genes account for milder forms of OCA: *OCA2* on chromosome 15 in OCA2; *TYRP1* on chromosome 9 in OCA3; and *MATP* gene on chromosome 5 in OCA4.

Tuberous sclerosis is an autosomal dominant disorder that results from mutations in genes at one of at least two loci: one on chromosome 9 (*TSC1*-hamartin) and the other on chromosome 16 (*TSC2*-tuberin). It is characterized by a number of cutaneous changes including angiofibromas, connective tissue nevi (shagreen patches), periungual fibromas, and hypopigmented macules (ash-leaf spots) (**Fig. 40-11**). Melanocytes and keratinocytes in these light-colored areas contain "effete" or poorly melanized small melanosomes. Angiofibromas, shagreen patches or connective tissue nevi, and periungual fibromas are other skin manifestations of the condition. Mental

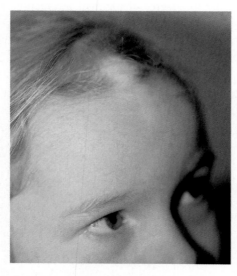

**FIGURE 40-10** ■ A white forelock and patch of unpigmented skin in young girl with piebaldism.

retardation, seizures, and renal and pulmonary involvement are the other major features of this condition that has very variable expression.

Hypomelanosis of Ito is the term given to the presence of hypopigmentation or hyperpigmentation distributed along the lines of Blaschko (**Fig. 40-12**). The biologic basis for this phenomenon is not understood. Individuals with these skin changes often have structural malformations and mental retardation. Almost two thirds of patients with this pattern of pigment disturbance and any other malformation or mental retardation are mosaic for detectable chromosomal aneuploidy. Mosaicism for X chromosome alterations, tetrasomy 12p, triploidy, trisomy 18, and chimerism are the more common abnormalities reported. It appears that it is the presence of two chromosomally distinct lines, rather than specific cytogenetic alterations that confers this striking pigment anomaly.

Individuals with hypopigmentation due to any cause need to be protected from excessive sun exposure.

## Hyperpigmentation

Neurofibromatosis type I (**Fig. 40-13**) is a relatively common (1/3000) autosomal dominant disorder caused by mutations in the *NF1* (neurofibromin) gene that resides on chromosome 17.

It is a disorder of neural crest cells, including the melanocyte. Affected individuals manifest pigment abnormalities including café-au-lait spots (brown macules and patches), usually numbering more than five and larger than 5 mm in children, 1.5 cm in adults; axillary, inguinal, and inframammary freckling (Crowe's sign) and a general increase in skin color (hypermelanosis). Pigment in these areas is packaged in giant melanosomes—a feature also common in café-au-lait spots not associated with neurofibromatosis. Over time, affected persons develop benign tumors, neurofibromas, which arise from Schwann cells and can occur along any myelinated nerve. These may be few or number in the hundreds. Severe complications include: plexiform neurofibromas—which are large disfiguring growths, pseudoarthrosis, mental deficiency (5% to 10%), sarcomatous degeneration of benign growths (malignant peripheral nerve sheath tumors), optic glioma, and leukemia (less than 1%). This is a condition which is extremely variable in its expression both within and among families.

The clinical features of McCune Albright syndrome (**Fig. 40-14**) are giant café-au-lait spots, polyostotic fibrous dysplasia, and endocrine abnormalities, primarily precocious puberty. It results from a postzygotic mutation in the *GNAS1* gene. Affected individuals are mosaic for this otherwise lethal dominant mutation. The severity and location of clinical features depends upon the proportion of normal to abnormal cells that are present. It is believed to be lethal in the fully heterozygous state; it is only tolerated by the organism if it is not present in all cells. Affected individuals who reproduce have no risk for affecting offspring, as embryos with the abnormal gene present in all cells cannot develop.

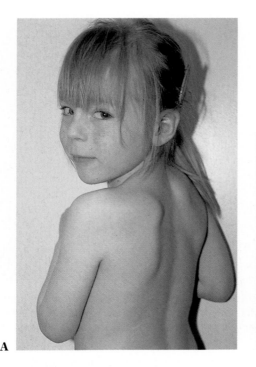

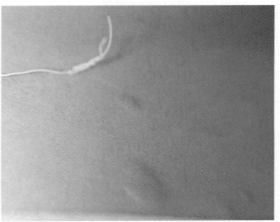

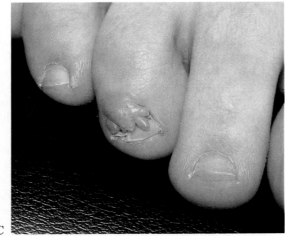

**FIGURE 40-11** ■ **(A)** A young girl with tuberous sclerosis; hypopigmented macules; angiofibromas on the cheeks. **(B)** Shagreen patches (collagenoma). **(C)** Periungual fibroma. *(B&C Reprinted from Sybert VP. Genetic Skin Disorders. New York: Oxford University Press; 1997.)*

Incontinentia pigmenti (IP) (Fig. 40-15) is an X-linked dominant condition caused by mutations in the *NEMO* gene affecting females almost exclusively. It is usually lethal prenatally in affected males. Newborns present with blistering distributed along the lines of Blaschko (see Dictionary/Index). Over weeks to months, these areas become hyperkeratotic and warty in appearance. This gradually subsides and hyperpigmentation develops, also along the lines of Blaschko, but not necessarily in or limited to the areas of blistering. This hyperpigmentation persists throughout childhood, but may fade to hypopigmented hairless skin in adult life. The severity of associated problems varies. These include central nervous system (CNS) abnormalities including seizures and mental retardation, retinal vascular dysplasia and visual defects, alopecia, hypodontia and peg-shaped teeth, nail

dysplasia, and skeletal abnormalities. Males with IP are usually mosaic due to postzygotic mutation or have Klinefelter syndrome (47, XXY) so that the presence of the additional X chromosome with a normal *NEMO* gene "rescues" them from the usual lethality in males. Mutations in a different region of the same gene give rise to an X-linked recessive condition in which affected males have a phenotype similar to hypohidrotic ectodermal dysplasia, coupled with immune defects.

## Disorders of Elasticity

Ehlers-Danlos syndrome (EDS) is the eponym given to a group of conditions, some of which share little in common. Recently, efforts have been made to limit application of this

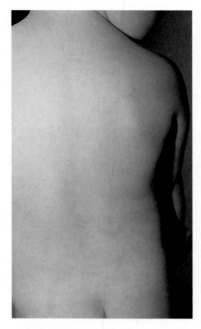

**FIGURE 40-12** ■ Streaky pigment variegation, along the lines of Blaschko in a patient with mosaicism for 46,XX/47,XX + rea (12).

eponym to those conditions in which fragility, thinness, and/or hyperelasticity of the skin is a primary finding.

The classical type of EDS is characterized by soft, velvety hyperextensible skin that is fragile, tears easily, and heals poorly with thin cigarette paper scars. There is easy bruising. Over time, elastosis perforans serpiginosa can become a significant management problem. Patients have marked ligament laxity. In some families, mutations in type 5 collagen (*COL5A1* or *COL5A2*) or type 1 collagen (*COL1A1*) have been identified. Individuals with the hypermobility type of

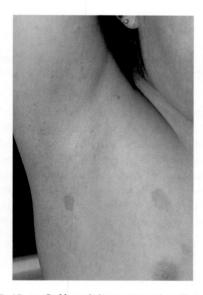

**FIGURE 40-13** ■ Café-au-lait spots and axillary freckling in neurofibromatosis. *(Reprinted from Sybert VP. Genetic Skin Disorders. New York: Oxford University Press; 1997.)*

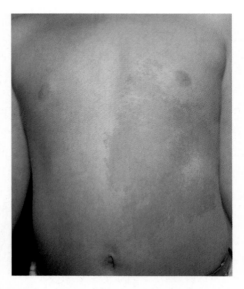

**FIGURE 40-14** ■ Giant café-au-lait in a patient with McCune–Albright syndrome. *(Reprinted from Sybert VP. Genetic Skin Disorders. New York: Oxford University Press; 1997.)*

EDS have essentially normal skin, but marked hyperextensibility of large and small joints. Electron microscopy of the skin shows abnormal collagen bundles in these conditions. The vascular type of EDS is autosomal dominant, as are the classical and hypermobility types. The skin in the vascular type of EDS is thin and taut, rather than velvety and soft. This is a disorder of type III collagen (*COL3A1*) that is distributed in the lining of vessels and viscera. Rupture of these is the major medical complication and death is common before age 50.

Cutis laxa is heterogeneous group of autosomal recessive and X-linked recessive conditions, which share laxity, not elasticity, of the skin. The skin is soft and progressively loses tone. Affected individuals have a prematurely aged "hound dog" appearance to the face. X-linked cutis laxa, also referred to as occipital horn syndrome, is caused by a defect in the *ATP7A* gene, whose product transports copper. These mutations result in secondary deficiency of copper-dependent enzymes. Internal involvement includes progressive hydronephrosis and bladder diverticula, emphysema and pulmonary blebs, and hernias. Intellect ranges from mild mental retardation to normal. Allelic mutations in *ATP7A* also cause Menkes syndrome, which is a much more severe disorder. Skin of affected males is thin, pale, with a prominent venus pattern. The hairs are fine, sparse, and fragile and demonstrate pili torti (twisting). Neurologic involvement is usually severe and progressive. Prenatal diagnosis is available for both X-linked cutis laxa and Menkes syndrome. Daily use of a dietary copper histamine supplementation when instituted shortly after birth may have some benefit in slowing progression of neurologic symptoms.

In pseudoxanthoma elasticum (PXE), there is progressive deterioration of elastic fibers in the dermis, choroid of the eye, and blood vessels. The skin becomes progressively

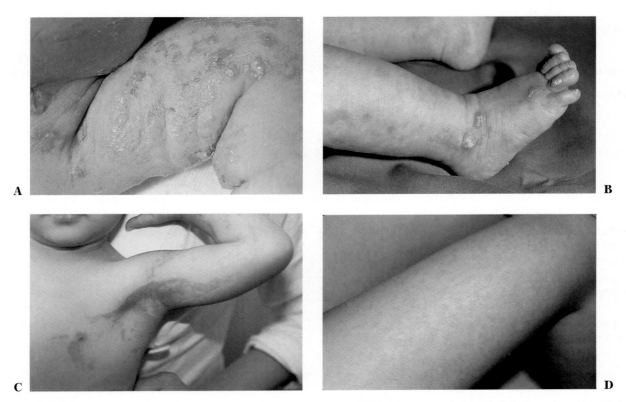

**FIGURE 40-15** ■ **(A–D)** Stages I to IV of incontinentia pigmenti. *(Reprinted from Sybert VP. Genetic Skin Disorders. New York: Oxford University Press; 1997.)*

involved by cobblestoned, yellowish plaques, especially at the nape and in the folds. These are clinically similar to solar elastosis. Progressive atherosclerotic disease, presumably due to calcified plaques developing on abnormal vessel walls, results in claudication, gastrointestinal (GI) bleeding, and stroke. Breaks in Bruch's membrane of the eye are seen as angioid streaks upon eye examination. This is a feature typical of the disorder. The changes in PXE are progressive. Making the diagnosis is unusual in childhood unless there is a positive family history and a high index of suspicion. Homozygosity or compound heterozygosity for mutations in the *ABCC6* gene underlie this autosomal recessive condition. Pedigrees with apparent autosomal dominant inheritance of PXE appear to be the result of pseudodominance.

## Disorders of Appendages

### Hair

Inherited defects in hair can affect the development of follicles, hair growth, and hair structure. Congenital alopecias are rare. They may be isolated or associated with other organ involvement. Most are autosomal recessive. A disorder of hair growth in early childhood is the loose anagen syndrome—a condition in which the anagen roots are structurally abnormal, the hairs are poorly anchored and easily plucked, and the growth period is reduced. Affected children have thin, short hair which "never needs to be cut." It tends to improve with time and by adult life hair may appear normal although

still relatively loosely anchored. Inheritance is uncertain. Structural hair shaft abnormalities are listed in Table 40-3.

### Nails

Isolated inherited disorders of nails are rare and most abnormalities are usually part of syndromes. Pachonychia congenita (P-C) (Fig. 40-16A) is a term used for two autosomal dominant conditions: type 1–Jadassohn–Lewandowsky and type 2—Jackson–Lawler. In P-C, the nail plates are thickened or may be small or absent. Nail changes may appear within the first few years of life or not until later. Not all nails are necessarily involved. Other physical findings include palmar–plantar hyperkeratosis, leukokeratosis of the oral mucosa (more common in P-C1), and follicular keratosis at the elbows and knees. Epidermal cysts, steatocystoma multiplex, and natal teeth are more typical of P-C 2. Mutations in keratins, keratins 6A and 16 in P-C 1 and keratins 6B and 17 in P-C 2, have been found.

Nail-patella syndrome (see Fig. 40-16B) is an autosomal dominant disorder marked by variable nail dystrophy with usually symmetric involvement. Skeletal abnormalities are also a feature and include hypoplasia to absence of the patellae, malformations of the elbows and scapulae, and iliac horns. Renal involvement ranges from glomerulonephritis to severe renal failure and occurs in up to a third of affected individuals. The causal gene, *LMX1B* (LIM-homeodomain protein), is linked to the ABO blood group on the long arm of chromosome 9.

**TABLE 40-3 ■ Hair Disorders**

| Name | Inheritance | Basic Defect | Microscopic Features | Associated Abnormalities |
|---|---|---|---|---|
| Monilethrix | AD | Mutations in type II hair keratins: hHb6 hHb1 | Beaded hairs; regular or irregular narrowing and widening of hair shaft | None |
| Pili annulati | AD | Unknown. Bands are due to air-filled cavities in cortex | Ringed hair; alternating bands of light and dark | None |
| Pili torti | XLR AD | Mutations in MNK1 (ATP7A) Unknown | Twisting along longitudinal axis of hair shaft | Menkes syndrome None |
| Pili trianguli et canaliculi (uncombable; spangled hair) | AD | Unknown | Grooved, triangular hair | None |
| Trichorrhexis invaginata | AR | Unknown | Nodal swelling of hair shaft; similar to bamboo | Netherton syndrome |
| Trichorrhexis nodosa | AD | Unknown | Fraying of medulla due to abnormal cuticle. Appearance of opposing broom heads | Argininosuccinic aciduria |
|  | AR Acquired | Unknown Argininosuccinate lyase deficiency |  | Trauma can be seen in any fragile hair |
| Trichothiodystrophy | AR | Decrease in disulfide bonds. Decrease in cysteine in hair | Thin fragile hairs with birefringent regions in polarized microscopy | Heterogeneous— may be associated with any of: Ichthyosis |
|  |  | Mutations in ERCC2/XPD and ERCC3/XPB in some with PIBIDS |  | Mental retardation Failure to thrive Short stature Infertility or maybe isolated |

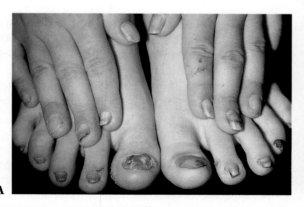 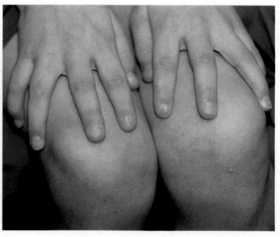

**FIGURE 40-16 ■ (A)** Nails in pachyonychia congenita. **(B)** Nails in nail-patella syndrome. *(Reprinted from Sybert VP. Genetic Skin Disorders. New York: Oxford University Press; 1997.)*

**TABLE 40-4 ■ Disorders Associated with Malignancy**

| Disorder | Mode of Inheritance | Gene | Major Dermatologic Findings | Associated Features | Typical Malignancy |
|---|---|---|---|---|---|
| Ataxia telangiectasia | AR | ATM | Progressive telangiectases on skin conjunctiva. Premature graying of the hair | Ataxia CNS degeneration Immunodeficiency | Lymphoreticular |
| Basal cell nevus syndrome | AD | PTCH | Basal cell nevi Palmar–plantar pits Epidermal cysts | Many, including odontogenic keratocysts and skeletal abnormalities | Basal cell carcinoma Medulloblastoma Ovary |
| Bloom syndrome | AR | BLM | Malar telangiectases | Immunodeficiency Growth failure Infertility in males | Many different organs |
| Cowden syndrome | AD | PTEN | Tricholemmomas Acral keratoses Palmar–plantar keratoses Oral papillomas | Thyroid abnormalities Fibrocystic breast disease GI polyps | Breast Ovary Thyroid |
| Dyskeratosis congenita | XLR AD ?AR | DKC1 TERC Unknown | Progressive reticular hyperpigmentation Nail dystrophy Oral leukoplakia | Bone marrow failure | Squamous cell cancer |
| Fanconi syndrome | AR | FACA FACC | Café-au-lait spots Patchy hyperpigmentation Sweet's syndrome | Bone marrow failure Radial ray defects Short stature | Hematopoietic Hepatocellular |
| Gardner syndrome | AD | APC | Epidermal inclusion cysts Fibromas Desmoid tumors | Intestinal polyps Mandibular osteomas | GI malignancies |
| MEN 2A/2B | AD | RET | Mucosal neuromas | Marfanoid habitus Ganglioneuromas of GI tract Pheochromocytoma | Thyroid |
| Peutz-Jeghers | AD | STK11 | Lentigines on lips, mucosa palms, soles, fingertips | GI polyposis | GI malignancy Ovary Testicle Uterus Pancreas |
| Rothmund-Thomson syndrome | AR | RECQL4 in some cases | Facial telangiectases Poikiloderma Alopecia | Short stature Radial ray defects Hypogonadism Cataracts | Squamous cell cancer |
| Xeroderma pigmentosa (many complementation groups) | AR | ERCC 2 ERCC3 ERCC5 XPCC XPAC | Progressive dyspigmentation Telangiectases Atrophy Progressive acinic changes | Neurologic involvement in XPA, XPC, XPD | Squamous cell cancer Basal cell cancer Malignant melanoma |

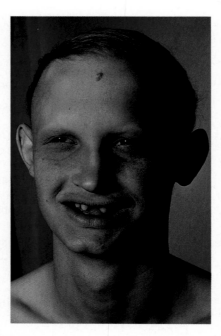

**FIGURE 40-17** ▪ A male with sparse hair; peg-shaped teeth, hypodontia, and the typical facies of hypohidrotic ectodermal dysplasia. *(Reprinted from Sybert VP. Genetic Skin Disorders. New York: Oxford University Press; 1997.)*

## Ectodermal Dysplasias

There are over 100 genetic conditions whose major findings involve alterations in two or more of the primary ectodermal derivatives—hair, teeth, sweat glands, and nails. Historically, the ectodermal dysplasias have been divided into those with relatively normal sweating—hidrotic and those with heat intolerance, hypohidrotic, or anhidrotic. The most common of the ectodermal dysplasias is X-linked recessive hypohidrotic ectodermal dysplasia (Christ–Siemens–Touraine syndrome), which is caused by mutation in the gene encoding ectodysplasin A *(EDA1)* (Fig. 40-17). Affected males may present with a collodion membrane at birth, have heat intolerance because of inability to sweat, hypodontia and peg-shaped teeth, and sparse hair. Female carriers may have patchy hair loss, patchy distribution of sweat glands, with minimal to significant tooth involvement.

## Hamartomas/Malignancies

A number of genetic skin conditions are marked by development of cutaneous and extracutaneous malignancy. Table 40-4 lists some of these.

## Suggested Readings

Beighton P, Paepe AD, Steinmann B, et al. Ehlers–Danlos syndromes: revised nosology, Villefranche, 1997. *Am J Med Genet.* 1998;77:31–37.

Byers PH. Disorders of collagen biosynthesis and structure. In: Scriver CR, Beaudet AL, Sly WS, et al., eds. *The Metabolic and Molecular Bases of Inherited Disease.* 8th ed. New York: McGraw-Hill; 2001:chap 205.

Callewaert B, Malfait F, Loeys B, et al. Ehlers–Danlos syndromes and Marfan syndrome. *Best Pract Res Clin Rheumatol.* 2008;22(1):165–189.

Chassaing N, Martin L, Calvas P, et al. Pseudoxanthoma elasticum: a clinical, pathophysiological and genetic update including 11 novel ABCC6 mutations. *J Med Genet.* 2006;42(12):881–192.

Ehrenreich M, Tarlow MM, Godlewska-Janusz E, et al. Incontinentia pigmenti (Bloch-Sulzberger syndrome): a systemic disorder. *Cutis.* 2007; 79(5):355–362.

Freire-Maia N, Pinheiro M. *Ectodermal Dysplasias: A Clinical and Genetic Study.* New York: Alan R. Liss; 1984.

Gronskov K, Ek J, Brondum-Nielsen K. Oculocutaneous albinism. *Orphanet J Rare Dis.* 2007;2:43. Available at http://www.OJRD.com/content/2/1/43.

Hu X, Plomp AS, van Soest S, et al. Pseudoxanthoma elasticum: a clinical, histopathological, and molecular update. *Surv Ophthalmol.* 2003;48: 424–438.

Juhlin L, Baran R. Hereditary and congenital nail disorders. In: Baran R, Dawber RPR, de Berker DAR, et al., eds. *Diseases of the Nails and Their Management.* 3rd ed. Oxford: Blackwell; 2001.

King RA, Hearing VJ, Creel DJ, et al. Albinism. In: Scriver CR, Beaudet AL, Valle ED, et al., eds. *The Metabolic and Molecular Bases of Inherited Disease.* 8th ed. New York: McGraw-Hill; 2001:chap 220.

Lamartine J. Towards a new classification of ectodermal dysplasias. *Clin Exp Dermatol.* 2003;28(4):351–355.

Neldner KH. Pseudoxanthoma elasticum. *Clin Dermatol.* 1988;6:1–159.

Oji V, Traupe H. Ichthyoses: differential diagnosis and molecular genetics. *Eur J Dermatol.* 2006;16(4):349–359.

Passeron T, Mantoux F, Ortonne J-P. Genetic disorders of pigmentation. *Clin Dermatol.* 2005;23(1):56–67.

Somoano B, Tsao H. Genodermatoses with cutaneous tumors and internal malignancies. *Dermatol Clin.* 2008;26(1):69–87, viii.

Sprecher E. Genetic hair and nail disorders. *Clin Dermatol.* 2005;23(1):47–55.

Steinmann B, Royce PM, Superti-Furga A. The Ehlers-Danlos syndrome. In: Royce PM, Steinmann B, eds. *Connective Tissue and Its Heritable Disorders.* New York: Wiley-Liss; 1992:351-407.

Stratigos AJ, Baden HP. Unraveling the molecular mechanisms of hair and nail genodermatoses. *Arch Dermatol.* 2001;137(11):1465–1471.

Sybert VP. Hypomelanosis of Ito: a description, not a diagnosis. *J Invest Dermatol.* 1994;103:1415–1435.

Sybert VP. *Genetic Skin Disorders.* New York: Oxford University Press; 1997.

Uitto J, Richard G. Progress in epidermolysis bullosa: from eponyms to molecular genetic classification. *Clin Dermatol.* 2005;23(1):33–40.

# CHAPTER 41

# Pediatric Dermatology

*Kimberly A. Horii, MD and Vidya Sharma, MBBS, MPH*

Skin disorders in infants and children may be different from the same diseases in older children or adults (**Figs. 41-1 and 41-2**). Certain skin conditions such as diaper dermatitis are typically seen only in infants; other conditions such as atopic dermatitis may appear different in children when compared with adults. Pediatric dermatology can be divided into neonatal dermatoses and dermatoses of infants and children. It is useful to describe a lesion by its morphology to develop a differential diagnosis of what the disorder might be.

## Neonatal Dermatoses (Birth to 1 Month)

A few lesions may be noted at birth or shortly thereafter (**Table 41-1**). In the newborn period, an infectious etiology for a skin eruption needs to be ruled out because some neonatal infections can be life threatening.

### Blistering (Vesiculobullous) Lesions

Blistering lesions can be mechanically induced or caused by infections.

- *Sucking blisters:* Usually seen as oval bullae on the hand or forearm thought to be caused by sucking in utero. They resolve rapidly.
- *Epidermolysis bullosa* (**Fig. 41-3**): A group of inherited disorders with fragile skin and bullous lesions that develop spontaneously or as a result of trauma.
- *Infections* (**Fig. 41-4**): Herpes simplex, congenital varicella, candidiasis, and congenital syphilis can present as blisters in the newborn. Herpes simplex is important to recognize because disseminated neonatal herpes infection can be fatal.

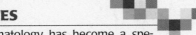

### SAUER'S NOTES

1. Pediatric dermatology has become a specialty unto itself.
2. Clinical appearances represent a different differential diagnosis than in adults.
3. Dermatopathology patterns have different meanings than in adults.
4. Numerous dermatology entities are specific for the pediatric age group.

### Pustular Lesions

Some pustular dermatoses are self-limited and require no treatment; others may be a result of an infection requiring therapy.

- *Candidiasis* (**Fig. 41-4**): Aside from blisters, candidiasis may also present with erythematous papules and pustules.
- *Erythema toxicum:* A common, benign, and self-limited condition of the newborn usually noted during the first few days of life. Erythematous macules, papules, and pustules may occur anywhere on the body.
- *Transient neonatal pustular melanosis* (**Fig. 41-5**): A benign, self-limited disorder characterized by sterile pustules that rupture and evolve into hyperpigmented macules.
- *Neonatal acne:* Papules and pustules develop at 2 to 4 weeks of age. It is self-limited and usually does not scar. Topical erythromycin or benzoyl peroxide may be helpful. Neonatal cephalic pustulosis is considered synonymous by some authors, and response to topical ketoconazole has been reported. The role of yeast is yet to be determined.
- *Milia:* Occurs commonly on the cheeks, nose, chin, and forehead. It presents as 1- to 2-mm white or yellow papules, which are frequently grouped. The lesions resolve without therapy.

### Birthmarks

Newborns may have many different types of birthmarks that can be categorized by color.

#### *White*

- *Albinism:* An uncommon inherited disorder with lack of pigment in the skin, hair, and eyes. A partial lack of pigmentation is termed *piebaldism* or *partial albinism.*
- *Ash leaf macules:* Lance-shaped hypopigmented macules on the trunk, arms, or legs, usually associated with tuberous sclerosis.
- *Nevus anemicus:* A solitary hypopigmented macule resulting from a localized vascular reaction. The surrounding borders classically blanch with pressure.

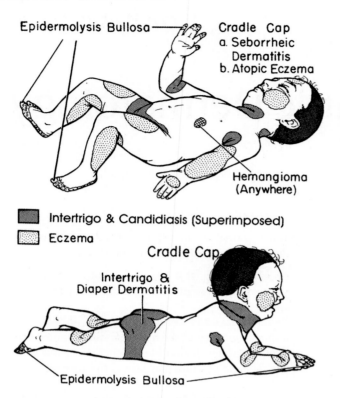

**FIGURE 41-1** ■ Pediatric dermograms (infancy).

■ *Nevus depigmentosus:* A unilateral hypopigmented patch with poorly defined borders.

*Brown*

■ *Café-au-lait spots* (**Fig. 41-6**): Light brown round or oval macules. These can be normal findings, but may be seen in association with neurofibromatosis type I. This condition should be suspected if six or more café-au-lait spots greater than 0.5 cm in diameter are present in association with other clinical findings.

■ *Congenital melanocytic nevus* (**Fig. 41-7**): A tan to dark brown well-circumscribed papule or plaque. Nevi vary in size from small to large, and often have associated hypertrichosis. Congenital nevi have the potential of developing into a melanoma depending on their size (especially >20 cm), location, border (irregular), color (especially black and multicolored), and texture (nodules).

■ *Dermal melanosis (Mongolian spots)* (**Fig. 41-8**): Deep brown, slate gray, or blue-black macules found mostly over the lumbosacral area and buttocks in darker pigmented infants. These are benign and self-limited.

■ *Epidermal nevus* (**Fig. 41-9**): Tan to brown verrucous linear lesions noted at birth. They may rarely have other associated neurologic or skeletal abnormalities.

*Vascular*

■ *Nevus simplex (Salmon patch)* (**Fig. 41-10**): Dull pink macules on the glabella, upper eyelids, nasolabial regions (also referred to as angel kisses), or nape of the neck (also referred to as a *stork bite or devil's bite*). Angel kisses usually fade when present on the face, but stork bites do not.

■ *Port-wine stain (capillary malformation)* (**Fig. 41-11**): A congenital vascular malformation composed of dilated capillaries. These are reddish purple macules or patches that do not involute. Laser therapy is a treatment option. Neurologic and ophthalmologic abnormalities (Sturge–Weber syndrome) may accompany a port-wine stain located on the face above the palpebral fissure.

■ *Hemangioma of infancy* (**Fig. 41-12**): Benign tumors of infancy composed of proliferating vascular endothelium. They grow rapidly in infancy, stabilize, and involute in childhood, most resolving by 10 years of age. They may be superficial, deep, or mixed. A new classification system separates hemangiomas based upon their configuration. Localized hemangiomas are symmetric and confined to a limited space. Segmental hemangiomas are large and appear to follow a geographic territory of the body (**Fig. 41-13**). Segmental hemangiomas can be associated with underlying anomalies and have been

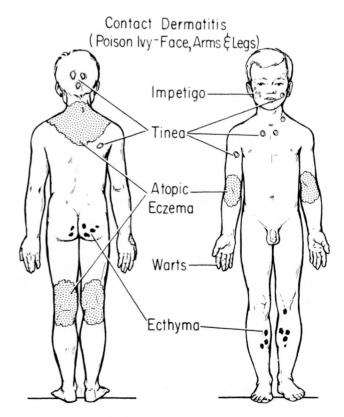

**FIGURE 41-2** ■ Pediatric dermograms (childhood).

**TABLE 41-1 ■ Neonatal Dermatoses (Birth to 1 Month)**

**Blistering (vesiculobullous lesions)**

Mechanical
Sucking blisters
Epidermolysis bullosa
Bullous ichthyosiform erythroderma (ichthyosis)

Infectious
Herpes simplex
Congenital varicella
Candidiasis
Congenital syphilis

**Pustular lesions**
Candidiasis
Erythema toxicum
Transient neonatal pustular melanosis
Neonatal acne
Milia

**Birthmarks**
White
Albinism
Piebaldism
Ash leaf macules
Nevus anemicus
Nevus depigmentosus

Brown
Café-au-lait spots
Congenital melanocytic nevus
Dermal melanosis
Epidermal nevus

Vascular
Nevus simplex (Salmon patch)
Capillary malformation (port-wine stain)
Hemangioma of infancy

Yellow
Nevus sebaceous

**Papulosquamous lesions**
Ichthyosis
Neonatal lupus erythematosus

associated with more complications and may require treatment more frequently. Numerous cutaneous lesions may be associated with hemangiomas in the viscera. Large facial hemangiomas may be associated with neurologic, ophthalmologic, and cardiac abnormalities (PHACE syndrome). Management may consist of observation alone, oral prednisolone, laser treatment, chemotherapy (interferon-α and vincristine), or surgery. Initial case series have also shown improvement with the use of propranolol.

*Yellow*

■ *Nevus sebaceous:* Noted at birth as a yellow orange oval or linear area of alopecia on the scalp. At puberty they become raised and warty. Basal cell carcinomas and squamous cell carcinomas can rarely develop within the nevus later in life. A benign warty tumor called *syringocystadenoma papilliferum* may occur in conjunction with a nevus sebaceous.

*Papulosquamous Lesions*

■ *Ichthyosis* (**Fig. 41-14**): Associated with dry, fishlike adherent scales. The rarer lamellar form and

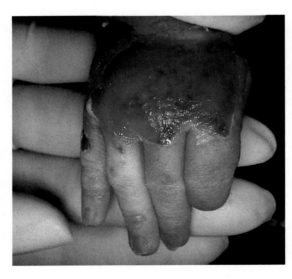

**FIGURE 41-3 ■** Epidermolysis bullosa. Junctional type.

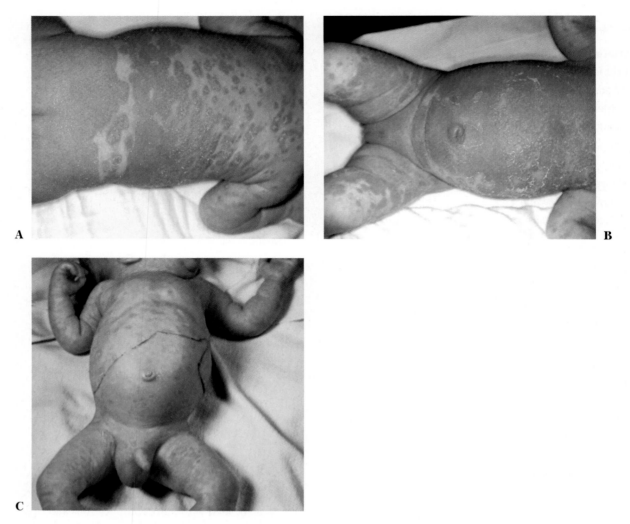

**FIGURE 41-4** ■ Candidiasis and syphilis. (**A and B**) Extensive candidiasis. (**C**) Congenital syphilis with hepatomegaly and splenomegaly.

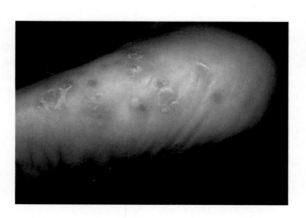

**FIGURE 41-5** ■ Transient neonatal pustular melanosis.

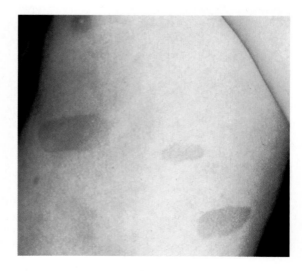

**FIGURE 41-6** ■ Café-au-lait lesions.

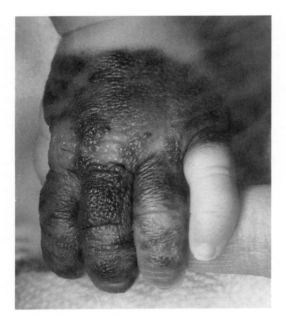

FIGURE 41-7 ■ Congenital melanocytic nevus.

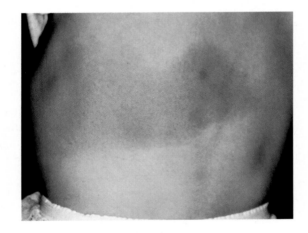

FIGURE 41-8 ■ Mongolian spot on back.

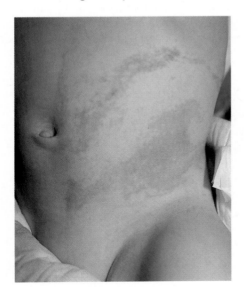

FIGURE 41-9 ■ Epidermal nevus.

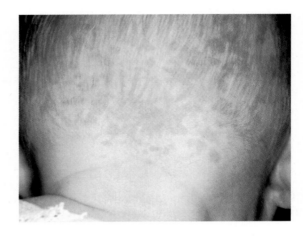

FIGURE 41-10 ■ Nevus simplex (Salmon patch).

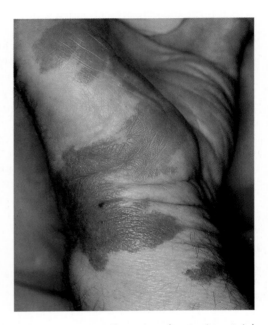

FIGURE 41-11 ■ Nevus flammeus (port-wine stain).

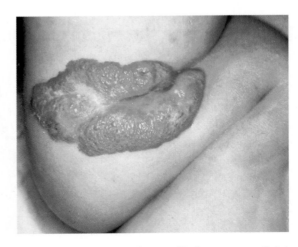

FIGURE 41-12 ■ Hemangioma of infancy—superficial.

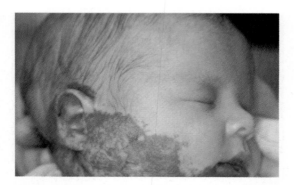

**FIGURE 41-13** ■ Segmented hemangioma on the lower extremity may be a sign of an underlying anomaly.

congenital ichthyosiform erythroderma are present at birth and may present with a shiny, tight layer of skin called a *collodion membrane.* Ichthyosis vulgaris, which is the commonest form, and X-linked ichthyosis are usually not present at birth.

■ *Neonatal lupus erythematosus* (Fig. 41-15): Characterized by congenital heart block and annular papulosquamous skin lesions on the forehead and cheeks. The skin lesions usually fade by 6 to 7 months of age while the heart block persists. Because this is maternally transmitted, the mother also needs to be evaluated for lupus. Anti-Ro or SSA and anti-La or SSB antibodies may be present in the mother or newborn.

## Dermatoses of Infants and Children

See Tables 41-2 and 41-3 for a summary of these dermatoses.

### Blistering Lesions (Vesiculobullous)

■ *Impetigo* (Fig. 41-16): Typically presents as small pustules that may develop into large, flaccid bullae (bullous impetigo). The pustules eventually rupture leaving erosions covered by a honey-colored crust. Impetigo is usually caused by *Staphylococcus aureus* and less commonly by *Streptococcus pyogenes.* Staphylococcal scalded skin syndrome is a desquamating disorder caused by an exfoliative toxin that results in perioral crusting and superficial desquamation most prominent in the intertriginous and flexural regions. In the newborn it is known as Ritter's disease.

■ *Viral blisters* (Fig. 41-17): Herpes simplex, varicella (chicken pox), and Coxsackie (hand–foot–mouth disease) can present with vesicles on an erythematous base.

■ *Bullous disease of childhood (linear IgA dermatoses):* Sausage-shaped bullae in a "string of pearls" configuration most commonly noted on the buttocks, groin, and lower extremities. It is usually a self-limited disease. Rarely, when treatment is needed, it responds well to dapsone. Direct immunofluorescence is positive for IgA noted at the dermal–epidermal junction.

■ *Dermatitis herpetiformis:* Recurrent crops of severely pruritic grouped vesicles or bullae on the extensor surfaces of the extremities, shoulders, and buttocks. The eruption is often associated with celiac disease and may improve with a gluten-free diet.

■ *Incontinentia pigmenti* (Fig. 41-18): An inherited disorder presenting with vesicles in a linear distribution during the first few months of life. The vesicles are replaced by a warty stage followed by a pigmented stage. There may be associated ophthalmologic and dental abnormalities.

### Pustular Lesions

■ *Acropustulosis of infancy:* Noted between birth and 2 years of age predominantly in African-American infants. Recurrent crops of pruritic papulopustules or vesiculopustular lesions develop on the palms,

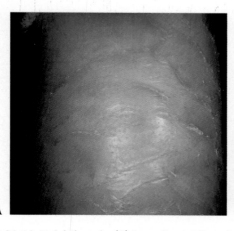

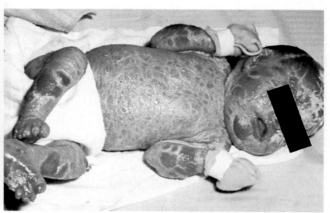

**FIGURE 41-14** ■ Ichthyosis. **(A)** Lamellar ichthyosis. **(B)** Harlequin fetus, fatal.

## TABLE 41-2 ■ Dermatoses of Infants and Children

**Blistering lesions**
Impetigo
Viral blisters
Bullous disease of childhood
Dermatitis herpetiformis
Incontinentia pigmenti

**Pustular lesions**
Acropustulosis of infancy
Impetigo
Candidiasis

**Papules/nodules**
Skin color
  Warts
  Molluscum contagiosum
  Keratosis pilaris
  Granuloma annulare
  Angiofibroma

Brown
  Melanocytic nevi
  Urticaria pigmentosa
Yellow papules
  Juvenile xanthogranuloma
  Nevus sebaceous

Red papules
  Papular acrodermatitis
  Papular urticaria
  Urticaria
  Erythema multiforme
  Pyogenic granuloma
  Viral exanthems
  Drug eruption

**Vascular lesions**
Blanching
  Spider angioma

Nonblanching
  Idiopathic thrombocytopenic purpura
  Henoch–Schönlein purpura
  Meningococcemia
  Vasculitis

## TABLE 41-3 ■ Dermatoses of Infants and Children

**Papulosquamous**
Psoriasis
Pityriasis rosea
Tinea versicolor

**Eczematous lesions**
Atopic dermatitis
Seborrheic dermatitis
Immunodeficiency
Allergic contact dermatitis
Diaper dermatitis

**Diseases affecting the hair**
Congenital/hereditary hair defects
Alopecia areata
Tinea capitis
Trichotillomania

**Diseases affecting the nails**
Congenital nail defects
Twenty-nail dystrophy
Psoriasis/atopic dermatitis
Warts
Paronychia

**Dermatoses owing to physical agents and photosensitivity dermatoses**
Sunburn
Thermal burn
Child abuse
Polymorphous light eruption
Phytophotodermatitis

soles, dorsum of hands, and feet. It is self-limited and often misdiagnosed as scabies.

■ *Impetigo:* (See earlier) may also be pustular.
■ *Candidiasis* (**Fig. 41-19**): Can present with pustules and erythematous papules in the diaper and intertriginous regions.

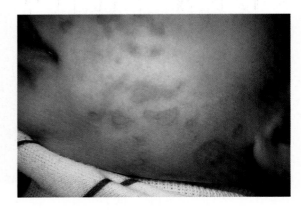

**FIGURE 41-15 ■** Neonatal lupus erythematosus.

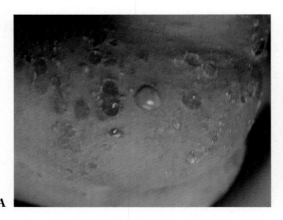
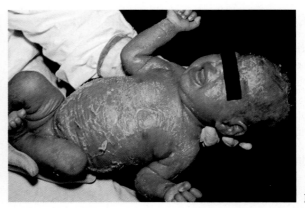

FIGURE 41-16 ■ Impetigo. (**A**) Impetigo. (**B**) Ritter's disease or Staphylococcal-scalded skin syndrome in a neonate.

*Papules/Nodules*

### Skin Color

- *Warts:* Verrucous papules caused by the human papillomavirus and transmitted by skin contact. They may resolve without therapy. In children, they are common on the face, hands, and feet. When they are noted in the genitalia, sexual abuse should be considered.
- *Molluscum contagiosum:* Viral disease caused by a member of the pox virus group. They present as single or multiple dome-shaped umbilicated papules found anywhere on the body. Spread by skin contact or autoinoculation, molluscum are more common in individuals with atopic dermatitis. They may dissipate without therapy.
- *Keratosis pilaris:* An autosomal dominant disorder characterized by minute follicular papules on the outer aspects of the arms, thighs, and cheeks. It is often seen in association with atopy and dry skin. Topical keratolytic creams may be helpful.

- *Granuloma annulare* (Fig. 41-20): Asymptomatic skin-colored or dull red papules that spread peripherally forming a ring with a normal appearing center. These are usually found on the dorsum of the hands and feet. The cause is unknown and spontaneous resolution without treatment occurs in months to years.
- *Angiofibroma:* Firm pink to skin-colored papules. They may be associated with tuberous sclerosis when seen in a symmetrical distribution on the face.

### Brown

- *Melanocytic nevi* (Fig. 41-21): Depending on the location of the nevus cells, these may be called junctional (at the border of the dermal–epidermal junction, usually flat and brown in color), intradermal (within the dermis, usually flesh colored and elevated), or compound nevi (both at the dermal––epidermal junction and in the dermis, usually elevated and brown). They occur anywhere on the body and may be flat, elevated, verrucous, or papillomatous. If they are black, multicolored, large (>6 mm), or have

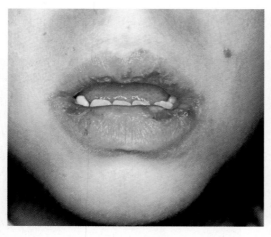
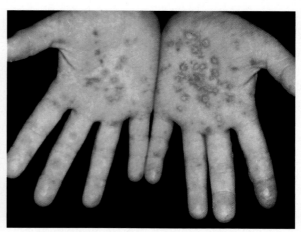

FIGURE 41-17 ■ Viral exanthem. (**A**) Erosions of the lips. (**B**) Blisters on the palms.

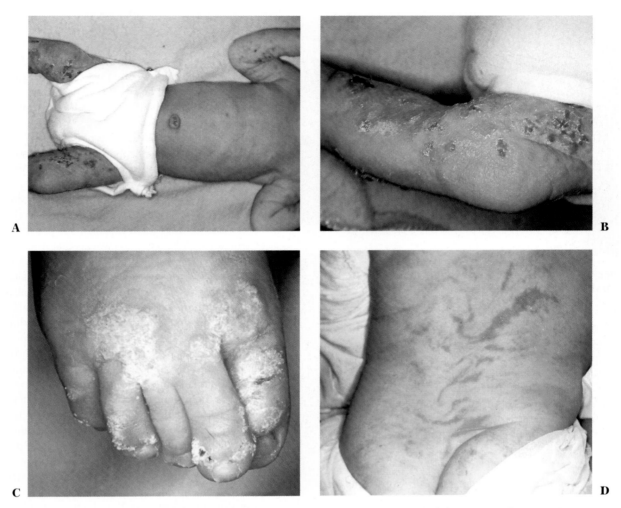

**FIGURE 41-18** ■ Incontinentia pigmenti. (**A and B**) Vesicular stage. (**C**) Warty stage. (**D**) Pigmented stage.

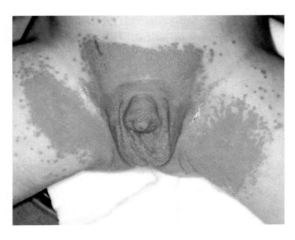

**FIGURE 41-19** ■ Candidal rash.

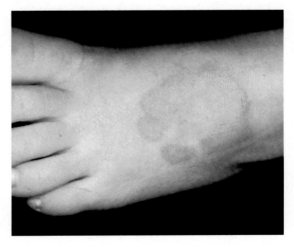

**FIGURE 41-20** ■ Granuloma annulare. On the dorsum of the foot.

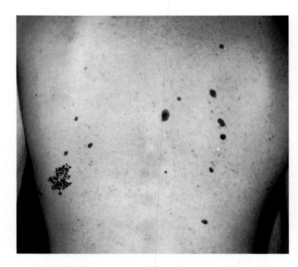

**FIGURE 41-21** ■ Melanocytic nevi. Junctional nevi on the back and speckled lentiginous nevus far left midback.

an irregular border, an excisional biopsy should be considered.

■ *Urticaria pigmentosa* (Fig. 41-22): Tan to brown macules and papules that urticate when stroked (Darier's sign). It usually has an excellent prognosis if there is no systemic involvement. Lesions eventually resolve without therapy. A positive tryptase test makes systemic involvement more of a concern.

### Yellow

■ *Juvenile xanthogranuloma:* Usually develops in the first year of life and disappears around 5 years of age. They present as either solitary or multiple small yellow papules on the scalp or body. There may be associated ocular involvement if multiple lesions are present.

■ *Nevus sebaceous:* See earlier.

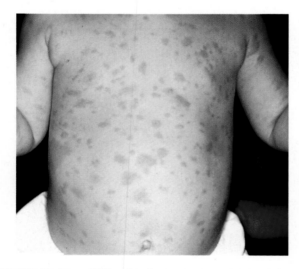

**FIGURE 41-22** ■ Urticaria pigmentosa. Urticaria pigmentosa in a 2-year-old patient (note the red, urticating lesion below the left nipple indicating a positive Darier's sign).

### Red

■ *Papular acrodermatitis (Gianotti–Crosti syndrome):* Nonpruritic flat-topped papules on the acral surfaces, especially elbows and knees. It was originally associated with the hepatitis B virus, but recently other viruses have been implicated. Usually it is benign and self-limited.

■ *Papular urticaria:* A delayed hypersensitivity reaction to a variety of arthropod bites. It presents as pruritic erythematous papules with a surrounding wheal. Recurrent crops occur in the summer.

■ *Urticaria:* Commonly seen in infants and children associated with an underlying infection or a reaction to a medication or food. It presents as pruritic, erythematous, and edematous wheals that migrate over a 24-hour period.

■ *Erythema multiforme (EM):* Acute hypersensitivity syndrome presenting with macular, urticarial, or vesiculobullous lesions commonly on the palms and soles. Target or "bull's eye" lesions are the hallmark of this condition with a central dusky hue and surrounding concentric erythema. It is commonly divided into EM minor, which is a benign, recurrent, and self-limited condition also involving one mucous membrane surface. EM minor is often associated with a recurrent herpes simplex virus infection. EM major presents with the involvement of at least two mucous membrane surfaces, widespread bullous lesions, and more systemic symptoms. EM major is frequently associated with mycoplasma pneumoniae infection or drugs.

■ *Pyogenic granuloma:* Bright red papule that bleeds easily. It may arise spontaneously or at sites of trauma. Excision is usually required.

■ *Viral exanthems:* Roseola, rubeola, rubella, adenovirus, erythema infectiosum, and enterovirus infections may present with erythematous macules and papules. Fever may also accompany the cutaneous manifestations.

■ *Drug eruption:* Multiple medications may cause a diffuse cutaneous eruption. Typically, morbilliform drug eruptions present with blanchable erythematous macules and papules.

## Vascular Lesions

### Blanching

■ *Spider angioma:* Small telangiectatic lesion on the cheeks, nose, dorsum of hands, or sun-exposed areas. Lesions are benign and often resolve spontaneously.

### Nonblanching (Petechiae and Purpura)

■ *Idiopathic thrombocytopenic purpura:* Low platelet disorder presenting with nonblanching petechiae and purpura especially on areas of trauma. Intravenous immunoglobulin is the treatment of choice.

- *Henoch–Schönlein purpura* (Fig. 41-23): Form of vasculitis presenting with petechiae followed by palpable purpura on the buttocks and lower extremities. Abdominal pain, joint swelling, and renal involvement may occur.
- *Meningococcemia:* Presents with nonblanching petechiae and purpura along with fever and signs of meningitis. Early diagnosis and treatment can be lifesaving.
- *Vasculitis:* Nonblanching palpable petechiae and purpura commonly found on the extremities. Associated causes can include underlying medication, infection, and rarely a collagen vascular disease.

### Papulosquamous

- *Psoriasis* (Fig. 41-24): Seen fairly frequently in children, especially "guttate psoriasis," which is often associated with an underlying streptococcal infection.

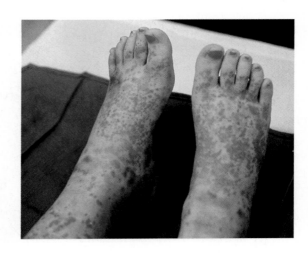

**FIGURE 41-23** ■ Henoch–Schönlein purpura.

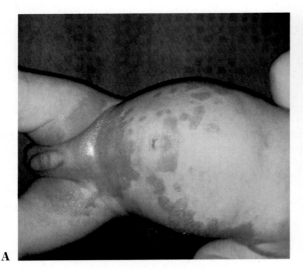

A

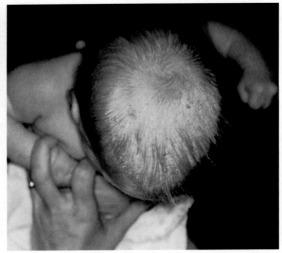

B

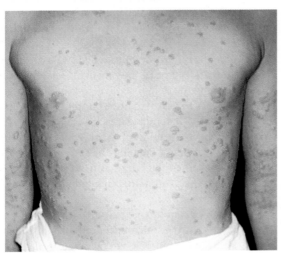

C

**FIGURE 41-24** ■ Psoriasis. (**A and B**) Psoriasis in a 2.5-month-old child. (**C**) Guttate psoriasis following a streptococcal pharyngitis.

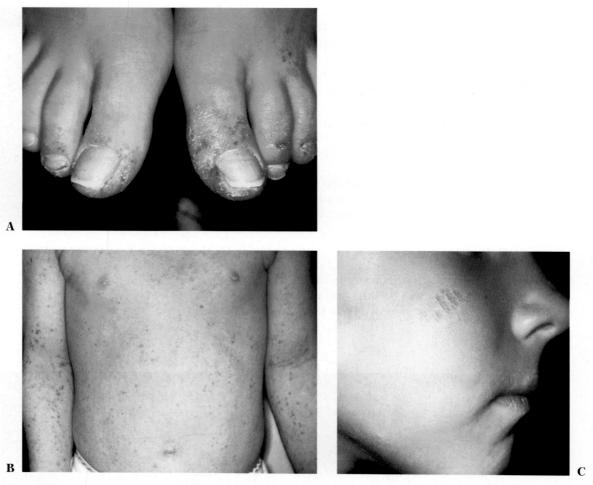

**FIGURE 41-25** ■ Atopic dermatitis. **(A)** Atopic dermatitis of the toes. **(B)** Atopic dermatitis of the chest and antecubital fossae in a 9-year-old child. **(C)** Hypopigmented patches on the cheeks (pityriasis alba).

- *Pityriasis rosea:* See Chapter 15.
- *Tinea versicolor:* See Chapter 15.

## Eczematous Lesions

- *Atopic dermatitis* (Fig. 41-25): Hereditary disorder usually beginning around 1 to 4 months of age. In infants, the involvement is usually of the face, scalp, trunk, and extensor extremities. Toddlers have involvement of flexural skin surfaces and adolescents have more severe involvement of the hands and feet. Individuals with atopic dermatitis may also have hypopigmented scaly patches on the cheeks and extensor arms referred to as *pityriasis alba.* First-line therapy continues to be emollients, antihistamines, and topical steroids. The topical calcineurin inhibitors are considered second-line therapeutic options for the treatment of children 2 years of age and older.
- *Seborrheic dermatitis* (Fig. 41-26): Scaly, erythematous eruption in the "seborrheic areas," which include the scalp, face, postauricular, groin, and intertriginous areas. It appears in infancy and usually

clears spontaneously. It is also seen in adolescents. Langerhans cell histiocytosis may be misdiagnosed as seborrheic dermatitis.

- *Immunodeficiency:* Severe combined immunodeficiency, Omenn's syndrome (familial reticuloendotheliosis with eosinophilia), HIV infection, and other rare immunodeficiencies can present with a widespread erythematous scaly eruption in early infancy.
- *Allergic contact dermatitis* (Fig. 41-27): The distribution and shape of these pruritic lesions are helpful in making the diagnosis. The lesions can range from vesicles to erythematous papules and eczematous plaques. Generalized reactions to poison ivy/oak are common in children. An eczematoid rash in the infraumbilical area may be seen in association with a "nickel" contact dermatitis to belt buckles and/or metal snaps on pants. Generalized "ID" reactions are not uncommon.
- *Diaper dermatitis* (Fig. 41-28): Irritant (secondary to stool or urine) or contact dermatitis is usually confined to the buttocks and perineal areas and typically

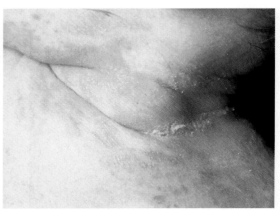

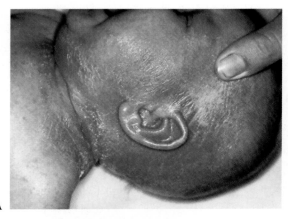

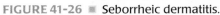

A                                                          B

FIGURE 41-26 ■ Seborrheic dermatitis.

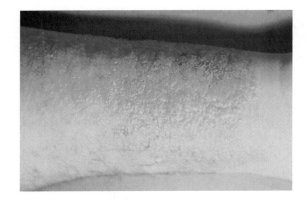

FIGURE 41-27 ■ Allergic contact dermatitis.

spares the creases. Pustular eruptions are often seen secondary to *Candida albicans* or staphylococcal infections. "Punched out" erosions can be seen in a severe form of irritant diaper dermatitis (Jacquet's dermatitis). Atopic dermatitis usually spares the diaper region.

### Disease Affecting the Hair

- *Congenital/hereditary hair defects* (Fig. 41-29): Congenital hair shaft defects can present with broken-off hairs, twisted, or spun-glass appearing hair. There is no satisfactory treatment for these conditions. Abnormal hair findings may be suggestive of other underlying disorders.
- *Alopecia areata* (Fig. 41-30): Common disorder presenting with the sudden appearance of patches of smooth, sharply defined alopecia. Short, tapered, "exclamation point" hairs tend to narrow as they enter the scalp. It is considered to be an

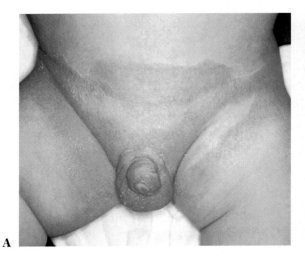

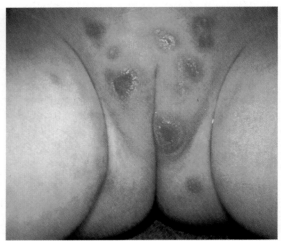

A                                                          B

FIGURE 41-28 ■ Diaper dermatitis. **(A)** Seborrheic diaper dermatitis. **(B)** Jacquet's diaper dermatitis.

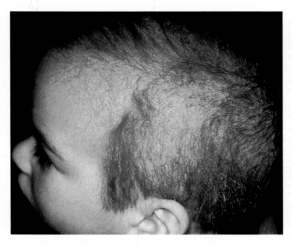

**FIGURE 41-29** ▤ Diffuse alopecia with ectodermal defect in a 3-year-old child.

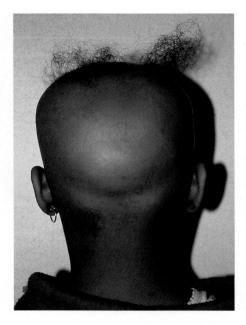

**FIGURE 41-30** ▤ Alopecia areata. Note completely smooth bald area.

autoimmune process involving the hair follicle and has been associated with thyroiditis. The prognosis depends on the extent of the hair loss (the less the better), the area involved, and chronicity. There may be associated nail pitting. Most commonly prescribed therapy remains topical or intralesional corticosteroids.

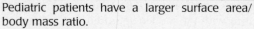

**SAUER'S NOTES**

Pediatric patients have a larger surface area/body mass ratio.

This necessitates more careful consideration for absorption of topical medications.

- *Tinea capitis* (Fig. 41-31): Common organisms are *Trichophyton tonsurans* (the most common cause of tinea capitis in the United States) and *Microsporum canis.* "Black dot" tinea, caused by *T. tonsurans,* often presents with broken-off hairs and minimal inflammation. Tinea capitis may be asymptomatic or can present with scale, pruritus, alopecia, or pustules. A kerion, which is an inflammatory, pus-filled, boggy mass with associated hair loss can be seen in more severe cases. Occipital lymphadenopathy is commonly noted in patients with tinea capitis. Fungal culture and potassium hydroxide mount can be diagnostic. Treatment is with oral griseofulvin for at least 2 months. Newer antifungals (fluconazole, itraconazole, and terbinafine) are also showing promise and may begin to replace griseofulvin.
- *Trichotillomania* (Fig. 41-32): Commonly seen between 4 and 10 years of age in both genders. Patients pluck, twirl, or rub hair-bearing areas either consciously or subconsciously as a result of a habit. It usually affects the scalp, but may also involve eyebrows and eyelashes. It is usually self-limited.

### Disease Affecting the Nails

- *Congenital nail defects:* Absent or poorly developed nails are associated with many syndromes, usually representing nail matrix disorders. Ectodermal dysplasias (Fig. 41-33) are syndromes associated with abnormal nails, skin, hair, and teeth.
- *Twenty-nail dystrophy:* Presents as thickened nails with exaggerated longitudinal ridges, noted in all nails of the hand (ten-nail dystrophy) (Fig. 41-34) or hands and feet (twenty-nail dystrophy). This dystrophy is self-limited and may resolve over time.
- *Psoriasis:* Nails may be thickened, shiny, and contain ridges or pitting with these conditions.
- *Warts:* Children frequently develop warts around (periungual) and under the nail (subungual). These warts can pose a therapeutic challenge.
- *Paronychia:* Usually presents as a red, painful, inflamed lesion around the nail fold, which may drain pus. It can be acute or chronic. *S. aureus* is the most common organism causing acute infection. The chronic form is often seen in thumb suckers, nail biters, and nail pickers and is commonly associated with *C. albicans.*

### Dermatoses Owing to Physical Agents and Photosensitivity Dermatoses

- *Sunburn:* On the first sunny days, parents tend to underestimate the effects of the sun rays and overexpose their children. Parents should be taught the ABCs of sun exposure. *Always* stay out of the sun

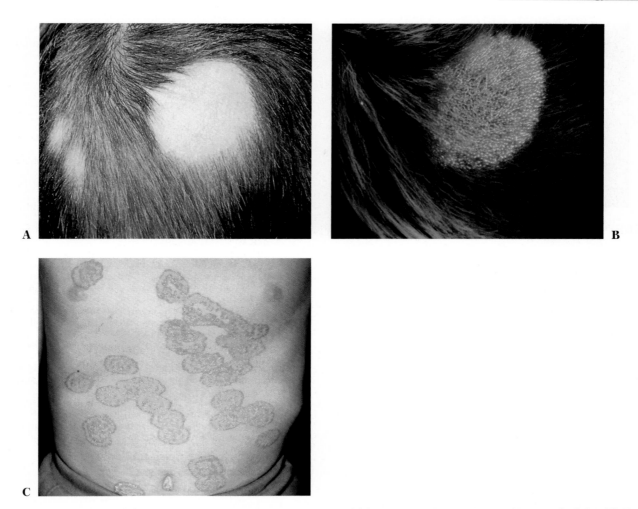

**FIGURE 41-31** ■ Tinea. (**A**) Tinea of the scalp due to *M. audouinii*. (**B**) Tinea hairs fluorescing under Wood's light. (**C**) Tinea of the body due to *M. canis*.

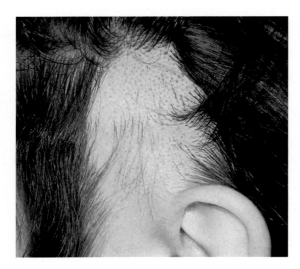

**FIGURE 41-32** ■ Trichotillomania of the scalp. Note there is not complete baldness and hairs are of varying lengths.

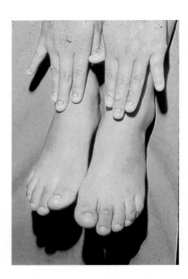

**FIGURE 41-33** ■ Ectodermal defect with hypoplasia of the fingernail and toenails.

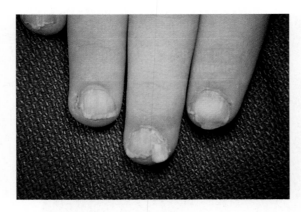

**FIGURE 41-34** ■ Ten-nail dystrophy.

between 10 AM and 4 PM. *B*lock the sun with sunscreens that protect against both UVA and UVB rays with a sun protection factor (SPF) of at least 30. *C*lothes, especially a hat and shirt, should be worn when outside. Adolescents should also be cautioned to avoid tanning salons.

- *Thermal burn:* Severe pain. May be partial thickness with erythema and blisters, or full thickness with loss of skin and subsequent scar formation.
- *Child abuse:* Well-demarcated atypical appearing purpura, erosions, or scars should raise the suspicion of possible child abuse.
- *Polymorphous light eruption (PMLE):* Idiopathic sensitivity to UV rays characterized by pruritic, eczematous, papulovesicular, or plaque-like lesions on sun-exposed areas such as the cheeks, ears, nose, neck, or dorsum of the hands. If no additional sunlight exposure occurs, lesions will involute spontaneously in 1 to 2 weeks. Broad-spectrum sunscreens providing protection against UVB and UVA are helpful.
- *Phytophotodermatitis:* Well-demarcated erythema (often linear) with residual hyperpigmentation on sun-exposed skin. This dermatitis is more common in the spring and summer in children who have

been exposed to a plant that contains furocoumarin psoralen, a photosensitizing agent. The hyperpigmentation can last for several months.

## Suggested Readings

Alvarez MS, Silverberg NB. Tinea capitis. *Cutis.* 2006;78:189–196.

American Academy of Pediatrics. Ultraviolet light: a hazard to children. *Pediatrics.* 1999;104:328–333.

Bruckner AL, Frieden IJ. Hemangiomas of infancy. *J Am Acad Dermatol.* 2003;48:477–493.

Carder KR. Hypersensitivity reactions in neonates and infants. *Dermatol Ther.* 2005;18:160–175.

Coloe J, Burkhart CN, Morrell DS. Molluscum contagiosum: what's new and true? *Pediatr Ann* 2009;38(6):321–325.

Dohil MA, Eichenfield LF. A treatment approach for atopic dermatitis. *Pediatr Ann.* 2005;34(3):201–210.

Dyer JA. Childhood viral exanthems. *Pediatr Ann.* 2007;36(1):21–29.

Eichenfield LF, Hanifin JM, Luger TA, et al. Consensus conference on pediatric atopic dermatitis. *J Am Acad Dermatol.* 2003;49:1088–1095.

Farvolden D, Sweeney SM, Wiss K. Lumps and bumps in neonates and infants. *Dermatol Ther.* 2005;18:104–116.

Fatahzadeh M, Schwartz RA. Human herpes simplex virus infections: epidemiology, pathogenesis, symptomatology, diagnosis, and management. *J Am Acad Dermatol.* 2007;57:737–763.

Garzon MC, Huang JT, Enjolras O, et al. Vascular malformations: part I. *J Am Acad Dermatol.* 2007;56:353–370.

Haggstrom AN, Drolet BA, Baselga E, et al. Prospective study of infantile hemangiomas: clinical characteristics predicting complications and treatment. *Pediatrics.* 2006;118(3):882–887.

Krakowski AC, Eichenfield LF, Dohil MA. Management of atopic dermatitis in the pediatric population. *Pediatrics* 2008;122(4):812–824.

Krol A, Krafchik B. The differential diagnosis of atopic dermatitis in childhood. *Dermatol Ther.* 2006;19:73–82.

O'Connor NR, McLaughlin MR, Ham P. Newborn skin: part I. common rashes. *Am Fam Physician.* 2008;77(1):47–52.

Paller AS, Mancini AJ. *Hurwitz Clinical Pediatric Dermatology.* 3rd ed. Philadelphia: Elsevier; 2005.

Schachner LA, Hansen RC. *Pediatric Dermatology.* 3rd ed. Philadelphia: WB Saunders; 2003.

Segal AR, Doherty KM, Leggott J, et al. Cutaneous reactions to drugs in children. *Pediatrics.* 2007;120(4):e1082–e1096.

Shin HT. Diaper dermatitis that does not quit. *Dermatol Ther.* 2005;18:124–135.

Strauss JS, Krowchuk DP, Leyden JJ, et al. Guidelines of care for acne vulgaris management. *J Am Acad Dermatol.* 2007;56:651–663.

Swerdlin A, Berkowitz C, Craft N. Cutaneous signs of child abuse. *J Am Acad Dermatol.* 2007;57:371–392.

Tromberg J, Bauer B, Benvenuto-Andrade C, et al. Congenital melanocytic nevi needing treatment. *Dermatol Ther.* 2005;18:136–150.

Weston WL, Lane AT, Morelli JG. *Color Textbook of Pediatric Dermatology.* 4th ed. St. Louis: Mosby Yearbook; 2007.

# CHAPTER 42

# General Principles of Skin Aging

*Deede Liu, MD, MS, Emily Stevens, BA, Daniel West, MD, and Daniel Aires, MD, JD*

## Introduction

The approach to the older patient is largely similar to the approach to any other patient. Differences arise mainly because some disorders increase in prevalence with increasing age. These disorders range from potentially life-threatening skin cancers to annoying but harmless benign neoplasms such as seborrheic keratoses.

Common skin conditions in elderly patients are shown in Figure 42-1.

## Incidence of Geriatric Skin Diseases

According to one study by Gip and Molin (see Suggested Readings), the 10 most prevalent dermatologic disorders in a large group of elderly Swedish patients are as follows (the numbers in parentheses refer to the total number of dermatologic disorders found in the 286 patients examined):

- Pigmented nevus (143)
- Discoloration of the toenails (133)
- Seborrheic keratosis (84)
- Plantar hyperkeratosis (36)
- Stasis dermatitis of the legs (31)
- Seborrheic dermatitis (27)
- Dermatitis of the legs (unspecified) (23)
- Marked atrophy of the skin (19)
- Xanthelasma (12) (Fig. 42-2)
- Capillary hemangiomas (10)

These investigators studied 286 patients over 60 years of age who were hospitalized in a Swedish geriatric clinic. Each patient underwent a full-body skin exam. Histopathologic,

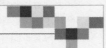

### SAUER'S NOTES

1. Aging is part of living.
2. There will be a never-ending attempt to be forever young, and the dermatologist will not be neglected in this pursuit.
3. The need to be helpful to our patients should not lead to unrealistic recommendations for fighting the inevitable changes of time.
4. We are physicians first and businessmen/women a distant second.

bacteriologic, or mycologic examinations were undertaken in some cases. In the 107 men, there were 231 skin diagnoses (2.2 per person), and in the 179 women, 372 skin diagnoses were made (2.1 per person). The number of skin diagnoses per person ranged from 1 to 5. No skin diagnoses were registered in 22 cases (8% of patients, 5 men and 17 women).

Based on common and concerning skin conditions in the elderly, we provide some general advice (Table 42-1). Understanding the most common dermatologic problems that are seen in elderly patients requires an appreciation of the mechanisms of aging in the skin. Thus, the next part of this chapter addresses the clinical and histologic features and prevention and treatment of intrinsic aging and photoaging.

### Intrinsic versus Extrinsic Skin Aging

Although much remains to be known, we present a brief overview of the science of aging skin since it provides a basis for the clinical changes discussed in more detail. Aging skin results from two forces: (1) intrinsic, or chronologic factors, and (2) extrinsic factors, such as sun damage.

#### Intrinsic Aging

Intrinsic factors cause the clinical, histologic, and physiologic changes observed in sun-protected aged skin. These changes include reductions in epidermal regeneration rate, rete ridge depth, dermal thickness, thermoregulatory ability, immune defense, wound healing, mechanical defense, sensory perception, sweat and sebum production, and vitamin D synthesis.

Clinical signs of intrinsic skin aging result mainly from thinning, fragility, and loss of elasticity. In the dermis, both intrinsic and extrinsic aging begin with fragmentation of the dermal collagen matrix. Collagen fragmentation is a normal process resulting from the actions of matrix metalloproteinases (MMPs). Fibroblasts typically keep the activity level of these collagen-degrading enzymes in balance with new collagen production. However, fibroblasts require attachment to unfragmented collagen in order to do this effectively. Once significant collagen fragmentation occurs, fibroblasts become less able to produce collagen and regulate MMPs. This leads to a self-perpetuating cycle of decreased fibroblast attachment to intact collagen, decreased collagen production, increased MMP activity, and increased collagen fragmentation.

A second underlying mechanism of intrinsic senescence involves telomere shortening. Telomere length is maintained

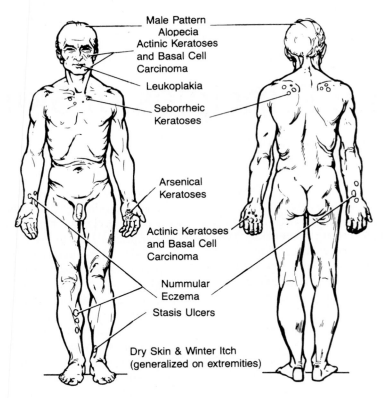

**FIGURE 42-1** ▪ Geriatric dermagrams.

in stem cells by the enzyme telomerase, which re-lengthens the DNA ends after each replication cycle. When inefficient duplication of telomeres occurs in dermal fibroblasts, senescence is the end result. Because many tumor cells express telomerase, it is thought that telomerase may play a role in preventing cancer.

Stem cell changes have recently been shown to play a key role in age-associated graying of hair. Hair pigmentation requires regular replenishment of hair melanocytes by stem cells residing in the follicular bulge. Age-related

changes in *PAX3* and *MITF* change the balance between melanocyte stem cell maintenance and differentiation and lead to the gradual loss of melanocyte stem cells, resulting in gray hair.

*Extrinsic Aging/Photoaging*

Most of what we see as aging is in fact extrinsic aging, due mainly to solar ultraviolet (UV) radiation exposure. This so-called photoaging resembles accelerated chronologic aging,

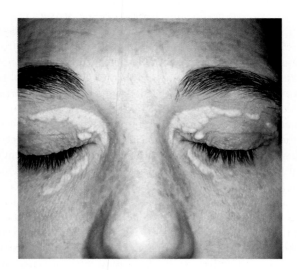

**FIGURE 42-2** ▪ Xanthelasma.

---

**TABLE 42-1** ▪ **General Skin Advice for Elderly Patients**

▪ Monthly self skin exams for new or changing lesions, especially if there is a history of previous skin cancers. May require assistance from family members or caregivers.

▪ Vitamin D$_3$ 800−1,000 IU supplement with meal unless there is a history of kidney stone; this pertains to elderly skin because elderly people generally get less sun.

▪ When cleansing, limit soap to strategic areas (groin, axillae, feet); avoid scrubbing and excessive hand-washing/bathing.

▪ Moisturize liberally with petrolatum or lactic acid and urea, especially in winter and/or dry climates.

▪ Clip toenails with squared-off ends to avoid ingrown toenails. Choose properly fitting shoes. Apply Vicks VapoRub daily to toenails for incipient Onychomycosis.

▪ Wear support hose for early signs of stasis dermatitis.

and it occurs via at least two well-documented mechanisms. First, solar UV irradiation generates deleterious reactive oxygen species such as superoxide anions, hydrogen peroxide, and singlet oxygen through NADPH oxidase activity. UV exposure also activates proinflammatory cytokine receptors in human skin, including those for epidermal growth factor, interleukin-1$\beta$, interleukin-6, interleukin-8, intercellular adhesion molecule-1, and tumor necrosis factor-$\alpha$. The increased inflammation further exacerbates oxidative stress. Second, it appears that UV irradiation decreases collagen production. It does this by upregulating multiple kinase-based signaling pathways as well as increasing expression and function of *AP-1*. *AP-1* is a nuclear transcription factor that shifts the balance between collagen degradation and production toward increased degradation by directly stimulating MMPs (*MMP-1, MMP-3, MMP-9*) and impeding collagen gene expression by dermal fibroblasts. In studies by Fisher et al., solar UV irradiation has been shown to reversibly reduce collagen production in young skin by approximately 80% within 24 hours after a single short exposure. In aged skin, it has been shown that decreased fibroblasts and elevated levels of partially degraded collagen act to reduce collagen synthetic activity.

On a cellular level, photoaging changes the structure and function of both the dermis and the epidermis. Photoaged epidermis, for example, can become either hyperplastic or atrophic. Histologic examination of severely photodamaged skin reveals atypical keratinocytes and loss of epidermal polarity, both of which can signify premalignant or malignant changes. In photoaged dermis, degraded and/or irregularly thickened collagen and elastic fibers can present clinically as wrinkling and yellow-brown discoloration. In addition, irregular dilation and increased fragility of dermal blood vessels can show up as telangiectasias and senile purpura.

In brief, sun damage causes the majority of age-related cosmetic and clinical problems on facial skin, including skin cancers, irregular pigmentation, rhytides, and increased skin fragility and coarseness.

## Histologic Changes

Histologically, the epidermis of aged skin demonstrates decreased numbers of all major cell types in the skin—keratinocytes, melanocytes, Langerhans cells, and fibroblasts. Accordingly, the function of these cell types is decreased. Keratinocytes, which form the basic barrier that confers the primary mechanical and immunologic defense to our skin, exhibit decreased proliferation, cell signaling, and response to growth factors with aging. These changes result in a reduction of the barrier function leading to increased skin fragility. The decrease in melanocytes, which results in decreased melanin synthesis for UV protection, is evident in the decreased number of nevi present as we age. Langerhans cells are antigen-presenting cells that play an important role in fighting skin infections and neoplasia. Reduced Langerhans cells result in increased rates of skin cancers and infections and decreased rates of contact dermatitis in the elderly. Reduced numbers of mast cells may also contribute to these changes.

The dermoepidermal junction of aged skin becomes flatter, which results in a lower threshold for separation and blister formation. Likewise, reductions in fibroblasts result in a thinned dermis with less collagen and mucopolysaccharide, especially hyaluronic acid. Capillary loops also shrink, resulting in decreased cutaneous blood flow. Appendages such as hair follicles, eccrine and apocrine glands, and pacinian and Meissner's corpuscles are similarly decreased, resulting in drier, less hairy, less sensitive skin.

## Prevention and Treatment

Primary photoprotection (reviewed in Chapter 7) is the most effective way to prevent photoaging. Even though this is obvious, not enough emphasis is given to this element of skin care. Multiple studies have demonstrated that daily liberal use of a broad-spectrum sunscreen that shields both UVA and UVB radiation with a high sun protection factor (SPF) reduces the number of new premalignant actinic keratoses (AKs) and hastens reduction of preexisting AKs in people at high risk for skin cancer.

With the precautions against solar UV radiation comes a risk of vitamin D deficiency, which is highly prevalent among many elderly patients. Vitamin D, which is naturally produced in the skin after sun exposure, is necessary for bone health, and emerging data indicates that it probably plays important roles in prevention of cancer, including skin cancer, and in prevention of autoimmune disease, such as multiple sclerosis. We do not recommend suntanning as a method of acquiring adequate levels of vitamin D. Instead, we recommend oral supplementation of vitamin D, which is widely available, as well as "smart sun" precautions such as applying sunscreen everyday, wearing sun-protective clothing including hats and gloves when doing outdoor activities like gardening and fishing, and also trying to stay out of the sun between 10:00 AM and 4:00 PM. These precautions can help prevent sunburns and reduce the risk for skin cancer.

### Retinoids

At this time, topical retinoids are the only longer-term treatment for photodamage. Tretinoin (all *trans*-retinoic acid) has well-documented rejuvenating effects on both chronologically aged and photodamaged skin. Recent work by Fisher has shown that through complex and not fully elucidated molecular pathways, retinoid compounds can cause deposition of new, nonfragmented collagen in both photodamaged and chronologically aged human skin, thereby markedly improving skin texture and appearance. Tretinoin has also been shown to block UV induction of nuclear transcription factors *AP-1* and NF-$\kappa$B as well as increases in interstitial collagenase and gelatinases in irradiated skin samples that were pretreated 48 hours prior to exposure. The restorative effects of tretinoin have also been demonstrated histologically in non–sun exposed, chronologically aged skin. Daily application of 0.025% tretinoin cream for 9 months in women aged 68 to 79 years resulted in thickened epidermal and granular cell layers with corresponding increased height in the dermoepidermal junction through the rete pegs, increased uniformity in keratinocyte density, and decreased melanocyte vacuolization. Dermal morphology showed new microvasculature and increased numbers and sizes of fibroblasts, collagen, elastin, microfibrils, and anchoring fibrils. Such changes suggest that tretinoin cream stimulated metabolic activation of chronologically aged skin in a similar fashion to that observed in photodamaged skin.

### Alpha-Hydroxy Acids

Alpha-hydroxy acids (AHAs), which include the compounds listed in Table 42-2, are known to increase epidermal thickness and dermal glycosaminoglycans and decrease hyperkeratinization. As such, AHA-containing products are employed for disorders such as ichthyosis, dry skin, and other disorders associated with retention of the stratum corneum or hyperkeratinization. Application of AHAs in higher concentrations can be useful in treating AKs, warts, and seborrheic keratoses.

### Estrogens

Estrogen deficiency, seen largely in postmenopausal women, causes wrinkling, dryness, atrophy, laxity, poor wound healing, hot flashes, and vulvar atrophy. Although data is sparse, there are reports of positive localized epidermal and dermal changes resulting from exogenous estrogen administration. These include increased skin surface lipid production and water-retention capacity, new collagen synthesis, and improved wound healing and quality of scarring. There are reports suggesting that postmenopausal HRT (hormone replacement therapy) may enhance the skin's thickness and barrier function. In light of recent data regarding chronic use of systemic estrogen supplementation, the risk-to-benefit ratio of HRT needs to be carefully evaluated by physicians and their patients.

### TABLE 42-2 ■ Alpha-Hydroxy Acids

- Glycolic acid
- Lactic acid
- Glycolic acid + ammonium glycolate
- $\alpha$-Hydroxyethanoic acid + ammonium $\alpha$-hydroxyethanoate
- $\alpha$-Hydroxyoctanoic acid
- $\alpha$-Hydroxycaprylic acid
- Hydroxycaprylic acid
- Mixed fruit acid
- Triple fruit acid
- Tri-$\alpha$-hydroxy fruit acids
- Sugarcane extract
- $\alpha$-Hydroxy and botanical complex
- L-$\alpha$-Hydroxy acid
- Glycomer in cross-linked fatty acids alpha nutrium

### Antioxidants

Antioxidants are reviewed in Chapter 7 and therefore will be discussed here only briefly. A well-balanced diet rich in fruits and vegetables is a good source for antioxidants. In regard to oral supplements, it should be noted that oral vitamin E has been shown to have deleterious effects, including reduced life expectancy.

Oral supplements containing ingredients such as L-proline, L-lysine, manganese, copper, zinc, quercetin, grape seed extract, and N-acetyl-D-glucosamine sulfate have been touted as potential wrinkle reducers. A supplement containing vitamin E, vitamin C, carotenoid, selenium, and proanthocyanidin showed the ability to decrease UV induction of MMPs.

Topical vitamin C prevents erythema following UV exposure. Studies have shown that vitamin C can upregulate collagen and tissue inhibitor of metalloproteinases (TIMP) synthesis as well as decrease wrinkles. Topical $CoQ_{10}$ has been shown to reduce wrinkles through its antioxidant properties. $\alpha$-Lipoic acid may have a role in the treatment of photoaging by reducing transcription factors, such as NF-$\kappa$B, that affect the production of cytokines.

### Interventional Treatments

More details on interventional treatments are discussed elsewhere, but a brief overview is included here.

Botulinum toxin A inhibits neuromuscular transmission by blocking acetylcholine release. Cosmetically, botulinum relaxes the underlying musculature of the face, lessening the appearance of wrinkles. Understanding underlying anatomy is important for optimal outcome.

Soft tissue augmentation, or "fillers," can partially offset age-associated subcutaneous atrophy. Maintenance is required every 6 to 12 months, depending on location, depth, and choice of filler. Immunogenicity can present a major drawback. Acellular dermal grafts from human cadavers show less immunogenicity than bovine collagen but have fallen out of favor since the development of newer lab-generated fillers. Both hyaluronic acid and calcium hydroxyapatite derivatives are less immunogenic, and calcium hydroxyapatite is also potentially more durable.

A variety of resurfacing techniques have been used to improve the appearance of aged skin. Microdermabrasion exfoliates the superficial epidermis, and microablation uses low-frequency radiofrequency via an electrode. The goal of therapy is to injure the superficial epidermis enough to activate cytokines, MMPs, and type I procollagen mRNA and trigger a healing cascade. Effects tend to be short-lived. Other radiofrequency devices aim to improve cheek and neck laxity via heat generation. Adverse affects range from burning and erythema to subcutaneous atrophy.

Laser systems treat multiple age-associated changes such as mottled pigmentation, wrinkling, and dermal atrophy. Fractionated-delivery laser systems have fewer side effects. Care must be taken to avoid ablating the surface of a potentially malignant pigmented lesion, thus allowing a deeper component to proliferate undetected.

## Tumorigenesis (Fig. 42-3)

Cumulative UV exposure rises with age, and the link between UV radiation exposure and the development of skin cancer is well established. Furthermore, there is a lag between exposure and tumor development. The combination of these factors leads to a dramatically increased incidence of many skin tumors in the elderly. Basal cell carcinomas (BCCs) and squamous cell carcinomas (SCCs), the two most common skin cancers, tend to occur on sun-exposed skin in older people with skin types 1 and 2. UVA and UVB both induce cyclobutane pyrimidine dimers (CPDs), which produce genetic alterations in DNA that are associated with BCCs and SCCs. Cutaneous melanomas have recently been shown to have a high proportion of UVB-signature mutations in tumor suppressor genes, including *TP53* and *CDKN2A*, and possibly also in oncogenes such as *BRAF* and *NRAS*.

### Premalignant Lesions

Clinically, AKs are flat or slightly elevated, pink, tan, or brownish, rough, scaly, adherent lesions. Though generally under 1 cm in size, AKs may get larger and even become confluent. As previously mentioned, these lesions occur mainly sun-exposed skin such as the face, ears, neck, and dorsum of the hands, especially in fair-skinned people. Cutaneous horns can arise in a proliferative variant of AK. If left untreated, up to 10% of these lesions may progress to SCC. Lesions with palpable induration, marked inflammation, or recurrence after treatment may merit further evaluation by biopsy. Shave biopsies are adequate as long as enough tissue is obtained to examine whether dermal invasion has occurred. Cryotherapy works well for single or scattered lesions. Treatment options for multiple and confluent lesions that cover a large surface area include topical 5-fluorouracil, imiquimod, and diclofenac, as well as photodynamic therapy with aminolevulinic acid and an activating light source.

Leukoplakia is the mucous membrane counterpart of AKs. It has a 20% to 30% progression rate to SCC and should be managed aggressively since SCC of the mucous membranes has a metastatic rate of 40% to 50% compared to 4% to 5% in the skin. Metastatic SCC has a poor prognosis as discussed in the following text.

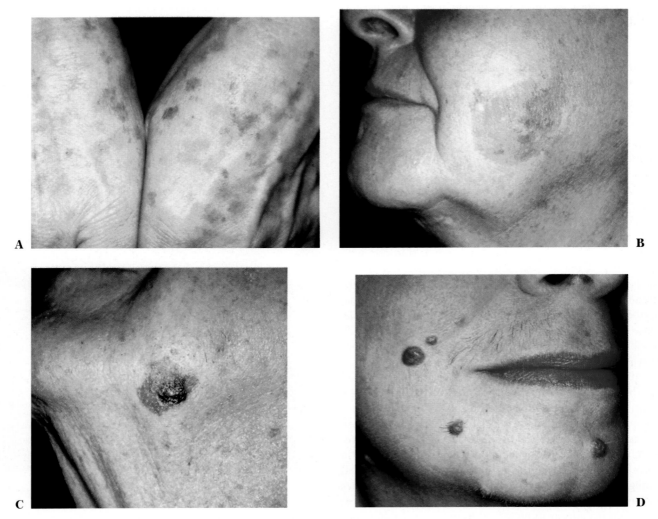

**FIGURE 42-3** ■ **(A)** Senile freckles on the dorsum of the hands. **(B)** Lentigo on the cheek. **(C)** Malignant melanoma in lentigo, on the jaw area. *(Syntex Laboratories, Inc.)* **(D)** Compound nevi on the face.

*Malignant Lesions*

BCC is the most common malignant skin cancer, and incidence increases with age. Although the risk of metastasis is very low, untreated tumors can become very locally destructive over time.

SCC is the second most common skin malignancy, and it too increases with age. The rate of metastasis is higher than that of BCC and lower than that of malignant melanoma. Although metastases are fairly uncommon, once the SCC becomes invasive to the lymph node, survival rates decline dramatically. Some types of SCC appear to be more aggressive than others. SCC from chronic injuries, burns, or scars, termed Marjolin ulcers, tend to be more aggressive, as do mucous membrane SCCs.

Common treatment options include surgical excision and electrodessication and curettage with or without subsequent adjuvant topical 5-fluorouracil or imiquimod treatment. Radiation therapy is generally reserved for elderly patients not able to tolerate surgery. New studies are showing that elderly patients with superficial SCCs or nodular or superficial BCCs who cannot tolerate surgery or elect not to undergo surgical excision may benefit from curettage followed by the application of imiquimod 5% cream five to seven times weekly for 6 weeks (BCCs) or a maximum of 16 weeks (SCCs). Patients wait 2 weeks after curettage before starting imiquimod to allow partial re-epithelialization. Recent studies have demonstrated clearance rates of 96% to 100% in the treatment of BCCs at 12 to 36 months follow-up; 80% to 100% clearance in the treatment of superficial SCCs at a mean of 31 months follow-up; and 71.4% clearance in the treatment of invasive SCCs at a mean of 31 months follow-up—all with excellent cosmetic outcomes and tolerance.

Merkel cells carcinomas (MCCs) are rare cutaneous tumors that account for less than 1% of cutaneous malignancies and are seen more common in the elderly. The mean age at diagnosis is 75 years and only 5% of cases occur before 50 years of age. These tumors usually present as shiny, solitary, dome-shaped, red or violaceous nodules or firm plaques on the head or neck. Risk factors for MCC include chronic immunosuppression, organ transplantation, B-cell lymphoma, erythema ab igne, and congenital ectodermal dysplasia. Once an MCC is diagnosed, wide local excision, if clinically feasible, and a referral to a surgical and medical oncologist as well as a radiation therapist is indicated.

The incidence of melanoma actually peaks before old age, but it, too, often presents in elderly patients. Any new mole in an older person should be carefully assessed, since new moles don't generally arise after age 40. The link between UV radiation exposure and melanoma is an area of active research. Lentigo maligna melanomas occur overwhelmingly in areas that have received the greatest cumulative exposure to sunlight, but no animal model has been developed to induce melanoma reliably with UV radiation alone, and other types of melanoma appear to be related to intense episodic exposure rather than total lifetime sun exposure.

## Common Benign Lesions

Actinic lentigines (liver spots) are hyperpigmented macules, typically arising on sun-exposed skin such as the face or dorsal hands, that result from an increase in melanocyte number. These benign pigmented lesions are seen in middle to late age and, to the chagrin of many patients, do not fade with time.

In severely photodamaged skin of the neck and chest, a mottled, reddish-brown discoloration known as poikiloderma of Civatte may be seen. Large, open comedones in the periorbicular area are also often seen in severely photodamaged patients. This is known as Favre–Racouchot syndrome (Fig. 42-4).

Seborrheic keratoses (known as "seborrheic warts" in Europe) (Fig. 42-5) typically appear as waxy, stuck-on, flesh-colored, tan, brown, or black papules on the head, neck, trunk, and extremities. These lesions are common in the elderly and are generally asymptomatic, so no treatment is required. However, if a lesion becomes inflamed or if a patient desires cosmetic destruction, cryotherapy generally works. Cryotherapy for these lesions is best performed at a lateral angle rather than head-on in order to minimize damage to surrounding tissue and decrease the potential for scarring. Another method is curettage followed by trichloroacetic acid. Although seborrheic keratoses usually have a characteristic appearance, they can sometimes be difficult to distinguish from malignant melanoma, especially when they become inflamed. Furthermore, they are generally not solitary. A biopsy should be performed if any doubt exists.

Dermatosis papulosa nigra (DPN) affects up to 35% of the African-American population in the United States and can also be seen in Asians. It is histologically the same as a seborrheic keratosis. Females are more frequently affected than males, and the incidence as well as the number and size of lesions increases with age, beginning in adolescence. Lesions

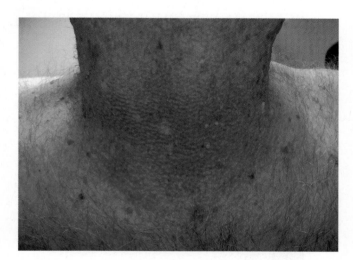

**FIGURE 42-4** ■ Poikilodermatous changes on the sides of the neck with sparing of the anterior neck where there was shading by the chin. This is typical of poikiloderma of Civatte and is a good way to gauge amount of sun exposure.

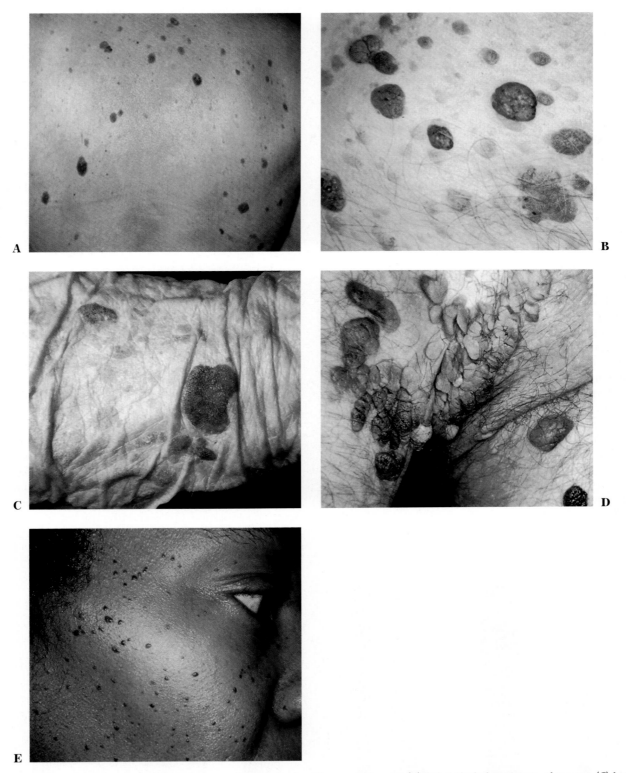

**FIGURE 42-5** ■ (**A**) Seborrheic keratoses over the back of a 71-year-old man. (**B**) Seborrheic keratoses, close-up. (**C**) Large seborrheic keratosis on the hand in an 84-year-old woman. (**D**) Multiple seborrheic keratoses of the crural area. (**E**) Seborrheic keratoses or dermatosis papulosa nigra on the face.

may be removed for cosmetic reasons, but the risk of keloid formation or hypopigmentation may outweigh the benefit.

Pedunculated fibromas (also known as acrochordons or skin tags) are extremely common on the neck and axilla. They are usually not a cause for concern and require no treatment unless they are inflamed or bothersome to the patient. Treatment options include cryotherapy or excision.

Benign vascular neoplasms, most notably cherry angiomas and venous lakes, occur in a significant proportion of elderly patients (see Chapter 27) and are typically found on the trunk, lips, and ears, respectively. Laser treatments have been used for these patients if lesions are cosmetically troublesome.

Sebaceous gland hyperplasia on the face is common. It is lobulated unlike most BCCs.

## Xerosis and Contact Dermatitis

Xerosis (**Fig. 42-6**), or dry skin, is characteristic of chronologically aged skin and can be attributed to intrinsic and extrinsic changes discussed earlier in this chapter. Dry skin can be asymptomatic or can present as irritation or pruritus, most commonly on the lower extremities and in winter (winter itch). Patients may also complain of drier mucous membranes. Should pruritus persist after xerosis is treated, it is important to consider an underlying systemic process, such as cutaneous T-cell lymphoma (CTCL) or a paraneoplastic syndrome. Biopsy can help. Generalized pruritus is discussed in more detail in Chapter 11.

Treatment of xerosis (**Table 42-1**) should include minimizing time spent immersed in water and avoidance of excess washing. In addition, we recommend using synthetic surfactant soaps, which are less drying, and limiting the application of soap to the hands, feet, face, groin, and axillae. Baths should be lukewarm, and harsh scrubbing should be discouraged. Fragrance-free and dye-free moisturizers should be applied immediately after bathing in order to minimize transepidermal water loss. Plain petroleum jelly ointment is effective if tolerated by the patient. Humectants containing ammonium lactate or urea are useful, especially in hyperkeratotic areas, but may sting if the area being treated is fissured or raw. Oral antihistamines may also be utilized with caution, due to their sedative effects, to relieve pruritus.

In elderly individuals, ACD (allergic contact dermatitis) is less common due to both decreased sensitization to new allergens and diminishing responses in previously sensitized patients. However, although the development of ACD may be delayed, the dermatitis may be more persistent once developed.

## Impaired Circulation and Ulcers

### Stasis Dermatitis

Stasis dermatitis (**Fig. 42-7**) is a common inflammatory skin condition of the calves and shins of middle-aged and elderly patients with chronic venous insufficiency and venous hypertension. It rarely occurs before the fifth decade of life. If a patient presents with stasis dermatitis before the fifth decade of life, the clinician should consider venous insufficiency secondary to trauma, surgery, or thrombosis. The prevalence of stasis dermatitis is 6% to 7% in patients over 50, and the risk steadily increases with age. In adults over 70, the prevalence of stasis dermatitis may be greater than 20%.

Patients with stasis dermatitis typically have a history of dependent leg edema resulting from comorbidities such as congestive heart failure or long-standing hypertension with diastolic dysfunction. A slight female prevalence has been reported, with some women experiencing earlier and more severe deterioration of lower extremity valvular function. This may be due to pregnancy-induced stress on the lower extremity venous system.

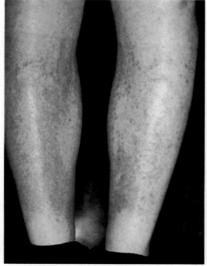
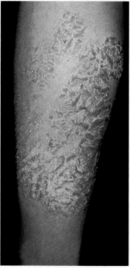
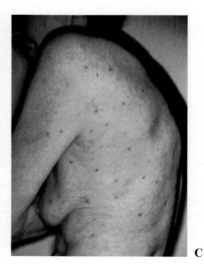

A     B     C

**FIGURE 42-6** ■ Xerosis. **(A)** Redness of winter itch on the legs. **(B)** Xerosis with secondary infection on the legs. *(Courtesy of Johnson & Johnson.)* **(C)** Senile pruritus in 74-year-old woman. *(Courtesy of Johnson & Johnson.)*

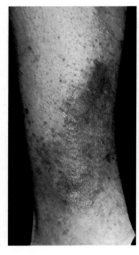 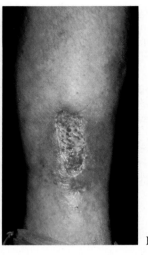

**FIGURE 42-7** ■ **(A)** Stasis dermatitis of the leg aggravated by contact allergy to neomycin. **(B)** Stasis ulcer of the leg with varicose veins.

Early stasis dermatitis typically presents as a gradual onset of pruritus affecting one or both lower extremities, sometimes accompanied by reddish-brown skin discoloration. In time, these early changes can progress to erythematous, swollen, scaling plaques. The medial ankle is most frequently and severely involved because of its relatively poor blood flow. Secondary bacterial or candidal infection can cause crusting. Lichenification, hyperpigmentation, edema, varicosities, atrophy, and induration can result from chronic scratching and rubbing. Severe chronic inflammation and thickening can lead to lipodermatosclerosis with its characteristic inverted champagne bottle appearance. The patient should be advised that these chronic changes generally persist despite treatment. The goal is generally to prevent worsening.

Treatment for stasis dermatitis focuses mainly on mitigating venous insufficiency. This involves leg elevation, compression stockings, elastic wraps, Unna boots, and/or end-diastolic compression boots. The patient's peripheral arterial circulation must be assessed before starting compression therapy because compressing a leg with compromised arterial circulation could cause claudication or even permanent ischemic damage.

In early stages, low-potency topical steroids and nonsteroidal calcineurin inhibitors (tacrolimus, pimecrolimus) can be helpful for reducing inflammation and pruritus in acute flares. However, high-potency topical corticosteroids carry risks of systemic absorption and steroid-induced atrophy.

Suspected cellulitis should always be treated with oral or intravenous antibiotics. Superficial bacterial infections should be cultured and may be treated empirically with topical mupirocin or an appropriate systemic antibiotic with activity against *Staphylococcus* and *Streptococcus* species. Alternatively they can be treated with wet-to-damp gauze dressings soaked with water or with a drying agent such as aluminum acetate, Domeboro, or a 1:1 water:white vinegar mix. Complications of chronic stasis dermatitis include increased incidences of allergic contact dermatitis, nonhealing lower extremity ulceration(s), cellulitis, lipodermatosclerosis, and id reactions on other parts of the body.

Allergic contact dermatitis commonly results from use of topical antibiotics such as neomycin and bacitracin. In addition, patients may become sensitized to rubber products found in some wraps and stockings. Topical corticosteroid allergy, while uncommon, should be considered when stasis dermatitis worsens despite seemingly appropriate prescription therapy. To minimize risk of allergies, patients with chronic but stable stasis dermatitis can be treated with bland topical emollients such as plain white petrolatum.

### Arterial Insufficiency

Manifestations of arterial insufficiency include erythema, local hair loss, ulcers, stellate scars, and atrophie blanche. Associated pain and gangrene are more common with arterial insufficiency than with venous insufficiency. Ulcers due to arterial insufficiency typically appear on the dorsal feet, toes, and lateral legs. Patients with diabetes are at an increased risk of complications. The treatment of ulcers due to arterial insufficiency should include consultation by a vascular surgeon and is beyond the scope of this chapter.

### Ulcers

As life expectancies have increased over the past several decades, the incidence of chronic venous leg ulcers, pressure ulcers, and diabetic ulcers in patients over 65 has steadily risen as well. Multifactorial age-related declines in skin repair and sensation can cause skin breakdown, which is then acerbated by excessive inflammatory responses, with associated proteolysis, vascular compromise, fibroblast dysfunction, and bacterial infection.

Pressure ulcers, sometimes misleadingly labeled decubitus ulcers or bedsores, occur most frequently in the buttocks and posterior heels of elderly and other bed-bound individuals. One and a half to three million Americans suffer from bedsores at an annual estimated cost of 3.6 billion dollars. As above, causes include poor circulation, decreased nerve sensation, skin atrophy, and the lack of strength, mobility, and mental capacity to turn oneself to redistribute pressure. Prophylactic measures are paramount. A bed-bound patient should be turned at least every 2 hours, and the bed needs to be kept clean and dry. Special cushion supporters and mattresses that can redistribute pressure are indicated. Surgical dressings such as Opsite, Duoderm, Tegaderm, and Polymem may be applied to incipient wounds. Vinegar soaks may be helpful in controlling potential bacterial infections, especially pseudomonas.

### Ulcer Colonization

Bacterial colonization of ulcers is common and does not impair wound healing or require treatment. For infected ulcers, silver sulfadiazine may increase the rate of healing. Before starting antibiotic treatment, a deep-tissue biopsy with quantitative cultures should be obtained during debridement. Do not use swabs of pus or necrotic tissue for culture results because these will only confirm surface contamination, not deep tissue infection. While awaiting results, one may begin empiric therapy for the most common organisms such as *S. aureus* and gram-negative bacilli (e.g., pseudomonas and anaerobes).

## Skin Infections

### Candidiasis

Although fungal infections are discussed in detail in Chapter 25, a brief summary is in order here. Candidiasis is the most common mycologic infection in the elderly, especially those who are obese, diabetic, debilitated, and/or chronic users of antibiotics. Debilitation can lead to increased bed rest and decreased cleansing, which greatly increases the risk. Cutaneous candidiasis typically crops up in the groin, inframammary folds, axillae, or inguinal areas. Treat with topical antifungal agents or with oral fluconazole if severe. Urinary and fecal incontinence can contribute to candidiasis, along with primary skin irritation and corrosion. Corrosion of skin due to urinary incontinence may require temporary use of an indwelling catheter.

### Onychomycosis

Onychomycosis is the major important and treatable change in the nails of the elderly. Onychomycosis increases with age, reaching 20% at 60 years with the great toenail, which is most commonly affected. Other risk factors include male gender, diabetes, smoking, family history, psoriasis, concurrent intake of immunosuppressive drugs, human immunodeficiency virus (HIV) infection, and peripheral vascular disease.

Dermatophytes are by far the most common cause of onychomycosis. Nondermatophyte molds can also be seen in the elderly (*Scopulariopsis brevicaulis, Hendersonula toruloidea, Scytalidium hyalinum*). *Scopulariopsis* tends to be found in conjunction with paronychia. This is of particular concern in immunocompromised patients, due to an associated increased risk of cellulitis.

Onychomycosis is difficult to treat permanently, especially in the elderly. Oral antifungals are notorious for having multiple drug interactions, and older individuals are more likely to be on multiple medications. Also, the metabolic capabilities in the elderly liver decline, making the medications less tolerable even without drug interactions.

Topical treatments are a safer alternative in the elderly and can work well even though onychomycosis is usually thought to be less easily treated than other superficial fungal infections. One safe and cheap method is application of Vicks VapoRub daily to the affected nails, including the base. Forty percent urea cream can be used as an adjunct, due to its keratolytic properties. The main disadvantage of this method is compliance, as complete clearance of an infection may take up to 16 months. However, a clear band of healthy nail has been seen in as little time as 2 months. Another topical treatment option is ciclopirox lacquer (Penlac). Ciclopirox has a broad range of antifungal activity as well as antibacterial and anti-inflammatory actions.

A simple but often overlooked issue in elderly patients, especially men, is foot hygiene. Many elderly patients have worn the same pair of occlusive shoes for literally decades. These shoes should be discarded.

Other common nail changes in the elderly include increased ridging and discoloration of the nail plate. Some patients with thinning nails may benefit from oral biotin supplementation.

### Scabies

*Sarcoptes scabiei* infection classically presents with excoriated papules on the flexor surfaces of wrists, interdigital webs, axillae, ankles, lower abdomen and back, pubic area, and perineum. Scabies transmission results mainly from close contact but can also occur via fomites. In chronic care facilities, vulnerability is usually limited to those with skin-to-skin contact such as health care workers. Although elderly persons who live independently can contract scabies, those in large care facilities are at a much higher risk. Scabies is often missed when itching is incorrectly attributed to dry skin or senile pruritus, especially in confused patients. In a 1-year Canadian study, 25% of surveyed institutions reported cases, with 11% reporting one or more infested health care workers. Mean number of infestations per outbreak was 18. All affected persons should be treated at the same time. Because of the large number of people involved, this can present a major management problem.

Elderly and immunocompromised patients are more likely to develop atypical presentations such as crusted scabies, also known as Norwegian scabies. This form can go unrecognized due to lack of itching and can spread. Norwegian scabies is associated with a much higher mite count: 2 million versus the more typical 10 to 15 mites per patient. Laboratory studies and treatments are the same as in normal adults and are discussed in detail in Chapter 17.

### Varicella-Zoster Virus

Viral skin infections are discussed in detail in Chapter 23. Varicella-zoster virus (Fig. 42-8), is mentioned here due to its elevated incidence of recurrence as herpes zoster (HZ) in the elderly. HZ has a lifetime prevalence of 10% to 20% and increases with age. Vaccination can help decrease morbidity and mortality of HZ. The Advisory Committee on Immunization Practices of the CDC (Centers for Disease Control and Prevention) recommends vaccination with the live attenuated virus (Zostavax) in adults over 60 years. Infections may be treated with a 7 to 10 day course of acyclovir, valacyclovir, and famciclovir. Treatment should start as soon as symptoms occur, preferably within 72 hours of onset. All three medications shorten the duration of acute pain, rash, viral shedding, and acute- and late-onset anterior horn complications.

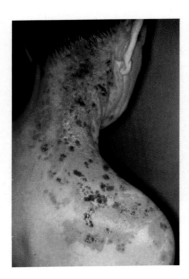

**FIGURE 42-8** ■ Herpes zoster of the shoulder and neck.

Twenty percent to forty percent of adults over age 60 develop neuropathic pain following HZ. This is termed "postherpetic neuralgia" or PHN. PHN can be severely debilitating and can last several months or years. Valacyclovir and famcyclovir decrease the incidence and severity of PHN, but they do not prevent it.

If PHN does occur, pain control is very important. One option is tricyclic antidepressants (TCAs). Nortriptyline and desipramine are relatively newer TCAs and are better choices for elderly patients than amitriptyline. The dose is generally 25 to 50 mg at bedtime, which is approximately half the dosage needed for antidepressant activity. Antiseizure medications have also been effective. These include gabapentin 600 mg two to six times daily and pregabalin 300 to 600 mg daily. These medications reduce the need for opioids and are synergistic with TCAs. Topical analgesics (5% lidocaine, lidocaine/prilocaine, capsaicin) can be added to any of the above treatments. In severe cases, opioids may be needed.

Postherpetic itch can be treated with antihistamines, but caution is advised when prescribing oral antihistamines to elderly patients as they are more likely to experience adverse reactions such as sedation, orthostatic hypotension, and urinary retention.

Several subtypes of HZ deserve special attention. Ophthalmic HZ involves the first division of the trigeminal nerve (CN V1). This branch is involved 20 times more often than CN V2 or V3. Ophthalmic HZ may lead to corneal scarring and secondary panophthalmitis with loss of vision. Characteristic signs include lesions on the tip of the nose (innervated by CN V1) and sensations of a foreign body in the eye. A second important subtype involves the facial nerve (CN VII), leading to Ramsay-Hunt syndrome, which can result in deafness. It can present with lesions in the external auditory meatus, pinna of the ear, and soft palate. This type is also associated with unilateral facial paralysis, aka Bell's palsy. A third important subtype of HZ is the disseminated form. Disseminated HZ involves more than three dermatomes or

more than 20 lesions outside of a single dermatome. It is more common in patients with lymphoproliferative disorders or advanced HIV. HZ can disseminate to internal organs leading to hepatitis, pneumonitis, meningoencephalitis, myelitis, or motor radiculopathy. All three of these important subtypes should be treated with IV acyclovir.

## Systemic Diseases with Cutaneous Manifestations

Cutaneous manifestations of systemic diseases, including malignancies, are discussed in Chapter 27. Some of these have aspects that are more common in elderly people.

### Metastatic Cancer

Only about 5% to 10% of patients with metastatic disease have cutaneous metastasis. Most of these are carcinomas. Of the cancers with cutaneous metastasis, lung cancer and breast cancer are the most common primary malignancies in men and women, respectively.

Metastases to the upper abdominal wall are usually from gastrointestinal (GI) tumors. Sister Mary Joseph nodule is a carcinoma metastasis to the umbilicus, most commonly from adenocarcinoma of the stomach. Lower abdominal wall metastases are more likely to be genitourinary (GU) tumors.

Cutaneous metastases are usually hard, fixed, subcutaneous or dermal nodules that may be of any color. Rarely, tumor cells may appear to have a zoster-like distribution due to perineural invasion. Ulceration is rare. The nodules may be solitary or multiple. A general rule is that any nodule with dermal or subcutaneous involvement of unknown origin should undergo biopsy. This is especially true if the nodules are hard or fixed.

### Paget's Disease

Paget's disease of the breast presents as a unilateral, pruritic, eczematous eruption of the nipple and areola indicative of underlying invasive ductal carcinoma or ductal carcinoma in situ.

### Signs of Internal Cancers

Internal cancers can present with cutaneous symptoms. These include paraneoplastic syndromes as well as other nonspecific lesions.

### Acanthosis Nigricans

Acanthosis nigricans (AN) is discussed in Chapter 38. It is characterized by pigmented velvety plaques on intertriginous areas and on the sides and nape of the neck. Acrochordons often arise within acanthotic plaques. AN can be caused by obesity, insulin resistance, or, less commonly, internal malignancy. Extensive AN has been linked with adenocarcinomas, particularly GI cancers. Severe AN may become verrucous and can be associated with papillomatous changes in the oral cavity.

The mechanism underlying AN is not yet known. An association with tumor-produced insulin-like growth factors

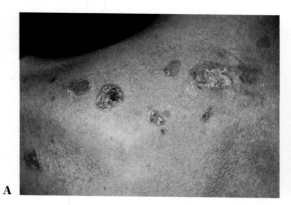
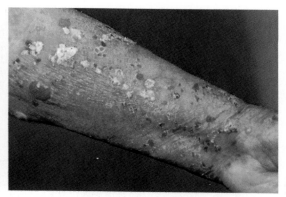

**FIGURE 42-9** ■ **(A)** Pemphigus vulgaris of the upper back area. **(B)** Pemphigus vulgaris of the forearm.

in the skin has been proposed. Another possible explanation is that elevated systemic transforming growth factor alpha (TGF-$\alpha$) induces epidermal growth factors, leading to acrochordons and AN. A similar explanation has been proposed for the sudden appearance of multiple rapidly growing seborrheic keratoses in the setting of an internal malignancy, also known as the sign of Leser–Trélat. The sign of Leser–Trélat is frequently seen along with malignancy-associated AN. However, both seborrheic keratoses and cancer are common in elderly people, so assessing the significance of Leser–Trélat is difficult.

### Clubbing

Fingertip clubbing may be associated with internal malignancy. Clubbing can be seen in 10% of patients with primary or metastatic lung cancer. This can also be seen in other pulmonary diseases. Clubbing is caused by subperiosteal bone formation of the phalangeal shaft. Associated symptoms such as joint swelling, synovitis, hyperhidrosis, and palmar erythema can mimic early rheumatoid arthritis.

### Dermatomyositis

Up to 25% of patients with adult-onset dermatomyositis have an internal malignancy. Dermatomyositis is most commonly associated with ovarian cancer, angiotropic lymphoma, urachal carcinoma, and prostate cancer. Cutaneous findings include heliotrope dermatitis, proximal nail fold telangiectasias, Gottron's papules, and cutaneous necrosis. An elevated erythrocyte sedimentation rate (ESR) is a common associated finding.

### Conditions Secondary to Cancer Treatment

In addition to skin conditions from active cancers, there are also changes that can occur as a result of prior cancer treatments. As cancer treatments become more effective and survivors live longer, the skin changes associated with these treatments are becoming increasingly common.

Radiodermatitis typically includes poikiloderma, telangiectasia, and atrophy. A more concerning symptom is non-healing ulceration. The increased risk of SCC in irradiated

skin makes regular skin examination important for these patients.

Radiation-induced morphea has been reported in breast cancer survivors. It is important to rule out recurrence of cancer with a biopsy. Morphea can be treated with local steroid injections, psoralens and ultraviolet A (PUVA), or UVA-1. Efficacy, however, is variable. The mechanism of action underlying PUVA may involve a reduction in cytokine activity, including TGF-$\beta$, which is a stimulator of fibroblast activity. If these less invasive therapies do not offer improvement, reconstructive plastic surgery can help reduce morphea-associated pain and disfiguration. Chapter 37 gives a more detailed description of morphea.

## Other Noteworthy Skin Issues in the Elderly

Other notable diseases that present more commonly in the elderly include pemphigus vulgaris (Fig. 42-9) and bullous pemphigoid (Fig. 42-10). These are discussed further in Chapter 18.

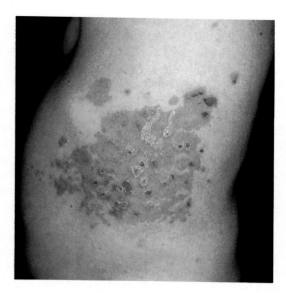

**FIGURE 42-10** ■ Pemphigoid on the lateral abdominal area.

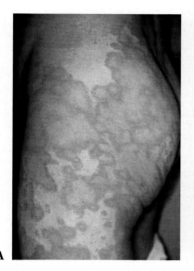 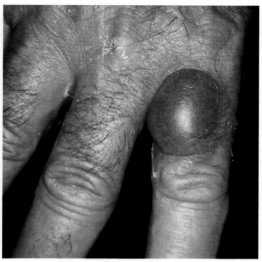

**FIGURE 42-11** ■ **(A)** Drug eruption from phenacetin. **(B)** Fixed bullous drug eruption due to tetracycline. *(Courtesy of Johnson & Johnson.)*

It is important to remember that elderly patients are often on many medications, some of which have cutaneous side effects (Fig. 42-11). Medications that increase photosensitivity are reviewed in Chapter 39. Photosensitizers especially relevant to the elderly include diuretics, nonsteroidal anti-inflammatory drugs (NSAIDS), phenothiazines, and antiarrhythmics. It is important to ask about blood thinners, as these can affect procedures performed in the office as well as contribute to easy bruising. Blood thinners, particularly warfarin, also have a number of drug interactions.

Changes in hair occur throughout life. Hair is discussed in detail in Chapter 32. Most older people experience a change in hair color, with eventual transition to gray or pure white. Male pattern alopecia can begin as early as late adolescence and tends to be progressive. Elderly patients who have not suffered typical male pattern alopecia often show a youthful hairline with diffuse thinning of scalp hair. This so-called senile alopecia can occur in both men and women. Diffuse hair loss also occurs in the axilla and pubic area. Excess facial hair is common in elderly women and can require treatment. Shaving facial hair blunts the otherwise tapered visible tip of the hair, but does not cause increased hair density or thickness.

Some conditions are seen less frequently in the elderly. These include atopic dermatitis, acne, pityriasis rosea, impetigo, syphilis, herpes simplex, warts, exanthems, chloasma, and sunburns. If acne is present, the patient should be asked about testosterone intake and corticosteroid drugs. Seborrheic dermatitis can become less bothersome with age but can worsen following a stroke or in the presence of Parkinson's disease.

## Suggested Readings

Brennan M, Bhatti H, Nerusu KC, et al. Matrix metalloproteinase-1 is the major collagenolytic enzyme responsible for collagen damage in UV-irradiated human skin. *Photochem Photobiol.* 2003;78(1):43–48.

Dancey AL, Waters RA. Morphea of the breast. Two case reports and discussion of the literature. *J Plast Reconstr Aesthet Surg.* 2006;59:1114–1117.

El-Mofty M, Mostafa W, Esmat S, et al. Suggested mechanisms of action of UVA phototherapy in morphea: a molecular study. *Photodermatol Photoimmunol Photomed.* 2004;20:93–100.

Feldser DM, Greider CW. Short telomeres limit tumor progression in vivo by inducing senescence. *Cancer Cell.* 2007;11:461–469.

Fisher G, Kang S, Varani J, et al. Mechanisms of photoaging and chronological skin aging. *Arch Dermatol.* 2002;138:1462–1470.

Geller AM, Zenick H. Aging and the environment: a research framework. *Environ Health Perspect.* 2005;113:1257–1262.

Gip L, Molin L. Skin diseases in geriatrics. *Cutis.* 1970;6:771.

Gonsalves WC, Chi AC, Neville BW. Common oral lesions: part I. Superficial mucosal lesions. *Am Fam Physician.* 2007;75:501–507.

Hall G, Phillips TJ. Estrogen and skin: the effects of estrogen, menopause, and hormone replacement therapy on the skin. *J Am Acad Dermatol.* 2005;53(4):555–568.

Harpaz R, Ortega-Sanchez IR, Seward JF. Prevention of herpes zoster. Recommendations of the Advisory Committee on Immunization Practices. *MMWR Recomm Rep.* 2008;57:1–30.

Hocker T, Tsao H. Ultraviolet radiation and melanoma: a systematic review and analysis of reported sequence variants. *Hum Mutat.* 2007;28(6):578–588.

Jones KR, Fennie K, Lenihan A. Evidence-based management of chronic wounds. *Adv Skin Wound Care.* 2007;20:591–600.

Jucgla A, Sais G, Berlanga J, et al. Hyperpigmentation of the flexures and pancytopenia during treatment with folate antagonists. *Acta Derm Venereol.* 1997;77(2):165–166.

Kaufman SC. Anterior segment complications of herpes zoster opthalmamicus. *Opthalmology.* 2008;115:S24–S32.

Kwangsukstith C, Maibach HI. Effect of age and sex on the induction and elicitation of allergic contact dermatitis. *Contact Dermatitis.* 1995;33(5):289–298.

Lambert EM, Dziura J, Kauls L, et al. Yellow nail syndrome in three siblings: a randomized double-blind trial of topical vitamin E. *Pediatr Dermatol.* 2006;23(4):390–395.

Lowe NJ, Meyers DP, Wieder JM, et al. Low doses of repetitive ultraviolet A induce morphologic changes in human skin. *J Invest Dermatol.* 1995;105(6):739–743.

Maldonado F, Tazelaar HD, Wang CW, et al. Yellow nail syndrome: analysis of 41 consecutive patients. *Chest.* 2008;134(2):375–381.

Mori K, Ando I, Kukita A. Generalized hyperpigmentation of the skin due to vitamin B12 deficiency. *J Dermatol.* 2001;28(5):282–285.

Nishimura EK, Granter SR, Fisher DE. Mechanisms of hair graying: incomplete melanocyte stem cell maintenance in the niche. *Science.* 2005;307(5710):720–724.

O'Donnell JA, Hofmann MT. Skin and soft tissues: management of four common infections in nursing home patients. *Geriatrics.* 2001;56:33–38.

Pavan-Langston D. Herpes Zoster. Antivirals and pain management. *Opthalmology.* 2008;115:S13–S20.

Penn I, First MR. Merkel's cell carcinoma in organ recipients: report of 41 cases. *Transplantation.* 1999;68(11):1717–1721.

Perrem K, Lynch A, Conneely M, et al. The higher incidence of squamous cell carcinoma in renal transplant recipients is associated with increased telomere lengths. *Hum Pathol.* 2007;38(2):351–358.

Ramsewak RS, Nair MG, Stommel M, et al. In vitro antagonistic activity of monoterpenes and their mixtures against 'toe nail fungus' pathogens. *Phytother Res.* 2003;17(4):376–379.

Rostan EF. Laser treatment of photodamaged skin. *Facial Plast Surg.* 2005;21(2):99–109.

Sato S. Iron deficiency: structural and microchemical changes in hair, nails, and skin. *Semin Dermatol.* 1991;10(4):313–319.

Scheinfeld N. Infections in the elderly. *Dermatol. Online J.* 2005;11:8.

Sinclair R. There is no clear association between low serum ferritin and chronic diffuse telogen hair loss. *Br J Dermatol.* 2002;147(5): 982–984.

Singh G, Haneef NS, Uday A. Nail changes and disorders among the elderly. *Indian J Dermatol Venereol Leprol.* 2005;71(6):386–392.

Stone SP, Buescher LS. Life-threatening paraneoplastic cutaneous syndromes. *Clin Dermatol.* 2005;23:301–306.

Tanaka K, Hasegawa J, Asamitsu K, et al. Prevention of the ultraviolet B-mediated skin photoaging by a nuclear factor kappaB inhibitor, parthenolide. *J Pharmacol Exp Ther.* 2005;315(2):624–630.

Theirs BH. Dermatologic manifestations of internal cancer. *CA Cancer J Clin.* 1986;36:130–148.

Vaziri H, Benchimol S. From telomere loss to p53 induction and activation of a DNA-damage pathway at senescence: the telomere loss/DNA-damage model of cell aging. *Exp Gerontol.* 1996;31:295–301.

Vorou R, Remoudaki HD, Maltezou HC. Nosocomial scabies. *J Hosp Infect.* 2007;65:9–14.

Wenk J, Schüller J, Hinrichs C, et al. Overexpression of phospholipid-hydroperoxide glutathione peroxidase in human dermal fibroblasts abrogates UVA irradiation-induced expression of interstitial collagenase/matrix metalloproteinase-1 by suppression of phosphatidylcholine hydroperoxide-mediated NFkappaB activation and interleukin-6 release. *J Biol Chem.* 2004;279(44):45634–45642.

# CHAPTER 43

# Obesity and Dermatology

*Noah S. Scheinfeld, JD, MD*

Obesity is defined as a weight or mass that exceeds the ideal weight or body mass index (BMI). A normal BMI is considered to be between 18.5 and 25. Overweight is defined by a BMI of 25 to 30. Obesity class I is defined by a BMI of 30 to 35, obesity class II is a BMI of 35 to 40, and obesity class III is defined as a BMI of 40 and above. The excess mass associated with obesity impacts and is related to several body systems that include (1) the cutaneous system and its subsystems (a) the epidermal system, (b) the follicular system, and (c) the adipose system; (2) the cardiovascular system; (3) the endocrine system; and (4) the nervous system. This review will assess the impact of obesity based on its effects on these systems.

## The Cutaneous System

### Obesity Leads to Alterations of Body Shape

Obesity alters foot shape and induces plantar hyperkeratosis, which should be considered a cutaneous stigma of morbid obesity. Weight can generate physical changes in the foot structure of children with lower footprint angles and a higher Chippaux-Smirak index. Obesity increases forefoot width and causes higher plantar pressure during standing and walking in both children and adults.

### Obesity Leads to Alterations of the Texture of the Skin

The main alterations to the texture of the skin involve the development of acanthosis nigricans, skin tags, striae, lymphedema, and stasis dermatitis. The changes in skin texture related to obesity can be due to etiologies other than obesity but are more common in the obese as compared with the general population.

#### Acanthosis Nigricans

Acanthosis nigricans (Fig. 43-1) is a cutaneous condition affecting localized areas of the skin (especially intertiginous areas in the axillary, inguinal and inframmary areas) under skin tags and then may disappear after pregnancy. It is commonly described as manifesting as brown velvety plaques on the skin. Other causes and relationships of acanthosis nigricans include malignancy and diabetes. Acanthosis nigricans can be associated with rare genetic syndromes.

Hyperpigmentation and apparent thickening of the skin correlate with histologic papillomatosis, and the apparent darkening is due to hyperkeratosis. The mechanistic basis of acanthosis nigricans includes (1) high levels of circulating insulin, (2) insulin resistance in keratinocytes, (3) stimulation of insulin-like growth factor (IGF) receptors in keratinocytes by insulin, and (4) IGF receptor induction of keratinocyte proliferation.

#### Skin Tags

Skin tags or acrochordons are common in patients who are obese. It is likely that this is due in large part to the association of skin tags with diabetes. Other conditions associated with skin tags include Birt–Hogg–Dube syndrome. Skin tags can arise during pregnancy but then disappear afterward. Some have stated that independent of diabetes, skin tags are not associated with obesity.

#### Striae

The tension of stretched skin results in the development of striae. While many patients who are obese have striae, not all patients who have striae are obese. Pregnancy and the growth spurt of adolescence can result in striae. The striae of pregnancy and obesity are usually permanent, while the striae related to growth spurts are sometimes transient.

The striae of obesity arise along cleavage lines perpendicular to the direction of greatest tension in areas with the most adipose tissue—the breasts, buttocks and lateral

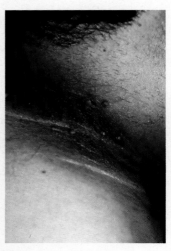

**FIGURE 43-1** ■ Acanthosis nigricans and skin tags on the side of the neck.

abdomen, and thighs. Striae are characterized by linear, smooth bands of atrophic-appearing skin that are sometimes initially erythematous, then purple, and finally white and depressed. Striae seem to be a type of dermal scarring with an aberrant healing response and replacement of collagen. Histologically, striae are marked by densely packed areas of thin, eosinophilic, collagen bundles, horizontal to the surface in a parallel fashion and lacking rete pegs, adnexal structures, and normal dermal undulations. In addition, hair follicles and other appendages are absent in striae.

### Lymphedema

Lymphedema manifests with pebbly skin on the legs. Due to the changes in circulation resulting in changes to the texture of the skin, lymphedema will be considered here and in the section on the cardiovascular system. Lymphedema is also referred to as elephantiasis nostra verrucosa (ENV). ENV and lymphedema can also occur due to the presence of parasites as is the case in filariasis, which obstructs the lymphatic vessels.

Lymphedema most commonly manifests on the shins and results from poor lymphatic return. Its etiology involves lymph accumulation and dilation of lymphatics. The initial manifestation is soft, pitting edema. The process can be furthered by recurrent bacterial lymphangitis and obstruction of the major lymphatic vessels. There can be hyperkeratosis and papillomas in the plaques of lymphedema.

### Stasis Dermatitis

Stasis dermatitis (**Fig. 43-2**) involves changes in circulation that result in changes in the texture of the skin and will be considered briefly here and in the section on cardiovascular

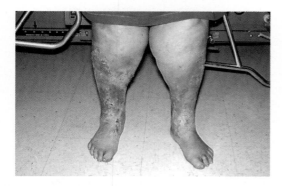

**FIGURE 43-2** ■ Stasis dermatitis.

disease. Stasis dermatitis manifests as brown-red scaly patches and plaques, most commonly on the shins. It is thought to occur due to decreases in the microcirculation that result from obesity, peripheral vascular disease, diabetes and coronary artery disease, and hyperlipidemia.

### Obesity Impairs the Integrity of the Skin

Loss of skin integrity leads to an increase in infections involving the skin and to dermatoses secondary to the breakdown of the skin itself. Changes involving the impairment of epidermal integrity are most pronounced in the skin folds. They are due to friction and other complex effects (neural changes, tension, pressure-related changes, etc.). Infections that are related to changes in epidermal integrity include cutaneous candidiasis (including erosio interdigitalis blastomycetica, candidal folliculitis, and tinea cruris). Vascular disease, diabetes mellitus, and obesity all play a role in the development of these infections.

### Intertrigo

Intertrigo is a common complication of the impairment of the integrity of skin that obesity causes. It occurs due to a combination of irritation and infection that results in an inflammatory dermatosis involving the body folds. There are more and deeper skin folds in obese patients. Factors that predispose obese patients to intertrigo include friction, maceration, moisture and warmth, sweating, and occlusion. Colonization of the skin and intertriginous areas with bacteria, yeast, and dermatophytes may exacerbate the intertrigo. Candidal colonization and infection is the most common pathogenic factor. Intertrigo manifests in the area below the abdominal pannus and in the genitocrural, subaxillary, gluteal, and submammary skin folds. Patients often complain of pruritus, irritation, and burning in areas where intertrigo manifests.

### Predisposition toward Traumatic Injury

The skin in obese individuals has a predisposition toward traumatic injury. There is an increase in the amount and severity of ulceration and tears in the skin of obese patients, particularly when they are hospitalized. Skin and wound problems that are common, yet more difficult to manage for obese patients, include pressure ulcers, decubitus ulcers, tracheostomy care (potentially resulting from ventilatory insufficiency), candidiasis, tape-related skin tears, incontinence, and lymphedema. Obesity increases the risk of skin breakdown because of immobility caused by underlying disease processes, sedation, improperly sized rooms and equipment, and inadequate staff numbers or staff who lack training in caring for such patients. These dermatoses of obesity often result from the caregiver's inability to mobilize the patient because of improperly sized rooms, inadequate staffing to rotate the patients, and inappropriate equipment (e.g., the lack of air beds). Obesity also appears to inhibit wound healing.

## The Follicular System

Obesity impacts the follicular system. Hidradenitis suppurativa is a recurrent, suppurative disease manifested by abscesses, fistulas, and scarring. Obesity is associated with hidradenitis suppurativa. The cause of hidradenitis is not certain, but some cases are related to genetic defects, in which case obesity is less of a factor in its development. The obese can expect to have a higher incidence of infections involving the hair follicle such as furunculosis, folliculitis, and carbunculosis.

## The Adipose and Fascial Systems

Alterations and increases in the quantity of adipose tissue are present in the obese and result in dermatoses. Important changes in the adipose system include cellulite and the appearance of the so-called buffalo hump associated with the use of corticosteroids. Other pathology involving the adipose and fascial systems include an increased risk of infection in the adipose and fascia associated with obesity (and its partner, diabetes). Dercum's disease (adiposis dolorosa) occurs in obese women and manifests with symmetrical, painful, circumscribed fatty deposits that can occur with weakness and psychiatric disturbances.

### Cellulite

Cellulite manifests as dimpled skin on the thighs of women. It is related to changes in the epidermis and dermis rather than the adipose tissue. It occurs on the thighs and buttocks of women who in most cases have no health problems and in some women who are not obese. It is rarely, if ever, noted in men.

Cellulite is thought to involve a multistep process. Incipient cellulite, identified by the mattress phenomenon, is related to the presence of focally enlarged fibrosclerotic strands partitioning the subcutis. Such strands possibly serve as a physiologic buttress against fat herniation, limiting the outpouching of fat lobules upon pinching of the skin. These structures might represent a reactive process to sustained hypodermal pressure caused by fat accumulation. Pronounced cases of cellulite likely involve a decrease in connective tissue growth in the face of progressive fat accumulation.

### Infections Involving the Adipose and Fascia

Infections involving the adipose and fascial systems in obese patients result in increases in the incidence of infectious cellulitis, gas gangrene, and necrotizing fasciitis relative to patients of normal weight.

## Medications, Obesity, and the Skin

Several medications can result in a redistribution of adipose tissue. The most important of these are oral corticosteroids, which induce Cushing's syndrome. Indinavir can cause a buffalo hump and diffuse lipomatosis. Many psychotropic medications such as selective serotonin reuptake inhibitors (SSRIs), atypical antipsychotics (e.g., risperidone), haloperidol, and anticonvulsants also can cause weight gain. Warfarin-induced skin necrosis is a condition related to a hypercoagulable state that occurs in patients started on warfarin who have deficiencies in protein C, protein S, and others. Warfarin-induced skin necrosis occurs most commonly on the breast, buttocks, and lateral thighs, with a ratio of women to men of 9:1.

## The Cardiovascular System

Obesity impairs the vascular supply. Changes associated with the cardiovascular system can result in pathology of the skin that includes stasis dermatitis, lipodermatosclerosis, varicose veins, lymphedema, and leg ulcerations. Obesity is associated with exaggerated blood pressure and systemic vascular resistance responses to stress. Normotensive obese patients demonstrate markedly impaired muscle and skin microcirculatory responses to stress. The increased propensity of obese individuals to develop hypertension under conditions of chronic stress may underlie obesity-related hypertension and cardiovascular disease.

### Leg Ulcerations

Leg ulcerations and varicose veins are more common in obese individuals than normal controls (although underlying peripheral vascular disease and coronary artery disease can cause leg ulcerations and varicose veins in patients of normal weight). The leg ulcerations of obesity can be a frequent consequence of the venous insufficiency associated with obesity. Leg ulcerations and varicose veins can be due in part to mechanical obstruction and valvular incompetence. Leg ulcerations can be associated with stasis dermatitis and occur most commonly on the lower leg. Such leg ulcerations can be due to the combination effects of obesity, venous insufficiency, and diabetes.

### Lipodermatosclerosis, Lymphedema, and Stasis Dermatitis

Decreases in the effectiveness of the circulatory system that correlate with obesity can result in lipodermatosclerosis, lymphedema, and stasis dermatitis. That is, while not all patients with lipodermatosclerosis and stasis dermatitis are obese, they are more likely to be obese. Lipodermatosclerosis results in inverse champagne bottle legs and hardened skin. The clinical appearance of stasis dermatitis and lymphedema was discussed previously. The stress put on the lymphatics by obesity and resultant impairment of the lymph valves underlies the development of lymphedema in the obese.

## The Endocrine System

Several changes in the endocrine system are associated with obesity. In particular, alterations of the insulin, adrenal, and thyroid systems can result in obesity and concomitant pathology of the skin.

## Insulin Resistance

The most important association of the endocrine system and obesity is diabetes. The increase of insulin levels and decreased cellular sensitivity to insulin increases the incidence of obesity and results in pathology such as acanthosis nigricans. Diabetes and obesity share many dermatoses in common as they occur together and are caused by and related to similar factors.

## Adrenal Insufficiency

Cushing's syndrome due to adrenal insufficiency is associated with centripetal obesity, moon facies, buffalo hump, supraclavicular fat pads, and abdominal striae. Cushing's syndrome can be endogenous due to internal suppression of the hypothalamic–pituitary–adrenal axis (HPA), resulting from pituitary basophilic tumors with adrenal cortical hyperplasia, or exogenous due to administration of corticosteroids. In endogenous cases, women are affected four times more frequently than men, with usual onset in the twenties and thirties. Cushing's disease refers to one specific cause, a non-cancerous tumor (adenoma) in the pituitary gland that produces large amounts of ACTH, which in turn elevates cortisol. Testing utilizes the dexamethasone suppression test. Obesity can be treated with liposuction.

## Hypothyroidism

Hypothyroidism is a result of a decrease in circulating thyroid hormone or rarely peripheral resistance to hormonal action. Its dermatologic manifestations include dry skin, obesity, macroglossia, swollen lips, cold hands and feet, brittle nails, and a mucinosis of the skin called myxedema. There can be a reduction of the basal metabolic rate. Hypothyroidism can respond to treatment with thyroid hormone, with a resultant resolution of the cutaneous findings.

# The Nervous System

The presence of adipose tissue affects sensitivity to pressure, pain, and temperature. Persons with extra adipose tissue have a higher pain sensitivity threshold than normal weight controls. This decreased sensitivity to pain can underlie the development of distal and pressure ulcers in obese persons. The older a person is, the higher pain sensitivity threshold. As obesity and diabetes often go hand in hand, the neuropathic changes of diabetes, tropic ulcers of the foot, are best considered alterations of the nervous system due to obesity.

## Temperature Regulation

The presence of adipose tissue alters temperature regulation. In anesthetized patients, body temperature decreases often, but overweight patients become less hypothermic. Adipose tissue insulates the body from a loss of body heat, and thermoregulatory reflexes may maintain normothermia in obese patients. It appears that core temperature is maintained in obese patients because their vasoconstriction threshold to a low environmental temperature is high. During cold application after injury, there is a clinically important direct relationship between adipose thickness and required cooling time that necessitates a longer cold application.

# Conclusion

This systemic approach toward obesity demonstrates the wide impact and systemic effects that obesity has on the skin. Obesity can be seen as a stressor on the skin that affects all aspects of the skin's structure including its vasculature, its nervous system, and its follicular system. As obesity is a worldwide problem whose incidence is increasing, dermatologists and generalists alike will have to assess and treat obesity-related pathology of the skin.

# Suggested Readings

Garcia Hidalgo L. Dermatological complications of obesity. *Am J Clin Dermatol.* 2002;3(7):497–506.

Scheinfeld NS. Obesity and dermatology. *Clin Dermatol.* 2004;22(4): 303–309.

Yosipovitch G, DeVore A, Dawn A. Obesity and the skin: skin physiology and skin manifestations of obesity. *J Am Acad Dermatol.* 2007;56(6): 901–916; quiz 917–920. Review.

# CHAPTER 44

# Skin Disease in Transplant Patients

*E.B. Olasz, MD, PhD and M. Neuburg, MD*

## Introduction

Since the first successful cadaver kidney transplant in 1962, the field of solid organ transplantation has undergone a remarkable journey, resulting in an ever-growing number of transplantations and increased transplant and recipient survival. The success of transplant survival is built on the advances in our understanding of physiology, immunology, improved surgical techniques, more efficient immunosuppressive treatments, and the multidisciplinary care of solid organ transplant recipients (OTRs). Longer recipient survival has led to an increased understanding of the consequences of long-term immunosuppression. Potent immunosuppressive drugs allow for long-term organ and patient survival. However, these drugs have numerous side effects, many of which manifest on the skin. These include direct effects from the individual drugs, immune-mediated effects from the grafted organ, and indirect effects of acute and chronic immunosuppression such as opportunistic infections and an increased incidence of skin cancers. The recognition of the accelerated and accentuated cutaneous carcinogenesis and the increased risk for cutaneous infections in OTRs opened the field of transplant dermatology. In 2001 the International Transplant Skin-Cancer Collaborative (ITSCC) was formed, joined by its European counterpart Skin Cancer in Organ Transplant Patients, Europe (SCOPE), in an effort to educate and care for the growing number of OTRs. The following sections outline the broad scope of skin diseases observed in OTRs.

### SAUER'S NOTES

1. Transplant patients will continue to increase in the foreseeable future and dermatologists need to help meet the challenge of their complex care.
2. Infections of the skin tend to be associated with less common organisms, to be more aggressive, and to be more recalcitrant to therapy.
3. Malignancies of the skin tend to be more common, more aggressive, and more apt to recur.
4. The skin is the window to other organ systems of the body. In this challenging group of patients, "this window" needs to be used to detect systemic infections and malignancies.

## Epidemiology

According to the United Network for Organ Sharing, over 28,000 solid organ transplants are performed in the United States each year and 74,000 worldwide. Approximately 250,000 solid OTRs are alive in the United States today, while over 90,000 people await transplantation. The overall five-year survival rate has steadily increased in the past 10 years, reaching 80% to 90% in kidney, 72% to 86% in liver, 70% in cardiac, and 42% in lung transplant recipients.

## Cutaneous Effects of Immunosuppressive Medications

The cutaneous adverse effects of commonly used immunosuppressive agents are detailed in the following text and summarized in Table 44-1.

**TABLE 44-1 ■ Cutaneous Adverse Effects of Commonly Used Immunosuppressive Agents**

| Drug | Common Cutaneous Side Effects |
|---|---|
| Corticosteroids | Cushing syndrome<br>Acne<br>Striae<br>Fragile skin |
| Cyclosporine | Hirsutism<br>Sebaceous hyperplasia<br>Gingival hyperplasia<br>Gynecomastia |
| Tacrolimus | Alopecia |
| Azathioprine | Hypersensitivity reaction |
| Mycophenolate Mofetil | Nonspecific eruptions<br>Acne |
| Sirolimus | Impaired wound healing<br>Acne/folliculitis<br>Edema |

Modified from Otley CC, Stasko T. *Skin Disease in Organ Transplantation*. New York: Cambridge University Press; 2008.

## Corticosteroids

### Cushing Syndrome

Cushing syndrome is caused by the administration of excess glucocorticoids as part of an OTR patient's immunosuppressive regimen. The patient may have any of the following typical physical stigmata: moon facies, facial plethora, supraclavicular fat pads, buffalo hump, truncal obesity, and purple striae. Individuals often complain of proximal muscle weakness, easy bruising, weight gain, hirsutism, and impaired wound healing. Reduction or discontinuation of glucocorticoid therapy should be managed by, or in conjunction with, the transplant physician due to the risks of (1) steroid withdrawal syndrome, (2) organ rejection, and (3) possible suppression of HPA axis with secondary adrenal insufficiency.

### Steroid Acne

Steroid acne presents with monomorphous, erythematous papules and pustules that appear relatively abruptly on the upper trunk, often sparing the face. The monomorphous nature and abrupt appearance distinguish steroid acne from acne vulgaris, which typically has a slower onset and is composed of acneiform lesions in different stages of development, usually involving the face. Cysts and comedones are common in acne vulgaris.

**Treatment.** In addition to the traditional treatments of acne vulgaris, including benzoyl peroxide wash or gel, topical or oral antibiotics, and topical retinoids, reduction of offending oral steroids, if possible, may have good results in treating steroid acne. Commonly, pityrosporum folliculitis is a cofactor in the development of steroid acne; therefore, treatment with appropriate topical antifungals should also be considered.

### Striae

Striae rubra distensae are linear bands of atrophic, cigarette paper-like skin, which are originally red and indurated, later becoming hypopigmented and atrophic. These may be widely distributed, especially over the abdomen, lower back, buttocks, and thighs.

**Treatment.** In the early erythematous stage, pulsed-dye laser has been shown to be somewhat helpful. After striae reach the late atrophic stage, treatment is very difficult. Topical retinoids, cryotherapy, and ablative laser resurfacing have been used with inconsistent results.

### Cutaneous Fragility and Ecchymosis

The skin may become thin and fragile. Spontaneous tearing may occur with trivial trauma. Purpura and ecchymoses are most commonly located on the dorsal forearms and dorsal hands. Avoidance of shearing trauma on the dorsal hands and forearms may help prevent the ecchymoses. Adhesive bandages should be removed with extreme care as skin may tear.

## Cyclosporine

### Hypertrichosis

Hypertrichosis is a cosmetically undesirable dose-dependent side effect of cyclosporine therapy, characterized by excessive hair growth not localized to the androgen-dependent areas of the body. It appears months after initiation of cyclosporine therapy in about 75% of patients. The cessation of cyclosporine therapy results in a progressive resolution of hypertrichosis. Laser-assisted hair removal or switching to tacrolimus may improve the hypertrichosis.

### Sebaceous Hyperplasia

Sebaceous hyperplasia is a well-known side effect of cyclosporine therapy, presenting within several years after starting treatment. About 10% to 15% of patients taking cyclosporine develop multiple small, yellowish umbilicated papules measuring 2 to 6 mm located usually on the central face. However, ectopic sites such as the oral mucosa may be affected as well. These lesions are benign but can be cosmetically bothersome to patients. Electrosurgery, laser treatment, shave excision, and photodynamic therapy (PDT) have been employed to treat sebaceous hyperplasia.

### Gingival Hyperplasia

Gingival overgrowth affects 30% to 50% of patients. It is first observed approximately 3 months following the initiation of cyclosporine therapy. Topical or systemic azithromycin may induce marked improvement. In some cases, periodontal surgery may be necessary. In addition, changing cyclosporine to tacrolimus has been reported to improve this condition.

## Tacrolimus

### Alopecia

Tacrolimus-induced hair loss presents in about 29% of patients as widespread hair thinning, occurring at a mean of 30 to 422 days after initiating tacrolimus. Rapid reversal of alopecia has been reported with the use of minoxidil. Reducing the dose of tacrolimus or switching to cyclosporine is helpful.

## Azathioprine

Azathioprine (AZA) has been reported to cause cutaneous hypersensitivity reactions including urticarial, maculopapular, and vasculitic eruptions. Less commonly reported side effects are mucositis, photosensitivity, and increased susceptibility to verrucae, herpes zoster, and Norwegian scabies. In addition, AZA has been shown in laboratory models to have direct carcinogenic effects.

## Mycophenolate Mofetil

Nonspecific cutaneous eruptions have been reported in 8% to 22% of patients on mycophenolate mofetil (MMF). Acne and peripheral edema, as well as exacerbation of dyshidrotic eczema, have been linked to MMF therapy.

## Sirolimus

### Infections and Pilosebaceous Eruptions

Infections and acne-like eruptions are common cutaneous side effects of sirolimus. More specifically, 34% of patients developed viral infections, 4% developed bacterial, and 16% of patients developed fungal infections. With predominance in men, inflammatory eruptions resembling acne were noted in 46% of renal transplant patients on sirolimus. Scalp folliculitis and hidradenitis suppurativa, as well as other skin eruptions resembling seborrheic dermatitis involving almost every body part, have also been reported. Topical and systemic antibiotics, benzoyl peroxide, and topical or systemic retinoids are recommended.

### Edema

Chronic edema, mainly affecting the lower legs (98%) was noted in more than half of OTRs (65%) treated with sirolimus. In some patients, upper extremity edema or angioedema involving the face and oral cavity was observed. The exact mechanism of sirolimus-induced edema is unknown, but it is thought to be due to vasculitis, lymphatic obstruction, or capillary obstruction. Sirolimus-induced edema is often resistant to diuretics; therefore, dietary restrictions, blood pressure control, and compression therapy are advised. Discontinuation of the inciting drug is often necessary. Depending on the severity of angioedema, airway support, antihistamines, glucocorticoids, and epinephrine may be required.

### Impaired Wound Healing

Sirolimus has been found to cause delayed wound healing, wound dehiscence, and superficial and deep wound fluid collections. The mechanism of impaired wound healing has been shown to be due to the inhibitory effect of sirolimus on fibroblast and endothelial cells through the blockade of growth factors, leading to anti-angiogenesis. Appropriate medical or surgical wound care, drainage of seromas, and in severe cases discontinuation of the drug are necessary. Temporary use of alternate immunosuppressive agents in anticipation of elective surgery is advised.

## Cutaneous Effects of the Transplanted Organ

### Graft Versus Host Disease (GVHD)

Although GVHD is most frequently associated with bone marrow or stem cell transplantation, it is also a rare but severe complication of solid organ transplantation. Transplanted solid organs contain a variable amount of lymphoid tissue, enabling the allografts to function as a mini bone marrow transplant and initiate an immunologically mediated and injurious set of reactions by cells genetically disparate to their host. In OTRs, GVHD is seen most frequently after liver transplantation, but the incidence of GVHD is highest after small bowel transplantation (about 5%), possibly owing to a large number of donor lymphocytes present in the gut. Risk factors for developing GVHD in liver transplant recipients include age greater than 65, closely matched HLA recipients, and a donor more than 40 years younger than the recipient.

The diagnosis of acute GVHD is established by clinical judgment, imaging studies, laboratory workup, and biopsy results. Skin involvement often precedes hepatic (except in liver transplant patients), hematologic, or gastrointestinal symptoms and presents from 2 days to 6 weeks post-transplant with an erythematous maculopapular eruption. The eruption has a predilection for the palms and soles and in severe cases can progress to generalized erythema with bullae and desquamation, often making it difficult to distinguish it from a severe drug eruption. Skin biopsy and the presence of other systemic symptoms including diarrhea, pancytopenia, and fever aid in confirming the diagnosis. When evaluating a maculopapular eruption in an OTR, in addition to GVHD, drug eruption, chemotherapy toxicity, and viral eruption should be considered in the differential diagnosis. The mortality rate of GVHD in OTRs is high (75% to 90%), with death usually resulting from overwhelming sepsis, gastrointestinal bleeding, pneumonia, or renal failure. Management of acute GVHD after solid organ transplantation requires a multidisciplinary approach. Current therapies include antilymphocyte regimens and various approaches resulting in either increased or decreased immunosuppression. New biologics including basiliximab, a chimeric mouse–human monoclonal antibody to the IL-2Rα receptor (CD25) of T cells, have been successfully used in some cases.

## Infectious Diseases of the Skin in OTR Patients

Due to their suppressed host immune defense mechanism, OTRs are more susceptible to bacterial, fungal, and viral infections. Most infections during the first month are related to surgical complications. Opportunistic infections typically occur from the second to the sixth month post-transplant. During the late post-transplant period (beyond 6 months), OTRs suffer from the same infections seen in the general community. Opportunistic bacterial infections seen in transplant recipients include those caused by *Legionella* spp., *Nocardia* spp., *Salmonella* spp., and Listeria monocytogenes. Cytomegalovirus (CMV) is the most common cause of viral infections. Herpes simplex virus (HSV), varicella zoster virus (VZV), Epstein–Barr virus (EBV), human papillomavirus (HPV), and others are also significant pathogens. Fungal infections caused by both yeasts and mycelial fungi are associated with the highest mortality rates. Mycobacteria, pneumocystis, and parasitic diseases may also occur. Due to the heightened risk of infection, the clinician should maintain an increased index of suspicion. More aggressive and earlier diagnostic approaches including skin biopsy with special stains, superficial and tissue culture, and diagnostic imaging modalities may be warranted. Many systemic antimicrobials require dose adjustments in the setting of renal insufficiency. Use of these drugs in renal transplant recipients should include comanagement by transplant nephrologists.

## Bacterial Infections

### Staphylococcal Infections

*Staphylococcus aureus* is a common pathogen and causes the majority of pyodermas and soft-tissue infections seen in solid OTRs. It often colonizes the anterior nares as well as superficial skin breaks and skin disruptions in these patients. Treatment of *S. aureus* colonization with topical mupirocin ointment has been shown to decrease the occurrence of *S. aureus* pyodermas including folliculitis, furuncles, carbuncles, impetigo, bullous impetigo, and ecthyma in certain nonimmunosuppressed patients. However, the same results in OTRs have not been proven. Topical treatment with clindamycin, mupirocin, retapamulin, or oral antibiotics according to sensitivities is recommended. Methicillin-resistant *S. aureus* is an increasing concern in OTRs (Fig. 44-1). Use of Vancomycin or treatment with Linezolid 600 mg b.i.d. may be employed if sensitivities are determined and infection is of significant concern.

### Streptococcus Infections

Group A beta-hemolytic streptococci can cause superficial pyodermas presenting as impetiginized skin and soft-tissue infections. Necrotizing fasciitis is a severe form of soft-tissue infection extending into the subcutaneous fat and deep fascia caused by beta-hemolytic streptococcus or a combination of non-group A streptococci and anaerobe bacilli. Pain out of proportion to clinical signs should raise the clinical suspicion of necrotizing fasciitis. Treatment includes clindamycin and gamma globulin in addition to extensive, emergency surgical debridement and intensive care monitoring.

Gram-negative bacteria, such as *Klebsiella pneumoniae*, *Escherichia coli*, *Pseudomonas aeruginosa*, *Proteus mirabilis*, and *Enterobacter*, may cause cellulitis in OTR patients,

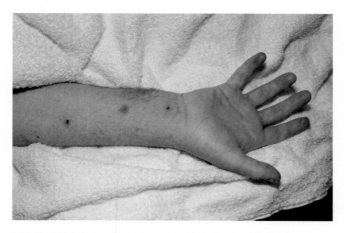

**FIGURE 44-1** ■ Heart transplant patient with 24-hour history of impetigo and swollen forearm, wrist, and hand. Culture was positive for CA-MRSA.

presenting with varying morphology including bullae, ulcers, or cutaneous necrosis with vascular involvement. Initial empiric coverage with gentamicin is helpful until tissue and blood cultures return.

### Nocardiosis

Nocardial infections have been reported primarily in renal and heart transplant patients, fewer than 4% of whom develop this type of infection. Nocardial infection is most commonly caused by *Nocardia asteroides*, a gram-positive, weakly acid fast bacterium. It can be directly introduced to the skin or more commonly spread by the hematogenous route from the lung. Primary cutaneous infection can present as abscesses, ulcers, granulomas, soft-tissue infection, mycetoma, or lymphocutaneous infection. Sulfonamides, either alone or in combination with trimethroprim, are the treatment of choice for nocardiosis. Antimicrobial therapy should be continued for a prolonged period after cure because there is a tendency to relapse and the optimal duration of therapy is not known.

### Bartonella Infection

Infection by *Bartonella henselae*, a gram-negative bacillus, has been reported in kidney, liver, and heart transplant recipients as early as 11 months and as late as 14 years after transplantation. The clinical manifestation of Bartonella infection in OTRs can vary greatly. Patients may present with the typical features of cat-scratch disease with regional lymphadenopathy and fever, but this will usually progress to a more severe, systemic illness if not treated promptly. Transplant recipients have also been reported to develop bacillary angiomatosis, the form of Bartonella infection caused by *B. henselae* and *B. quintana*, commonly seen in individuals with HIV infection. Patients with bacillary angiomatosis present with red-to-violaceous, dome-shaped friable papules and nodules, ranging in size from a few millimeters up to 2 to 3 cm in diameter. Culture of the organism from the skin or a lymph node may be difficult to obtain and requires an incubation period of as long as 30 days. For this reason, polymerase chain reaction of the tissue specimen may be preferable. The antibiotics of choice are erythromycin 250 to 500 mg PO four times daily or doxycyline 100 mg two times daily, continued for 3 months.

### Vibrio vulnificus

*Vibrio vulnificus*, a gram-negative rod, may contaminate shellfish and oysters. Infection occurs either through ingestion or direct inoculation through open wounds from seawater mainly along the Atlantic seacoast. Skin lesions begin within 24 to 48 hours after exposure as erythematous plaques and rapidly progress to hemorrhagic bullae, subsequently becoming necrotic ulcers. Aggressive early surgical debridement is mandatory. Mortality is not insignificant. It is important to remember that infection with *V. vulnificus* can lead to sepsis in immunocompromised hosts and these patients should be cautioned about eating uncooked shellfish. Treatment with Doxycyline 100 mg twice daily is recommended.

## Fungal Skin Infections

Fungal skin infections in OTR patients include classical dermatomycosis, opportunistic fungal infections, and infections with rare fungal pathogens. Fungal infections in solid OTRs continue to be a significant cause of morbidity and mortality. *Candida* spp. and *Aspergillus* spp. account for most invasive fungal infections. The incidence of fungal infection varies with the type of solid organ transplant. Liver transplant recipients have the highest reported incidence of Candida infections while lung transplant recipients have the highest rate of Aspergillus infections.

The classic superficial fungal infections, such as tinea cruris, corporis, and pedis, are seen in up to 50% of OTR patients and are most commonly caused by *Trichophyton rubrum*. Onychomycosis is also a frequent finding. Onychomycosis more commonly involves multiple toe- or fingernails in OTRs, and more importantly it is frequently caused by molds, such as *Scopulariopsis* species. In an immunosuppressed host this fungus may cause subcutaneous infection or fatal systemic infection. Proximal white subungual onychomycosis is a pathognomic sign of immunosuppression, involves the nail plate adjacent to the proximal nail fold, and is produced by *T. rubrum* and *T. megnini*. In addition to topical antifungal medications, treatment with terbinafine for extensive superficial fungal infections is a good option because the potential for drug interactions with immunosuppressants is minimal.

## Opportunistic Infections

Opportunistic fungal infections in OTRs may be caused by fungi normally occurring in our environment that do not typically cause infection in a normal host, such as *Candida, Aspergillus, Cryptococcus, Zygomycetes,* and *Scedosporium* spp. In a severely immunocompromised host these saprophytes can cause serious infections. *Candida* species are found in the human gastrointestinal tract, from the oropharynx to the anus, in the female gynecologic tract, and on the skin. Small numbers of yeast colonies are normally present, increasing in number when the normal microbial flora is altered by antibiotics or when there is a defect in immune competence. Thrush (candidiasis of the oral mucosa) is the most common fungal infection in transplant patients, affecting up to 64% of patients. Treatment with oral fluconazole 200 mg on the first day, then 100 mg once daily for at least 2 weeks to decrease the likelihood of relapse, is recommended. Candida infection may also involve the skin folds and nails and can cause chronic paronychia. Additionally, it can present as Candida folliculitis or appear granulomatous, as seen in mucocutaneous candidiasis. Disseminated candidiasis is one of the most common serious opportunistic mycoses in severely immunocompromised patients.

Invasive aspergillosis remains among the most significant opportunistic infections in OTRs. The incidence of invasive aspergillosis varies from relatively low rates in renal transplant recipients to approaching 15% in lung transplant recipients. Mortality rates in transplant recipients with Aspergillus

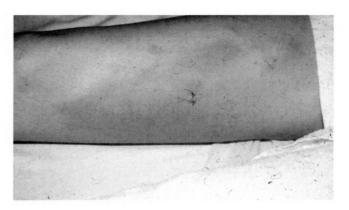

**FIGURE 44-2** ■ Cryptococcal cellulitis in a renal transplant that was diagnosed by culture and viewing fungal organisms in tissue.

infections have ranged from 68% to 92%. An estimated 9.3% to 16.9% of deaths in the first post-transplant year have been considered to be attributable to invasive aspergillosis. Primary cutaneous aspergillosis is rare and most cases occur at the site of intravenous cannulas. Infection presents with erythematous nodules, and hemorrhagic bullae or ulcers. Pulmonary involvement is usually present in invasive Aspergillus infection, with associated cutaneous involvement in only 10% of cases. Biopsy of the skin lesion may establish the diagnosis, and tissue culture will provide definitive diagnosis. Lipid formulation of Amphotericin B is the drug of choice for treatment of aspergillosis. Voriconazole and the new echinocandins have also proven to be useful.

Cutaneous *Cryptococcus* spp. (Fig. 44-2) infection occurs secondarily in up to 15% of patients with disseminated disease as described in renal, liver, and lung transplant patients. Skin infection occurs most commonly on the head and neck, presenting with variable morphology, such as molluscumlike lesions, ulcers, papules, pustules, nodules, acneiform eruptions, and cellulitis. Initial intravenous Amphotericin B followed by oral fluconazole is the standard treatment.

Infection with other opportunistic fungi, including *Mucorales* spp. (Fig. 44-3) dematiaceous and nondematiaceous fungi also pose a real threat to immunosuppressed patients. In addition, these patients are at increased risk to develop infection by rare or endemic fungi, including *Sporothrix schenckii, Histoplasma capsulatum,* and *Coccidioides immitis,* and *Blastomyces* and *Penicillium* species. Geographic location and travel history of the patient can be crucial when taking a complete medical history from these patients.

## Viral Diseases

Viral infections cause a wide variety of complications in solid OTRs, some of them are life threatening. Approximately 10% of patients have chronic or progressive infection with HBV, HCV, CMV, EBV, or papillomavirus. Such viral infections may cause injury to the infected organ (the liver in the case of

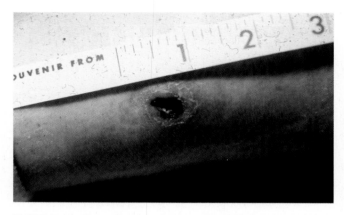

**FIGURE 44-3** ■ Ulcer on the inner calf of a heart transplant patient that showed mucormycosis on tissue stains from a skin biopsy at the ulcer's edge.

the hepatitis viruses and the retina in the case of CMV) or contribute to the development of cancer (e.g., hepatocellular carcinoma following HBV or HCV infection, lymphoma due to EBV, and squamous cell cancer due to papillomavirus).

### Herpes Simplex Virus-1 and -2

The majority of HSV infections in OTRs are reactivation of latent infections, typically occurring in the first 3 months post-transplantation. The lesions commonly present with typical grouped vesicles in a localized distribution in the perioral, anogenital, or digital area. However, with increasing immunosuppression, chronic large ulcers, widespread vesicular eruption, eczema herpeticum, or disseminated visceral infection (hepatitis, pneumonitis, encephalitis) may occur. Infection can be diagnosed by isolation of the virus from lesional smears. Treatment with valacyclovir, famciclovir, or acyclovir is recommended. Intravenous acyclovir should be considered in severe infections.

### Varicella Zoster Virus

Primary infection with VZV via the airborne route causes varicella (chickenpox). Reactivation of VZV in the dorsal root ganglia, and subsequent replication in the epithelial cells produces the characteristic vesicular eruption of herpes zoster. Unlike HSV infections that usually occur in the immediate post-transplant period, VZV reactivation usually occurs after day 100 in OTRs. Herpes zoster in transplant recipients can follow one of three clinical patterns. In most instances, the patients develop a dermatomal skin eruption similar to what is seen in immunocompetent patients; however, the risk of dissemination is higher (40%). Less commonly, OTR patients develop varicella-like eruption with no obvious primary dermatomal eruption, a syndrome that is termed "atypical generalized zoster." Finally, some patients may develop subclinical reactivation of latent VZV, with no evidence of cutaneous lesions. Cutaneous complications in immunocompromised children include bullous or hemorrhagic varicella lesions,

necrotizing fasciitis, purpura fulminans, and bacterial super-infections. Complications related to herpes zoster may include postherpetic neuralgia, cutaneous scarring, and bacterial superinfections. Hematogenous dissemination of VZV to the eye can cause acute retinal necrosis and blindness. Fewer than 5% of transplant patients experience a second episode of herpes zoster. A positive Tzanck test confirms diagnosis of either VZV or HSV. Detection of viral antigen on a smear from the base of a vesicle is diagnostic. Treatment is with the same drugs as approved for HSV. Varicella vaccination is currently recommended prior to transplantation in children and adolescents. The vaccination has been used post–renal transplantation with no adverse affects to the vaccine and a 66% rate of seroconversion.

### Epstein–Barr virus

Primary cutaneous EBV-associated post-transplant lymphoproliferative disease (PTLD) is the most common cutaneous manifestation of EBV infection in OTRs. Disease localized to the skin is rare and presents with polymorphic lesions characterized by maculopapular eruption, single or multiple erythematous nodules or ulcers.

### Cytomegalovirus

The most important pathogen affecting transplant recipients is CMV, with infection occurring mainly after the first month post-transplant. CMV can present as primary infection, reinfection, or reactivation of latent disease. Classically, CMV presents with fever, constitutional symptoms, visceral disease including colitis, esophagitis, hepatitis, laboratory evidence of bone marrow suppression, and rarely pneumonitis. Cutaneous manifestations are variable and rare, often with delayed diagnosis. Multiple skin morphologies have been reported, including maculopapular eruption, petechiae, vesiculobullous lesions, indurated hyperpigmented nodules, and plaques. Ulceration, particularly involving the genital, perineal, and perianal areas, as well as necrosis of mucosal membranes, can occur in more severe cases. However, none of these appearances is pathognomonic for CMV. Despite the morphologic cutaneous variances, all exhibit uniform histologic appearance, including typical vascular endothelial cytopathic changes with intracytoplasmic and intranuclear inclusions affecting skin capillaries. Definitive diagnosis relies on histopathologic examination. Treatment of clinical CMV disease usually requires administration of intravenous ganciclovir for 2 to 4 weeks; clearance of viremia should be documented before intravenous therapy is discontinued.

### Human Herpesvirus-8

Human herpesvirus (HHV8), a gamma herpesvirus, is associated with Kaposi sarcoma (KS), Castleman disease, and primary effusion lymphoma. KS, by far the most common HHV8-associated disease (Fig. 44-4), has been observed most frequently in patients suffering from acquired immunodeficiency syndrome (AIDS). Solid organ recipients show an

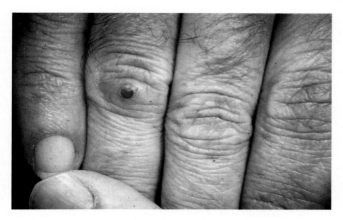

FIGURE 44-4 ■ Purple papule on the dorsal finger in a renal transplant patient was proven Kaposi sarcoma by biopsy. This tumor and similar other ones dissipated when immunosuppression was decreased. Kaposi sarcoma is by far the most common HHV-8 disease in solid transplant recipients.

increasing incidence of KS. According to the Cincinnati Transplant Tumor Registry up to 6% of all de novo cancers following solid organ transplantation are KS. The risk of developing this type of malignancy for renal recipients is approximately 500 times more than that seen in the nontransplant population. The clinical presentation of Kaposi sarcoma in transplant recipients is often limited to the skin, although visceral Kaposi sarcoma has been described. The lesions present as red-purple, infiltrated macules, plaques, and nodules that vary in number and size depending on the level of immunosuppression. In most transplant patients KS is located predominantly on the lower legs, similarly to the classical form of KS, and often associated with lymphedema. Mucosal lesions show a predilection for the nasal mucosa and hard palate.

A diagnosis of KS should be established by skin biopsy, which should be taken from the center of the most infiltrated plaque. The main approach to managing transplant-associated Kaposi sarcoma is to reduce or even discontinue immunosuppressive therapy. The addition of rapamycin in place of other immunosuppressant medication, in particular cyclosporine, has been associated with regression of KS. Isolated KS lesions can be treated with surgical excision or cryotherapy. Radiotherapy should be avoided due to the risk of additional cutaneous malignancies. Systemic immunotherapy or chemotherapy can be considered for indolent, disseminated KS.

### Molluscum Contagiosum Virus

In contrast to the general population, molluscum contagiosum virus (MCV) infection is commonly found in the adult OTR patients in addition to the pediatric transplant recipients, where the incidence has been reported to be 6.9%. Molluscum lesions present as 1 to 3 mm pink papules with a characteristic central umbilicated keratinous plug. In addition, giant molluscum lesions larger than 1 cm may occur in OTRs as well. Diagnosis is easily made based on the characteristic appearance.

Treatment of cosmetically disturbing lesions with cryotherapy is recommended. Reduction of immunosuppression is the most efficacious treatment but is rarely required.

### Human Papillomavirus

There is a wide diversity of high levels of HPV, in particular, the epidermodysplasia verruciformis (EDV)–type HPV (HPV 5 and 8) detected in cutaneous warts, dysplastic keratoses, and squamous cell carcinomas (SCCs) in solid organ recipients. The epidemiologic data and the high prevalence of HPV DNA in premalignant and neoplastic skin lesions in OTRs may suggest an etiologic role of HPV in NMSC oncogenesis even though the exact mechanism is still unknown. Common warts present as skin colored or pink verrucous (verruca vulgaris) or flat topped (verruca plana) papules, which upon close examination characteristically disrupt the normal dermatoglyphics. As opposed to the general population, common warts appear predominantly on sun-exposed sites, tend to be more numerous or grouped, and display fewer tendencies for spontaneous regression in OTRs. More importantly, in immunocompromised patients, HPV-induced lesions have the potential for malignant transformation, particularly on sun-exposed areas (**Fig. 44-5**). Therefore, rapidly enlarging hyperkeratotic verrucae should be biopsied to rule out malignant transformation. HVP-induced anogenital in situ and invasive SCC is ten times more common in transplant recipients. Screening of the anus and cervix with Pap test and lesional biopsy is warranted.

Treatment of viral warts is similar to that in general population and includes conventional ablative therapies, such as cryotherapy, topical application of 40% salicylic acid and pulsed-dye laser treatment. In certain cases, intralesional injection of bleomycin may be attempted. Patients with extensive warts should be managed by reduction of sun exposure, sunscreen use, reduction of immunosuppression, and close follow-up to detect the development of malignant lesions. Therapy for condyloma acuminatum includes topical podophyllotoxin applied twice daily on 3 consecutive days per week for 4 to 5 weeks. Use of imiquimod 5% cream, a topical

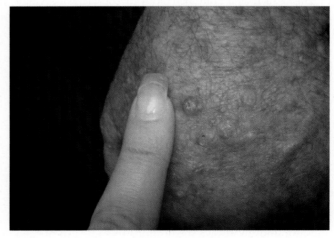

FIGURE 44-5 ■ Multiple squamous cell carcinomas on the elbow of a renal transplant patient.

immune modulator, in OTR patients is still controversial. Small studies with the use of imiquimod cream in OTRs showed moderate efficacy for condyloma without deleterious effects on the transplanted organ. For genital warts, it is recommended once daily three times a week for 16 weeks. Surgical removal of the genital wart may be a first option if there are a few small warts or a large number of warts over a large area. Several other modalities are available, including local excision, laser therapy, cryotherapy, and electrosurgical excision. Recurrence is frequent and close follow-up is recommended.

## Mycobacterial Diseases

Solid OTRs are at risk for mycobacterial infections because of their depressed cell-mediated immunity and the effects of chronic corticosteroid administration. *M. tuberculosis* infection occurs in approximately 1% of solid OTRs in North America and Europe. Solid OTRs are at increased risk for both primary and reactivation infection. Disseminated disease is also more common in this population than in nonimmunocompromised populations. There is a 30% mortality rate associated with *M. tuberculosis* infection in transplant recipients. *M. tuberculosis* is acquired primarily by inhalation of aerosolized droplets containing the organism. This leads to infection of the respiratory tract and occasional subsequent dissemination via the lymphatic system or bloodstream. Atypical mycobacteria comprise slow-growing organisms including *M. marinum*, *M. kansasii*, *M. avium*–intracellulare complex, and *M. ulcerans* and rapid-growing organisms including *M. fortuitum*, *M. chelonae*, and *M. abscessus*. The spectrum of cutaneous manifestations of *M. tuberculosis* and atypical mycobacteria is diverse and range from indurated plaques, to nodules, to ulcers, at times with purulent drainage. Similarly to the general population, infection with *M. marinum* usually occurs following exposure to fish tank water and presents with nodules on the hands and arms often with a sporotrichoid spread. Solid organ transplantation recipients should be warned of the hazards of infection from home fish tanks. Failure to respond to standard antimicrobial therapy should raise the question of infection with an unusual organism such as a nontuberculous mycobacterium. Aspiration or biopsy of lesions for histopathologic testing, staining for mycobacteria, and mycobacterial culture are essential for diagnosis. Tissue culture may be delayed up to 6 weeks due to the slow-growing nature of most mycobacterial species. Importantly, the tuberculin skin test is positive in only one quarter to one third of solid organ transplantation recipients with tuberculosis; therefore, serologic testing using the interferon-gamma assay specific to *M. tuberculosis* may prove to be a better option. Treatment of mycobacterial infections is complex and depends on the infecting organism and the severity of the infection. For tuberculosis, therapeutic guidelines are similar to the general population. However, special consideration should be made regarding drug interactions between certain antimycobacterial agents, such as rifampicin and rifambutin and immunosuppressive medications that are also metabolized via cytochrome P-450 enzymes, such as cyclosporine, sirolimus, and tacrolimus. In most cases of atypical my-

cobacterium infections, a course of antibiotics is necessary. These include rifampicin, ethambutol, isoniazid, minocycline, ciprofloxacin, clarithromycin, azithromycin, and co-trimoxazole. Usually treatment consists of a combination of drugs. *M. marinum* species are often resistant to isoniazid. Treatment with other antibiotics should be for at least 2 months. *M. kansasii* should be treated for at least 18 months. *M. chelonae* is best treated by clarithromycin in combination with another agent. Sometimes surgical excision is the best approach.

### Benign Tumors Occurring in Increased Frequency in OTRs

Verrucal keratoses (**Fig. 44-6**) present in large numbers in transplant patients as gray-white flat or hyperkeratotic papules mainly on sun-exposed sites. Consistent use of moisturizers, topical urea products, or topical retinoids may improve appearance and texture, but these lesions are often resistant to topical therapy. Liquid nitrogen may be used to treat individual bothersome lesions.

### Skin Cancer in Organ Transplant Recipients

Skin cancer encompasses 42% of all post-transplant malignancies. Population-based standard incidence ratios for SCCs are increased 65- to 250-fold and for basal cell carcinomas (BCCs) 10- to 16-fold in OTRs compared with nontransplanted patients (**Table 44-2**). Within 20 years of transplantation, approximately 40% to 50% of white patients in most western countries and 70% to 80% of white Australians will have developed at least one nonmelanoma skin cancer (NMSC). An increased incidence of melanoma in transplant patients has been reported, but recent studies have failed to confirm these findings. Kaposi sarcoma has been reported in excess among OTRs, especially from patient populations in which the disease is endemic, such as patients of Mediterranean, black African, or

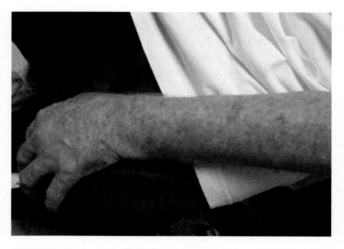

**FIGURE 44-6** ■ Multiple hyperkeratotic tumors over the extensor forearm in a renal transplant patient. Frequent observation, aggressive therapy, and biopsy when necessary are needed to control these premalignant tumors.

**TABLE 44-2** ■ **Population-Based Standard Incidence Ratios of Skin Cancer in Transplant Patients Compared to the General Populations**

| Skin Cancer | Incidence Ratio in Transplant Patients Compared to the General Population |
|---|---|
| SCC | 65–250 |
| SCC of lip | 20 |
| BCC | 10–16 |
| Melanoma | 1.6–3.4 |
| Kaposi sarcoma | 84 |

**TABLE 44-3** ■ **Risk Factors for NMSC in Solid Organ Transplant Patients**

| | General Population | Transplant Population |
|---|---|---|
| Increasing age | ++ | ++++ |
| Fair skin, light hair, light eyes | ++ | ++++ |
| Sun exposure | ++ | ++++ |
| History of previous skin cancer | 50% risk of second cancer | >70% risk of second skin cancer |
| Intensity and length of immunosuppression | N/A | Positive correlation |

Caribbean origin. In addition, Merkel cell carcinoma (MCC) appears to be more common in OTRs and has a high mortality rate. Lymphomas affect up to 5% of all OTRs, but purely cutaneous lymphomas are rare. Other types of skin cancer, such as atypical fibrous histiocytoma and dermatofibroma protuberans have been reported, but due to the rarity of these tumors, increased incidence in OTRs has been difficult to quantify.

### Incidence of Skin Cancer by Allograft Type

Cardiac OTRs are reported to have a higher incidence of NMSC in comparison to other OTRs, which is attributed to the significantly higher doses of immunosuppressant medications used to prevent allograft rejection in this subset of OTR patients. It has been postulated that another possible factor is that heart OTRs are generally 15 years older at transplantation than renal OTRs, and therefore are at a higher risk for skin cancer. The time interval between transplantation and development of skin cancer was found to be much shorter in heart OTRs (3.9 years) compared to the renal OTRs (8.6 years). There are few studies concerning skin cancer in liver, pancreas, or lung OTRs, but it has been suggested that the incidence of NMSC in liver OTRs is less than in heart or kidney OTRs because the level of immunosuppression is lower and the drug regimens differ from those employed for other solid OTRs.

### Incidence of Skin Cancer by Age

Although older transplant patients develop more skin cancer, probably due to higher cumulative sun exposure before transplantation, younger transplant recipients have a higher risk relative to others of their same age. The reversal of SCC/BCC ratio compared to the general population was found to be even more pronounced in children than in adult OTRs (2.8:1 vs. 1.7:1).

### Evaluation of OTR Patients for Risk Factors

When evaluating an OTR patient, careful history taking about risk factors for transplant-associated dermatologic problems is crucial. There are multiple well-defined risk factors for ultraviolet-induced skin cancer in the general population that are accentuated in transplant patients, including increasing age, skin type, history of extensive ultraviolet exposure, and a history of previous NMSC (Table 44-3). Additional risk factors include blue or gray eyes, a Celtic background, infection with HPV, and a low CD4 count. Cancer risk appears to be higher for heart transplant recipients who are maintained on high levels of immunosuppression and lower for kidney and liver transplant patients who require less immunosuppression. The duration and intensity of immunosuppression positively correlates with the risk for skin cancer and cutaneous infections. Exposure to chronic immunosuppression severely depresses specific components of host immunity including both antitumor immune surveillance and antimicrobial host defense. The link between immunosuppression and cancer formation is further evidenced by observed decrease in skin cancer formation with reduction or cessation of immunosuppressive therapy. This has prompted an expert consensus panel to recommend reductions in immunosuppressive medication for those patients with numerous or life-threatening skin cancers. Additionally, there has been recent evidence that some immunosuppressive agents, most notably azathioprine, have direct procarcinogenic effects, whereas others may have anticarcinogenic properties, as shown with sirolimus. Nevertheless, determining the relative contribution of the individual immunosuppressive drug to the development of skin cancer has been difficult to quantify.

### Actinic Keratosis

Actinic keratosis (AK) is a partial thickness proliferation of atypical keratinocytes confined to the epidermis, with the potential to progress to invasive SCC. AKs present as pink, rough, scaly papules on sun-exposed sites, with a predilection for the bald scalp, face, ears, dorsal hands, and forearms. Diffuse AKs of the lower vermillion lip is called actinic cheilitis and presents with diffuse scaling as well as erythematous, keratotic, or nonhealing erosions. Within the first 5 years of immunosuppression, about 40% of OTRs may develop AKs. Similar to the general population, fair skin and extensive sun exposure predisposes to the development of AKs. However, in transplant patients, AKs not only appear with increased frequency, but also appear earlier, in greater numbers, and progress more rapidly to invasive SCC. Because of the increased risk for malignant transformation, early and aggressive treatment of lesions is recommended.

**Treatment.** There are a wide variety of treatment options that need to be tailored to the patient risk factors for skin cancer, the number, and anatomic location of these lesions. For low-risk patients with a limited number of AKs, the recommended treatment is cryotherapy of the individual AKs. For best results, cryotherapy should be applied for 15 to 20 seconds with two freeze–thaw cycles. Curettage, electrosurgery, carbon dioxide laser, and surgical excision are less common treatment options. For areas with diffuse, severe actinic damage and a large number of AKs, the best approach is to perform "field therapy" with topical 5-fluorouracil (5-FU), topical diclofenac, PDT, or imiquimod cream. Topical 5-FU, as 5% (Efudex), 1% (Fluoroplex), or 0.5% (Carac) preparations are recommended twice or once daily, respectively, up to 4 weeks as tolerated. Patients should be counseled about the expected side effects including moderate to severe erythema, irritation, burning, and occasional erosions. Patients also should avoid sun exposure and wear sunscreen as ultraviolet light may increase side effects. Topical Solaraze (3% diclofenac in 2.5% hyaluronic acid base) is used twice daily for 60 to 90 days. It has been shown to be moderately efficacious to the face and scalp in the general population, and in one case series in OTRs. PDT involves the application of a photosensitizing agent, aminolevulinic acid (ALA) and a light of a specific wavelength to activate the phototoxic reaction, which produces controlled cell death of dysplastic or malignant cells via free oxygen radical release. The clearance rate of AKs in OTR patients has been shown to be similar to that of the general population. Recommended incubation times with ALA vary from 1 to 4 hours depending on the anatomic area. Destruction of thicker AKs by cryotherapy or curettage is recommended prior to PDT. Topical imiquimod has been shown to reduce AKs in renal transplant patients. No detrimental effects were shown to the renal allograft with three times per week use for 16 weeks on a 60 cm$^2$ area. Imiquimod should be used with caution in transplant patients because of the theoretical risk of excessive immune system stimulation resulting in allograft rejection. Other modalities, including topical retinoids, ablative lasers, chemical peels, and dermabrasion, have been used to treat AKs. Most importantly, regular use of high SPF sunscreen should be recommended, as it has been shown to reduce the development of AKs and increase the rate of remission of existing AKs in transplant patients.

### Basal Cell Carcinoma

BCCs are most common in the heart transplant population where they develop 15 years earlier compared to the general population. In the general population the incidence of SCC is less than that of BCC, with an SCC/BCC ratio of about 1:4.

It is well recognized that the SCC/BCC ratio is reversed in transplant recipients. BCCs have a predilection for sun-exposed areas and appear as erythematous, slightly scaly plaques (superficial type), pearly translucent telangectatic papules which may ulcerate (nodular and infiltrative type), or shiny scar like plaques (morpheaform type). Most importantly, BCCs in transplant patients do not seem to display increased "aggressive" behavior. Metastasis is extremely rare. Treatment is similar to nonimmunosuppressed patients and listed in Table 44-4.

### Squamous Cell Carcinoma

SCC is the most common skin cancer in the organ transplant population and may have a somewhat different presentation and clinical course compared to the general population. SCCs tend to occur in a younger age, typically first appearing 3 to 8 years after transplantation. They may develop in large numbers and follow an aggressive clinical course, resulting in significant morbidity and mortality. Approximately 6% to 9% of SCCs metastasize, most often during the 2 years after excision, with a 50% 3-year disease-specific survival in those patients with metastasis. SCCs in OTRs most frequently occur in chronically sun-damaged areas and often present as red, pink scaly, hyperkeratotic papules and plaques within a field of diffuse keratotic lesions that may include verrucae, verrucal keratoses, porokeratoses, and AKs, making it difficult to distinguish clinical borders. The most common locations for SCC in OTRs include the scalp, face, ears, neck, dorsal forearms, and hands. The history of a chronic, nonhealing lesion, which may be painful or bleeding, aids the diagnosis. Physical examination should include careful examination of the surrounding skin, assessment of the fixed nature of the lesion, facial nerve examination (for facial lesions), and palpation of regional lymph nodes to evaluate for invasive tumor and metastasis. It is important to identify clinical features of high-risk tumors (Table 44-5) because these lesions have an aggressive clinical course and may require a cooperative management by dermatologists and transplant physicians, as well as surgical, medical, and radiation oncologists. In situ SCC and low-risk SCC are managed similarly to that in general population, while high-risk SCCs need excision with intraoperative margin evaluation by Mohs micrographic surgery with or without reduction of immunosuppression and chemoprevention with oral retinoids (Table 44-4). If a tumor shows high-grade atypia or a pattern of perineural invasion, postoperative adjuvant radiation therapy may be indicated. Sentinel lymph node biopsy may provide some aid in evaluation and management, but there are no studies demonstrating survival benefit. Patients with high-risk tumors are usually subjected to preoperative staging examination with PET/CT. Chemoprevention with oral retinoids (acitretin 10 to 50 mg daily) has been shown to reduce the incidence of precancerous and SCC lesions while on therapy, but severe side effects and the rebound phenomenon pose serious limitations to therapy. Chemotherapies used for prevention are investigational. Similarly, individual case reports of success with the new class of

**TABLE 44-4** ■ **Treatment Options for AK, BCC, and SCC in Transplant Patients**

| Treatment | Actinic Keratosis | Basal Cell Carcinoma | Squamous Cell Carcinoma | Comments |
|---|---|---|---|---|
| **Destructive** | | | | |
| Cryosurgery | First line of individual lesions | Only for superficial BCC | Only for in situ SCC | Lack of margin control Scarring |
| Electrodessication and curettage | Not indicated | For low-risk BCC | For low-risk SCC | Lack of margin control Scarring |
| **Topical** | | | | |
| 5-Fluorouracil | Individual or field treatment | For superficial BCC | Not FDA approved | Rare contact hypersensitivity Application site reaction |
| Imiquimod | Individual or field treatment | For superficial BCC | Not FDA approved | Potential risk of immune activation Local inflammation and irritation |
| Diclofenac | Individual or field treatment | Not FDA approved | Not FDA approved | Potential risk to effect renal function |
| Retinoids | Field treatment | Not Indicated | Not Indicated | Chronic irritation |
| Photodynamic therapy | Field treatment | For superficial BCC | Not indicated | Provider controlled |
| Chemical peel | Field treatment | Not indicated | Not indicated | Medium-to-deep peels needed |
| **Excisional** | | | | |
| Excision with postoperative margin evaluation | Not indicated | For low-risk lesions | For low-risk lesions | 4-mm margin Re-excision |
| Mohs micrographic surgery | Not indicated | For high-risk lesion | For high-risk lesions | Needs specialized provider Removal of skin cancer with maximal tissue preservation |
| **Systemic** | | | | |
| Oral retinoids | Field treatment | Chemoprevention | Chemoprevention | Retinoid side effect Rebound |
| Systemic chemotherapy | Not indicated | Adjuvant | Adjuvant | Significant adverse effects |
| Reduction of immunosuppression | Adjuvant | Adjuvant | Adjuvant | |
| Radiotherapy | Not indicated | Poor surgical candidates In-transit metastasis | Poor surgical candidates In-transit metastasis | Radiation dermatitis Recurrence |

biologic agents used in an off-label manner occasionally appear in the literature, but no controlled case series have been published.

## Malignant Melanoma

Malignant melanoma (MM) is the most aggressive skin tumor and commonly presents as an atypical pigmented lesion. The incidence of MM in transplant patients compared to the general population is debated. Prior studies have shown variable rates ranging from no increase to an eight-fold increase in incidence. Risk factors for development of MM are similar to the general population and include those with fair skin, red or blonde hair, blue eyes, history of sunburns, atypical nevi, numerous nevi, and a personal or family history of MM. MM in transplant patients appears most commonly on the trunk, followed by the upper arms. Transplant recipients with a history of MM before transplantation may have a high incidence of recurrence after transplantation. In addition, MM is one of the most common donor-transmitted cancers in OTRs. Current treatment recommendations are based on the guidelines established for

**TABLE 44-5 ■ Characteristics of High-Risk SCCs**

- Rapid growth or recurrence
- Ulceration
- Location: forehead, temple, ear, nose, lip, mid face, genitalia
- Large size
  - >1.0 cm cheeks, forehead, neck, and scalp
  - >0.6 cm other areas of face
  - >2.0 cm trunk and extremities
- Poor differentiation
- Deep invasion (fat, muscle, cartilage, bone)
- Perineural/neural invasion

**TABLE 44-6 ■ Recommended Follow-Up Intervals for Organ Transplant Patients**

| Clinical Exam and History | Follow-Up Intervals (Months) |
| --- | --- |
| No history of skin cancer, no risk factors | 12–24 |
| No history of skin cancer, positive risk factors | 6–12 |
| Actinic keratosis or viral warts | 3–6 |
| One BCC or SCC | 3–6 |
| Multiple NMSC | 3 |
| High-risk SCC | 3 |
| Metastatic SCC | 1–3 |

the general population; in addition, a decrease in the level of immunosuppression should be attempted in collaboration with the transplant team.

## Other Malignant Skin Tumors in OTRs

### Merkel Cell Carcinoma

MCC is a rare neuroendocrine tumor with very high mortality rate and greater than 10-fold increased incidence rate in organ transplant patients. Clinically, these lesions appear as rapidly growing, firm, red-to-violaceous nodules with a shiny surface and overlying telangiectasia. Distribution is similar among OTRs and the general population and includes the head and neck, followed by the upper extremities and the trunk. Five-year disease-specific survival in transplant patients is reported to be 46%. Management is similar to that of general population and includes excision, with or without sentinel node mapping, followed by radiotherapy or chemotherapy if needed.

Other rare cutaneous neoplasms reported in OTRs include atypical fibroxanthoma, malignant fibrous histiocytoma, leiomyosarcoma, sebaceous carcinoma, microcystic adnexal carcinoma, angiosarcoma, and dermatofibrosarcoma protuberans. None of these have been reported to occur with significantly increased frequency in OTRs.

### Education and Management of OTRs

It is imperative to repetitively educate patients about the importance of sun protection, which should include the use of sunscreen with SPF greater than 30, avoidance of direct sun exposure in the midday, and sun protective clothing. The goal of education and preventive treatments is to decrease future skin cancer formation. Early recognition and treatment of skin cancers is important in this population. The patients should be risk stratified and undergo regular surveillance

with a frequency based on their skin cancer risk (Table 44-6). A multidisciplinary approach involving the transplant team and oncologist in caring for patients with life-threatening skin cancers is highly recommended.

## Suggested Readings

Ablashi DV, Chatlynne LG, Whitman JE Jr, et al. Spectrum of Kaposi's sarcoma-associated herpesvirus, or human herpesvirus 8, diseases. *Clin Microbiol Rev.* 2002;15:439.

Berg D, Otley CC. Skin cancer in organ transplant recipients: epidemiology, pathogenesis, and management. *J Am Acad Dermatol.* 2002;47(1):1–17; quiz 18–20.

Dantal J, Soulillou JP. Immunosuppressive drugs and the risk of cancer after organ transplantation. *N Engl J Med.* 2005;352(13):1371–1373.

Euvrard S, Kanitakis J, Claudy A. Skin cancers after organ transplantation. *N Engl J Med.* 2003;348(17):1681–1691.

Fishman JA. Infection in solid-organ transplant recipients. *N Engl J Med.* 2007;357(25):2601–2614.

Harwood CA, McGregor JM, Swale VJ, et al. High frequency and diversity of cutaneous appendageal tumors in organ transplant recipients. *J Am Acad Dermatol.* 2003;48(3):401–408.

Harwood CA, Proby CM. McGregor JM, et al. Clinicopathologic features of skin cancer in organ transplant recipients: a retrospective case-control series. *J Am Acad Dermatol.* 2006;54(2):290–300.

Nindl I, Gottschling M, Stockfleth E. Human papillomaviruses and non-melanoma skin cancer: basic virology and clinical manifestations. *Dis Markers.* 2007;23(4):247–259.

Neuburg M. Transplant-associated skin cancer: role of reducing immunosuppression. *J Natl Compr Canc Netw.* 2007;5(5):541–549.

Otley CC, Berg D, Ulrich C, et al. Reduction of immunosuppression for transplant-associated skin cancer: expert consensus survey. *Br J Dermatol.* 2006;154(3):395–400.

Otley CC, Stasko T. *Skin Disease in Organ Transplantation.* New York: Cambridge University Press; 2008.

Snydman DR. Infection in solid organ transplantation. *Transpl Infect Dis.* 1999;1(1):21–28.

Stasko T, Brown MD, Carucci JA, et al. Guidelines for the management of squamous cell carcinoma in organ transplant recipients. *Dermatol Surg.* 2004;30(4 pt 2):642–650.

Stockfleth E, Ulrich C, Meyer T, et al. Epithelial malignancies in organ transplant patients: clinical presentation and new methods of treatment. *Recent Results Cancer Res.* 2002;160:251–258.

# CHAPTER 45

# Tropical Diseases of the Skin

*Francisco G. Bravo, MD and Salim Mohanna, MD*

A chapter on tropical diseases is a must in this era of globalization. By tropical diseases, one may think of diseases limited to the tropical and subtropical areas of the world. The term actually implies the study of infectious diseases endemic to specific areas of the world, not always located in the tropics (i.e., human T-cell lymphotropic virus [HTLV]-1 in Japan). Once a domain of European doctors traveling to colonies in the 19th century, tropical disease now has implications for every specialty in medicine, including, of course, dermatology. Traveling, either for tourist, business, or military purposes or just as immigrants in search of a better future for their families, has expanded the limits of where diseases discussed in this chapter can be seen. Let's keep an open mind and not forget to ask where the patient was born and where he or she is coming from.

## Viral Diseases

### HTLV-1

The HTLV-1 is a retrovirus of the subfamily Oncovirinae, with the ability to infect CD4 cells and induce different degrees of immunosuppression. An estimated 10 to 20 million persons are infected with the virus worldwide. There are multiple endemic areas in the world, in Africa (Gabon, Zaire, Ivory Coast), Asia (Japan, Iran), and Australia (the aborigines group). In the American continent its presence is well established in Caribbean countries such as Jamaica, Trinidad, Barbados, and Haiti. In South America, countries affected include Brazil, Colombia, and Peru. In the United States, Canada, and Europe, the incidence of seroprevalence is low, but when one looks at specific migratory populations, the number can increase dramatically.

The infection was disseminated to the Americas from three different sources: early migration of Mongoloid population to the American continent in ancient times, the trade of African slaves in the 19th century, and migration of the Japanese as a labor force in the 19th and 20th centuries.

#### Presentation and Characteristics

The most common routes of transmission are breast-feeding, sexual contact, and blood transfusions. As opposed to human immunodeficiency virus (HIV) infection

(the other well-known retrovirus), most HTLV-1–infected patients will remain asymptomatic for the rest of their lives and no more that 5% will develop some clinical manifestations.

HTLV-1 infection can induce disease due to an altered immune system (infective dermatitis, crusted scabies, and disseminated dermatophyte infections), autoimmunity (tropical spastic paraparesis, uveitis), and neoplasia (leukemia/lymphoma). Most dermatologists may have heard of cutaneous T-cell lymphomas, but, in fact, cutaneous disease due to immune dysfunction may be more common.

- Infective dermatitis was first described in Jamaican children in 1966. Louis La Grenade described its relation to HTLV-1 infection in 1970. The clinical picture is that of a chronic, eczematous dermatitis affecting the scalp and intertriginous areas, such as the neck folds, axillae, and groin (Fig. 45-1). On the face it may follow a seborrheic dermatitis–like distribution. The main affected population is children, although the disease may be seen in adulthood. An important component is the constant degree of superinfection by *Staphylococcus aureus* and *β*-hemolytic Streptococcus. This condition can be described as an "oozing, honey-crusted seborrheic dermatitis or intertrigo," as an "always

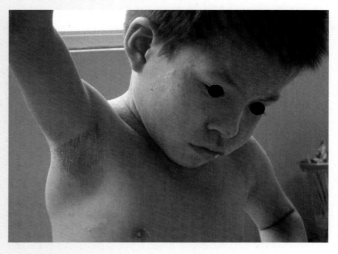

**FIGURE 45-1** ■ Infective dermatitis, showing an eczematous rash involving the face and axillae.

impetiginized scalp psoriasis," or as "atopic dermatitis with predominant scalp involvement." This is, in fact, a viral-induced dermatitis and a model for atopic dermatitis. Most patients with infective dermatitis clear when treated with antibiotics, but the disease recurs when the treatment is discontinued, adopting a chronic course. Many affected children will go into remission when reaching puberty, in a way similar to atopic patients. Some consider infective dermatitis a marker for a higher risk of developing lymphoma.

- Crusted scabies have been described in populations that are known to be endemic for HTLV-1, such as Australian aborigines. Also, in places with high prevalence, like Lima and Peru, most cases are related to the retrovirus infection, even more commonly than immunosuppression secondary to HIV infection or chronic steroid therapy.
- Pruritus, xerosis, and ichthyosis are considered by some researchers as the most common HTLV-1 manifestations, although they are not very specific.
- Adult T-cell leukemia/lymphoma was linked to HTLV-1 in the Japanese population in 1977 and is actually seen in all endemic areas. Between 25% and 40% of cases will have cutaneous involvement. Five subtypes have now been recognized including acute leukemia, chronic leukemia, lymphoma, smoldering, and a purely cutaneous form. The skin lesions may vary: a number of cases will be indistinguishable from mycosis fungoides and others will present with a more varied morphology including papules, nodules, tumors, and even erythroderma and ichthyosiform eruptions.

## Dengue

### Presentation and Characteristics

Dengue, or breakbone fever, is one of the most prevalent viral diseases in the world, causing a systemic illness expressed as a neurologic infection, an acute febrile disease with arthropathy, or a hemorrhagic fever. It is caused by an RNA flavivirus, with four described serotypes. It is present around the world (one hundred million cases per year), in tropical and subtropical areas of Africa and Asia, and it is also becoming an increasing public health problem for some countries in South and Central America.

The disease is transmitted by the bite of mosquitoes belonging to the genus *Aedes*, mainly *A. aegypti*, which is also a carrier of yellow fever. Dengue is present most commonly in urban areas with poor sanitary systems. The mosquitoes thrive whenever they find open water reservoirs. Aedes is also the main living reservoir for the virus.

The disease may adopt various clinical forms, from mild to classic to a more severe and dangerous hemorrhagic form, the so-called dengue hemorrhagic fever (DHF). Whereas the classical form is more common in new arrivals to endemic areas, the more severe DHF is more likely to affect children, residents of endemic areas, and those who have already had dengue in the past.

### Clinical Appearance

The classical form starts as a sudden fever, lasting 2 to 5 days, and is associated with headache, intense myalgias and arthralgia, and retro-orbital pain. Cutaneous involvement varies, from facial flushing to a more diffuse macular or maculopapular morbilliform eruption. The erythematous areas become confluent, leaving small spared areas of normal skin, similar in a way to what is seen in pityriasis rubra pilaris, although lacking its roughness; this image is described as "white islands on a red sea" (**Fig. 45-2**). The main area of involvement is the trunk, with the eruption spreading centrifugally toward the extremities. Petechial eruptions affecting the lower extremities are also seen. Pruritus may be present, and a later state of desquamation may follow.

DHF presents with a more severe course, including vomiting, facial flushing, perioral cyanosis, and weakness with cool and clammy extremities. Hemorrhagic complications, such as gastrointestinal (GI) and genital bleeding, appear, and the patient may go into a dengue shock syndrome. This state may have a mortality rate as high as 10% if not given the appropriate support.

### Hemorrhagic Fevers

These febrile diseases result from infection by viruses from these viral families: Arenaviridae, Bunyaviridae, Filoviridae, and Flaviviridae. Not all viruses in these families cause hemorrhagic fever. These viruses have a higher occurrence in tropical areas, such as South America, Africa, and the Pacific Islands. Clinical manifestations of hemorrhagic fever include capillary permeability, leukopenia, and thrombocytopenia. Hemorrhagic fever is manifested by sudden onset, fever, headache, generalized myalgia, backache, petechiae, conjunctivitis, and severe prostration. Intensive supportive care is necessary for most cases of hemorrhagic fevers.

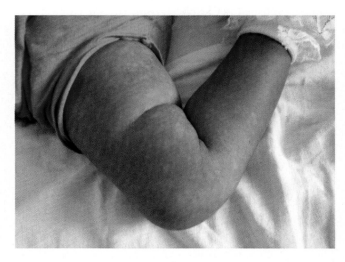

**FIGURE 45-2** ■ Dengue rash in a baby: "white islands in a red sea."

# Bacterial Infections

## Bartonellosis, Including Carrion's Disease and Bacillary Angiomatosis

Until the AIDS (acquired immunodeficiency syndrome) era, bartonellosis was one of those exotic diseases only studied for board examinations. The first description of *Carrion's disease* was made at the beginning of the 20th century and came from endemic areas in the Peruvian Andes; the causal agent was identified as *Bartonella bacilliformis*. The bacteria, a gram-negative rod, was transmitted from the natural reservoirs to humans by the bite of mosquitoes belonging to the *Lutzomyia* family.

### Presentation and Characteristics

The disease has two characteristic phases, one systemic and another purely cutaneous. The first phase, known as Oroya fever, produces an impressive bacteremia and parasitism of the reticuloendothelial system, in which microorganisms may be seen inside red blood cells on peripheral smears. The clinical picture is a systemic disease with fever, malaise, and high susceptibility to other bacterial infections, such as salmonellosis.

The most distinct and relevant phase for the dermatologist is the eruptive phase, known as verruga peruana. It may follow the bacteremia or it may present de novo. Characteristically, an eruption of multiple papules, nodules, and tumors appears over a period of weeks. The more superficial lesions have an angiomatous appearance, resembling pyogenic granulomas (**Fig. 45-3**). The natural course of the disease is toward spontaneous involution, although antibiotic treatment may induce a more prompt remission.

At the beginning of the 1980s, some patients with AIDS presented with a clinical picture very similar to the eruptive phase of verruga peruana. This new disease was named *bacillary angiomatosis*. The histologic descriptions of the eruptive lesions of bacillary angiomatosis were identical to those described in verruga peruana, which was the only bartonellosis known at the time. The initial thought was to associate this new entity with catscratch disease. At a later time, isolation of a gram-negative rod from the lesions led to classifying it under a new family of bacteria called *Rochalimaea*. Genetic studies demonstrated a close relation between Rochalimaeas and Bartonellas, resulting in a new grouping under the term *Bartonella*. The new species include *B. henselae*, *B. quintana* (both cause bacillary angiomatosis, catscratch fever, and systemic disease associated with fever), and *B. elizabethae*, which causes septicemia and endocarditis in alcoholics.

Bacillary angiomatosis is now recognized as a disease characteristic of immunosuppressed patients of all kinds, although it has been reported in immunocompetent patients. The most likely natural reservoir is domestic animals such as cats. It is cosmopolitan, as opposed to verruga peruana, which is still endemic to Andean areas of Peru and Ecuador.

## Anthrax

Anthrax is an infection caused by *Bacillus anthracis*, an encapsulated gram-positive bacteria capable of surviving up to 20 years in dry grass. The disease is more common in people working with cattle. The infection is acquired either by contact through the skin or by inhalation of spores. The cutaneous lesion, called malignant pustule, is usually located in exposed areas of the skin, especially the face, neck, arms, or hands and is usually solitary. One to five days after the inoculation, a papule grows. A blister then forms on an edematous base that eventually breaks, leaving a hemorrhagic crust. Redness and edema may be very marked (**Fig. 45-4**). General symptoms appear on the third or fourth day; the condition may result in severe toxicity and even lead to death.

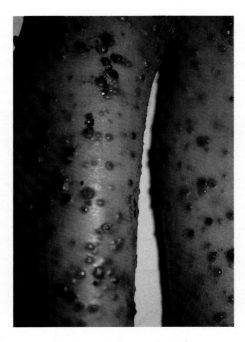

**FIGURE 45-3** ■ Angiomatous papules of verruga peruana.

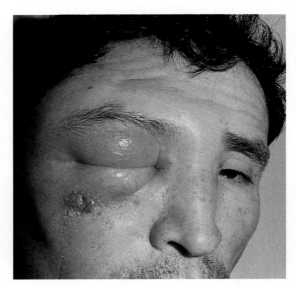

**FIGURE 45-4** ■ Anthrax, 48 hours after infection.

*Treatment*

Treatment options include penicillin, doxycycline, and quinolones.

## Rhinoscleroma

*Presentation and Characteristics*

Rhinoscleroma, also known as scleroma, is a chronic disease of very slow progression that is potentially fatal. It is caused by *Klebsiella rhinoscleromatis* (Frish bacillus). Three stages have been recognized:

- The initial stage is that of rhinitis. The first symptoms are generally nasopharyngeal; the lesions grow slowly, and often the patient does not seek medical attention for years. This is an exudating stage, with symptoms similar to those of a common cold, including headache and difficulty in breathing. There is a very purulent, fetid secretion with crusts and occasional epistaxis.
- The second stage is proliferative, characterized by obstruction and infiltration of nasal tissues by a friable granulomatous tissue. By extending into the pharynx and the larynx, it may cause hoarseness. Later, during a nodular period, the nose increases in size, adopting a "tapir" shape. Respiration becomes difficult, and it may be necessary to do a tracheotomy.
- The third stage is fibrotic sclerosis (Fig. 45-5), and although associated with partial improvement and occasionally a spontaneous cure, it usually results in a marked distortion of the anatomic structures. Invasion of the bone and nasal sinuses, with eventual destruction of bone tissue may occur. The diagnosis is based on the clinical and histologic picture and the presence of the Frish bacillus.

*Treatment*

Treatment includes antibiotics such as tetracycline, azithromycin, cephalosporins, and trimethoprim. It does not respond to sulfa or penicillin. When using tetracycline, 2 g/d should be given for a period of 6 months.

## Nonvenereal Treponematoses

Different species of the spirochete *Treponema* cause different infections in humans. *T. pallidum* causes venereal syphilis. *T. carateum* and *T. pertenue* cause pinta and yaws, respectively. Endemic syphilis or bejel is caused by *T. pallidum endemicum.*

Pinta has been restricted to lowland tropical areas of Central and South America. Transmission occurs during childhood by direct contact with lesions from infected individuals, but it is not transmitted by sexual contact. Patients go through three different stages, with early, secondary, and late lesions. The primary lesion is an erythematous papule that becomes scaly, psoriasiform, and even liquefied. It is usually located on lower extremities and becomes dyschromic with time. Secondary lesions appear about 2 months after the primary lesion. They are multiple and similar to the primary lesion, although smaller. The most prominent change is again the dyschromia, with hyper/ hypopigmentation mixed in single lesions. The late lesions consist of extensive areas of hypopigmentation and achromia, resembling vitiligo (Fig. 45-6). Pinta should be suspected in patients from endemic areas with extensive dyschromias. Treatment is based on penicillin therapy. The changes in color do not reverse with antibiotic therapy.

Yaws, also called "pian" or "frambesia," is a contagious, nonvenereal disease that mainly occurs in children younger than 15 years. It is endemic to all tropical areas around the world, from Central and South America, to Africa, Asia, Australia, and the Pacific Islands. The clinical manifestations go through the three classical stages of early, secondary, and late lesions. The primary lesion is a chancroid in appearance, whereas the secondary lesions are papillomatous verrucous, similar to condylomas. In skin they resemble raspberries, giving origin to the French name, "frambesia." Bone involvement can be rather destructive, ending in severe deformities and mutilations. Tertiary lesions can be gumma-like and

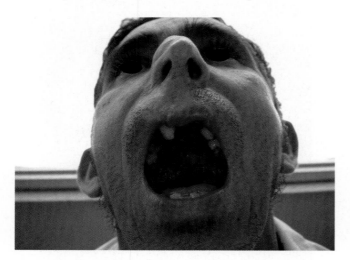

**FIGURE 45-5** ■ Rhinoscleroma, showing deformity of the nose and ulceration of the palate.

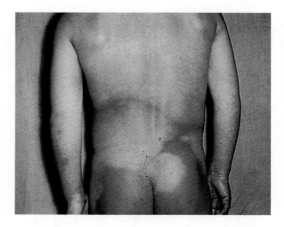

**FIGURE 45-6** ■ Pinta, showing hyper- and hypopigmented lesions.

achromic, as in pinta, and can produce palmoplantar hyperkeratosis. Treatment is based on the use of penicillin.

Bejel is still reported in the Middle East, the African Sahara, and some areas of the tropical belt. Like yaws, it is a disease of infants and children. The clinical manifestations are similar to the mucosal lesions of secondary syphilis, with a condylomatous appearance. Tertiary lesions are similar to yaws.

## Mycobacterial Infections

Tuberculosis and leprosy are diseases caused by mycobacteria. They are discussed in Chapter 21.

### Mycobacterium marinum Infection (Swimming Pool Granulomas)

*Mycobacterium marinum* (formerly called *Mycobacteria balnei)* infection is characterized by the presence of an indolent verrucous papule that later evolves into a plaque or a nodule with central scarring that may eventually ulcerate.

#### Presentation and Characteristics

It is commonly located on the extremities, especially at points of trauma (hands, elbows) that are in contact with fresh water, salt water, or marine animals such as fish or turtles. The incubation period ranges from 2 to 6 weeks. Patients may present with a papule or nodule that subsequently ulcerates (Fig. 45-7). The lesion is usually solitary, and there is no systemic reaction. Satellite lesions may appear and may simulate a localized granuloma or sporotrichotic lymphangitis. Both visualization of the bacteria on skin tissue and its isolation by culture are rather difficult.

#### Treatment

Minocycline seems to be the drug of choice. Alternatives drugs include rifampin plus ethambutol, tetracyclines, trimethoprim/sulfamethoxazole, clarithromycin, and fluoroquinolones. The duration of therapy is empiric, with rec-

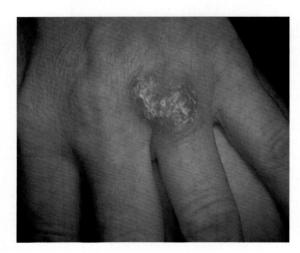

**FIGURE 45-7** ■ Swimming pool granuloma.

ommendations to continue therapy for several weeks following clinical resolution of lesions. Surgical excision, or thermal therapy, has been employed with relative success.

### Mycobacterium ulcerans Infection (Buruli Ulcer)

This mycobacterial infection was first described in southern Australia as Bairnsdale ulcer and later in Africa (from the Buruli valley in Uganda) and South America. In west and central Africa, it is considered a public health problem. This is, in fact, the third most common worldwide mycobacterium infection in immunocompetent patients, after only tuberculosis and leprosy.

#### Presentation and Characteristics

The bacteria lives in the environment and is acquired by humans through contamination of traumatic wounds. The classical clinical presentation is an ulcer, located most commonly on extremities. The cavity extends laterally, undermining the edges of the lesion, so the defect is always larger than what is seen at first glance. The ulceration will continue to enlarge and produce marked destruction and mutilation of the affected areas. The morbidity of the disease is directly related to the skin lesion, with no systemic disease.

On histology, the pattern is of massive necrosis of fatty tissue. With stains such as Ziehl–Neelsen, a huge amount of bacteria is seen in the necrotic areas, in quantities only comparable to lepromatous leprosy. The necrosis is a direct effect of a bacterial toxin, mycolactone, which is a soluble polyketide.

#### Diagnosis

The diagnosis is made on the basis of the clinical and histologic findings. The bacteria are difficult to isolate, although it can be done on special mycobacterial media. New diagnostic techniques such as polymerase chain reaction (PCR) will allow early diagnosis in smaller lesions. Surgical excision of the whole necrotic area is considered the treatment of choice.

### Rapidly Growing Mycobacteria (*Mycobacterium fortuitum* group)

This group includes a series of microorganisms causing chronic infections after traumatic surgical, cosmetic, or therapeutic inoculation. A growing number of cases are being reported in South America and around the world as late complications of liposuction or mesotherapy. Mycobacterium species implicated include *M. fortuitum, M. abscessus,* and *M. chelonae.*

#### Presentation and Characteristics

Patients present with cold abscesses at the site of trauma, injection, or surgery, weeks to months after the precipitating event (Fig. 45-8). Upon draining, a purulent fluid may be obtained. Direct examination shows the presence of acid-fast staining bacilli. Unless treated, the lesion becomes chronic, with fistula formation and progressive infiltration of surrounding tissues. Although these groups of bacteria are

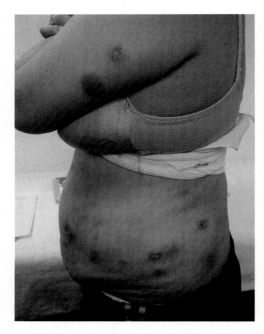

**FIGURE 45-8** ■ Multiple draining abscesses due to *Mycobacterium chelonae,* after mesotherapy.

called rapid growers, their isolation requires special media and low temperatures. *M. abscessus* is able to grow for more than a year in distilled water; contamination of surgical material or injectable substances is considered a potential source of infection when dealing with epidemic outbreaks.

### Treatment

Treatments of choice include clarithromycin and quinolones. Amikacin can be used in deep-seated infections

## Parasitic Diseases

### Protozoal Dermatosis

### Leishmaniasis

Leishmaniasis is an infectious process caused by intracellular parasites of the *Leishmania* genus. The disease is transmitted from natural reservoirs to humans by mosquito bites.

***Presentation and Characteristics.*** The different forms of cutaneous disease are produced by species of *Leishmania* specific for certain regions in the world, like those seen in the Middle East (*L. tropica*), Central America (*L. mexicana*), and South America (*L. peruviana* and *L. braziliensis*). There is even an endemic area of leishmaniasis in the state of Texas. Different names are given to the disease depending on the geographical location: Oriental sore in Asia, Chiclero's ulcer in Mexico, Uta in the Andes, and Espundia in the Amazon basin.

The classical cutaneous lesion consists of a round, isolated ulceration, with slightly elevated and indurated borders (Fig. 45-9). Common locations are areas of the body not covered by clothing and therefore exposed to the mosquito bite

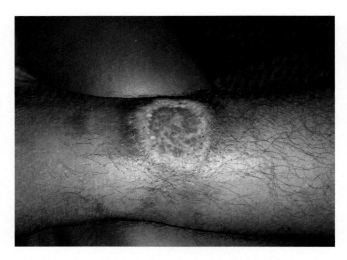

**FIGURE 45-9** ■ Round ulceration with slightly elevated borders typical of cutaneous leishmaniasis.

such as the face, neck, and extremities. The lesion itself is painless and tends to regress spontaneously.

The variety known as mucocutaneous leishmaniasis, which is cased by *L. braziliensis*, is characterized by its ability to produce, after a dormant period, an ulceration on the mucosae of the nasal septum. This can progress externally, mutilating the whole nose and nasolabial area (Fig. 45-10). When the progression is on the mucosal side, it may destroy the palate, producing a granulomatous infiltration of the pharynx, the larynx, and even the upper respiratory airway.

The tissue destruction seen in leishmaniasis is in fact a result of the great inflammatory reaction induced by the parasite, rather than the virulent effect of the microorganism

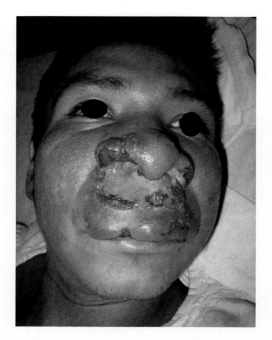

**FIGURE 45-10** ■ Nasal ulceration and upper lip infiltration and destruction typical of mucocutaneous leishmaniasis.

itself. In an early lesion, a heavy infiltration of histiocytes, many of them engulfing the *Leishmania* organism, is mixed with lymphocytes and plasma cells. The more organized the granulomas, the less likely *Leishmania* is seen on the biopsy specimens.

**Diagnosis.** Diagnostic methods include direct examination of aspirate from the ulcer, culture in specific media, skin biopsy, and PCR techniques. The leishmanin test, an intradermal reaction to fragments of the parasite, is useful when working up a diagnosis in someone who is just an occasional visitor to endemic areas. The high sensitivity of the test makes it very useful to rule out rather than to confirm the diagnosis.

**Treatment.** Treatment, when indicated, is based on use of antimonial preparations and, in difficult cases, of amphotericin B. Always consider leishmaniasis in the differential diagnosis of chronic cutaneous ulcerations, especially when there is a history of living in or traveling to endemic areas, some of which are very popular among the adventure tourist. A significant number of soldiers involved in the Middle East war have developed the disease.

### African/American Trypanosomiasis

African trypanosomiasis or "sleeping sickness" is transmitted to humans by bites of infected tsetse flies. A painful and indurated trypanosomal chancre appears in some patients 5 to 15 days after the inoculation of the parasite and resolves spontaneously over several weeks. Transient edema is common and can occur in the face, hands, feet, and other periarticular areas. Pruritus is frequent, and an irregular maculopapular rash is often present. This rash is located on the trunk, shoulders, buttocks, and thighs and consists of annular, blotchy, erythematous areas with clear centers, called trypanids. Eventually, the parasitic invasion reaches the central nervous system (CNS), causing behavioral and neurologic changes (giving rise to the name sleeping sickness).

American trypanosomiasis or Chagas disease is transmitted by a reduviid, *Triatoma infestans* (kissing bug). Infections occur when the bug breaks into the skin, mucous membranes, or conjunctivae. They then become contaminated with bug feces containing infective parasites. When the organisms enter the skin, an indurated area of erythema and swelling (chagoma), accompanied by local lymphadenopathy, may appear. The Romaña sign, which consists of unilateral, painless edema of the palpebrae and periocular tissues, occurs in cases of entry through the conjunctiva. These initial local signs may be followed by malaise, fever, anorexia, and edema of the face and lower extremities. Some patients may also develop a rash that clears in several days. Cardiac involvement is the most frequent and serious defined manifestation of chronic Chagas disease. Treatment is unsatisfactory, with only two drugs (nifurtimox and benznidazole) available for this purpose.

Unfortunately, both drugs lack efficacy and often cause severe side effects.

### Amebiasis, Including Free-living Amebas and Entamoeba histolytica

Free-living amebas are usually associated with disease of the CNS. The infection is acquired by swimming in ponds and streams with still water. There are two types of meningoencephalitis produced by these organisms. The *Naegleria* species cause an acute form, with no skin manifestations. The subacute, granulomatous form is produced by two genera, *Acanthamoeba* and *Balamuthia*. *Acanthamoeba* infection is known to induce chronic ulcerative lesions in AIDS patients and, rarely, isolated, centrofacial plaques in immunocompetent hosts. In the 1990s, a new variety, named *Balamuthia mandrillaris*, was recognized as the causative agent of many cases of free-living amoeba granulomatous meningoencephalitis around the world, especially in South America and Australia. Cases have been reported in the United States, mainly in the states of California and Texas.

The classical presentation will include a primary skin lesion, in the form of a central face plaque, of granulomatous appearance, usually located on the nose but also in the trunk and extremities. In the months following the cutaneous involvement, all patients develop focal CNS symptoms, marking the beginning of necrotizing encephalitis. Except for few cases reported in the last few years, the outcome is always fatal. However, the early recognition of the skin lesion as a marker of the infection may allow early treatment with a combination of antiparasitic and antifungal drugs, with subsequent improvement of the survival rates.

*Entamoeba histolytica* can produce cutaneous lesions, most commonly in the anal margin and genital region (**Fig. 45-11**) but also beyond those areas, such as in the abdominal wall. The lesions are large cutaneous ulcerations, vegetative lesions, and even abscesses. They are, characteristically, extremely painful.

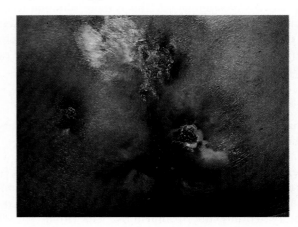

**FIGURE 45-11** ■ Cutaneous amebiasis with deep ulcers on the buttocks, due to *Entamoeba histolytica*. *(Courtesy of Dr. A. Gonzalez-Orchoa.)*

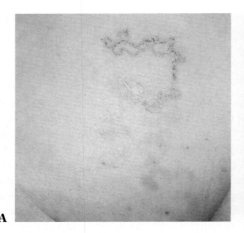
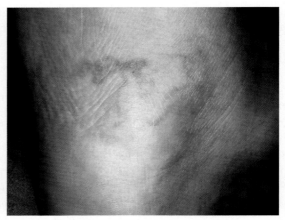

A                                          B

**FIGURE 45-12** ■ **(A)** Larva migrans. **(B)** Creeping eruption of larva migrans on the sole.

## Helminthic Dermatosis (Roundworm)

### Cutaneous Larva Migrans

**Presentation and Characteristics.** This is a disease caused by hookworms, usually parasites of dogs and cats. The ova are excreted through the feces, and they remain viable in sandy, moist ground. The larva penetrates the skin of bathers or people who walk on the contaminated ground. Usually, the "culprits" are *Ancylostoma duodenale, Necator americanus,* and other hookworms. Clinically, the parasite causes a serpentine, erythematous, papular, pruritic eruption in the skin (Fig. 45-12). The parasite is usually ahead of the tract. Vesicles, excoriations, and crusts are present.

**Treatment.** Treatment includes topical thiabendazole or albendazole by mouth, 200 mg twice a day for 3 days.

### Larva Currens

As opposed to cutaneous larva migrans, in which lesions move over a period of days, the cutaneous form of *strongyloidiasis* moves over a period of hours, which is the reason for the "currens" denomination. This is more common in immunosuppressed patients, in whom multiple tracts are seen. At the present time, ivermectin is the treatment of choice, 200 μg/kg, and in these immunosuppressed patients, it can actually be life saving.

### Gnathostomiasis

This condition was described initially as a parasite of large felines by Owen in 1886.

**Presentation and Characteristics.** Several species of *Gnathostoma* are capable of causing the disease, most commonly *G. spinigerum.* Clinically, it produces a nodular, migratory, eosinophilic panniculitis. The adult parasite normally inhabits the stomachs of domestic animals such as dogs and cats. The eggs are excreted in the stools of these animals. They then reach the rivers, hatch in the

water, and are ingested by crustaceans of the *Cyclops* species, where they develop into a second larval stage. Fish later ingest the *Cyclops* organisms, forming a third larval stage in their muscular tissue. Humans, who are not the definitive host, could develop the characteristic panniculitis of this disease from eating contaminated raw fish, in the form of seviche or sushi. The parasite migrates through the tissues, most commonly to the skin, but it may go to any of the internal organs. Clinically, after a variable incubation period of 4 weeks to 3 years, patients develop the classical symptom of a pruritic, migratory, edematous panniculitis (Fig. 45-13).

**Treatment.** Treatment alternatives include albendazole 200 mg, twice daily for 2 to 3 weeks or ivermectin 200 μg/kg in a single dose that can be repeated every 2 weeks.

### Filariasis

Three species of filarial parasites commonly inhabit the lymphatic system of humans: *Wuchereria bancrofti* and *Brugia*

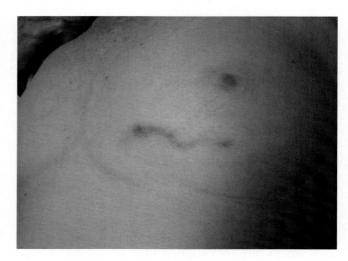

**FIGURE 45-13** ■ Gnathostomiasis showing superficial and deep patterns of migration.

*malayi* in Asia and tropical Africa and *Brugia timori* on the Indonesian archipelago.

**Presentation and Characteristics.** The major symptoms of filariasis relate to damaged lymphatics. Acute lymphangitis and lymphadenitis may affect limbs, breasts, and genitalia. Urticaria may be part of the clinical presentation. Late changes are due to obstruction of lymphatics, giving origin to different forms of elephantiasis with massive edemas. Some patients with elephantiasis develop a crusty, verrucous skin change.

**Diagnosis.** Diagnosis is reached by the presence of microfilaria in blood smears and by serologic testing.

**Treatment.** Treatment with diethylcarbamazine (6 mg/kg daily for 12 days) remains the treatment of choice for the individual with active lymphatic filariasis, although albendazole (400 mg twice daily for 21 days) has also demonstrated macrofilaricidal efficacy.

## Onchocerciasis

Onchocerciasis is a chronic infestation of the skin by *Onchocerca volvulus*. This is a microfilarial nematode whose natural hosts are humans and flies from the genus *Simulium*.

The disease was first described in Africa and later in Central America. Recently it has been reported in the northern countries of South America.

**Presentation and Characteristics.** The transmission occurs when flies become infected by biting infected people. After a short period of maturation, the microfilaria moves to the buccal apparatus of the insect and enters the skin of a noninfected human with the next blood meal. The infective forms become adults in 6 to 8 months inside cutaneous nodules called onchocercomas, where they start to produce microfilarias. These nodules are firm, often flattened or bean-shaped, usually movable, and nontender. They can be up to several centimeters in diameter. Other clinical presentations include acute and chronic papular forms, facial erythema, facial livedoid discoloration, facial aging, and prurigo-like eruption on the buttocks and extremities. Later signs are extensive lichenification and dyschromia similar to vitiligo. Ocular involvement is due to the direct invasion of eye structures by the microfilaria, causing uveitis, conjunctivitis, keratitis, optical nerve atrophy, and glaucoma. It may evolve into complete and permanent loss of vision, thus the reason for naming the disease "river blindness."

**Diagnosis.** Diagnosis is easy to confirm, either by direct scraping or histologic analysis of skin lesions in which adult forms and microfilarias are identified.

**Treatment.** Ivermectin is extremely effective, even as a single-dose therapy.

## Trematodes Dermatosis (Flukes)

### Cercarial Dermatitis

*Cercarial dermatitis* or swimmer's itch is caused by the penetration of the skin by schistosoma of birds or mammals. The cercaria is found in bodies of fresh water. It can penetrate the skin of a mammal and, if the host is receptive, reach the bloodstream and spread to other organs. In humans, who are not the definitive host, the cercariae are unsuccessful in reaching the blood. They are retained in the epithelial layers and finally destroyed, resulting in dermatitis. Clinically, pruritic macules, papules, hemorrhages, and excoriations develop in the exposed areas. This resulting dermatitis is a product of the sensitization to the cercarial proteins. In massive or repeated infestations, the signs and symptoms are consequently more severe.

Cercarial dermatitis should be distinguished from *seabather's eruption*. The latter is an eruption that generally occurs in the area under swimwear after bathing in the ocean. However, it may also be seen in the axilla, neck, and flexor areas (Fig. 45-14). It is pruritic and papular and occurs within hours of leaving affected waters. Occasionally, the skin eruption is complicated by fatigue, malaise, fever, chills, nausea, and GI complaints. These episodes appear to be more severe after repeated attacks. The condition is caused by the cnidarian larvae of *Linuche unguiculata* (thimble jellyfish). This larva has been found in water samples, and, in affected patients, high immunoglobulin G (IgG) levels specific to *L. unguiculata* have been demonstrated. Symptomatic treatment is accomplished with antihistamines, topical corticosteroids, and even oral steroid therapy. A self-limiting condition, it lasts up to 12 days.

### Schistosomiasis and Bilharziasis

Schistosomiasis and bilharziasis occur when humans come into contact with water infested by the flukes belonging to the genus *Schistosoma*. The disease manifests itself by the immune response to invading and migrating larvae. Cercarial dermatitis refers to the clinical picture elucidated

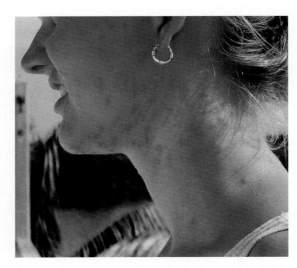

**FIGURE 45-14** ■ Seabather's eruption, caused by thimble jellyfish off the coast of Belize. *(Courtesy of Dr. Kate Schafer.)*

by the penetration of cercaria into the skin. The clinical findings are those of an acute pruritic, papular rash at the site of the cercarial penetration, accompanied by a prickling sensation. Treatment of cercarial dermatitis and acute schistosomiasis should be directed toward treating the symptoms. Chronic schistosomiasis can be effectively treated with a single dose of praziquantel, with artemisinin as an alternative treatment.

## Dermatosis Caused by Arthropods

### Human Scabies

#### Presentation and Characteristics

This disease is transmitted through prolonged personal contact and less often by clothing and bed linens. The mite's location is in a "burrow" in the stratum corneum where it deposits its eggs. An allergic sensitization to the mite and/or its products causes the clinical picture. Itching appears 2 to 4 weeks after the infestation and is classically more severe at night. As a clinical finding, the burrow is pathognomonic and diagnostic. The remaining lesions are secondary to scratching, secondary infection, and allergic reaction. The burrow is a skin-colored, tortuous, elevated line of 1 to 1.5 cm in length. It is usually found in the finger webs, flexor surfaces of the wrists, nipples, and elbows (Fig. 45-15). In children, the lesions can be vesicular and located on the face, palms, and soles.

#### Diagnosis

The diagnosis is confirmed by a scraping preparation of the skin and identification of the parasite.

#### Treatment

One 8-hour application at night of permethrin, 5% solution or cream, is considered the standard treatment today. The gamma isomer of hexachlorobenzene (lindane), 1% in a vanishing cream, was used for years, but it is used less commonly today because of its toxicity and should not be used in pregnant women or infants. With both medications, a second application is made after 1 week. Note that this application should cover the entire body very thoroughly. Areas not to be missed include the umbilicus, genital area, and the area under the nails. Ivermectin, 200 $\mu$g/kg, in a single dose has been found to be very effective. A 6% sulfur precipitate in Vaseline for 3 consecutive days is employed in infants and pregnant women. The nails should be cut short and scrubbed vigorously. Clothing and bed linen should be washed thoroughly.

#### Variations

Norwegian scabies, also known as crusted scabies, is the same disease but in an immunosuppressed individual. Typically, extensive, crusted hyperkeratotic plaques are seen but itching may not be as prominent. The direct examination of scrapings shows a massive infestation, and the patient is much more contagious. Treatment should include exfoliants such as 20% urea or 20% salicylic acid in an ointment base. Nodular scabies consists of brown or red firm nodules on the penis, scrotum, or buttocks. Such lesions may persist for months despite specific scabicidal treatment. Their prolonged course is the result of a delayed allergic reaction that does not require a viable mite to be present.

### Animal Scabies

In this disease, very similar to papular urticaria, the mites invade human skin but they do not become established in it. There are varieties from dogs, sheep, birds, and so forth. Excoriated, crusted papules can be seen and pruritus can be very severe, especially in the evening.

### Arachnidism

#### Latrodectism

*Latrodectus mactans* are small, dark spiders called "black widows." They have a black or brown underside with a red,

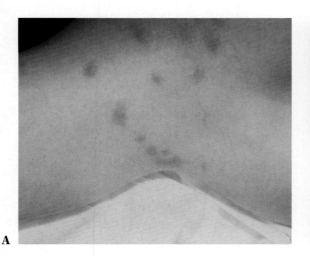
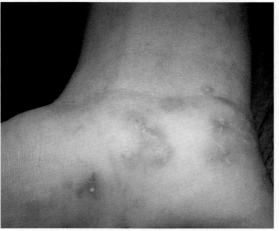

**FIGURE 45-15** ■ **(A)** and **(B)** Scabies.

orange, or white hourglass marking on the back. They are commonly found near protected places such as the undersides of stones and logs, in the angles of doors, windows, and shutters, and in outhouses. Their venom is neurotoxic; they usually bite on the genitalia or buttocks. Pain develops within about an hour, with accompanying reddening and swelling. Systemic symptoms include muscle cramping, rigidity, and later weakness, sweating, bradycardia, hypothermia, and hypotension. The mortality rate is about 5% in children.

***Treatment.*** Treatment includes intravenous 10% calcium gluconate and corticosteroids. However, the most effective therapy is systemic antivenom.

### Loxoscelism

*Loxosceles reclusus* is found in the United States, and *Loxosceles laeta* is found in Central and South America. The *Loxosceles* spiders are light brown to chocolate in color, with nocturnal habits, and are commonly found seeking warmth in discarded clothing.

***Presentation and Characteristics.*** Usually affected areas include the arm and thigh of adults or the face in children. Pain develops 2 to 8 hours after the bite. The lesion becomes indurated and red, with a central blister and subsequent necrosis that can be quite large (Fig. 45-16). The necrotic area eventually becomes mummified. Around the 14th day, the eschar may slough off.

Rarely, general symptoms include fever, chills, vomiting, petechiae on the skin, as well as thrombocytopenia and hemolytic anemia, especially in children. Treatment is with antivenom, corticosteroids, and dapsone, which may be very effective in limiting the size and extension of the necrosis.

### Diseases Caused by Chiggers

These mites, also known as *harvest mites*, are the cause of the infestation known as trombiculiasis. It is seen worldwide, although most frequently in tropical areas. The disease is acquired while walking through vegetation, and the affected area is usually exposed skin depending on the type of clothing worn. The offending chigger is the larval stage of the mite, 0.25 to 0.4 mm in diameter, orange to red in color, and with three pairs of legs. It gets fixed to the skin by its buccal apparatus and starts a process of liquefying and sucking the skin elements. As a consequence, it produces a type of papular urticaria and multiple red itchy papules that are sometimes purpuric and are extremely pruritic (Fig. 45-17).

### Treatment

Topical treatment is with steroids and antipruritic lotions. Occasionally this condition requires systemic antibiotic therapy as well as systemic steroids.

### Diseases Caused by Nigua

Tungiasis is a human infestation produced by *Tunga penetrans*, a sand flea that thrives on moist, sandy ground near pigsties and cowsheds. It is widely distributed in tropical and subtropical areas of South America and Africa. It is known by various names (*pique, nigua, bicho dos pes*). It is commonly acquired when walking barefoot in contaminated areas, including residential gardens recently fertilized with cattle manure.

### Presentation and Characteristics

The infection is produced by the female flea, which burrows into the skin between the toes and near the nail. The flea inserts her body full of eggs, to die at a later time. The initial clinical manifestation is a black dot representing the burrow full of eggs that can later be seen on top of a papule or vesicle (Fig. 45-18). The walls of the burrow are horny tissue from the epidermis itself. The lesion becomes infected or simply produces a foreign body reaction that terminates in suppuration and opening of the cavity. Coalescing lesions may form a honeycomb plaque. This may serve as a port of entry for a more severe infection and even gangrene.

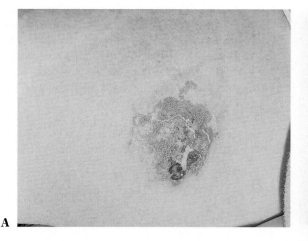
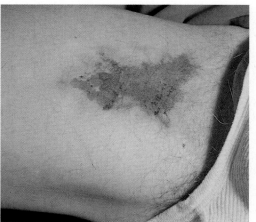

**FIGURE 45-16** ■ **(A)** Spider bite (*Loxosceles laeta*), with erythema, central necrosis, and blister formation. **(B)** Spider bite (*L. laeta*), with vertical extension of necrosis due to gravity.

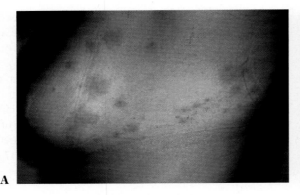

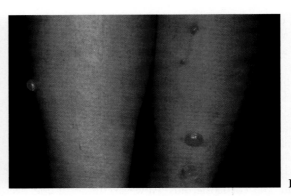

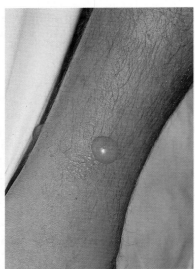

**FIGURE 45-17** ■ **(A)** Chigger bites collected under the bra. **(B)** Bullous chigger bites on the legs. **(C)** Chigger bite blister formation.

### Treatment

The best treatment is the extraction of all insect parts. The best prevention is to wear closed shoes in high-risk areas.

### Paederus Dermatitis

*Blister beetle dermatitis,* or *paederus dermatitis,* is caused by contact with the body fluids of *Paederus irritans,* a member

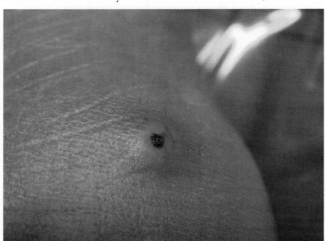

**FIGURE 45-18** ■ *Tunga penetrans* on the heel: classic morphology of a black dot at the center of a pustule.

of the order Coleoptera, family Staphylinidae. These blister beetles are closely related to the Spanish fly, the producer of cantharidin. An increased incidence has been seen in Peru and Ecuador during years of presentation of the El Niño phenomenon. The same disease, following an identical cycle during El Niño years, is seen in other continents like Africa. In Kenya, different species of *Paederus,* mainly *P. crebinpunctatis* and *P. sabaeus,* are responsible for the disease (*Nairobi fly*). Clinically, an initial burning is felt followed by erythema and, later, the appearance of a blister, usually in a linear fashion ("latigazo" or whiplash) in exposed parts of the body (Fig. 45-19). The vesication is produced by paederin, a protein from the exoskeleton of the insect.

### Treatment

Treatment includes compresses, topical corticosteroids, and in some serious cases, oral prednisone and antibiotics.

## Deep Fungi

### Histoplasmosis

This disease is caused by *Histoplasma capsulatum.* Found throughout the world in temperate areas, *H. capsulatum* is a saprophytic fungus that grows in the soil, prevalently in the soil of caves inhabited by bats. The disease is transmitted by

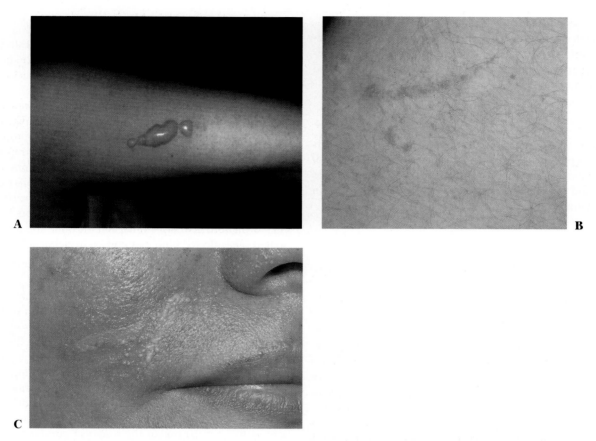

**FIGURE 45-19** ▪ **(A)** Blister beetle bullous reaction on the arm. **(B, C)** Beetle dermatitis, whiplash effect (latigazo).

the inadvertent inhalation of the spores. Epidemics have occurred while exploring infested caves or cleaning sites where chicken excrement (guano) may be present.

*Presentation and Characteristics*

A benign clinical form mimicking a common cold may leave a calcified nodule in the lung similar to that of tuberculosis. In its most severe form, the disease can disseminate, involving the reticuloendothelial system. Most cutaneous cases are seen in patients with AIDS. In such patients the disease is seen in its most severe form. Lesions can be papules, plaques, ulcerations (Fig. 45-20), umbilicated lesions, mimicking molluscum contagiosum, and deep-seated nodules, mimicking cellulitis or panniculitis. Primary cutaneous histoplasmosis occurs and is caused by direct inoculation. It is a nodular or indurated chancroid ulcer with accompanying lymphadenopathy. Occasionally, an allergic response has been seen appearing as urticaria or as erythema annulare centrifugum.

*Diagnosis*

The diagnosis is accomplished by demonstrating the presence of small, intracellular *H. capsulatum* in sputum, bone marrow, or biopsy specimens. Serology can be helpful.

*Treatment*

Treatment is with ketoconazole or itraconazole.

## Coccidioidomycosis or San Joaquin Valley Fever

This disease is caused by *Coccidioides immitis*, a soil inhabitant. Infection in both humans and animals is acquired by the inhalation of fungus-laden dust particles or, rarely, through a primary infection of the skin.

*Presentation and Characteristics*

The severity of coccidioidomycosis can range from very mild, simulating a common cold, to an acute disseminated

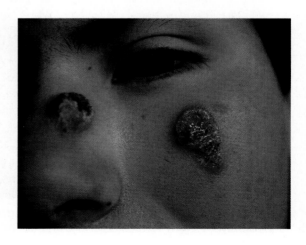

**FIGURE 45-20** ▪ Ulceration due to histoplasmosis.

fatal disease, especially in patients with AIDS. An allergic reaction with erythema multiforme or erythema nodosum occurs in some cases. The basic symptoms of malaise and fever may suggest coccidioidomycosis if the patient has traveled through an endemic area.

### Diagnosis

Diagnosis is made by potassium hydroxide (KOH) mounts of sputum or isolation of the fungus in a culture. Colonies of the coccidioidomycosis fast-growing phase are dangerous to handle and the greatest care should be implemented when manipulating cultures.

### Treatment

Treatment includes amphotericin B, ketoconazole, and itraconazole.

## Chromoblastomycosis

Chromoblastomycosis is a chronic cutaneous mycosis, characterized by a distinct clinical presentation and the presence of the so-called sclerotic bodies on tissue cuts. A great variety of fungi are able to cause the disease, including *Phialophora verrucosa, Fonsecaea pedrosoi, Fonsecaea compacta, Cladosporium carrionii, Rhinocladiella aquaspersa,* and *Botryomyces caespitosus.* The disease has been reported worldwide, with most cases coming from the tropical and subtropical areas of South America and Africa. Some fungi have a preference for certain climates. *F. pedrosoi* is most common in wet and humid areas within the torrid zones, whereas *C. carrionii* prefers the dry and semidesert regions of the tropical–intertropical zones.

### Presentation and Characteristics

The most common affected areas are the lower extremities, although in some geographic locations, like the arid plains of Venezuela, the upper girdle (shoulder, arm, back) is the prevalent site of infection.

The primary process occurs at the site of inoculation, most probably through traumatized skin. The fungus is acquired from the environment, where it lives as a saprophyte of wood, vegetable debris, or soil. The disease is not transmitted from person to person. The primary lesion is exophytic, presenting as a papule, a nodule, or a tumor. The lesions multiply and tend to coalesce, forming plaques with a verrucous surface (**Fig. 45-21**). Ulceration may develop, but there is no fistula formation, as in mycetoma, and the bone and muscle are spared. The affected limb may end up in elephantiasis.

### Diagnosis

The diagnosis is easily made by direct examination with KOH of scrapings from the lesion. The morphology adopted by the fungus is a cluster of oblong, round cells with thick walls and flattened abutting surfaces, divided by septation in more than one plane. They are known as *sclerotic bodies* or *muriform cells.* The histopathology shows pseudocarcinomatous hyperplasia with a granulomatous suppurative reaction in the dermis. The sclerotic bodies have a brown color and are easily identified because their size (4 to 12 mm) makes them appear similar to "copper pennies." Species identification is only possible after culture isolation on Sabouraud's media, after 4 to 6 weeks.

### Treatment

Treatment options include surgical excision when the lesion is small. Pharmacologic agents, reported to be useful but

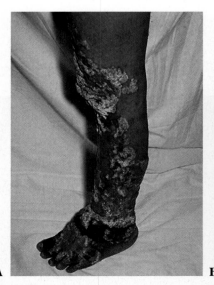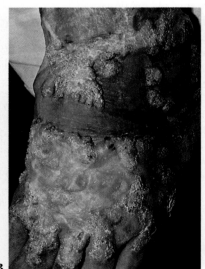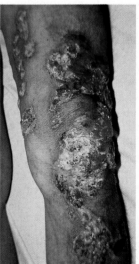

**FIGURE 45-21** ■ Chromoblastomycosis: cauliflower like leg lesion (**A**), with a close-up of the foot (**B**) another case of Chromoblastomycosis with verrucous surface and ulcerations (**C**).

probably not curative by themselves, include 5-flucytosine, itraconazole, and saperconazole.

## Mycetoma or Maduromycosis

Also known as Madura foot, mycetoma is a chronic subcutaneous infection with a distinct clinical picture of edema with fistula formation and draining of grains. The disease is caused by at least 20 different species of fungi (eumycetoma) and actinomycetes (actinomycetoma). Among the true fungi are *Madurella mycetomi, Madurella grisea, Pseudallescheria boydii, Acremonium kiliense, Leptosphaeria tompkinsii, Exophiala jeanselmei, Neotestudina rosati, Curvularia lunata, Aspergillus nidulans, Fusarium moniliforme,* and *Phialophora cyanescens.* Actinomycetomas may be caused by *Actinomadura madurae, Streptomyces somaliensis, Nocardia asteroides,* and *Nocardia braziliensis.* The disease has a worldwide distribution. Originally described in India, with a high incidence in the region of Madura, it is typically seen in dry, tropical areas. Endemic areas include Sudan, India, Somalia, Mexico, and the Amazon region. Whereas in Mexico cases are predominantly due to *Nocardia* species, in South America the predominant agent is *M. grisea.*

### Presentation and Characteristics

The organisms gain entry into the body due to trauma, and the disease is most common in adult males who work outdoors barefoot or who expose large areas of the skin, as stevedores do. The clinical picture manifests over a period of months or years as a nodule that later evolves into edematous areas with marked fibrosis, followed by the formation of a fistula that drains or expels "grains" (**Fig. 45-22**). Lesions are commonly located on the extremities, either on the feet or the shoulder. Bone involvement is characterized by periosteal erosion and proliferation as well as the development of lytic lesions; otherwise, there is no systemic involvement.

### Diagnosis

The presence of grains in the context of the clinical picture of edema and fistula formation favors mycetoma. Morphology of the grains may give an idea of the specific etiologic agent, but precise identification will require culture isolation. Dark grains are usually due to fungi and white to yellow grains can be either due to actinomyces or fungi.

### Treatment

Treatment depends on the organism isolated. For cases where actinomycetes are isolated, therapeutic agents that have been used include streptomycin, dapsone, sulfamethoxazole/ trimethoprim, rifampin, and amikacin. Eumycetoma is more difficult to treat, with some response to oral imidazoles reported, including ketoconazole, itraconazole, voriconazole, and posaconazole. Surgery should be considered for more advanced cases.

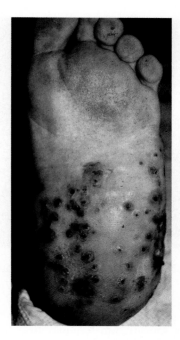

**FIGURE 45-22** ■ Mycetoma. The black granules are more indicative of a fungal rather than an actinomycotic etiology.

## Sporotrichosis

Sporotrichosis is a mycotic infection produced by the environmental fungus *Sporothrix schenkii.* It has a worldwide distribution, although hyperendemic areas do exist, for example in the Peruvian Andes. It is commonly associated with trauma from a rose thorn and is an occupational hazard for florists and gardeners.

### Presentation and Characteristics

The classical picture (about 70% of cases) is the so-called lymphocutaneous or sporotrichoid pattern characterized by a primary lesion, mostly an ulcerated plaque, followed by several satellite lesions, either papular, nodular, or crusted, in a linear distribution, following the lymphatic drainage (**Fig. 45-23**). It is commonly located on an extremity and, in children, on the face. There is a second type of presentation with only one isolated lesion, either a plaque, a nodule, or an ulcer (**Fig. 45-24**). This is known as the fixed cutaneous form of sporotrichosis. Rarely, the infection can disseminate to involve multiple sites and organs. The most common extracutaneous sites are joints.

### Diagnosis

The fungus is rarely seen on direct examination or on tissue cuts, even with special stains. When visible, it has a levaduriform morphology. However, the fungus easily grows on Sabouraud's media, which is the easiest and most reliable method for diagnosis. The intradermal reaction

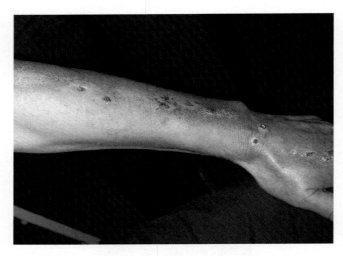

**FIGURE 45-23** ■ Sporotrichosis, classical sporotrichoid pattern.

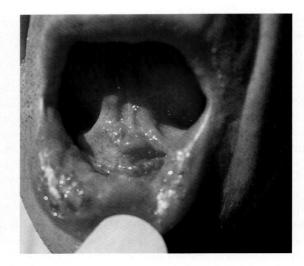

**FIGURE 45-25** ■ An infiltrative, deforming lesion of paracoccidioidomycosis.

known as the sporotrichin test may help to confirm the diagnosis.

### Treatment

Treatment options include the use of potassium iodide solution and itraconazole. Therapy should be prolonged for 2 weeks after achieving total clinical remission.

## Paracoccidioidomycosis

As opposed to sporotrichosis and chromoblastomycosis, in which the disease is located at the inoculation site, paracoccidioidomycosis is a systemic disease with hematogenous spreading from a primary pulmonary focus.

The infection has a specific geographic distribution through Central and South America. The agent, *Paracoccidioides brasiliensis*, is a dimorphic fungus with special preference for tropical and subtropical forest with mild temperature and high humidity.

### Presentation and Characteristics

The infection is acquired by inhalation, with a primary lesion in the lung. From there, it may take one of two forms:

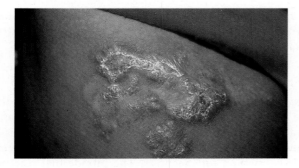

**FIGURE 45-24** ■ Sporotrichosis, fixed lesion.

an aggressive form with an acute severe pneumonia and rapidly progressive systemic disease or a relentless course with chronic pulmonary disease. The typical patient is a middle-aged male agricultural worker. These patients may present to the dermatologist with involvement of the mucosae and skin. Lesions on the lips, buccal mucosae, gums, palate, and pharynx are infiltrating, ulcerated plaques and nodules, with subsequent destruction and scarring deformities (Fig. 45-25).

On the skin the lesions vary widely. They may begin as small acneiform pustules 2 to 3 mm in size that later ulcerate, or they can adopt a pattern related to the affected lymph nodes. A cold abscess may develop. In some instances multiple symmetric papules, either with verrucous or umbilicated surfaces, may be present. On soles, they could be easily misinterpreted as warts (Fig. 45-26), whereas on the face, they may look like molluscum contagiosum.

### Diagnosis

The size of the fungus and its characteristic morphology allow easy identification on sputum preparations and scrapings from the mucosal and cutaneous lesions. It is easy to recognize the blastospores with multiple budding giving the "pilot wheel" appearance (Fig. 45-27). Identical structures are seen on histologic examination of the affected tissues. The reaction pattern seen on biopsy is a granulomatous reaction with multiple giant cells, some of them engulfing the budding elements. The fungus will grow on Sabouraud's medium in 4 or more weeks, as a mold at 20°C to 26°C and as a yeast at 34°C to 37°C.

### Treatment

Treatment choices have evolved, from sulfonamides to ketoconazole up to the new triazoles (itraconazole and fluconazole). At present, itraconazole is considered the drug of

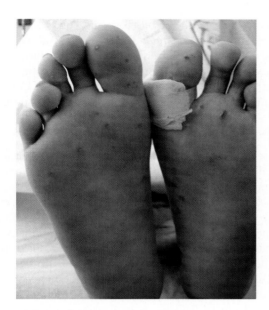

**FIGURE 45-26** ■ Wartlike lesions of paracoccidioidomycosis on the soles.

choice because of the lower doses required, shorter period of treatment, and fewer side effects.

## Lobomycosis

This chronic skin infection is produced by *Lacazia loboi* (formerly *Loboa loboi*), a large fungus with a levaduriform morphology. The disease is endemic in tropical areas of South America.

### Presentation and Characteristics

The disease is acquired by primary inoculation from the environment through traumatized skin. The clinical lesions take years to develop. The classical clinical manifestation is the formation of nodules with a keloid appearance, usually located on the extremities, ears, face,

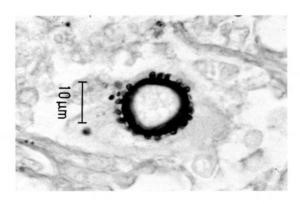

**FIGURE 45-27** ■ A Grocott methenamine silver (GMS) stain in tissue demonstrating the blastospore with the characteristic "pilot wheel" appearance. *(Courtesy of Dr. James Fishback, University of Kansas Medical Center.)*

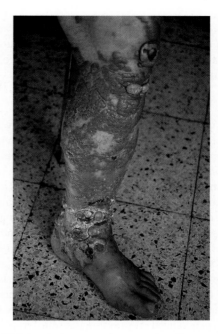

**FIGURE 45-28** ■ Lobomycosis: compare the smooth surface with what is seen in chromoblastomycosis.

and neck, with the scalp spared in most cases. Other primary lesions include infiltrated plaques, gummas, ulcers, and verrucoid nodules (Fig. 45-28). The histology consists of a massive histiocytic infiltrate, without the pseudocarcinomatous hyperplasia commonly seen in chromoblastomycosis. This is the reason why in lobomycosis the nodules tend to have a smooth surface, as opposed to the verrucous surface of chromomycosis. The morphology of the fungus is quite distinctive, as globose, lemon-shaped buds, 9 to 10 mm in diameter, organized in short and long chains of uniform beads. The organism is easily seen in KOH preparations from lesions. The fungus has not been grown in culture media.

### Treatment

The only effective treatment is wide surgical excision. Recurrence is very common. A recent report suggests that the combination of itraconazole and clofazimine, or posaconazole alone may be of some benefit.

## Noninfectious Miscellaneous Dermatosis

### Pityriasis Alba

This is very common in children and consists of hypopigmented, poorly defined, scaly macules and plaques found on the face and upper outer arms. It is believed to be a mild form of atopic eczema. Lesions are first noticed after exposure to sunshine where the surrounding sun-affected skin appears quite tan.

### Treatment

Treatment consists of topical 1% hydrocortisone cream at night and sunscreens during the day. Topical tacrolimus has been used as an alternative treatment.

### Papular Urticaria

This term defines an exuberant reaction to arthropod bites. Initially there is an irritated weal, and, later, an intensely pruritic papule develops at the site of the bite. There may be a central hemorrhagic puncture, a vesicle, or even a blister, especially in children. A linear array of the lesions is a common characteristic (Fig. 45-29). The number and localization of the lesions depends on the type of exposure and feeding habits of the arthropod. New bites may exacerbate quiescent old bites. Because of scratching, lesions can become infected and crusted. Localization of the affected areas helps reveal the causative arthropod. Involvement of the legs suggests fleas, involvement of the waist and thighs suggests chiggers, involvement of the abdomen and arms suggests sarcoptic mange of dogs, and a generalized eruption suggests bird mites.

### Treatment

Treatment consists of oral antihistaminics, topical corticosteroids, and fumigation of the dwelling.

### Miliaria

Also known as *prickly heat, sudamina,* or *lichen tropicus,* this condition results from the obstruction of the sweat ducts caused by a combination of extreme heat and humidity. Depending on the level of obstruction, different clinical pictures can be seen. In the so-called *miliaria crystallina,* obstruction is very superficial, resulting in tiny vesicles. In *miliaria rubra,* the obstruction is deeper and clinically more pruritic. The

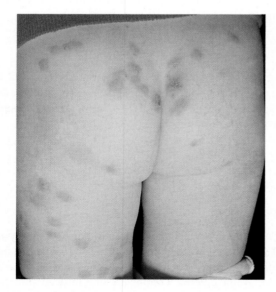

FIGURE 45-29 ■Papular urticaria: note how lesions group in a linear array, three or four in a row.

lesions have an erythematous base and consist of tiny, red papules. In *miliaria profunda* there can be associated anhydrosis, compensatory hyperhydrosis, and so-called *tropical asthenia.* Secondary infections are common. Treatment consists of a cooler environment, loose clothing, fluids by mouth, and antibiotics where indicated for secondary infection.

### Pemphigus Foliaceus (Fogo Selvagem)

Fogo selvagem is an endemic type of pemphigus foliaceus, described in the Amazonic regions of Brazil and to a lesser degree in other countries in South America. It is clinically identical to the common type of pemphigus foliaceus, except for the young age of the population affected and its common presentation in families. Genetic as well as environmental factors have been implicated in the pathogenesis. Field studies have demonstrated that healthy populations from endemic areas have circulating antibodies against desmoglein 1. The areas of prevalence are regions of wild jungle that have become agricultural. The disease may take a self-limited course or, most likely, progress to a generalized form that otherwise is identical to the cosmopolitan forms of pemphigus. The patient may become erythrodermic. The disease follows a chronic course; treatment is based on high-dose corticosteroid therapy as well as other forms of immunosuppressive therapy.

## A Final Word

The globalization of present times has made the word "exotic" useless. The patient that one might see in a clinic in a midwestern city may have just returned from a trip to the Amazon—less than a 23-hour flight—and the little ulceration he has on his right arm may not be just a simple impetigo but a cutaneous form of leishmaniasis or another heretofore remote condition. A global world means global patients and, thus, requires global thinking. A sufficient history for the dermatology patient should include questions about the faraway places to which he or she may have traveled and the surroundings to which he or she may have been exposed. In jet age dermatology, just looking may no longer be enough.

## Acknowledgements

We are grateful to Dr. Beatriz Bustamante, Dr. Carlos Seas, and the Leishmania Group of the Instituto de Medicina Tropical Alexander von Humboldt of the Universidad

---

**SAUER'S NOTES**

1. Ignore the plethora of diseases related to tropical climates in this globalized world and you will run the risk of missed diagnoses.
2. Where your body has been may have a lot to do with where your health is going.
3. Once again the skin is at the forefront of early signs of disease, when it is at its most treatable stage.

Peruana Cayetano Heredia for allowing us to use some of their clinical photos.

## Suggested Readings

Bravo F, Sanchez MR. New and re-emerging cutaneous infectious diseases in Latin America and other geographic areas. *Dermatol Clin.* 2003;21(4): 655–668.

Canizares O, Harman R. *Clinical Tropical Dermatology.* 2nd ed. Boston: Blackwell Scientific; 1992.

Cieslak TJ, Eitzen EM Jr. Clinical and epidemiologic principles of anthrax. *Emerg Infect Dis.* 1999;5(4):552–555.

Cockerell CJ. The causative agent of bacillary angiomatosis. *Int J Dermatol.* 1992;31:615–617.

Fisher AA. *Atlas of Aquatic Dermatology.* Orlando, FL: Grune & Stratton; 1978.

Grevelink SA, Lerner EA. Leishmaniasis. *J Am Acad Dermatol.* 1996;34: 257–272.

Koff AB, Rosen T. Nonvenereal treponematoses: yaws, endemic syphilis, and pinta. *J Am Acad Dermatol.* 1993;29(4):519–535; quiz 536–538.

Lotti T, Hautmann G. Atypical mycobacterial infections: a difficult and emerging group of infectious dermatosis. *Int J Dermatol.* 1993;321:499–501.

Lucchina LC, Wilson ME, Drake LA. Dermatology and the recently returned traveler: infectious diseases with dermatologic manifestations. *Int J Dermatol.* 1997;36:167–181.

Lupi O, Tyring SK. Tropical dermatology: viral tropical diseases. *J Am Acad Dermatol.* 2003;49(6):979–1000.

Munayco CV, Grijalva CG, Culqui DR, et al. Outbreak of persistent cutaneous abscesses due to *Mycobacterium chelonae* after mesotherapy sessions, Lima, Peru. *Rev Saude Publica.* 2008;42(1):145–149.

Negroni R. Paracoccidioidomycosis. *Int J Dermatol.* 1993;32:847–859.

Schaller KF. *Colour Atlas of Tropical Dermatology and Venerology.* New York: Spinger-Verlag; 1994.

Steen CJ, Carbonaro PA, Schwartz RA. Arthropods in dermatology. *J Am Acad Dermatol.* 2004;50(6):819–842, quiz 842–844.

Tyring S, Lupi O, Hengge U. *Tropical Dermatology.* Philadelphia: Elsevier; 2006.

Vetter RS, Visscher PK. Bites and stings of medically important venomous arthropods. *Int J Dermatol.* 1998;37:481–496.

Walsh DS, Portaels F, Meyers WM. Buruli ulcer (Mycobacterium ulcerans infection). *Trans R Soc Trop Med Hyg.* 2008;102(10):969–978.

Werner AH, Werner BE. Sporotrichosis in man and animal. *Int J Dermatol.* 1994;33:692–700.

# CHAPTER 46

# Sports Medicine Dermatology

*Rodney S.W. Basler, MD*

Parallel to the burgeoning interest of the general population in establishing personal fitness programs, sports-related conditions of the skin resulting from injury, infection, and exacerbation of preexisting dermatosis are presenting with increasing frequency in the offices of dermatologists across the country. In addition, athletes at all levels of competition from junior high school through professional sports are in need of the services of dermatologic practitioners who are well-informed in this subset of cutaneous problems. By classifying the various categories of dermatologic issues related to sports medicine into these groupings, a problem-oriented approach to dermatology and sports medicine emerges that will enable the clinician to evaluate these problems in a direct organized manner (Table 46-1).

## Athletic Injuries

The integument, positioned at the interface between the athlete and the sporting environment, experiences disruption both from acute and long-term application of sports-related external forces. Preventing these injuries, or treating them aggressively to bring about an immediate resolution, greatly enhances a participant's ability to quickly return to workouts and competition.

### Friction Injuries

#### Abrasions

***Presentation and Characteristics.*** Abrasions occur when the granular and keratinized cells of the outer layers of skin are abruptly removed from the underlying dermis or "true skin." This trauma exposes the lower papillary and reticular dermis, causing punctate bleeding from the severed arterials of the dermal papilla. These pinpoint areas of bleeding within a larger patch of tissue exudate produce the appearance of a lesion referred to in the vernacular as a "raspberry" or "strawberry."

***Treatment.*** The treatment of acute abrasions, as with all other forms of injury, is determined by its severity. Minor abrasions can be treated by gentle cleansing with a mild detergent or soapless cleanser such as Cetaphil antibacterial bar. A trick used by many trainers is to have a can of mentholated shaving gel in their treatment kit, which also works well for cleansing minor lesions and precludes the

**TABLE 46-1** ■ **Classification of Dermatologic Issues Related to Sports Medicine**

**Injury**
Friction
Abrasions
  Acute traumatic
  Turf burn
  Chronic
    Calluses
    Blisters
    Chafing
    Jogger's nipples
Pressure
  Tennis toe
  Acne mechanica
  Talon noir
Ultraviolet damage

**Infections**
Bacterial
  Impetigo
  Occlusive folliculitis
  Bikini bottom
  Pitted keratolysis
Fungal
  Tinea cruris
  Tinea pedis
Viral
  Plantar warts
  Herpes gladiatorum
  Molluscum contagiosum

**Preexisting Dermatosis**
  Physical urticaria
  Eczema

need for having clean water on the sideline, although the latter is usually present for preventing dehydration. Bacitracin ointment and a dry dressing can then be applied.

This provides a moist environment promoting healing with a minimum of scarring. Larger abrasions, especially those that have been contaminated by the environment, require more aggressive immediate care. Treatments must minimize additional trauma, and aggressive scrubbing, especially with cleansers such as hydrogen peroxide or povidone iodine (which may be cytotoxic), should be avoided. A large "pistol-type" or plunger syringe should be used to irrigate the lesion. Nontoxic surfactant cleansers are the wash of choice.

Proper cleansing is followed by the application of a hydrocolloid or semiocclusive hydrogel dressing that provides a moist healing environment allowing for epithelial migration and prevents the formation of crust or eschar (Fig. 46-1) These artificial barriers can remain in place for 5 to 7 days, and may be covered with padding and tape to allow for continued participation in practice or competition.

***Prevention.*** Preventing abrasions requires little more than a commonsense approach to protecting skin potentially exposed to acute trauma. Areas at risk should be covered with protective equipment such as sliding pads, long-sleeved shirts, long socks, "biker" shorts, or a self-adhesive bandage such as Coban.

### Turf Burn

***Presentation and Characteristics.*** Turf burn is a related injury that develops when an athlete, most commonly a football or soccer player, has an exposed area of skin slide across artificial turf. Interestingly, the injury is also seen, with some frequency in an ancillary group of athletes, particularly at a collegiate or professional level, namely cheerleaders. As the name implies, the injury results as much from the generation of heat in the skin as from friction, producing an injury that is part abrasion and part burn; artificial turf has a lower coefficient of friction than natural grass, especially when wet.

***Treatment.*** Because the injury is not as deep as seen with most acute traumatic abrasions, treatment can be less aggressive with cleansing of the area and the application of an antibiotic ointment such as mupirocin or silver sulfadiazine (Silvadene).

***Prevention.*** As with other forms of abrasion, turf burns are best prevented by having specialized equipment, athletic tape, or Coban applied to areas of potential injury.

### Chronic Friction Injury

#### Calluses

***Presentation and Characteristics.*** Calluses present as thick hypertrophied stratum corneum without the characteristic puncta noted with clavi or "hard corns." They represent a compensatory protective response that forms a keratin shield between the outer layers of the skin and an article of equipment, by far the most common being athletic shoes. There often is a history or recently appearing clinical evidence of an anatomic defect underlying the callus. Significant calluses also may be observed on the palmar surface of the hands of golfers, oarsmen, tennis players (Fig. 46-2), and gymnasts. The latter usually consider calluses to be a competitive advantage, and for that reason, generally do not treat them.

***Treatment.*** Because calluses often represent a protective mechanism of the skin, treatment is usually not necessary. The main reason to approach the lesions is to prevent the formation of painful blisters near the edges of the calluses. Careful paring, usually after soaking, followed by smoothing with a pumice stone or file, usually eliminates the calluses.

***Prevention.*** To a certain extent, calluses are not preventable, and there is no particular reason for concern, unless they interfere with athletic performance or blister formation is a problem. Modification of footwear and the addition of gloves for tennis players and weightlifters are sometimes helpful.

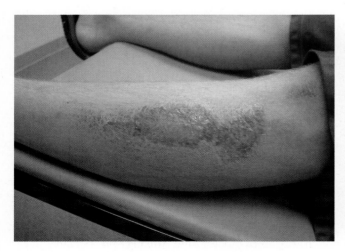

**FIGURE 46-1** ■ A resolving deep abrasion treated with hydrocolloid dressing.

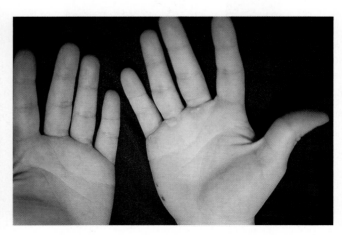

**FIGURE 46-2** ■ Calluses on the hand of high school tennis player.

### Blisters

***Presentation and Characteristics.*** The appearance of a tender vesicle or bullae, sometimes tinged with blood, over the site of the application of applied force does not usually represent a diagnostic quandary (Fig. 46-3). Unfortunately, especially when unroofed, these lesions cause significant pain and tenderness to the athlete, and may seriously curtail the length or level of competitive activity. During a recent playing of the US Open tennis tournament, it was noted that more participants visited the first aid tent for skin-related problems than for all other injuries combined, and the great majority of the problems were blisters.

***Treatment.*** As with most injuries, treatment depends on the size and location of the blister. Small blisters are usually self-limiting and respond to conservative management. It has been shown that the optimal approach to the epidermal "roof" is to leave it intact when possible. The blister should be drained three times at 12-hour intervals for the first 24 hours by using a flamed needle or scalpel. The blister is then covered with a hydrocolloid membrane or tape, either of which can be left in place for 5 to 7 days, allowing for repair of the epithelim.

***Prevention.*** In general, to help prevent blisters, athletes should increase the length and intensity of exercise workouts gradually, especially when breaking in new shoes or rackets. Early studies in the military proved, unequivocally, that moisture is a major contributory factor, and needs to be minimized, especially over the feet. Newer acrylic-composition socks are designed to wick perspiration from the skin at the same time that they diminish friction and should be changed every 30 to 60 minutes if they become drenched in sweat. Some athletes also find the application of petroleum jelly or Aquaphor over pressure points to be of considerable benefit.

### Chafing

***Presentation and Characteristics.*** Chafing is produced by the mechanical friction between the skin covering two apposing body parts or between the skin and an article of clothing. It is a common problem, familiar to participants of nearly all sports, and presents as bright red, inflamed, abraded patches that are sensitive to the touch. In extreme cases, bleeding may be noted from the area of involvement. Although it is annoying and distracting, the condition usually does not lead to cessation of play. The upper inner thighs and axillae represent the most common distribution, and excess muscle or fat may contribute to the problem.

***Treatment.*** The application of both a lubricating ointment such as triple antibiotic and Aquaphor relieves the symptoms and helps prevent further friction injury.

***Prevention.*** Merely changing the athletic clothing to a fabric that generates less friction may bring about very significant improvement. Any adjustment in the area of involvement that eliminates or diminishes the friction applied to the skin surface ameliorates chafing. As already mentioned, the application of petrolatum or Aquaphor may be very helpful. To decrease moisture, which may play a causative role, some athletes favor absorbent powders.

### Jogger's Nipples

***Presentation and Characteristics.*** A painful problem caused by long-term friction applied to a specific body part is the erosions that occur over the areolae and nipples of certain athletes. In extreme cases, the resulting injury may even cause hemorrhage into the clothing or uniform covering the area of involvement. Because the condition is particularly common in long-distance runners, it is usually referred to as *jogger's nipples*. Because most women athletes wear some type of soft protective sports bra, the problem is more common among men than women.

***Treatment.*** Treatment is essentially the same as for all forms of superficial abrasion. The application of an antibiotic ointment covered by a simple dressing such as a Band-Aid is usually sufficient.

***Prevention.*** The most obvious preventative action, of course, is to simply have athletes who are prone to this condition run without a shirt. However, for obvious reasons, this may not be practical. Changing to a softer fabric of running shirt, especially one that does not have a logo, may be beneficial. Friction-reducing ointments may also be helpful, but often are rubbed off over time. Affixing a piece of tape cut exactly to the size and shape of the areola is probably the best preventative measure.

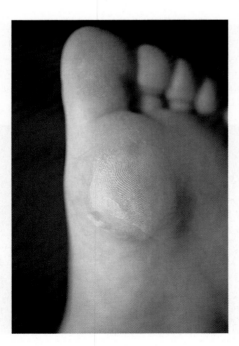

**FIGURE 46-3** ■ A large blister on the foot of a high school tennis player.

## Pressure Injuries

### Subungual Hemorrhage

**Presentation and Characteristics.** The appearance of pooled blood under the plate of the great toenail (Fig. 46-4) is a manifestation of acute bleeding resulting from the repeated forceful contact of the anterior nail plate with the front part of the athletic shoe. Although the injury can be caused by shoes that are too short, it usually results from too small of a toe box. Although tennis players are more commonly affected than participants in other sports (giving rise to the epithet *tennis toe*), the injury is also noted in other sports with the associated terms *jogger's toe* and *skier's toe*. Although acute cases may cause some pain and tenderness, symptoms are usually minimal and it is not necessary to shorten an exercise or competition schedule.

**Treatment.** In the acute phase, blood may be drained from beneath the nail with the time-honored flamed paperclip, or with a Geiger cautery if one is available. Soaking in warm water brings about some palliative benefit, as well, and tends to be more popular with affected athletes.

**Prevention.** Trimming the great toenail, in a straight tangential plane to the shortest point that it does not cause discomfort, is of major benefit. Careful attention to properly fitting shoes, especially ones with a generous toe box, is also recommended. Unfortunately, some athletes who are particularly prone to this condition notice some degree of involvement regardless of attempts to eliminate the problem.

### Acne Mechanica

**Presentation and Characteristics.** Acne mechanica is a papulopustular eruption in the areas beneath heavy padding of certain contact sports, especially football and hockey. It varies in clinical presentation from acne vulgaris in that there is more inflammation, particularly around the papules, and the pustules appear to be more deep seeded. As first described by Mills and Klugman, the condition is produced by

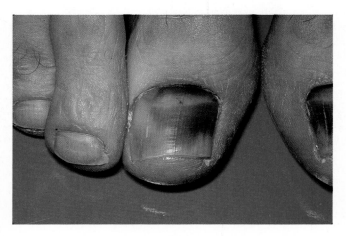

**FIGURE 46-4** ▪ A subungual hematoma in a high school tennis player.

the combined factors of pressure, occlusion, friction, and heat. As would be expected, skin changes are most dramatic during the season when the equipment is worn and tend to spontaneously resolve after the season concludes.

**Treatment.** Acne mechanica responds to a certain, although lesser, extent to entities used to treat acne vulgaris. Rigorous cleansing with a moderately abrasive cleanser, and the use of a back brush, is recommended after each practice session or game. The application of an astringent or keratolytic agent, such as adapalene or retinol, may also be of considerable benefit. Because physical factors play an important role in pathogenesis, systemic antibiotics seem to be of considerably less help in treating the condition than in treating acne vulgaris, but may still be used, even if with only limited success.

**Prevention.** The simplest form of prevention of acne mechanica is the wearing of a clean, absorbent, cotton T-shirt under the equipment causing the problem, especially the shoulder pad in football players. The procedures and medications recommended for treatment might also be considered as part of prevention.

### Talon Noir

**Presentation and Characteristics.** The skin change referred to as *talon noir* or *black heel* involves the skin over the calcaneal portion of the foot, and demonstrates asymptomatic color change due to blue to black punctate petechiae, especially on the posterolateral aspect of the heel. In uncommon cases, the condition may also be seen on the palms of weight lifters, golfers, or tennis players, where it is referred to as *black palm*. For reasons that are not entirely clear, talon noir is seen almost exclusively in older teenagers and young adults.

**Treatment.** No treatment is available or actually warranted for this essentially cosmetic condition. It usually comes to the attention of caregivers only because of the concern of the patient or their family, of the possibility of it representing a malignant melanoma.

**Prevention.** Although there is probably little that can be done to prevent black heel, properly fitting shoes may contribute to fewer problems during subsequent seasons.

### Ultraviolet Damage

**Presentation and Characteristics.** Photoinjury to the skin is characterized by the all too familiar, painful, erythematous to deep red, to even violaceous changes that occur in exposed skin secondary to overexposure to ultraviolet rays of the sun. In extreme cases, vesicles, bullae, and even systemic symptoms may accompany this reaction. Participants in nearly all of the outdoor sports are at risk, especially protracted activities, such as fishing, general water sports, and golfing. Long-term ultraviolet damage includes premature aging, premalignant keratosis, and actual cutaneous malignancy, all of which are among the most preventable diseases to afflict the integument.

***Treatment.*** Although treatment definitely takes a backseat to prevention when dealing with solar injury, nearly all people who participate in any form of outdoor sports and lack deep natural melanotic pigmentation have experienced some level of sunburn. For the milder cases, topical application of an emollient moisturizing agent, with or without minimum potency corticosteroids, usually suffices to bring about significant palliation of symptoms. Systemic over-the-counter anti-inflammatories such as aspirin and ibuprofen are also of value, as are the more potent anti-inflammatories such as prescription nonsteroidal anti-inflammatories and corticosteroids with more severe photoinjury. Many practitioners and patients prefer spray steroids to cover the involved areas because they preclude the need of further irritation and discomfort from application. Usually a short course, generally 5 to 7 days, of treatment is adequate in nearly all cases.

***Prevention.*** The prevention of actinic damage of the skin in the general population is one of the most important and rigorously pursued challenges to face dermatologists. The basic recommendations of limiting outdoor athletic exposure to the hours before 10:00 AM and after 4:00 PM are sometimes impractical, but must be stated. Covering all exposed areas as much as possible with opaque clothing is equally important, but also sometimes not possible. Headcovering with a brim rather than a cap is advised, but represents protection no greater than a sun protective factor (SPF) of 2 unless a headcovering specifically for sunprotection is used. Sunscreen remains our most valuable line of defense, and should optimally be applied 20 to 30 minutes before sun exposure and every 2 to 4 hours during sun exposure, according to the amount of water or perspiration that is diluting the product. An SPF of at least 15 is required and a product with combined UVB and UVA protection is recommended. Of course, sunscreen must be applied even on cloudy days because the damaging rays can penetrate even through the clouds cover.

## Infections

### Bacterial Infections

#### Impetigo

***Presentation and Characteristics.*** Superficial bacterial infection such as pyoderma or impetigo is a hazard of all contact sports. If community-acquired methicillin-resistant *Staphylococcus aureus* (CA-MRSA) is suspected, a sulfa-based systemic antibiotic should be empirically started, or clindamycin if there is a sulfa allergy. Incision and drainage has been shown to be the procedure of greatest value in all types of bacterial abscesses. As with many of sports-related infections, wrestling probably puts its participants at greatest risk, and bacterial skin infections may reach epidemic proportions among wrestling teams and at large wrestling meets. Any thin-roofed vesicle or bullae with purulent fluid or honey-crusted plaque on exposed areas of skin, particularly those extending from a mucous membrane, are suspects

for this type of infection. These may progress rapidly to sharply marginated erosions, sometimes with points of bleeding. Large furuncles or abscesses may rapidly appear with CA-MRSA infections.

***Treatment.*** Treatment should be aggressive, straightforward, and immediate with systemic antibiotics being the main line of defense. The application of a compress made of warm water and antibacterial cleanser eliminates much of the surface bacteria, and the application of an antibacterial cream usually hastens healing as well.

***Prevention.*** Any athlete suspected of carrying bacterial infection must be prohibited from competition. In wrestling, careful and regular sterilization of the mats with an appropriate disinfectant is also a necessity. Showering with an antibacterial soap immediately after competition often prevents infection in athletes as well.

### Occlusive Folliculitis

***Presentation and Characteristics.*** Occlusive folliculitis is seen under heavy, protective padding in sports such as football and hockey, much in the same way as is acne mechanica. The deep infection of the follicles with furuncle production and the lack of more superficial inflammatory papules (Fig. 46-5) differentiate these entities. In addition, the area of involvement is more limited and coincides exactly with overlying equipment.

***Treatment.*** As with other bacterial infections, aggressive systemic antibiotic therapy is warranted in occlusive folliculitis, although it may need to be prolonged over several weeks or

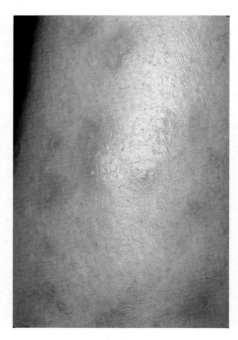

**FIGURE 46-5** ■ Occlusive folliculitis under the thigh pad of a collegiate football player.

months during which the causative equipment is in contact with the skin. The topical application of antibiotics used to treat acne, such as clindamycin or erythromycin, with or without benzoyl peroxide, is also of considerable benefit.

**Prevention.** The application of an absorbent powder over the areas of involvement may be of considerable value. The causative equipment or padding should be removed as quickly as possible after a workout, and any clothing or equipment that comes into direct contact with the skin should be kept as clean as possible, even disinfected if necessary.

### Pitted Keratolysis

**Presentation and Characteristics.** Pitted keratolysis is a superficial infection of the stratum corneum accompanied by the hallmark pungent odor, which has contributed to its alternative designation of *toxic sock syndrome*. Examination of the bottom of the foot shows macerated skin, often with a faintly erythematous border and characteristic "punched out" areas. It is only mildly symptomatic to the athlete.

**Treatment.** The application of over-the-counter acne gels, such as 10% benzoyl peroxide may, in themselves, be curative for this condition. If this does not represent adequate treatment, prescription acne medicines such as benzoyl peroxide–clindamycin and benzoyl peroxide–erythromycin products are particularly beneficial.

**Prevention.** Careful washing of the feet with an antibacterial soap, followed by towel drying and air-drying, is a common-sense approach to the problem. Absorbent powders inside the stocking and the regular application of a 20% aluminum chloride solution also help prevent the condition.

## Fungal Infections

### Tinea Pedis

**Presentation and Characteristics.** *Athlete's foot* and *jock itch* indicate the close association of fungal infections with sports. The macerating effect of perspiration in nearly every athletic environment reduces the natural barrier of the epidermis, allowing invasion of fungal elements. Toe webs are usually the first, and generally the most common, site of infection, with spread to the keratin over the soles and lateral aspects of the feet. Marginated erythema and scaling, often with vesicle formation, are noted in areas of involvement. Unilateral distribution is also helpful in differentiating this entity from dyshidrotic eczema. Dystrophic onychomycosis may represent a reservoir of organisms that later spread over the skin.

**Treatment.** Topical antifungal creams, such as terbinafine and clotrimazole, may be effective in some early superficial cases, but systemic antifungals, such as griseofulvin, fluconazole, itraconazole, or terbinafine, are often required for treatment. When topical medications are used in the toe webs,

solutions, sprays, and gels seem to work better than creams or ointments. If there is a deep commensal infection of the toe web where the infection seems to be potentiated with bacterial overgrowth, strong systemic medications such as ciprofloxacin may be indicated.

**Prevention.** Any procedure that helps keep the stratum corneum dry, thereby maintaining the natural physical barrier of fungal invasion, is beneficial in preventing this infection. The application of a foot powder or aluminum chloride in patients who show significant maceration is definitely helpful, and the use of shower thongs in the locker room may help those prone to chronic recurrent infections. The long-term administration of a systemic antifungal, such as fluconazole or itraconazole with a dosage as low as 200 mg/mo, may be highly effective for prophylaxis.

### Tinea Cruris

**Presentation and Characteristics.** Another time-honored epithet that underscores the association of fungal infection with athletes is *jock itch*. Although this infection presents in the groin, the source of infection is usually an indolent infection of the feet or toenails. When the causative organism is a dermatophyte, the involved area shows erythema and scaling, with a sharp margination, and rarely progresses to the genitals because of the fungistatic effect of sebum in this area. Fungal infections also lack the deep red coloration and satellite lesions seen when yeast is involved. Individual lesions may look particularly innocuous and imitate nummular eczema in wrestlers.

**Treatment.** Early localized infections may respond to prescription, or even over-the-counter, topical antifungals, such as miconazole or terbinafine. Some clinicians favor the older iodochlorhydroxyquin HC preparation. Systemic antifungals may be required in stubborn, persistent cases, and high-dose (250 mg b.i.d.) terbinafine may be required in particularly virulent infections in wrestlers, especially in the hair.

**Prevention.** Immediate showering after any exercise session with careful attention to removing soap and towel drying intertriginous regions is strongly recommended. The daily change of sports briefs and attention to choosing those made of an absorbent fabric is also helpful. Absorbent powders in the groin as well as axillae may also prevent infection in these areas, particularly in susceptible wrestlers. Fluconazole at a dosage of 200 to 400 mg/wk throughout the entire season may preclude missing important meets because of active fungal lesions.

## Viral Infections

### Plantar Warts

**Presentation and Characteristics.** Cutaneous invasion by the human papillomavirus, particularly of the skin of the feet, is relatively common among athletes. The macerating effect of perspiration is a contributing factor as with other forms of infection. In addition, the moist environment of the locker room, especially the showers, provides for a most hospitable environment for causative viruses to live and reproduce. Any area of the plantar portion of the foot may be involved with a very tender hyperkeratotic papule present, often revealing small black dots when the superficial portion is removed. Confluence of individual papules may result in relatively large mosaic warts, and lesions over the weight-bearing portions of the foot may cause considerable morbidity, especially in long-distance runners.

**Treatment.** In treating these localized viral infections, a conservative approach to therapy is recommended, particularly one that allows for continued practice and competition during therapy. If maceration appears to be a major contributory factor, the application of a 20% aluminum chloride solution or even stronger mixtures containing 10% to 25% formalin often bring about complete resolution with no morbidity. Some physicians and trainers favor the topical application of 50% trichloroacetic acid solution under a 40% salicylic acid plaster, applied once or twice weekly, followed by vigorous paring. Aggressive ablative therapy, such as excision, electrodessication, or laser treatment, holds no curative advantage, and carries a significant risk of short-term disability and even permanent scarring.

**Prevention.** Wearing shower thongs in the locker room decreases the likelihood of coming into contact with the causative virus, while foot powders diminish maceration. The regular application of a 20% aluminum chloride solution may also be of considerable preventative value.

### Herpes Gladiatorum

**Presentation and Characteristics.** As implied by its name, this superficial viral infection of the skin is noted almost exclusively in wrestlers, although it may sometimes be seen in other forms of contact and noncontact sports, including basketball. The head, neck, and upper extremities, which are exposed during periods of contact, are usually those noted, with the appearance of grouped vesicles on an erythematous to violaceous base (**Fig. 46-6**). Dermal edema is usually present, and burning and tenderness are noted by the athlete.

**Treatment.** Systemic antivirals are, of course, the primary entity in the arsenal for treating this infection, and should be started immediately when symptoms occur, even before actual skin lesions are noted. Local improvement can be accelerated by unroofing the vesicles and applying benzoin topically, then injecting localized lesions intralesionally with a dilute triamcinolone solution.

**Prevention.** Athletes with a history of recurrent herpes lesions may greatly benefit from the prophylactic use of acyclovir or valacyclovir. Adequate dosage usually is 400 mg/d of acyclovir or 500 mg/d of valacyclovir. These medications

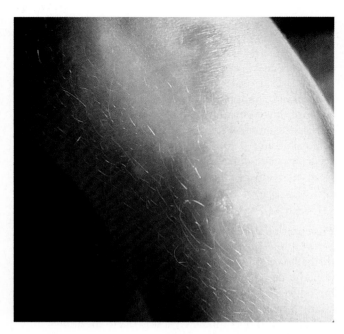

**FIGURE 46-6** ■ Herpes gladiatorum in a collegiate wrestler.

should be started before the training season begins, and continued through the course of the competitive schedule. Any athlete with active herpes must be prohibited from competition during the stage of intact or draining vesicles, usually requiring a quarantine period of 4 to 6 days, until all lesions are dry.

### Molluscum Contagiosum

**Presentation and Characteristics.** Again, the venues of competitive wrestling seem to offer the primary athletic source of infection with the large pox virus that causes molluscum contagiosum. Less commonly, these lesions may also be seen in swimmers, and it has been speculated that the solutions used to sterilize pool water are not adequate to completely eliminate the virus. In addition, many athletes may be infected in nonsports arenas, such as "coed wrestling." Small, grouped, waxy papules are usually seen on exposed areas of skin with individual papules showing a central umbilication in some cases. A linear distribution of lesions referred to as *pseudo-koebnerization* may also be noted, especially in wrestlers.

**Treatment.** Lesions are easily removed by curettage, even though this leads to superficial abrasions that may preclude contact for a short period of time. Curettage may be easily carried out following the application of a topical anesthetic gel. Liquid nitrogen and tape striping with highly adhesive tape may also be effective.

**Prevention.** The prohibition of competition by infected participants is a necessity, and removal of localized individual lesions at their first appearance also helps prevent self-inoculation.

## Preexisting Dermatoses

### Physical Urticarias

**Presentation and Characteristics.** The physical urticarias, particularly cholinergic urticaria, are most commonly diagnosed through history, although they have a distinctive form of papular erythema with a more punctate dermal edema than seen with acute allergic urticaria. The erythematous papules are smaller and more distinct, and wheal formation is much less pronounced. The inner aspects of the arms and legs as well as the lateral flanks are common areas of involvement. By history, factors that induce physical urticaria are those indigenous to athletic endeavor, such as rapid temperature changes, especially cold to hot, physical exertion, and emotional stress. Cold urticaria and aquagenic urticaria also fall into this category and can be disabling to swimmers. Pressure urticaria usually appears under articles of athletic equipment.

**Treatment.** Because of its antiserotonin effect, cyproheptadine is particularly helpful in the physical urticarias. A dosage of 4 mg at bedtime may, in fact, be essentially curative in milder cases. Unfortunately, this antihistamine is quite sedating, and taking the drug the night before a morning competition may leave the athlete in less than prime condition, especially in terms of competitive alertness. Combination therapy with $H_1$-$H_2$-inhibiting antihistamines usually works better than a single-drug regimen. In especially difficult cases, corticosteroids, sometimes on a long-term alternate-day schedule, may be required to eliminate the problem. Athletes being administered this course of treatment must be aware of the fact that the older, less specific means of steroid screening may reveal this use of corticosteroids, causing them to test positive.

**Prevention.** The use of prophylactic antihistamines, especially cyproheptadine, as noted, is probably the best precaution to take for athletes who are prone to developing physical urticaria. Otherwise, elimination of the problem may be particularly difficult, short of complete cessation of athletic activity. If the reaction is seen secondary to changes in the temperature, gradual warming or cooling the body may diminish the severity to a limited extent.

### Atopic Eczema

**Presentation and Characteristics.** Most atopes have a lifelong history of skin sensitivity with the characteristic flexural (**Fig. 46-7**) and facial involvement, and are well aware of their problem. Poorly marginated erythema and scaling in the commonly involved areas associated with persistent itching and evidence of excoriation are the hallmark of this condition. Unfortunately, increased body heat and perspiration, which are found in nearly all forms of athletic endeavor, generally exacerbate the condition.

**Treatment.** The treatment of sports-induced eczema is essentially the same as that for any patient with atopic eczema,

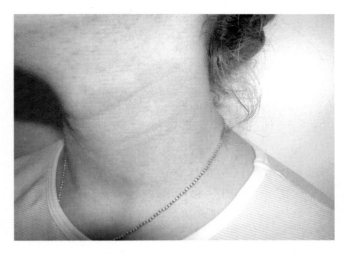

**FIGURE 46-7** ■ Eczema of the neck flaring mid-season in an atopic collegiate tennis player.

although there may be a need to be more aggressive in athletes during their competitive seasons. Topical corticosteroids in emollient cream or ointment bases are the traditional first line of defense, with the newer immunomodulators, tacrolimus and pimecrolimus, more beneficial in patients who have a long-standing history of atopic eczema. Tacrolimus and pimecrolimus may have a significant drawback, however, in that they usually impart a sensation of heat in the skin during periods of exercise, which the athlete may find annoying or distracting. Systemic corticosteroids over varying lengths of time may ultimately be required to bring the condition under control to a point that it does not interfere with athletic performance.

**Prevention.** Short, tepid showers, using an oil- or cream-based soap immediately following exercise periods to remove sweat are recommended, and should be followed with lubrication with an emollient cream or lotion, or a bath oil. Any of the medications used for treatment may also be considered to be preventative, including the use of antihistamines throughout the course of the season. It is particularly important for patients suffering from eczema to have the condition under the best possible control in the off season so as to preclude the need for aggressive therapy once conditioning becomes more intense.

## Conclusion

Well-informed, up-to-date medical practitioners who deal with problems of the integument need to have a basic understanding of the care and prevention of cutaneous injuries that pertain to recreational and competitive athletes. Most skin problems that arise in the course of training or general fitness regimens can be treated aggressively and directly, and prevented through thoughtful planning and preparation. When treated in an immediate and knowledgeable manner, very few of the skin conditions that arise as a result of sports participation need interfere with an active lifestyle or the pursuit of lofty competitive goals.

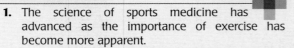

## SAUER'S NOTES

1. The science of sports medicine has advanced as the importance of exercise has become more apparent.
2. Dermatology needs to keep up with this explosion of information in order to keep the athlete off the couch and in the game.

## Suggested Readings

Basler RSW. Skin lesions related to sports activity. *Prim Care.* 1983;10: 479–494.

Basler RSW. Sports related injuries in dermatology. In: Callen JP, ed. *Advances in Dermatology.* St Louis: Mosby; 1988:4, 29–50.

Basler RSW. Skin injuries in sports medicine. *J Am Acad Dermatol.* 1989;21: 1257–1262.

Basler RSW. Acne mechanica in athletes. *Cutis.* 1992;50:125–128.

Basler RSW. Managing skin problems in athletes. In: Mellion MB, Walsh W, Shelton GL, eds. *Team Physician's Handbook.* 3rd ed. Philadelphia: Hanley & Belfus; 2002:311–325.

Basler RSW, Basler DL, Basler GC, et al. Cutaneous injuries in women athletes. *Dermatol Nurs.* 1998;10:9–18.

Basler RSW, Basler GC, Palmer AH, et al. Special skin symptoms seen in swimmers. *J Am Acad Dermatol.* 2000;43:299–305.

Basler RSW, Garcia MA. Acing common skin problems in tennis players. *Phys Sportsmed.* 1998;25:37–44.

Basler RSW, Garcia MA, Gooding KS. Immediate steps for treating abrasions. *Phys Sportsmed.* 2001;29:69–70.

Bergfeld WF. Dermatologic problems in athletes. *Clin Sports Med.* 1982;1:3.

Eiland G, Ridley D. Dermatological problems in the athlete. *J Orthop Sports Phys Ther.* 1996;23:388–402.

Levine N. Dermatologic aspects of sportsmedicine. *Dermatol Nurs.* 1994;6: 179–186.

# CHAPTER 47

# Cutaneous Signs of Bioterrorism

*Megan Kinney, MHAM, BS, Steven R. Feldman, MD, PhD,*
*Jeffrey N. Lackey, MD, and Scott A. Norton, MD, MPH*

The world changed on the day we now know as "9/11." In this new era, physicians in the United States and worldwide have an additional responsibility to know the fundamentals of recognizing and diagnosing an outbreak associated with biologic agents. In this regard, the dermatologist has a particularly important role because most illnesses that arise from biologic agents can have a cutaneous component.

The Centers for Disease Control and Prevention (CDC) has identified six biologic agents as Category A agents, which pose the greatest risk for use in terrorism (Table 47-1). The assessment of risk is based on the ease of production, ease of dissemination, rate of subsequent person-to-person transmission, lethality, and psychosocial effects (literally, how terrified the community will be). These six agents are smallpox, anthrax, botulism, tularemia, plague, and viral hemorrhagic fevers.

In some, for example, smallpox, skin involvement is the most dramatic feature of the disease. In others, cutaneous manifestations are not a central feature, but it is possible, even likely, that the diagnosis of the index case will be made from cutaneous findings, whether they are subtle or obvious. For this reason, an in-depth discussion of the most dermatologically important of these agents, smallpox and anthrax, follows. The other four agents will be briefly discussed highlighting their cutaneous findings.

Category B and C agents, second- and third-highest priority, respectively, are presented in Tables 47-2 and 47-3.

## Smallpox

The patient with smallpox presents a terrible picture, unequalled in any other disease. A picture that fully justifies the horror and fright with which smallpox is associated in the public mind.

William Osler from *The Principles and Practice of Medicine*

### Historical Aspects

The World Health Organization (WHO) regards smallpox, also called *variola,* as humankind's deadliest disease. Indeed, smallpox has caused perhaps 10% of all human deaths and, even during its waning years in the 20th century, smallpox killed half a billion people. One third of its victims die. Survivors are usually maimed for life with pocked scars or blindness. Because of the mortality and morbidity associated with smallpox, people long sought ways to prevent, ameliorate, or cure the disease. Fortunately for humankind, smallpox had several characteristics that made it amenable to eradication: there is no subclinical carrier state in humans, the disease is not transmitted by food or water, and there are no animal reservoirs or vectors. The disease occurs only in humans and, during the smallpox era, it was readily diagnosed on a clinical basis alone. A person who survived a bout of smallpox achieved lifelong immunity, but most important, smallpox was preventable through vaccination.

The cowpox vaccine, which Edward Jenner used, and the vaccine that replaced it (one derived from the closely related vaccinia virus) confer near-complete immunity against smallpox. A concerted global vaccination program, led by the health organizations and governments around the world, used the vaccine to quell this disease. The last naturally occurring cases were in Bangladesh and Somalia during the mid-1970s, and a few years later the WHO proclaimed the eradication of smallpox. Shortly afterward, all laboratory stocks of variola virus were destroyed except for a few facilities that maintained small amounts of the virus, putatively for research purposes. There is worrisome speculation, however, that stocks of virus are in unmonitored hands. In addition, the ability to synthesize viral genomes in vitro brings these concerns to a new level as the altered or engineered viral strains could have virulence-enhancing properties. Consequently, there is a risk, at least theoretically, that smallpox might recur. If so, the reappearance of this disease will mark one of the most catastrophic medical, public health, and criminal events that our species has witnessed. For this reason, it is worth bringing smallpox out of the history books and into our current textbooks.

### Presentation and Characteristics

#### Virology

Smallpox is caused by the variola virus, a member of the *Orthopoxvirus* genus within the poxvirus family. This genus also includes cowpox, vaccinia, monkeypox, and a few other viruses that cause mostly nonhuman disease. The poxvirus family has two other genera, one with the familiar molluscum contagiosum, and the other with the zoonotic disorders of orf and milker's nodules. All members in the poxvirus

**TABLE 47-1** ■ **CDC Category A Agents: Biologic Agents Most Likely to Be Used in Terrorism or Warfare***

| Disease | Pathogen | Likely Presentation When Used as a Bioweapon | Cutaneous Manifestations | % of Patients in a Bioterrorism Setting Who Have Cutaneous Manifestations |
|---------|----------|----------------------------------------------|--------------------------|--------------------------------------------------------------------------|
| Smallpox | *Variola*, an orthopoxvirus | Classic illness described in chapter | Exanthem followed by classic vesiculopustular eruption predominantly on acral surfaces; "pearls of pus" | All |
| Anthrax | *Bacillus anthracis*, an aerobic encapsulated spore-forming gram-positive rod | Inhalational disease starts with flulike presentation and progresses | Edematous papule or plaque evolving into an ulcer surmounted by a black eschar | Roughly 50% |
| Plague | *Yersinia pestis*, an aerobic gram-negative rod with safety-pin bipolar staining | Fever, weakness, and rapidly developing pneumonia with dyspnea, chest pain, and bloody cough, leading to respiratory failure, shock, and rapid death | Bubonic form from fleabites produces painful tender enlarged lymph nodes (buboes); pneumonic plague may cause DIC with purpura | Not known |
| Tularemia | *Francisella tularensis*, an aerobic pleomorphic gram-negative coccobacillus | Hemorrhagic bronchopneumonia with fever | If acquired transcutaneously, then an ulceroglandular or lymphocutaneous presentation | Not known |
| Botulism | Toxin produced by the anaerobic gram-positive rod, *Clostridium botulinum* | Rapid onset of symmetric descending flaccid, paralysis starting in bulbar muscles; afebrile, normal mental status, and no sensory deficits | Facial nerve paralysis, dilated pupils, dry oral mucosa | Presumably most |
| Viral hemorrhagic fevers | Examples include arenaviruses (e.g., Lassa), filoviruses (Marburg and Ebola) | Flulike illness with fever, myalgias, and extreme fatigue; severe cases have uncontrolled internal and orofacial bleeding | Petechiae, purpura, and hemorrhage | Presumably most |

*Biologic warfare is defined as the intentional use of microorganisms or toxins to produce death or disease in humans, animals, or plants.

*Abbreviation:* DIC, disseminated intravascular coagulation.

family are DNA viruses that replicate within the host cell's cytoplasm, unlike nearly all other viruses that replicate inside the nuclei.

### Clinical Disease

Smallpox is transmitted primarily in a respiratory manner by droplets from close contact with infected individuals. Fomite transmission, for example, from skin crusts can occur but it is rare. It is feared that weaponized smallpox, on the other hand, will be spread long distances through aerosolization of the virus.

Smallpox has three clinical stages. The first, the incubation phase, starts when a person is initially infected with the virus. Incubation lasts approximately 12 to 14 days (range: 7 to 17 days) and during this time, individuals are unaware that they are infected. They feel well, have no clinical manifestations, and cannot transmit the virus to others. The second stage, the prodrome, begins with a sudden high fever (typically 102°F to 105°F) accompanied by severe headache and backache. During the prodrome, the patient is viremic, appears toxic, is often prostrate with pain, and may be delirious. After 2 to 4 days, the prodrome ends with a slight defervescence and the appearance of an oropharyngeal enanthem. This marks the beginning of the eruptive stage and now the patient is infectious. The classic exanthem has several distinctive features (Fig. 47-1). Individual lesions evolve gradually through several morphologic forms over 14 to 18 days. Lesions progress from macules to papules to vesicles to umbilicated vesicles to pustules to crusted scabs, with each form lasting 1 to 2 days. An important diagnostic feature of

TABLE 47-2 ■ **Category B Agents: Second-Highest Priority Biologic Agents to Be Used in Terrorism or Warfare**

| Agents/Diseases | Pathogen | Likely Presentation When Used as a Bioweapon | Cutaneous Manifestations |
|---|---|---|---|
| Brucellosis (undulant fever) | *Brucella* species | Flulike symptoms (fever, sweats, headaches, back pains, and physical weakness) | May cause wound infection |
| Epsilon toxin | *Clostridium perfringens* | Pulmonary edema leading to renal failure and cardiovascular collapse* | None |
| Food safety threats | *Salmonella* species *Escherichia coli* 0157:H7 *Shigella* | GI symptoms | "Rose spots" in typhoid fever (*Salmonella typhi*)[†] |
| Glanders | *Burkholderia mallei* | Pulmonary: malaise, headache, pleurisy[†] | Inoculation nodule and lymphadenitis, ulcerated nodule, mucous membrane ulceration with granulomatous reaction[†] |
| Melioidosis | *Burkholderia pseudomallei* | *Pulmonary*: symptoms of mild bronchitis to severe pneumonia, but normal sputum | Inoculation through breaks in the skin may form nodule |
| | | *Bloodstream*: Usually affects immunosuppressed patients and leads to septic shock | Pustules or subcutaneous abscesses (10–20%); in children, suppurative parotitis[†] |
| | | *Chronic Suppurative*: Organ abscesses throughout the body | |
| Psittacosis | *Chlamydia psittaci* | Fever, chills, headache, muscle aches, dry cough, pneumonia | Horder spots (pink macules similar to typhoid rose spots), acrocyanosis, superficial venous thrombosis, splinter hemorrhages, erythema multiforme, erythema nodosum[†] |
| Q Fever | *Coxiella burnetti* | Pneumonia with nonproductive cough due to aerosolization and inhalation of organism; high fever, vomiting, diarrhea | Occasionally can cause erythema nodosum and erythema annulare centrifugum[†] |
| Ricin toxin | From *Ricinus communis* (castor beans) | *Inhalation*: Sudden onset congestion, respiratory distress (possibly leading to respiratory failure), flulike symptoms (fever, nausea, muscle pain) | Allergic reaction: Erythema, vesication, irritation, and pain may occur |
| | | *Ingestion*: mucosal ulceration and hemorrhage leading to severe GI distress; splenic, hepatic, and renal bleeding*[,‡] | |
| Staphylococcal enterotoxin B | From specific strains of *Staphylococcus aureus* | *Inhalation*: Flulike symptoms, respiratory distress, chest pain, cough | None |
| | | *Ingestion*: food poisoning symptoms (nausea, vomiting, abdominal cramping, diarrhea)*[,‡] | |
| Typhus | *Rickettsia prowazekii* | Malaise, myalgias, headaches, fever, chills; neurologic symptoms such as meningismus and coma may develop | Centrifugally spreading eruption that spares the palms and soles; begins as erythematous, nonconfluent, blanching macules that become maculopapular and petechial |

*(continued)*

**TABLE 47-2** ■ *(continued)*

| Agents/Diseases | Pathogen | Likely Presentation When Used as a Bioweapon | Cutaneous Manifestations |
|---|---|---|---|
| Viral encephalitis | Togaviridae (Eastern equine encephalitis, Venezuelan equine encephalitis, and Western equine encephalitis viruses)[§] Flaviviridae (Japanese encephalitis, St. Louis encephalitis, West Nile Virus) Bunyaviridae, Arenaviridae, Paramyxoviridae[¶] | Decreased consciousness, seizures, focal neurologic signs, encephalitis,[§] fever, headache, flulike symptoms, nausea, vomiting, diarrhea[¶] | Facial/periorbital edema, jaundice, flushing, lymphadenopathy, alopecia, palatal vesicular or petechial-eruption, cutaneous morbilliform or petechial eruption may be present[¶] |
| Water safety threats | *Vibrio cholerae* (cholera) *Cryptosporidium parvum* (cryptosporidiosis) | Nausea, vomiting, headache, diarrhea (described as rice-water stool in cholera) | Skin infection through open wound and hemorrhagic bullous lesions have occurred with *Vibrio*, but are very rare |

From the CDC Web site unless otherwise indicated.

*Marks JD. Medical aspects of biologic toxins. *Anesth Clin North Am* 2004;22:509–32, vii.

[†]Lupi O, Madkan V, Tyring SK. Tropical dermatology: bacterial tropical diseases. *J Am Acad Dermatol.* 2006;54:559–578.

[‡]Henghold WB. Other biologic toxin bioweapons: ricin, staphylococcal enterotoxin B, and trichothecene mycotoxins. *Dermatol Clin.* 2004;22:257–262, v.

[§]Donaghy M. Neurologists and the threat of bioterrorism. *J Neurol Sci.* 2006;249:55–62.

[¶]Bossi P, Tegnell A, Baka A, et al. Bichat guidelines for the clinical management of viral encephalitis and bioterrorism-related viral encephalitis. *Euro Surveill.* 2004;9:E21–E22.

smallpox is that at any one time, all lesions are in the same morphologic stage of development in the region of the body. In contrast, chickenpox lesions progress rapidly and asynchronously; thus, all morphologic forms (e.g., papules, vesicles, pustules, and crusts) are typically present at any moment in the same region of the body.

Another distinction between classic smallpox and chickenpox is that in the former disease, lesions are most abundant on acral surfaces (face, palms, and soles), whereas in the latter, lesions are most abundant centrally (on the trunk). Furthermore, the delicate lesions of classic chickenpox are described as "dewdrops on a rose petal," but firm smallpox lesions can be described as "pearls of pus"—they are deep-seated, globose, opalescent papules and pustules (Fig. 47-2). The smallpox patient is infectious from the onset of the

enanthem until all scabs have separated, roughly 20 to 25 days later. Historical records show that the disease killed roughly 30% of unvaccinated individuals, and produced pocks (depressed facial scars) on most survivors. In people who received vaccinations less than 10 years before exposure to smallpox, historical case fatality rates were 1% to 3%.

*Types of Smallpox*

About 90% of patients with smallpox present with classic disease (see Fig. 47-1) in which individual pustules are either discrete (surrounded by normal-appearing skin) or coalesce perhaps with one or two neighboring pustules. Two variants of smallpox, the hemorrhagic type and the malignant (or flat) type, have especially poor prognoses. *Hemorrhagic smallpox* is characterized by disseminated intravascular coagulation (DIC)

**TABLE 47-3** ■ **Category C Agents: Third-Highest Priority Biologic Agents to Be Used in Terrorism or Warfare**

| Disease | Pathogen | Likely Presentation When Used as a Bioweapon | Cutaneous Manifestations |
|---|---|---|---|
| Nipah encephalitis | Nipah virus | Fever, headache, mental distortion (drowsiness, giddiness, confusion), possible respiratory illness, neurologic deficits | None |
| Hantavirus pulmonary syndrome | Hantavirus | Fatigue, fever, myalgias, headaches, dizziness, vomiting, diarrhea, shortness of breath | Rash is uncommon |

From the CDC Web site unless otherwise indicated.

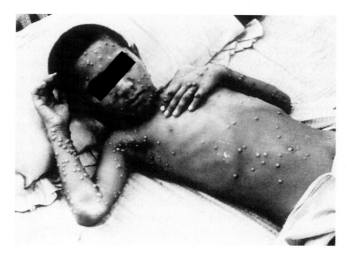

**FIGURE 47-1** ■ The classic exanthem of smallpox (variola major) shows pustules with uniform morphology, more prominent on acral surfaces. In the past, one third of unvaccinated individuals who acquired smallpox died of the disease. The survivors were usually marked with pitted scars called *pocks,* and many were blinded by smallpox as well. *(Courtesy of the James H. Graham, MD & Gloria F. Graham, MD Dermatopathology Library.)*

and purpura. It seems to occur more frequently in pregnant women. *Malignant smallpox* is characterized by innumerable flat lesions that cover the entire skin, producing an edematous appearance that resembles anasarca. This form produces neither classic pustules nor scabs. Both of these variants, hemorrhagic and malignant smallpox, have mortality rates of more than 95%.

## Diagnosis

Naturally occurring disease has not existed since 1977, and there is no absolute confirmation that stocks of smallpox

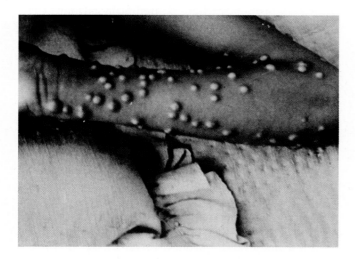

**FIGURE 47-2** ■ Smallpox lesions can be described as "pearls of pus"—they are firm, deep-seated, globose, opalescent papules, and pustules. *(Courtesy of the James H. Graham, MD & Gloria F. Graham, MD Dermatopathology Library.)*

**TABLE 47-4** ■ **Differential Diagnosis for Febrile Patient With Vesicles and Pustules**

Chickenpox

Disseminated herpes zoster

Disseminated herpes simplex

Impetigo

Pustular drug eruptions

Erythema multiforme

Enteroviral infections (especially hand, foot, and mouth disease)

Infected arthropod bites

Contact dermatitis

Monkeypox

Molluscum contagiosum (in immunocompromised patients)

virus are in the hands of anyone who would use them. Therefore, practitioners confronted by a patient with fever and pustules should remind themselves to look for alternative explanations. The CDC has an algorithm for the evaluation of suspected smallpox and offers the differential diagnosis shown in Table 47-4. The algorithm *Evaluating patients for smallpox: acute, generalized vesicular or pustular rash illness protocol* is available on the CDC's Web site (www.bt.cdc.gov/agent/smallpox/diagnosis/pdf/spox-poster-full.pdf).

A thousand years ago and today, the disease that most closely resembles smallpox is chickenpox. A typical presentation of chickenpox will not resemble smallpox, but as a variant presentation, one perhaps with a few more acral lesions and a higher temperature. If faced with a patient in whom smallpox is in the differential diagnosis, the physician should institute the same infection control precautions used for chickenpox or other respiratory diseases, then review the key clinical differences between the two diseases (Table 47-5), consult the CDC algorithm, and attempt to establish the

**TABLE 47-5** ■ **Clinical Presentations of Classic Chickenpox and Smallpox**

| Chickenpox | Smallpox |
|---|---|
| Mild or no prodrome | Febrile prodrome |
| Superficial vesicles | Deep pustules |
| "Dew drops on a rose petal" | "Pearls of pus" |
| Individual lesions evolve rapidly | Individual lesions evolve gradually |
| Lesions with different morphologies | Lesions with same morphology |
| Central predominance | Acral predominance |
| Spares palms and soles | Involves palms and soles |
| Patient is rarely toxic | Patient is usually toxic or moribund |

diagnosis of some other disease (Table 47-4). In other words, by ruling in chickenpox or another disease, one can rule out smallpox. Disseminated herpes simplex and disseminated herpes zoster may also resemble smallpox. There are ongoing, scattered, small outbreaks of zoonotic monkeypox in equatorial Africa; this is a poxvirus infection that also resembles smallpox.

Although clinical judgment is important, laboratory confirmation of the cause of a patient's febrile, vesicopustular eruption is critical. In the past, electron microscopic examination was used to look for the classic brick- or dumbbell-shaped cytoplasmic virions of poxviruses. Viral culture was an effective but slow diagnostic technique. Today, PCR, DFA, immunohistochemical techniques, and in situ hybridization offer alternative—and more rapid—means to differentiate among poxviruses and herpesviruses.

According to the CDC algorithm, if one cannot rule out smallpox, then local public health authorities must be notified. One should continue to follow the algorithm. If an index case of smallpox were confirmed by laboratory studies, the entire clinical approach to a patient with fever and a rash would change dramatically. The clinical situation changes from one in which one must look for other causes to one in which we assume the patient may have smallpox. Unvaccinated health care workers who are exposed to a patient with smallpox can take reassurance in the rapid efficacy of the smallpox vaccine. It works so quickly that postexposure vaccination, even up to 4 to 5 days after exposure, prevents the disease from progressing through the 12-day asymptomatic incubation stage into the symptomatic or infectious stages of the disease. Furthermore, recent studies show that remote vaccination (i.e., smallpox vaccination several decades earlier) seems to confer longer lasting immunity than originally believed.

## Vaccination

The smallpox vaccine is clearly the most successful immunization ever devised. Once the World Health Organization declared smallpox's demise, there was no further need to continue to vaccinate populations. In the United States and most other developed nations, compulsory vaccination against smallpox ceased in the early 1970s. Since shortly after the attacks of September 11, 2001, however, smallpox vaccination has been made available once again for certain emergency response personnel, law enforcement officials, medical staff, and the military. In 2003, the CDC recommended vaccination for persons who might be first-responders after a smallpox outbreak. Each state and territory was advised to maintain a smallpox response team that includes vaccinated individuals. Some of these teams would undoubtedly consist of dermatologists for their expertise in skin biopsies and diagnosis. The vaccine was initially believed to confer immunity for 3 to 10 years but now that immunity is felt to last perhaps for decades.

Since there are many relative contraindications to vaccination, it is usually not necessary to vaccinate unless there has been a history of recent exposure. Because the vaccine contains a live virus, it should not be administered to persons who are pregnant or immunocompromised. Voluntary vaccination is not recommended for individuals with a history of heart disease or multiple risk factors for heart disease as there is risk for developing myopericarditis. Use of steroid eye drops, nonemergency vaccination of patients under 18 years, and emergency vaccination of patients under age 1 year are also contraindications.

People with atopic dermatitis, active or quiescent—or who have a remote history of atopic dermatitis—should not be vaccinated because of the risk of eczema vaccinatum (**Fig. 47-3**, top left). In this condition, the specific immunologic defects associated with atopic dermatitis render these individuals vulnerable to a virulent and unchecked replication of the live vaccinia virus over the entire skin. Eczema vaccinatum can be fatal. Another possibly fatal condition is progressive vaccinia (**Fig. 47-3**, bottom left, top right). In this condition, a severely immunocompromised person is vaccinated (or inadvertently infected with vaccinia) and is unable to mount an immune response to control the live virus. Vaccinia infection can spread inexorably through the compromised person's skin and organs.

Institutions that administer the smallpox vaccine should maintain a vigilant monitoring program to examine the postvaccination response. The desired, normal response to vaccination is a "Jennerian pustule," an exuberant, umbilicated pustule at the vaccination site. Vaccination programs should instruct PATIENTS on hygiene practices to prevent autoinoculation and contact infection. If there is a laboratory-confirmed case of smallpox, vaccination guidelines would be modified to emphasize widespread protection of the potentially exposed population.

## Treatment

Research evaluating new treatments for both smallpox and adverse vaccination reactions is continually ongoing. CDC recommendations include supportive therapy and antibiotics for any secondary bacterial infections. Other treatment regimens include postexposure vaccination (with greatest efficacy if given within 1 to 3 days after exposure), vaccinia immune globulin (VIG), and cidofovir (or cidofovir analogs); these are updated regularly on the CDC's Web site.

## Anthrax

Anthrax is one of the oldest diseases known to humankind. It is a naturally occurring bacterial disease caused by the aerobic gram-positive rod, *Bacillus anthracis*. Typically, anthrax occurs in rural areas where it is associated with domesticated ruminants (sheep, cattle, and goats). Its historical importance includes several "firsts." It was the first bacterium seen under the microscope, the first organism to satisfy Koch's postulates, the first bacterial disease to have an effective vaccine, and the first bioterrorism agent of the 21st century.

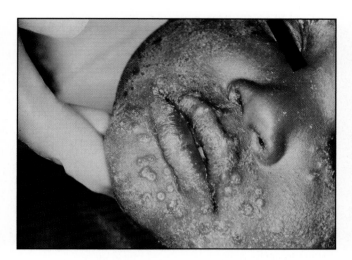

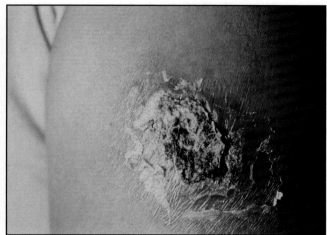

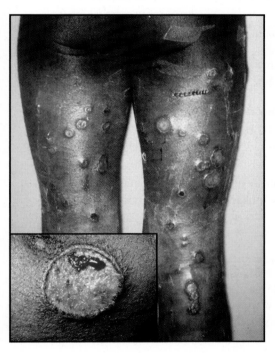

**FIGURE 47-3** ■ Smallpox vaccine reactions. Eczema vaccinatum (*top left*). Necrotizing vaccinia (*top right*). Progressive Vaccinia in AIDS (*bottom left*). (*Courtesy of the James H. Graham, MD & Gloria F. Graham, MD Dermatopathology Library.*)

When exposed to harsh environmental conditions, the rods of *B. anthracis* transform into spores that can remain dormant in soil for decades, impervious to heat, cold, desiccation, and solar radiation. These hardy spores are 1 to 2 μm in diameter and can be easily aerosolized and inhaled. *Wool-sorter's disease* is the name for the occupational illness caused by the inhalation of anthrax spores aerosolized during the handling of unprocessed wool and animal hides. The mortality rate of untreated inhalational anthrax exceeds 90%. Thus, easy weaponization of this highly lethal agent makes it one of the most feared biologic weapons. During the Cold War, several nations produced massive quantities of weaponized anthrax, evidence of which became well known after a mishap at a Soviet bioweapons facility. A cloud of anthrax spores was accidentally released and dozens of people downwind in the town of Sverdlosk died from inhalational anthrax.

Perhaps 95% of naturally occurring anthrax manifests as cutaneous disease, usually in agrarian settings. The Sverdlosk disaster, however, led to the notion that weaponized anthrax caused only inhalational illness. The letter-borne anthrax incidents of late 2001 in the United States, however, showed otherwise: only 11 of the 22 victims had inhalational disease. The other 11 had cutaneous anthrax.

## Clinical Features

Cutaneous anthrax develops when spores enter minor, often unnoticed, breaks in the skin of a mammal (such as a human). The most typical sites are exposed surfaces of the

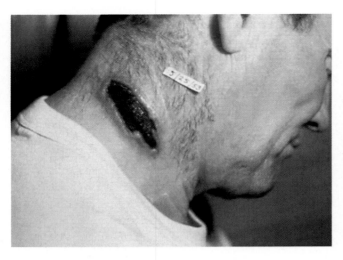

**FIGURE 47-4** ■ Lesion of cutaneous anthrax on the neck. Note the central black eschar surrounded by a red rim. The word anthrax derives from the Greek term for burning coal, anthracis. *(Courtesy of the Public Health Image Library of the Centers for Disease Control and Prevention.)*

**TABLE 47-6** ■ **Differential Diagnosis for Cutaneous Anthrax**

### Differential Diagnosis of Eschar and Ulceration

| | |
|---|---|
| Cutaneous anthrax | Cutaneous diphtheria |
| Brown recluse spider bite | Orf/Milker's nodule |
| Coumadin necrosis | Plague |
| Cutaneous leishmaniasis | Rat bite fever |
| Cutaneous tuberculosis | Pyoderma gangrenosum |
| Ecthyma gangrenosum | Staphylococcal ecthyma (especially due to methicillin-resistant *S. aureus*) |
| Glanders | Streptococcal ecthyma |
| Heparin necrosis | Tropical ulcer |
| | Tularemia |

Antiphospholipid antibody syndrome ulcers

Opportunistic fungal infections (e.g., due to aspergillosis or mucormycosis)

Scrub typhus, tick typhus, and rickettsialpox

### Differential Diagnosis for Ulceroglandular Syndromes

| | |
|---|---|
| Cat scratch disease | Melioidosis |
| Chancroid | Plague |
| Glanders | Staphylococcal |
| Herpes simplex infection | Streptococcal adenitis |
| Lymphogranuloma venereum | Tuberculous adenitis |
| | Tularemia |

hands, legs, and face (Fig. 47-4). In the hospitable environment, the spores are activated; they revert to rods and begin producing toxins. A dermal papule, often resembling an arthropod bite reaction, develops over several days and soon evolves into a painless edematous ulcer with a central black eschar. One to several lesions may appear, depending on the manner of inoculation. There may be regional lymphadenitis, malaise, and fever. Individual lesions often look pustular, leading to the phrase "malignant pustule." Nevertheless, they contain no pus. In fact, histologic examination of cutaneous anthrax shows edema and necrosis with no inflammatory infiltrate. This is because anthrax is a toxin-mediated disease, an important point because antibiotic treatment of anthrax kills the bacteria but does not alter the course of already-produced toxins.

## Diagnosis

Dermatologists played a pivotal role in the diagnosis of anthrax in the letter-borne anthrax incidents of autumn 2001 and will likely be called upon again in the future. The acute onset of a painless edematous noduloulcerative lesion with a black eschar should invoke the clinical diagnosis of cutaneous anthrax. Other entities to consider are listed in Table 47-6. The CDC requests that practitioners notify local or state health departments before attempting a laboratory diagnosis of cutaneous anthrax. The American Academy of Dermatology's *Cutaneous Anthrax Management Algorithm* (available at www.aad.org/professionals/educationcme/bioterrorism/CutaneousAnthrax.htm) leads one through the proper steps to swab exudates for gram stain and culture, to obtain biopsy specimens for histopathology and immunohistochemical staining, and to draw blood samples for culture and serology.

Patients with inhalational anthrax often present with a flulike illness that rapidly progresses into a severe illness.

Inhalational anthrax can be confirmed by examination, culture, or PCR of blood or aspirated pleural fluid. A distinctive radiographic feature of inhalational disease is a widened mediastinum without evidence of a primary pulmonary disorder such as pneumonia.

## Treatment

Naturally occurring anthrax is susceptible to penicillin and doxycycline but weaponized anthrax may have been engineered to be resistant to these antibiotics. Therefore, a fluoroquinolone such as ciprofloxacin is recommended for initial treatment of confirmed or suspected anthrax, even in pregnant women and children in whom this class of antibiotic is rarely administered. Once drug sensitivities have been established, the patient may be switched to another antibiotic as clinically indicated. As mentioned, antibiotics kill activated *B. anthracis* rods but do not reverse the effects of toxins that have been produced. Surgical alteration of the cutaneous lesions may exacerbate the injury and therefore is not recommended unless antibiotics are started concurrently.

Although cutaneous anthrax is usually an uncomplicated and readily treatable infection, public health ramifications warrant hospitalization. Standard universal precautions are appropriate, but specific measures against secondary respiratory transmission are unnecessary. Unlike smallpox, anthrax cannot be transmitted from person to person; it is acquired only via exposure to spores, not to the activated bacilli found in people with clinical disease.

## Prophylaxis

Anthrax vaccine absorbed (AVA) is the FDA-approved vaccine in the United States and is used regularly by veterinarians, laboratory workers, and animal handlers. The US military uses this vaccine to prevent combat-related exposure to aerosolized anthrax spores, although this remains controversial. The vaccine is administered at 0, 2, and 4 weeks and 6, 12, and 18 months with yearly boosters. If an outbreak were to arise, this complex schedule would cause difficulties in maintaining supplies and vaccinating the public. Therefore, continued research in creating a better vaccine is of utmost importance.

## Botulism

Although a bioterrorism attack involving botulism has never occurred, it is considered an ideal bioweapon. Aerosolization of botulinum toxin would be the most likely method of release in a bioterrorism attack, but other methods such as intentional injection of the toxin by adding it to injectable medications, foodborne botulism by adding it to a food-source, and water contamination could also pose a threat.

Botulism occurs when a neurotoxin from *Clostridium botulinum* is absorbed through mucosal membranes or via a wound. *Clostridia* are anaerobic, gram-positive bacilli that form extremely hardy spores. They are found in soil, salt and fresh water sediments, and in the gastrointestinal tract of many animals. There are six clinical syndromes of botulism that include foodborne, infant, wound, adult intestinal toxemia, inhalational, and iatrogenic.

## Clinical Features

This section focuses on the clinical features of wound botulism as this is most relevant to the dermatologist. This would not be the primary syndrome in a bioterrorist attack, but it is likely that aerosolized botulinum toxin would infect open wounds. In a nonbioterrorist setting, wound botulism is sometimes seen among intravenous drug users who use a technique of injecting black tar heroin subcutaneously called "skin popping." In an incidence reported by the CDC, the "black tar heroin" (a brown-to-black-colored form of crudely processed heroin commonly from Mexico) is probably contaminated with spores when the heroin is "cut" with dirt or boot polish. Through tissue necrosis and the formation of an abscess, an anaerobic environment is created where *Clostridia* can thrive. As a bioweapon, contamination of wounds with the neurotoxin could also lead to the same result. As with the other syndromes, cranial nerve dysfunction and descending paralysis ensue.

## Diagnosis

The standard method of diagnosis is the mouse bioassay. This method is slow, labor-intensive, and uses live animals. Other options available are real-time PCR (a good option for wound botulism), rapid mass spectrometry (equal sensitivity to the mouse assay), and ELISA testing (a fast screening technique that is less sensitive).

## Treatment

Treatment is mostly supportive, although antitoxin may be given to prevent progression of the paralysis. Cleaning the infected wound and avoiding antibiotics (unless treating secondary infections) is also advised as they may inhibit the neuromuscular junction further.

## Vaccine

A vaccine for laboratory personnel in contact with *C. botulinum* has been available since the early 1960s. Doses are given at 0, 2, and 12 weeks with an annual booster.

## Tularemia

Like botulism, there is no recorded use of tularemia in a bioterrorist attack. Even so, the United States maintained it as a biologic weapon until 1970 and other countries have maintained it as well. If tularemia were to be used as a biologic weapon, aerosol release would be the most probable method leading to an outbreak of pleuropneumonitis, but there would likely be some instances of cutaneous manifestations as aerosolized bacteria might enter broken skin or mucocutaneous surfaces. This cutaneous clinical presentation is described here.

Tularemia is caused by *Francisella tularensis*, an aerobic, intracellular, gram-negative coccobacillus that does not form spores, but instead survives for weeks in water, soil, hay, animal hides, and carcasses. Although tularemia is often called rabbit or deerfly fever because of historically common routes of transmission, the most common vectors today are ticks. Contact with blood or tissues from infected animals, ingestion of contaminated water or meat, and inhalation of aerosols may also transmit the infection. Though tularemia is most often associated with rabbits, squirrels, beavers, rodents, and other small animals are also reservoirs for the disease.

## Clinical Features

Tularemia is characterized by seven clinical syndromes including ulceroglandular, glandular, oculoglandular, oropharyngeal, typhoidal, pneumonic, and septic syndromes. Ulceroglandular tularemia is the most common presentation in nature and is the most relevant presentation to the dermatologist. A tender or pruritic papule will mark the site of inoculation (most commonly on an exposed extremity) approximately 2 to 5 days after cutaneous exposure. This papule will enlarge to form a sharply demarcated ulcer with a

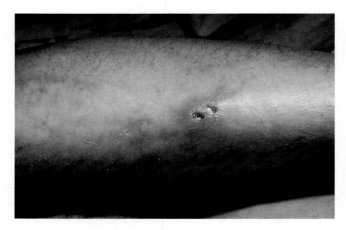

**FIGURE 47-5** ■ This sharply demarcated tularemia ulcer formed from a pruritic papule at the site of inoculation. It may evolve into a black eschar. *(Courtesy of the James H. Graham, MD & Gloria F. Graham, MD Dermatopathology Library.)*

yellowish exudate (Fig. 47-5). Eventually it develops a necrotic base and may form a black eschar. Regional lymphadenopathy is also present. Ulcers may persist for months and heal leaving a scar.

In addition to the ulceroglandular form itself, "tularemids" are secondary skin eruptions that may appear on the face or extremities in any of the seven clinical forms of tularemia. They can range from papular or macular to petechial, vesicular, or pustular and generally emerge in the second week. Erythema nodosum, erythema multiforme and Sweet's syndrome have also been described as nonspecific secondary manifestations.

## Diagnosis

Serology is the most frequent method of diagnosis, though other methods are available. Other methods include fluorescent-labeled antibodies for microscopic examination of tissues or smears; culture of tissue, blood, exudates, and sputum samples; and histologic examination of tissue. The latter would show a neutrophilic infiltrate early in the disease and a granulomatous response later.

## Treatment and Postexposure Prophylaxis

The CDC offers different recommendations for individual cases or mass casualty settings. In isolated cases, streptomycin or gentamicin is recommended for adults, children, and pregnant women. In the setting of a mass casualty, doxycycline and ciprofloxacin are recommended for both treatment and postexposure prophylaxis. Prophylactic treatment for close contacts and isolation precautions are not necessary as there is no person-to-person transmission.

## Vaccine

A live-attenuated vaccine is available for laboratory personnel who frequently work with the bacterium.

## Plague

It is estimated that 200 million deaths throughout the course of history have been attributed to plague. Because of its high mortality and the panic associated with outbreaks of the disease, it is of great concern as a bioweapon. In fact, during World War II, Japanese army units used plague-infected fleas as bioweapons against civilian Chinese populations.

Plague is caused by *Yersinia pestis*, belonging to the Enterobacteriaceae family, is a gram-negative coccobacillus usually transmitted by flea bite or through inadvertent percutaneous inoculation after handling an infected animal. The three forms of the disease are bubonic, pneumonic, and primary septicemic plague.

If the bacterium were used as a bioweapon today, it would most likely be used in an aerosolized form leading to primary pneumonic plague. This manifestation of the disease is rare in the United States and should raise suspicion of bioterrorism.

### Clinical Features

Historically, bubonic plague is the most common form. It begins as a skin pustule at the inoculation site and progresses to local or regional lymphadenitis. The swollen, tender lymph nodes are referred to as buboes. The disease may then spread through the lymphatic system. Necrosis of the involved nodes may result in septicemia or secondary yersinial pneumonia. In the pneumonic and septicemic forms, the patient may develop cyanosis, petechiae, purpura, and ecchymoses, also know as "Black Death."

### Diagnosis

Culture of bubo aspirate, CSF, blood, or sputum is the standard method of diagnosis. Direct microscopy of the bubo aspirate, direct immunoflourescence assay, serology, and PCR are also possible. These methods are hazardous to personnel so a novel immunohistochemical assay to identify *Y. pestis* in formalin-fixed, paraffin-embedded tissues has been developed similar to an assay used in animal models.

### Treatment

It is recommended to isolate any patient with suspected plague for at least 72 hours. Antibiotics should be started immediately upon suspicion of this diagnosis. The CDC recommends the use of IV or IM injection of streptomycin, but due to limited availability, gentamicin may also be used. In a mass causality setting, oral doxycycline is the treatment of choice. Ciprofloxacin may also be used orally.

### Prophylaxis

If a plague outbreak were to occur, patients with symptoms, such as fever, should receive IV antibiotics immediately as postexposure prophylaxis. Those in close contact with infected individuals, but without symptoms, are recommended to take a 7-day course of doxycycline. The plague vaccine was discontinued in 1999, but research is in progress to develop a new vaccine.

## Viral Hemorrhagic Fevers

The CDC classifies viral hemorrhagic fevers as "a group of illnesses that are caused by several distinct families of viruses." The term describes a multiorgan system syndrome generally leading to hematologic collapse and is characterized by acute onset of fever associated with malaise, fatigue, dizziness, loss of strength, diarrhea, and headache. Bleeding under the skin, from internal organs, or from body orifices is also common. Over 25 viruses from four families (filoviridae, flaviviridae, bunyaviridae, and arenaviridae) can cause viral hemorrhagic fevers. The Marburg, Ebola, Lassa, Junin, and Marchupo viruses are of special note because the former Soviet Union had weaponized these viruses. Our discussion will mainly focus on two filoviruses– Ebola and Marburg.

### Clinical Features

Viral hemorrhagic fevers are characterized by acute onset of fever associated with malaise, fatigue, dizziness, loss of strength, diarrhea, and headache. Bleeding under the skin, from internal organs, or from body orifices is also common. Hemorrhagic signs such as petechiae, epistaxis, hematemesis, puncture site bleeding, and bleeding gums manifest themselves in most infected individuals. Progression to DIC is also possible.

Other cutaneous signs commonly may arise. A morbilliform eruption, for example, may appear approximately 5 days after a filovirus infection. Generally, the eruption is located on the extremities or trunk and begins in patches that later coalesce and desquamate. Burning and paresthesias may also be associated with the disease whether or not an eruption is apparent.

### Diagnosis

Evaluating patients with viral hemorrhagic fevers can be hazardous for health care personnel because collected tissues and fluids can easily transmit the infection. Ebola has been diagnosed through culturing the virus, RT-PCR, sequencing technology, ELISA, and indirect fluorescent antibody testing. The limitation of serologic testing is that the individuals generally die before the diagnosis is made. In the 1995 Ebola outbreak in Kikwit, Congo/Zaire, skin biopsies were taken postmortem from infected individuals, and immunohistochemical staining detected the Ebola virus with the same accuracy as the ELISA method.

### Treatment

Strict infection control measures and supportive care are the only treatments for viral hemorrhagic fevers. In Junin hemorrhagic fever, convalescent serum with specific antibodies has successfully treated this infection. Ribavirin has been effective in treating some individuals with Lassa fever. Neither has been effective with filoviruses. There are currently no recommendations for postexposure prophylaxis interventions. Vaccines are available for yellow fever and Argentine hemorrhagic fever.

## Suggested Readings

Arora, S. Cutaneous reactions in nuclear, biological, and chemical warfare. *Indian J Dermatol Venereol Leprol.* 2005;71:80–86.

Bossi P, Tegnell A, Baka A, et al. Bichat guidelines for the clinical management of anthrax and bioterrorism-related anthrax. *Euro Surveill.* 2004;9(12):E3–E4.

Carucci JA, McGovern TW, Norton SA, et al. Cutaneous anthrax management algorithm. *J Am Acad Dermatol.* 2002;47:766–769.

CDC Bioterrorism Web site: http://www.bt.cdc.gov/bioterrorism/

Cieslak TJ, Christopher GW, Ottolini MG. Biological warfare and the skin II: viruses. *Clin Dermatol.* 2002;20(4):355–364.

Cieslak TJ, Talbot TB, Hartstein BH. Biological warfare and the skin I: bacteria and toxins. *Clin Dermatol.* 2002;20(4):346–354.

Cronquist SD. Tularemia: the disease and the weapon. *Dermatol Clin.* 2004;22:313–320.

Dellavalle RP, Heilig LF, Francis SO, et al. What dermatologists do not know about smallpox vaccination: results from a worldwide electronic survey. *J Invest Dermatol.* 2006;126(5):986–989.

Fenner F, Henderson DA, Arita I, et al. *Smallpox and Its Eradication.* Geneva: World Health Organization; 1988.

Guarner J, Shieh WJ, Greer PW, et al. Immunohistochemical detection of *Yersinia pestis* in formalin-fixed, paraffin-embedded tissue. *Am J Clin Pathol.* 2002;117(2):205–209.

Henghold WB. Other biologic toxin bioweapons: ricin, staphylococcal enterotoxin B, and trichothecene mycotoxins. *Dermatol Clin.* 2004; 22:257–262.

Jacobs MK. The history of biologic warfare and bioterrorism. *Dermatol Clin.* 2004;22:231–246.

Lupi O, Madkan V, Tyring SK. Tropical dermatology: bacterial tropical diseases. *J Am Acad Dermatol.* 2006;54:559–578.

Marks JD. Medical aspects of biologic toxins. *Anesth Clin North Am.* 2004; 22(3):509–532.

McGovern TW, Christopher GW, Eitzen EM. Cutaneous manifestations of biological warfare and related threat agents. *Arch Dermatol.* 1999; 135:311–322.

Meffert JJ. Biological warfare from a dermatologic perspective. *Curr Allergy Asthma Rep.* 2003;3:304–310.

Noeller, TP. Biological and chemical terrorism: recognition and management. *Cleve Clin J Med.* 2001;68:1001–1016.

Nuovo GJ, Plaza JA, Magro C. Rapid diagnosis of smallpox infection and differentiation from its mimics. *Diagn Mol Pathol.* 2003;12(2):103–107.

Reissman DB, Whitney EA, Taylor TH, Jr., et al. One-year health assessment of adult survivors of Bacillus anthracis infection. *J Am Med Assoc.* 2004;291:1994–1998.

Salvaggio MR, Baddley JW. Other viral bioweapons: Ebola and Marburg hemorrhagic fever. *Dermatol Clin.* 2004;22:291–302.

Seward JF, Galil K, Damon I, et al. Development and experience with an algorithm to evaluate suspected smallpox cases in the United States, 2002–2004. *Clin Infect Dis.* 2004;39:1477–1483.

Slifka MK, Hanifin JM. Smallpox: the basics. *Dermatol Clin.* 2004;22:263–274.

Villar RG, Elliot SP, Davenport, KM. Botulism: the many faces of botulinum toxin and its potential for bioterrorism. *Infect Dis Clin North Am.* 2006;20:313–327.

Wenner KA, Kenner JR. Anthrax. *Dermatol Clin.* 2004;22:247–256.

Wollenberg A, Engler R. Smallpox, vaccination and adverse reactions to smallpox vaccine. *Curr Opin Allergy Clin Immunol.* 2004;4(4):271–275.

# Dermatoses of Pregnancy

*J. K. Shornick MD, MHA*

The dermatoses of pregnancy can be extremely confusing. Several reported entities have not survived the scrutiny of time. It is doubtful whether perpetuating their inclusion in any current classification scheme serves any useful purpose. In the end, the vast majority of rashes specific to pregnancy can be relegated to one of four categories: pemphigoid gestationis (PG; herpes gestationis), pruritic urticarial papules and plaques of pregnancy (PUPPP), prurigo of pregnancy, and cholestasis of pregnancy.

Needless to say, the pregnant woman is subject to the entire repertoire of the dermatologist's trade. Often the first challenge is to decide whether pregnancy is relevant to the current condition or not.

## Terminology

The generally accepted current classification of skin diseases specific to pregnancy is listed in Table 48-1.

## Pemphigoid Gestationis (Herpes Gestationis)

PG is the prototype of rashes specific to pregnancy. It is almost always associated with pregnancy. There are, however, multiple reports of PG in association with choriocarcinoma or trophoblastic tumors in women. There are no reports of a PG-like disease in association with choriocarcinoma in men. Thus, PG appears to be exclusively associated with the presence of placentally derived tissue.

Although the least common pregnancy-related dermatoses (occurring in approximately 1:50,000 pregnancies), PG is the most clearly defined skin condition, and the most important to exclude. It remains idiopathic, although it is invariably associated with pregnancy (or trophoblastic tissue), carries a genetic predisposition, and is immunologically mediated.

### SAUER'S NOTE

The chapter author has done an impressive job of summarizing a very complex group of illnesses. Review of this chapter will help all those concerned with care of the pregnant patient.

## Presentation and Characteristics

### Clinical Appearance

- First onset may occur during any pregnancy, generally during the second or third trimester. Explosive onset in the immediate postpartum period can occur in up to 25% of cases.
- Clinical lesions vary from intensely pruritic urticarial plaques to pemphigoid-like tense blisters (Fig. 48-1). One often sees rapid evolution from the urticarial phase to clustered or arcuate tense blisters. Patients with only urticarial lesions and no progression to blisters have been reported.
- Intense, relentless pruritus is invariable.

**TABLE 48-1 ■ Classification of Dermatoses of Pregnancy***

| Classification | Synonyms or Variants |
|---|---|
| Pemphigoid gestationis | Herpes gestationis |
| Pruritic urticarial papules and plaques of pregnancy (PUPPP) | Polymorphic eruption of pregnancy |
| | Toxemic rash of pregnancy |
| | Toxic erythema of pregnancy |
| | Late-onset prurigo of pregnancy |
| Prurigo of pregnancy | Prurigo gestationis (Besnier) |
| | Early onset prurigo of pregnancy |
| | Papular dermatitis of pregnancy |
| | Pruritic folliculitis of pregnancy |
| | Linear IgM disease of pregnancy |
| Cholestasis of pregnancy | Obstetric cholestasis |

1. Prurigo gravidarum
2. Jaundice of pregnancy

*Preferred terminology is noted in bold.

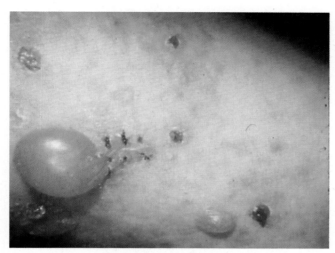

**FIGURE 48-1** ■ Urticarial plaques and tense bullae on the thighs of a patient with herpes gestationis.

### Distribution

Onset occurs in the periumbilical area in 50% of patients, but may also first appear on the palms, soles, or extremities. Facial involvement is rare and mucosal involvement essentially nonexistent.

### Course

- Exacerbation at delivery occurs in approximately 75% of patients and may be dramatic.
- Generally recurs during subsequent pregnancies, although "skip pregnancies" have been reported. Flares associated with menstruation or oral contraceptives are also reported.
- Spontaneous resolution over weeks to months following delivery is the rule, although case reports of protracted disease are available.
- There is no increased maternal risk in association with PG.
- Newborns may be affected up to 10% of the time, presumably through passive transfer of the PG IgG.
- There is an increased risk of premature delivery associated with PG (32% before 38 weeks, 16% before 36 weeks).

### Laboratory Findings

- Routine laboratory results are normal. Mild peripheral eosinophilia may occur, but is not clearly clinically relevant.
- Histopathology classically shows a subepidermal blister with eosinophils. Eosinophils are uncommon in PUPPP and suggest one should at least consider PG in the differential diagnosis.
- Direct immunofluorescence showing complement, with or without IgG deposited in a smooth, linear band along the dermal–epidermal junction, is the diagnostic sine qua non, occurring in essentially 100% of cases. Split specimens show staining on the epidermal fragment. Indirect immunofluorescence reveals an IgG1 capable of avid complement activation. Titers of the PG antibody are low and historically do not correlate with the extent or severity of skin involvement. Recent, more sensitive immunoblotting and enzyme-linked immunoassays (NC16a ELISA, now commercially available) may challenge that assessment.

### Cause

- The PG antigen is a subcomponent of collagen XVII, a 180-kDa collagenous, transmembrane glycoprotein with its N-terminal end embedded within the intracellular component of the hemidesmosome and its C-terminal component located extracellularly. The extracellular portion contains 15 collagenous domains interspersed by 16 noncollagenous domains. Antibodies from patients with bullous pemphigoid, mucous membrane pemphigoid, lichen planus pemphigoides, and linear IgA disease all react to specific antigens along the extracellular component of BP180. The 16th noncollagenous A domain (NC16A) lies immediately adjacent to the basal cell membrane and is the target in PG. NC16A is also known as BP180 and BPAg2.
- Pathophysiologically, the PG antibody fixes to the BMZ, triggering complement activation via the classical complement pathway. Chemoattraction and degranulation of eosinophils follow. It is the release of proteolytic enzymes from eosinophilic granules, which appears to dissolve the bond between epidermis and dermis.
- Up to 80% of PG patients carry HLA-DR3, approximately 50% have HLA-DR4, and 40% to 50% have the simultaneous presence of both. HLA-DR3 shows linkage disequilibrium with the C4 null allele, and a corresponding increase in the C4 null allele has also been reported. However, neither HLA-DR3 nor HLA-DR4 is requisite for the development of PG, and there is no obvious correlation between the presence of antigen and the extent or severity of disease.
- All patients demonstrate anti-HLA antibodies. Whether this represents phenomenon or epiphenomenon remains to be seen, but their strikingly high incidence implies the universal presence of placental compromise.
- Special stains of PG placenta have suggested a primary immunologic reaction in the villous stroma of chorionic villi, leading to the suggestion that PG is actually a primary disease of placental tissue, with secondary involvement of the skin. This hypothesis is attractive from many viewpoints, but remains to be clarified.
- Antithyroid antibodies are also increased; although their clinical relevance is unclear; the majority of patients are clinically euthyroid. On the other hand, the risk of autoimmune thyroid disease, especially

Grave's disease, is clearly increased in those with a history of PG.

## Differential Diagnosis

The primary differential in PG is between PUPPP and a wide variety of diseases irrelevant to pregnancy. Urticaria and arthropod bites can be difficult to differentiate. Immunofluorescence or Elisa is the key to separating PG from the rest but is hardly reasonable in all cases of pruritic rashes during pregnancy. Most typically, the relentless progression of unbearable itch associated with urticarial lesions, rapidly progressing to tense blisters, is characteristic of PG.

## Treatment

- PG is sufficiently rare that treatment guidelines are all driven by expert opinion.
- Because PG is not associated with significant maternal or fetal risk and because it tends to remit spontaneously postpartum, it is imperative not to create significant risk from therapy.
- Topical steroids and antihistamines are rarely of benefit.
- Systemic steroids, beginning at 0.5 mg/kg/d, remain the cornerstone of effective therapy. Many patients improve during the later part of pregnancy, only to flare at the time of delivery. Because profound flares at the time of delivery are common, one should be prepared to initiate or increase steroids during the immediate postpartum period.
- There has been no clear evidence that PG is associated with increased fetal morbidity or mortality (other than premature birth), although that impression certainly remains from a review of individual case reports.
- There is no evidence that systemic steroids decrease the risk of premature delivery.
  - Alternative therapies, including the use of rituximab for recalcitrant disease as reccomended in some case reports.

## Pruritic Urticarial Papules and Plaques of Pregnancy (Polymorphic Eruption of Pregnancy)

Polymorphic eruption of pregnancy (PUPPP) is the most common of the specific dermatoses of pregnancy, estimated to occur in 1:130 to 1:300 pregnancies. It is idiopathic, defined clinically, has negative immunofluorescence, and tends to not recur during subsequent gestations.

## Presentation and Characteristics

### Clinical Appearance

- Most cases (75% to 85%) develop during the first pregnancy, but first onset after multiple pregnancies has been reported.

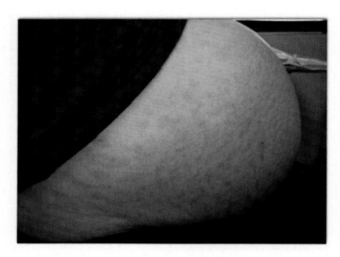

**FIGURE 48-2** ■ Urticarial plaques over the abdomen in the striae of a woman with PUPPP.

- There is an abrupt onset of intensely itchy urticarial or papular lesions, often within abdominal striae in the last month of pregnancy (Fig. 48-2) or immediate postpartum period. Rapid spread to the trunk and extremities is characteristic.
- Fine vesicles are present in up to 40% of cases, but there are no tense blisters.

### Distribution

There is a curious tendency for lesions to develop first within abdominal striae, although this is certainly not universal. The face and mucosal surfaces are almost always spared.

### Course

- Spontaneous resolution within days of delivery is the rule.
- Generally does not recur during subsequent gestations.
- No maternal risks or complication noted, except for an increased incidence of excessive weight gain and fetal twinning.

### Laboratory Findings

- Laboratory investigations are normal.
- Histopathology is nonspecific and typically devoid of eosinophils. The presence of eosinophils, however, does not exclude PUPPP.
- Direct and indirect immunofluorescence are negative. An increase in activated T cells within dermal infiltrates has led to speculation that PUPPP may be a consequence of a delayed T-cell hypersensitivity to skin antigens.
- HLA typing shows no disease associations.

## Differential Diagnosis

Because no definitive marker exists for PUPPP, the diagnosis is clinical and made by exclusion. As with PG, the differential is typically between incidental hives, viral exanthems, and PG. Immunofluorescence, though not indicated in all cases, is the key to distinguishing PG.

### Treatment

Potent topical steroids and antihistamines may provide symptomatic support. Systemic steroids are quite helpful, although not always necessary.

## Prurigo of Pregnancy

This group of rashes is less common than PUPPP (estimated to occur in between 1:300 and 1:450 pregnancies) and by far the most confusing. Several variations have been reported. Confusion persists regarding the entities reported without histopathology or routine laboratory investigations and prior to the advent of immunofluorescence. The unifying feature of this group is that there is no diagnostic clarity, only a similar clinical pattern. No doubt, this group will be subdivided with time.

### Presentation and Characteristics

#### Clinical Appearance

- The classical presentation occurs during the second or third trimester with discrete or clustered scratch papules, predominantly on the extensor surfaces. Lesions may or may not be follicular.
- There may be pustules, but not blisters.

#### Distribution

Generally on the extensor surfaces, sparing the face and mucosal surfaces.

#### Course

- Generally self-limited, the symptoms resolve over weeks to months postpartum.
- No fetal or maternal risks have been reported.
- Recurrence during subsequent pregnancies is variable.

#### Laboratory Findings

- Liver function tests (by definition) are normal. Other laboratory findings have been inconsistently described.
- Histopathology is typically nonspecific. Whether inflammation tends to be follicular or not depends on whether poorly described variants are included in this group.
- Immunofluorescence is characteristically negative.

### Differential Diagnosis

By definition, laboratory investigations and immunofluorescence are noncontributory. With no defining marker and only a nonspecific clinical pattern to unite the reported variants, there is little guidance to separate prurigo of pregnancy from atopy or diseases coincident to pregnancy.

### Treatment

Treatment is symptomatic; no morbidity or mortality has been associated with this group.

## Cholestasis of Pregnancy (Obstetric Cholestasis)

Jaundice occurs in approximately 1 in every 1,500 pregnancies. Cholestasis of pregnancy (CP) is the second most common cause of gestational jaundice, viral hepatitis being more common. CP accounts for approximately 20% of cases of obstetric jaundice, although the frequency varies both geographically and seasonally.

The incidence of CP varies in different racial groups. It seems to be highest in Chile-Bolivia (6% to 27%) and Sweden (1% to 1.5%) and lowest among blacks and Asians. CP occurs in approximately 1:1,000 pregnancies in the United States. The defining features of CP are

- generalized pruritus, with or without jaundice, with no history of exposure to hepatitis or hepatotoxic drugs;
- the absence of primary lesions;
- elevated serum bile acids;
- disappearance of signs and symptoms following pregnancy; and
- recurrence during a subsequent gestation (does not always occur).

There is, however, a broad spectrum of clinical presentations.

CP is not really a primary *dermatosis* of pregnancy because the defining feature is pruritus associated with cholestasis but without dermatologic primary lesions. The literature on CP is unusually inconsistent.

### Presentation and Characteristics

#### Clinical Appearance

- Typically presents during the last trimester of otherwise uneventful pregnancies. Onset as early as 8 weeks has been reported.
  - ❑ Increased incidence of twin pregnancies.
- Intense, generalized pruritus, worse at night and often worst on the palms and soles.
- Skin findings are all secondary.

#### Distribution.

Symptoms are typically worse on the trunk, palms, and soles.

#### Course

- Symptoms may wax and wane, with or without changes in liver function tests.

- Up to 50% of patients may develop signs of hepatitis—dark urine, light-colored stools, or jaundice—usually within 4 weeks of presentation.
- Recurrences during subsequent gestations occur in 60% to 70% of cases. Recurrences are also common with the use of oral contraceptives.
- Signs and symptoms disappear within weeks of delivery.
- Failure of pruritus to stop within days of delivery or the persistence of elevated liver function tests suggest underlying hepatic or primary biliary disease.
- If intrahepatic cholestasis lasts for weeks, vitamin K absorption may be impaired, leading to a prolonged prothrombin time. Without exogenous vitamin K, fetal prothrombin activity may lead to an increased incidence of intracranial hemorrhage. The prothrombin time should be monitored and intramuscular vitamin K administered as necessary.
- Meconium staining and premature labor occurs in 20% to 60% of cases. Fetal distress and increased stillbirths are also reported, with mortality in some series as high as 13%.
  - Fetal risk does not appear to be correlated with laboratory abnormalities.
- Most authors argue for increased fetal monitoring after 30 weeks, with delivery upon signs of meconium staining or fetal stress. Others argue for delivery at 38 weeks for mild symptoms, 36 weeks for severe cases.
- There appears to be a tendency for these women to develop cholelithiasis or gallbladder disease at increased rates later in life.

## Laboratory Findings

- Hepatic ultrasonography is normal. Liver biopsy is not indicated.
- In those without jaundice, elevated serum bile acids may be the only identifiable laboratory abnormality (prurigo gravidarum). Conjugated (direct) bilirubin is increased, but rarely above 2 to 5 mg/dL. Alkaline phosphatase, GGT, and cholesterol are unreliable during pregnancy, but AST typically remains below four times normal, even in those with CP.

- Serum abnormalities confirm the presence or absence of disease. Whether or not serum levels correlate with disease severity is disputed.

## Cause

- CP remains multifactorial. The existing literature is confusing and contradictory but points towards an estrogen (or progesterone) dependent decompensation of genes encoding for hepatobiliary transport proteins.
- Onset in association with a urinary tract infection has been reported in up to 50% of cases, although the causative relationship between the two is unclear.
- Current CP immunogenetic research is largely directed at the transport genes ABCB4 and MDR3 and the bile salt export pump ABCB11 and BSEP.

## Differential Diagnosis

Increased bile acid salts are the sine qua non and are typically 3 to 100 times normal.

## Treatment

- Phototherapy, phenobarbital, and cholestyramine are the historical treatments and remain viable options. Expert opinion suggests these therapies improve maternal morbidity without improving fetal outcome. Cholestyramine is also associated with increased malabsorption of fat soluble vitamins.
- Ursodeoxycholic acid (15 mg/kg/d) is generally considered the treatment of choice. Its use appears to both control symptoms and decrease the risk of adverse fetal outcome(s).

## Suggested Readings

Kondrackiene J, Kupcinskas L. Intrahepatic cholestasis of pregnancy-current achievements and unsolved problems. *World J Gastroenterol.* 2008;14(38):5781–5788.

Powell AM, Sakuma-Oyama Y, Oyama N, et al. Collagen XVII/BP180: a collagenous transmembrane protein and component of the dermoepidermal anchoring complex. *Clin Exp Dermatol.* 2005;30:682–687.

# CHAPTER 49

# Nutritional and Metabolic Diseases and the Skin

*Brian J. Hall, MD*

Nutrition will always play an important role in the maintenance and protection of the skin. As more is being discovered about the foods we eat and more attention is being paid to different vitamins and minerals, we will undoubtedly find out more important information regarding nutrition and its role in skin maintenance as well as skin disease. Also, problems associated with developing countries are becoming more important as more people continue to migrate to the United States from abroad. Due to the increasing elderly population in the United States, adequate nutritional intake among the elderly will continue to be a very important subject for clinicians to be attentive to. Diet is many times inadequate in elderly populations and does not contain enough variety to provide elderly patients with all of the nutrients that they need. Also, as Americans have enjoyed an excess of food in recent times, one of our biggest problems is obesity and the medical problems it creates for them. The skin is not immune to these problems. We will also discuss how different metabolic diseases can have profound effects on the skin.

## Vitamin Deficiencies

### Vitamin A Deficiency

*Presentation and Characteristics*

Vitamin A deficiency is mainly a disease limited to the developing countries. One of the first signs of deficiency is night blindness, and it is the leading cause of blindness in developing countries. The most striking characteristic of the skin associated with vitamin A deficiency is phrynoderma. It is marked by follicular hyperkeratosis with spinous papules at the end of hair follicles. It is symmetrically distributed and often initially located at the extensor surfaces of the thighs and forearms. Many times this hyperkeratosis causes the patient's skin to appear like toad skin and it sometimes occurs on a background of dry and rough skin that may feel like sandpaper or nutmeg grater. The worst cases often plague children of preschool age. Other signs of deficiency include keratomalacia, pruritis, broken fingernails, and keratinization of mucous membranes. Even mild deficiencies can have a profound effect on a child's immune system and can increase the child's chances of dying from other childhood illnesses such as measles.

*Treatment*

Skin lesions recover impressively with retin-A cream. Nutritional state can be improved with cod liver oil, palm oil, carrots, sweet potatoes, leafy green vegetables, fruits, and a variety of meats such as liver. Daily oral supplements can be given for vitamin A deficiency and are listed in dosages depending on age: children 3 years or younger—600 $\mu$g (2,000 IU); children aged 4 to 8 years—900 $\mu$g (3,000 IU); children aged 9 to 13 years—1,700 $\mu$g (5,665 IU); children aged 14 to 18 years—2,800 $\mu$g (9,335 IU); and all adults—3,000 $\mu$g (10,000 IU).

*Prevention*

Eating a healthy diet with plenty of fruits and vegetables and a variety of other foods is the best prevention for vitamin A deficiency. Besides the foods listed in the previous section, fortified milk, whole milk, chicken, beef, and eggs are also rich in vitamin A.

### Vitamin A Excess

*Presentation and Characteristics*

Hypervitaminosis A presents with dry, coarse, scaly skin, hair loss, seborrhea, yellow discoloration of the skin, peeling of skin, fissures of the lips, pruritis, sore tongue or mouth, increased sensitivity to sunlight, and low-grade fever.

---

**SAUER'S NOTES**

As foreign travel and the global economy expand, vitamin and mineral abnormalities are a group of illnesses in which all specialists need to develop awareness.

---

*Treatment*

Elimination of sources of vitamin A and/or carotenoid in the diet or from supplementation.

*Prevention*

The liver of certain animals such as polar bear, husky, and seal are unsafe to eat due to their extraordinarily high vitamin A content. This fact has been known to Inuit for centuries and even to European explorers since the middle 16th century. It is also extremely important not to take more than the recommended daily allowance (RDA) of this vitamin because the amount over and above the RDA is one of the narrowest of all vitamins and minerals. Especially with recent emphasis on vitamin A and beta-carotene as anticancer agents, accidental chronic overdose (through oral supplementation) is a possible problem. Excessive ingestion of carotenoids (which can cause carotoderma—discussed in the next section) is nontoxic and does not cause hypervitaminosis A because the conversion of carotene to vitamin A is too slow.

## Carotenemia

*Presentation and Characteristics*

Carotenemia is a benign skin condition most often seen in light-skinned patients who have ingested large amounts of foods rich in vitamin A precursors. Carotenemia commonly occurs in vegetarians and young children. This causes a yellow discoloration of the skin excluding the eyes and oral mucosa (Fig. 49-1). It is important to distinguish this condition from more serious conditions such as jaundice. In dark-skinned individuals, the palms and soles may have yellow discoloration, but not the rest of the body. This condition more commonly occurs in children with liver disease, hypothyroidism, or diabetes mellitus. Hypothyroidism, diabetes mellitus, hepatic diseases, anorexia nervosa (AN), and renal diseases may be associated with carotenemia unassociated with the ingestion of carotene. Mothers may induce carotenemia by giving their infants large amounts of carrots in commercial infant food preparations.

*Treatment*

Since carotenemia is a benign condition, it can be treated with dietary modification alone.

*Prevention*

A lower or more moderate carotene diet will prevent recurrence.

## Vitamin B$_2$ (Riboflavin) Deficiency

*Presentation and Characteristics*

Riboflavin deficiency is associated with perlèche or angular stomatitis (Fig. 49-2), atrophic glossitis (magneta-colored cobblestone tongue), and inflammation of the oral mucosa. A seborrhea-like follicular keratosis may also be observed. It can be generalized, but the areas of the face, chest, abdominal wall, extremities, and genital areas are most severely and consistently affected. On the face it can resemble shark skin and the genital area can show redness with a fine, powdery desquamation.

*Treatment*

Treatment consists of taking riboflavin 6 to 30 mg PO q.d. until symptoms resolve.

*Prevention*

Prevention involves eating foods high in riboflavin, such as milk, cheese, yogurt, meat, and vegetables (especially spinach, asparagus, and broccoli).

## Vitamin B$_3$ (Niacin) Deficiency

*Presentation and Characteristics*

Pellagra is the common term used to refer to niacin deficiency and includes the "three D's" of dermatitis, diarrhea, and dementia. There is sometimes a fourth D referred to because, if left untreated for an extended period of time, death

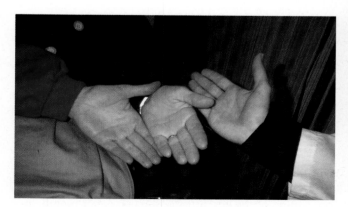

**FIGURE 49-1** ▪ Carotenemia in a patient due to ingestion of large amounts of carrots.

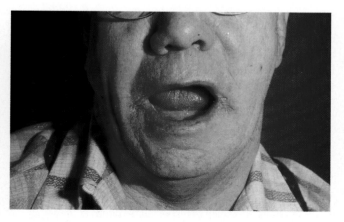

**FIGURE 49-2** ▪ Perlèche in any elderly patient such as this one would necessitate a workup for a vitamin B deficiency.

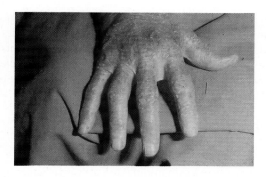

FIGURE 49-3 ▪ A patient with pellagra on the dorsal hands, which is almost always involved, demonstrating hyperkeratosis with redness and superficial scaling.

can result. The diarrhea and dementia are only found in advanced cases. The dermatitis is a symmetrical photodermatitis, affecting sun-exposed areas, areas of friction, or areas of pressure. The patient may report a burning sensation or pain early on. The initial erythema can also subside and darken to a brown color and become brittle, rough, hyperkeratotic, or scaly over time. Almost all patients will have involvement of the dorsal hands (**Fig. 49-3**). The rash begins in the neck and appears as a broad symmetric hyperpigmented scaly and erythematous collar that has the appearance of a scarf tied around the neck, which then tapers downward, hence the common name "Cassal's necklace." The skin rash heals centrifugally with a line of demarcation remaining actively inflamed after the center of the lesion has desquamated.

### Treatment

Treatment is supplementation with niacinamide either orally or IV. The usual oral dosage is 0.5 g daily and the usual dosage of an injection is 50 to 100 mg b.i.d. for a period of 3 months. Skin lesions can be covered with emollients, and since sun protection is important during the recovery phase, sunscreen should be applied to all exposed body areas. Since most patients with pellagra also suffer from other vitamin deficiencies, treating the patient with a high-protein diet rich in B-vitamins is also necessary to restore the patient to health. Long-term addition of milk, eggs, and meat is many times necessary to help with recovery. Also, the addition of peanuts, green leafy vegetables, whole or enriched grains, brewer's dry yeast, and meats can enhance niacin uptake in the acute phase of recovery.

### Prevention

Niacin deficiency is rare in Western society. It mainly affects societies whose main dietary intake is maize (which has a low tryptophan content) and millet or sorghum (both of which interfere with tryptophan metabolism due to their high leucine content). Since most of their diet was maize, the Native Americans discovered that they could prevent pellagra by adding lime (an alkali) that makes niacin more available. It is hypothesized that pellagra is caused by not only niacin deficiency but also lack of either tryptophan or one of the vitamin cofactors. However, pellagra does sometimes affect chronic alcoholics, or patients with gastrointestinal disorders or patients with severe psychiatric disturbances in more developed societies like the United States. The main way to prevent pellagra is to have a diet with adequate calories and protein.

## Vitamin B$_6$ Deficiency

### Presentation and Characteristics

As far as the skin is concerned, a deficiency can paint a similar clinical picture as pellagra since B$_6$ is needed by the body to produce its own B$_3$ vitamin. Although extremely rare, the skin is one of the first organs to show signs of B$_6$ deficiency and can include nails that are uneven (transverse ridging), scaly facial eruptions resembling seborrheic dermatitis, painful, edematous glossitis, angular cheilitis, and generalized stomatitis. Multiple skin disorders including eczema, acne, and seborrheic dermatitis have been associated with B$_6$ deficiency.

### Treatment

Pyridoxine 50 to 100 mg PO q.d. is usually sufficient for adults.

### Prevention

Vitamin B$_6$ is actually present in most foods, so deficiency is quite rare. As with most vitamin deficiencies, make sure the patient takes in a variety of foods especially poultry, fish, liver, eggs, meat, vegetables, and grains. For patients taking pyroxidine-inactivating drugs such as anticonvulsants, cycloserine, hydralazine, corticosteroids, and penicillamine, the use of pyridoxine in the amount of 50 to 100 mg PO q.d. is recommended. For patients taking isoniazide, a dose of 30 to 50 mg of pyridoxine q.d. is advised.

## Vitamin B$_{12}$ Deficiency

### Presentation and Characteristics

Clinically, a patient with a B$_{12}$ deficiency may present with skin hyperpigmentation (especially over the dorsum of the hands and feet with a concentration over the interphalangeal joints and terminal phalanges), vitiligo, perlèche (angular cheilitis), or glossopyrosis (burning mouth syndrome) that can later result in a focal or diffuse smooth, painful glossitis and hair changes.

### Treatment

Treatments can vary but both IM and oral routes are acceptable. IM administration usually involves initial loading doses followed by monthly maintenance doses. One dose of 1,000 $\mu$g q.d. × 2 weeks followed by a maintenance dose of 1,000 $\mu$g q 1 to 3 months is one example. Oral supplementation is usually 1,000 to 2,000 $\mu$g PO q.d. × 2 weeks with a maintenance therapy of 1,000 $\mu$g q.d. for life.

### Prevention

Since $B_{12}$ is present only in animal foods and cannot be synthesized by the body, a proper diet including fish, meat, poultry eggs, milk, and milk products is necessary to prevent deficiency. For vegetarians, fortified cereals help prevent deficiency.

## Biotin (Vitamin H) Deficiency

### Presentation and Characteristics

Classically in neonates it presents as a universal alopecia with an extensive bran-like erythematous desquamation that is more pronounced in intertriginous areas. Within 3 to 5 weeks of deficient biotin intake the patient will clinically exhibit seborrheic dermatitis, dry skin, and hair thinning that can progress to total scalp or even universal alopecia (**Fig. 49-4**) over several months. Other associated signs include: fine and brittle hair without abnormalities of the shaft, fungal infections (especially with *Candida albicans*), and rashes including periorificial dermatitis with mild, scaly erythema and crusted erosions. Some patients also exhibit keratoconjunctivitis or blepharitis.

### Treatment

Treatment with 10 to 20 mg PO q.d. is normally adequate, although quantities up to 40 mg have been used and tolerated by patients.

### Prevention

Prevention depends on the cause, and there are a variety of causes for biotin deficiency. Metabolic causes (biotinidase deficiency or holocarboxylase/multiple carboxylase deficiency) cannot be prevented by diet. For deficiencies caused by anticonvulsants a switch to another anticonvulsant medication that does not interfere with absorption must be made or the patients should be supplemented with biotin. For prolonged antibiotic therapy as the cause, the patient should receive biotin supplementation as well if antibiotic therapy must be continued. Otherwise, discontinuation of antibiotic

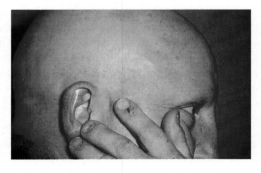

**FIGURE 49-4** ■ A patient with alopecia universalis. A patient with alopecia, alopecia totalis, or alopecia universalis should raise suspicion for a deficiency in biotin, zinc, or an essential fatty acid in the proper setting. Hair loss of any type can be a sign of poor nutrition.

therapy is advised. Patients should also be advised not to consume large amounts of raw eggs as raw egg whites because they both contain avidin. Avidin in large amounts can bind biotin and prevent absorption in the intestine. A dietary deficiency is quite rare, but foods high in biotin include most vegetables, some fruits, chicken, eggs, and milk.

## Vitamin C Deficiency (Scurvy)

### Presentation and Characteristics

The most distinctive skin finding in scurvy is follicular hyperkeratosis with coiled, corkscrew hairs growing out of the follicles on the upper arms, back, buttocks, and lower extremities. Later patients can get hemorrhagic petichiae in a perifollicular location, ecchymoses, spongy bluish-purple gingivae that may become massively swollen, bleeding of gums, and, in extreme cases, bleeding of all mucous membranes.

### Treatment

Treatment is vitamin C 300 to 1000 mg preferably divided into doses of 100 mg throughout the day for at least 1 week and then 400 mg per day until complete recovery.

### Prevention

Prevention of scurvy can be accomplished merely by providing a moderate amount of fruits and vegetables in the diet. Foods exceptionally high in vitamin C include bell peppers, brussel sprouts, papaya, broccoli, oranges, strawberries, cantaloupe, kiwifruit, cauliflower, and kale.

## Mineral Deficiencies/Excesses

### Iron Deficiency

### Presentation and Characteristics

Some of the skin signs of iron deficiency include pruritis, brittle nails, nails with vertical stripes, koilonychias (spoon-shaped nails), angular stomatitis, a smooth and swollen tongue that can develop a burning sensation, dryness of the throat and mouth, brittle and dry hair, possible increased hair shedding, and pale skin if the patient is anemic.

### Treatment

Oral iron therapy is the treatment of choice in most patients; however, the underlying cause of iron deficiency needs to be determined. Iron sulfate 325 mg PO t.i.d. is given for up to 2 months after the anemia has been corrected.

### Prevention

Including iron-rich foods or iron-fortified flour, bread, or cereals in the diet is the best prevention. Foods high in iron include red meat, liver, eggs, leafy green vegetables, and legumes. Oral iron supplementation is sometimes recommended during periods of increased requirement such as lactation or pregnancy.

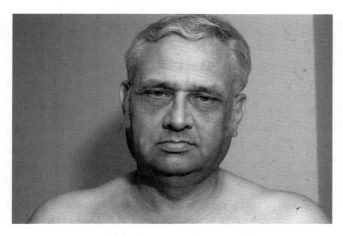

**FIGURE 49-5** ■ A patient with hemochromatosis demonstrating bronzing of the skin.

## Iron Excess (Hemochromatosis)

### Presentation and Characteristics

The classic triad of hemochromatosis is hyperpigmentation, cirrhosis, and diabetes mellitus. Skin hyperpigmentation is one of the earliest signs of the disease and is therefore very important for the physician to recognize. It is most pronounced on sun-exposed areas, especially the face (**Fig. 49-5**).

### Treatment

Therapeutic phlebotomy is the treatment of choice, and skin hyperpigmentation is often substantially alleviated. For patients not able to tolerate therapeutic phlebotomy due to extreme anemia, Desferal (Deferoxamine) is used to chelate the excess iron.

### Prevention

Hereditary hemochromatosis cannot be prevented. Secondary hemochromatosis can be due to several factors such as diet, anemia, chronic liver disease, blood transfusion, iron intake, and long-term kidney dialysis. Prevention depends on the factor that caused the disease.

## Folate Deficiency

### Presentation and Characteristics

Although best known for causing megaloblastic anemia that slowly progresses over months and delays maturation of granulocytes and megakaryocytes, pure folate deficiency has also been known to cause hyperpigmentation of the skin and mucous membranes similar to what is seen in $B_{12}$ deficiency. Hyperpigmentation is accentuated particularly on the dorsal surfaces of the fingers, toes, as well as in the creases of the palms and soles of patients. The pathogenesis is unknown, but it does clear with appropriate treatment.

### Treatment

Treatment consists of oral or IV folic acid supplements on a short-term basis until anemia resolves, and a diet rich in green leafy vegetables and citrus fruits. In cases of intestinal malabsorption, lifelong replacement therapy may be necessary.

### Prevention

Prevention involves a high intake of folate-rich foods especially in high-risk patients (i.e., pregnant women, the elderly, celiac patients, cancer patients, alcoholics). For the general population, eating a well-balanced diet and including foods high in folate such as green leafy vegetables, liver, beans, certain fruits (especially oranges and satsumas), brewer's yeast, and fortified breads and cereals is recommended.

## Zinc Deficiency

### Presentation and Characteristics

Acrodermatitis enteropathica, which is an autosomal recessive disorder affecting the intestinal absorption of zinc, clinically presents as the triad of diarrhea, alopecia, and a periorificial and acral rash. Clinically it will present in infants that become photophobic and develop a vesiculobullous dermatitis on the hands, feet, periorificial areas, and many times quite dramatically in the diaper area 4 to 6 weeks after weaning. Conjunctivitis and blepharitis may also be seen. Acute zinc deficiency from dietary insufficiency will show the same clinical picture with eczematous eruptions of the hands, feet, and anogenital areas. Flat, grayish, bullous lesions surrounded by red-brown erythema will cover the finger flexural creases and palms. Hair growth is slow, with thinning of scalp hair that can lead to alopecia totalis. Angular stomatitis and paronychia also occur. In chronic cases, lesions are seen on areas subject to repeated pressure or friction such as the elbows, knees, and knuckles. These lesions are well demarcated, thickened, and brownish, and may develop lichenification and scaling. Nails show Beau's lines (deep transverse depressions). This condition has been associated with total parental nutrition (TPN) and cystic fibrosis.

### Treatment

Oral zinc in a dose of 2 mg/kg for acrodermatitis enteropathica can resolve clinical manifestations within 2 weeks. However, the infant should remain on oral zinc supplementation therapy for life. For dietary zinc deficiency, increasing intake of foods rich in zinc content is suitable for mild deficiency. For a more severe zinc deficiency, zinc picolinate or zinc gluconate can be taken orally and dosing will vary depending on the severity of the deficiency.

### Prevention

Eating a well-rounded diet and including foods that are high in zinc is the best means of prevention. Foods high in zinc include veal liver, red meats, sesame seeds, pumpkin seeds, yogurt, green peas, shrimp, and green leafy vegetables.

## Copper Excess (Wilson's Disease)

### Presentation and Characteristics

Skin pigmentation and a bluish discoloration at the base of the fingernails (azure lunulae) have been described in patients with Wilson's disease. Patients can also have the following skin manifestations secondary to hepatic insufficiency and cirrhosis (which can progress to fulminant hepatic failure): ascites and prominent abdominal veins, spider nevi, palmar erythema, digital clubbing, and jaundice.

### Treatment

Treatment with copper chelators such as penicillamine, trientine, and zinc acetate is the best therapy to prevent a fatal outcome in these patients.

### Prevention

Genetic counseling is recommended for persons with a family history of Wilson's disease.

## Selenium Deficiency

### Presentation and Characteristics

Although best known for causing cardiomyopathy, selenium has been documented in at least one case to cause xerosis, erythematous scaly papules and plaques on the cheeks, hips, thighs, and popliteal areas as well as erosions in the diaper area, and short, thin, light-colored hair.

### Treatment

Supplementation with sodium selenite is reported to resolve symptoms. One study found that Brazil nuts alone were just as efficacious as sodium selenite in raising selenium levels in patients who were selenium deficient.

### Prevention

Eating a balanced diet and including selenium-rich foods is the best prevention. Foods high in selenium include Brazil nuts, tuna, salmon, shrimp, mushrooms, and halibut.

# Protein Deficiency (PEU or Protein Energy Undernutrition)

## Kwashiorkor

### Presentation and Characteristics

Skin changes are characteristic and progress over a few days. The definition of kwashiorkor is a total body weight of 60% to 80% of the expected weight according to age and height (body mass index [BMI]) with either edema or hypoalbuminemia. The patient will classically have a diffuse, fine reddish-brown scale resembling "flaky paint." Frequently, erosions on areas of friction and vesicles or bullae also occur. Areas of hypo- and hyperpigmentation are also common along with lightening of the hair and "flag sign," which is alternating areas of lighter and darker hair pigmentation.

This reflects inconsistent states of nutritional intake in the patient. Many times the edema can mask the underlying muscle and subcutaneous tissue atrophy, hence the importance of detecting the cutaneous signs of the disease. Many of the findings are not specific, which makes for a very broad differential diagnosis and many times clouds the clinical picture. Temporal recession and hair loss from the back of the head can occur, likely secondary to pressure when the child lies down. In some cases, loss of hair can be extreme. Hair can also become softer and finer and appear unruly. The eyelashes can undergo the same change, having a so-called "broomstick appearance". Nail plates are thin and soft and may be fissured or ridged. Atrophy of the papillae on the tongue, angular stomatitis, xerophthalmia, and cheliosis can also occur. Depigmentation of hair causes it to be reddish-yellow to white. Curly hair often becomes straightened. Skin changes are characteristic and progress over a few days. The skin becomes dark and dry, and then splits open when stretched, revealing pale areas between the cracks (also known as "crazy pavement dermatosis" or "enamel paint skin"). This feature is seen especially over pressure areas. In contrast to pellagra, these changes seldom occur on sun-exposed skin. Kwashiorkor typically presents with a failure to thrive, edema, moon facies, a swollen abdomen (potbelly), and a fatty liver. Other nutritional deficiencies often coexist such as vitamin C deficiency, anemia, and niacin deficiency. The poor nutritional state of the patients puts them at increased risk for calciphylaxis, which can ultimately produce ischemia and necrosis of skin.

### Treatment

Treatment is similar for both kwashiorkor and marasmus with the goal of therapy to restore the patient's normal body composition and nutritional state. In severe marasmus or kwashiorkor, there are two phases of treatment. The first involves correcting fluid and electrolyte imbalances, treating infections with antibiotics that specifically do not interfere with protein synthesis, and addressing any other related medical problems. The second phase involves slowly replenishing the essential nutrients to prevent taxing the patient's weakened system. Tube feedings can be implemented for certain patients if needed; however, oral refeeding is preferred. If diagnosed in time, both marasmus and kwashiorkor can be treated with complete resolution of symptoms, with the exception of retarded growth and development in more severe cases.

### Prevention

The most important prevention strategy for improving nutritional education among communities who are prone to both of these types of protein energy undernutrition (PEU) is public health measures and reduction of poverty. There is also a form of secondary PEU that can be due to multiple factors including drugs that interfere with macronutrient absorption; other disorders that affect GI function such as enteritis, enteropathy, and pancreatic insufficiency; wasting disorders such as AIDS, cancer, and renal failure; and any conditions that increase metabolic demands such as infections, hyperthyroidism, pheochromocytoma, burns, or other critical illnesses. Treatment of secondary PEU obviously varies widely depending on the underlying etiology.

### Marasmus

*Presentation and Characteristics*

Marasmus may have no cutaneous findings. However, inconsistent skin findings include fine, brittle hair, alopecia, impaired growth, and fissuring of the nails. Occasionally, marked growth of lanugo is noted. Many times kwashiorkor and marasmus coexist. Marasmus is caused by a lack of protein and calories. Edema is absent in marasmus. Many times signs of vitamin A deficiency exist due to a lack of carrier protein and zinc deficiency. Loss of skin elasticity, failure to develop body fat, muscle wastage, loss of muscle tone, mental dullness, and growth arrest are many times present. Skin ulcerations may occur. The hair can be sparse with a reddish tinge. In adults there may be prominent follicular hyperkeratosis.

*Treatment*

See Kwashiorkor section.

*Prevention*

See Kwashiorkor section.

## Eating Disorders

Dermatologic changes in anorexia nervosa (AN) and bulimia nervosa (BN) may be the first signs that an eating disorder is present; therefore, it is extremely important for the physician to understand the cutaneous signs of eating disorders. Many times these two eating disorders coexist, and it has been estimated that approximately 50% of AN patients also practice bulimia.

### Bulimia Nervosa

*Presentation and Characteristics*

Acne is usually mild or moderate and is common in both BN and AN. In clinic the patient will many times be normal or above normal weight. The most classic signs include hypertrichosis, Russell's sign (scarring on knuckles or back of hand due to self-induced vomiting), perimylolysis (decalcification of teeth due to gastric acid exposure from chronic vomiting), and self-induced dermatitis. Isolated signs are not predictive of a patient having an eating disorder, but any cluster of or combination of multiple signs in any patient who has a distorted perception of body weight can justify clinical suspicion of an eating disorder. Other signs include enlargement of the submandibular and parotid glands, which indicates frequent vomiting. Xerosis with mild hyperpigmentation, also called "dirty skin," is another frequent sign, but it is more common in patients with a longer duration of the disease. Occasionally, drug eruptions from laxatives, diuretics, herbal remedies, or

diet pills can be seen. Signs from drug consumption can sometimes be specific and include finger clubbing due to senna, photosensitivity due to thiazide diuretics, urticaria due to phenolphthalein, and fixed drug eruption from laxatives. Purpura, edema, and subconjunctival hemorrhage are also quite common in cases of BN. Limb coldness and compulsive washing are also concomitant signs. Acne is usually mild or moderate and is common in both BN and AN. The lesions are more often localized on the face and back and are frequently excoriated. However, since acne has such a high incidence among adolescents, it is difficult to make a distinction between those who developed acne previous to and those who developed acne during the period of the eating disorder. Also, interestingly acne can be a risk factor for anorexia in psychologically vulnerable patients who may choose dieting to control their acne. Carotenemia can be found in both AN and BN, but it is more common in BN due to ingestion of carotene-rich vegetables. Acrocyanosis, although uncommon, may occur and is more prevalent among the severely ill patients. Livedo reticularis and, more rarely, acute cutaneous ischemia may also develop. There may be dry mucous membranes, xerosis, and less frequently xerophthalmia. In some cases, caries, dental enamel erosions, and tooth abscess can be seen due to self-induced vomiting.

*Treatment*

Depending on the severity of the disease and the patient's nutritional state, the patient may need to be hospitalized for a period of time. However, most cases of bulimia can be treated outside the hospital. Psychotherapy is very helpful in most cases. Also, many times, antidepressants are of help in these patients specifically Prozac, which is the only FDA-approved drug for treatment of bulimia. Consulting a dietician is very helpful to educate the patient about eating a healthy diet and to help design a plan to meet the patient's nutrition and weight goals. Treatment can be difficult and many times requires multidisciplinary care, but most bulimics do recover. However, some find that they can have relapses during periods of stress.

*Prevention*

Although there is no true way to prevent bulimia, early detection especially by a pediatrician or a dermatologist can help prevent the disease from progressing, and this may be the most important way in which physicians can help patients with this disease. Questions about eating habits and satisfaction with appearance can sometimes help reveal valuable clinical clues in suspect age groups and certain patient populations.

### Anorexia Nervosa

*Presentation and Characteristics*

Xerosis, lanugo hair (a soft, downy body hair that grows in patients as a result of the body trying to insulate itself due to loss of body fat), and telogen effluvium are common skin manifestations in AN. Pruritis, hypercarotenemia, edema, acrocyanosis, nail dystrophy, and angular stomatitis are occasionally associated with anorexia, while scurvy and pellagra are rarer. Also, erythema ab igne, self-phlebotomy, dermatitis artefacta, and trichotillomania are many times found in these patients. Also perniosis (a rare vasculitis from prolonged exposure to cold conditions) and pompholyx have been reported in some cases. Other general skin signs associated with the starvation and malnutrition associated with AN are interdigital intertrigo, seborrheic dermatitis, follicular hyperkeratosis, striae distensae, gingivitis, depapillated tongue, aphthae, alopecia, opaque hair, pili torti, onychoschizia, and nail fragility. Also, Raynaud's phenomenon following the onset of AN has been reported.

### Treatment

Depending on the severity of the disease, the patient may need to be hospitalized in order to correct abnormalities such as electrolyte imbalances, dehydration, or psychiatric problems. There are many day programs or residential programs as well as clinics dedicated just to eating disorders that are helpful in the treatment of AN. Just like bulimia, a multidisciplinary approach involving dieticians, psychologists, medical personnel, and possibly psychiatric medications (even though there are no FDA-approved drugs for anorexia) can be helpful. Psychiatric drugs can many times help patients deal with anxiety or depression that may be concomitant. One of the most difficult aspects of the disease is convincing patients that they need treatment. Those that do seek treatment have a tough time preventing relapse and periodic appointments with medical personnel especially during times of stress can be extremely helpful.

### Prevention

Just like bulimia there is no true way to prevent the disease. The best prevention may be detecting the disease early on so that it does not progress into full-blown anorexia. Asking patients about their eating habits and satisfaction with appearance are good screening questions.

## Alcohol Abuse

### Presentation and Characteristics

During acute alcohol ingestion, flushing is the most common skin manifestation affecting about half of Asians, 80% Native Americans, and about a quarter of Caucasians. Chronic drinkers who have cirrhosis exhibit the cutaneous manifestations of spider angiomas, palmar erythema, jaundice, petichiae, salivary gland hypertrophy, and Dupuytren's contracture. Even in the absence of cirrhosis about 18% of chronic alcoholics have palmar erythema and spider angiomas. Dupuytren's contracture is also quite common even in the absence of cirrhosis. Hypoalbuminemia from cirrhosis can lead to edema and ascites. Dilated superficial veins over the abdomen (caput medusae) can be a good clinical clue that a patient has portal hypertension. The following diseases are also listed as occurring more frequently in alcoholics: lichen planus, spontaneous

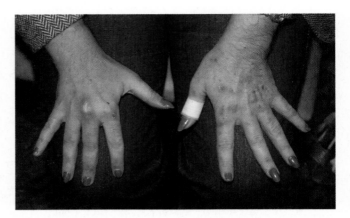

**FIGURE 49-6** ■ A patient with porphyria cutanea tarda involving the hands commonly associated with alcoholism. Bullae and scarring are seen over the dorsal hands and fingers.

skin necrosis, disseminated superficial porokeratosis, necrolytic migratory erythema (without glucagonoma), reactive angioendotheliomatosis, and arteriovenous malformations. Alcohol has also been found to induce and aggravate the disease of rosacea. "Breakouts" of pustular and granulomatous lesions can appear after consumption of even small amounts of alcohol, although they are more common after drinking bouts. Telangiectasias in the central portion of the face tend to develop with greater frequency and severity in rosacea patients who drink heavily.

Excessive alcohol consumption is also the most common factor associated with development of porphyria cutanea tarda (PCT; **Fig. 49-6**). Alcohol appears to unmask an underlying inherited defect in the enzyme uroporphyrinogen decarboxylase. In PCT, vesicles and bullae appear on sun-exposed areas such as the face, dorsa of the hands, and forearms. The resulting erosions and ulcers become covered with crusts, heal slowly over weeks, and may leave atrophic scars and milia.

Alcohol also tends to precipitate hemochromatosis due to its facilitation of the absorption of iron. A pigmented erythema on the lower extremities has been reported to be present in up to 40% of alcoholics under 60 years of age. Alcohol can interfere with the absorption, digestion, and metabolism of vitamins and other nutrients. Even in alcoholics who are not malnourished, vitamin deficiencies are common. Vitamins B and C are the most common vitamins to be deficient in chronic alcoholics. An alcoholic lingual syndrome that consists of a thickened tongue with atrophic mucosa, "lacquer" edges, and an often brown covering has been reported in late-stage alcoholics. Chronic alcoholics also tend to look older and have a "dull expression." Clinically the facial skin can look corrugated, wrinkled, and flabby with a lack of elasticity.

### Treatment

Treatment depends on whether the patient is alcohol dependent or not. If the patient is dependent on alcohol, then abstinence must be a part of treatment. Cognitive behavioral therapy is often used to help patients deal with the disorder.

**SAUER'S NOTES**

Anorexia nervosa, bulimia nervosa, and alcoholism are pernicious problems throughout the world. Early detection is recognized as an important aspect of therapy. Skin signs can help provide early diagnosis and appropriate referral of these patients.

Several medications have been approved for treatment, including antabuse, campral, and naltrexone. Alcoholics Anonymous is a voluntary, international self-help organization founded in 1935 that uses a 12-Step program to assist alcoholics in achieving and maintaining sobriety and is the single most effective therapy.

### Prevention

Knowing and recognizing a family history and early intervention are the best ways to prevent alcohol use or abuse from progressing to alcoholism.

## Essential Fatty Acid Deficiency

### Presentation and Characteristics

There are several different skin manifestations that are associated with essential fatty acid deficiencies (EFADs). These were discovered by studying patients on long-term parenteral nutrition that did not contain adequate amounts of essential fatty acids, by a study on infant formulas that contained varying amounts of linoleic acid (omega-6), and by studying varying case reports in the literature. Through these studies it has been found that EFAD can lead to hemorrhagic dermatitis, skin atrophy, generalized scaly dermatitis that can resemble congenital ichthyosis, dry skin, keratosis pilaris, edema, scalp dermatitis, alopecia, depigmentation of hair, and hemorrhagic folliculitis. The patient's history will involve either long-term total parenteral nutrition devoid of omega-3 (linolenic acid) or omega-6 (linoleic acid) fatty acids or infant formula devoid of either of these two essential fatty acids. However, most infant formula companies have now added these essential fatty acids to their formulas.

**TABLE 49-1 ■ Criteria for Clinical Diagnosis of Metabolic Syndrome**

| Measure (Any Three of Five Constitute Diagnosis of Metabolic Syndrome) | Categorical Cutpoints |
| --- | --- |
| Elevated waist circumference*,† | ≥102 cm (≥40 in) in men |
| | ≥88 cm (≥35 in) in women |
| Elevated triglycerides | ≥150 mg/dL (1.7 mmol/L) |
| | or |
| | On drug treatment for elevated triglycerides‡ |
| Reduced HDL-C | <40 mg/dL (1.03 mmol/L) in men |
| | <50 mg/dL (1.3 mmol/L) in women |
| | or |
| | On drug treatment for reduced HDL-C‡ |
| Elevated blood pressure | ≥130 mm Hg systolic blood pressure |
| | or |
| | ≥85 mm Hg diastolic blood pressure |
| | or |
| | On antihypertensive drug treatment in a patient with a history of hypertension |
| Elevated fasting glucose | ≥100 mg/dL |
| | or |
| | On drug treatment for elevated glucose |

*To measure waist circumference, locate top of right iliac crest. Place a measuring tape in a horizontal plane around abdomen at level of iliac crest. Before reading tape measure, ensure that tape is snug but does not compress the skin and is parallel to floor. Measurement is made at the end of a normal expiration.

†Some US adults of non-Asian origin (e.g., white, black, Hispanic) with marginally increased waist circumference (e.g., 94–101 cm [37–39 in] in men and 80–87 cm [31–34 in] in women) may have strong genetic contribution to insulin resistance and should benefit from changes in lifestyle habits, similar to men with categorical increases in waist circumference. Lower waist circumference cutpoint (e.g., ≥90 cm [35 in] in men and ≥80 cm [31 in] in women) appears to be appropriate for Asian Americans.

‡Fibrates and nicotinic acid are the most commonly used drugs for elevated TG and reduced HDL-C. Patients taking one of these drugs are presumed to have high TG and low HDL.

Adapted from www.americanheart.org/presenter.jhtml?identifier=764.

**TABLE 49-2 ■ WHO/Fredrickson Classification of Primary Hyperlipidemias**

| Disorder | Principle Plasma Abnormality (Corresponding Fredrickson Classification) | Clinical Features | Estimated Frequency |
|---|---|---|---|
| Heterozygous familial hypercholesterolemia TC>7.5, LDL>5.0, TG<2.3 | +LDL only (inherited abnormality of the LDL receptor) [IIa] | Tendinous xanthomas (Fig. 49-7) Corneal arcus Premature CAD Family history of hypercholesterolemia | 0.2% of general population 5% of MI survivors <60 yr old Autosomal codominant |
| Familial defective apolipoprotein B | +LDL (inherited abnormality of apoprotein B interferes with binding to LDL receptor) [IIa] | Same clinical features as heterozygous familial hypercholesterolemia | Same frequency as heterozygous familial hypercholesterolemia |
| Familial combined hyperlipidemia TC>7.0, LDL>4.0, HDL<1.0, TG>3.5 | 1/3: LDL only [IIa] 1/3: VLDL only [IV] 1/3: LDL and VLDL [IIb] | Apo-B overproduction is common Usually >30 yr old Often overweight Usually no xanthomas Premature CAD Different generations have different lipoprotein abnormalities | 0.5% of general population 15% of MI survivors <60 yr old Autosomal dominant |
| Polygenic hypercholesterolemia TC>6.5, LDL>4.0, TG<2.3 | +LDL [IIa] | Premature CAD No xanthomas Possible family history of hypercholesterolemia | Unknown |
| Familial hypertrigl-yceridemia (2.3–10 mmol/L) | +VLDL only (high VLDL production, decreased lipoprotein lipase activity) [IV] | Often overweight >30 yr old Often diabetic Hyperuricemic May or may not have premature CAD Determined by family history and HDL-C | 1% of general population 5% of MI survivors <60 yr old Autosomal dominant |
| Severe hypertrigl-yceridemia (TG >10 mmol/L) | +Chylomicrons and VLDL (high VLDL production, decreased lipoprotein lipase activity) [V] | Usually middle-aged Often obese Often hyperuricemic Usually diabetic Risk for recurrent pancreatitis | Unknown |
| Familial hypoalpha-lipoproteinemia reduced HDL (<0.78 mmol/L in males; <0.90 mmol/L in females) | Decreased apo A-1 production | Premature CAD | 1% of general population 25–30% of patients with premature CAD Autosomal recessive |
| Dysbetalipoproteinemia (TC 9–14 mmol/L; TG 9–14 mmol/L) | +IDL, +Chylomicron remnants (Defective apo E2/2) [III] | Yellow palmar creases Palmar xanthomas Tuberoeruptive xanthomas (Fig. 49-8) Premature CAD | Uncommon 3% of MI survivors Autosomal recessive |

Adapted with permission from GPNotebook at www.gpnotebook.co.uk/medwebpage.cfm?ID=x20020617063512021840.

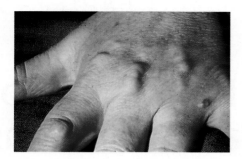

**FIGURE 49-7** ■ A patient with tendinous xanthomas involving the hand. These are associated with heterozygous familial hypercholesterolemia.

### Treatment

It was once thought that topical application of linoleic acid (safflower or sunflower) oil could reverse signs/symptoms of EFAD; however, more recent reports in the literature have shown that topical application of these oils was unable to reverse symptoms. Treatment with dietary EFAs or Intralipid (parenteral lipid) is the treatment of choice.

### Prevention

Prevention involves fortifying all parenteral nutrition therapies with parenteral lipid as well as making sure that infant formula contains adequate amounts of essential fatty acids. Good sources of omega-3s include walnuts, wheat germ oil, flaxseed oil/canola oil, fish liver oils/fish eggs, human milk, organ meats, and seafood/fatty fish like albacore tuna, mackerel, salmon, and sardines. Good sources of omega-6s include corn oil, peanut oil, cottonseed oil, soybean oil, and many other plant oils.

## Metabolic Diseases

### Metabolic Syndrome (Syndrome X)

#### Presentation and Characteristics

Metabolic syndrome is defined by a set of risk factors that include abdominal obesity, increased blood glucose, and/or insulin resistance, dyslipidemia, and hypertension. Several different specific definitions of the disease have been developed by different health organizations in the past, but all seem to address those same five issues, just with varying defining criteria. The most recent criteria proposed by the American Heart Association and the National Heart, Lung, and Blood Institute published in 2005 are listed in Table 49-1. Since most patients with metabolic syndrome tend to be obese, cutaneous signs and symptoms would be the same as those described in Chapter 43.

### Treatment

Treatment involves patient education. Patients are instructed to diligently check their lipid levels, watch for signs of diabetes, have their blood pressure monitored, and exercise regularly. Probably the most important overall treatment is exercise in addition to an overall change to a healthier lifestyle. It has been

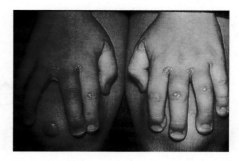

**FIGURE 49-8** ■ A patient with tuberous xanthomas on the knees and hands. These are associated with dysbetalipoproteinemia.

suggested that patients should have somewhat specific goals including weight loss to achieve a desirable weight (i.e., BMI < 25 kg/m$^2$), increased physical activity with a goal of at least 30 minutes of moderate-intensity activity on most days of the week, and healthy eating habits that include reduced intake of saturated fat, trans fat, and cholesterol.

### Prevention

With an estimation that more than 50 million Americans are afflicted with this disease, its prevention will continue to become more important. Prevention and treatment go hand in hand for metabolic syndrome. The mainstay for prevention is the same as treatment, with an emphasis on the maintenance of a healthier lifestyle.

### Abnormal Lipid Metabolism

Xanthomatoses—See Table 49-2.

## Suggested Readings

Glorio R, Allevato M, De Pablo A, et al. Prevalence of cutaneous manifestations in 200 patients with eating disorders. *Int J Dermatol.* 2000;39(5):348–353.

Grundy SM, Cleeman JI, Daniels SR, et al. Diagnosis and management of the metabolic syndrome: an American Heart Association/National Heart, Lung, and Blood Institute Scientific Statement. *Circulation.* 2005;112(17):2735–2752 [Epub 2005 Sep 12].

Gupta MA, Gupta AK, Haberman HF. Dermatologic signs in anorexia nervosa and bulimia nervosa. *Arch Dermatol.* 1987;123(10):1386–1390 [Review].

Heath ML, Sidbury R. Cutaneous manifestations of nutritional deficiency. *Curr Opin Pediatr.* 2006;18(4):417–422.

Kanekura T, Yotsumoto S, Maeno N, et al. Selenium deficiency: report of a case. *Clin Exp Dermatol.* 2005;30(4):346–348.

Kannan R, Ng MJ. Cutaneous Lesions and vitamin B$_{12}$ deficiency: an often-forgotten link. *Can Fam Physician.* 2008; 54(4):529–532.

McLaren DS. Skin in protein energy malnutrition. *Arch Dermatol.* 1987;123 (12):1674–1676a [Review].

Nagaraju M, Adamson DG, Rogers J. Skin manifestations of folic acid deficiency. *Br J Dermatol.* 1971;84(1):32–36.

Olumide YM. Nutritional dermatoses in Nigeria. *Int J Dermatol.* 1995; 34(1):11–16.

Oumeish OY, Oumeish I. Nutritional skin problems in children. *Clin Dermatol.* 2003;21(4):260–263.

Sanchez MR. Alcohol, social behavior disorders, and their cutaneous manifestations. *Clin Dermatol.* 1999;17(4):479–489.

Schneider JB, Norman RA. Cutaneous manifestations of endocrine-metabolic disease and nutritional deficiency in the elderly. *Dermatol Clin.* 2004; 22(1):23–31.

Strumia R. Bulimia and anorexia nervosa: cutaneous manifestations. *J Cosmet Dermatol.* 2002;1(1):30–34.

Tyler I, Wiseman MC, Crawford RI, et al. Cutaneous manifestations of eating disorders. *J Cutan Med Surg.* 2002;6(4):345–353 [Epub 2002 Apr 15].

# CHAPTER 50

# Where to Look for More Information about a Skin Disease

*John C. Hall, MD*

"Doctor, I saw a patient yesterday who was diagnosed as having epidermolysis bullosa. I understand this is quite a rare condition. Where can I find the latest information on this subject?" This is the type of question frequently asked of a teaching dermatologist. A computer gives you references, and some databases provide information about a dermatosis. But, assuming these are not readily available, there are other sources.

## Print Resources

First, the inquiring physician or student should check out the Dictionary–Index of this book. Even for rare conditions, there is at least a definition of the disease. The Suggested Readings at the end of each chapter can also point one in the right direction for books or papers on a given subject.

Second, there are several comprehensive general texts on dermatology that include rare diseases. The following are suggested.

- Arndt KA, LeBoit DE, Robinson JK, et al. *Cutaneous Medicine and Surgery*. Philadelphia: WB Saunders; 1995.
- Bolognia JL, Jorizzo LJ, Rapini, RP. *Dermatology*. 2nd ed. Elsevier. e-Edition available.
- Burgdorf WHC, Plewig G, Wolff H, et al. *Braun-Falco's Dermatology*. New York, NY: Springer; 2008.
- Champion RH, Burton JL, Burns DA, et al. *Rook/Wilkinson/Ebling Textbook of Dermatology*. Vol 4. 6th ed. Cambridge, MA: Blackwell; 1998.
- Demis DJ, Dahl M, Smith EB, et al. *Clinical Dermatology*. Vol 4. Philadelphia: JB Lippincott (revised annually).
- *Diseases of the Skin: A Color Atlas and Text*. 2nd ed. Mosby; 2005.
- Edwards L. *Genital Dermatology Atlas*. Hagerstown, MD: Lippincott Williams and Wilkins; 2004.
- Goodheart HP. *Goodheart's Photoguide to Common Skin Disorders*: Diagnosis and Management, 3rd ed. Philadelphia: Lippincott Williams and Wilkins; 2009.
- Jablonski, NG. *Skin: A Natural History*. University of California Press; 2006.
- Odum RB, James WD, Berger TG. *Andrew's Diseases of the Skin: Clinical Dermatology*. 10th ed. Philadelphia: WB Saunders; 2006.
- Trozak D. *Dermatology Guide for Primary Care: An Illustrated Guide*. Humana Press; 2006.
- White GM, Cox NH. *Diseases of the Skin*. St. Louis: Mosby; 2005.
- Wolff K, Goldsmith LA, Katz SI, et al. *Fitzpatrick's Dermatology in General Medicine*. 7th ed. New York, NY: McGraw-Hill, Available as e-Edition.

## Online Resources

The National Library of Medicine, 8,600 Rockville Pike, Bethesda, MD 20014 (www.nlm.nih.gov), has very good information on different medical sites. Other useful Web sites include the following.

- A.B. Ackerman's Atlas Online at www.derm101.com
- American Academy of Dermatology at www.aad.org
- British Association of Dermatologists (clinical practice guidelines) at www.bad.org.uk
- Dermatologic Clinics at www.derm.theclinics.com
- Dermatology Slide Atlas at www.med.unc.edu/derm/atlas/welcome.htm
- Evidence-based Dermatology at http://ebderm.org
- *Internet Journal of Dermatology* at www.ispub.com
- The *Journal of American Academy of Dermatology* at www.eblue.org.
- Medical Dermatology at www.labordedermatology.com
- National Organization for Rare Disorders at http://www.rarediseases.org/
- Skin Cancer Foundation at www.skincancer.org
- University of Iowa, Dermatology Dictionary DermPathTutor at www.tray.dermatology.uiowa.edu/home.

The following journals are highly pertinent and are available online.

- *Acta Dermato-Venereologica*, 6 issues per year. Published by Taylor & Francis Group.

- *American Journal of Clinical Dermatology,* 6 issues a year. Published by Adis International.
- *American Journal of Contact Dermatitis,* published by W.B. Saunders. Although this journal is no longer published, you can continue to view the contents of this Web site and order reprints from 2002 and earlier.
- *American Journal of Dermatopathology,* 6 issues a year. Official journal of the International Society of Dermatopathology.
- *Archives of Dermatology,* a monthly journal published by the American Medical Association, Chicago. It is indexed in both the June and December issues.
- *British Journal of Dermatology,* published monthly by Blackwell Synergy.
- *Clinics in Dermatology,* 6 issues a year. Published by Elsevier.
- *Cutis,* a monthly magazine for the general practitioner, published by Reed Medical Publishers.
- *Dermatologic Surgery,* a journal published by Blackwell Synergy.
- *Dermatologic Therapy,* published by Blackwell Synergy.
- *Dermatology Online Journal,* Senior editor Barbara Burrall, M.D., published by Arthur C. Huntley.

- *Internet Journal of Dermatology,* Editor-in-chief Madeleine Duvic, M.D.
- *Journal of the American Academy of Dermatology,* a monthly journal published by the American Academy of Dermatology.
- *Journal of Cutaneous Pathology,* 10 issues a year. Official publication of the American Society of Dermatopathology. Published by Blackwell Synergy.
- *Journal of Dermatological Treatment,* 6 issues a year. Published by Taylor & Francis Group.
- *Journal of Drugs in Dermatology,* official publication of the International Society for Dermatologic Surgery.
- *Journal of Investigative Dermatology,* a monthly journal published on behalf of the Society for Investigative Dermatology by Blackwell Publishing.
- *Journal Watch Dermatology,* from the publishers of *The New England Journal of Medicine,* the Massachusetts Medical Society. It is published biweekly on the web and monthly in print.
- *Pediatric Dermatology,* published bimonthly by Blackwell Synergy.
- *Practical Reviews in Dermatology,* Johns Hopkins School of Medicine, Oakstone Publishing. Updated monthly and available online.

# DICTIONARY—INDEX

**Introduction** The purpose of the dictionary portion of this index is to define and classify some of the rarer dermatologic terms not covered in the text. Some very rare or unimportant terms have purposely been omitted, but undoubtedly some terms that are *not* rare and *are* important have also been omitted. Most of the histopathologic terms have been defined. If you think this is confusing, consider the source. Suggestions or corrections from the reader will be appreciated.

Acantholytic dermatosis, transient (Grover's disease) (TAD). Characterized by intensely pruritic, small, firm, reddish-brown, papules mainly on the upper torso, aggravated by sweating. Seen predominantly in white, older men. Histologically, there is acantholysis of the epidermis. There is also a persistent form that is called persistent acantholytic dermatosis (PAD). It has been associated with bone marrow transplantation, underlying malignancy, chronic renal failure, radiation therapy, AIDS and excessive heat, sweating or occlusion. Also with eczema, asteatosis, allergic contact dermatitis and non-specific irritation.

Acanthosis nigricans, 391t

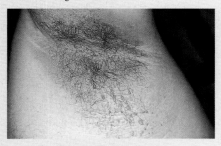

Pseudoacanthosis nigricans of the axilla.

Acne, 8, 24, 41, 152–158, 152f–154f, 158f
  conglobata, 152
  fulminans, 152
  hidradenitis suppurativa, 152
  instruction sheet, 154–156
  inversa, 152
  neonatal, 425, 427t
  rosacea, 158–159, 158f
  scars of, 152, 155, 156–157, 158f
  treatment of, 154, 157–158
Acne keloidalis nuchae. Seen mainly in African American men (ten times more common in dark skinned people than Caucasians). It causes up to 0.5% of all dermatology cases in African Americans. Usually in the occipital scalp and posterior neck. Papules and pustules

form hairline keloidal papules and plaques that can be tender, disfiguring and result in scaring alopecia. Topical or intralesional steroids, long term antibiotics, and in severe cases surgery is used for treatment. A prolonged course of Accutane has also been used by some authors.

Acne mechanica, 490t, 493
Acne necrotica miliaris, 202t, 205
Acne varioliformis. A chronic inflammatory disorder in adults on the scalp, the forehead, the nose and the cheeks, and rarely the trunk, characterized by the presence of papulopustular lesions that heal within a few days, leaving a smallpox-like scar. Recurrent outbreaks can continue for months and years.

Acquired brachial cutaneous dyschromatosis (ABCD). Usually bilateral, usually female, Caucasian, middle-aged patients with asymptomatic, common, acquired geographic gray brown patches interspersed with hypopigmented macules on dorsal forearms. It is not associated with estrogens but may be associated with angiotensin converting enzyme inhibitors.

Acquired ichthyosis, 395, 395f
Acquired immunodeficiency syndrome (AIDS), 35, 270. *See also* Human immunodeficiency virus
Acquired perforating disease (APD). Intensely pruritic papular eruption that may be hyperkeratotic or form a crater, which tends to koebnerize. Usually on the trunk and extremities and skin biopsy will help confirm the diagnosis. Associated with renal failure, diabetes mellitus, hepatitis, hyperparathyroidism, hypothyroidism, AIDs, atopic dermatitis, herpes zoster, scabies, and as a paraneoplastic disorder, 398
Acquired progressive kinking, 345
Acral erythema. Intense redness of palms and soles with dysesthesia and occasionally blisters. Associated with anticancer chemotherapy, 100t
Acral lentiginous melanoma, 314, 314f
Acrochordons, 284–285. *See also* Fibromas, pedunculated
Acrocyanosis. Characterized by constant coldness and bluish discoloration of the

fingers and the toes, which is more intense in cold weather and on dependence by dangling the legs over a chair or bed. Seen more often in women.
Acrodermatitis chronica atrophicans. A chronic, biphasic disease seen most commonly in western Europe. The first phase begins with an erythematous patch on an extremity, which, in weeks or months, develops the second phase of skin atrophy. The cause is believed to be a mixed infection with group B arboviruses, transmitted by the wood tick *Ixodes ricinus*. It is a penicillin-sensitive bacterium or spirochete. Can be a chronic late stage of Lyme disease.

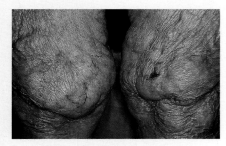

Acrodermatitis chronica atrophicans on the legs.

Acrodermatitis continua of Hallopeau, 351, 351f
Acrodermatitis enteropathica. Condition of zinc deficiency manifested by inflammatory periorificial and acral dermatitis, alopecia, and diarrhea. When zinc was added to pediatric formulas and to hyperalimentation regiments it became rare. Autosomal recessive.
Acrodermatitis, papular, of childhood. *See* Gianotti-Crosti syndrome
Acrodynia. Mercury poisoning usually in infants. Itching, painful swelling, pink, cold, clammy hands and feet with hemorrhagic puncta. Stomatitis and loss of teeth occur. Greater than 0.001 mg per liter mercury is found in the urine.
Acrokeratoelastoidosis. Different size, symmetric, horny, glossy translucent papules on the knuckles, thenar eminences, hypothenar eminences, dorsa and sides of the fingers and margins of the hands.

**529**

Acrokeratoelastoidosis. (*continued*)
May also involve the tibia, anterior ankles, malleoli, Achilles tendon, dorsal feet, and dorsal toes.

Acrokeratosis, paraneoplastic (Bazex's syndrome). A specific sign of cancer of the upper respiratory and upper digestive tracts characterized by plum-colored acral skin lesions, paronychia, nail dysplasias, and keratoderma, 391t

Acrokeratosis verruciformis of Hopf. A rare disease affecting the dorsa of the hands and the feet characterized by flat warty papules. Probably hereditary. Differentiate from *flat warts* and from *epidermodysplasia verruciformis*.

Acromegaly. Hyperpituitary condition causing gross thickening of the skin with characteristic facies, enlarged hands, feet, digits, hyperhidrosis, hypertrichosis, and hyperpigmentation.

Acropustulosis of infancy. Tiny pustules or vesicles on the distal extremities that occur within the first year of life and are intensely pruritic. Spontaneous resolution usually occurs within the first 2 or 3 years of life, 430, 431t

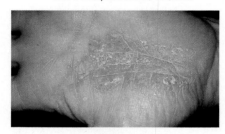

Acropustulosis.

Actinic dermatitis, chronic (Actinic reticuloid). Persistent erythema of the face, hands, and other exposed areas. CD8+ cells infiltrate the skin due to sensitivity to UVA, UVB and even visible light. Especially in elderly men it is associated with increased contact allergies. Strict UVA, UVB and visible light protection is difficult but beneficial. May become generalized and difficult clinically and histologically to tell from cutaneous T-cell lymphoma (mycosis fungoides). Contact dermatitis is a common association.

Actinic granuloma. *See* Annular elastotic giant cell granuloma

Actinic keratosis, 281t, 282t, 289f, 291–293, 467, 470t

Actinic prurigo. *See* Prurigo, actinic

Actinomycosis, 202t, 218

Acute hemorrhagic edema (Finkelstein disease, AHE). Benign cutaneous leukocytoclastic vasculitis in children under two years of age. Polycyclic plaques with a dark necrotic center in a medallion, target or cockade configuration sparing the trunk. Resolves in 1 to 2 weeks without sequelae and can be postinfectious.

Addison's disease, 383, 393

Adenoma sebaceum (Pringle's disease), 299, 400, 401f

Adhesion disorders, 415, 415f, 416t

Adiposis dolorosa (Dercum's disease). A lipoma-like disorder characterized by irregular and painful deposits of fat in the subcutaneous tissue of the trunk and limbs, more common in women than in men.

Africa tick bite fever. Occurs in clusters of patients especially in South Africa in game hunters and tourists visiting endemic areas such as the eastern Caribbean. Five to seven days after a bite is the abrupt onset of fever, nausea, headache, myalgias and neck pain. The bites are often multiple and consist of a black, hemorrhagic eschar surrounded by a red halo and tender regional lymphadenopathy. Life threatening complications are rare and doxycycline 100 mgs twice a day for 7 days is the treatment of choice. It is caused by the bite of the Amblyomma tick.

Aicardi-Goutières syndrome. Itchy, red, swelling of the fingers, toes, earlobes that mimics chilblains. The hands and feet are puffy and cold. This is accompanied by intracranial calcifications and numerous neurologic complications.

AIDS. *See* Acquired immunodeficiency syndrome

Ainhum. Essentially a tropical disease of blacks that results in the amputation of a toe or toes because of constricting bands.

Albinism, 417, 425

Albright's hereditary osteodystrophy. Multiple areas of cutaneous ossification, skeletal abnormalities, abnormalities of the parathyroid gland, mental retardation, and shortening of the metacarpal bones.

Albright's syndrome. Large hyperpigmented macules, precocious puberty in females, and polyostotic fibrous dysplasia. The macules have a jagged border like the coast of Maine, unlike café-au-lait macules that usually have a smooth, or coast of California, border, 418

Alkaptonuria. *See* Ochronosis

Allergic granulomatosis (Churg-Strauss syndrome). The combination of transitory pulmonary infiltrations of Loeffler's syndrome, asthma, blood eosinophilia, and nodular purpuric or erythema multiforme-like skin lesions. Target organs beside skin and lung include kidney, upper respiratory tract, and central nervous system, 135

Alopecia. From the Greek *alopekia*, meaning "hair loss." 100t, 339–346, 340t, 342t
androgenetic pattern, 340
areata, 35, 73–74, 337–341, 340t, 342–343
central centrifugal cicatricial, 372
cicatricial, 344–346

cicatrisata, 206
congenital triangular alopecia. Probably under reported, idiopathic, triangular-shaped temporal area of hair loss. Present at birth or in the first year of life that can be bilateral. (See Congenital triangular alopecia).
drugs causing, 342t
frontal fibrosing, cicatricial frontoparietal alopecia mainly in postmenopausal women associated with nonscarring alopecia of the eyebrows.
lipedematous. Rare nonscarring permanent hair loss seen mainly in older black women. Diffuse and mainly on the vertex with a thickened boggy scalp. On lateral radiographic exam the scalp is twice as thick due to increased thickness of subcutaneous fat. On biopsy the hair shaft is replaced by lamellar fibroplasias and hairs cannot grow more than 2 cm and break easily (see lipedematous alopecia).
lymphocytic cicatricial, 344
male-pattern, 453f
moth eaten scalp, 221
neutrophilic cicatricial, 344
nonscarring diffuse, 340–342
nonscarring patchy, 342–344
scarring, 344–345
syphilis related, 342

Alopecia neoplastica. Infiltrated metastatic cancer to the scalp causing loss of hair. Breast cancer is often the underlying malignancy.

Alpha-1-antitrypsin deficiency. *See* Panniculitis, alpha-1-antitrypsin deficiency.

Alternariosis. Plant pathogens that rarely cause human cutaneous infection in patients that are immunocompromised. It can be caused by primary innoculation or endogenous spread after inhalation. Solitary or grouped papules, plaques or macules mainly on the lower extremities. Staining of tissue and culture are needed for diagnosis and medical as well as surgical therapy is often indicated.

Amebiasis, 477, 477f

Amyloidosis.
cutaneous amyloidosis is a rare condition that can be suspected clinically but should be proven by histologic examination. Amyloid is a protein-carbohydrate complex, which on histologic section assumes a diagnostic stain when treated with certain chemicals. Several biochemical varieties have been delineated. Amyloidosis can be systemic or localized.
localized amyloidosis (lichen amyloidosis). The skin only is involved. Clinically, this dermatosis appears as a patch of lichenified papules seen most commonly on the anterior tibial area of the legs. These pruritic lesions can be differentiated from lichen simplex chronicus or hypertrophic lichen

planus by biopsy. Some authors feel the amyloid deposits are due to keratinocyte breakdown products caused by scratching and lichen amyloidosis is, therefore, a variant of lichen simplex chronicus.

primary systemic amyloidosis. This peculiar and serious form of amyloidosis commonly involves the skin along with the tongue, the heart, and the musculature of the viscera. The skin lesions appear as transparent-looking, yellowish papules or nodules, which are occasionally hemorrhagic. Commonly (40%) "pinch purpura" which is ecchymosis due to minor trauma. This is often seen on the eyelids. This form is familial.

secondary amyloidosis. Secondary amyloid deposits are very rare in the skin but are less rare in the liver, the spleen, and the kidney, where they occur as a result of certain chronic infectious diseases, and in association with multiple myeloma.

Androgenetic pattern hair loss, 340

Anetoderma. *See* Atrophies of the skin, macular atrophy

Angioedema, acquired. May be associated with urticaria (*see* Chap 12), other illnesses especially B-cell lymphoproliferative disease (AAE-I) or an autoantibody directed against the C1 inhibitor molecule (AAE-II), 101t

Angioedema, hereditary. Rare autosomal dominant form of angioedema that may be associated with respiratory and gastrointestinal symptoms. Low level or dysfunctional inhibitor of the first component of complement is the cause.

Angioendotheliomatosis, malignant (intravascular large cell lymphoma). Usually fatal B cell intravascular lymphoma in the skin (lower dermal and subcutaneous blood vessels) and central nervous system. Erythematous telangiectatic plaques or nodules especially on the lower extremities.

Angiofibromas. Asymptomatic skin-colored or pinkish-brown asymptomatic telangiectatic papules usually symmetrically scattered over the central face. When multiple they have been considered pathognomonic for tuberous sclerosis but have been reported with multiple endocrine neoplasia type 1 (MEN1), 400

Angiohistiocytoma, multinucleate cell. *See* Multinucleate cell angiohistiocytoma

Angioleiomyoma. Rare, usually acral, solitary, asymptomatic, subcutaneous, 1 to 4 cm nodule. To be differentiated from angiomyolipoma, which is usually renal and associated with tuberous sclerosis.

Angiolipoleiomyoma (angiomyolipoma). Well-circumscribed, asymptomatic,

subcutaneous, rare tumor associated with renal disease and rarely extracutaneous sites may occur especially in the kidney.

Angioimmunoblastic lymphadenopathy with dysproteinemia. Fever, night sweats, hepatosplenomegaly and generalized lymphadenopathy. Fifty percent with skin findings that are most often a transient morbilliform eruption. Plaques, purpura, and urticarial lesions also occur. It is a subtype of T-cell lymphoma, which may be primary or, according to some authors, triggered by a drug allergy or viral infection.

Angiokeratomas, 294
    Fabry's form, 294
    Fordyce form, 294
    Mibelli's form, 294

Angiolymphoid hyperplasia with eosinophilia (Kimura's disease). A rare benign condition, usually seen on the face, characterized by a solitary or, less frequently, multiple dermal or subcutaneous nodules. There is a blood eosinophilia and there are eosinophils in the histologic infiltrate. Some consider Kimura's disease to be the systemic form only with deeper, larger lesions. When you biopsy be prepared to stop some often impressive bleeding. It has been associated with human herpes virus 8.

Angioma serpiginosum. Characterized by multiple telangiectases, which may start from a congenital vascular nevus but often arise spontaneously. This rare vascular condition is to be differentiated from *Schamberg's disease, Majocchi's disease,* and *pigmented purpuric dermatitis of Gougerot and Blum.*

Angioma, targetoid hemosiderotic. Solitary benign tumor in adults on the trunk or extremities. Violaceous papule with an ecchymotic evanescent ring. It may be caused by trauma.

Angioma, tufted. *See* Tufted angioma (Progressive capillary hemangioma or Nakagawa's angioblastoma). Rare vascular tumor usually on the trunk, slow growing with a tendency to resolve. Usually develops within the first year of life but not present at birth. One third are tender and form dusky reddish-blue subcutaneous plaques or nodules that may be annular with depression resembling a "doughnut." Surrounding skin may be hyperhidrotic or have increased vellus hairs. It can be associated with Kasabach-Merritt syndrome.

Angiosarcoma. Malignancy of vascular tissue usually seen on the face and scalp of elderly male patients, or at the site of chronic lymphedema when it is referred to as Stewart-Treves syndrome. Exertion, an increase in ambient

temperature or a tilting of the head below the heart for 5 to 10 seconds (head-tilt maneuver) can accentuate redness on the face and aid in early diagnosis.

Anhidrosis. The partial or complete absence of sweating, seen in ichthyosis, extensive psoriasis, scleroderma, prickly heat, vitamin A deficiency, one form of ectodermal dysplasia, and other diseases. Partial anhidrosis is produced by many antiperspirants.

Anhidrotic asthenia, tropical. Described in the South Pacific and in the desert in World War II. Soldiers showed increased sweating of the neck and face and anhidrosis (lack of sweating) below the neck. It was accompanied by weakness, headaches, and subjective warmth and was considered a chronic phase of prickly heat.

Anhidrotic ectodermal dysplasia, 8

Annular atrophic plaques of the face (Christianson's disease). Rare sclerotic annular plaques mainly on the face. Chronic, progressive, recalcitrant to treatment with unknown cause. May be a variant of scleroderma.

Annular elastotic giant cell granuloma (Actinic granuloma). Rare, in fair complexion, middle-aged or older patients. Asymptomatic (rarely intense pruritus) large (20-25 cm) plaques on the trunks and upper extremities. Chronic but may spontaneously remit after years. It may occur with alcoholic liver disease, diabetes, temporal arteritis, and sun bed radiation exposure. May be a variant of granuloma annulare on sun damaged skin.

Annular lichenoid dermatitis of youth. Persistent erythematous macules and papules that are round with a reddish-brown border and hypopigmented centrally especially in the groin and flanks. Phototherapy, topical corticosteroids and systemic corticosteroids were effective but relapse recurred after therapy withdrawal. Histopathology is characteristic.

Anonychia. Absence of all or part of one or several nails. Congenital in diseases such as Apert's syndrome, cartilage-hair dysplasia syndrome, dyskeratosis congenita, Ellis-van Creveld syndrome, nail-patella syndrome, Goltz syndrome, progeria, hypohydrotic ectodermal dysplasia, incontinentia pigmenti, Turner's syndrome, trisomy 13, and trisomy 18. Acquired in diseases such as lichen planus, Stevens-Johnson syndrome, epidermolysis bullosa, and trauma. It can also be seen in a simplex form associated with digital, hand or foot abnormalities.

Anthralin. A proprietary name for dihydroxy-anthranol, which is a strong reducing agent useful in the treatment of

**Anthralin.** (*continued*)
chronic cases of psoriasis. Its action is similar to that of chrysarobin. It causes troublesome staining and can be irritating. Short contact anthralin therapy (SCAT) is less irritating.

**Anthrax.** A primary chancre-type disease caused by *Bacillus anthracis,* occurring in persons who work with the hides and the hair of infected sheep, horses, or cattle. A pulmonary form is known. It has the potential for use as a bioterrorist agent, 473–474, 473f, 500t, 504–507, 506f, 506t

**Antimalarial agents.** Dermatologically active agents include quinacrine (Atabrine), chloroquine (Aralen), and hydroxychloroquine (Plaquenil). Their mode of action is unknown, but these agents are used in the treatment of chronic discoid lupus erythematosus, lymphocytic infiltrate of Jessner, lichen planus, polymorphous light eruption and others. Eye exams by an ophthalmologist should be done at 6 to 12 month intervals to check for retinal damage except with quinacrine. Liver enzyme elevation should also be monitored.

**Antiphospholipid antibody syndrome.** Hypercoagulable state related to the presence of lupus anticoagulant and anticardiolipin antibodies. Cutaneous necrosis, vasculitis, thrombophlebitis, and ecchymoses occur. Recurrent inflammatory vascular thrombosis of veins and arteries can occur throughout the body and treatment is based on anticoagulation. Recurrent fetal loss and thrombocytopenia can also occur

**Antisynthetase syndrome.** Antibodies are produced against histidyl-transfer ribonucleic acid synthetase (Jo-1). Mechanic's hands is the characteristic skin sign of the disease which can also have involvement of skeletal muscle, lungs, heart, liver and kidneys.

**Apert syndrome.** Craniosynostosis, symmetric severe syndactyly and numerous abnormalities of the skin, skeleton, brain and visceral organs. Skin signs include resistant acne, hyperhidrosis, interrupted eyebrows, excessive forehead wrinkling, lateral plantar hyperkeratosis, skin dimpling over joints, and oculocutaneous hypopigmentation.

Aphthous stomatitis, 361–362, 361f

**Aphthous ulcers.** *See* Canker sores

**Aplasia cutis congenita.** Rare condition showing absence of skin at the time of birth. It presents with ulcerations, especially on the scalp that heal with scars.

Apocrine adenomas, 299–300, 300f

Apocrine epitheliomas, 300, 300f

**Aquagenic syringeal acrokeratoderma.** Rare symmetric palmar, hyperpigmented plaques and papules that become more prominent on exposure to water.

**Aquagenic wrinkling of the palms (aquagenic syringeal acrokeratoderma, aquagenic palmoplantar acrokeratoderma, transient reactive papulotransluscent acrokeratoderma, aquagenic keratoderma).** Rapidly forming, transient, edematous, white plaques on the palms after exposure to water (hand in bucket sign) that may be asymptomatic, pruritic or burning. Associated with cystic fibrosis, atopy, and hyperhidrosis.

Arachnidism, 480–481, 480f

**Argyll Robertson pupils.** Small irregular pupils that fail to react to light but react to accommodation. This is a late manifestation of neurosyphilis, particularly tabes dorsalis.

Argyria, 383

**Arsenic.** Inorganic arsenic preparation include Fowler's solution and Asiatic pills and were used in the treatment of resistant cases of psoriasis. Can cause arsenical pigmentation, actinic keratoses, Bowen's disease, squamous cell carcinoma, and underlying malignancies (especially lung and bladder). Other sources are well water and industrial sources such as pesticides, sheep dips, metal ores, and fabric dyes. Organic arsenic agents include neoarsphenamine and Mapharsen, used formerly in the treatment of syphilis.

Arsenical keratosis, 290, 291

Arsenical pigmentation, 383

**Arteritis, temporal (giant cell arteritis).** Inflammation of the cranial arteries most commonly the temporal artery that may show overlying swelling, erythema, tenderness and pain in the temporal scalp. Blindness may occur due to involvement of the retinal artery. Blindness may be prevented with systemic corticosteroids.

**Arthus phenomenon.** Characterized by local anaphylaxis in a site that has been injected repeatedly with a foreign protein.

Ash-leaf macule, 384, 401

**Ashy dermatosis.** Also known as erythema dyschromicum perstans. An uncommon pigmentary disorder characterized by ash-colored macules that slowly increase in size and number. The border may be erythematous. Could be a variant of *erythema perstans*. It is more common in natives of Central and South America.

**Asymmetric periflexural exanthem of childhood (APEC).** *See* Unilateral laterothoracic exanthem

**Ataxia-telangiectasia(Louis-Barr syndrome).** Clinically shows oculocutaneous telangiectasia, progressive cerebellar ataxia, recurrent sinopulmonary infections, increased incidence of malignancy, x-ray hypersensitivity, and autosomal recessive inheritance.

**Athlete's nodules.** Benign, symmetric, asymptomatic, firm, flesh-colored, intradermal, 0.5 to 4.0 cm nodules that are sports-related and acquired. Most often over knuckles, knees pretibial area or dorsal aspect of the feet or any areas of chronic friction depending on the activity. Different terms used are knuckle pads (marble players, boxers) on dorsal fingers, surfer's nodules or knots (surfers) on dorsal feet and running shoe nodules or Nike nodules (joggers) on the dorsal aspect of the feet. Morphologically and histologically similar to collagenomas. Treatment is cessation of trauma, high-potency topical corticosteroids, intralesional corticosteroids, and excision. There is the potential for scarring, keloid formation, and recurrence.

Atopic dermatitis, 117, 386, 387t, 399–400, 408t, 436f–437f

Atrophie blanche, 35, 141, 449

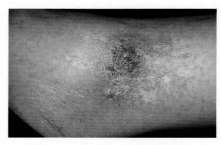

Atrophie blanche on the ankle.

Atrophies of the skin
Acquired atrophies
Inflammatory

*Acrodermatitis chronica atrophicans.* A rare idiopathic atrophy in older adults, particularly women, characterized by the presence of thickened skin at the onset, with ulnar bands on the forearm, changing into atrophy of the legs below the knee and of the forearms. In the early stages this is to be differentiated from scleroderma. High doses of penicillin may be effective. It may be a late stage of Lyme disease especially noted in Europe.

*Atrophie blanche (segmental hyalinizing vasculopathy).* A form of cutaneous atrophy characterized by scar-like plaques with a border of telangiectasis and hyperpigmentation that cover large areas of the legs and the ankles, mainly of middle-aged or older women. May ulcerate and biopsy shows a vasculopathy. Treatment is with anticoagulants.

*Atrophoderma, idiopathic, of Pasini and Pierini.* Similar to morphea (localized scleroderma) but without induration.

The round or irregular depressed atrophic areas are asymptomatic and appear mainly on the trunk of young females.

*Folliculitis ulerythematosa reticulata.* A very rare reticulated atrophic condition localized to the cheeks of the face; seen mainly in young adults.

*Hemiatrophy.* May be localized to one side of the face or may cover the entire half of the body. Vascular and neurogenic etiologies have been proposed, but most cases appear to be a form of *localized scleroderma.*

*Lichen sclerosus et atrophicus (kraurosis vulvae, kraurosis penis, and balanitis xerotica obliterans{penis}).* An uncommon atrophic process, mainly of women, which begins as a small whitish lesion that contains a central hyperkeratotic pinpoint-sized dell. These 0.5-cm or less whitish macules commonly coalesce to form whitish atrophic plaques. The most common localizations are on the neck, shoulders, arms, axillae, vulva, and perineum. Many consider kraurosis vulvae, kraurosis penis, and balanitis xerotica obliterans(penis) to be variants of this condition. Can be very pruritic and 5% risk of associated squamous cell carcinoma when occurring in adult female genitalia.

*Macular atrophy (Anetoderma of Jadassohn).* A very rare condition characterized by the appearance of circumscribed reddish macules that develop an atrophic center that progresses toward the edge of the lesion, seen mainly on the extremities. May be seen after acne, varicella, syphilis, pilomatrichoma, and other inflammatory skin diseases. There is a primary form that may be associated with systemic lupus erythematosus, vitiligo, alopecia areata, hypothyroidism associated with antithyroid antibodies, and primary Addison disease.

*Poikiloderma atrophicans vasculare (Jacobi).* This rare atrophic process of adults is characterized by the development of patches of telangiectasis, atrophy, and mottled pigmentation on any area of the body. This resembles chronic radiodermatitis clinically and may be associated with dermatomyositis, lupus erythematosis or scleroderma. May precede the development of a lymphoma and some generalized cases are already mycosis fungoides (cutaneous T-cell lymphoma{CTCL}).

*Secondary atrophy.* From inflammatory diseases such as syphilis, chronic discoid lupus erythematosus, leprosy, tuberculosis, scleroderma, etc.

*Ulerythema ophryogenes.* A rare atrophic dermatitis that affects the outer part of the eyebrows, resulting in redness, scaling, and permanent loss of the involved hair.

Noninflammatory

*Linear atrophy, striae albicantes* or *distensae stretch marks.* On the abdomen, thighs, and breasts associated with pregnancy, Cushing's disease, obesity, systemic and topical corticosteroids, adolescence, abuse of androgens, idiopathic, and rapid weight gain.

*Macular atrophy (anetoderma of Schweninger-Buzzi).* Characterized by the presence of small, oval, whitish depressions or slightly elevated papules, which can be pressed back into the underlying tissue. Associated with antiphospholipid antibodies and thrombotic events.

*Secondary atrophy.* From sunlight, x-radiation, injury, and nerve diseases.

Senile atrophy. Often associated with senile pruritus, senile purpura, and winter itch in the elderly.

Congenital atrophies. Associated with other congenital ectodermal defects.

Atrophoderma of Moulin. Hyperpigmented, linear atrophoderma which follows lines of Blaschko beginning during childhood or adolescence. Usually preceeding inflammation.

Atypical cutaneous lymphoproliferative disorder (ACLD). Widespread, pruritic papules and plaques, often hyperpigmented (rarely hypopigmented) seen in the later stages of HIV infection. The pathology mimics cutaneous T-cell lymphoma (CTCL) but is usually composed of CD8 (+) cells and only rarely progresses to true CTCL.

Auspitz's sign, 160

Autoeczematous dermatitis, 136

Autoeczematization. *See* Id reaction

Autoerythrocyte sensitization syndrome (Gardner-Diamond syndrome, psychogenic purpura). Bizarre, tender ecchymotic lesions mainly in young females. May be associated with psychological disturbance. Skin lesions reproduced with intradermal injection of whole blood or red blood cell fractions.

Autoimmune bullous disease, 115–116

Autoimmune polyendocrinopathy-candidiasis-ectodermal dystrophy syndrome (APECED). Multiple endocrinopathies in association with chronic mucocutaneous candidiasis. Up to one third have keratitis. The endocrinopathies can develop after childhood. It is due to the AIRE (autoimmune regulatory) gene autosomal recessive defect.

Baboon syndrome, 101t. *See* Chapter 9 under Dermatoses and Drugs That Cause Them

Bacterial infection, 473–475, 473f, 474f, 494–495, 494f

Balanitis, fusospirochetal, 365

Balanitis circumscripta plasmacellularis (balanitis of Zoon). Erythematous papules and plaques on the glans penis in uncircumcised males that is benign and that may resolve after circumcision. A similar condition in females is called *vulvitis circumscripta plasmacellularis.* It has a characteristic histopathology on biopsy.

Balanitis xerotica obliterans, 365

Bamboo hairs. *See* Netherton's syndrome (trichorrhexis invaginata).

Bannayan-Riley-Ruvalcaba syndrome. Also called Riley-Smith, Bannayan-Zonana, or Ruvalcaba-Mybre-Smith syndrome. Rare autosomal dominant with macrocephaly, genital melanotic macules and hamartomatous intestinal polyposis is the classic triad. Numerous other skin, eye, musculoskeletal and nervous system abnormalities are reported.

Bannayan-Zonana syndrome. Macrocephaly, hypotonia, developmental delay, hamartomas such as intestinal polyposis, lipomas and vascular malformations. Pigmented penile macules are common.

Bartonellosis, 473, 473f

Bart's syndrome. Congenital localized absence of skin (CLAS) of the lower extremities, skin and/or mucous membrane blistering, and nail absence and/or deformity. Probably a form of dominant dystrophic epidermolysis bullosa.

Basal cell carcinoma, 305–308, 305f, 407, 468

Basal cell nevus syndrome. A rare hereditary affliction characterized primarily by multiple genetically determined basal cell carcinomas, cysts of the jaws, peculiar pits of the hands and the feet, calcification of the falx cerebri, and developmental anomalies of the ribs, the spine, and the skull, 423t

Bazex's syndrome. *See* Acrokeratosis, paraneoplastic

Bazin's disease. *See* Erythema induratum.

Beckwith-Wiedemann syndrome. Consists most prominently of EMG (exophthalmos-macroglossia-gigantism). Many other characteristics including renal malformations and embryonal tumors with 20% mortality. To be differentiated from Proteus syndrome and CLOVE syndrome.

Behçet's syndrome, 128, 134, 362

Bejel. The name given to syphilis as it occurs among Arabs, 474, 475

Berloque dermatitis. Similar to the *melanosis of Riehl* and can result from contact with toilet waters containing oil of bergamot or other essential oils, followed by exposure to sunlight, causing a dermatitis that appears to drip down the neck, like a pendant (berloque).

Bier spots. Small irregular white macules seen in a dependent or externally compressed limb. They disappear upon elevating the limb or relieving the compression and are felt to be due to microvessel vasoconstriction due to lack of oxygen. Not a sign of significant vascular disease.

Bilharziasis, 479

Biologic false-positive reaction, 222

Bioterrorism, cutaneous signs of, 499–509, 500t, 503f, 505f, 506t, 508f

Biotinidase deficiency. Seen in children with partial or complete alopecia, rash, and infection. The rash is periorificial around the mouth, eyes, nose and back. It is eczematous, desquamating and mimics seborrhea. Neurologic manifestations include hypotonia, lethargy, seizures, developmental delay and depression (adults). Oral biotin treats the condition and prevents hearing and vision loss seen in up to 50% of untreated patients.

Birthmarks, 425–427, 427t, 427f–430f

Birt-Hogg Dube syndrome. Multiple fibrofolliculomas which are benign, hard papules, 1-3 mm, flesh-colored, common, hair follicle derived tumors especially on the nose, earlobes, forehead, and temples associated with pulmonary cysts, spontaneous pneumothorax, renal tumors, and adenomas of the colon.

Bites

Insect bite reactions may be exaggerated in HIV+ patients and in certain malignancies such as chronic lymphocytic leukemia, acute lymphoblastic leukemia and acute monocytic leukemia, mantle cell lymphoma, large cell lymphoma and myelofibrosis. Many patients do not recall a bite and in some cases this may represent an insect bite-like reaction.

Björnstad syndrome. Pili torti with congenital deafness in a variable hereditary pattern.

Black dermographism, 383

Black dot ringworm. Tinea of the hair caused by *Trichophyton tonsurans*. These endothrix fungi do not produce fluorescent hairs under the Wood's light and usually occur in children when broken short hairs are seen ("black dot tinea"), 257

Black heel (talon noir). Black asymptomatic macules on the posterior or lateral aspect of the heel in the area where the skin is thickly keratinized. Related to

trauma in such sports as tennis and basketball.

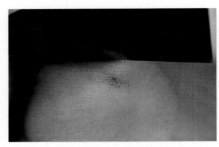

Heel exhibiting black heel (talon noir) in a tennis player.

Black palm (tache noir). Similar to black heel but on the palms of golfers, gymnasts, mountain climbers, tennis players, and weight lifters.

Black tongue, 363, 364f

Blackheads, 8, 17

Blaschko's lines. A cutaneous pattern of distribution followed by many skin disorders described in 1901 by Alfred Blaschko. The origin of these lines is not known.

Blastomycosis

North American, 260–266, 260f

South American (see paracoccidioidmycosis)

Blastomycosis-like pyoderma. Seen mainly in immunosuppressed patients at sites of injuries, tattoos, venous stasis and foreign body reactions. Verrucous plaques studded with pustules usually culture staph aureus and biopsy shows neutrophilic abscesses with pseudoepitheliomatous hyperplasia.

Blau syndrome. Rare autosomal dominant disorder usually in childhood with iritis, granulomatous arthritis, and a skin rash. Tiny generalized red dots reveal granulomas on biopsy and usually spontaneously resolve.

Bleomycin sulfate injection, 97t

Blister beetle dermatitis. Beetles of the family *Meloidae* contain cantharidin, which on contact with the skin causes the formation of a tense, itching, burning bulla. *See* Paederus dermatitis

Blistering distal dactylitis. Painful, tense blister on a red base over the anterior fat pad of one (due to Group A, beta-hemolytic streptococci) or two (due to staphylococci aureus) fingers usually between 2 and 16 years of age usually without systemic symptoms. Responds to antibiotics.

Bloom's syndrome, 423t

Blue nevus, 296

Blue rubber-bleb nevus syndrome (BEAN syndrome). Rare distinctive gastrointestinal and cutaneous vascular malformations. Gastrointestinal bleeding may occur and rarely other organs are involved. Usually present at birth or early infancy with soft compressible asymptomatic red to blue tumors. Occasionally painful or with overlying

hyperhidrosis. Blue macular or pinpoint blue-black areas may be seen. Deeper subcutaneous tumors without overlying skin changes are especially associated with gastrointestinal disease. Disease often progressive and may be associated with other tumors.

Bockhart's impetigo. A very superficial bacterial infection of the hair follicle.

Body odor, 8. *See also* Bromhidrosis

Bohn's nodules (gingival cysts). Innocuous, resolving (weeks to months) white papules in 50 to 80% of newborns on vestibular or lingual surfaces of the alveolar ridge or the palate.

Bolognia's sign. Eccentric foci of hyperpigmentation on clinical examination of pigmented tumor or with dermoscopy which indicates the need for a biopsy to rule out a malignant melanoma.

Borreliosis. *See* Lyme disease

Botox. *See* Botulinum toxin

Botryomycosis. Rare, chronic, granulomatous, abscess with granules mimicking actinomycosis but actually due to bacterial masses most often caused by staphylococcus aureus and pseudomonas aeruginosa among many others.

Botulinum toxin (BT), 44, 44f

Botulism, 500t

Bowel-associated dermatoarthritis syndrome. Seen in 20% of small bowel bypass patients and occasionally in inflammatory bowel disease. Intermittent neutrophilic pustules in crops with arthritis and increased cryoglobulins.

Bowen's disease, 298, 299f

Brachio-oculo-facial syndrome. Rare disorder caused by malformation of brachial arches. Malformed lip, nose, and ears result. Also lacrimal duct obstruction, brachial cleft sinus, linear neck scars, microphthalmia, auricular and lip pits, cysts of the scalp, high arched palate dental anomalies, cardiac anomalies, and renal anomalies have also been reported.

Brachioradial pruritus. Localized idiopathic, pruritus on the outer upper arms mainly over the elbow area. Sun exposure may be a causative factor.

Branchio-oto-renal syndrome (Melnick-Fraser syndrome). Preauricular pits, renal and ureteral anomalies, hearing loss, and branchial cleft cysts.

Brittle nail syndrome. Affects 20% of the population with women having double the incidence of men. Consists of onychoschezia (lamellar transverse splitting of the distal nail plate) and onychorrhexis (longitudinal nail plate thickening or ridging). Due to dryness and, although difficult to treat, may respond to 2.5 mgs biotin orally each day or topical 50% urea (Kerastik).

Bromhidrosis. The odor of the body that is associated with sweating, commonly called

"B.O." Freshly secreted sweat has no odor, but an odor develops when the sweat becomes contaminated with bacteria. Methods used to decrease sweat are curative, 6

Bromoderma. A dermatosis, usually pustular-like, due to the ingestion of bromides. *See also* Drug eruptions

Bronze diabetes. *See* Hemochromatosis

Brooke-Spiegler syndrome. Autosomal dominant association of trichoepitheliomas (usually on the face) and cylindromas (usually on the scalp). Other tumors (especially eccrine spiroadenomas) may also occur.

Brucellosis. The human infection of undulant fever is infrequently accompanied by a nondescript skin eruption. However, after delivering an infected cow, a high percentage of veterinarians experience an itching, red, macular, papular, or pustular dermatitis on the contaminated arms and hands that lasts for a few days to 3 weeks without systemic illness.

Bubble hair, 345

Buerger's disease, 135

Bullous congenital ichthyosiform erythroderma, 413t

Bullous disease of childhood, 430, 431t

Bullous impetigo, 184

Bullous pemphigoid, 35, 186

Bullous pyoderma, 391t

Burn
 sun, 431t, 438–440
 thermal, 431t, 440
 turf, 490t, 491

Burning mouth syndrome. Common, chronic, painful oral mucosae seen mainly in postmenopausal women with no apparent abnormalities visible.

Burning tongue, 363

Burrow's solution. A solution of aluminum acetate that in its original formula contained lead. A lead-free Burrow's solution for wet dressings can be made by adding Domeboro tablets or powder to water to make a 1:20 or 1:10 solution, 179, 272, 480

Buschke-Löwenstein. Virally induced giant condyloma of the penis that may progress to invasive squamous cell carcinoma. It is considered a subtype of verrucous carcinoma. *See* Verrucous carcinoma

Buschke-Ollendorf syndrome. A syndrome consisting of connective tissue nevi and osteopoikilosis of the hands, feet, pelvis, and long bones.

Bywaters Lesions. Tiny, painless, proximal nailfold blood clots that can occur on the ends of digits where they are painful. Most closely associated with rheumatoid arthritis.

CADASIL syndrome (cerebral autosomal dominant arteriopathy with subcortical infarcts and leukoencephalopathy).

Familial arteriopathy with migraines, strokes and early onset multi-infarct dementia. Skin biopsy of normal skin with electron microscopy can be diagnostic.

Café-au-lait spots, 281t, 283t, 284t

Calcifying epithelioma, 300, 301f

Calcinosis cutis, 386

Calcinosis. *Localized calcinosis* can occur in many tumors of the skin and following chronic inflammatory lesions, such as severe acne. *Metabolic calcinosis* may or may not be associated with an excess of blood calcium and is divided into universal calcinosis and circumscribed calcinosis.

Calciphylaxis. Sudden onset cutaneous necrosis and gangrene due to blood vessel and tissue calcification in association with hyperparathyroidism, longterm renal dialysis, renal transplantation, and rarely AIDS or autoimmune disease. Usually fatal(parenteral sodium thiosulfate infusions may be lifesaving) and almost always with marked renal disease, 358

Callus. A hyperkeratotic plaque of the skin due to chronic pressure and friction, 491, 491f

Cancer. *See* Tumors

Candidal intertrigo, 212, 262, 263f, 264f

Candidal paronychia, 262

Candidal vulvovaginitis, 263, 264

Candidiasis, 242, 251t, 254, 255, 262, 263f, 278, 425, 427t, 428f

Canker sores (aphthous ulcers), 361, 361f

Capillary hemangiomas, 441

Carbuncle, 202t, 207, 208f

Carcinoid syndrome. A potentially malignant tumor of the argentaffin chromaffin cells of the appendix or the ileum. Some of these tumors or their metastases produce large amounts of serotonin (5-hydroxytryptamine), which causes transient flushing of the skin accompanied by weakness, nausea, abdominal pain, diarrhea, and sweating. The redness usually begins on the head and the neck and then extends down on the body. These episodes last from several minutes to a few hours. Repeated attacks of the erythema lead to the formation of permanent telangiectasias and a diffuse reddish purple hue to the skin. The diagnosis can be made by the finding of over 25 mg of 5-hydroxyindoleacetic acid in a 24-hour urine sample, 391t

Carcinoma en cuirasse. Thickened indurated plaque over large areas of the thorax which may have a peau d'orange appearance that is seen most often with metastatic breast cancer.

Carcinoma erysipelatoides. Rare cutaneous metastasis usually from breast cancer with erythema, tenderness, increased temperature, spreading border and often eventually vesiculation. Unlike

erysipelas, which it resembles, there is no systemic toxicity.

Carcinoma, verrucous. *See* Verrucous carcinoma

Carcinosarcoma. Rare malignant neoplasm with both epithelial (usually basal cell cancer) and mesencyhmal (usually sarcoma) components. Especially head and neck or older men and may be aggressive with metastasis.

Cardio-facio-cutaneous syndrome. Ectodermal defects especially hair (wooly, friable hair and alopecia), skin lesions in 95% (especially follicular keratin plugging resembling keratosis pilaris), typical facial dysmorphism, cardiac defects, psychomotor retardation and growth failure. Probable autosomal dominant and associated with increased parental age.

Carney Complex. Myxomas (heart, skin, breast), spotty pigmentation (lentigines, blue nevi), endocrinopathies (Cushing's syndrome, acromegaly, sexual precocity) and schwannomas.

Carotenemia. Buildup of carotene or similar yellow-orange pigment in the blood and keratin layer of the skin. Stains skin a characteristic yellow. Harmless condition due to eating large amounts of foods such as carrots and tomatoes (lycopenemia due to similar pigment called lycopene). It can be seen in hypothyroidism.

Carrion's disease, 473

Caseation necrosis. Histologically, this is a form of tissue death with loss of structural detail leaving pale eosinophilic, amorphous, finely granular material. It is seen especially in tuberculosis, syphilis, granuloma annulare, and beryllium granuloma.

Caterpillar dermatitis (erucism). An irritating chemical is released when the hairs of some species of caterpillars penetrate the skin. The onset of irritation is quite immediate. Red macular lesions, then urticarial papules, and occasionally vesicles develop in areas exposed. Mild lesions can be gone in 12 hours, but more extensive cases can take several days to resolve. In these more severe cases, there occasionally can be constitutional symptoms of restlessness and headache. Therapy is not very effective or necessary. Scotch tape placed over the affected skin might pull out some of the bristle-like hairs.

Cat-scratch disease. Manifested by inflammation at the site of a cat scratch or bite obtained a few days previously. Malaise, headache, low-grade fever, chills, generalized lymphadenopathy, and splenomegaly occur. A maculopapular rash or erythema nodosum-like eruption occurs occasionally. Caused by *Bartonella henselae*, formerly *Rochalimaea henselae*, 462

Causalgia, A condition characterized by burning pain aggravated by touching the neuralgic site.

Cellulitis, 141, 209
eosinophilic. *See* Eosinophilic cellulitis

Central centrifugal cicatricial alopecia (CCCA), 372

Chagas disease, 477

Chalazion. A small, pink, usually painless cyst of the meibomian glands of the eyelid. It may resolve without treatment.

Chancre, 214. *See also* Primary chancre-type diseases
monorecidive. A relapsing form of syphilis characterized by the development of a lesion reduplicating the primary sore
primary, 214

Chancre-type, primary disease. *See* Primary chancre-type diseases.

Chancroid, 202t, 210, 214, 214f, 267t

CHAND. Curly hair, ankyloblepharon and nail dysplasia. Rare, congenital, and autosomal dominant.

Charcot joints. A type of joint destruction in patients with central nervous system syphilis of the paretic type.

Chédiak-Higashi syndrome. A fatal syndrome in children characterized by pigmentary disturbances, photophobia, pyogenic infections, excessive sweating, pale optic fundi, splenomegaly, and lymphadenopathy, 383

Cheilitis glandularis, 364

Cheilitis, granulomatous. Recurrent idiopathic swelling of one or both lips. Biopsy shows noncaseating granulomatous inflammation. It can be part of Melkersson-Rosenthal syndrome when associated with a scrotal tongue (lingua plicata) and facial paralysis. Treatment is difficult.

Cheyletiella dermatitis. A very pruritic papulonecrotic or papulovesicular eruption at the site of contact with cats, dogs and rabbits. The animal host may be asymptomatic. Treatment of the animal who is the host of the Cheyletiella mites is curative.

Chickenpox, 503t

Chiclero ulcers, 476

Chigger bites, 210, 482f

Chilblain lupus erythematosus of Hutchinson. Subtype of lupus erythematosus with cold induced, red, ulcerative symmetrical lesions on the ears, nose, digits, knees and elbows.

Chilblains. Also called *pernio*. A cutaneous reaction, either acute or chronic, from exposure to excessive cold.

Child abuse. Cutaneous signs of this abuse include linear bruising, loop marks, buckle marks, pinch marks, blunt trauma lesions, burns, traumatic alopecia, human bites, and genital tears, 394t, 404

CHILD syndrome. Rare disease present at birth showing congenital hemidysplasia, ichthyosis, and limb defects. Occurs almost exclusively in females.

Childhood granulomatous periorificial dermatitis. Possibly a granulomatous form of perioral dermatitis (periorificial dermatitis) in children except it is more common in darker skinned children and it can have extra-facial lesions.

Chimerism. When an individual is composed of two genetically different types cells. Occurs in healthy individuals but can be pathogenic. Dermatologic diseases where chimerism plays a role are pigmentary disorders, genital ambiguity, pityriasis lichenoides or polymorphic eruptions of pregnancy and autoimmune disorders such as scleroderma. Microchimerism occurs at birth where fetal cells are transferred to the mother in fetal chimerism or when maternal cells pass into the fetus in maternal chimerism. Chimerism can occur after bone marrow or hematopoietic stem cell transplant. Spontaneous chimerism from the amalgamation of 2 zygotes in the same embryo is called tetragametic chimerism.

Chloasma (Melasma), 380–381, 380f

Cholestasis, pregnancy with, 510t, 513

Cholinergic urticaria, 6

Chromhidrosis. The excretion of colored sweat, usually brownish, grayish, bluish, or yellowish. On the face, axillae, and breast areolae it is apocrine in nature and do to increased lipofuscin. It is not associated with underlying disease and the etiology is unknown. Eccrine chromhidrosis is due to injestion of dyes or certain drugs. Pseudochromhidrois is due to extrinsic exposure to dyes, paints or bacteria

Chromoblastomycosis, 484, 484f

Chronic actinic dermatitis, 408t, 409, 409f

Chronic infantile neurologic cutaneous and articular syndrome (CINCA, infantile onset multisystem inflammatory disease). Rare neonatal onset of periodic fever, arthropathy, neurologic abnormalities, ocular anomalies, and deafness. The skin has an urticarial, pink, migratory, maculopapular eruption on the face, torso, and extremities in episodic time intervals usually with a negative family history.

Chrysarobin. A reducing agent that hastens keratinization when it is applied to the skin. It can be incorporated into petrolatum or chloroform but must be used with great caution and in mild strength such as 0.25% to 3%. This was mainly used in treatment of resistant cases of psoriasis and tinea cruris.

Churg-Strauss syndrome. *See* Allergic granulomatosis

Cicatricial alopecia, 344, 372

Cicatricial pemphigoid, 185

CLAPO syndrome. Capillary malformation of the lower lip, Lymphatic malformation of the face and neck, Asymmetry of the face and limbs, Partial or generalized overgrowth.

Clarke-Howell-Evans syndrome. Familial hyperkeratosis of the palms and soles associated with carcinoma of the esophagus, squamous cell carcinoma in the skin, larynx, bronchus and oral leukoplakia. Type A has tylosis between ages 5-15 with painful fissuring. Type B is less commonly associated with underlying malignancies, has sharply delimited edges, and uniform thickness of keratosis.

Clear cell acanthoma, 298

Clear cell hidradenoma, 301

Clear cell papulosis. Rare, under three years of age on the trunk with multiple, white papules with characteristic large, basal layer, and clear cells on histopathology.

CLOVE syndrome. Congenital lipomatous overgrowth, vascular malformations and epidermal nevi. Must be differentiated from Proteus syndrome.

Clutton's joints. A symmetric serous synovitis of the knee joints with hydrarthrosis due to congenital syphilis.

Cobb syndrome. Skin angioma usually of the trunk in a dermatomal distribution associated with underlying spinal cord angioma.

Coccidioidomycosis, 483–484

Cockayne syndrome. Rare, autosomal recessive syndrome with great variability of type and severity of signs and symptoms which may include cachectic dwarfism, deafness, cutaneous photosensitivity without sun-induced neoplasms, thick skull, retinal pigmentation, intracranial calcification, mental deficiency, and characteristic facial features.

Collagen vascular diseases, 385–389, 385f, 387t–388t, 389f

Collagenomas. Rare, benign connective tissue nevi (hamartomas) that can be familial, part of tuberous sclerosis as a shagren patch, associated with other various abnormalities, or acquired (eruptive collagenomas).

Collodion baby, 414t

Colloid milium. There are four types of this disease. The juvenile form is rare and apparently disappears around puberty. Clinically on the face and dorsum of the hands, one sees cream-colored or yellowish 1- or 2-mm firm papules. The second type is the adult or acquired form, which is apparently related to the exposure of the skin to the sun and petroleum products. The clinical picture resembles the juvenile form. The third type is nodular colloid degeneration which is one or several larger (up to 5 cm) nodules felt to be related to sun exposure on the face, trunk, and scalp. A fourth type shows pigmented "caviar-like" papules in secondary ochronosis due to chronic topical hydroquinone use.

Coma bullae. Drug induced (especially barbiturates), hypoglycemic or central nervous system induced coma can produce bullae, erythema, violaceous plaques, necrosis or erosions usually, but not exclusively, on pressure sites.

Comedones, 17

Complex regional pain syndrome (Reflex sympathetic dystrophy). A syndrome that results from an injury (50% or greater after a bone fracture especially a Colles' fracture) usually on a limb. Severe pain is not limited to simple peripheral nerve and is disproportionate to the inciting event. Skin findings include edema, hyperhidrosis or anhidrosis, pallor, erythema, coolness and nail dystrophy. Diagnosis is difficult and treatment is of limited success.

Compound nevus, 294, 295f

Computer calluses. Trauma induced skin thickening occurs with chronic use of computers such as computer palm, mouse finger and mousing callus (on wrist over the pisiform prominence when wrist has friction with table.

Condyloma acuminata (venereal warts). Genital viral warts. When types 16, 18 (as well as other subtypes) involved is a precursor of cervical cancer (common), penile cancer (rare) and anal cancer (most common in gay HIV patients). Usually sexually transmitted.

Condylomata lata, 221, 224f

Confluent and reticulated papillomatosis of Gougerot-Carteaud. Pruritic, pigmented, truncal papules especially between the breasts and umbilicus. May become verrucous, erythematous, and reticulated.

Congenital ectodermal defect, 446

Congenital ichthyosiform erythroderma, 413t, 414f. *See also* Ichthyosis

Congenital melanocytic nevus, 426, 427t, 429f

Congenital triangular alopecia (Brauer nevus, temporally limited alopecia). Very rare permanent triangular patches on one or both frontotemporal scalp regions beginning at 3 to 5 years of age.

Congo red test. An intravenous test used to diagnose generalized amyloidosis. An intradermal skin test using Congo red solution will stain localized amyloid nodules red.

Connective tissue nevus (see collagenomas). Hamartomas of connective tissue present as 1) familial cutaneous collagenomas 2) Shagren patch of tuberous sclerosis 3) eruptive collagenomas and 4) isolated collagenomas.

Conradi Hunermann disease, 413t, 415f

Contact dermatitis, 9, 15, 21f, 22, 78–84, 79f–81f, 184, 448

Contraction, 56

Corn. A small, sharply circumscribed, often painful hyperkeratotic lesion that may be either hard with a central horny core or soft, as commonly seen between the toes. Underlying bone protuberances are causative (can be very painful). No tiny clotted capillaries as in warts. Normal skin markings are preserved.

Corticosteroids, 24, 32t, 36, 369
  drug eruptions from abuse of, 94f

Cosmeceuticals, 74–77

Cosmetics, 21f, 67–77

Costello syndrome. Formally considered a variant of Noonan syndrome and synonymous with cardiafaciocutaneous syndrome. It can be separated on clinical and genetic findings. Approximately 50% of patients will have verrucous papules with a characteristic histopathology that occurs on the abdomen, face, axillae, knees elbows, vocal cords, face and anus between 2 and 15 years old. The neck, hands and feet have loose redundant skin. Other skin markers include vascular birth marks, acanthosis nigricans, pigmented acral nevi, hyperpigmentation, hyperkeratosis, thin deep set nails, thick eyebrows, and sparse curly scalp hair. Mental retardation with a sociable personality as well as cardiac abnormalities, musculoskeletal abnormalities, abnormal facies, and increased risk of malignant tumors.

Cowden's disease. Autosomal dominant disease associated with multiple trichilemmomas of the face and multiple papules of the oral mucosa, causing a cobblestone appearance, as well as visceral malignancies, especially cancer of the breast in females, 386t

Coxsackievirus infections, 237–238

Crabs. *See* Pediculosis

Creeping eruption, 35

CREST syndrome (Calcinosis cutis, Raynaud's phenomenon, Esophageal dysfunction, Sclerodactyly, Telangiectasias), 386, 388t

Crohn's disease. An inflammatory granulomatous disease of the bowel. Cutaneous manifestations include pyoderma gangrenosum, exfoliative dermatitis, erythema multiforme, Stevens-Johnson syndrome, urticaria, herpes zoster, palmar erythema, cutaneous (metastatic) Crohn's disease, and necrotizing vasculitis.

Crouzon's disease. Autosomal dominant (but often spontaneous) craniofacial dystrophy with exophthalmos, craniosynostosis, maxillary hypoplasia, orbitostenosis, hooked nose, and acanthosis nigricans.

Crowe's sign, 418

Cryoglobulinemia. Purpura, livedo reticularis, and ulcers, especially on the lower extremities caused by a complex of proteins that precipitate on cooling in vitro. It can be primary or associated with underlying cancer, collagen vascular diseases, infection, and thromboembolic disease. Hepatitis C may be associated and interferon alpha may be therapeutic.

Cryotherapy, 406

Cryptococcosis (torulosis). A worldwide disease caused by a yeast-like fungus, *Cryptococcus neoformans*. It characteristically invades the central nervous system via the respiratory tract. Variable skin lesions are uncommon.

Crystal storing histiocytosis. Phagocytosis of immunoglobulin crystals of the kappa chain in organs throughout the body which rarely includes the skin. Infiltrated skin colored or erythematous plaques can precede an underlying cancer which is most often multiple myeloma but can be an immunocytoma, amyloidosis or a clofazimine drug induced reaction. Diagnosis is made by biopsy with characteristic histology findings.

CTCL. *See* Cutaneous T-cell lymphoma

Cullen's sign. Bruising around the umbilicus seen in acute hemorrhagic pancreatitis, ectopic pregnancy or blunt trauma and is due to retroperitoneal bleeding.

Cushingoid appearance, 24

Cushing's syndrome, 391t, 393

Cutaneous horn, 17, 291

Cutaneous T-cell lymphoma (CTCL), 125, 328–335, 373t

Cutis laxa, 420–421

Cutis marmorata. *See* Livedo reticularis

Cutis marmorata telangiectatica congenita. Uncommon sporadic congenital syndrome with persistent cutis marmorata, telangiectasia, phlebectasia, ulceration, atrophy, and undergrowth of involved skin.

Cutis verticis gyrata. A rare abnormality of the posterior scalp in which the skin is thrown into waves and folds resembling the cerebral convolutions of the brain. Usually a symmetric primary form affects males in childhood or puberty and is often associated with neurologic, psychiatric, and chromosomal diseases. Usually asymmetrical acquired variety occurs later in life. It may be associated with cylindromas, neurofibromas, intradermal nevi, other benign tumors, amyloidosis, acromegaly, hyperthyroidism, myxedema, and as part of a paraneoplastic syndrome.

Cyclic neutropenia. A form of agranulocytosis characterized by a periodic decrease in neutrophilic leukocytes. Skin lesions include severe ulcerative gingivitis and stomatitis.

Drug reaction, granulomatous interstitial. Rare drug reaction with characteristic histology that mimics interstitial granuloma annularae. Infiltrative plaques on medial thighs and inner arms is the classic presentation. It can occur weeks to months after drug exposure and take weeks to months to resolve.

Duhring's disease, 394. *See also* Dermatitis herpetiformis

Dyschromatosis, brachial acquired cutaneous. *See* Acquired brachial cutaneous dyschromatosis

Dyshidrosis (pompholyx). A syndrome characterized by pinhead-sized, very pruritic blisters on the palms of the hands, fingers, and feet. Some authors think stress can play a causative role. If the cause is known, this term should not be used. Considered by many to be a subtype of atopic eczema.

Dyskeratosis, benign. A histopathologic finding of faulty keratinization of individual epidermal cells with formation of corp ronds and corp grains. Seen in Darier's disease and occasionally in familial benign chronic pemphigus.

Dyskeratosis congenita. With pigmentation, dystrophia unguis, and leukokeratosis oris, this is a rare syndrome characterized by a reticulated pigmentation, particularly of the neck, dystrophy of the nails, and a leukoplakia condition of the oral mucosa. Increased sweating and thickening of the palms and soles may occur, 423t

Dyskeratosis, malignant. A histopathologic finding in Bowen's disease and also in squamous cell carcinoma and actinic keratosis in which premature and atypical keratinization of individual cells is seen.

Dysplastic nevus syndrome, 294

Dystrophia unguium mediana canaliformis, 354

Ebola, 500t

EBV. *See* Epstein-Barr virus

Ecchymoses, 139. *See also* Purpura

Eccrine angiomatous hamartoma. Rare, benign, painful hyperhidrotic proliferation of eccrine tissue with vascular stroma. Present at birth or early childhood. Surgical excision may be required due to severity of pain.

Eccrine epithelioma, 301, 301f

Eccrine glands, 6

Eccrine hidradenitis. *See* Palmoplantar eccrine hidradenitis

Eccrine poroma, 301, 301f

Eccrine spiradenoma, 301, 301f

Eccrine squamous syringometaplasia. Clinically and etiologically similar to neutrophilic eccrine hidradenitis but with different specific histopathology. Painful erythematous plaques or macules seen especially on the groin, axilla, palms and soles in bone marrow transplant patients due to high dose chemotherapy.

Eccrine syringofibroadenoma (ESFA), 300

ECHO (Entire cytopathic human orphan), 238

Echovirus exanthem, 238

Ecthyma, 202t, 204–206, 204f

Ecthyma gangrenosum. Rapidly developing painful necrotic escharotic gangrenous plaques usually in the intertriginous areas. Seen in patients with sepsis that is usually due to pseudomonas.

Ectodermal dysplasias, 424, 424f

Ectodermal dysplasia-skin fragility syndrome. Rare genodermatosis caused by defective plakophilin, which is a component of desmosomes. Generalized red skin at birth becomes fragile. Progressive plantar keratoderma, nail dystrophy and alopecia are also a part of this syndrome.

Ectodermosis erosiva pluriorificialis. A synonym for Stevens-Johnson syndrome.

Eczema

atopic. *See* Atopic eczema

craquelé. A French term for cracked appearing skin, especially seen on the legs when skin is very dry.

housewives', 85

infantile, 20f, 85, 85f, 86f, 90–91

nummular, 19f, 22, 91, 92f, 103t

winter, 22

Eczematous eruption, 101t

Eczematous lesions, 431t, 436–437, 436f–437f

Ehlers-Danlos syndrome, 419

Ehrlichiosis, 218

Elasticity disorders, 419–421

Elastoderma. Acquired, localized laxity of the skin. Dense aggregates of eosinophilic material are present in the dermis.

Elastofibroma dorsi. Rare benign firm subcapsular tumor in elderly women that may be necessary to remove due to pain and difficulty in movement. Abduction of the arms may be necessary to see this subcutaneous tumor with freely movable normal underlying tissue.

Elastosis perforans serpiginosa. A rare asymptomatic disease in which keratotic papules occur in a circinate arrangement around a slightly atrophic patch, usually on the neck. May be seen in association with scleroderma, renal disease, Ehlers-Danlos syndrome, osteogenesis imperfecta, Marfan's syndrome, Rothmund-Thompson syndrome, acrogeria, and especially Down's syndrome.

Electrocautery, 53

Electrocoagulation, 53

Elephantiasis nostras verrucosa. Nonfilarial gross enlargement of a body region (usually a limb) due to recurrent streptococcal lymphangitis resulting in dermal woody fibrosis and epidermal papillomatosis and hyperkeratosis causing a dramatically enlarged, firm deformity. Treatment is difficult with compression dressings and long term antibiotics most often used.

ELISA (Enzyme-linked immunosorbent assay), 509

EM. *See* Erythema multiforme

Embolic nodules. Emboli can come from a left atrial myxoma, fat from bone marrow after bone trauma, or from arteriosclerotic plaques with or without vascular surgical procedures, appear as distal, papular, hemorrhagic, sometimes painful areas in the distribution of the vessel involved, 135

Emollients, 28, 30, 67, 69–71, 91, 110, 122, 124

Encephalocraniocutaneous lipomatosis (ECCL). Unilateral lipomas of the face and scalp associated with cerebral and ophthalmologic malformation on the ipsilateral side. Sporadic and very rare in newborns.

Endometriosis. The presence of extracutaneous endometrial tissue. Rarely found in skin usually in abdominal scars related to pelvic surgery (especially caesarean sections). Tumoral nodules are painful and bleed during menstrual cycles and if primary usually occur near the umbilicus.

Entamoeba histolytica, 477

Entire cytopathic human orphan. *See* ECHO

Eosinophilic cellulitis (Well's syndrome). Characterized by the sudden onset of pruritic, red, infiltrated, urticaria-like patches, which persist for 3 to 4 weeks and can recur. Characteristic histopathology with an infiltrate of eosinophils and "flame figures."

Eosinophilic fasciitis (Shulman's syndrome). Acute onset of induration, tenderness, swelling, and erythema of one or more extremities resulting in sclerodermatous skin changes. Believed by some to be a variant of scleroderma with a diagnosis confirmed by deep biopsy into the fascia showing significant inflammation with eosinophils.

Eosinophilic polymorphic pruritic eruption associated with radiation (EPPER). Excoriated papules, wheals, and vesicles with eosinophilic infiltrate, generalized pruritus and is seen in association with radiation therapy mainly for cervical cancer. It spares the palms, soles, and mucous membranes.

Eosinophilic ulcer of the oral mucosa. Uncommon, self-limited ulcer that may be initiated by trauma. Histopathology is usually characteristic. One third are painful and the commonest location of the ulcer is the tongue, buccal mucosa, and lip.

Epidermal nevus. Usually benign overgrowth of epidermal tissue. Can develop into squamous cell carcinoma. Rarely associated with underlying bone, central nervous system, eye or kidney abnormalities (epidermal nevus syndrome), 426, 427t, 429f

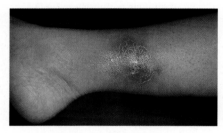

Erythema induratum.

associated with underlying cancer and the skin has the appearance of grains of wood, 134

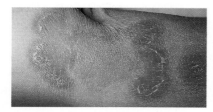

A. Erythema perstans on the elbow
(*Drs. H. Shair and L. Grayson*).

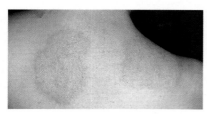

B. Erythema perstans on the back.

Erythema toxicum neonatorum. An evanescent skin eruption in newborns usually occurring within 48 hours after birth and lasting about 3 days; consists of erythema, papules, macules, and occasional pustules.

Erythermalgia. *See* Erythromelalgia

Erythrasma, 209–210

Erythroderma
bullous congenital ichthyosiform, 413t
ichthyosiform, T cell. *see* Sézary syndrome

Erythrodermia desquamativa. Term for Leiner's disease

Erythrokeratodermia progressive symmetrica (progressive symmetric erythrokeratodermia). Rare autosomal dominant persistent hyperkeratotic erythematous plaques especially on the head, extremities and buttocks. It appears during the first year of life and is progressive for a few years and then may remit or remain stationary. Fifty percent of patients have involvement of the palms and soles.

Erythrokeratodermia variabilis. Rare, chronic, autosomal dominant usually developing months after birth. Red to brown patches that change from minutes to hours to days. Also variable keratotic brownish plaques and keratoderma of the palms and soles may occur.

Erythromelalgia or erythermalgia. A rare disorder of the hands and feet most common in middle age; characterized by swelling, redness, burning pain that is activated by exertion or heat and is refractory to treatment.

Erythromelanosis follicularis faciei. Hyperpigmentation, follicular plugging, and well demarcated erythema on the face especially in men.

Erythropoietic protoporphyria, 408t, 410

Erythrose pigmentaire peribuccale. A rare condition of middle-aged women, characterized by diffuse brownish red pigmentation about the mouth, the chin, and the neck with or without a slight burning sensation.

ESFA. *See* Eccrine syringofibroadenoma

Espundia, 476

Essential pruritus, 125

Excisions, 55, 55f

Excoriation, 15

Exfoliative dermatitis, 101t, 192–194, 194f, 382
primary, 192–193
secondary, 193–194, 194f

Exostosis, subungual. *See* Subungual

Expanded polytetrafluoroethylene facial implants (e-PTFE implants), 47–48, 48f

External otitis, 128–129

Eye makeup, 73

Fabry's disease, 399

Factitial dermatitis, 198–199, 198f, 199f

FAMI. *See* Fat autograft muscle injection

Familial benign chronic pemphigus, 185

Fanconi anemia. Uncommon autosomal recessive associated with bone marrow failure, and predisposition to myeloid leukemia, squamous cell carcinomas of the oral mucosa and female genitalia as well as liver neoplasms. Dyspigmentation is a common feature with café-au-lait macules, hyperpigmented macules, and guttate hypopigmented macules. Sweet's syndrome, cutaneous amyloidosis, and generalized hyperpigmentation from iron overload after repeated red blood cell transfusions have also been reported skin findings.

Fanconi syndrome, 423t

Fasciitis, nodular. Painful, tender, rapidly growing, soft-tissue mass usually on an extremity and usually less than 3cm. Reactive, inflammatory, benign and can be excised or possibly treated by intralesional corticosteroids. Histopathological examination may lead to an erroneous diagnosis of a malignancy. Proliferative fasciitis is a similar condition that can be differentiated by histology.

Fat autograft muscle injection (FAMI), 45–46, 45f

Fat necrosis of the newborn. Rare indurated, well demarcated subcutaneous nodules and plaques over the arms, legs, cheeks, buttocks or trunk within the first few weeks of life. Usually occurs following a complicated pregnancy and may be associated with hypercalcemia. Usually resolves without sequela.

Fat necrosis, subcutaneous. *See* Subcutaneous fat necrosis

Fat necrosis, subcutaneous, with pancreatic disease. Histologic picture is quite characteristic.

Fatal granulomatous disease of childhood. A very rare, X-linked disease of mainly males characterized by eczematous lesions in infancy with progressive chronic granulomatous bacterial infections.

Favre-Racouchot syndrome. The term for multiple comedones on the high cheek and temple areas in older persons due to chronic sun exposure, 446

Felty syndrome. Triad of arthritis, leucopenia and splenomegaly. Increased leg ulcers (22%), rheumatoid nodules (76%), and mortality (25%) related to increased infections with sepsis.

Fetal alcohol syndrome. Approximately 40% of newborns of alcoholic mothers develop mental retardation, skeletal abnormalities, and cardiac abnormalities. The cutaneous markers are hemangiomas, hypertrichosis, and nail dysplasias with thinning.

Fiberglass dermatitis. Irritant contact dermatitis with itching papules, erythema, vesicles, desquamation, and excoriations. Dorsal hands, fingers and forearms present mainly in workers using reinforcement filling in printed circuit boards. One of the commonest occupational dermatoses.

Fibrokeratoma, acquired digital. Tumor occurring in adults on fingers or toes; mimics a rudimentary supernumerary digit but without nerve tissue.

Fibroma, recurrent infantile digital. Fibrous nodules that occur at birth or sometimes during childhood on the fingers and toes; may spontaneously involute and then recur.

Fibromas, pedunculated, 284–285, 285f

Fibrosarcoma, 301

Fibrosis, postirradiation. Gradual onset of dermal atrophy, fibrosis and telangiectasia at a radiation site. Worse with an increase in radiation dose.

Fibroxanthoma, atypical. Relatively uncommon, malignant (metastasis is rare), raised nodular lesion that occurs most often on the head and neck at chronically sun-exposed or irradiated sites. Treated with Mohs surgery to attempt to avoid frequent local recurrence.

Filariasis, 478–479

Filoviruses, 500t

Finger pebbles (Huntley's papules). Fine asymptomatic flesh colored grouped micropapules on the dorsum of the fingers associated with diabetes mellitus.

Fish-Odor syndrome (trimethylaminuria). Rare metabolic disease with malodor of the body similar to that of decaying fish. Serious psychosocial problems relate to the malodor. Free urinary trimethylamine should be checked both on a normal and restricted diet. Dietary restriction of choline containing foods such as eggs, peas, beans, marine fish, liver and kidney should be tried. Large quantities of milk, brussel sprouts, and vegetables of the Brassica family should be avoided. Other therapeutic modalities include

Fish-Odor syndrome. (*continued*)
lactulose, metronidazole, neomycin sulfate, activated charcoal, and copper chlorophyllin.

Flagellate erythema. Erythematous centripetal linear streaks (zebra-like stripe eruption) on the trunk and proximal extremities in a centripetal distribution. Seen in association with systemic bleomycin therapy and dermatomyositis.

Flea bites, 218, 481, 481f

Flow cytometry, 13

Flukes. *See* Trematodes dermatosis

Fluorinated corticosteroids, 35

Fluoroscopy-induced chronic radiation injury. Acquired vascular, morphea-like or ulcerated area seen at the site of usually multiple fluoroscopic procedures that is seen over the scapula, back or lateral trunk below the axilla.

Foams, 33

Focal dermal hypoplasia (Goltz syndrome). X linked dominant syndrome showing cribriform atrophy with an increase or decrease in pigment often along Blaschko lines. Eye, skeletal, teeth, nail, and soft tissue abnormalities may occur.

Focal epithelial hyperplasia. Benign condition possibly caused by HPV 13 or 22 consisting of asymptomatic, multiple, mucosal papules especially in young females especially in Native Americans, Eskimos (where it is more common in adults) and South Africans. Seen on the inner upper and lower lips, buccal mucosa, and tongue with a variable course lasting a few months to years. Important to differentiate from condyloma to avoid implications of sexual transmission and abuse. Ablative therapy such as laser, cryotherapy, and surgical excision have been used with variable results.

Follicular plugs, 17

Folliculitis, 202t, 205–206, 205f
decalvans, 202t, 206
deep, 202t, 206
scalp, 202t, 205–206, 205f
superficial, 202t, 205
treatment of, 205, 206

Folliculitis, eosinophilic pustular. Recurrent extremely pruritic crops of sterile pustules. Has a characteristic histologic appearance and is seen most often in association with HIV positive patients. There is an adult variant and an infancy variant not associated with immunosuppression.

Folliculitis, hot tub. A bacterial folliculitis with inflammatory nodules caused by *Pseudomonas aeruginosa* in people exposed to poorly chlorinated hot tubs, jacuzzis, whirlpools, and swimming pools.

Folliculitis, perforating, of the nose. A folliculitis of the stiff hairs of the nasal mucocutaneous junction that penetrates deeply through to the external nasal skin. Unless the basic pathology is understood and corrected by plucking the involved stiff hair, the condition cannot be cured. The external papule can simulate a skin cancer.

Fordyce's disease, 299, 363

Foreign body granuloma. *See also* Granuloma, foreign body

Forme fruste, 24

Formaldehyde, 72

Formulary, 27–34, 32t

Foshay test. A 48-hour intradermal test that, if positive, indicates that the person has or has had *tularemia*.

Fox-Fordyce disease. A rare, intensely pruritic, chronic papular dermatosis of the axillae and the pubic area in women. The intense itching is due to the closure of the apocrine gland pore with rupture of the duct and escape of the apocrine sweat into the surrounding epidermis. Treatment is difficult.

Frambesia. *See* Yaws

Freckles, 296, 303, 445, 445f

Frey's syndrome. Auriculotemporal nerve syndrome where gustatory stimuli cause facial flushing or sweating in the distribution of the auriculotemporal nerve. Usually due to trauma to the parotid gland in adults.

Friction injuries, 490–492, 491f

Frostbite. Exposure to cold can cause pathologic changes in the skin that are related to the severity of the exposure but vary with the susceptibility of the person. Other terms in use that refer to cold injuries under varying conditions include *trench foot, immersion foot, pernio,* and *chilblains.*

Fungal infections, 246–265, 462–463
antifungal agents for, 250t–251t
candidiasis as, 262–264, 263f–264f
deep, 260–265, 261f–265f
North American blastomycosis as, 260–261, 260f
onychomycosis as, 347–350, 348f, 349f
sporotrichosis as, 264–265
superficial, 246–265, 248f, 249t, 250t, 250t–251t, 252f–254f, 256f, 257f, 259f, 260f, 263f–265f
tinea of beard as, 206, 247t, 258t, 258–259, 259f
tinea of feet as, 246–250, 248f, 249t, 249f, 250t
tinea of groin as, 249t, 250t, 254–255, 254f
tinea of hands as, 249t, 250t, 251–253, 253f
tinea of nails as, 249t, 250t, 253–254, 253f
tinea of scalp as, 249t, 250t, 256–258, 256f, 259t
tinea of smooth skin as, 249t, 250t, 255–256, 256f

Furrowed tongue, 364

Furuncle, 202t, 207, 207f, 494

Fusospirochetal balanitis, 365

Futcher's line. *See* Voigt-Futcher line

Gangosa. A severe ulcerative and mutilating form of yaws that affects the palate, pharynx, and nasal tissues.

Gangrene. symmetrical peripheral. A rare syndrome associated with a multitude of underlying medical problems. Disseminated intravascular coagulation occurs in most cases. Probably synonymous with purpura fulminans.

Gardner's syndrome. An autosomal dominant trait with osteomas, fibrous and fatty tumors, epidermoid inclusion cysts of the skin, and multiple gastrointestinal polyps, 423t

General paresis. A psychosis due to syphilitic meningoencephalitis.

Genital herpes, 230–232, 232f, 233t, 267

Genital melanotic macule. Benign, hyperpigmented, asymptomatic, well, demarcated macule seen in the genitalia of men, and women. It's not associated with underlying illness and histologically looks like a lentigo.

Genodermatoses, 412–424, 413t–414t, 414f, 415f, 416t, 417f–421f, 422t, 422f, 423t
adhesion disorders with, 415, 416t, 417f
appendages disorders with, 421–424, 422t, 422f
hair in, 422, 422t
nails in, 422–423, 423f
ectodermal dysplasias with, 424, 424f
elasticity disorders with, 419–420
cutis laxa as, 420
Ehlers-Danlos syndrome as, 419
pseudoxanthoma elasticum as, 420
hamartomas/malignancies with, 423t, 424
keratinization disorders with, 412–415, 413t–414t, 414f, 415f
ichthyoses as, 412, 413t–414t, 414f
palmar-plantar keratodermas as, 412, 415f
pigmentation disorders with, 417–419, 417f–419f
hyperpigmentation as, 418–419, 418f, 419f
hypopigmentation as, 417–418, 417f–418f

Gentian violet. A dye that destroys gram-positive bacteria, yeast, and some fungi.

Geographic tongue, 360, 360f

German measles (Rubella), 237

Gianotti-Crosti syndrome. (papular acrodermatitis of childhood, *see* Chap. 33). Characterized by the acute onset of symmetrical, red or flesh-colored, flat-topped papules, usually 2 to 3 mm in diameter, mainly on the face and limbs. Nonpruritic, they last about 3 weeks. The cause is a virus, sometimes of the hepatitis type.

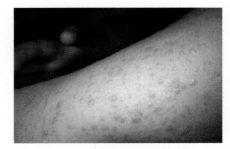

Gianotti-Crosti syndrome on the upper outer arm

Giant cell fibromas. Uncommon, benign, oral cavity, asymptomatic, solitary papule usually less than 1cm and probably a reactive process to trauma or inflammation.

Giant cell arteritis, 144t

Glanders. Gram negative bacterial (Burkholderia, formerly called Pseudomonas mallei) infection usually acquired from horses seen mainly in Asia, Africa, and South America. Four clinical manifestations can appear after an incubation period of 1 day to 2 weeks: 1) nodule with lymphangitis at the site of inoculation and the nodule eventually breaks down and ulcerates 2) mucous membrane ulceration and granulomatous formation 3) sepsis with cutaneous papules and pustules, 4) pulmonary disease with malaise, headache, and pleurisy. Treated with sulfadiazine.

Gleich syndrome. Rare episodic angioedema with eosinophilic (60 to 70%) in peripheral blood and tissue, fever, weight gain due to fluid retention, hypoalbuminemia, swollen lymph nodes, increased LDH but no visceral organ involvement, and a benign course. There is no specific treatment. Myeloproliferative disease, allergic processes, parasitic infections, autoimmune diseases, Wells syndrome, and hypereosinophilic syndrome are in the differential diagnosis.

Glomangiomas, 303

Glomus body, 302

Glossitis

Moeller's, 364

rhomboidea mediana, 364, 364f

Gloves and Socks syndrome (GSS). *See* Papular-purpuric "Gloves and Socks" syndrome

Glucagonoma syndrome. A glucagon-secreting islet cell neoplasm of the pancreas results in a polymorphous skin eruption characterized by superficial epidermal necrosis with fragile blister formation (necrolytic migratory erythema). The perioral area and intertriginous areas are frequently involved. Thin, brown, superficial crusts with peripheral scaling that occurs on annular erythematous edema with "map-like" margins that can be seen around the edges of the eruption.

Gnathostomiasis, 478

Gnatophyma. Rare variant of rosacea where changes similar to rhinophyma occur except on the chin.

Goltz syndrome. *See* focal dermal hypoplasia

Gonorrhea, 202t, 217, 218f

Gonorrheal dermatosis. *See* Keratoderma blennorrhagicum

Gottron papules. Flat reddish papules on the knuckles seen in 30% of the patients with advanced dermatomyositis, 389f, 389t

Gottron sign, 389t

Graft-*versus*-host disease (GVHD). Both the acute and chronic forms are accompanied by erythematous lesions that may develop into an erythroderma, with bullae and necrolysis (can be a mimic of TEN). The chronic type can eventuate into sclerodermatous-like lesions with ulcerations or lichen planus-like eruptions. Nails and hair can be affected. Clinical situations in which this disease can occur are: small bowel, pancreas-spleen, lung-heart, lung, heart, liver, and bone marrow transplants, non-irradiated whole blood transfusions to immunocompromised patients, and neonates that are immunocompromised after in utero transfusions. Liver disease and bowel disease with diarrhea complete the usual triad of disease, 461

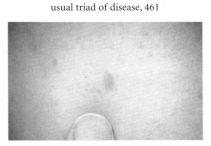

A. Acute GVHD mimicking lichen planus.

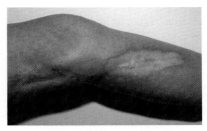

B. Chronic GVHD mimicking scleroderma

Graham-Little Syndrome (Piccardi-Lassueur-Graham-Little Syndrome). Multifocal cicatricial scalp alopecia, non-scarring alopecia of the axillae and/or groin, and keratotic perifollicular papules.

Grain itch. Due to a mite, *Pediculoides ventricosus*, that lives on insects that attack wheat and corn. This mite can attack humans working with the infested grain and cause a markedly pruritic papular, and papulovesicular eruption.

Granular cell schwannoma, 302

Granular cell tumor. See granular cell schwannoma

Granular parakeratosis. Especially in women in 5th and 6th decades and intertriginous areas with reddish brown and often asymptomatic papules that coalesce into macerated plaques. Mimics Hailey-Hailey disease and reported to clear with topical tretinoin.

Granuloma

epithelioid, 174

foreign body. A granulomatous reaction seen in the dermis due to the introduction, usually by trauma, of certain agents such as lipids, petrolatum, paraffin, indelible pencil, silica and silicates (talc), suture, hair, and zirconium from certain deodorants, 174

histiocytic, 174

mixed inflammatory, 174

necrobiotic, 174

silica, 175

swimming pool, 475, 475f. *See also* Swimming pool granuloma

Granuloma annulare, 36, 176–177, 176f, 431t, 432, 433f

Granuloma faciale. Typically occurs as brownish papules or plaques, multiple or single, usually on the face, in middle-aged or older persons (usually men). Asymptomatic, benign, often recalcitrant to therapy and probably represents a form of localized vasculitis. Dapsone, intralesional corticosteroids, and cryosurgery are sometimes beneficial.

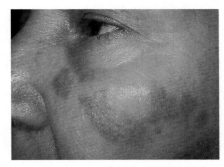

Granuloma faciale (*Dr. J. DeSpain*).

Granuloma gluteale infantum. Purplish, pink nodules in the diaper area in infants or in women wearing garments for incontinence. May be related to prolonged use of fluorinated topical corticosteroid preparations or to candidiasis.

Granuloma inguinale, 202t, 213, 213f

Granuloma, lethal midline. See Lethal midline granuloma

Granuloma pyogenicum, 296, 302, 302f

Granulomatosis

allergic. *See* Allergic granulomatosis

lymphomatoid. *See* Lymphomatoid granulomatosis

Granulomatous cheilitis. *See* Cheilitis, granulomatous

Granulomatous dermatitis (interstitial granulomatous dermatitis with arthritis). Most often in middle aged women with rheumatoid arthritis. Burning, symmetric, erythematous to violaceous nodules or plaques or linear cords ("rope sign") especially axillae, trunk and inner thighs. Biopsy is needed to make correct diagnosis. Topical corticosteroids, dapsone, and hydroxychloroquine have all been used as effective therapy.

Granulomatous disease of childhood, chronic. An X-linked recessive disorder of leukocyte function characterized by indolent infections of the skin, as well as lymph nodes, lungs, liver, spleen, bone, and bone marrow. 60%–70% of cases have cutaneous disease. Diagnostic pigmented lipid macrophages, found in skin and visceral granuloma.

Granulomatous slack skin syndrome. *See* Slack Skin syndrome

Granulomatous vasculitis, 144t

Grey-Turner's sign. Bruising of the flanks usually seen in acute hemorrhagic pancreatitis due to retroperitoneal bleeding.

Griscelli syndrome. Variable immunodeficiency associated with partial albinism. Characteristic histology of hair and skin is seen.

Grover's disease. *See* Acantholytic dermatosis, transient

Guttate psoriasis, 435, 435f

GVHD. *See* Graft-*versus*-host disease

Habit tic deformity, 354, 354f

Hair collar sign. A circle of elongated hyperpigmented hair around a congenital nodule seen in infants with cephalocele, meningocele, hypertrophic brain tissue, membranous aplasia cutis, and congenital dermatofibrosarcoma protuberans.

Hairy leukoplakia of tongue, 364

Halitosis, 363

Hallermann-Streiff syndrome. Usually mutational, rare, craniofacial dysostoses with bird-like facies, facial telangiectasias, face, and scalp atrophy, alopecia (characteristically along suture lines), skeletal and ocular abnormalities.

Halo nevus, 295f, 296

Hamartoma, congenital smooth muscle. Rare, usually present at birth, hyperpigmented or skin-colored, benign, patch or plaque.

Hamartomas, 424

Hand-foot-and-mouth disease, 363

Hanifin/Rajka criteria, 90t

Harlequin fetus, 413t, 430f

Hamartoma syndrome, generalized basaloid follicular. Multiple tan papules that usually present in childhood especially face, scalp, neck, and trunk. Rare, autosomal dominant and can be associated with milia, comedones, and acrochordons. Hypertrichosis, hypohidrosis, and palmoplantar pits are also part of the syndrome. Autoimmune disorders such as myasthenia gravis, alopecia universalis, systemic lupus erythematosus, and antiphospholipid antibodies have been rarely associated. Solitary tumors are not hereditary.

Haverhill Fever. *See* Rat bite fever

Hay-Wells syndrome. Autosomal dominant syndrome with ankyloblepharon, ectodermal dysplasia, and/or cleft lip or cleft palate.

Heck disease. See focal epithelial hyperplasia.

Helminthic dermatoses (Roundworms), 178, 478, 478f

Hemangioendothelioma, Kaposi-form, 302, 303. *See* Kaposiform hemangioendothelioma

Hemangioendothelioma, retiform. Rare low-grade angiosarcoma that really metastasizes but frequently recurs. Non-descript clinical lesion but with a characteristic histology.

Hemangioma, 294, 294f, 302
angiokeratoma, 294
as birthmarks, 292
capillary, 296f, 294
senile, 296
spider, 294f, 294
spindle cell. Benign subcutaneous and dermal, firm, red-blue nodules that occur mainly in children and young adults especially on the distal extremities. Satellite nodules develop in the same anatomical region. Histology is diagnostic.
superficial, 291–293
targetoid hemosiderotic. Simple benign acquired brown to violaceous papulonodule with pale ring surrounded by a ring of ecchymosis. May be due to trauma and resolves spontaneously. Characteristic histology.
treatment of, 292, 293, 294
varix, 294
venous lake, 294
verrucous, congenital hyperkeratotic, usually unilateral, bluish nodules associated with deep vascular tumors involving skin and subcutaneous tumors. On the legs most commonly and worsens with age so early deep excision is preferable.

Hemangioma of infancy, 426–427, 427t, 429f

Hemangiomatosis, benign neonatal. Multiple widespread hemangiomatosis usually confined to the skin and lips. They increase rapidly in number and size (up to 2cm) during the first 2 months with regression usually occurring within the first 6 months. Usually no treatment is required. Not inherited.

Hemangiomatosis, diffuse neonatal. Severe condition with over 50% mortality. Multiple cutaneous mucosal and visceral hemangiomas especially in the liver. Not inherited. Therapy with systemic corticosteroids radiation therapy, embolization, subcutaneous interferon, partial hepatic resection, embolization, and hepatic artery ligation have all been attempted with varying success.

Hemangiopericytoma, 302

Hematoma, 139
subungual, 352, 352f

Hemochromatosis. A rare hereditary metabolic disease characterized by a deposit of hemosiderin in the glandular tissues, and hemofuscin in the connective tissues, the spleen, and the smooth muscles. Diabetes mellitis often develops and the skin develops a bronze discoloration. "Bronze diabetes."

Hemophagocytic lymphohistiocytosis. Rare rapidly progressive, often fatal illness with characteristic histology and presents as fever, pancytopenia and hepatosplenomegaly. Up to 65% of patients may have skin manifestations which include transient generalized maculopapular eruption, petechial, and purpuric macules, and morbilliform erythema.

Henoch-Schönlein purpura, 139, 399, 431t, 435, 435f. *See* Chapters 12 and 13

Hepatitis C. Viral infection of the liver associated with porphyria cutanea tarda, lichen planus, essential mixed cryoglobulinemia, Sjögren's syndrome, urticaria, pruritus, prurigo nodularis, membranoproliferative glomerulonephritis, leukocytoclastic vasculitis, necrolytic acral erythema, antiphospholipid syndrome, and rarely polyarteritis nodosa.

Hermansky-Pudlak syndrome. Autosomal recessive, oculocutaneous albinism, excessive bleeding (due to platelet storage pool deficiency), fatal (usually by 4th to 5th decade) pulmonary fibrosis (due to lysosomal accumulation of ceroid lipofuscin), and granulomatous colitis (10%–20%). High frequency in northwest Puerto Rico.

Herpangina. A name applied to a coxsackievirus infection that occurs on the mucous membranes of the mouth in children. Fever and malaise accompany this acute infection, which lasts approximately 2 weeks, 238

Herpes gestationis. Rare vesicular bullous disease associated with pregnancy. Intensely pruritic and may be associated with fetal complications. It is autoimmune in origin with the third component of complement deposited in the basement membrane with the direct immunofluorescent technique, 510–511, 511f

Herpes gladiatorum, 496, 496f

Herpes simplex virus, 36
mucous membrane disease with, 362

Herpes simplex virus 1 (HSV-1), 230, 231f, 232f

Herpes simplex virus 2 (HSV-2), 230–232, 232f, 233t, 236

Herpes zoster, 36

Herxheimer reaction. An acute reaction characterized by fever and aggravation of existing cutaneous lesions following the administration of penicillin for syphilis. In patients with central nervous system syphilis, neurologic findings may be aggravated. In patients with cardiovascular syphilis, the reaction may be fatal, but some observers doubt the occurrence of this severe form of Herxheimer reaction.

Hibernoma, 302

Hidradenitis. *See* Idiopathic recurrent palmo-plantar hidradenitis

Hidradenitis suppurativa, 6, 152, 208

Hidradenoma papilliferum, 300

Hidrocystoma. Benign tumor of the face that is cystic, quite small, may have a slight bluish discoloration and can be a derivative of the eccrine or apocrine sweat gland. Accentuated by a warm environment.

Higoumenakia sign. Enlargement of the sternoclavicular joint due to osteitis and periostitis of congenital syphilis.

Hirschsprung disease, 417

Hirsutism, 338–339, 338t

Histiocytic necrotizing lymphadenitis. Benign, self limiting with cervical lymphadenopathy, fever, leukopenia, elevated sedimentation rate and 30% with skin manifestations mimicking drug eruption, rubella, lymphoma or subacute cutaneous lupus erythematosus, especially in young women. Diagnosis is made by lymph node biopsy.

Histiocytoma, 293, 293f, 301

Histiocytoma, generalized eruptive. Widespread symmetric asymptomatic numerous dark red or bluish papules. Appear in crops and spontaneously resolve. It is seen mainly in adults.

Histiocytoma, malignant fibrous. Subcutaneous soft tissue sarcoma is usually of the lower extremities. It may recur and metastasize and wide excision is the treatment of choice. Atypical fibroxanthoma is a less aggressive variant on sun-exposed skin.

Histiocytoma, progressive nodular. A normolipemic proliferative histiocytic syndrome with cutaneous tumors of two types: superficial xanthomatous papules and deep nodules.

Histiocytosis, benign cephalic. Rare histiocytic eruption of infants associated with erythematous pustules mainly on the face, neck or shoulders. There is no visceral involvement. Lesions often involute. Racquet-shaped organelles and S-100-staining cells are absent.

Histiocytosis, congenital self-healing. Rare congenital, generalized, papules, vesicles or nodules with no or mild systemic symptoms with spontaneous resolution of all skin lesions. Pathology shows S100, CD+ cells, and coexistence of laminated dense bodies and Birbeck granules.

Histiocytosis X. Also known as an L-cell (Langerhan's cell histiocytosis) granulomatosis, this includes Letterer-Siwe disease, Hand-Schüller-Christian disease, and eosinophilic granuloma. Characteristic racquet-shaped organelles of Langerhans cells are found on electron microscopy and histiocytes are S-100 positive.

Histoplasmosis. Histoplasmosis is endemic in the Midwestern United States and is caused by *Histoplasma capsulatum,* a soil saprophyte. Inhalation of the spores produces an asymptomatic pulmonary infection that rarely goes on to produce disseminated disease. The secondary skin lesions are multiform, consisting of granulomatous ulcers, purpura, impetiginized lesions, and abscesses, 482–483, 483f

HIV. *See* Human immunodeficiency virus

Hives, 132. *See also* Urticaria

HLA. The term originally meant human leukocyte antigen. It is now known to be the major histocompatibility antigen (MHC) in humans. They have significant implications for immune function including regulation of CD4 (T-helper cells) and CD8 (killer cells).

Hodgkin's disease. *See* Lymphoma

Homocystinuria. Marfanoid body characteristics with malar rash, large facial pores, livedo reticularis, tissue paper scars on the hands, sparse fine hair, and superficial thrombophlebitis. Elevated plasma levels of homocysteine cause increased platelet adhesiveness with resulting deep vein thromboses, pulmonary emboli, and thromboses in cerebral, peripheral and coronary arteries. Autosomal recessive due to defect in cystathione synthetase.

Hookworms, 478, 478f

Hot foot syndrome. Painful, tender nodules on plantar, weight bearing sites caused by pseudomonas exposure from walking in hot tubs or wading pools. Usually self-limited in 2 weeks but may require systemic fluoroquinolones.

Hound dog appearance, 420

Housewives' hand dermatitis, 81

HPV. *See* Human papillomavirus

HSV-1. *See* Herpes simplex virus 1

HSV-2. *See* Herpes simplex virus 2

HTLV-1 (Human T-cell lymphotropic virus, type 1). Virus associated with human T-cell leukemia lymphoma syndrome and tropical spastic paresis. Endemic in Japan, Caribbean base, South and Central America and southeastern USA. Less than 4% of seropositive patients have overt disease. 0.025% of USA blood donors are seropositive. Latent period may be up to 30 years, 471–472

Human immunodeficiency virus (HIV), 240–245, 241f–245f, 307

Human papillomavirus (HPV), 235

Hunter's syndrome. Rare x-linked recessive mucopolysaccharidosis characterized by short stature, stiff joints, claw-like hands, deafness, hepatosplenomegaly, cardiomegaly, unusual facies, and symmetrical ivory-white papulonodules that form reticular ridges over the upper trunk and proximal extremities.

Hutchinson's sign. Extension of pigment onto the lateral and proximal nail fold from a subungual melanoma. Also in herpes simplex where involvement of the nasal tip indicates involvement of the nasociliary branch of the ophthalmic nerve and warrants careful monitoring of the eye for consequent sequalae.

Hutchinson's teeth. Changes in the teeth of patients with congenital syphilis characterized especially by narrowing of the upper incisors with a central depression of the cutting edge.

Hutchinson's triad. The occurrence in patients with congenital syphilis of ocular keratitis, deafness, and dental defects.

Hyalinosis cutis et mucosae. *See* Lipoid proteinosis

Hyaluronic acid, injectable, 46

Hydroa aestivale. This rare recurrent vesicular dermatosis occurs in the summer on the exposed areas of the body. It is more common in young males and usually disappears at the age of puberty. The erythema, urticaria-like lesions, vesicles, and crusted lesions develop following sun exposure and are aggravated by continued exposure. When the vesicle shows a central depression, as in a vaccination, the eruption is called *Hydroa vacciniforme.*

Hydroa vacciniforme. *See* Hydroa aestivale. A severe form of hydroa vacciniforme has been associated with non-Hodgkin's lymphoma. Ebstein-bar virus has been suggested as possibly the causative agent.

Hydrocortisone, 35

α-hydroxy acids, 75

β-hydroxy acids, 75–76

Hypereosinophilic syndrome. Eosinophilia of $1.5 \times 10$ cells/L for at least 6 months with systemic involvement without any other identifiable cause of eosinophilia. Urticaria, angioedema, erythematous papules, and nodules are the commonest cutaneous manifestations.

Hyperhidrosis of the palms. Increased sweating of the palms can be a challenging therapeutic problem. Drysol, Drionic, and botulism injections all have their advocates and transthoracic sympathectomy has been used but can cause concomitant morbidity. Subcutaneous suction curettage after tumescent anesthetic distention or excision of sweat glands are more permanent surgical therapies. Usually improves with age.

Hyperhidrosis. Primary (idiopathic) form usually involves the palms, soles, and axillae. Social and psychological problems can be significant. Certain-Dri and Drysol are aluminum chloride preparations that can be helpful. Iontophoresis (Drionic) with tap water has been used. Botulism toxin has been tried with some success but it needs to be repeated and is painful. Anticholinergic (probanthine) drugs can be taken orally but have other side effects. Beta blockers have been used and are occasionally helpful. Sympathectomy is not always helpful and is fraught with numerous complications. Underlying illnesses that need to be considered are lymphoma (night sweats) and other underlying malignancies, infectious etiologies, and hyperthyroidism. Usually improves with age.

Hyper-IgE syndrome. Autosomal dominant with "cold" staphylococcal abscesses of the skin, atopic dermatitis, lung infection with pneumatoceles, increased serum IgE, defective granulocyte chemotaxis, osteoporosis, retained teeth, prominent forehead, broad nasal bridge, and rough facial skin with prominent pores.

Hyper-IgM immunodeficiency syndrome (HIM). Rare x-linked recessive with increased IgM and IgD and decreased IgA, IgG and IgE. Recurrent pyogenic infections treated with intravenous gamma globulins, and recalcitrant severe oral ulcers, and recalcitrant widespread warts are part of the syndrome.

Hyperimmunoglobulin D syndrome. Laboratory diagnosis depends on at least 2 vitamin D levels greater than 100mg/ml at least 1 month apart. Normal levels of vitamin D have been reported also. It is autosomal recessive with 50% of patients of Dutch ancestry. Mutations occur in the mevalonate kinase (MVK) gene. The first attack is often prior to 1 year of age and lasts 3 to 7 days with a 4 to 8 week asymptomatic period. The attack consists of fever, polymorphic (especially macules) erythematous skin with vasculitis on biopsy, tender cervical lymphadenopathy abdominal pain, 50% splenomegaly, and sometimes aphthous oral or vaginal ulcers.

Hyperkeratosis follicularis en cutem penetrans (Kyrle's disease). A rare, usually non-pruritic eruption, worse on the extremities, of discrete papules with a central keratotic plug. Deeper erythematous papules can leave atrophic scars.

Hyperkeratosis lenticularis perstans (Flegel's disease). Rare disease with tiny keratotic papules usually on the lower extremities in middle aged persons. May have a red halo, and removal leaves pinpoint bleeding site. Can involve oral mucosa.

Hyperpigmentation, 24, 101t, 136, 418–419, 419f
Hypertrichosis, 101t, 339
Hypertrichosis lanuginosa acquisita, 391t
Hypertrophic scar, 293
Hypokeratosis (circumscribed acral hypokeratosis). Idiopathic, well-circumscribed, acquired, solitary, asymptomatic, depressed areas with a raised border on the palms and rarely the soles especially on the hypothenar and thenar prominences. Probably a reaction pattern to various stimuli such as human papilloma virus or trauma.
Hypomelanosis of Ito, 384, 418
Hypopigmentation, 24, 383, 417–418, 417f–418f
Hypoplasia, focal dermal (Goltz syndrome). Rare syndrome usually seen in females with linear hypoplastic skin lesions and vertical striations of long bones. Digit and eye abnormalities also occur.

Ichthyoses, 412, 413t–414t, 414f
Ichthyosiform erythroderma, 426f, 427t
Ichthyosis, 395, 395f
Ichthyosis vulgaris, 391t
Id reaction (autoeczematous reaction). This phenomenon is characterized by an erythematous, vesicular, or eczematous eruption that occurs in disseminated parts of the skin. Most commonly id reactions are seen to follow inflammatory fungal infections of the feet, stasis dermatitis with or without venous ulcers, inflammatory fungus infections of the scalp (kerion), and severe contact dermatitis of the hands., 212. *See also* Dermatophytid; Epidermophytid; Trichophytid; Candidid refers to various organisms involved in the etiology.
Idiopathic guttate hypomelanosis (annular depigmented macules). Small macular, whitish, sharply marginated, approximately 0.5-cm lesions found on sun-exposed extremities, mainly the legs, but never on the face. Related to excessive sun exposure in genetically predisposed persons. Therapy is not necessary or effective.
Idiopathic recurrent palmoplantar hidradenitis. Tender multiple red nodules on the palms and soles that occurs in children and spontaneously involutes in 2-21 days without sequelae. May be related to heat or trauma and has a characteristic histopathology when biopsied.
Idiopathic thrombocytopenic purpura, 431t, 434–435
IgA pemphigus, 188
Immediate pigment darkening, 404
Immersion foot. *See* Frostbite
Immunofluorescence, 12
Immunohistology, 12, 12f
Impetigo, 203–204, 204t, 205f, 430–431, 431t, 432, 431f, 494
Impetigo herpetiformis, 186
Incontinentia pigmenti, 185, 383, 419, 421f, 430, 431t, 433f

Indirect immunofluorescence, 186, 187t
Industrial dermatoses, 78
Infantile pedal papules. Relatively common, usually asymptomatic, flesh-colored papules and tumors seen on the medial aspect of the feet in infants. It occasionally extends onto the heels. Most common at 1 year of age and disappear at 2 to 3 years of age. Benign and require no therapy.
Infectious eczematoid dermatitis, 202t, 211–212, 211f
Inflammatory bowel disease, 394–395, 394f
Insect bites. *See* Bites
Intensed pulsed light (IPL), 41–42, 41f, 42f
Iododerma. A dermatosis due to the ingestion of iodides, usually of a pustular nature.
IPL. *See* Intensed pulsed light
Itch, 5. *See also* Pruritus; Scabies
    swimmer's, 178, 479
    Winter, 22, 179, 448, 448f
Itch-scratch cycle, 196

Jacquet's diaper dermatitis. Granulomatous erosive, diaper dermatitis in school age children with chronic urinary and/or fecal incontinence. May mimic condyloma acuminatum.
Janeway nodes. Palmar-plantar, fingers and plantar toes with painless, irregular, hemorrhagic, nonblanchable papules seen with acute bacterial endocarditis.
Jarisch-Herxheimer reaction. *See* Herxheimer reaction
Jellyfish, 479
Jessner's syndrome (lymphocytic infiltrate of Jessner). Benign lymphocytic infiltration of the skin, mainly of the face, resembling deep chronic discoid lupus erythematosus.

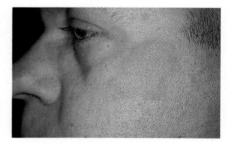

Jessner's benign lymphocytic infiltration of the skin.

Job's syndrome (HIES). Hyperimmunoglobulin E, recurrent infections. Rare, congenital.
Jogger's nipples. Painful erosions of nipples in runners, especially braless females, and when hard, irritating clothing is worn, 490t, 492
Jogger's toe. Subungual hematoma and hyperkeratosis in runners due to repeated trauma due to front of the toe box of the shoe. Tight lacing, high and long toe box, and nail trimming straight and close may all be helpful.

Junctional Epidermolysis Bullosa-Pyloric Atresia syndrome. Rare autosomal recessive with atresia of the gastric antrum or pylorus and bullous disease of the skin and oral mucosa.

Junctional nevus, 294, 295f

Jüngling's disease. *Osteitis fibrosa cystica* of the small long bones, particularly of the fingers, due to sarcoidosis.

Juvenile xanthogranuloma, 431t, 434

Juxta-articular nodes. Syphilitic gummatous tumors occurring in the corium or subcutaneous layer of the skin in the region of the joints.

Kaposiform hemangioendothelioma. Usually seen on the trunk and develops at birth or in neonates in the first few months of life with approximately 25% mortality rate due to tumor infiltration or Kasabach-Merritt syndrome. Destructive bone changes are not uncommon. Treatment is for as other infantile hemangiomas. Transcatheter embolization and surgical excision may be required.

Kaposi's sarcoma, 243–244, 243f, 302, 302f

Kasabach-Merritt syndrome. Rare syndrome of thrombocytopenia, bleeding and petechiae and association with rapidly enlarging, tufted angioma or Kaposiform hemangioendothelioma.

Kassowitz-Diday's law. The observation that successive children of a syphilitic mother will become progressively less infected with syphilis or not be infected at all.

Kawasaki disease, 36. *See also* Mucocutaneous lymph node syndrome

Kawasaki's syndrome, 36, 392

Keloid, 15, 17f, 23f, 39f, 293–294, 293f, 374–375, 375f

　treatment of. Intralesional corticosteroids, 585-nm pulsed dye laser, 30 second liquid nitrogen cryosurgery and silicon gel sheets for 12 to 24 hours each day for at least 2 months.

Keratinization disorders, 412–415, 413t–414t, 414f–415f

Keratoacanthoma, 298, 308f, 309f

Keratoacanthoma centrifugum marginatum. A rare variant of keratoacanthoma that shows progressive peripheral growth with coincident central healing.

Keratoconjunctivitis sicca, 364

Keratoderma blennorrhagicum. A rare chronic inflammatory dermatosis with horny pustular crusted lesions mainly on the palms and the soles; occurs in conjunction with gonorrheal infection of the genital tract and Reiter's syndrome.

Keratoderma climactericum. Circumscribed hyperkeratotic lesions of the palms and the soles of women of the menopausal age. These lesions resemble psoriasis, and the majority of cases are considered to be this disease.

Keratoderma, epidermolytic palmoplantar (EPPK of Vörner). Diffuse, yellowish, hyperkeratotic, thickening of the palms and soles. Familiar or sporadic and has a characteristic shape and erythematous line of demarcation. May be hyperhidrotic and rarely with blisters. Autosomal dominant variant called Unna-Thost has a slightly different histopathology.

Keratolytics, 27

Keratoplastic agents, 27

Keratoses, stucco. Discrete, flat, keratotic papules, "stuck on" to the skin in elderly persons especially over legs, ankles, and tops of the feet. They can be removed by scratching without causing bleeding. Probably a type of seborrheic keratoses.

Keratosis, 100t

　actinic, 20, 281t, 282t, 283t, 289–291, 467–468, 470t

　arsenical, 290, 291, 298

Keratosis follicularis spinulosa decalvans. Rare familial disease with diffuse keratosis pilaris scarring scalp alopecia, photophobia, facial erythema, and palmoplantar keratoderma.

Keratosis Ichthyosis and Deafness. *See* KID syndrome

Keratosis lichenoides chronica. Rare, chronic, progressive, violaceous, lichenoid papules arranged in linear plaques. May be a variant of lichen planus.

Keratosis pilaris rubra. Variant of keratosis pilaris with accompanying redness over the face, extensor upper arms, extensor thighs and buttocks. No atrophy or hyperpigmentation. Seen mainly in children before puberty.

Keratosis pilaris, 431t, 432

KID syndrome. Keratitis, ichthyosis and deafness in a congenital syndrome affecting ectodermal tissue.

Kikuchi-Fujimoto disease (histiocytic subacute necrotizing lymphadenitis with granulocytic infiltration). Painless lymphadenopathy (mainly cervical), leukopenia, fever, myalgias, sore throat, increased LDH, seen more commonly in women with a mean age of 30 years. 40% have cutaneous lesions that may be exudative erythema, facial rash or erythematous papules, plaques or nodules. Histology examination is diagnostic.

Kimura's disease. *See* Angiolymphoid hyperplasia with eosinophilia

Kindler syndrome. A rare condition presenting simultaneous manifestations of both poikiloderma congenitale and epidermolysis bullosa. The four major features are acral blisters, poikiloderma, atrophy, and photosensitivity.

Kissing bug, 477

Klippel-Trenaunay-Parkes-Weber syndrome. Hemihypertrophy of arm or leg associated with varicosities and nevus

flammeus (or hemangioma) with an arteriovenous malformation.

Knuckle pads. Nodules over metacarpal phalangeal and interphalangeal joints. It may be associated with trauma, Dupuytren contracture, camptodactyly, induratio penis plastica, acrokeratoelastoidosis, degenerative collagenous plaques of the hands or Touraine's hereditary polyfibromatosis (knuckle pad disease).

Koebner phenomenon. The ability of the skin to react to trauma by the production of lesions of a previously existing skin disease. This phenomenon occurs in patients with skin diseases such as psoriasis, lichen planus, flat warts (pseudokoebnerization), and lichen nitidus, 160, 162, 169f, 393

KOH preparation, 10

Koplik's spots, 363

Kwashiorkor. Severe dietary protein deficiency seen mainly in poorly developed countries but also in developed countries in infants with protein poor diets (rice milk diets in infants). Diffuse "flaky paint" dermatitis with desquamation as well as stunted growth, decreased stamina, vomiting, diarrhea, anorexia, edema, steatosis, anemia and increased susceptibility to infection. Coma, stupor and fatalities can occur related to infection.

Kyrle's disease. *See* Hyperkeratosis follicularis en cutem penetrans

Labial melanotic macule (solitary labial lentigo). Pigmented macules (often singular) on the lower lip (most common), tongue or intraoral mucosa. Biopsy shows a lentigo.

LAMB syndrome. **L**entigines, **a**trial myxoma, **m**ucocutaneous myxomas, and **b**lue nevi.

Lamellar ichthyosis, 413t

Langerhans cell, 4

Lanugo hair, 337

Larva migrans, 478, 478f

Lasers, 38–41, 39f–41f

　carbon dioxide, 38–39, 39f

　neodymium:yttrium aluminum garnet (Nd:Yag), 39, 40f

　pulsed dye, 39, 40f

　Q-switched, 39, 40f

Lassar's paste. Zinc oxide paste (U.S.P.) containing 25% zinc oxide, 25% starch, and 50% petrolatum.

Latrodectism, 480–481, 481f

Laugier-Hunziker syndrome. Rare disorder of numerous pigmented macules mainly on the lower lip, hand, palate, and tips of the fingers. No underlying gastrointestinal polyposis. Occur in 3rd to 5th decade and may also be seen on the nails (may be a linear band), soles, abdomen, neck, thorax, floor of the mouth, gums, and the labial commissures.

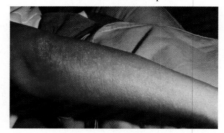

White monotonous papules on the forearm in lichen nitidis

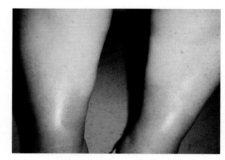

Lipodermatosclerosis of the lower extremities with wine bottle deformity

Lipogranuloma. Fat necrosis of breast tissue commonly due to trauma.

Lipogranulomatosis subcutanea (Rothmann-Makai syndrome). Characterized by subcutaneous nodules mainly on the legs, tender to touch, lasting 6 to 12 months. Seen mainly in children. Patients are afebrile.

Lipoid proteinosis (Urbach-Wiethe disease). Autosomal recessive disease in which infiltration of glycoprotein causes hoarseness, induration of the tongue, and nodular lesions on the eyelids, elbows, knees, hands, and face.

Lipoma, 288, 301

Lipomatosis. Encephalocraniocutaneous. *See* Encephalocraniocutaneous lipomatosis, benign symmetric, Symmetric accumulation of normal fatty tissue on the neck, upper back, proximal arms, and shoulders. Rare, mainly males (15:1) especially in alcoholics but malignancies and metabolic syndromes have been reported. Gives a "pseudoathletic" appearance.

Liposarcoma, 301
  Malignant tumor of fat with 20%–40% recurrence rate and 30%–50% metastasis rate. Usually on the lower extremities and usually intramuscular especially in patients 40–60 years of age.

Liposuction, 44, 44f

Lipotransfer, 45–46

Livedo reticularis. A reddish blue mottled discoloration of the skin of the extremities, which can be divided into three forms: (1) *cutis marmorata,* which develops following exposure to cold and disappears on warming the skin; (2) *idiopathic form* not related to temperature changes; and (3) a *secondary form* associated with various types of vascular disease (vasculitis and vasculopathy), 141, 143f

Lobomycosis, 487, 487f

Lofgren's syndrome. Erythema nodosum and bilateral arthritis usually heralding sarcoidosis.

Loose anagen syndrome, 340t, 342

Loxoscelism, 481

LSC. *See* Lichen simplex chronicus

Lucio's phenomenon. Necrotizing vasculitic lepromatous leprosy with painful hemorrhagic ulcers and severe systemic disease that may be fatal.

Lupus erythematosus, 36, 101t, 111, 385–386, 385f, 386t, 402, 402f, 408t
  acute cutaneous, 385–386, 387t
  Chilblain. *See* Chilblain lupus erythematosus
  chronic cutaneous, 385–386, 385f, 387t
  neonatal, 386
  subacute cutaneous, 385–386, 385f, 387t
  systemic, 149, 159, 386, 386t
  vulgaris, 215, 215t

Lupus erythematosus tumidus. This is felt by some authors to be a variant of chronic cutaneous lupus erythema-

tous. It is characterized by marked photosensitivity and seen most often in sun exposed areas. Erythema and edema respond adequately to topical corticosteroids and systemic antimalarials but recurrence is common after therapy is stopped. Direct immunoflourescence is usually negative and histology is moderately specific.

Lyell's disease. *See* Toxic epidermal necrolysis

Lyme disease, 228–229, 397

Lymephobia, 229

Lymphadenoma. Cutaneous lymphadenoma is a rare, benign, slowly enlarging, adult-onset tumor usually on the head that does not recur after surgical excision. Pathologic examination is diagnostic.

Lymphangioma, 302

Lymphangitis, sclerosing, of the penis. Cord-like lesion in the coronal sulcus that usually resolves within 2 months, is sudden in onset, and usually is asymptomatic.

Lymphedema. This may be *congenital (Milroy's disease)* or *acquired.* Acquired lymphedema of unknown cause can occur in young women, and it can occur following chronic or recurrent cellulitis and lymphangitis *(elephantiasis nostras).* The classic form of lymphedema is the elephantiasis associated with filariasis of the tropics.

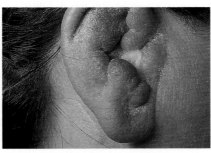

Lymphedema (elephantiasis nostras) of the ear (*Dr. M. Feldaker*).

Lymphocytic cicatricial alopecia, 344

Lymphogranuloma venereum, 274–275, 275f, 506t

Lymphogranulomatosis benigna. *See* Sarcoidosis

Lymphoma, 243, 297, 298t, 303, 396. *See also* Marginal zone B-cell lymphoma

Lymphoma, intravascular large cell. *See* Angioendotheliomatosis, malignant

Lymphomatoid granulomatosis. A serious vasculitis, primarily of the lungs. Skin lesions occur in more than one third of patients, mainly erythematous papules, plaques, and subcutaneous nodules, which may ulcerate. Approximately 15% develop lymphoma.

Lymphomatoid papulosis. Self-healing, erythematous, maculopapular lesions that occasionally ulcerate. Mimics pityriasis lichenoides et varioliformis acuta of Mucha and Habermann.. Clinically these look benign, but histologically

they appear malignant. The more chronic form may become a lymphoma, but most cases run a benign course. Persistently agminated papules are usually a precursor to cutaneous lymphoma.

Macula cerulea. *See* Tache bleuatre.

Macule, melanotic. *See* Genital melanotic macule; Labial melanotic macule

Madelung's disease. Rare syndrome of symptomatic benign lipomatosis. Usually in the cervical region giving a "horse collar" appearance. Adult onset (30–60 years old) and increased in males (15:1).

Maduromycosis. *See* Mycetoma

Maffucci's syndrome. Multiple enchondromas (Ollier's disease) and subcutaneous hemangiomas with up to 30% of patients developing chondrosarcomas.

Majocchi's granuloma. A deep, nodular, inflammatory, mycotic infection due to dermatophyte fungi, especially *T. rubrum.*

Malacoplakia. Rare condition of accumulation of phagocytic macrophages usually in immunocompromised patients. Usually involves the genitourinary tract but can involve the skin in mainly the perineal areas. Michaelis-Gutmann bodies are electron dense intracytoplasmic laminations seen in macrophages.

Malherbe's tumor

Malignant granular cell schwannoma, 302

Malignant melanoma, 283, 284t, 297, 445f, 469–470

Mal perforans ulcer, 17

Mantoux. *See* Tuberculin tine test

Marginal zone B-cell lymphoma (Immunocytoma). The commonest primary cutaneous B-cell lymphoma. Still quite rare. Low grade with good overall outcome. Characteristic histopathology. Medium sized indolent nodules on the trunk, upper extremities and scalp. Responds to x-ray but relapse is common in the skin and extra nodal sites such as the orbit, salivary glands, and breast.

Marshall's syndrome. Pediatric Sweet's syndrome (acute neutrophilic dermatosis) and cutis laxa due to loss of dermal elastic tissue. Associated with Alpha-1 antitrypsin deficiency.

Mascara, 73

McCune-Albright syndrome. Sexual precocity with polyostotic fibrous dysplasia, café-au-lait spots, pituitary adenomas, adrenal hypercorticolism, hyperthyroidism, and osteomalacia, 380, 382f

McKusick syndrome (cartilage hair hypoplasia). Autosomal recessive with short stature, short limbs, hair abnormalities and immunodeficiency associated with an increased risk of infections and malignancy (especially leukemia and non-Hodgkin's lymphoma)

Measles (Rubeola), 236–237

Mechanic's hands. Hyperkeratotic, lichenified, fissured dermatitis over radial sides of the hands and inner edge of the feet. Similar to calloused hands seen in manual laborers. Most closely associated with antisynthetase syndrome but can also be seen in polymyositis, systemic lupus erythematosus, systemic scleroderma, and overlap syndromes.

Mediterranean Fever, Familial. Autosomal recessive syndrome of recurrent febrile episodes of peritonitis, pleuritis, and joint synovitis. Erysipelas-like skin lesions occur most commonly but bullae, pyoderma, panniculitis, and vasculitis may be seen. Predominantly in Arabic, Turkish, Armenian, and Sephardic Jewish people.

Melanocytosis, familial genetic. Diffuse brown hyperpigmentation with raindrop hypopigmentation caused by failure of melanocytes to deliver melanin to the surrounding keratinocytes. Probably autosomal dominant with characteristic histopathology.

Melanonychia. Longitudinal, hyperpigmentation of nailbeds in lines along the long axis due to a normal variant in darkly pigmented patients, PUVA therapy, infliximab, neoplasm, HIV, chemotherapy, and antimalarials. Transverse, hyperpigmentation in transverse lines across nails due to radiation therapy, infliximab, zidovudine, antimalarials, and chemotherapy.

Melanosis, Becker's (Becker's nevus). Large localized mottled hypermelanotic noncongenital, and hypertrichotic patches, located especially on the upper back; not associated with underlying structural abnormalities and without cancer potential.

Melanosis of Riehl. A brownish pigmentation of the skin on the sun-exposed areas of the body that have come into contact with certain tars.

Melanotic macule. *See* Genital melanotic macule; Labial melanotic macule

Melanotic macule of the nail unit. The commonest cause of a pigmented longitudinal streak of the nail plate. Caused by an increase in melanin production by the melanocytes of the nail matrix. It must be biopsied especially in fair skinned patients to rule out a malignant melanoma.

Melasma. *See* Chloasma

Melioidosis. An infectious disease of rodents and humans with abscesses and pustules of the skin and other organs, similar to glanders.

Melkersson-Rosenthal syndrome. Idiopathic facial swelling, facial nerve palsy, and lingua plicata (fissured tongue, scrotal tongue).

Menkes' Kinky Hair syndrome. Impaired metabolism of copper (serum Cu below 25% of normal), x-linked, hair shaft abnormalities (pili torti, monilethrix), stretchable skin (especially over the hands), central nervous system abnormalities, and failure to thrive.

Merkel cell cancer. Highly malignant (approximately 33 % mortality at 3 years), rare, reddish, dome-shaped tumor of neuroendocrine origin, usually seen on the face. As many as 90% have 3 or more of the AEIOU (asymptomatic/lack of tenderness, expanding rapidly, immune suppression, older than 50 years, ultraviolet exposed site on a fair complexion patient) criteria.

Metabolic syndrome. Polycystic ovaries, insulin resistance, hirsutism, acanthosis nigricans, obesity, skin tags, acne, abnormalities of periods often with amenorrhea. Also associated with increased triglycerides and LDL cholesterol. Some studies show an increase in psoriasis.

Meyerson's nevus. An eczematous halo clinically and histologically described in benign nevocellular nevi, atypical nevi, and congenital nevi.

Meyerson's phenomenon. Transient, eczematous dermatitis around nevi, seborrheic keratoses, basal cell carcinomas, squamous cell carcinomas, and dermatofibroma associated with the appearance of these tumors. Affects healthy individuals, is rare, and has no proven etiology. The tumors stop forming after the inflammation dissipates. Seborrheic keratoses may decrease in number.

Microcystic adnexal carcinoma. Locally aggressive adnexal malignancy. Often recurs after radiation or surgery. Mainly affects the central face with a slow growing cystic papule or plaque that infiltrates deeply into surrounding structures. It is a difficult clinical diagnosis since it is so nonspecific. Often with sensory changes such as numbness, tenderness or paresthesias. Characteristic pathology.

Microscopic polyangiitis. A microscopic form of MPO-ANCA-positive vasculitis now separated from classic polyarteritis nodosa. There is an absence of immunoglobulin and complement localization in vessels. There is often a severe progressive course with necrotizing and crescentic glomerulonephritis and pulmonary capillaritis. Approximately 30% have skin lesions with palpable purpura, erythematous macules, and livedo reticularis mainly seen on the lower extremities.

Mid-dermal elastolysis. Rare acquired disease well-circumscribed fine wrinkling and/or papular protrusions especially on the trunk, neck, and arms. It especially affects middle-aged women after prolonged artificial or natural ultraviolet exposure. Histopathological exam is diagnostic with loss of elastic tissue in the mid-dermis.

Milker's nodules. A viral disease contracted from the infected udders of cows. The lesions, usually on the hands, consist of brown-red or purple firm nodules that subside in 4 to 6 weeks, conferring immunity.

Minimal erythema dose(MED), 404

Mitochondrial DNA syndromes. A group of genetic diseases that may appear at any age. Growth retardation, myopathy, seizures, renal failure, eye disease, and occasionally skin disease. Symmetrical cervical lipomas and poikiloderma are the commonest skin manifestations. Defects of mitochondrial DNA can be acquired and be related to aging and many diseases.

Mole. *See* Nevus

Mondor disease. Thrombophlebitis as subcutaneous veins on the anterolateral thoracoabdominal wall. Palpable, visible, tender, painful cords in the mammary areas from the axilla to the subcostal margin. Three times more common in women. It is usually benign and self-limited but underlying conditions especially breast cancer must be ruled out. Inciting events including trauma, surgery, infection, increased physical activity, and pendulous breasts.

Monkeypox. Viral infection transmitted in the United States mainly from prairie dogs that were kept as pets. Fever, malaise, lymphadenopathy, headache, backache and fatigue with pox lesions 2 to 4 days later at first around bite or scratch and then generalized papules to vesicles to pustules. These progress to erosions and crusts and heal without scarring and no significant long term morbidity or mortality.

Monoclonal antibodies. Specific antibodies produced from a hybrid cell. This hybrid cell results from the fusion of nuclear material from two cells. Used for therapy for cancer, psoriasis, autoimmune bullous disease, and many other diseases.

Monosymptomatic hypochondriacal psychosis (MHP), 196–198, 197f

Morbilliform, 24

Morgellon's disease. Cutaneous dysthesia caused by perceived invasion of foreign material. Long strips of keratotic debris is reported to be pulled out by the patient. Olanzapine and pimozide have been shown to be helpful therapeutic agents. There are well financed, well formed, very formidable consumer groups at work here as with other similar diseases.

Morphea, 388t

Morphea, postirradiation. Occurs 1 month to 3 years after supervoltage radiation for malignancy (usually breast cancer and subcutaneous lymphoma). Usually but not always, confined to radiation port. Treatment is difficult but usually slow improvement occurs. Clinically and histologically similar to morphea.

Morcicatio buccarum et labiorum (morcicatio). Habitual excessive cheek and lip biting that becomes a fixed neurosis in patients that may be unaware of the habit. Misdiagnosis of pemphigus, lichen planus or leukoplakia is common. Biopsy is distinctive.

Mosaic "fungus." Not a fungus but an artifact commonly found in KOH slide preparations taken from the feet and the hands. They consist of beaded lines outlining epidermal cell borders and are due to precipitation of KOH.

Mucinosis. When fibroblasts produce an excess amount of acid mucopolysaccharides (mucin), that may replace the connective tissue elements. This occurs in myxedema and localized pretibial myxedema. *See also* Myxedema, localized

follicular (alopecia mucinosa). This rare disease is characterized by one or more symptomatic, well-circumscribed, indurated, slightly erythematous plaques with loss of hair. The most common site is the face. The plaques involute spontaneously after several months. Some cases are associated with a T-cell lymphoma.

papular. A rare cutaneous fibromucinous disease with a monoclonal serum protein of cathodal mobility. Clinically seen as localized or generalized papules, plaques, or nodules.

mucinosis, reticular erythematous (REM). Erythematous papules and plaques mainly on the chest of middle-aged women. Worsens with sun exposure. Characteristic mucin and lymphocytic infiltrate around vessels and follicles. Thyroid disease should be considered.

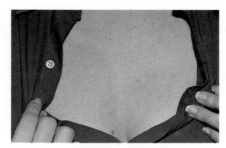

Reticular erythematous mucinosis (REM).

Muckle-Wells syndrome. Rare autosomal dominant with urticaria-like eruptions in infancy associated with progressive perceptive deafness, limb pain, periodic fever, malaise, and amyloid nephropathy.

Mucocutaneous lymph node syndrome. (Kawasaki's disease). A self-limited febrile illness seen mainly in children, with conjunctivitis, dryness and redness of lips, reddening of palms and soles with later characteristic digital skin desquamation, polymorphous exanthema of the trunk, and swelling of cervical lymph nodes. May be associated with coronary artery aneurysms, 392

Mucormycosis. Nodules and ulcerations caused by *Mucor* or *Rhizopus* fungi in patients that are uremic, diabetic, or otherwise immunocompromised. May also occur under adhesive tape. Rare cause of necrtotizing fasciitis.

Muir-Torre syndrome. Rare genodermatosis (autosomal dominant) of sebaceous neoplasms (adenomas, especially sebaceous adenoma, epitheliomas, carcinomas) and visceral cancer (especially genitourinary and gastrointestinal) with prolonged survival.

Multicentric reticulohistiocytosis. Rare condition of numerous reddish or yellow papules on the dorsal hands (especially nail folds and distal interphalangeal joints), ears, and bridge of the nose. Associated with arthritis mutilans, and one fourth of patients have an underlying cancer. The histiocytic infiltrate is characteristic on pathology and may involve internal organs. May be treated successfully with alkylating agents systemically.

Multinucleate cell angiohistiocytoma. Rare red-brown grouped papules especially in middle-aged and elderly females. Innocuous and may spontaneously dissipate. Confused with Kaposi's sarcoma and angiofibromas but histopathology is characteristic.

Multiple endocrine neoplasia IIB, 393

Multiple minute digitate hyperkeratosis. Rare skin condition of multiple, tiny, spiky projections and dome shaped keratotic papules on the face, extremities

and trunk. It can occur on the palms. Reports have been made in association with numerous underlying malignant and benign conditions.

Multiple mucosal neuroma syndrome, 393

Mycetoma, 485, 485f

Mycobacterial infections, 202t, 215–219, 216f–218f, 475–476, 475f

leprosy as, 202t, 216–218, 217f, 218f

tuberculosis of skin as, 202t, 215–216, 216f–218f, 215t

Mycology, 246–265, 248f, 249t, 250t, 250t–251t, 252f–254f, 256f, 257f, 259t, 260f–265f

Mycosis fungoides (CTCL or cutaneous T-cell lymphoma), 36, 298t, 304

Myelosis, 304

Myiasis. Infestation of the skin with flies (*Diptera*), usually the larva. This has been used to debride chronic necrotic skin ulcers.

Myofibromatosis, infantile. Commonest fibrous tumor of infancy. Fifty percent present at birth and 90% present in first 2 years of life. Benign and usually with good prognosis. Usually solitary on the extremities and may recur after excision. Rare, congenital, hard pink purple nodules in the skin, bone, heart, lung, gastrointestinal tract and central nervous syndrome. Cutaneous solitary or multiple lesions without visceral involvement has a good prognosis with spontaneous regression common. When visceral disease is present it is often fatal in the first few months of life. It can be autosomal recessive or autosomal dominant.

Myxoid cyst, 358

Myxoma, 301

Myxosarcoma, 301

Nail(s), 7, 347–359, 349f–358f

anatomy of, 347, 348f

brittle, 355, 355f

diseases of, 421, 422f, 431t, 438, 439f, 440f

enamels, 74

green, 254

habit tic deformity of, 354, 354f

ingrown, 353–354, 353f

internal diseases of, 431t, 438, 439f, 440f

longitudinal melanonychia of, 355–356, 356f

median canaliform dystrophy of, 354

onychocryptosis of, 353–354, 353f

onychomycosis of, 347–350, 349f, 350f

pincer, 352–353, 353f

pits, 351

psoriasis of, 351–352, 351f

racket, 354

rough, 354, 355f

squamous cell carcinoma with, 357–358, 357f

subungual hematoma of, 352, 352f

tinea, 247t, 253–254, 253f

trachyonychia of, 354, 355f

tumors of, 356–358, 357f, 358f

twenty-nail dystrophy. Longitudinal striations with distal splitting of all the nail plates, may be a variant of lichen planus, 431t, 438

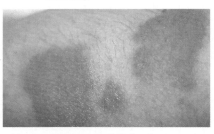

Neutrophilic acute febrile dermatosis (Sweet's syndrome) (*Dr. J. DeSpain*).

occur without underlying signs of other organ involvement, can be seen with osteopoikilosis in the Buschke-Ollendorf syndrome, or as shagreen patches in tuberous sclerosis. Biopsy shows increased amounts of collagen bundles and elastic fibers.

depigmentosus, 426
dysplastic syndrome, 294, 295–296, 303
epidermal. *See* Epidermal
halo, 295f, 296
intradermal, 294
junctional, 291t, 294, 295f, 303
linear epidermal, 297, 298f
lipomatosus superficialis, 301
Mongolian spots, 303
pigmented, 441
resting, 294
sebaceous, 299, 299f
speckled lentiginous. *See* Nevus spilus
Spitz, 296

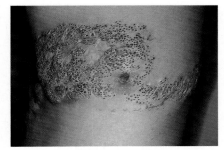

Nevus comedonicus on the abdomen.

targetoid, seen in children and young adults. Target-like shape with rings of clear skin or lighter brown pigments. Benign and often dissipates over 6 to 12 months.
Nevus cell tumors, 281t, 294–297, 295f, 296f, 303
Nevus depigmentosus. Non-progressive hypopigmented macule in children that may begin at birth (19.4%) or after the age of 3 (7.4%). It may be segmental (40%) and is due to a decrease number of melanocytes and decreased pigment. It is not associated with underlying abnormalities.
Nevus flammeus, 429f
Nevus lipomatosis cutaneous superficialis. Rare idiopathic hamartoma with dermal adipose tissue not connected to underlying fat. There are two main types. The multiple types are soft, benign, non-tender yellow papules and plaques that are often linear, zosteriform, systematized and often along lines of skin folds. They can occur anytime of life but often congenital and occur mainly on the upper thighs, buttocks, and pelvic girdle and lumbar areas. The solitary type can occur anywhere usually 30–60 years of age.
Nevus sebaceous (Jadassohn), 299, 299f, 427, 427t, 431t, 434
Nevus simplex, 426, 427t, 429f
Nevus, speckled lentiginous (Nevus spilus). Congenital light brown lentigo with

scattered spots of junctional nevi. Very rarely one of the junctional nevi is a precursor of malignant melanoma, 296f
Nevus spilus. *See* Nevus, speckled lentiginous
Nicolau syndrome (embolia cutis medicamentosa). Intra-arterial and periarterial intramuscular injection resulting in acute painful induration, ecchymosis, livedo with fibrin thrombi occluding vessels and resulting in hemorrhagic infarcts. Heparin and systemic corticosteroids are suggested treatments. Infection (rarely necrotizing fasciitis), paresthesias, myositis, abscess, muscle atrophy, palsies, scars or sphincter incontinence can result, 102t
Nigua, 481
Nikolsky's sign. The Nikolsky's test is positive in patients with pemphigus and toxic epidermal necrolysis and demonstrates acantholysis histologically. The test is performed by pulling the ruptured wall of the blister back into the apparently normal skin, or by rubbing off the epidermis near the bullae with slight friction and producing a moist surface that results in extension of the blister.
Nocardiosis. Various species of *Nocardia* can cause cutaneous, pulmonary, and systemic infection. The cutaneous lesions of the subcutaneous tissue and bones are clinically similar to maduromycosis.
Nodes, Heberden's. Sometimes tender, firm bony outgrowths of the distal interphalangeal joints of the fingers of patients with osteoarthritis.
Nodes, Osler's. Transient, red, painful, nodules located on the palms and the soles in patients with chronic bacterial endocarditis.
Nodular chondrodermatitis of ear, 303
Nodular fasciitis. *See* Fasciitis, nodular
Nodular melanoma. *See* melanoma, nodular
Nodular panniculitis. *See* panniculitis, nodular
Nodular vasculitis, 129
Nodules, 14, 16f, 431t, 432–434, 433f, 434f
Nodules, athlete's. see athlete's nodules.
Nodules, weathering of the ear. Asymptomatic fairly common, multiple, white smooth nodules along the free margin of the helix seen mainly in elderly males with marked sun damage.
Noma (cancrum oris). Mainly 1 to 4 year old children especially in sub-Saharan Africa in association with poverty, malnutrition and HIV. Begins as an oral erosion or black area of perioral or facial skin. Untreated, it progresses to extensive, grotesque, ulcerative, destructive, gangrenous, vegetative growth with destruction of underlying tissue. The children are often shunned by their society. There is a 70 to 90% death rate. It is polymicrobic due mainly to fusobacterium necrophorum and *Prevotella intermedia*. Debridement especially early in its course

and systemic penicillin and metronidazole are therapies of choice.
Nonbullous congenital ichthyosiform erythroderma, 413t, 414f
Nonthrombocytopenic purpura, 139
Nontropical pyomyositis. Similar to tropical pyomyositis but in temperate climates in debilitated elderly patients in association with diabetes mellitus, HIV infection, connective tissue disease, and underlying malignancy.
North American blastomycosis(blastomycsis), 260–261, 260f
Notalgia paresthetica, 130. *See also* Pruritic hereditary localized patch on the back. Rarely a sign of a sensory neuropathy.
Nummular eczema, 19f, 22, 91–93, 92f, 102t, 212, 442f

Obliterans, arteriosclerosis. A degenerative change mainly in the arteries of the extremities; most commonly seen in elderly men. Leg ulcers and gangrene can result from these vascular changes.
Obliterans, thromboangiitis. *Buerger's disease* is an obliterative disease of the arteries and the veins that occurs almost exclusively in young men. It mainly involves the extremities and produces tissue ischemia, ulcers, and gangrene.
Obstetric cholestasis, 510t, 513–514
Occipital Horn syndrome, 420
Occlusive dressing therapy, 139
Ochronosis. A rare hereditary metabolic disorder characterized by a brownish or blackish pigmentation of cartilages, ligaments, tendons, and intima of the large blood vessels due to the deposit of a polymer of homogentisic acid. The urine in ochronosis turns black, particularly in the presence of alkali; hence the term *alkaptonuria. See also* pigmentary disorders. There is an exogenous form at the site of chronic topical hydroquinone application (see Chapter 9), 102t
Ointments, 28, 30–33, 32t
Oleomas. Subcutaneous granulomas due to injection of sesame seed oil used for tissue augmentation or as a slow release substance for anabolic steroids. Usually in bodybuilders.
Olmsted's syndrome. Very rare; consists of congenital keratoderma of the palms and soles, onychodystrophy, constriction of digits, and periorificial keratoses. Can be confused with acrodermatitis enteropathica.
Omenn's syndrome. Combined immunodeficiency. Rare, congenital. A type of severe combined immunodeficiency with lymphocytosis and leukocytosis with eosinophilia. Often fatal in childhood with a chronic skin eruption mimicking severe seborrhea, lymphadenopathy, hepatosplenomegaly, recurrent infections, fever, and failure to thrive. Humoral and cellular immunity are both defective, 436

now believed to be a distinct entity. One chronic form of parapsoriasis, *parapsoriasis guttata,* can resemble guttate psoriasis, pityriasis rosea, or seborrheic dermatitis. This condition does not itch and persists for years. A variant of this type of parapsoriasis is *pityriasis lichenoides chronica* (Juliusberg), which is a form of guttate parapsoriasis with slightly larger scaly areas. Another chronic form of parapsoriasis, *parapsoriasis en plaque,* is characterized by nonpruritic or slightly pruritic scaly brownish patches and plaques. A significant percentage of patients that are given this last diagnosis develop mycosis fungoides, 165

Parasitic diseases, 476–480, 476f–479f
   amebiasis as, 477, 477f
   bilharziasis as, 479–480
   Chagas' disease as, 477
   entamoeba histolytica as, 477
   filariasis as, 478–479
   gnathostomiasis as, 478, 478f
   helminthic dermatoses as, 478–479, 478f
   larva migrans as, 478, 478f
   leishmaniasis as, 476–477, 476f
   onchocerciasis as, 479
   protozoal dermatoses as, 476–477, 477f
   schistosomiasis as, 479–480
   trematodes dermatosis as, 479–480, 479f
   trypanosomiasis sudamericana as, 477

Parasitophobia, 179
Paronychia, 350–351, 431t, 438
Parry-Romberg's syndrome. Facial hemiatrophy in a child with or without sclerodermatous skin changes.
Pasini and Pierini atrophoderma. *See* Atrophies of the skin
Patch test, 9
PCT. *See* Porphyria cutanea tarda
PDT. *See* Photodynamic therapy
Pearly penile papules. Noninflammatory, orangish, innocuous, acral angiofibromas located in a symmetrical ring around the glans of the penis.
Peau d' orange, 24
Pediculosis, 179, 180–182, 181f
Pedunculated fibromas, 281t, 284–286, 287f, 448
Peeling skin syndrome. Very rare autosomal recessive disease, which usually presents at birth or later in childhood. Asymptomatic exfoliation of skin that can be generalized, acral only or face only. The stratum corneum peels at the subcorneal or intracorneal level for a life time and treatment is difficult with emollients seeming to be the most beneficial.
PELVIS syndrome. Perineal hemangiomas, external genital malformations, lipomyelomeningocele, viscerorenal abnormalities, imperforate anus and skin tag. Infants with large perineal hemangiomas should have spinal and pelviperineal imaging done.
Pemphigoid, 35, 103t

cicatricial. Localized scarring cutaneous pemphigoid with mucous membrane disease most notably of the eye. It usually presents first to an ophthalmologist, which results in progressive loss of vision and ultimately blindness. Direct immunofluorescence studies mimic pemphigoid.
localized cicatricial (Brunsting-Perry). In elderly patients, recurrent blisters are seen, most commonly of the head and neck. Histology and immunofluorescence are similar to cicatricial mucosal pemphigoid, but there is no mucous membrane involvement in this form. Heals with scarring.
Pemphigoid gestationis. *See* Herpes gestationis
Pemphigus
   erythematosus, 187
   foliaceous, 187, 488
   herpetiformis. A generalized bullous eruption which resembles dermatitis herpetiformis clinically and histologically, but resembles pemphigus by responding to steroids and immunosuppressive drugs and having a pemphigus direct immunofluorescent pattern, 187
   IgA, 188
   paraneoplastic, 188
   vegetans, 187
   vulgaris, 187–189, 190f, 190
Pemphigus neonatorum, 203
Pemphigus nodularis. Uncommon variant of pemphigoid with prurigo nodularis-like nodules with or without blisters. Histopathology of prurigo nodularis but the direct immunofluorescence is compatible with bullous pemphigoid.
Penile horn. Thick, dry, keratinized epithelium overlying a previously existing lesion on the glans of the penis. Usually preceded by chronic preputial inflammation and long-standing phimosis in individuals who undergo adult circumcision. The underlying tumor can be benign epidermal hyperplasia, warts, keratoacanthoma and, up to 1/3, with a squamous cell carcinoma.
Perforating skin disorders. Several dermatoses exhibit epidermal perforation as a histologic feature. Many represent transepithelial elimination. Four diseases are essential perforating disorders: elastosis perforans serpiginosa, reactive perforating collagenosis, perforating folliculitis, and Kyrle's disease.
Periadenitis mucosa necrotica recurrens, 363, 363f
Perianal streptococcal dermatitis. Sharply demarcated painful erythema usually in children that may lead to pain, painful defecation, pruritus, tenesmus, constipation, rectal bleeding, and anal discharge. Usually Group A beta hemolytic streptococci (rarely staphylococcus aureus) is causative.
Perianal pyrimidiform protrusion (see perianal protrusion, infantile). Exophytic flesh

colored to pink soft tissue swelling along the median rafe in the genital area in children especially females. Associated with diarrhea or constipation and may resolve when gastrointestinal normalcy is restored. May be confused with condyloma accuminata.
Periarteritis nodosa, 135
Perifolliculitis capitis abscedens et suffodiens. (dissecting cellulitis of the scalp). Draining dissecting pustular sinuses and abscesses in the scalp. Part of the follicular occlusion triad that also includes cystic acne and hidradenitis suppurativa.
Perineal erythema. See recurrent toxin-mediated perineal erythema.
Perineal protrusion, infantile (see pyradimal pyrimidoform profusion). A pyradimal soft-tissue protrusion with a tongue-like lip and velvety surface located in the midline just anterior to the anus in neonates. It can be genetic, functional after diarrhea, constipation or other irritation or associated with lichen sclerosis et atrophicus. It usually resolves with time and therapy of any underlying condition with rarely a need for surgical intervention.
Perioral dermatitis. Common and mainly seen in women with pinhead sized papules and pustules and some accompanying desquamative erythema. Often with a perioral halo meeting the lips only at the corners of the mouth. First improves with topical corticosteroids and then worsens with topical corticosteroids. Improves within 2 to 4 weeks of oral tetracycline or erythromycin. Topical clindamycin and erythromycin as well as topical metronidazole have been used with some success. Rarely occurs around the eyes, nares and even perirectal so some authors feel it should be called periorificial dermatitis. There is a more chronic granulomatous form
Pernio. See Chilblain; Frostbite
Persistent pigment darkening, 404
Petechiae, 15, 139, 141
Peutz-Jeghers syndrome, 395, 423t
PHACES syndrome. Large facial hemangiomas especially in female infants associated with posterior fossa brain abnormalities (most often Dandy-Walker type malformations). Other anomalies are ocular, cardiac, and vertebral maldevelopment.
Phacomatosis pigmentokeratotica. Rare syndrome with simultaneous occurrence of organoid epidermal nevus and speckled lentigines nevus.
Phacomatosis pigmentovascularis. Rare syndrome of simultaneous occurrence of nevus flammeus and pigmented nevus, nevus pigmentosas, mongolian spot, nevus spilus, nevus verrucosus or nevus anemicus.

PIBIDS. Photosensitivity, ichthyosis, brittle hair (trichothyrodystrophy), intellectual impairment, delayed development, and short stature.

Piedra. The word is Spanish for stone and refers to a fungal infection of the hair shaft forming gritty adherent nodules. Black piedra is caused by Piedraia hortae and appears mainly on scalp hairs in tropical countries as dark hard nodules. White piedra is caused by Trichosporun beigelii and other Trichosporum species and appears as white nodules on scalp hair in tropical and temperate regions. The disease mimics the nits of pediculosis capitis but can be distinguished by KOH examination of the hair shafts. Treatment is accomplished by antifungal azole shampoos and oral agents.

Piezogenic papules. Herniation of fat into the dermis that are painful or asymptomatic seen only on standing on the lateral or medial heel. 2–5 mm and flesh colored.

Pigmentation, idiopathic eruptive macular. Spontaneously regressing (months to years), idiopathic, asymptomatic, brown, confluent macules. No previous inflammation, no drug association, on the trunk, neck and proximal extremities in children and adolescents. Basal cell layer hyperpigmentation and prominent dermal melanocytes and no increase in mast cells on skin microscopy.

Pilonidal sinus. Cavity lined by epithelial or granulation tissue often containing hair. Usually sacrococcygeal but can occur in other hair-bearing areas. It can be occupational in the interdigital areas of the hands of barbers, milkers, sheep shearers and dog groomers. Treatment is surgical and control of secondary bacterial or fungal infection.

Pincer nails. Transverse curling of the nail along its longitudinal axis. It may arise as a developmental abnormality but may be acquired due to subungual exostosis, osteoarthritis, onychomycosis, traumatic acroosteolysis, epidermal cysts, and psoriasis. It is painful and may require nail surgery. See under chapter on nails, 352–353, 353f

Pink disease. See Acrodynia

Pityriasiform. Used in naming many skin diseases to describe fine, tiny scale.

Pityriasis amiantacea. A distinct morphologic entity characterized by masses of sticky, silvery, overlapping scales adherent to the hairs and scalp. When the thick patch of scales is removed, the underlying scalp is red and oozing and often has a foul odor. The underlying cause can be tinea, pyoderma, neurodermatitis, or psoriasis.

Pityriasis lichenoides chronica (Juliusberg). A form of guttate parapsoriasis. See Parapsoriasis.

Pityriasis lichenoides et varioliformis acuta (Mucha-Habermann). An acute disease that appears as a reddish macular generalized eruption that may have mild constitutional signs including fever and malaise. Vesicles may develop and also papulonecrotic lesions. This disease gradually disappears in several months. Histologically, it is characterized by a vasculitis that differentiates it from the parapsoriasis group of diseases. It may improve with UVB therapy or oral antibiotics (tetracycline, erythromycin). There is a febrile ulceronecrotic form that can involve the liver and gastrointestinal tract and be fatal. Methotrexate, dapsone and systemic corticosteroids may be life-saving., Some authors think pityriasis lichenoides chronica is a chronic form of this disease.

Pityriasis rubra pilaris. Papulosquamous psoriasiform eruption that often begins in the scalp and progresses to an erythroderma with islands of normal skin. Keratoderma of the palms and soles ("keratotic sandal") is common. Clinically mimics psoriasis and histological examination may help in differentiation. It has a bimodal distribution in the first and fifth decades. Retinoids and methotrexate are the mainstays of therapy which is not always satisfactory.

Pityriasis simplex faciei (pityriasis alba). A common disorder of children seen predominantly in the winter as a well-localized, scaly, hypopigmented, oval patch on the cheeks, upper outer arms, and upper outer legs. The end result is hypopigmentation of the area, but the normal pigment returns when the eruption clears up (usually in the summer, however, an initial tan may make it temporarily more prominent). We believe this condition to be a mild form of atopic eczema.

Plantar fibromatosis (Ledderhose disease). The equivalent of Dupuytren's contracture (palmar fibromatosis) except it occurs on the plantar surface of the foot. Abnormal fibrous tissue replaces the plantar aponeurosis. Contractures are rare but there are slowly growing, sometimes painful, flesh-colored, fixed nodules especially on the central or medial sole of the foot. It can be bilateral and, if painful, intralesional corticosteroids or surgery for more aggressive disease is indicated. Recurrence is common.

Plasmacytoma. Rare cutaneous B-cell lymphoma. Erythematous papules and plaques. Death from disseminated disease occurs in a minority of patients.

Plica polonica. Rare disorder where scalp hair shafts become irreversibly entangled into a matt of malodorous encrusted, sticky, moist mass. Predisposng factors include pediculosis capitis, pyoderma, poor hygiene, and deficient hair care. Removal of the plait of hair is necessary for therapeutic improvement. Some ethnic groups consider it a sign of health and recommend it to be left in place ("polish plat," "Rasfarian hair style,").

Plummer-Vinson syndrome. A syndrome characterized by dysphagia, glossitis, hypochromic anemia, and spoon nails in middle-aged women. The associated dryness and atrophy of the mucous membranes of the throat may lead to leukoplakia and squamous cell carcinoma

Podoconiosis (non-filarial endemic elephantiasis of the lower legs). Asymmetric, bilateral elephantiasis nostras of the lower extremities seen in the highlands of Africa, Central and South America, and Indonesia due to walking barefoot on volcanic soil where small amounts of silica are absorbed through the feet and obstruct the lymphatics.

POEMS syndrome.(**P**olyneuropathy,**O**rganomegaly,**E**ndocrinopathy,**M**-protein, and **S**kin changes). Cherry-type and subcutaneous hemangiomas, hyperpigmentation, and hypertrichosis are reported in this syndrome. Glomeruloid hemangioma may be quite specific.

Poikiloderma congenitale. A rare syndrome characterized by telangiectasis, pigmentation, defective teeth, and bone cysts; may be similar to dyskeratosis congenita.

Poliosis. Localized loss of hair pigment. It has been associated with vitiligo, regrowth of hair in alopecia areata, piebaldism, tuberous sclerosis, malignant melanoma, intradermal nevi, congenital pigmented nevi, halo nevi, and Waardenburg syndrome.

Polychondritis, relapsing. Inflammation of cartilage most often involving the auricle of the ear but that may also involve inflammation of the eye, joints, nose, and most significantly heart valves or upper respiratory tract. The ear will demonstrate recurrent attacks of redness, pain, and swelling.

Polycystic ovary syndrome (Stein-Leventhal). Amenorrhea and large polycystic ovaries, hirsutism (2/3), obesity (1/2) and insulin resistant hyperinsulinemia. Great variations in this syndrome make diagnosis and classification difficult.

Polyfibromatosis. Rare syndrome with multiple cutaneous fibrotic conditions (Dupuytren's contracture, keloids, Peyronie's disease, plantar fibromatosis).

Polymorphic eruption of pregnancy. *See* Pruritic urticarial papules and plaques of pregnancy

Pool toes. Erythematous, tender areas seen from friction against the cement bottom of pools at the beginning of swimming season. Treat by wearing protective footwear, avoiding contact with the bottom of the pool or be observed since protective calluses usually form with time.

Porokeratosis. Begins as a small, slightly elevated, wart-like papule that slowly enlarges, leaving an atrophic center with a keratotic, ridge-like border (coronoid lamellae). The small individual lesions may coalesce, this is the Mibelli type, and squamous cell cancers can arise (1-2% especially if very hyperkeratotic) in these tumors. A disseminated form (disseminated superficial actinic porokeratosis of Chernowski,DSAP) develops in middle-aged persons on sun-exposed limbs. Three other types are linear porokeratosis, porokeratosis punctuate palmaris et plantaris, and porokeratosis palmaris plantaris et disseminate. Histopathology may be characteristic.

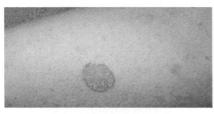

Porokeratosis of the leg.

Potassium permanganate. An oxidizing antiseptic usually used as a wet dressing in the concentration of 1:10,000.

Prausnitz-Küstner reaction. A demonstration of passive sensitization of the skin of a nonsensitive person. This is accomplished by the intradermal injection of serum from a sensitive patient into the skin of a nonsensitive person. After 24 to 48 hours, the allergen to be tested is injected intracutaneously into the previously injected site on the nonsensitive person's skin. Passive transfer of the sensitivity is manifested by the formation of a wheal.

Prayer marks. Lichenification and hyperpigmentation seen mainly in Muslims over bony prominences that experience repeated, extended pressure during times of prayer.

Precalcaneal congenital fibrolipomatosus (podalic papules, bilateral congenital fatty heel pads). Congenital, bilateral nonpulsatile, nontender, soft, skin color, elastic nodules between 0.5 and 1.5cm. Covered with normal epidermis, they are unattached to underlying tissue and do not transilluminate. Usually no therapy is necessary but surgery has been done if there is impairment of function.

Progeria. Extremely rare autosomal dominant mutation condition. Noticed early in life with characteristics of the elderly but no mental changes. Most patients die between 10 and 15 years of age. A factor may be a defect of hyaluronic acid.

Progressive symmetric erythrokeratodermia. *See* Erythrokeratodermia progressive symmetrica

Prolidase deficiency. Rare hereditary syndrome affecting protein degradation. Resistant skin ulcers of the lower extremities are the commonest and most troublesome finding. Scar formation, xerosis, telangiectasias, purpura, poliosis, telangiectasias, and erythematous rash are among many other manifestations.

Proliferating trichilemmal cysts (proliferating pilar tumor). Locally aggressively, rapidly growing, scalp (90% of time) tumors usually in women. Rare malignant transformation.

Protein kinase inhibitors. Anitcancer agents that are selective inhibitors of signal transduction molecules. Research in dermatology is being done for possible treatment for melanoma, nonmelanoma skin cancer, dermatofibrosarcoma protuberans, Merkel cell carcinoma, Kaposi's sarcoma, and systemic mastocytosis. Tyrosine kinase inhibitors are the commonest but threonine and serine can also be inhibited as well as combinations of all three(dual treatment). Histidine kinases are also in development.

Proteus syndrome. Sporadic, progressive, congenital, rare condition which includes hemihypertrophy, epidermal nevi, macrodactyly, scoliosis, exostoses, and a variety of benign hamartomatous skin and sift tissue tumors. Elephant man (John Hermick) exhibited this syndrome even though some authors incorrectly diagnosed neurofibromatosis.

Prototothecosis. Very rare chronic cutaneous infections with a nonpigmented algae (usually Prototheca wickerhamii) having protean clinical manifestations.

Prurigo. This term is used more commonly in Europe. It lacks a precise definition but implies itchy bumps.

  actinic. A chronic photodermatitis seen in native Americans and Hispanics.

Prurigo nodularis. A rare chronic dermatosis, usually of middle-aged women, consisting of discrete nodular pruritic excoriated papules and tumors scattered over the arms and the legs. This can be a warning sign of anemia, liver disease, renal disease, underlying cancer, and human immunodeficiency virus infection.

Prurigo pigmentosa. Rare inflammatory pruritic papules mainly over the upper trunk healing with netlike hyperpigmentation. Pathology is nonspecific. Reportedly mainly in the Japanese literature.

Pruritic hereditary localized patch on the back (notalgia paresthetica). A rather common, benign problem manifested by a single patch of approximately 4 to 8 cm, usually lichenified, on the back. Frequently, the person rubs the area on the door jam or similar scratching post. May be slightly hyperpigmented. Can rarely be associated with impingement on a spinal nerve.

Pruritic papular eruption. Papular, chronic, symmetrical, pruritic eruption in HIV (+) patients without other identifiable cause of pruritus. Common in HIV (+) patients and often seen early in the infection.

Pruritic urticarial papules and plaques of pregnancy (PUPPP syndrome). Most common gestational dermatoses (1 in 200 pregnancies) especially in the third trimester with first pregnancy and more common with twins. Very pruritic papules and plaques beginning in stretch marks on the abdomen (usually spares the periumbilical area) then spreads to the extremities. No perinatal risk to the mother or neonate. Treat with topical or occasionally systemic corticosteroids, 510t, 512–513

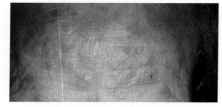

Pseudolymphoma of Spiegler-Fendt.

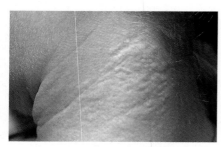

Pseudoxanthoma elasticum of the neck.

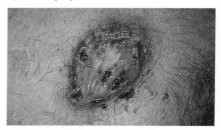

Pyoderma gangrenosum above the nipple.

Radiation recall dermatitis (see Chapter 9). Inflammatory dermatitis at a previously irradiated skin site precipitated by certain medications usually on the first exposure. Clinical features can be erythema, urticarial-like lesions, blisters, necrosis, and ulceration. Medications include gemcitabine, actinomycin D, paclitaxel, doxorubicin, tamoxifen, simvastatin, interferon alpha 2-b, and anti-tuberculous drugs.

Ragweed dermatitis, 9

RAPADILINO syndrome. A subset of Rothmund-Thompson syndrome with RAdial hypoplasia/aplasia, PAtellar hypoplasia/aplasia, cleft of highly arched PAlate, Diarrhea and DIslocated joints, Little size, Limb malformation, slender Nose and NOrmal intelligence.

Rat bite fevers. The bite of a rat can cause *sodoku* and *Haverhill fever*. Sodoku, caused by *Spirillum minus*, is manifested by a primary-type chancre and later by an erythematous rash. Haverhill fever (epidemic arthritic erythema), caused by *Streptobacillus moniliformis*, is characterized by joint pains and an erythematous rash.

Raynaud's disease. Over 3 years of Raynaud's phenomena without underlying disease.

Raynaud's phenomena, 388t, 403. Vascular constriction to cold (especially core body temperatures) resulting in painful color changes of the fingers and toes from red to white to violaceous. Seen most commonly in scleroderma (alone or as part of CREST syndrome) and systemic lupus erythematosus. In its most severe form ulcers and gangrene of the fingertips can occur. Calcium channel blockers and phosphodiesterase inhibitors have been used with some success. Less conventional therapies include TENS units, sildenafil, and acupuncture.

Recombinant DNA technology. A manipulation of specific genetic information from one organism or cell to another.

Recurrent toxin-mediated perineal erythema. Differentiated from Kawasaki syndrome (usually < 2y/o) by age range (usually 3-6 y/o), commonly recurrent, rare heart or platelet abnormality, no cervical lymphadenopathy, rare conjunctival injection, no fever, no polymorphous exanthem, always perineal erythema and known result of streptococcal or staphylococcal infection. Both have oral mucous membrane changes and a strawberry tongue.

Reed syndrome. Autosomal dominant condition with cutaneous and uterine leiomyomas.

Reflex sympathetic dystrophy. see Complex regional pain syndrome.

Refsun's disease. Ichthyosis with progressive neurologic degeneration. Diagnosis by measuring decreased phytanic acid levels.

Reiter's syndrome, 134

Renal failure, chronic, 399

Rendu-Osler-Weber disease, 294

Resorcinol. This agent is similar in its properties and use to salicylic acid, 34

Restrictive dermopathy. Very rare fatal (shortly after birth) autosomal recessive syndrome of very thin, friable, translucent, skin that is associated with arthrogryposis multiplex, microstomia, and microagnathia.

Reticulate acropigmentation of Dohi. Localized hyperpigmented and hypopigmented macules. Autosomal dominant.

Reticulate acropigmentation of Kitamura. Presents in the 1st three decades of life as reticulated hyperpigmentation on extensor, distal extremities, and can affect the face and neck. May develop slight depressions. May have palmar pits. Autosomal dominant or sporadic.

Reticulohistiocytoma, giant-cell. The localized form consists of one or a few asymptomatic large intracutaneous nodules, which may involute with time. The generalized form (*see* Multicentric reticulohistiocytosis) is characterized by many nodules over the body, especially around the fingers, usually associated with a destructive arthritis.

Reticulohistiocytosis, self-healing (Hashimoto-Pritzker disease). Neonatal eruption resolving in the first year of life. S-100 histiocytes and Birbeck granules are present.

Reticulosis, pagetoid (Woringer-Kolopp disease; localized epidermotropic reticulosis). Clinically represented by a single very slowly enlarging warty, plaque-type skin lesion without internal organ involvement. A disseminated type resembles mycosis fungoides. Histologically there is an extensive epidermal infiltration with atypical-appearing mononuclear cells.

Rheumatic fever. Immune response to group A streptococcal infection (usually pharyngitis) that causes carditis, polyarthritis, chorea (has become very rare), and rare skin changes consisting of subcutaneous nodules or erythema marginatum (transient blanching, serpiginous, rapidly spreading erythema especially on the trunk).

Rheumatic vasculitis, 144t

Rheumatoid arthritis, 110t

Rheumatoid neutrophilic dermatitis. Very rare dense dermal neutrophilic dermatoses without vasculitis seen in rheumatoid arthritis mainly in women. Erythematous papules, plaques and rarely vesicles that may be tender appear mainly on the elbows, extensor forearms and dorsal hands. Less often lesions appear on the trunk, palms and soles. They resolve spontaneously and may recur.

It has a poor response to systemic corticosteroids and this is not necessarily associated with a worsening of arthritis or systemic symptoms.

Rheumatoid nodules. Seen in 25% of patients (especially white men) with rheumatoid arthritis (RA). Firm, asymptomatic (except feet or palms) 0.5 to many cm, especially in areas of mild repetitive trauma. A late manifestation of RA is most common with an increased rheumatoid factor titer. Treatment of RA does not affect the nodules and treatment is usually not necessary. Diagnosis is usually made clinically but biopsy is helpful.

Rheumatoid nodulosis. Subcutaneous nodules and associated cystic bone lesions in patients with mild rheumatoid arthritis especially in males 30 to 60 years of age. Usually hands and feet, self-limited, and responds to NSAIDs or hydroxycholoroquine.

Rheumatoid vasculitis. Seen in 1 to 5% of rheumatoid arthritis patients and may cause painful punched out leg ulcers. Rarely (<1%) with systemic involvement which may have significant morbidity and mortality.

Rhinoscleroma, 474, 474f

Rhinosporidiosis. The fungus *Rhinosporidium seeberi* causes a raspberry-like papillomatous tumor of the nares of the nose.

Richner-Hanhart's syndrome. Photophobia, mental retardation, painful palmoplantar keratoderma, usually appearing in the first year of life. Due to a deficiency of tyrosine aminotransferase and may improve with restriction of dietary tyrosine and phenylalanine.

Rickettsial diseases, 202t, 218

Rickettsial pox, see Bacterial disease chapter

Riehl's melanosis, 383. *See* Melanosis of Riehl

Ringworm, 257. *See also* Tinea

Ritter's disease, 203, 430, 432f

River blindness, 479

Rocky Mountain spotted fever, 218, Be suspicious of this disease early because delay in tetracycline (usually doxycycline) or chloramphenicol can have a fatal outcome. A tick bite with unexplained fever, toxicity, nausea, vomiting, muscle pain, and severe headache especially in the South Atlantic United States (Delaware, Maryland, Washington DC, Virginia, North Carolina, South Carolina, Georgia, Florida) should prompt therapy before waiting for the appearance of the rash (3–7days) or laboratory confirmation (weeks). The Pacific Region (Washington, Oregon, California) and the South Central Region (Oklahoma, Louisiana, Arkansas, Texas) are other endemic areas. North Carolina and Oklahoma are the commonest states with 35% of all cases. Children under

aimed at education and protection. Facial ulcerations may also occur.

Tripe palms. Rare thickened velvety palms with accentuated dermoglyphics associated with underlying cancer (pulmonary is the most common).

Triple response of Lewis. A physiologic vascular response that occurs following scratching of the skin or injection of histamine and other related compounds that consists of (1) an immediate red flush due to local capillary dilation, (2) wheal formation due to increased capillary permeability, and (3) an erythematous flare due to reflex dilation of arterioles. *See also* Dermographism

Tropical pyomyositis. Rare abscesses arising mainly in the large muscles of the limbs and trunk. Primarily found in humid areas in Central Africa and Central America but also in the Amazon rainforest. Usually caused by *Staphylococcus aureus* in otherwise healthy children and young adults. Progressive pain, induration and enlargement occur over 1 to 2 weeks. Sepsis and even death in 1 to 2% of patients. Fever, leukocytosis and sed rate elevation occur with normal or only slightly elevated CPK. Scanning techniques help in diagnosis and in defining extent of disease. Treatment is intravenous antibiotics and abscess drainage.

Tropical ulcer (tropical pagedenic ulcer). Rapidly growing, painful, sloughing ulcer usually on the lower leg in undernourished children or rural laborers who tend to injure their leg. Most common in hot tropical regions. Polymicrobic with fusobacterium, anaerobic microorganisms (Baccilus fusiformis) and spirochetes (Treponema vincenti). May reach the muscle and periosteum. Treatment is tetracycline and metronidazole.

Troisier's Sign. An enlarged lymph node (Virchow's node) in the supraclavicular fossa due to metastasis from an abdominal malignancy. The spread of the cancer occurs via the thoracic duct.

Trousseau's syndrome. *See* Thrombophlebitis, superficial migratory

T.R.U.E. Test (Glaxo), 9, 77

Trypanosomiasis, 477

Tuberculin tine test (Mantoux), 9

Tuberculoid leprosy, 216f, 217

Tuberculosis of the skin, 36, 202t, 215–216, 215f–217f, 215t

Tuberous sclerosis, 299, 400–402, 401f, 418, 419f

Tufted angioma. Rare skin and subcutaneous slowly growing benign tumors that will occasionally self-involute. Often painful, tender and with hyperhidrosis and can develop the Kasabach-Merritt syndrome. They are dull, red, brown-red or purple patches or plaques that usually present prior to 5 years of age, may be multifocal and can develop in port-wine stains. *See* Angioma, tufted

Tularemia. The most common form is the ulceroglandular form with its primary chancre-type lesion and regional and generalized lymphadenopathy. Caused by *Pasteurella tularensis*. Other forms are oculoglandular, glandular, and typhoidal, 500t

Tumors, 14, 16f, 280–336

Tungiasis. Caused by skin penetration of the pregnant female of the Tunga penetrans flea. A white to yellow-gray, papulonodule with a brown-black central tip forms as the flea begins to produce eggs and enlarges up to 1 cm by a phenomenon called physiogastry. Seen in Central and South America, sub-Saharan Africa and central Asia. Treatment is surgical excision.

Turf burn, 490t, 491

Twenty-nail dystrophy, 431t, 438

Tyrosinemia Type II (see Richer-Hanhart syndrome) (keratosis palmoplantar circumscriptus). Rare autosomal recessive syndrome of bilateral hyperkeratosis of the palms and soles (Richer-Hanhart syndrome) and (if tyrosine and phenylalanine are not restricted from the diet) mental retardation. Due to hepatic deficiency of hepatic tyrosine aminotransferase (TAT).

Tzanck smear. Cells scraped with a 15 Bard Parker blade from the floor of fresh bullae of pemphigus. These cells are altered epithelial cells, rounded, and devoid of intercellular attachments. Similar multinuclear giant cells seen in herpes simplex and herpes zoster. Smear is left to dry and stained with Giemsa for one minute and examined after drying under high magnification after applying a drop of emersion oil and coverslip.

Ulcerative colitis, 394–395, 394f

Ulcerative lichen planus of the sole. Rare variant of lichen planus especially in females often accompanied by loss of toenails and scarring alopecia in addition to chronic, painful, progressive, ulcerations of the soles with histopathology indicative of lichen planus which may be present on other areas of the skin as well.

Ulcers, 15
  chiclero, 476
  decubitus, 210
  infected, 202t, 210–211
  mal perforans, 17
  nonhealing leg, 137t
  phagedenic, 210
  pyodermic, 137
  stasis, 136–138

Ulerythema ophryogenes. *See* Atrophies of the skin

Ultraviolet light, 404–411, 405t, 406f, 408t, 408f–411f, 410t

Uncombable hair syndrome ("Cheveux incoiffables," pili canaliculi, pili canaliculi et trianguli). Congenital, slowly growing, frizzy, scalp hair that is fragile and difficult to brush or comb. Rarely associated with ectodermal dysplasia. Electron microscopy may show a longitudinal groove (may also be seen on light microscopy) and a triangular, kidney bean or oval shape, 345, 422t

Unilateral laterothoracic exanthem (ULE). Also called asymmetric periflexural exanthem of childhood (APEC). Maculopapular or eczematous unilateral exanthem of childhood (mean age of onset 24 months) mean duration exanthem 5–6 weeks with regional lymphadenopathy. Probable viral origin. Spreads from the axilla and has an increased incidence in females (2:1). Unique eccrine lymphocytic infiltrate on biopsy.

Urea. 27, 30, 71–72, 77, 85, 124, 138, 151, 154, 159, 354, 355, 412, 480

Uremic pruritus. A difficult problem of extreme pruritis associated with renal failure. May be helped by ultraviolet radiation, cholestyramine, oral charcoal, or lidocaine infusions. Consult the literature for cautions on different therapeutic interventions.

Urticaria, 36, 104t, 106–107, 106f, 131–133, 141, 182, 296, 434
  physical, 497

Urticaria pigmentosa, 296, 431t, 434, 434f

Uta, 476

Vaccinia. Generalized viral exanthema seen as a rare complication of smallpox vaccine. It usually resolves after a benign course. A generalized maculopapular eruption which often vesiculates and becomes umbilicated in a febrile moderately ill patient.

Van der Woude syndrome. Rare autosomal dominant with symmetric congenital lower lip pits that may have a salivary discharge. May be associated with hypodontia, bifid uvula, syngnathia, symblepharon, ankyloblepharon, polythelia, megacolon, auricular septal defect, congenital heart disease, syndactyly, equinovarus foot deformity, and sternal abnormalities.

Varicella. *See* Chickenpox

Varicella-zoster virus (VZV), 232–234, 233f, 241, 450–451, 451f

Varicelliform, 25

Varioliformis, 25

Varix. *See* Venous Lake

Vascular steal syndrome. In hemodialysis patients with arteriovenous fistulas, distal to the fistula a hernia can result in pain at rest, coolness, numbness, paresthesias, cyanosis, loss of distal pulses, muscle atrophy of the thenar muscles, paralysis, and gangrene of the digits and hand. Treatment is prompt surgical shunt ligation. Symptoms can develop from 1 week to 1 month after the fistula has been created.